FETAL AND NEONATAL CARDIOLOGY

Walker A. Long, M.D.
Senior Clinical Research Scientist
Clinical Research Division
Wellcome Research Laboratories
Research Triangle Park, NC

Research Assistant Professor
Division of Pediatric Cardiology
School of Medicine
University of North Carolina
Chapel Hill, NC

With Forewords by
William H. Tooley, M.D.
and
Dan G. McNamara, M.D.

1990

W. B. SAUNDERS COMPANY

Harcourt Brace Jovanovich, Inc.
Philadelphia   London   Toronto
Montreal   Sydney   Tokyo

W. B. SAUNDERS COMPANY
Harcourt Brace Jovanovich, Inc.

The Curtis Center
Independence Square West
Philadelphia, PA 19106

Library of Congress Cataloging-in-Publication Data

Fetal and neonatal cardiology.

1. Heart—Abnormalities.   2. Infants (Newborn)—
Diseases.   3. Fetal heart—Diseases.   4. Pediatric
cardiology.   I. Long, Walker A. [DNLM: 1. Cardiovascular
Diseases—In Infancy & Childhood.   2. Fetal Diseases.
3. Heart Defects, Congenital.   4. Infant, Newborn,
Diseases. WS 290 F419]

RJ269.F47   1989   618.3'261   88–11671

ISBN 0–7216–1887–1

Editor: William J. Lamsback
Designer: Maureen Sweeney
Production Manager: Bill Preston
Manuscript Editor: Roger Wall
Illustration Coordinator: Walt Verbitski
Indexer: Angela Holt
Cover Designer: Jim Gerhard

Fetal & Neonatal Cardiology   ISBN 0–7216–1887–1

Last digit is the print number: 9   8   7   6   5   4

To my father, William Lunsford Long, Jr., M.D.,
whose great spirit, brilliance, and compassion still shine brightly
in the hearts of his colleagues, students, patients, and family
25 years after his death

&

To my father-in-law, Harry Emerson Dascomb, M.D.,
a scholar and a gentleman,
the diagnostician's diagnostician,
the physician's physician,
the finest teacher, and the finest man I know.

CONTRIBUTORS

Lindsey D. Allan, MD, FRCP
Senior Lecturer in Paediatric Cardiology, British Heart Foundation Research Centre for Perinatal Cardiology, Guy's Hospital, London, England.
  FETAL ARRHYTHMIAS

Page A. W. Anderson, MD
Professor of Pediatrics, and Assistant Professor of Physiology, Duke University School of Medicine, Durham; Attending Physician, Duke University Medical Center, Durham, North Carolina.
  MYOCARDIAL DEVELOPMENT

Annalisa Angelini, MD
Research Fellow, Istituto di Anatomia e Istologia Patologica, Padova, Italy.
  DEVELOPMENTAL CARDIAC ANATOMY

Ron Auslender, MD
Senior Physician, Department of Obstetrics and Gynecology, Carmel Hospital, Haifa, Israel.
  FETAL ELECTROCARDIOGRAPHY

Gerald Barber, MD
Assistant Professor of Pediatrics, University of Pennsylvania School of Medicine, Philadelphia; Director, Cardiopulmonary Exercise Laboratory, and Assistant Physician, The Children's Hospital of Philadelphia, Pennsylvania.
  VOLUME LOADS EXCEPT TAPVD

S. Kenn Beeman, MD
Chief, Resident Surgery, Vanderbilt University Affiliated Hospitals, Nashville, Tennessee.
  NEONATAL LEFT VENTRICULAR OUTFLOW TRACT SURGERY

D. Woodrow Benson, Jr., MD, PhD
Professor, Northwestern University Medical School, Chicago; Attending Cardiologist, Children's Memorial Hospital, Chicago, Illinois.
  ELECTROCARDIOGRAPHY

Watson A. Bowes, Jr., MD
Professor of Obstetrics and Gynecology, School of Medicine, University of North Carolina at Chapel Hill; Attending Physician, North Carolina Memorial Hospital, Chapel Hill, North Carolina.
MATERNAL DISEASES AFFECTING THE FETAL CARDIOVASCULAR SYSTEM; MATERNAL THERAPY AFFECTING THE FETAL CARDIOVAS-CULAR SYSTEM

Richard L. Bucciarelli, MD
Professor of Pediatrics and Chief, Division of Neonatology, University of Florida College of Medicine, Gainesville; Attending Physician, Shands Hospital, Gainesville, Florida.
CARDIAC ENZYMES

Catherine Bull, MRCP
Senior Lecturer in Paediatric Cardiology, Institute of Child Health, London; Honorary Consultant Cardiologist, Hospital for Sick Children, London, England.
TOTAL ANOMALOUS PULMONARY VENOUS DRAINAGE

Andrew Bush, MD, MRCP
British Heart Foundation Research Fellow, Departments of Paediatric Cardiology and Respiratory Physiology, Brompton Hospital, London, England.
BRONCHOPULMONARY DYSPLASIA AND THE HEART

Aldo R. Castañeda, MD
William E. Ladd Professor of Child Surgery, Harvard Medical School, Boston; Surgeon-in-Chief, Children's Hospital, Boston, Massachusetts.
NEONATAL REPAIR OF TETRALOGY OF FALLOT; NEONATAL REPAIR OF TRANSPOSITION OF THE GREAT ARTERIES

Nancy C. Chescheir, MD
Assistant Professor, Department of Obstetrics and Gynecology, School of Medicine, University of North Carolina at Chapel Hill; Attending Physician, North Carolina Memorial Hospital, Chapel Hill, North Carolina.
MANAGEMENT OF HYDROPS FETALIS

Alvin J. Chin, MD
Assistant Professor of Pediatrics, University of Pennsylvania School of Medicine, Philadelphia; Director, Noninvasive Laboratories, Division of Cardiology, and Associate Physician, The Children's Hospital of Philadelphia, Pennsylvania.
VOLUME LOADS EXCEPT TAPVD

Ronald I. Clyman, MD
Associate Professor of Pediatrics, University of California, San Francisco; Associate Staff, Cardiovascular Research Institute, University of California, San Francisco; Director, Neonatal Research, Mt. Zion Hospital and Medical Center, San Francisco, California.
DEVELOPMENTAL PHYSIOLOGY OF THE DUCTUS ARTERIOSUS; MEDICAL TREATMENT OF PATENT DUCTUS ARTERIOSUS IN PREMATURE INFANTS

Neal H. Cohen, MD, MPH
Professor and Vice Chairman, Department of Anesthesia, University of California, San Francisco; Director, Intensive Care Unit, University of California Hospital and Clinics, San Francisco, California.
ANESTHESIA FOR NEONATAL CARDIAC SURGERY

John G. Coles, MD, FRCS(C)
Assistant Professor of Surgery, School of Medicine, University of Toronto; Attending Physician, Division of Cardiovascular Surgery, The Hospital for Sick Children, Toronto, Ontario, Canada.
NEONATAL SURGERY FOR CRITICAL PULMONARY STENOSIS

Stephen R. Daniels, MD, MPH
Assistant Professor of Pediatrics (Cardiology) and Environmental Health (Epidemiology and Biostatistics), University of Cincinnati College of Medicine; Attending Cardiologist, Children's Hospital Medical Center, Cincinnati, Ohio.
EPIDEMIOLOGY

Peter Danilo, Jr., MPhil, PhD
Senior Research Scientist, Department of Pharmacology, Columbia University College of Physicians and Surgeons, New York, New York.
DEVELOPMENTAL ELECTROPHYSIOLOGY

Susan W. Denfield, MD
Fellow, Pediatric Cardiology, The Lillie Frank Abercrombie Section of Pediatric Cardiology, Baylor College of Medicine and Texas Children's Hospital, Houston, Texas.
NEONATAL POSTOPERATIVE CARDIAC INTENSIVE CARE

Donald B. Doty, MD
Clinical Professor of Surgery, School of Medicine, University of Utah, Salt Lake City; Chairman of Cardiovascular and Thoracic Surgery, LDS Hospital, Salt Lake City, Utah.
NEONATAL SURGICAL PALLIATIONS

C. Elise Duffy, MD
Associate Professor, Northwestern University Medical School, Chicago; Attending Cardiologist, Children's Memorial Hospital, Chicago, Illinois.
ELECTROCARDIOGRAPHY

Martin J. Elliott, MBBS, MD, FRCS
Senior Lecturer in Paediatric Cardiology, Institute of Child Health, London; Honorary Senior Lecturer in Cardiac Surgery, Royal Postgraduate Medical School, Hammersmith Hospital, London; Consultant, Cardiothoracic Surgeon, The Hospital for Sick Children, London, England.
NEONATAL REPAIR OF TOTAL ANOMALOUS PULMONARY VENOUS CONNECTION

Stephen J. Elliott, MB, FRCP(C)
Assistant Professor of Pediatrics, Division of Neonatology, Department of Pediatrics, Baylor College of Medicine, Houston, Texas.
NEONATAL HYPERTENSION

David J. Fisher, MD
Associate Professor of Pediatrics, Physiology and Biophysics, Baylor College of Medicine, Houston; Associate in Pediatrics, Texas Children's Hospital, Houston, Texas.
CARDIOMYOPATHIES

Derek A. Fyfe, MD, PhD
Assistant Professor and Director, Echocardiography, Medical University of South Carolina, College of Medicine, Charleston, South Carolina.
ATRIOVENTRICULAR BLOCK

Arthur Garson, Jr., MD
Professor of Pediatrics and Medicine, Baylor College of Medicine, Houston; Chief, Pediatric Cardiology, Texas Children's Hospital, Houston, Texas.
TACHYARRHYTHMIAS

Paul C. Gillette, MD
Professor of Pediatrics and Surgery, Director, Pediatric Cardiology, and Director, South Carolina Children's Heart Center, Medical University of South Carolina College of Medicine, Charleston, South Carolina.
ATRIOVENTRICULAR BLOCK

Thomas P. Graham, Jr., MD
Professor of Pediatrics and Director of Pediatric Cardiology, Vanderbilt University School of Medicine, Nashville; Attending Physician, Vanderbilt University Medical Center, Nashville, Tennessee.
CONOTRUNCAL ABNORMALITIES

Howard P. Gutgesell, MD
Professor of Pediatrics and Director, Pediatric Cardiology, University of Virginia Medical School, Charlottesville, Virginia.
PULMONARY VALVE ABNORMALITIES; CONOTRUNCAL ABNORMALITIES

John W. Hammon, Jr., MD
Professor of Surgery, Department of Cardiac/Thoracic Surgery, School of Medicine, Vanderbilt University, Nashville; Attending Physician, Vanderbilt University Medical Center, Nashville; Chief, Cardiac and Thoracic Surgery, Veterans Administration Hospital, Nashville, Tennessee.
NEONATAL LEFT VENTRICULAR OUTFLOW TRACT SURGERY

Thomas N. Hansen, MD
Associate Professor of Pediatrics and Head, Division of Neonatology, Department of Pediatrics, Baylor College of Medicine, Houston, Texas.
NEONATAL HYPERTENSION

Herbert S. Harned, Jr., MD
Professor of Pediatrics, School of Medicine, University of North Carolina at Chapel Hill; Attending Physician, North Carolina Memorial Hospital, Chapel Hill, North Carolina.
TERATOGENIC AGENTS

Sheila G. Haworth, MD, MRCPath, FRCP, FACC
Reader in Paediatric Cardiology, Institute of Child Health, London; Honorary Consultant in Paediatric Cardiology, The Hospital for Sick Children, London, England.
PULMONARY VASCULAR DEVELOPMENT

G. William Henry, MD
Associate Professor of Pediatrics, School of Medicine, University of North Carolina at Chapel Hill; Chief, Division of Pediatric Cardiology, North Carolina Memorial Hospital, Chapel Hill, North Carolina.
NEONATAL POSTOPERATIVE CARDIAC INTENSIVE CARE

Siew Yen Ho, MPhil, PhD
Senior Lecturer, Cardiothoracic Institute, London, England.
DEVELOPMENTAL CARDIAC ANATOMY

James C. Huhta, MD
Professor of Pediatrics and Obstetrics and Gynecology, University of Pennsylvania School of Medicine, Philadelphia; Director of Cardiology, The Children's Hospital of Philadelphia, Philadelphia, Pennsylvania.
FETAL DIAGNOSIS OF CONGENITAL HEART DISEASE; PATENT DUCTUS ARTERIOSUS IN THE PRETERM NEONATE; STRUCTURAL HEART DISEASE IN THE LOW BIRTHWEIGHT NEONATE

Roger A. Hurwitz, MD
Professor of Pediatrics (Cardiology) and Radiology (Nuclear Medicine), Indiana University School of Medicine, Indianapolis, Indiana.
RADIONUCLIDE ANGIOCARDIOGRAPHY

Alastair A. Hutchison, MBChB, FRACP
Assistant Professor of Pediatrics, University of Florida College of Medicine, Gainesville; Neonatologist, Shands Hospital, Gainesville, Florida.
PATHOPHYSIOLOGY OF HYDROPS FETALIS

William Jackson, MD
Assistant Professor of Pediatrics, Wayne State University School of Medicine, Detroit; Attending Physician, Children's Hospital of Michigan, Detroit, Michigan.
NEONATAL CARDIAC INFECTIONS

Gregory L. Johnson, MD
Professor of Pediatrics, University of Kentucky College of Medicine, Lexington; Attending Pediatrician and Pediatric Cardiologist, Albert B. Chandler Medical Center of the University of Kentucky, Lexington, Kentucky.
CLINICAL EXAMINATION

Richard A. Jonas, MD
Assistant Professor of Surgery, Harvard Medical School, Boston; Associate in Cardiovascular Surgery, Children's Hospital, Boston, Massachusetts.
NEONATAL REPAIR OF TETRALOGY OF FALLOT

Enid R. Kafer, MD (Sydney), FRACP, FFARCS
Professor of Anesthesiology and Director of Neuroanesthesiology, School of Medicine, University of North Carolina at Chapel Hill; Attending Physician, North Carolina Memorial Hospital, Chapel Hill, North Carolina.
NEONATAL GAS EXCHANGE AND OXYGEN TRANSPORT; BLOOD GASES

Vern L. Katz, MD
Assistant Professor of Obstetrics and Gynecology, School of Medicine, University of North Carolina at Chapel Hill; Attending Physician, North Carolina Memorial Hospital, Chapel Hill, North Carolina.
MATERNAL DISEASES AFFECTING THE FETAL CARDIOVASCULAR SYSTEM; MATERNAL THERAPY AFFECTING THE FETAL CARDIOVASCULAR SYSTEM

Ernest A. Kiel, MD
Assistant Professor, Pediatric Cardiology, University of Arkansas for Medical Sciences, Little Rock; Attending Physician, University of Arkansas for Medical Sciences and Arkansas Children's Hospital, Little Rock, Arkansas.
AORTIC VALVE OBSTRUCTION

James K. Kirklin, MD
Professor of Surgery, University of Alabama School of Medicine, Birmingham, Alabama.
NEONATAL CARDIOPULMONARY BYPASS; NEONATAL PATENT DUCTUS SURGERY

Zuhdi Lababidi, MD
Professor of Pediatric Cardiology and Director of Pediatric Cardiology, University of Missouri—Columbia School of Medicine; Attending Physician, University of Missouri Hospital and Clinics, Columbia, Missouri.
NEONATAL CATHETER PALLIATIONS

George Lister, MD
Associate Professor of Pediatrics and Anesthesiology, Yale University School of Medicine, New Haven; Director, Pediatric Intensive Care Unit, Yale-New Haven Hospital, New Haven, Connecticut.
BLOOD GAS AND ACID-BASE ALTERATIONS IN NEONATAL CONGESTIVE HEART FAILURE

Walker A. Long, MD
Research Assistant Professor, Division of Pediatric Cardiology, School of Medicine, University of North Carolina at Chapel Hill; Attending Physician, North Carolina Memorial Hospital, Chapel Hill; Senior Clinical Research Scientist, Clinical Research Division, Wellcome Research Laboratories, Research Triangle Park, North Carolina.
DEVELOPMENTAL PULMONARY CIRCULATORY PHYSIOLOGY; PNEUMOPERICARDIUM; PERSISTENT PULMONARY HYPERTENSION OF THE NEWBORN SYNDROME (PPHNS)

John E. Mayer, Jr., MD
Assistant Professor of Surgery, Harvard Medical School, Boston; Associate in Cardiac Surgery, Children's Hospital, Boston, Massachusetts.
NEONATAL REPAIR OF TRANSPOSITION OF THE GREAT ARTERIES

Jeffrey P. Moak, MD
Assistant Professor of Pediatrics and Physiology, Baylor College of Medicine, Houston; Associate in Pediatric Cardiology, Texas Children's Hospital, Houston, Texas.
TACHYARRHYTHMIAS

Gonzalo Moscoso, MD
Fetal and Perinatal Pathology Unit, King's College Hospital, King's College School of Medicine and Dentistry, London, England.
DEVELOPMENTAL CARDIAC ANATOMY

Hrudaya Nath, MD
Professor of Radiology, University of Alabama School of Medicine, Birmingham; Attending Physician, University of Alabama Hospital, Birmingham, Alabama.
CHEST RADIOGRAPHY; ANGIOGRAPHY

Catherine A. Neill, MD, FRCP
Associate Professor of Pediatrics, Johns Hopkins University School of Medicine, Baltimore; Pediatric Cardiologist, Johns Hopkins Hospital, Baltimore, Maryland.
GENETICS AND RECURRENCE RISKS OF CONGENITAL HEART DISEASE

Michael R. Nihill, MS, BS, MRCP, FAAP, FACC, MSC
Associate Professor of Pediatrics, Baylor College of Medicine, Houston; Associate in Pediatric Cardiology, Texas Children's Hospital, Houston, Texas.
CARDIAC CATHETERIZATION

Jacqueline A. Noonan, MD
Professor and Chairman, Department of Pediatrics, University of Kentucky School of Medicine, Lexington; Chief, Division of Pediatric Cardiology, University of Kentucky Medical Center, Lexington, Kentucky.
CHROMOSOMAL ABNORMALITIES; SYNDROMES

Albert D. Pacifico, MD
John W. Kirklin Professor of Cardiovascular Surgery, University of Alabama School of Medicine, Birmingham; Director, Division of Cardiothoracic Surgery, University of Alabama at Birmingham Medical Center, Birmingham, Alabama.
REPAIR OF ATRIOVENTRICULAR SEPTAL DEFECTS

Julian T. Parer, MD, PhD
Professor, Department of Obstetrics, Gynecology, and Reproductive Sciences, and Associate Staff, Cardiovascular Research Institute, University of California, San Francisco; Attending Physician, University of California Hospitals and Clinics, San Francisco, California.
FETAL ELECTROCARDIOGRAPHY

Lowell W. Perry, MD
Senior Attending Cardiologist, Children's Hospital National Medical Center, Washington, DC; Clinical Professor of Child Health and Development, George Washington University School of Medicine, Washington, DC; Clinical Professor of Pediatrics, Georgetown University School of Medicine, Washington, DC.
COARCTATION; INTERRUPTED AORTIC ARCH

Joseph B. Philips, III, MD
Associate Professor of Pediatrics, University of Alabama School of Medicine, Birmingham; Medical Director, Newborn Nurseries, University Hospital, University of Alabama at Birmingham, Alabama.
TREATMENT OF PPHNS

William Pinsky, MD
Professor and Vice Chairman of Pediatrics, Wayne State University School of Medicine, Detroit; Chief of Pediatric Cardiology, Children's Hospital of Michigan, Detroit, Michigan.
NEONATAL CARDIAC INFECTIONS

Francisco J. Puga, MD
Professor of Surgery, Mayo Medical School, Mayo Foundation, Rochester; Staff Consultant, Saint Marys Hospital and Rochester Methodist Hospital, Rochester, Minnesota.
CONGENITAL HEART SURGERY: PRESENT AND FUTURE

Marlene Rabinovitch, MD
Professor of Pediatrics and Pathology, University of Toronto; Director of Cardiovascular Research, The Hospital for Sick Children, Toronto, Ontario, Canada.
VASCULAR PATHOLOGY OF PPHNS

P. Syamasundar Rao, MD
Professor of Pediatrics and Director, Division of Pediatric Cardiology, University of Wisconsin Medical School, Madison; Attending Physician, University of Wisconsin

Hospital and Clinics, Meritor/Madison General Hospital, and St. Marys Hospital Medical Center, Madison Wisconsin.
TRICUSPID ATRESIA; OTHER TRICUSPID VALVE ANOMALIES

Thomas A. Riemenschneider, MD, MBA
Professor of Pediatrics, Epidemiology, and Biostatistics, and Associate Dean, Case Western Reserve University School of Medicine, Cleveland; Associate Pediatrician, Rainbow Babies and Children's Hospital of University Hospitals, Cleveland, Ohio.
PERICARDIAL DEVELOPMENT

Bertrand A. Ross, MD
Assistant Professor and Director, Pediatric Exercise Physiology, Medical University of South Carolina College of Medicine, Charleston, South Carolina.
ATRIOVENTRICULAR BLOCK

David J. Sahn, MD
Professor of Pediatrics and Radiology and Chief, Division of Pediatric Cardiology, University of California, San Diego Medical Center, San Diego, California.
FETAL ECHODOPPLER AND COLOR FLOW MAPPING

Mark E. Sand, MD
Major, USAF, MC, Department of the Air Force, USAF Medical Center, Keesler, Keesler Air Force Base, Mississippi.
REPAIR OF ATRIOVENTRICULAR SEPTAL DEFECTS

Stephen P. Sanders, MD
Assistant Professor of Pediatrics, Harvard Medical School, Boston; Associate in Cardiology and Director, Cardiac Noninvasive Laboratory, Department of Cardiology, Children's Hospital, Boston, Massachusetts.
ECHOCARDIOGRAPHY

Adam Schneeweiss, MD
Director, Geriatric Cardiology Research Foundation, Geneva, Switzerland, and Tel-Aviv, Israel.
NEONATAL CARDIOVASCULAR PHARMACOLOGY

John W. Seeds, MD
Associate Professor, Department of Obstetrics and Gynecology and Department of Radiology, School of Medicine, University of North Carolina at Chapel Hill; Director of Prenatal Diagnostic Services, North Carolina Memorial Hospital, Chapel Hill, North Carolina.
FETAL DISTRESS; MANAGEMENT OF HYDROPS FETALIS

Elliot A. Shinebourne, MD, FRCP
Consultant Paediatric Cardiologist, Brompton Hospital, London, England.
BRONCHOPULMONARY DYSPLASIA AND THE HEART

Richard T. Smith, Jr., MD
Assistant Professor of Pediatrics, Baylor College of Medicine, Houston; Associate in Pediatric Cardiology, Texas Children's Hospital, Houston, Texas.
TACHYARRHYTHMIAS

Benigno Soto, MD
Professor of Radiology, University of Alabama School of Medicine, Birmingham; Professor of Radiology, Division of Cardiac Radiology, University of Alabama Hospital, Birmingham, Alabama.
CHEST RADIOGRAPHY; ANGIOGRAPHY

Jaroslav Stark, MD, FRCS
Consultant Cardiothoracic Surgeon, The Hospital for Sick Children, London, England.
NEONATAL REPAIR OF TOTAL ANOMALOUS PULMONARY VENOUS CONNECTION

Norman S. Talner, MD
Professor of Pediatrics (Cardiology) and Diagnostic Imaging, Yale University School of Medicine, New Haven; Attending Physician, Yale-New Haven Hospital, New Haven, Connecticut.
BLOOD GAS AND ACID-BASE ALTERATIONS IN NEONATAL CONGESTIVE HEART FAILURE

George A. Trusler, MD, FRCS(C)
Professor of Surgery, School of Medicine, University of Toronto; Chief, Division of Cardiovascular Surgery, The Hospital for Sick Children, Toronto, Ontario, Canada.
NEONATAL SURGERY FOR CRITICAL PULMONARY STENOSIS

Herbert G. Whitley, MD
Pediatric Cardiologist, Department of Pediatrics, Fitzsimons Army Medical Center, Aurora, Colorado.
COARCTATION; INTERRUPTED AORTIC ARCH

FOREWORD

A multidisciplinary interchange among obstetrics, neonatology, pediatric cardiology, and pediatric heart surgery has evolved in most medical centers to manage the fetus and newborn infant with known or potential heart or lung disease. This text might be looked upon as a manifestation of this recent progress in both patient care and research on the developing circulation.

Improved skill in obtaining and interpreting the ultrasonographic record as well as advances in echocardiographic technology has had much to do with establishing the discipline of perinatal cardiology. Within a few years, we have progressed from fairly crude prenatal continuous wave Doppler detection of no more than fetal heart rate to the current highly sophisticated range-gated pulsed Doppler, by which the cardiologist can identify cardiac anomalies and arrhythmias early in fetal life.

New definitions for relationships among physicians and patients are emerging. Huhta states it well in Chapter 15:

> Prenatal screening (by echocardiography) for congenital heart disease . . . means a new physician-patient relationship—namely that between the doctor and the fetus. Regardless of gestational age or state or federal laws . . . , once the fetus is identified as a person in need of medical care, then the need for a *personal physician* exists. The participation of obstetricians, neonatologists, pediatric cardiac surgeons, and pediatric cardiologists in decisions about management of the mother and her unborn child is mandatory from the time of fetal diagnosis . . . of heart disease.

To carry examples of this professional collaboration further, the obstetrician usually alerts the neonatologist to prepare to manage the very premature infant. These patients, of course, are likely to have an open ductus and respiratory distress. Before current echocardiographic technology was available to view the ductus and the direction and volume of blood flow through it, the pediatric cardiologist was very much involved in the clinical bedside decision whether or not a ductus was open and to what extent it contributed to the respiratory problem.

The neonatologist today usually serves as primary physician in charge and becomes "cardiologist for the ductus" after the echocardiogram is performed, making the decision about pharmacologic or surgical closure and dealing with all the extracardiac consequences of any ductal treatment. Some pediatric cardiologists might view this role for the neonatologist as requiring them to give up turf, but it is required in the best interest of the patient.

There are many unmet needs in basic research, clinical investigations, advances in technology, standards for neonatal and fetal echocardiography facilities, and training requirements to practice this new discipline of perinatal cardiology.

Readers themselves will recognize in this book areas in which research and development are needed. Clinicians from the several disciplines involved are reminded daily of unmet needs whenever their efforts fail to remedy the clinical problem at hand.

Some unmet needs include the following:

1. *Easily available information on the effect of maternal pharmacologic therapy on the cardiovascular systems of the fetus and newborn.* There is an extensive review of this subject in Chapter 11 by Katz and Bowes. Busy physicians need to know without too much time-consuming research and reading which drugs have (1) a deleterious effect on the fetus, (2) a questionable effect, (3) no known effect, and (4) no available information on their effect.

2. *Development of new drugs.* These drugs would be directed specifically to the fetus, i.e., those that preferentially cross the placenta or drugs that can be instilled into the amniotic fluid.

3. *Improved imaging technology.* Sahn in Chapter 14 states that the technology in ultrasonography needs improvement for fetal echocardiography and that few Doppler systems and practically no flow imaging systems are optimized for fetal study.

Further needs in echocardiography include improved imaging for certain common malformations. Huhta points out the limitations in fetal echocardiographic diagnosis of anomalies of the pulmonary veins and systemic veins entering the heart. Also, fetal identification of ventriculo-arterial connection (for example, transposition of great arteries) is not yet completely reliable. Ventricular septal defect and atrial septal defect may also be difficult to identify in the fetus.

With more sophisticated technology in ultrasonography, prices are due to increase for equipment, and thus higher fees may be charged by the institutions that must purchase new equipment. There is an unmet need for better technology, to be sure, but at lower prices.

4. *Quality control.* From the standpoint of quality control, there is a need for standardized criteria for fetal echocardiographic units, including equipment, technicians, and professional staff. Except for the obstetrician who is expert at screening for signs of fetal cardiac abnormality, it is no longer simply ideal but *mandatory* for the echocardiographic study to be either performed or supervised, and certainly interpreted, by a clinician who is trained in pediatric cardiology and who has first-hand knowledge of the patient. In my experience, studies performed or interpreted by individuals who are not trained and experienced in pediatric cardiology and who have limited clinical information on the patient are usually incomplete or erroneously interpreted or both.

5. *Electrophysiology.* Danilo in Chapter 4 points out the need for further research on how fetal and neonatal development modulates cardiac electrophysiology and the response of the heart and circulation to cardioactive drugs.

6. *Genetic and familial factors in etiology of congenital heart defects.* Neill in Chapter 10 in Part 2 points out the wide variance in reports of incidence of congenital heart anomalies in the offspring of a parent (mother or father) who has existing or surgically repaired congenital heart disease. A large cooperative prospective study from several centers should be able to settle this question within a few years time.

The authors of these chapters and the editor who planned for and consolidated them deserve much credit for putting out this major work in one volume. It will be of interest and practical value to practitioners and investigators involved in the care of patients with perinatal heart disease. The chapter authors point out the necessity for close collaboration and cooperation among the several disciplines involved. In some instances, for the benefit of the patient new or expanded roles of involvement will be called for, and in others, because of new developments, some areas of traditional responsibility will be better delegated to other specialties. This text also serves as a stimulus to future investigators to carry out further research in prevention and treatment of perinatal cardiac problems.

DAN G. MCNAMARA, M.D.
Baylor School of Medicine
Houston, Texas

One of the great triumphs of medicine in the twentieth century is the dramatic drop in infant mortality. Much of the credit for this improvement goes to the advances in hygiene and nutrition that occurred in the century's first decades. The neonatal death rate which was more than 10 per cent in 1900, fell to 2 to 3 per cent by midcentury. By the 1950s, with the lower risk of death from infection and malnutrition, the attention of those concerned with the care of newborn infants focused on the origins, prevention, and treatment of developmental abnormalities. This change led to an enormous increase in the amount of research performed on the anatomy, physiology, and biochemistry of the fetus and newborn infant. The new knowledge that was acquired allowed a more rational approach to the diagnosis and treatment of many of the problems of newborn infants. Obstetricians started to view fetuses as well as mothers as patients. Some pediatricians began to specialize in the diseases of the newborn infant and created special units for the care of their patients. With the introduction of neonatal intensive care and the expanded interest in developmental phenomena, death from respiratory failure in infants with birthweights over 1000 grams was less common, and it became possible to repair even the most complex congenital lesions. In developed countries, infant mortality decreased to less than 1 per cent. The advancements in perinatal medicine made in the last 3 decades stem in large part from our increased understanding of the cardiopulmonary system.

Fetal and Neonatal Cardiology relates the most recent advances in basic research to the clinical problems associated with the developing cardiovascular system. The text has three parts. The first chronicles the advances made in our understanding of developmental structure and function in the three and one-half centuries since Harvey described the course of both the fetal and adult circulations. Here we learn of the cellular and biochemical events accompanying the anatomic changes that occur during gestation. Particular emphasis is placed on the regulation of the pulmonary circulation as it advances from the fetal to the newborn state. The interdependence of the respiratory and the cardiovascular systems with metabolic needs of the fetus and newborn is noted, and the factors favoring neonatal hypoxia are stressed.

The second part of the book deals with prenatal cardiology. The genetics and recurrence rates of congenital heart disease and the direct and indirect effects of maternal disease and their treatments on the developing fetus are reviewed. In addition to the alterations in the heart rate and ECG patterns that accompany fetal stress, the use of echocardiographic imaging and flow-velocity determinations to provide information on fetal cardiovascular well-being are highlighted. The authors discuss the emerging use of these methods for the intrauterine diagnosis of cardiac lesions and point out the ethical problems that intrauterine recognition of congenital heart disease creates.

The third part of the book has four sections. Section 1 brings us up-to-date on both the traditional and the new methods used in the diagnosis of cardiovascular status. Although two-dimensional echocardiography has in many instances supplanted cardiac catheterization for anatomic diagnosis, the authors point out that catheterization and angiography are still necessary for precise pressure and cardiac output measurements and to determine oxygen concentrations in different vascular channels; these more traditional procedures are carefully described. The uses of clinical examination, electrocardiography, chest radiographs, cardiac enzymes, blood gases, and radionucleotide studies are considered. Section 2 concerns the cardiovascular disorders of the prematurely born infant. The special role of patency of the ductus arteriosus in cardiopulmonary stability and the effect of bronchopulmonary dysplasia on cardiac function receive special attention. The final two sections present in detail the pathophysiology and clinical presentations of all the major cardiovascular disorders of the newborn and their treatments. The critical interactions of surgeons, cardiologists, anesthesiologists, and intensive care specialists in achieving the present level of success in surgical management of many complex congenital malformations of the heart are stressed. However, the limitations of current therapies for both the short- and long-term are also discussed. Intrauterine surgery and heart and lung transplants are acknowledged as possibilities for the future, but the ethical dilemmas they create and their possible long-term adverse consequences, on both the individual patient and society, are also carefully considered.

Fetal and Neonatal Cardiology fulfills the valuable function of reviewing our current knowledge and providing comprehensive literature reviews on all the important areas in the field. It is a pleasure to read. I think it very fortunate that Dr. Long undertook to produce this timely addition to the neonatology literature. *Fetal and Neonatal Cardiology* will be an important addition to the libraries of all neonatologists and pediatric cardiologists.

WILLIAM H. TOOLEY, M.D.
University of California
at San Francisco
San Francisco, California

PREFACE

In 1984 the need for this book became obvious to me. During the preceding 10 years, the advances in understanding, diagnosis, and medical and surgical therapy for the unborn and newborn with cardiovascular problems were virtually revolutionary, and yet no single source was available that even attempted to summarize briefly those widespread advances, much less comprehensively review them. This book was conceived to fill that need, and substantial efforts have been made in an attempt to ensure that the book fulfills its purpose. For example, over a year was invested in developing the book before a single word of text was written or a contributor contacted, and a second year was invested in revising the manuscript once it was assembled at Research Triangle Park. However, the disadvantage of such deliberate work is that it takes time. One innovation was the use of each contributor's electronic word processing files to typeset the galleys; this approach saved a substantial amount of time during production.

The book is organized into three parts. Part 1 deals with the structural and functional development of the cardiovascular system from a clinical perspective; clinicians who are not cognizant of the information presented in Part 1 and who care for sick fetuses or neonates put themselves and their patients at a disadvantage. Part 2 covers the very rapidly developing field of fetal cardiology. The physiology, diagnosis, and treatment of important fetal cardiovascular problems are reviewed in detail. Part 3 discusses neonatal cardiology and is divided into four sections. Section 1 provides comprehensive descriptions of the diagnostic methods commonly used in neonates who may have cardiovascular disorders. Section 2 describes in detail the major cardiovascular problems that occur in premature infants. Section 3 offers comprehensive descriptions of the major cardiovascular problems of term infants. Section 4 presents a comprehensive review of the medical and surgical therapies available for management of neonatal cardiovascular disorders.

The book is extensively illustrated with figures that are intended both to inform and delight the reader. Encyclopedic citation of the published literature was intended and often accomplished. Both because we too frequently overlook our tremendous debt to the many brilliant, creative, and courageous men and women who have gone before us and established the field in which we work and because it is difficult to understand the present and envision the future without knowledge of the past, each chapter begins with a historical perspective. Such perspectives are a standard feature of many fine textbooks; however, in this book the reader will find the results of extensive sleuthing to determine who was the first to recognize a given disorder or to perform a given procedure in the fetus or newborn infant.

The contributors to this book are a heterogeneous group of scholars who share several characteristics. All have a passion for investigation and for excellence in clinical care. Most represent the "young turks" of fetal medicine, pediatric cardiology, neonatalogy, and pediatric cardiac surgery, those who are making many of the advances heralded in this book. These younger scholars were sought out so that perinatal cardiovascular research and clinical care could be described by new voices, voices with the enthusiasm, vigor, and innovative ideas necessary to create the improved standard of clinical care that ill unborn and newborn infants deserve. The few more senior scholars who contribute to the book were certainly the "young turks" of their own generation, and it remains quite difficult for even the most youthful and productive of the younger scholars to keep pace with the current investigative efforts of these "old turks."

Ultimately, of course, it is the reader who will determine whether the book succeeds or fails in its task. From my own perspective the book accomplishes what was intended and delineates what has become a new field of multidisciplinary cardiovascular research and clinical care—perinatal cardiology. The fetus and the newborn infant are really only slightly different incarnations of the same organism, the developing human being, and experts from many different backgrounds will continue to push back the frontiers in perinatal cardiologic research and clinical care. It would be a surprise to the editor if the book does not live on in future editions long after all those involved in this first edition are forgotten, carried forward and greatly improved upon by editors and contributors who are themselves unborn today.

WAL
Research Triangle Park
August 10, 1988

ACKNOWLEDGMENTS

This book would not have been possible without the help of many different people. First, I wish to acknowledge the many distinguished teachers I have had. Harry E. Dascomb inspired me to go into medicine and taught me the clinical method. Robert L. Ney taught me internal medicine. Floyd W. Denny taught me pediatrics. Ernest N. Kraybill taught me neonatology. Herbert S. Harned, Jr., and his associates and Robert T. Herrington and Stewart A. Schall taught me pediatric cardiology. Edward E. Lawson taught me research. Ten thousand sick children and adults taught me courage and stoicism as well as the natural history of disease and the results of therapy.

Second, I have had the privilege of pursuing clinical problems at the bench. Moving back and forth from the bench to the bedside is one of the best ways to remain critical and current, both scientifically and clinically, and was essential in putting together this book. My interest in research began with Harry E. Dascomb, who taught me that research is a true and enduring passion. Without research support, a dual existence at the bench and bedside would not have been possible. Stalwart supporters of my research include Dr. Arnold Lupin and the Physicians New Orleans Foundation, who were early to see promise in my strange ideas, and the Wellcome Research Laboratories, which continue to contribute generously.

Third, a book such as this could not exist without the cooperation, enthusiasm, and patience of the contributing authors, all of whom graciously tolerated my editorial suggestions.

Fourth, without the consistent encouragement of the staff at W. B. Saunders, this book could not have become a reality. All of those involved along the way contributed significantly to the book's development, and I thank them.

Finally, my lovely wife Wendy Dascomb Long and our fine children Joshua Forrest Pescud Long, Millie Dascomb Long, and Hadley Pirkko Long kindly tolerated many lonely evenings and long weekends while this book was in preparation. I can only hope that as a result of this book many children from other families will grow up to gain more than they have lost.

CONTENTS

PART 3 Neonatal Cardiology

COLOR FIGURES

CHAPTER 14
COLOR FIGURES

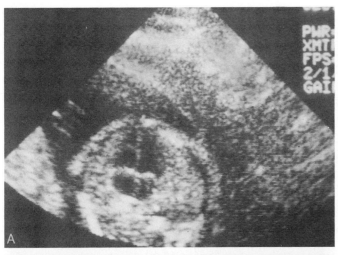

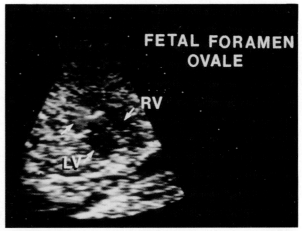

Color Figure 2

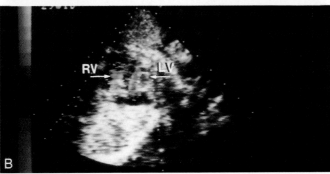

Color Figure 1

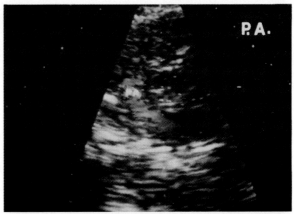

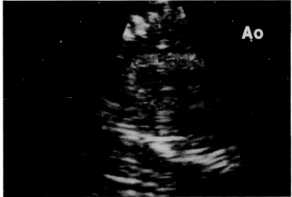

Color Figure 1. *A*, Four chamber view of 16-week fetus shows high resolution of both ventricles and endocardium in AV valve structures. *B*, In comparison with Figure 1*A*, 29-week fetus imaged in a four chamber view shows that resolution of the flow mapper is not as high as the dedicated obstetric scanner. The color echos overlap the tissue echos as a function of distorted balance between the lateral resolution for imaging and the lateral resolution for Doppler. LV = left ventricle; RV = right ventricle.

Color Figure 2. Low velocity flow across the foramen ovale imaged as a plug of blood going from the right to the left atrium away from the transducer is shown in blue at the arrow. LV = left ventricle; RV = right ventricle.

Color Figure 3. Both the fetal pulmonary artery with a broad curvature (upper panel) and the aortic arch with a tighter curvature (lower panel) are imaged in this 31-week human fetus. Ao = aorta; PA = pulmonary artery.

Color Figure 3

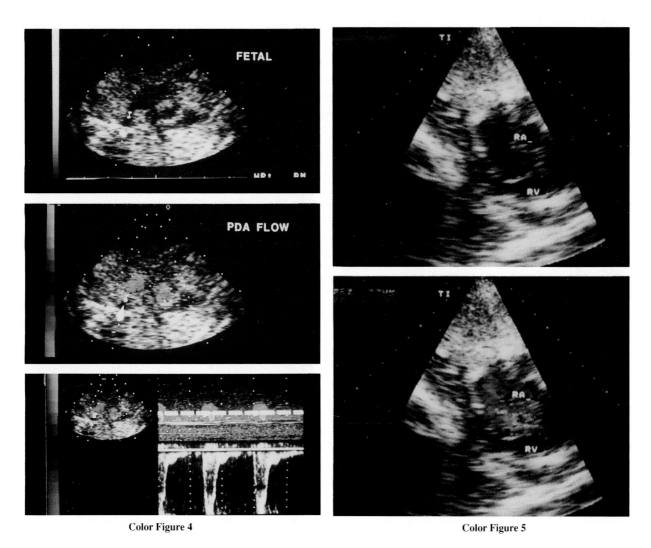

Color Figure 4   Color Figure 5

Color Figure 4. Echo visualization (upper panel), flow mapping (middle panel), and pulse Doppler sampling (lower panel) of the distal ductus arteriosus at its insertion in the aorta are seen in this 31-week human fetus. The high flow velocity in the ductus (110 cm/sec, highest in the human fetus) caused ductal aliasing in the middle panel.

Color Figure 5. The same fetus as shown in Figure 14–4, here on a flow map that illustrates right atrial dilatation (upper panel) and wide open tricuspid insufficiency filling the right atrium (lower panel). RA = right atrium; RV = right ventricle; TI = tricuspid insufficiency.

CHAPTER 25
COLOR FIGURES

Color Figure 6. Color flow mapping of the atria demonstrating a right-to-left shunt across a patent foramen ovale. Blue indicates flow away from the transducer. a = anterior; LA = left atrium; RA = right atrium; s = superior; SVC = superior vena cava.

Color Figure 7. Parasternal long axis view of the left ventricle with color flow mapping that demonstrates a midmuscular ventricular septal defect. The speckled, green apperance of the jet indicates turbulence. a = anterior; l = left; LA = left atrium; LV = left ventricle; RV = right ventricle; VSD = ventricular septal defect jet.

Color Figure 8. *A*, Parasagittal plane view for visualizing the ductus arteriosus. Color flow mapping illustrates the typical location of the flow jet along the superior wall of the main pulmonary artery. Again, the speckled appearance of the jet is due to aliasing. *B*, Continuous wave Doppler in a restrictive, persistent ductus arteriosus (PDA) showing high velocity, continuous flow. a = anterior; DA = ductus arteriosus; Dsc Ao = descending aorta; LPA = left pulmonary artery; MPA = main pulmonary artery; s = superior.

Color Figure 9. Doppler color flow map illustrating tricuspid regurgitation. The regurgitant jet is blue, indicating flow away from the transducer. The red signal in the left atrium is pulmonary venous flow. l = left; LA = left atrium; r = right; RA = right atrium; RV = right ventricle; s = superior.

Color Figure 10. *A*, Color flow mapping of the aortic arch from the suprasternal notch in a newborn with critical aortic stenosis. Note that flow is toward the transducer (red) in both the ascending aorta and the proximal descending and transverse aorta, indicating that the right ventricle supplies blood flow as far proximal as the right innominate artery. Flow in the descending aorta distal to the insertion of the ductus arteriosus (arrow) is away from the transducer (blue). *B*, The same view in this infant following balloon dilation of the aortic valve, indicating that flow in the proximal descending aorta is now anterograde (blue). a = anterior; s = superior.

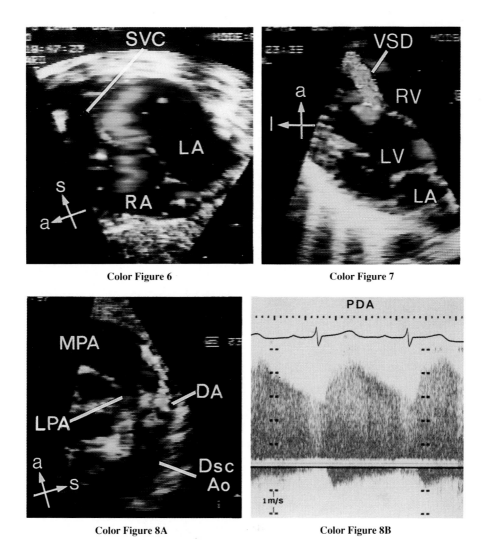

Color Figure 6

Color Figure 7

Color Figure 8A

Color Figure 8B

Color Figure 9

Color Figure 10A

Color Figure 10B

PART 1

Developmental Structure and Function

1 DEVELOPMENTAL CARDIAC ANATOMY

Siew Yen Ho

Annalisa Angelini

Gonzalo Moscoso

*I seem to have been only as a boy playing on the seashore, and
diverting myself in now and then finding a smoother pebble or a
prettier shell than ordinary, whilst the great ocean of truth lay all
undiscovered before me.*

Sir Isaac Newton

Despite quantum leaps of improvement in investigative technology, relatively little is known about the precise early development of the human embryonic heart. Of necessity, the normal developmental process is extrapolated mainly from animal studies or else is fraught with postulations based on hypothetical pathogenetic mechanisms derived from congenitally malformed hearts. Nonetheless, the works of investigators such as Born,[10] Tandler,[69] and Mall[41] are viewed as classics. As pointed out by Steding and Seidl,[67] the understanding of cardiac development would be simplified if embryologists (including biologists and anatomists) and cardiologists (including surgeons and pathologists) could conduct a dialogue in a common language. The diversified nomenclature was reviewed by O'Rahilly.[47] He also recorded sequentially the events in human cardiogenesis. Since most accounts of congenital cardiac malformations include a summary of cardiac development up to completion of septation, it would seem opportune to deviate from the mainstream and devote this chapter to further development beyond septation and look at the anatomy of the heart from this stage to birth. It is from this stage of development that technical advances are increasingly utilized in studies. We will assume from the outset that the reader has a knowledge of normal neonatal and adult cardiac anatomy.

The precise point in time for completion of septation is uncertain but probably lies between 37 and 44 days of gestation.[47,68] From then on, the shape and form of the fetal heart are moulded in response to the hemodynamics of the intracardiac circulation. For this reason it is necessary first to review the pathways of the fetal circulation together with those changes associated with the transference of gaseous exchange from the placenta to the lungs at the time of birth.

We are grateful to Professor Robert Anderson for his guidance and critical review of this manuscript. We are indebted to Mrs. Christine Anderson and Mrs. Rachel Marinos for their help in the preparation.

THE FETAL CIRCULATION

Information on the human fetal circulation is primarily inferred from physiologic studies in other mammals, such as the sheep or goat, or from examination of postmortem human fetal material, although recent developments in fetal echocardiography will soon give us the opportunity to study the developing human heart directly. Existing studies on the fetal and neonatal pulmonary circulation have been extensively reviewed by Rudolph.[56] One is faced with considerable difficulties in relating quantitative studies, even in animals, to the physiologic status of the fetus at the time of investigation. In earlier investigations, the fetal animals were exteriorized so as to measure flow through the various vessels.[19,20,31] Anesthesia and manipulation of the vessels in such investigations were likely to have affected the distribution of flow to the various regions of the body. Improved techniques of investigation were later employed by Rudolph and Heymann.[58] They introduced catheters into fetal lamb vessels via a small uterine incision. Since the fetus was maintained in its natural environment, they argued that the distribution of cardiac output was unaltered. To translate directly cardiac output figures from animal studies into ones for the human fetal circulation is not, however, without its drawbacks. Be that as it may, comparison of these figures with angiographic and echocardiographic studies on human fetal hearts has ascertained that in all essential respects the *course* of circulation is identical.[3,7,40,60,61]

Some of the anatomic differences between the fetal and adult circulation were described as early as 1628 by Harvey.[28] One of the distinctive differences is the presence of intra- and extracardiac shunts in fetuses. Left and right circuits work in parallel, with communications at the levels of the venous duct, the fossa ovalis, and the arterial duct. The course of the fetal circulation can conveniently be described as starting with the umbilical vein from the placenta (Fig. 1–1). A portion of the blood perfuses the liver by way of the hepatic capillary circulation and then proceeds via the hepatic veins to the inferior vena cava.

3

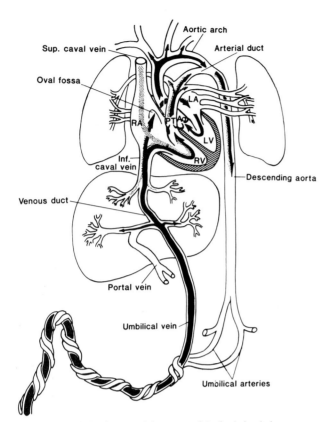

Figure 1–1. Diagram of the course of the fetal circulation.

A significant proportion (40 to 60 per cent) bypasses the liver via the venous duct, which connects the left branch of the portal vein to the common hepatic vein at the junction of the latter with the inferior vena cava. The blood returning via the umbilical vein joins the blood that returns from the lower half of the fetal body in the inferior vena cava.

The inferior vena caval return to the heart is separated into two streams owing to the anatomic relationship between the inferior vena cava and the borders of the fossa ovalis of the atrial septum. The free edge of the septum (the crista dividens) is situated opposite the entrance of the inferior vena cava. As a consequence, more than half of the inferior vena caval return is said to pass directly through the fossa ovalis into the left atrium and then into the left ventricle.

The remainder passes into the right atrium, where it mixes with blood returning from the upper part of the body via the superior vena cava and with blood returning from the coronary sinus. It is reported that very little of the superior vena caval return crosses the fossa ovalis to the left atrium.[52] The right atrial blood mainly passes into the right ventricle and the pulmonary trunk. A portion of the blood from the right ventricle goes to the lung, while the remainder passes through the arterial duct into the descending aorta. Here, it is joined by output carried from the left ventricle by the aortic arch.

This pattern of circulation ensures that the more well-oxygenated umbilical venous blood returning from the placenta is supplied to the coronary and cerebral circulations rather than to the organs of the body. Less well-oxygenated blood is diverted to the placental circulation, where reoxygenation occurs. This diversion is achieved by shunts (two extracardiac and one intracardiac), which, under normal circumstances, become nonfunctional after birth. These shunts occur at the venous duct, the fossa ovalis, and the arterial duct. The venous duct serves as a low resistance channel that bypasses the hepatic capillary circulation so that a significant portion of the relatively well-oxygenated blood is able to enter the heart directly. The position of the dividing crest of the atrial septum ensures that much of this flow is streamed through the fossa ovalis into the left atrium and left ventricle. The ascending aorta then distributes this flow to the myocardium, brain, head, and upper extremities. Less well-oxygenated blood is passed to the right ventricle through the right atrium and then ejected into the pulmonary trunk. The arterial duct serves to connect the pulmonary trunk with the descending aorta, returning the blood to the placenta.

POSTNATAL CHANGES IN CIRCULATION

The changeover of fetal to neonatal circulation is inextricably linked to the functional development of the pulmonary vascular bed. Immediately following birth, the infant takes its first breath of air and is then separated from the placenta. With the first breath, there is a dramatic increase in blood flow to the lungs accompanying a reduction in pulmonary vascular resistance. The alterations in pulmonary arterial pressure and vascular resistance are due to a combination of the response of the arterial walls to the changes in gas composition of the blood[16,36] and to bradykinin, which acts as a potent vasodilator of pulmonary blood vessels.[13]

Concomitant with the decrease in pulmonary vascular resistance is an increase in systemic vascular resistance. The direction of blood flow through the arterial duct changes to become primarily left to right (from aorta to pulmonary trunk). This shunt generally lasts through the first day of life, but may persist for several days until the arterial duct becomes occluded. A right-to-left shunt or bidirectional shunt is uncommon except in situations associated with hypoxemia. The physiologic basis for the closure of the arterial duct has been extensively reviewed.[29] Unlike the situation in the lamb, the human duct is not closed immediately.[51] The timing of functional closure varies widely according to different investigators,[2,6,14,25,53,63] but it is generally agreed that the normal duct is closed by the end of the first year. Patency after that time should be considered persistent.[12] About 80 per cent of normal ducts will have closed by the third month after birth.[14,63]

Another fetal shunt that closes concomitantly with the circulatory change is the fossa ovalis. Early investigators thought that the closure of the fossa ovalis was a consequence of the interruption of the placental circuit, which reduced the relative volume of blood entering the right

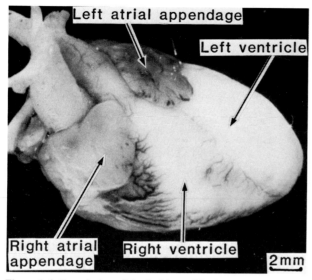

Figure 1–2. Frontal view of the fetal heart (20 weeks' gestation) showing the dominance of the atrial appendages.

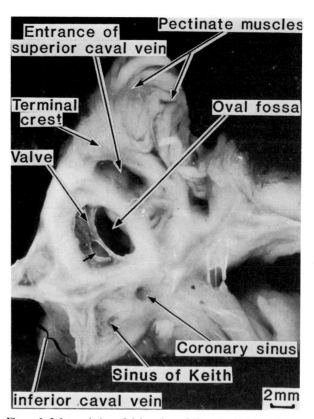

Figure 1–3. Internal view of right atrium of 10-week-old fetus. The oval fossa valve is membranelike. The smaller defect (arrow) is an artifact.

atrium as compared with that entering the left.[49] Later work, however, demonstrated that during the first few hours of extrauterine life the amount of blood returning from the lungs to the left atrium is much greater than that in the fetus. Increased pulmonary venous return raises the left atrial pressure and aids in the functional closure of the fossa ovalis. Functional closure is thought to be effected by about the twelfth week,[14] although probe patency occurs in more than 25 per cent of normal adult hearts.[63] Of greater concern is premature closure of the fossa ovalis during gestation, which can result in hypoplasia of the left heart.[37,46]

The precise mechanisms that control the flow of blood through the venous duct are not clear. The flow of blood through the liver is probably regulated by the constrictions and dilations of the venous duct. After birth, with the clamping of the placenta, the empty umbilical vessels contract. Following the cessation of flow in the umbilical vein, a decrease in pressure in the portal sinus results in muscular contracture of the sinus wall near the origin of the venous duct.[43] Anatomic closure is effected by proliferation of connective tissue strips in the lumen of the duct. Within about 2 months the venous duct becomes a fibrous strand superficially embedded in the wall of the liver.[6]

FUNCTIONAL ANATOMY

The growth of the fetal heart is accomplished by an increase in number of muscle fibers. Further growth in postnatal life is due to enlargement of elements of existing muscle fibers.[22] In the first 6 months of development the fetal heart is proportionately larger and heavier than the rest of the fetus. There is rapid growth of the fetus as a whole in the last 3 months of intrauterine life. From the third trimester to the first 6 months after birth, the ratio of heart to body weight declines to 1:200.[64] This ratio is then altered little throughout life under normal conditions.

In the early postseptational period, the shape of the ventricular mass resembles a cone, but in later states the apex becomes more rounded. The external appearance of the fetal heart in the late development bears much similarity to that of the postnatal heart. After birth, the base of the heart widens as the atria and heart valves enlarge.

The Atria

The atrial appendages dominate the atrial appearance more so in fetal hearts than in the newborn or adult hearts. The broad triangular shape of the right atrial appendage can be readily distinguished from the crenelated shape of the narrowed left appendage (Fig. 1–2).

Compared with the other cardiac chambers, the right atrium is a relatively prominent chamber in intrauterine life. The prominence of the right atrium reflects its function as a receiver of all venous return to the heart, which includes the systemic return as well as the oxygenated return via the umbilical vein. The right atrium consists of two portions derived from different segments of the embryonic heart tube. The smooth-walled component (which receives the systemic veins and the coronary sinus) is of sinus venosus origin. This part is separated from the other portion—the trabeculated part—by a muscle band, the terminal crest, from which pectinate muscles arise (Fig. 1–3). Stretched between the pectinate muscles are areas of atrial wall consisting of only endocardium and

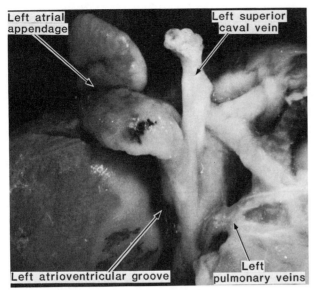

Figure 1–4. View from the left of a 20-week-old fetal heart showing the course of the persistent left superior caval vein between the appendage and the pulmonary venous component of the left atrium. Under normal circumstances this vein regresses to form the ligament of Marshall.

epicardium. It is thought that this webbed arrangement gives the right atrium the distensibility it requires to accommodate the entire venous return in fetal life.[22] The trabeculated wall of the right atrium is able to enlarge in concertina fashion. A further area that may also enable the right atrium to distend is the subeustachian sinus of Keith, which was designated the posteroatrial appendage by His. This area is situated posteroinferiorly just underneath the eustachian valve of the inferior vena cava.

The superior and inferior vena cavae enter the fetal and newborn heart at a sharper angle than they do later in life as the chest grows.[72] Inferior vena caval return is directed upward and toward the atrial septum by the eustachian valve, which is usually a prominent shelflike structure in the fetus but may vary considerably in form. Inadequate resorption may lead to multiple perforations and produce the extensive netlike structures—Chiari networks—found in some adult hearts.

Also prominent in the fetus and newborn is a right atrial structure described by Franklin[24] as the crista dividens, which is essentially the anterior rim of the fossa ovalis. As described previously, the function of this crest is believed to be to divide the inferior vena caval return into left and right atrial streams.

After atrial septation, the left horn of the sinus venosus is shifted to a position across the external aspect of the dorsal left atrial wall and forms the definitive coronary sinus. The left common cardinal vein regresses to form the oblique vein (or ligament) of Marshall (Fig. 1–4). In some newborn hearts it is possible to pass a probe from the coronary sinus to the much reduced proximal part of the oblique vein.

Unlike the right atrium, the left atrium has no thinned-out nonmuscular areas, but it is essentially a thin-walled chamber. It extends dorsally and inferiorly in relation to the right atrium so that it is in a prime position to receive inferior vena caval blood through the fossa ovalis. The relatively large fetal dimension of the left atrium as assessed echocardiographically suggests high left atrial flow.[3] The dilation and hypertrophy of the left atrium in postnatal life are associated with increased pulmonary venous return and closure of the fossa ovalis. Marked left atrial enlargement in postnatal life, however, is usually indicative of lesions of the mitral valve.

The Fossa Ovalis

The fossa ovalis is one of the essential pathways in fetal circulation that is closed after birth. The fossa ovalis was well described by Galen in his "Opera Omnia," but since then, the term has been used with a variety of meanings. This problem has been reviewed by Patten.[49] To most anatomists and physiologists, the fossa ovalis is taken to be the rounded opening in the definitive interatrial septum of the fully formed fetal heart. The opening is surrounded by a muscular rim derived from the secondary septum, clearly visible from the right atrial aspect.

The opening of the fossa ovalis is partially closed on the left aspect by a thin curtain, which is the persisting part of the primary septum. The thin septum acts like a valve and is adequately patent anteriorly to allow shunting of inferior vena caval blood into the left atrium (Fig. 1–5A). The valvelike motion of the thin septum can be observed during fetal life by concurrent M-mode and cross-sectional echocardiographic techniques.[3] In the ninth week of development, the area of the functional orifice is roughly the same as that of the inferior vena caval orifice.[39] At term, however, the functional orifice has diminished by 60 per cent in comparison to the inferior vena caval orifice.[50]

The valve of the fossa ovalis has excessive fullness and is "cut too large" for the opening it covers.[49] It balloons into the left atrium when right atrial pressures are high. After birth, with increasing pulmonary venous return to the left atrium, the valve is pushed against the rim of the fossa ovalis. Gradually, the slackness disappears, and the valve becomes stretched across the rim, with its anterior free margin in close contact with the septum (Fig. 1–5B). A probe may be passed obliquely through this free margin from right atrium to left atrium (probe patency). This free margin remains nonadherent to the septum in the neonatal period. With growth of the atrial chambers, the size of the fossa ovalis becomes relatively small, and the valve is less conspicuous when seen from its left atrial aspect. Following functional closure, the valve changes in histologic appearance. Initially a predominantly muscular structure, it subsequently seems to be a more robust and fibrous structure, which is less moveable by the eighth or ninth month.[49] The valve with its immediate muscular rim becomes the true interatrial septum.

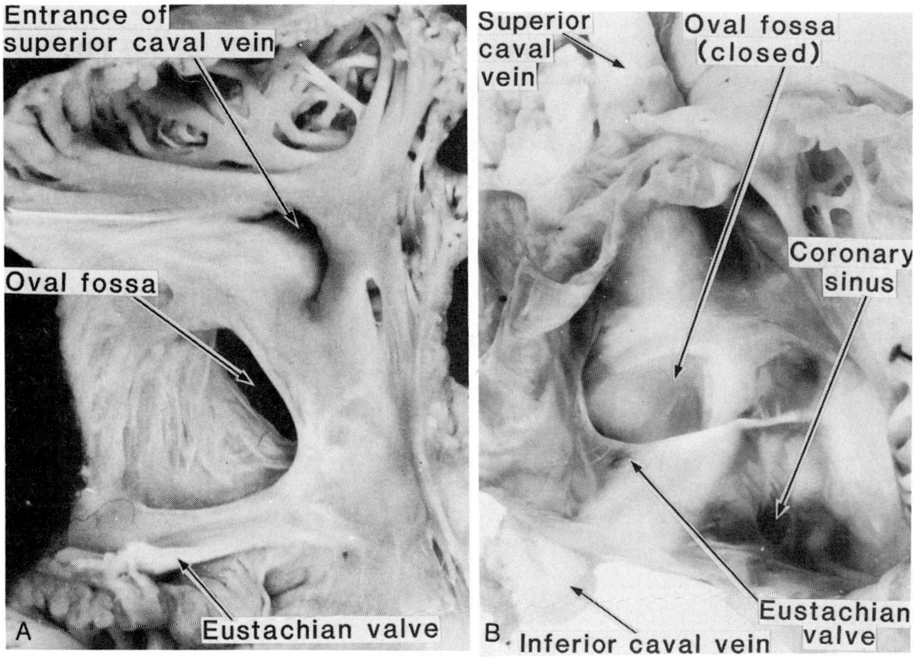

Entrance of superior caval vein

Oval fossa

A

Eustachian valve

Superior caval vein

Oval fossa (closed)

Coronary sinus

B Inferior caval vein

Eustachian valve

Figure 1–5. Right atrial views of the oval fossa of a 33-week-old fetus (*A*) compared with a 2-day-old neonate (*B*). Note that the valve in (*A*) is more substantial than that seen in Figure 1–3. In (*B*) the valve has closed off the oval fossa. In this heart there is also persistence of a large Eustachian valve.

The Ventricles and Atrioventricular Valves

In the younger fetus, in comparison to the one approaching term, more of the front of the ventricular mass is composed of left ventricle. Even in the younger fetus, however, the right ventricle has an ellipsoidal shape compared with the cylindrical shape of the left ventricle. The definitive "wraparound" relationship of the ventricles is less apparent in early development. The main portions of the ventricles are then side by side (Fig. 1–6). The apex of each ventricle is pointed in the young fetus, and the ventricular mass can have a bifid apical portion accentuated by the course of the interventricular coronary arteries (Fig. 1–7*A* and *B*). The apices in some hearts appear to have a spiral relationship when viewed from the ventricular tip (Fig. 1–7*C*). The left apex is anterosuperior in relation to that of the right. In later development the spiral relationship is no longer apparent, as the left apex dominates as the cardiac apex and the interventricular boundary shift from a median position toward the left.

Scanning electron microscopic studies have revealed the origin of the ventricular trabecular network.[67] The trabeculations are not formed, as previously thought, by protrusions from the inner myocardium.[67] The endocardium undergoes a process of rupture, and the trabeculations are remnants of strands between the ruptures. The coarse right ventricular trabeculations, as distinct from the fine left trabeculations, are a consequence of the differences in ventricular growth patterns. Differentiation between right and left ventricular trabeculations can be made from the seventh week of gestation[44] and occasionally earlier (Fig. 1–8). The right trabeculations have a radiating pattern. Left ventricular trabeculations, in particular, undergo a "thinning-down" process of the individual strands between 9½ weeks and 11 weeks of gestation. The trabeculations are more extensive in younger hearts than in older hearts. With increase in fetal age the trabecular portions become limited toward the apical ventricular portions (Fig. 1–9). The characteristic septal trabeculation of the right ventricle, the septomarginal trabeculation, is recognizable as a distinctive band from the early postseptation stage (Fig. 1–10).

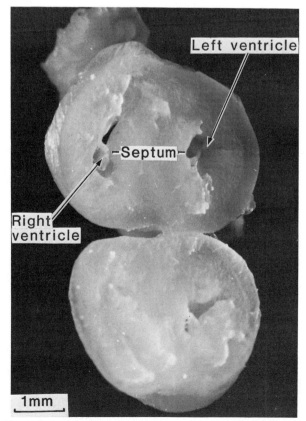

Figure 1–6. The ventricular mass of a 10-week-old fetal heart cut in short axis sharing the side-by-side ventricular relationship. Note the thick ventricular septum.

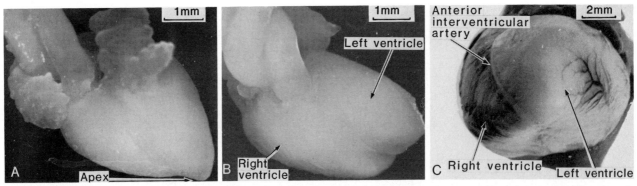

Figure 1–7. Frontal view of two hearts of 9 weeks' (*A*) and 10 weeks' gestation (*B*) and apical view of a heart of 20 weeks' gestation (*C*) to show the range of shapes of the ventricular mass.

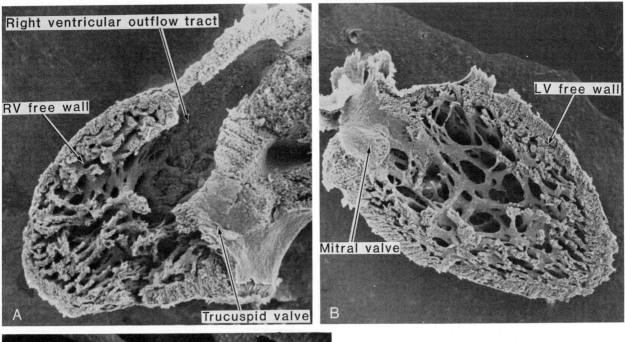

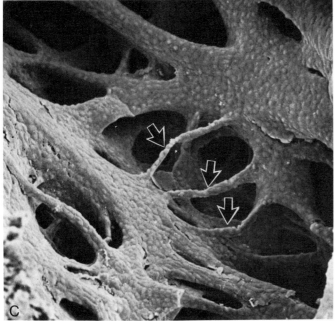

Figure 1–8. A series of scanning electron micrographs showing the ventricular trabeculation characteristics in a 6-week-old fetal heart (*A* and *B*) and a 10-week-old fetal heart (*C*). Dissection of the right ventricle in (*A*) shows the radial trabecular arrangement. The left ventricular trabeculations (*B*) in the free wall have a less distinct arrangement and are finer at the apex. A close-up view of the left ventricular trabeculations (*C*) shows thinning down of some of the strands (arrows) (Magnification: *A* and *B* × 40; *C* × 240).

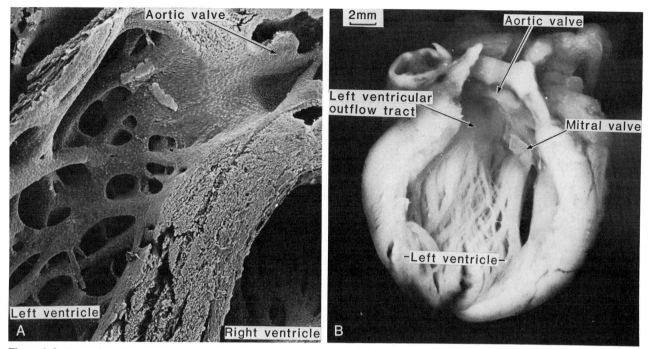

Figure 1–9. A scanning electron micrograph of the left ventricular outflow tract (*A*) in a 10-week-old fetal heart viewed from the back shows the trabeculations extending to underneath the aortic valve. Left ventricular view of a 20-week-old fetal specimen (*B*) shows the lack of trabeculations in the outflow tract (Magnification: *A* × 78).

Some of the more massive trabeculations are connected to the ventricular surfaces of the primordia of the atrioventricular valves. In the early days of development, soon after septation, the papillary muscles are still not well defined, and the valve leaflets appear to be supported by a single bunch of trabeculations. The leaflets appear like gelatinous sheets attached directly to muscular struts. The putative mitral valve has an appearance not unlike the parachute formation described as a malformation (Fig. 1–11*A*). With further development the valvar ends of the

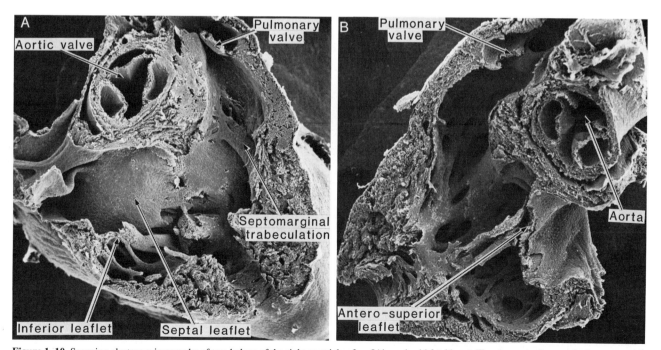

Figure 1–10. Scanning electron micrographs of two halves of the right ventricle of an 8½-week-old fetal heart. The view onto the ventricular septum (*A*) shows the differentiation of the septomarginal trabeculation. The septal leaflet of the tricuspid valve has not yet delaminated from the septum, although the inferior leaflet is already formed. The free wall half (*B*) shows the well-formed anterosuperior leaflet (Magnification: *A* and *B* × 53).

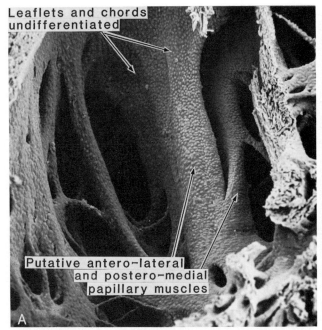

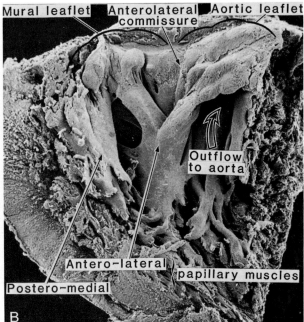

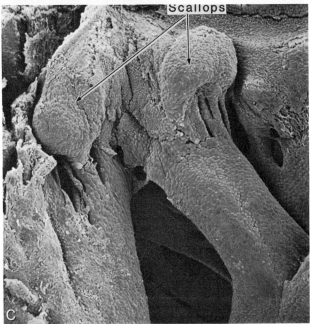

Figure 1–11. The development of the mitral valve in a 10-week old (*A*) and a 13-week-old (*B* and *C*) fetal heart. The papillary muscle primordium is beginning to separate into two masses in (*A*). The tendinous chords are undifferentiated at this stage. A view into the left ventricle from a posterior incision in (*B*) shows the appearance of tendinous chords and the arrangement of the papillary muscle groups. A close-up view of the mural leaflet in (*C*) shows the scallop formation (Magnification: *A* × 82; *B* × 30; *C* × 88).

trabeculations regress to become tendinous chords (Fig. 1–11*B* and *C*). The other ends are retained as primordia for the papillary muscles. Separation into distinct papillary muscle groups becomes obvious from 13 weeks' gestation. The close arrangement of the papillary muscles of the mitral valve gives it the optimal mechanical advantage. On the tricuspid side, the medial papillary muscle is visible in early development, but the septal leaflet is not fully delaminated from the septal surface until late development. The membranous septum of the heart is not divided into its two components, the atrioventricular and interventricular portions, until the septal leaflet is fully delaminated. This process may last into the neonatal period.[3] Our initial observations suggest that "maturation"

of the valves begins from the posteroinferior parts of the heart and progresses anterosuperiorly. This progression is particularly obvious in the delamination of the septal leaflet of the tricuspid valve. The definitive tricuspid and mitral valves show the same variation within normal limits to those seen in the neonate.

The mutual relationships of the atrioventricular valves are very similar throughout development and life. Just as in the newborn, the fetal tricuspid valve orificial circumference is larger than that of the mitral valve.[64] The developing valve tissue contains delicate vascular channels that may become engorged to form "blood cysts." The vascular channels usually disappear in later stages of development. The free edges of the leaflet may show

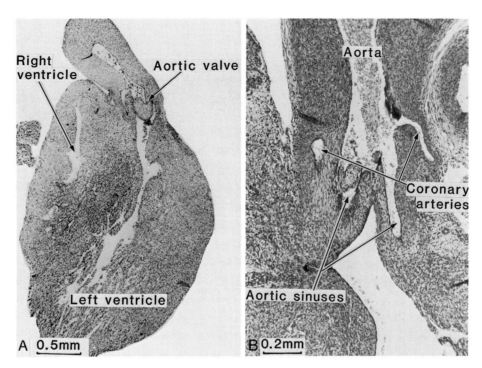

Figure 1–12. Photomicrographs of the aortic outflow tract of an 8½-week-old fetal heart (A) and the aortic root of a 10-week-old fetus (B).

gelatinous thickenings, which become more pronounced in postnatal life.

The Arterial Valves

The pulmonary valve is slightly larger than the aortic valve,[64] and this relationship is maintained at birth and beyond until pathologic processes are superimposed during adult life. In the fetus the arterial valves are well differentiated before the atrioventricular valves are fully formed (see Fig. 1–10). In younger fetuses the semilunar leaflets appear fairly thick (Fig. 1–12A), but these become less thick with growth of the heart. Nodules of Arantius, thickenings on the semilunar leaflets, are thought to be an alteration due to aging, but these have also been seen in

fetal hearts.[22] The coronary arteries arise high from the aortic sinuses (Fig. 1–12B).

The Arterial Duct and Great Arteries

In fetal circulation, blood that does not pass right to left through the fossa ovalis goes into the right ventricle and is then ejected into the pulmonary trunk. From the pulmonary trunk the flow is divided into flow to the lungs and flow through the arterial duct into the descending aorta. Information derived mainly from assays of fetal animals has indicated that there is a large flow through the arterial duct into the descending aorta.[57,58]

Our recent studies on a series of 16 formalin-fixed and three fresh postmortem human fetuses ranging from 11 to

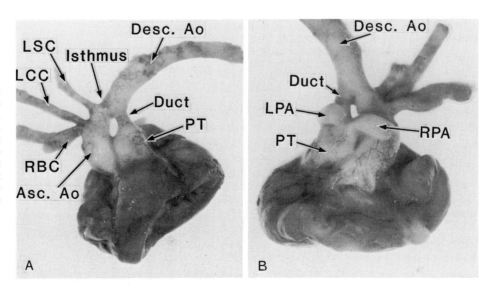

Figure 1–13. Front (A) and back (B) views of the great arteries and the aortic arch of a 23-week-old fetus. Asc. Ao = ascending aorta; Desc. Ao = descending aorta; LCC = left common carotid artery; LPA = left pulmonary artery; LSC = left subclavian artery; RBC = right brachiocephalic artery; RPA = right pulmonary artery; and PT = pulmonary trunk.

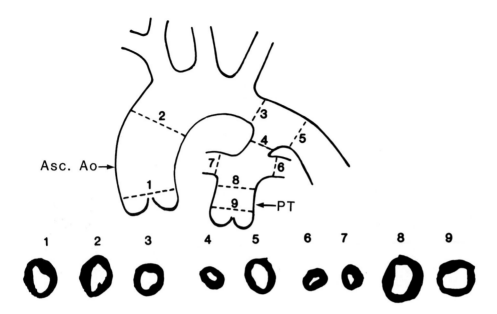

Figure 1–14. Diagram showing the levels of sectioning of the vessels and the sections studied from one of the hearts (23 weeks' gestation). Asc. Ao = ascending aorta; PT = pulmonary trunk.

33 weeks' gestation indicate some differences from the animal studies[5] (Fig. 1–13). It could be argued that formalin fixation might affect the calibers of elastic and muscular vessels differently and that isolation of the specimen might cause premature contraction of the arterial duct. Be that as it may, isolation would, to our mind, have a similar effect on the duct as exteriorization of the fetal animal.

Despite these drawbacks, our findings show that in humans the luminal cross-sectional area of the right pulmonary artery is larger than that of the duct in 14 of 19 specimens and that although the left pulmonary artery is always smaller than the right, it is larger than the duct in 9 of 19 specimens (Figs. 1–14 and 1–15). The isthmus is also larger than the duct in the majority of specimens (14

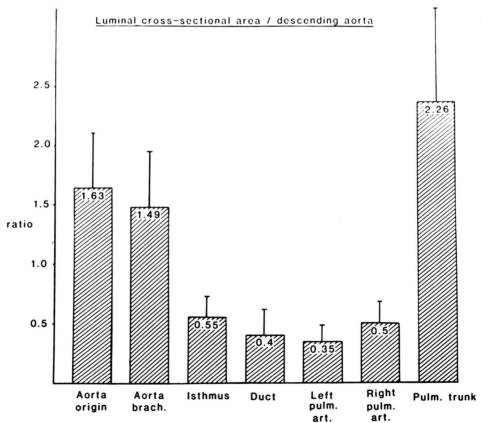

Figure 1–15. Histogram of the measurements obtained from 19 specimens.

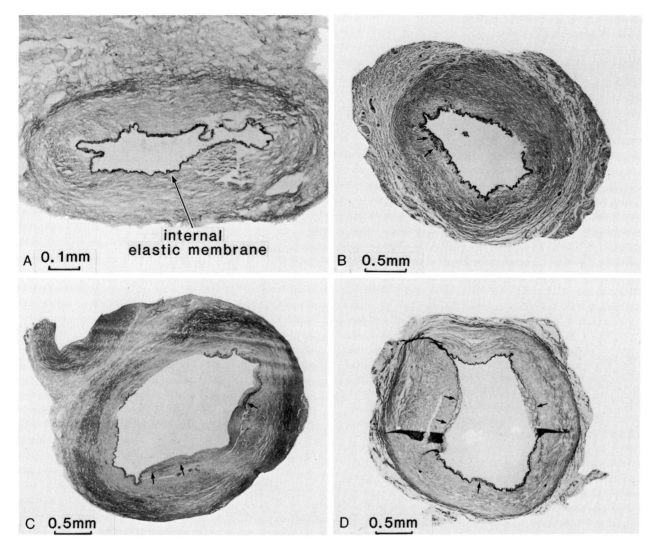

Figure 1–16. A series of histologic sections through the arterial ducts of 15-week- (*A*), 26-week- (*B*), and 33-week- (*C*) old fetuses and a 2-day-old infant (*D*). The elastic membrane is a single intact layer in the youngest fetus but multilayered and disrupted in the older specimens.

of 19). If the theory that flow is proportional to the relative size of a vessel[35,54] holds true, then the flow through the isthmus and the pulmonary arteries in humans would seem to be larger than that estimated in fetal lambs. This study could be interpreted to suggest a greater role for the isthmus in fetal circulation than has traditionally been thought.

That the arterial duct not only stopped growing but also became smaller and eventually shrivelled in the infant was noted by Galen. Since then, several theories for its anatomic closure have been proposed. These include compression by the left bronchus following the onset of inspiration,[34] traction by the left recurrent laryngeal nerve,[15] a flap-valve at the junction of the aorta and the arterial duct,[66] and thrombosis, as believed by many German authors.[12] With the advent of microscopy and improvements in histologic techniques, the generally accepted mechanism of closure is muscular contraction

accompanied by an alteration in the structure of the ductal wall. For this, the studies of Costa in 1930 (see reference 12) remain a classic. Even in early fetal life the ductal wall is thicker than that of the aorta. Because the ductal wall is essentially a muscular vessel, it is histologically distinct from the pulmonary artery and aorta. The internal elastic membrane is a continuous single layer in the youngest ducts but becomes disrupted and split into several layers with maturation. The vessel wall further thickens with the development of the intimal protuberances, which provide the characteristic wrinkled appearance of its luminal aspect (Fig. 1–16). Connective tissue caps may appear atop the protuberances, further occluding the lumen. With muscular contracture the intimal mounds eventually meet and fuse across the lumen. The muscle fibers then degenerate and become replaced by dense collagen, elastic tissue, and hyaline material, and the duct shrinks to become a cordlike structure.

RESPONSE TO ABNORMAL MORPHOLOGY

The Morphologic Significance of Flow Pathways

Experimental studies on animals have shown that the heart tube has the tendency to form segments and become loop shaped independently of blood flow.[27] Blood shapes the heart. Lack of flow through a chamber results in its underdevelopment, or hypoplasia, although its form remains recognizable. The spiraling courses of two blood streams in 34-to-38-hour-old chick embryos before cardiac septation[11] classically demonstrate the predetermined destiny of the flow pattern. It would seem that the heart septates independently of the manner of flow through the heart tube.[70] That the moulding of the fetal heart is inextricably linked to changes in the manner in which blood flows through the chambers is a reasonable assumption. Physiologic studies in animal preparations[55] have shown that most heart defects do not have an adverse effect on the developing fetus. This concept is supported by the observation that most infants with congenital heart diseases are normally developed and of normal weight at birth. Furthermore, a study of spontaneous abortuses[71] has shown that heart defects in isolation are not likely to lead to fetal loss, since the prevalence of defects was similar to that among live-borns.

The reason for the tenacity of the malformed fetal heart lies in the pattern of intrauterine circulation. By having two parallel circuits whereby part or all of the systemic venous return has two alternative pathways, the effects of most abnormal communications between the circuits and/or between the obstructions are minimized. The fetus is still provided with a normal blood supply for gas exchange and nutrients. An interatrial communication in the form of the fossa ovalis is a normal and necessary feature of the fetal circulation. It permits blood to pass from right atrium to left atrium. In congenital defects of the interatrial septum (manifested as a larger communication than the usual fetal fossa ovalis), there will be a proportionally larger flow into the left heart, but the total flow reaching the aorta remains unaltered. In the case of an isolated atrial septal defect, the increased workload on the right heart only occurs after birth when left atrial pressures rise with increased pulmonary venous return and left-to-right shunt occurs. Even so, atrial septal defect is extremely well tolerated in infancy and childhood. If there is associated stenosis of the mitral valve, a strain will be placed on the fetal circulation. In this situation, left atrial pressure will be increased, and flow through the right ventricle and arterial duct will be increased. This increased workload on the right side of the fetal heart will result in dilated pulmonary arteries at birth.

A fossa ovalis defect has been described in association with almost every form of congenital heart disease. Its presence may dramatically alter the natural history of the associated lesion. For instance, its association with complete transposition (concordant atrioventricular and discordant ventriculoarterial connections) will allow mixing of systemic and pulmonary circulations in postnatal life and thus improve the immediate prognosis.

Holes between the ventricles have no hemodynamic significance in the fetal circulation, since both ventricles eject blood into the aorta, the right ventricle doing so through the arterial duct. After birth, the ventricular septal defect becomes an alternative exit route for left ventricular ejection. The time of onset of symptoms and their severity are related to the size and location of the defect and to the pressure differences between the two ventricles. The defect may remain clinically silent until pulmonary vascular resistance falls some time after birth. Pulmonary vascular resistance is important in determining the magnitude of left-to-right shunt in the neonatal period.[18,53] In the presence of large ventricular septal defects, the change of pattern of the fetal pulmonary arteries to thin-walled structures with increased lumens and consequent decline in pulmonary vascular resistance appears to be delayed. Increased pulmonary venous return results in an enlarged left atrium and left ventricle and a compensatory increase in left ventricular muscle mass within the first 3 months of life.[32]

Fallot's tetralogy has a similar fetal hemodynamic pattern to isolated ventricular septal defects. The anatomic basis of Fallot's tetralogy is an anterosuperior deviation of the outlet septum, creating muscular subpulmonary stenosis and at the same time a ventricular septal defect and aortic override. The pulmonary outflow obstruction, be it muscular or valvar or both, is of little consequence, since the lungs are underutilized in fetal life. The changeover to neonatal circulation results in venous blood being ejected from the right ventricle into the overriding aorta. As the lungs become expanded, the obstruction of the pulmonary arterial supply becomes increasingly apparent. The outflow stenosis may be more severe when there is infundibular muscular contracture. Right ventricular hypertrophy develops secondary to the right outflow tract obstruction.

Persistent Arterial Duct

The role of the arterial duct in fetal circulation cannot be overemphasized, since it allows right ventricular flow to reach the aorta via the pulmonary trunk. Marked narrowing, obliteration, or absence of the duct (especially in the absence of other shunting defects proximal to it) creates serious problems in the fetal circulation. The right ventricular output will be forced through the high resistance fetal pulmonary bed. On the other hand, its persistent patency after birth provides a shunt from the high pressure aorta to the decreasing pressure of the pulmonary artery. A large shunt results in increased work for the left ventricle, and hypertrophy of the left ventricle is usual. Persistent patency is recognizable as an entity histologically.[26]

The Growth of the Ventricular Walls

Data largely based on fetal lamb studies have suggested that the right ventricle is larger than the left ventricle, supposedly because of greater right ventricular blood flow.[57] Ventricular wall thickness grows to match the amount of work a ventricle is required to do.[23] The right ventricle has been thought to increase in weight in the latter part of gestation, eventually becoming as thick as or slightly thicker than the left ventricle at birth. De la Cruz et al,[21] however, made measurements of normal unfixed hearts in the range of 6 months' prematurity to 12 years and found the right ventricle to be always thinner than the left. The development of high-resolution ultrasound cross-sectional imaging systems has made it possible to follow the anatomy of fetal cardiac development from about the sixteenth week of gestation.[2] Making use of such techniques, Sahn et al[59] followed fetuses from the second half of pregnancy and found the right ventricle consistently slightly larger than the left ventricle before birth. In contrast, using echocardiographic assessments together with direct measurements, St. John Sutton et al[60,61] found that right ventricular thickness did not differ from septal or left ventricular wall thickness at any point in gestation. The increases in thickness were linear from 20 weeks to term. These researchers contended that their observations did not support the theory of right ventricular dominance, in terms of either weight or wall thickness, in the human fetus.

The ventricular status immediately after birth is also controversial. By weighing the ventricular components of 231 hearts, Keen[33] found that the right ventricle atrophies immediately after birth. Its weight was shown to decrease by about 20 per cent during the first month of life in response to a transient decrease in workload as pulmonary vascular resistance falls. Keen also critically reexamined the work of Muller[45] and came to similar conclusions despite differing views expressed by others,[38,48,62] who had inferred their conclusions from the same source. During the same period, left ventricular mass increases at an accelerated rate[64] in response to rising systemic resistance and pressure. The cardiac apex is then formed by the left ventricle. Boellaard's[9] study on the microscopic diameter of cardiac muscle fibers in the postnatal period up to 10 months showed reduction in diameter of right ventricular fibers and a considerable increase in fiber diameter of the left ventricle. After its early postnatal atrophy, the right ventricle attains its original weight at birth by 6 months of age; thereafter there is a stable weight relationship between the two ventricles that continues into adult life.

With regard to the ventricular septum, Maron et al[42] found that disproportionate thickening of the ventricular septum with respect to the left ventricular free wall was a common finding, especially in young fetuses. The septal-free wall ratio decreases with the age of the fetus and approximates unity in the newborn.

Closure of Interventricular Defects

Small ventricular septal defects are particularly prone to closure without intervention. It has been estimated that 75 to 80 per cent of smaller defects close spontaneously, the majority in the first 2 years of life. In a clinical study of 84 infants with congestive heart failure due to large ventricular septal defects observed for up to 12 years, Somerville[65]

found a reduction in the size of the defect in 56 patients and complete closure in 11. The mechanism that closes most ventricular septal defects is adhesion of tags cleaved from the tricuspid valve leaflets to the septum, aided by a fibrotic process.[4] An aneurysm of the ventricular septum marks the site of closure in many patients. In other patients a prolapsed aortic leaflet may partially close the defect. While closure or reduction in size of a ventricular septal defect is usually beneficial to the patient, it is occasionally less desirable. For instance, the process that closes the defect may encroach upon the conduction axis. Somerville[65] discussed the changing cardiac form in a variety of lesions. Of the 84 infants with ventricular septal defect observed, six developed features of tetralogy of Fallot in a course similar to a patient described by Becu et al.[8] The pulmonary outflow tract obstruction was progressive owing to hypertrophy of the outlet muscle bundles in response to right ventricular hypertension.

References

1. Abbott ME (1927): In Olser W, McCrae T (eds): Modern Medicine. Philadelphia, Lea & Febiger.
2. Allan LD, Joseph MC, Boyd EGCA, Campbell S, Tynan M (1982): M-mode echocardiography in the developing human fetus. Br Heart J 47:573–583.
3. Allwork SP, Anderson RH (1979): Developmental anatomy of the membranous part of the ventricular septum in the human heart. Br Heart J 41:275–280.
4. Anderson RH, Lenox CC, Zuberbuhler JR (1983): Mechanisms of closure of perimembranous ventricular septal defects. Am J Cardiol 52:341–345.
5. Angelini A, Allen LD, Anderson RH, Thiene G, Ho SY (1986): The role of the aortic isthmus in fetal circulation: A preliminary morphometric study. 5th Meeting of the Working Group on Embryology and Teratology, Gottingen, 1986.
6. Arey LB (1954): Fetal Circulation and Changes at Birth. Developmental Anatomy. Philadelphia, WB Saunders, pp 387–389.
7. Barclay AE, Franklin KJ, Prichard MML (1944): The Foetal Circulation and Cardiovascular System and the Changes That They Undergo at Birth. Oxford, Blackwell Scientific Publications.
8. Becu L, Ikkos D, Ljungquist A, Rudhe U (1961): Evolution of ventricular septal defect and pulmonary stenosis with left to right shunt into classic tetralogy of Fallot. A case report with clinical, angiographic and anatomic correlations. Am J Cardiol 7:598–607.
9. Boellaard JW (1952): Uber Umbauvorgange in der rechter Herzkammerwabd wahrend der Neugeboren und Sauglingsperiode. Z Zellforsch 41:101–111.
10. Born G (1889): Beitrage zur Entwicklungsgeschicht der Singetierherzen. Arch Mikrosk Anat 33:284–378.
11. Bremer JL (1932): The presence and influence of two spiral streams in the heart of the chick embryo. Am J Anat 49:409–440.
12. Cassels DE (1973): The Ductus Arteriosus. Springfield, Charles C Thomas.
13. Campbell AGM, Dawes GS, Fishman AP, Hyman AI, Perks AM (1968): The release of bradykinin-like pulmonary vasodilator substance in foetal and newborn lambs. J Physiol 195:83–96.
14. Christie A (1930): Normal closure time of the foramen ovale and the ductus arteriosus. An anatomic and statistical study. Am J Dis Child 40:323–326.
15. Chevers N (1845): Observations on the permanence of the ductus arteriosus and constriction of the thoracic aorta, and on the means by which the duct becomes naturally closed. Lond Med Gaz 36:187.
16. Cook CD, Drinker PA, Jacobson HN, Levison M, Strang LB (1963): Control of pulmonary blood flow in the foetal and newly born lamb. J Physiol 169:10–29.
17. Costa A (1930): La minuta struttura e le trasformazioni involutive

del dotto arterioso di Botallo nella specie umana. Cuore e Circulaz 14:546–568.

18. Dammann JF Jr, Ferencz C (1956): The significance of the pulmonary vascular bed in congenital heart disease. III. Defects between the ventricles or great vessels in which both increased pressure and blood flow may act upon the lungs and in which there is a common ejectile force. Am Heart J 52:210–231.

19. Dawes GS, Mott JC, Widdicombe JG (1954): The fetal circulation in the lamb. J Physiol 126:563–587.

20. Dawes GS, Mott JC (1964): Changes in O_2 distribution and consumption in fetal lambs with variations in umbilical blood flow. J Physiol 170:524–540.

21. de la Cruz MV, Anselmi G, Romero A, Monroy G (1960): A qualitative and quantitative study of the ventricles and great vessels of normal children. Am Heart J 60:675–690.

22. Dische MR (1972): Observations on the morphological changes of the developing heart. Cardiovasc Clin 4:175–191.

23. Ford LE (1976): Heart size. Circ Res 39:297–303.

24. Franklin KJ (1948): Cardiovascular Studies. Springfield, Charles C Thomas.

25. Gerard G (1900): De l'obliteration du canal arteriel: Les theories et les faits. J de l'Anat et Physiol 36:323–357.

26. Gittenberger de Groot AC (1977): Persistent ductus arteriosus: Probably a primary congenital malformation. Br Heart J 39:610–618.

27. Goerttler K (1955): Ueber Blutstromwirkung als Gestaltungsfaktor fur die Entwicklung des Herzens. Biet Path Anat Allgem Path 115:33–56.

28. Harvey W (1628): Movement of the Heart and Blood in Animals. Translated from the original Latin by K.J. Franklin. Oxford, Blackwell Scientific Publications, 1957, pp 44–60.

29. Heymann MA, Rudolph AM (1975): Control of the ductus arteriosus. Physiol Rev 55:62–77.

30. Hort W (1953): Quantitative histologische Untersuchungen an wachsenden Herzen. Virchows Arch (Pathol Anat) 323:223–242.

31. Huggett AStG (1927): Foetal blood gas tensions and gas transfusion through the placenta of the goat. J Physiol 62:373–384.

32. Jarmakani JMM, Graham TP Jr, Canent RV Jr, Spach MS, Capp MP (1969): Effect of site shunt of left heart volume characteristics in children with ventricular septal defect and patent ductus arteriosus. Circ 40:411–418.

33. Keen EN (1955): The postnatal development of the human cardiac ventricles. J Anat 89:484–487.

34. King WT (1842): On the open state of the ductus arteriosus after birth. Lond Edin Month J Med Sci 11:83.

35. Krediet P, Klein HW (1981): Synopsis of normal cardiac development. In Pexeider T (ed): Mechanisms of Cardiac Morphogenesis and Teratogenesis: Perspectives in Cardiovascular Research. Vol 5. New York, Raven Press, pp 7–16.

36. Lauer RM, Evans JA, Aoki M, Kittle CF (1965): Factors controlling pulmonary vascular resistance in fetal lambs. J Pediatr 67:568–577.

37. Lev M, Arcilla R, Rimoldi HJA, Licata RH, Gasul BM (1963): Premature narrowing or closure of the foramen ovale. Am Heart J 65:638–647.

38. Lewis T (1914): Observation on ventricular hypertrophy with special reference to preponderance of one or other chamber. Heart 5:367–403.

39. Licata RH (1954): The human embryonic heart in the ninth week. Am J Anat 94:73–125.

40. Lind J, Stern L, Wegelius C (1964): Human Foetal and Neonatal Circulation. Springfield, Charles C Thomas.

41. Mall FP (1912): On the development of the human heart. Am J Anat 13:249–298.

42. Maron BJ, Verter J, Kapur S (1978): Disproportionate ventricular septal thickening in the developing normal human heart. Circ 57:520–526.

43. Meyer WW, Lind J (1966): The ductus venosus and the mechanism of its closure. Arch Dis Child 41:597–605.

44. Moscoso GJ, Whimster WF, Anderson RH (1986): Development of the ventricles and atrioventricular valves during fetal life—a preliminary study. 5th Meeting of the Working Group on Embryology and Teratology, Gottingen, 1986.

45. Muller W (1883): Die Massenverhaltnisse des menschlichen Herzens. Hamburg und Leipzig, Leopold Voss.

46. Naeye RL, Blanc WA (1964): Prenatal narrowing or closure of the foramen ovale. Circ 30:736–742.

47. O'Rahilly R (1971): The timing and sequence of events in human cardiogenesis. Acta Anat 79:70–75.

48. Patten BM (1930): The changes in circulation following birth. Am Heart J 6:192–205.

49. Patten BM (1931): The closure of the foramen ovale. Am J Anat 48:19–44.

50. Patten BM, Sommerfield WA, Paff GH (1929): Functional limitations of the foramen ovale in the human foetal heart. Anat Rec 44:165–178.

51. Prec KJ, Cassells DE (1955): Dye dilution curves and cardiac output in newborn infants. Circ 11:789–798.

52. Rigby ML, Shinebourne EA (1981): Growth and development of the cardiovascular system: Functional development. In Davis JA, Dobbing J (eds): Scientific Foundations of Paediatrics. London, William Heinemann Medical Books, Ltd, pp 373–389.

53. Rudolph AM (1965): The effects of postnatal circulatory adjustments in congenital heart disease. E. Mead Johnson Award Address. October 1964. Pediatrics 36:763–772.

54. Rudolph AM (1970): The changes in the circulation after birth: Their importance in congenital heart disease. Circ 41:343–359.

55. Rudolph AM (1974): Congenital Diseases of the Heart. Chicago, Year Book Medical Publishers.

56. Rudolph AM (1979): Fetal and neonatal pulmonary circulation. Ann Rev Physiol 41:383–395.

57. Rudolph AM, Heymann MA (1967): The circulation of the fetus in utero: Methods for studying distribution of blood flow, cardiac output and organ blood flow. Circ Res 21:163–184.

58. Rudolph AM, Heymann MA (1970): Circulatory changes during growth in the fetal lamb. Circ Res 26:289–299.

59. Sahn DJ, Lange LW, Allen HD, Goldberg ST, Anderson C, Giles H, Haber K (1980): Quantitative real-time cross-sectional echocardiography in the developing normal human fetus and newborn. Circ 62:588–592.

60. St John Sutton MG, Gewitz MH, Shah B, Cohen A, Reichek N, Gabbe S, Huff DS (1984): Quantitative assessment of growth and function of the cardiac chambers in the normal human fetus: A prospective longitudinal echocardiographic study. Circ 69:645–654.

61. St John Sutton MG, Raichlen JS, Reichek N, Huff DS (1984): Quantitative assessment of right and left ventricular growth in the human fetal heart: A pathoanatomic study. Circ 70:935–941.

62. Scammon RE (1923): A summary of the anatomy of the infant and child. Abt's Pediatrics. Philadelphia, WB Saunders, pp 257–444.

63. Scammon RE, Norris EH (1918): On the time of the postnatal obliteration of the fetal blood passages (foramen ovale, ductus arteriosus, ductus venosus). Anat Rec 15:165–170.

64. Schulz D, Giordano DA (1962): Hearts of infants and children. Arch Pathol 74:464–465.

65. Somerville J (1979): Changing form and function in one ventricle hearts. Herz 4:206–212.

66. Strassman P (1902): Der verschluss des ductus arteriosus. Beitr Path 6:98–117.

67. Steding G, Seidl W (1980): Contribution to the development of the heart. Part I. Normal development. Thorac Cardiovasc Surg 28:386–409.

68. Streeter GL (1951): Developmental horizons in human embryos: Description of age groups XIX, XX, XXI, XXII, and XXIII. Contrib Emb 34:165–196.

69. Tandler J (1912): The development of the heart. In Keibel F, Mall FP (eds): Manual of Human Embryology. Philadelphia, JB Lippincott, pp 534–570.

70. Tondury G (1980): Development of the human heart. In Graham G, Rossi E (eds): Heart Disease in Infants and Children. London, Edward Arnold (Publishers) Ltd, pp 13–25.

71. Ursell PC, Byrne JM, Strobino BA (1985): Significance of cardiac defects in the developing fetus: A study of spontaneous abortuses. Circulation 72:1232–1236.

72. Walmsley T (1929): The heart. In Sharpey-Schafer E, Symington J, Bryce TH (eds): Quain's Elements of Anatomy. Vol 4. London, Longman's Green & Co.

2 MYOCARDIAL DEVELOPMENT

Page A. W. Anderson

The myocardium undergoes many changes in its structure and function during the fetal and newborn periods. How these changes are interrelated and controlled remain, in large part, to be resolved. A major physiologic change with maturation is the enhancement in the ability of the myocardium to generate force and to shorten. This change and how birth alters ventricular function as well as structural and functional changes of the myocardium during fetal and newborn periods will be considered.

ANATOMY

The structure of the myocardium undergoes significant maturational changes prior to birth. However, the stimulus of birth must induce some of the transition of the myocardial cell from the immature form to that of the adult. The work of the right and left ventricles suddenly changes with the transition from fetal to neonatal life. Cardiac output increases significantly with birth. Moreover, the right and left ventricles now function in series, with the right ventricle ejecting blood against a low afterload, while the left ventricle ejects against a higher afterload. In apparent response to these changes, the relative proportion of the ventricular mass composed of right and left ventricles changes.[10,87] Left ventricular weight increases relative to body weight, while right ventricular weight stays relatively the same or decreases. This change is reflected in the left ventricular freewall thickness's increasing significantly while minimal changes occur in the right.

The increase in left ventricular mass is related to an increase in cell number and size. After birth, hyperplasia is prominent initially, and then cell size increases, i.e., hypertrophies, with binucleation occurring.[10,51] This process appears to differ between the right and left ventricle. For example, the left ventricular myocyte number increases more rapidly than that of the right.

Myocyte

Maturational changes occur in the size, shape, and architecture of the ventricular myocyte at birth.[10,44,51,54,55, 63,72,77,87,97] Of note, the level of maturation in these properties at the time of birth varies widely among species. These differences appear to be related to the level of maturation and function of the animal at birth, e.g., the lamb as compared with the rat pup. The ultrastructure of the ventricular myocyte of the lamb is quite mature in the last week of gestation (e.g., T-tubules are present), while that of the rat does not achieve the same level of maturation until the end of the first week of postnatal life.

In addition to variations in the developmental timing of these changes from species to species, differences appear to occur in the timing of these changes in the cells of the right and the left ventricle; the left ventricle matures more quickly following birth. During this maturation, myocardial cell shape changes. The immature cells are more rounded, with a smoother outline. As they develop, immature myocardial cells acquire the irregular shape of the adult cell with its stepped changes along its lateral borders at the location of the intercalated disk.

With these changes in shape, the cell also becomes longer and acquires a larger cross-sectional area, e.g., going from 30 to 40 μm in length and 5 to 10 μm in cross-sectional diameter to 100 μm or longer in length and 20 to 30 μm in width. Part of the stimulation of this cell growth may be related to the sympathetic nervous system. It is of interest to note that in many species the number of α-adrenoceptors is highest in the newborn, with this number usually falling to very low levels in the adult myocardium.[26,35,119] The circulating norepinephrine levels are also usually at their highest in the neonatal period. Relating these aspects of the sympathetic nervous system to cell growth is based on the findings that α_1 stimulation induces cell growth in tissue culture and that this growth is prevented with α_1 antagonists.[99–101]

Myofilaments

Myofibrils and sarcomeres are present during fetal life. In the newborn, the characteristics of the sarcomere differ somewhat from those of the adult in that the A-I bands are frequently irregular, the Z-band disk is thicker and more variable, and the M-band is acquired with maturation. At the time of birth, the orientation of the myofibrils within the architecture of the ventricular myocyte depends on the species examined. For example, in the fetal lamb and guinea pig myocyte, the myofibrils may be organized as they are in the adult cell—in long parallel rows from one end of the cell to the other. When the cell architecture is most immature, the myofibrils are chaotically organized and often not oriented in the same direction as the long axis of the cell. Following the orientation of the fibrils with the long axis of the cell, the myofibrils are found arranged in a subsarcolemmal shell surrounding a large central mass of nuclei and mitochondria. This arrangement may persist for weeks following birth in some

The author wishes to thank Annette Oakeley for her kind assistance in preparing and illustrating the manuscript and Patrick Donovan for his patient researching of the material.

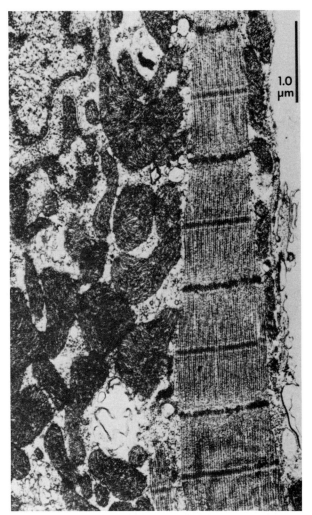

Figure 2–1. Electron micrograph of a longitudinal section obtained from an isolated ventricular cell from a 3-week-old rabbit heart. A single myofibril lies adjacent to the cell surface to the right. The mitochondria and nucleus occupy the central portion of the cell.

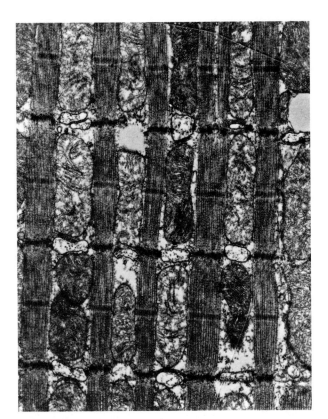

Figure 2–2. Electron micrograph of a longitudinal section obtained from an adult rabbit ventricular myocyte. The alternating rows of mitochondria and myofibrils typify the arrangement in the adult cell. T-tubules are regularly seen at each Z-line (see arrow).

species, such as the rabbit (Fig. 2–1). Ultimately, the myofibrils become distributed across the cell, as in the adult (Fig. 2–2).

The organization of the myofibrils in the developing heart is further disordered by the process of sarcomerogenesis. Fragmented myofilaments undergoing the process of sarcomere formation and addition are scattered throughout the cell. This process results in the maturational increase in the myofilament content of the myocyte.

The developmental changes in the organization of the myofibrils, the increase in the proportion of cell volume containing myofilaments, and the completion of the process of sarcomerogenesis have been used to explain the maturational increase in the ability of the myocardium to contract during the fetal and newborn periods.

Mitochondria

The cell volume containing the mitochondria increases with development. However, this increase is most rapid following birth. The timing of this increase is common to all mammals despite marked differences among species in other characteristics of cell maturation at birth. For example, the cell organization of the fetus may be quite mature at birth, including the presence of a transverse tubular system, yet the volume of the cell containing mitochondria does not undergo a rapid increase until following birth. This increase is striking and can exceed the developmental increase in the myofibrillar content of the cell.

This postnatal mitochondrial increase is most likely related to the changes in myocardial metabolism that occur during the days following birth. During this period, metabolism becomes primarily oxidative, with long chain fatty acids becoming the primary energy substrate, as in the adult heart. Long chain fatty acids are not a significant substrate in the fetal heart. The depressed ability of the immature myocardium to utilize this substrate may result from a deficiency in myocardial carnitine, and a delay in the maturation of the activity of carnitine palmitoyl CoA transferase and that of palmitoyl CoA synthetase.[112,118] The maturation of this system appears to be related, in part, to structural changes within the mitochondrion. In the fetus, the cristae of the mitochondrion are sparse and widely spaced, while in the first days following birth, the cristae become dense and closely packed.[54,102]

The location of the mitochondria within the cell architecture also changes with development. In the most immature myocardium, mitochondria are scattered chaotically

with the myofibrils throughout the cell, while with increasing maturity, they are found in the central portion of
the cell surrounded by the myofilaments. Ultimately, in
the adult, the mitochondria become distributed in a highly
ordered arrangement among the myofilaments (Fig. 2–2),
a process that may require weeks following birth to be
achieved. In the adult cell, the mitochondria surround each
myofilament with the mitochondria above, below, and to
each side of the sarcomeres. This arrangement would appear to be most efficient for coupling the sarcomere to its
source of energy.

The changes in the appearance, number, and size of the
mitochondria, coupled with the developmental acquisition
of a more highly ordered relationship of the mitochondria
to the myofilaments, are consistent with the importance
of the mitochondria in the transition of the myocardial
metabolism following birth.

Acquisition of the Transverse Tubular System

The transverse tubular system (T-system) is acquired
with maturation in most mammalian species, including
humans. The sarcolemma extends by way of the T-system
as invaginations into the cell (Fig. 2–3).[103] The ontogeny
of the T-system is not known. Its acquisition occurs at different stages of maturation and at different rates among
various species. In those that are relatively mature at birth,
e.g., the lamb, transverse tubules are present in the fetal
myocardium, while in others, e.g., the rat, mouse, rabbit,
and dog, this system is absent in the fetal myocardium and
is acquired in the days or weeks following birth.

In view of the importance of the sarcolemma in the
process of excitation-contraction coupling, the large developmental increase in cell volume that occurs in most
species could have a significant effect on the relationship
between surface area of sarcolemma and cell volume. The
acquisition of the T-system and its addition of sarcolemma
to that of the surface sarcolemma have been considered
sufficient to keep the cell surface-volume ratio constant
during the maturational increase in cell size. Thus, the
acquisition of the T-system appears to be a consequence of
the cells becoming wider, thicker, and longer. As a result,
as the cell hypertrophies in response to development, no
change occurs in the cell surface-volume ratio.[103,44]

Phylogenetic studies support this relationship between
cell size and diameter and the acquisition of the transverse
tubular system.[103] For example, the T-system is not found
in some species with small adult ventricular cells, while in
species whose adult cells are large, the T-system is absent
in the small immature cells but present in the large adult
cells. In that in cardiac muscle the sarcolemma making up
the transverse tubular system has not been shown to differ
from the surface sarcolemma, the transverse tubules serve
as a means of avoiding significant intracellular ionic gradients from the sarcolemma to the cell center, which would
be expected to exist in cells that hypertrophy during development. The presence of the glycocalyx on the T-sytem
sarcolemma ensures that binding sites for calcium and
other ions are present, thus allowing the T-system sarcolemma to participate, like the surface sarcolemma, in the

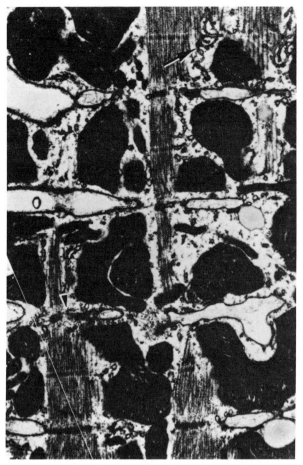

Figure 2–3. Slightly oblique longitudinal section of an adult myocyte.
T-tubule profile can be seen invaginating from the cell surface that lies
to the left. Intermediate filaments are associated with the sarcoplasmic
surface of the T-tubules (black and white triangles). The glycocalyx is
seen in the lumen of the T-tubules. Longitudinal sarcoplasmic reticulum is seen at the arrow.

modulation of cytosolic calcium. The acquisition of the
T-system does not appear to change the physiologic
properties of the myocardium qualitatively. For example,
modulation of myocardial activator calcium as manifested
by postextrasystolic potentiation occurs in the absence of
a T-system. The T-system may be considered, then, to be
the mechanism by which the process of activation affects
myofilaments that are far from the surface sarcolemma in
a similar manner to the myofilaments that lie just beneath
the surface sarcolemma.

Sarcoplasmic Reticulum

The sarcoplasmic reticulum (SR) is a specialized form
of the endoplasmic reticulum.[103] The SR is important in
the modulation of calcium that bathes the myofilaments
during contraction. A range of studies have demonstrated
that the SR serves as a release site for activator calcium,
an uptake site for removal of calcium from the cytosol,
and a storage site of calcium.[24,46,64,65] The SR is composed
of longitudinal, junctional, and corbular components (Fig.
2–3), which have a prominent, repetitive, well-organized

relationship to other cell structures in the adult. The longitudinal SR extends from one end of the sarcomere to the other, surrounding the thick filaments, and is rich in the ATP-dependent calcium pump and its associated protein, phospholamban. The lumen of this network is connected directly to the junctional and corbular SR, which are located at the level of the Z-line or Z-disk. The lumens of the junctional and corbular SR are filled with densely staining material that contains calsequestrin, a protein with a high affinity for calcium, and their cytosolic surfaces have foot processes. In contrast, the lumen of the longitudinal SR appears empty of calsequestrin, and its surface has no foot processes. The junctional SR foot processes extend toward the closely related surface sarcolemma. These specialized couplings between the sarcolemma and the junctional SR are thought to transduce the effects of activation to bring about calcium release, as the SR calcium release channel is located in this region of the SR.[67]

Although the junctional, corbular, and longitudinal SR are present across the broad range of development, the special relationship that this system has to the myofibrils and the structural appearance of its components changes with development. In the neonatal rabbit, the fixed repetitive relationship of the corbular SR to the sarcomeres is frequently absent.[72] In addition, the dense material inside the corbular SR can be found to continue into the longitudinal SR, while the dense coat on the cytosolic surface of the SR can be found to continue onto the surface of the longitudinal SR.[72] This obscuring of structural demarcations may indicate that functional differentiation is acquired with development.

Specialized couplings between the junctional SR and the sarcolemma, i.e., peripheral couplings, are present prior to the acquisition of the transverse tubular system, and with its formation, internal couplings are also acquired. In the adult, internal couplings are many times more frequent than peripheral couplings,[79] suggesting that with maturation the majority of the couplings are acquired in the transverse tubular system. In the case of the rabbit, the ratio of junctional SR membrane area per unit myofibrillar volume increases from fetal to newborn life and then remains constant from the day after birth through neonatal growth.[78] This day of birth increase suggests that cytosolic calcium modulation through the SR may be enhanced with birth, while subsequently the contribution of this structure to contraction remains unchanged. The generalness of the timing of these relationships remains to be established across species.

Further evidence that the SR and its contributions to the modulation of calcium are changed with development is provided by the findings that the volume fraction of SR increases through late gestation and following birth.[44] An increase in smooth endoplasmic reticulum subsequent to birth has also been described,[77] as has an increase in the ability of the SR to pump calcium with development.[70,73] A large portion of this maturational increase occurs perinatally. A developmental increase in the calcium-sensitive ATPase activity of the SR has been observed in the rabbit during late gestation and from the newborn to

the adult; in the guinea pig an increase has been noted from fetal to neonatal life.[73]

Although the presence of the components of the SR would allow the basic processes controlling calcium to be similar from late gestation through neonatal life, the developmental increase in the amount of the SR, its ability to pump calcium, and the maturational changes in the appearance and organization of the SR all suggest that the effectiveness of the SR in releasing calcium, taking it up, and storing it is enhanced quantitatively with maturation. Consequently, the immature myocardial cell may be more likely to have a greater dependence on extracellular sources of calcium, and so contraction will be more dependent on sarcolemmal-based systems and the transsarcolemmal movement of calcium with activation.

Cytoskeleton

The cytoskeleton is the intracellular structure that provides the myocardial cell its shape and organization (Fig. 2–3).[23,74,75,81,104,109] Its presence in the adult myocyte appears to integrate and to unify the contractile actions of the myofilaments so that they maintain their relationship to the membrane systems that control cytosolic calcium and the mitochondria that serve as sources of energy.

The organization of the cytoskeleton and its relationship to the organelles change in the course of development. For example, in the neonatal rabbit, the myofibrils are linked as a thin shell underneath the sarcolemma, and a central mass of nuclei and mitochondria are present, which appear to prevent the cytoskeleton from linking sarcomeres through the center of the cell.[72] In contrast, the adult cell is compartmentalized by the cytoskeleton, which connects sarcomeres from one side of the cell to another while organizing the cell into transverse compartments. In the immature myocardium, the centrally placed noncontractile structures appear to produce an internal load when the myofilaments contract. The presence of an internal load that is greater in the immature myocyte than in the adult would contribute to the observed slower sarcomere shortening in the neonatal myocyte.[72] Furthermore, the developmental change in the organization of the cytoskeleton and the isoforms of the cytoskeletal protein may result in the maturational increase in the compliance of the myocardium[74] (see the section Passive Stress-Strain Relationship). The assessment of such developmental effects remains to be performed.

PHYSIOLOGY

Passive Stress-Strain Relationship

Cardiac muscle, like all biologic tissues, undergoes strain when stress is applied to it (Fig. 2–4). The relationship between the deformation of the tissue, e.g., the length of change in a papillary muscle, and the stress (force) applied to it is nonlinear. The extent of the change in length in cardiac tissue can be quite large as compared with that of other biologic tissues. As noted in Figure 2–4, the curvilinear or exponential relationship between length and extending force demonstrates that initially large increases in length can be achieved with small increases in tension, while with continued extension of the muscle, a region of the relationship is achieved in which large increases in tension are required to produce small increases in length. This physical relationship, which describes the passive properties of the myocardium, i.e., the myocardium at rest, undergoes significant maturational changes.

Isolated Myocardium

In comparing myocardium obtained from the fetal, neonatal, and adult heart, the relationships between muscle length and extending force are qualitatively similar. However, the fetal myocardium is stiffer or less compliant than that of the adult.[28,37] A large portion of this maturational change appears to occur within the first few days of postnatal life in the sheep. When these maturational changes were examined in the cat, the resting tension was significantly greater in the early neonatal preparations than in adult preparations, while myocardium from 2- to 3- week-old kittens fell between these two extremes. This developmental increase in compliance of the isolated muscle is reflected in the intact ventricle (see the next section, Intact Heart).

The structural basis of this decrease in myocardial stiffness is unclear. For example, the connective tissue content is higher in the older animal than in the neonate.[37] Indeed, the extracellular matrix that makes up the connective tissue in the cardiac muscle increases quantitatively during fetal and neonatal growth.[18,19,77] For example, in the rodent the initial formation of the network occurs within the first few days after birth, with little organized collagen being found at birth.

In view of the clear developmental changes in the stiffness of the myocardium, other explanations appear necessary. For example, the changes in different types of collagen with development could produce the observed maturational changes in myocardial compliance, for different collagens have different elastic properties. Alterations in the amount and proportion of collagen types I, II, III, and V with maturation have yet to be well described.

Additional explanations for developmental changes in the stiffness of the myocardium could lie in the development of the extracellular matrix. Developmental changes occur in the sites on the ventricular cell surface that recognize and allow for attachment of fibronectin, laminin, and the collagens.[18] For example, neonatal cells attach well to all types of collagen, laminin, and fibronectin, whereas adult cells attach well to only type IV collagen and laminin. Furthermore, the site of attachment in the adult appears to be located at the ends of the cell near the Z-disk, while such a localization of the attachment site does not appear to be present in the immature cell. These maturational changes in the extracellular matrix and its cell attachments could contribute to the maturational decrease in stiffness.

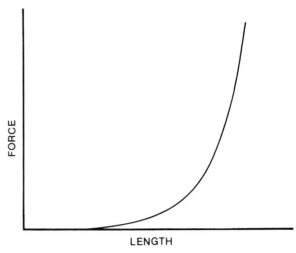

Figure 2–4. The typical relationship between extending force and the length of an isolated piece of myocardium is illustrated.

An additional explanation for the developmental increase in myocardial compliance could have a cytoskeletal basis (see Anatomy). In relaxed adult cardiac muscle isolated from its extracellular matrix and membranes, extension of the fiber demonstrates a different stress-strain relationship, indicating that the physical properties of the cytoskeleton influence myocardial compliance. Thus, maturational changes in cytoskeletal organization and the isoform expression of cytoskeletal proteins could affect compliance significantly.

Intact Heart

The compliance of both the right and left ventricles increases with maturation. The right and left ventricles of the fetal lamb heart are less compliant than those of the 1-week-old neonate, while those of the neonate are less compliant than the ventricles of the adult heart.[87]

During the weeks following birth, marked alterations in the relative contributions of the right and left ventricles to ventricular mass occur, with the right ventricular mass becoming relatively less compared with that of the left. During this process, the right ventricle becomes more compliant than the left. As a consequence, in vitro changes in right ventricular volume have a greater effect on left ventricular filling in the fetal heart than in the adult heart.[87]

In the adult heart, mechanical interaction between the ventricles has been demonstrated.[12,92] An increase in right ventricular volume or afterload interferes with left ventricular filling; for example, increasing ventricular diastolic pressure to 15 mmHg or higher will significantly decrease the volume introduced into the contralateral chamber in response to a filling pressure of 5 mmHg. In vitro studies have demonstrated that this impairment in filling is most marked in the fetal heart, less so in the 1- to 2-week-old, and least in the adult. Although this in vitro interaction has not been proved in vivo in the hearts of the fetus and neonate, ventricular interaction is likely to have more profound effects in the fetal and newborn heart in

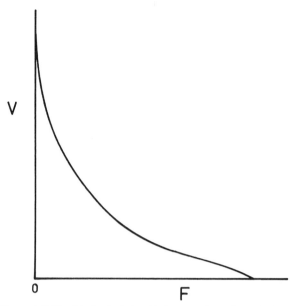

Figure 2–5. The idealized relationship between shortening velocity and the force borne during shortening (i.e. afterload) for cardiac muscle. The fastest velocity is obtained at zero load and is related to the rate of cross-bridge interactions. When the load is so great as to prevent shortening, the force waveform is termed isometric and depends on the number of cross-bridge attachments. F = force; V = shortening velocity.

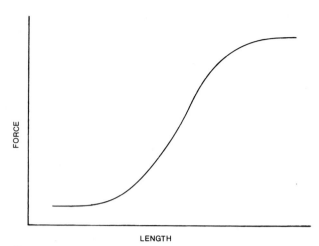

Figure 2–6. The effect of preload (i.e., muscle length) on the ability of the myocardium to develop force. Preload must be applied to cardiac muscle to enable the myocardium to develop force. This relationship is common to adult and fetal isolated myocardium. If length is extended far enough (not portrayed here), the ability of the muscle to generate force stops increasing and instead falls.

light of the relatively lower compliance of the immature myocardium.

In the immature heart, this interrelationship will be very sensitive to changes in right ventricular diastolic or systolic loading pressures. An increase in right ventricular afterload will result in an increase in right ventricular end-diastolic volume, which will compromise left ventricular filling and thus stroke volume. On the other hand, the neonatal fall in pulmonary artery pressure may contribute significantly to the neonatal enhancement in left ventricular filling and therefore stroke volume. The relative stiffness of the right ventricle will have other hemodynamic effects: For example, right-to-left shunting occurs at the atrial level when pulmonary artery pressure is raised in the isolated neonatal heart,[111] and in the open-chested neonatal lamb volume loading can produce right-to-left atrial shunting.[1] Thus, as an anticipated consequence of the passive properties of the myocardium, diseases that increase right ventricular preload, e.g., papillary muscle dysfunction, or those that increase right ventricular afterload, e.g., persistence of pulmonary hypertension, will have a greater effect on neonatal left ventricular function than on adult left ventricular function.

Contractile Properties

The Basis of Myocardial Contraction

This section discusses the basic aspects of contraction that are common to the heart over a broad range of development. These processes can explain the dependence of the force of contraction and shortening velocity on muscle length (preload), inotropy, and the load borne during the contraction (afterload).

Force and Velocity. The general characteristics of the relationship between force and shortening velocity of the myocardium are illustrated in Figure 2–5. In summary, the maximum velocity of muscle shortening is obtained at zero load. With an increase in load (afterload), the velocity of muscle shortening decreases. When the load is so great that no external shortening occurs, the contraction is considered to be isometric. The force developed by the myocardium can be altered by changing muscle length (preload) (Fig. 2–6) and the experimental conditions. The latter include alterations of the milieu of the myocardium, such as exposure to sympathomimetic agents. These alterations represent changes in the inotropy of the myocardium, as they act without a change in preload.

Contractile Apparatus. The processes that control contraction appear to be the same in the fetal and the adult heart. The sarcomere with its interdigitating thick and thin filaments, containing myosin and actin, respectively, is the basic contractile unit. The interaction between these filaments results in force development through cross-bridge attachments. The greater the number of cross-bridges, the greater the force developed. The increase in cytosolic calcium concentration that occurs with activation allows this interaction. Although activation is all-or-none in cardiac muscle, the increase in cytosolic calcium is modulated (see the section Inotropy), so that the force developed can vary from contraction to contraction. This effect of calcium concentration is a consequence of the regulatory proteins tropomyosin, troponin T, troponin I, and troponin C, which are located on the thin filament.[76] The troponin complex is bound to tropomyosin by troponin T. Troponin I inhibits the force producing cross-bridge interactions, while troponin C, through its binding calcium, overcomes this inhibition of cross-bridge formation.

The Force-Interval Relationship. In cardiac muscle the force or velocity of shortening is affected by altering the rate and pattern of stimulation[47] in the absence of a change in preload or afterload. Postextrasystolic potentiation is an example of this force-interval relationship (Fig. 2–7). These physiologic properties are present across a wide range of development, from late gestation to adulthood,[3,7,28,49,66] and can be found to some extent in all mammalian myocardium.

These alterations in the force of contraction result from variations in activator calcium and so represent changes in inotropy. Recent studies using the aequorin luminescence signal have confirmed the presence of these changes in calcium,[114] e.g., potentiation in the luminescence signal is present in the postextrasystolic contraction. This potentiation in activator calcium concentration is thought to be a consequence of a combination of transsarcolemmal movement of calcium during the extrasystole and postextrasystole and enhanced release of calcium from intracellular stores, i.e., the sarcoplasmic reticulum (SR) and more specifically the junctional and corbular components of the SR.[16,24,42,46,68] The contributions of sarcoplasmic reticulum release of calcium to postextrasystolic potentiation have been explored with the use of ryanodine, an agent that is thought to affect the calcium release channel of the SR.[67,114] In the presence of ryanodine, postextrasystolic potentiation of force and of the luminescence signal is abolished.

The restitution of contractility following contraction (Fig. 2–8) is another aspect of the force-interval relationship that depends on the control of activator calcium.[47] In the adult myocardium contractility is depressed immediately after a contraction and then increases gradually with time until the force is equal to that of the previous contraction (Fig. 2–8), e.g., the most premature extrasystole develops little force. These changes in contractility that occur after the contraction are markedly accelerated in the presence of ryanodine.[114]

The knowledge that postextrasystolic potentiation and restitution of contractility are based on changes in cytosolic calcium and that these relationships are affected by the SR make the force-interval relationship of value in exploring developmental changes in the control of activator calcium.

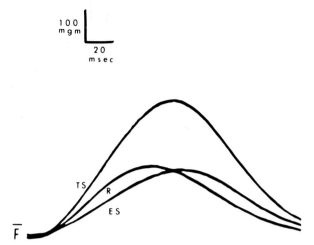

Figure 2–7. Postextrasystolic potentiation. Force as a function of time for the contraction at the basic rate, an extrasystole, and a postextrasystole are illustrated. The extrasystole develops the smallest force, while the potentiated, or postextrasystolic, contraction develops the greatest. These changes in force are the result of changes in activator calcium concentration. ES = extrasystole; F = force; TS = postextrasystole; R = response at basic rate.

Isolated Myocardium

Among the many physiologic changes that the myocardium undergoes with development is a maturational increase in its ability to contract and to develop force. A sudden increase in force-generating ability does not occur with birth. This ability (corrected for cross-sectional area) increases as development proceeds from the fetus to the neonate to the adult.

The maturational increase in contractile force can be related to several of the structural changes noted in the earlier discussion of myocardial anatomy. The maturational increase in the myofibrillar content of the myocardium will allow an increase in the number of cross-bridge attachments and thus greater force. The maturational increase in the orderliness of the myofibrillar arrangement within the myocyte could also contribute to the maturational increase in force development. As to whether the calcium sensitivity of the contractile apparatus could be

Figure 2–8. The restitution of contractility at two different stages of development. ΔS, The amount of sarcomere shortening in an extrasystole, is plotted against the time interval between the application of the extrasystolic stimulus and the stimulus that elicited the previous contraction for two different cells obtained from rabbit ventricular myocardium. Dashed line = restitution for a cell from a 3-week-old rabbit heart; solid line = restitution for a cell from an adult rabbit heart.

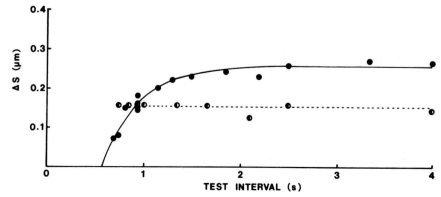

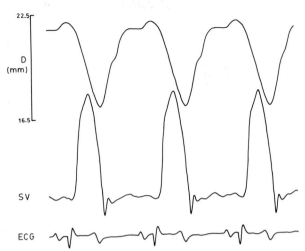

Figure 2–9. Data obtained from a chronically instrumented fetal lamb describing left ventricular filling and ejection. From the top of the illustration downward: left ventricular minor axis dimension, ascending aortic flow, and electrocardiogram. D = left ventricular minor axis dimension; ECG = electrocardiogram; SV = ascending aortic flow.

changing, the relationship between force and the calcium bathing the myofilaments has been described in fetal as well as adult myocardium.[34] Of interest in this study, fetal myofilaments appeared to be more sensitive to calcium, the opposite of what would be anticipated to explain the maturational increase in force development.

Maturational changes in the membrane systems that control calcium would provide another explanation for the increase in the ability of the myocardium to develop force. If activator calcium concentration is increased with maturation, the sensitivity of the contractile apparatus to calcium need not change. The cell could simply operate over a different portion of the force/pCa relationship. The extent to which cytosolic calcium increases with activation depends on the sarcolemma and the sarcoplasmic reticulum and how they have been altered by preceding events, e.g., exposure of the muscle to an agent that alters inotropy, such as a sympathomimetic agent. Evidence for

maturational changes in these systems is provided in the sections Anatomy and Inotropy.

The maturational increase in the ability of the myocardium to develop force over the stages of development from late gestation to the adult does not appear to be related to changes in the basic processes that control contraction. Rather, quantitative changes in the components of these processes are likely to be the basis for this maturational increase.

Intact Heart

Ventricular filling, pressure development, and ejection in the heart of the intact fetus are similar in many ways to those in the neonate and the adult. Figures 2–9 and 2–10 illustrate filling and ejection for the fetal right and left ventricles.

Some of the properties of ejection appear to differ between the fetal right and left ventricle; for example, see the ventricular dimension waveform and the pressure and flow waveforms of the ascending aorta and main pulmonary artery during systole in Figures 2–9 to 2–11. Similar differences are present in the neonate and in the adult.

When ejection measures such as stroke volume are used to examine the ability of the developing heart to eject blood, significant maturational increases are the expected result because of the growth of the heart and the increase in needs of the body. When left ventricular output (corrected for body weight) is used as the measure, little difference is noted between the left ventricular output of the sheep fetus during late gestation and that of the lamb 6 weeks following birth. However, as will be considered later in the chapter, a marked increase in ventricular output occurs with birth.

Pressure development in the fetal left ventricle appears similar to that of the adult. For example, the peak first derivative of left ventricular pressure ($[dP/dt]_{max}$), a measure of the ability of the ventricle to contract, which is in part dependent on preload and afterload, has the same range of values in the fetal lamb as it does in the adult

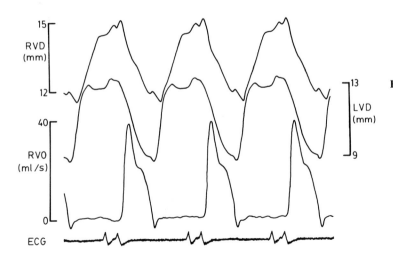

Figure 2–10. Data obtained from a chronically instrumented fetal lamb illustrating right and left ventricular dimension waveforms and main pulmonary artery flow. The right ventricular dimension and left ventricular dimension were measured from the ventricular septum to the endocardial free wall of each ventricle. The differences noted between right and left ventricular filling and ejection are typical for the fetal lamb. ECG = electrocardiogram; LVD = left ventricular dimension; RVD = right ventricular dimension; RVO = main pulmonary artery flow.

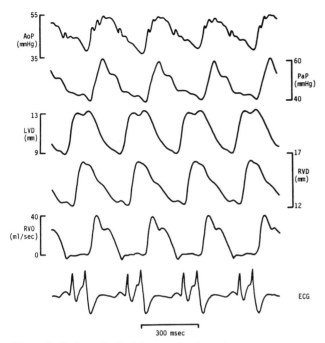

Figure 2–11. Data obtained from a chronically instrumented in utero fetal lamb during normal sinus rhythm. From the top of the illustration downward: aortic pressure, pulmonary artery pressure, left ventricular dimension (obtained as in Fig. 2–10), right ventricular dimension, main pulmonary artery flow, and electrocardiogram obtained using atrial electrodes. Note the similarity in the differences between the aortic and pulmonary artery pressure waveforms and those in the systolic portion of the left and right ventricular dimension waveforms. AoP = aortic pressure; ECG = electrocardiogram; LVD = left ventricular dimension; PaP = pulmonary artery pressure; RVD = right ventricular dimension; RVO = main pulmonary artery flow.

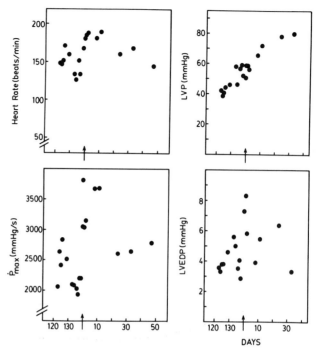

Figure 2–12. Hemodynamic data obtained from a lamb instrumented at 123 days of gestation and delivered vaginally at 140 days of gestation. On each abscissa, days of gestation are to the left of the arrow and days following birth are to the right. LVEDP = left ventricular end-diastolic pressure; LVP = left ventricular peak systolic pressure; $\dot{P}_{max}$ = the peak first derivative of left ventricular pressure.

ewe (e.g., 1500 to 3000 mmHg/s). Of note, this range is the same as that observed in the child and in the adult human. However, a significant increase in $[dP/dt]_{max}$ occurs with birth, as discussed in the section Inotropy.

The peak systolic pressure generated by the left ventricle increases throughout late gestation and following birth (Fig. 2–12), while with birth a rapid fall in right ventricular peak systolic pressure occurs.

The Effect of Birth

The ability of the isolated myocardium to contract, in response to pacing at a constant rate, does not appear to change significantly from late gestation to immediately following birth. However, striking differences in function are manifest in vivo.[3,5] Among these, the outputs of the right and left ventricles are increased.[90] The relative increase is greater for the left ventricle, which is in part related to the relative contributions of the right and left ventricle to cardiac output in the fetus. The mechanisms that bring about the enhancement in ventricular output with birth are yet to be clarified; for example, in some instances left ventricular output is more than tripled. As will be considered in subsequent sections, an increase in pulmonary venous return, an enhancement in inotropy, an increase in heart rate, and the diastolic and systolic inter-

actions of the right and left ventricles may all be potential contributors to this enhancement.

In the weeks following birth, while left ventricular systolic pressure and end-diastolic volume continue to increase, left ventricular output (corrected for body weight) returns to the fetal level and lower (Figs. 2–12 and 2–13). In addition, the birth-associated increase in $[dP/dt]_{max}$ and the changes in other measures of inotropy return to the fetal levels (Figs. 2–12 and 2–14). These findings suggest that the reserves of the heart are to a large extent expended in response to birth and that in the subsequent days these reserves are restored. Consequently, disease states that affect the mechanisms that bring about the neonatal enhancement in cardiac output or those that place demands for a further increase in cardiac output will have a more marked effect in the first days following birth than during the subsequent weeks.

Frank-Starling Relationship

The Frank-Starling relationship is characterized by the effect of ventricular end-diastolic volume on ventricular output. In that this preparing or loading of the ventricle occurs prior to activation, it is termed "preload." The effect of preload on ventricular contraction was first described in the isolated heart, where Frank demonstrated that as ventricular end-diastolic volume was increased over a broad range, the ability of the ventricle to contract

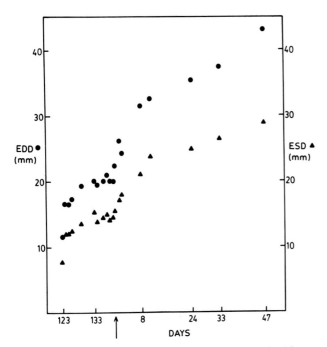

Figure 2–13. Left ventricular minor axis dimension data obtained from a lamb instrumented and studied in utero prior to vaginal delivery at 140 days of gestation. Birth is indicated by the arrow with days of gestation on the left and days following birth on the right. EDD = left ventricular end-diastolic dimension; ESD = left ventricular end-systolic dimension.

and to develop pressure increased. Ultimately, this relationship achieved a plateau, and then with a further increase in ventricular volume, the ability to develop pressure fell.

At the level of the sarcomere, the sliding filament theory continues to explain the length dependence of force development (although this preload dependence has

also been attributed to changes in the sensitivity of the myofilaments to calcium concentration). Sarcomere length, which describes the overlap of the thick and thin filaments, is crucial in force development, as has been described in skeletal muscle. When the sarcomere is stretched so that the thick and thin filaments no longer overlap, no cross-bridge attachments can be made; consequently, force cannot be developed. At the optimal overlap of the thick and thin filaments, the maximum number of cross-bridge attachments can be made and peak force can be developed. When the sarcomere length is so short that double overlap of the thin filaments occurs, the ability of the sarcomere to develop force is decreased.

Isolated Myocardium

The Frank-Starling relationship is present in the immature myocardium. Isolated myocardium from the fetal heart, including that of humans, illustrates this property.[37] With an increase in muscle length, force development is enhanced for fetal myocardium, as it is for neonatal and adult myocardium (see Fig. 2–6). As would be anticipated from the maturational increase in the ability of the myocardium to develop force, when the fetal relationship between muscle length and force (corrected for cross-section area) is plotted, this relationship falls below that of the adult.[28,37] Regardless of this maturational difference, the basic process that results in the Frank-Starling relationship is present in fetal and neonatal myocardium.

Intact Heart

In the intact heart, preload is a consequence of ventricular filling. In the fetal right and left ventricles, diastole is marked by periods of rapid filling, slow filling, and presystolic enhancement of ventricular end-diastolic volume

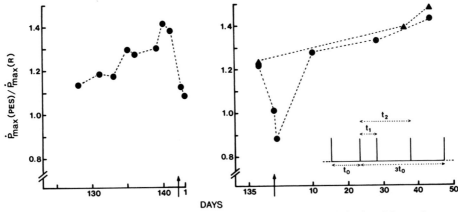

Figure 2–14. Postextrasystolic potentiation (the peak first derivative of the postextrasystole/peak first derivative of the previous systole at the basic rate) is illustrated for two chronically instrumented lambs. The data in the left-hand panel were obtained from a lamb delivered by cesarean section at 142 days of gestation and that in the right-hand panel from a lamb delivered vaginally at 138 days of gestation. The abscissa in each panel is divided by an arrow representing birth: days of gestation are to the left of the arrow and days following delivery are to the right. The insert describes the pacing pattern used to obtain these data. Two systoles were introduced in a pause in the basic pacing rate, the extrasystole was elicited following the interval t_1 with the postextrasystole following the interval of t_2. During maturation, postextrasystolic potentiation increased. At the time of birth, postextrasystolic potentiation fell in a manner similar to that induced by an infusion of isoproterenol in the fetal lamb (see Fig. 2–18). t_1 = first time interval; t_2 = second time interval. (Reproduced with permission from Anderson PAW, Glick KL, Manring A, Crenshaw CC Jr [1984]: Developmental changes in cardiac contractility in fetal and postnatal sheep: In vitro and in vivo. Am J Physiol 247:[3 Pt 2]H371–H379.)

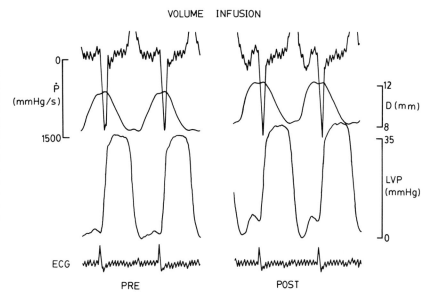

Figure 2–15. Data obtained from a chronically instrumented fetal lamb illustrating the effects of a volume infusion. The data on the left-hand side of the illustration were obtained prior to the infusion (pre) and that on the right following the infusion (post). The waveforms from the top of the illustration downward are the first derivative of left ventricular pressure, left ventricular minor axis dimension, left ventricular pressure, and the electrocardiogram. The heart rate was the same during each period. D = left ventricular minor axis dimension; ECG = electrocardiogram; LVP = left ventricular pressure; $\dot{P}$ = the first derivative of left ventricular pressure.

in response to atrial contraction (see Figs. 2–9 to 2–11). These characteristics of diastolic filling are similar to the classical description of ventricular filling in the adult heart. Of interest, in the fetal heart the end-diastolic dimension of the right ventricle is larger relative to that of the left ventricle (as measured from the septum to the endocardial surfaces of the right and left ventricular free walls.)[4] In addition, differences appear to exist in the relative rates of right and left ventricular filling.

Similar to the effects of preload on force development in isolated myocardium, when the maximum rate of rise of left ventricular pressure ($[dP/dt]_{max}$) is used to assess the effects of changing end-diastolic volume, $[dP/dt]_{max}$ is increased when end-diastolic volume is increased (Fig. 2–15).

When other measures of ventricular function such as stroke volume and ventricular output are used to assess the effects of preload in the fetal heart, the results are less certain.[2,4,5,40,49,90,107,108] An initial study suggested that the Frank-Starling relationship does not exist in the fetal heart, while subsequent studies have concluded that the fetal right and left ventricles have little functional reserves in the Frank-Starling relationship. In essence, the fetal heart can be considered to be operating at the peak of this relationship, since the withdrawal of blood, which produces a fall in atrial pressure, decreases ventricular output, while an increase in atrial pressure over the resting level produces little increase in output. Other fetal studies provide evidence that changes in end-diastolic volume significantly affect stroke volume (Fig. 2–16).

The differences among these studies may be a consequence of the variables used to assess a change in end-diastolic volume; for example, when an indirect measure of end-diastolic volume changes significantly while stroke volume changes little, the interpretation would be that the Frank-Starling relationship is absent, yet end-diastolic volume might have changed little. Recalling the exponential or curvilinear relationship between pressure and end-diastolic volume present in the heart, a large change

in diastolic pressure may produce little change in end-diastolic volume. The relatively low compliance of the fetal myocardium would bring about this effect at modest filling pressures (see the section Passive Stress-Strain Relationship). Indeed, maturational increases in myocardial compliance have been suggested as a cause of the

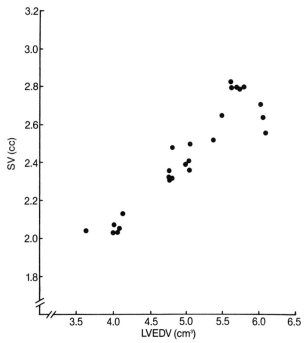

Figure 2–16. The relationship between fetal left ventricular stroke volume and end-diastolic volume obtained from a chronically instrumented fetal lamb. A range of left ventricular end-diastolic volumes was obtained by altering the pacing interval. Left ventricular end-diastolic volume was computed by measuring three left ventricular dimensions. LVEDV = left ventricular end-diastolic volume; SV = stroke volume.

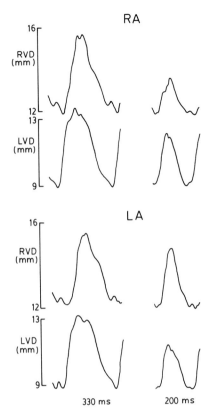

Figure 2–17. Right ventricular minor axis dimension and left ventricular minor axis dimension obtained during right atrial pacing (the upper half of the illustration) and during left atrial pacing (the lower half of the illustration). The data on the left-hand side of the illustration were obtained at a pacing interval of 330 ms and those on the right at a pacing interval of 200 ms. Regardless of the site of atrial pacing, both right and left ventricular end-diastolic dimensions fell with the increase in rate. However, a differential effect on end-diastolic dimension was induced by the site of atrial pacing. An increase in rate using right atrial pacing resulted in a greater fall in right ventricular end-diastolic dimension, while left atrial pacing produced a greater fall in left ventricular end-diastolic dimension. These effects are those typically seen in the chronically instrumented fetal lamb. LA = left atrial pacing; LVD = left ventricular minor axis dimension; RA = right atrial pacing; RVD = right ventricular minor axis dimension.

apparent developmental acquisition of the Frank-Starling relationship.[88] When ventricular dimensions are used to assess the effect of preload on fetal right or left ventricular stroke volume, a significant and positive relationship between end-diastolic volume and stroke volume is found in the fetal heart. The relationship between fetal ventricular end-diastolic volume and stroke volume is revealed by examining systoles during variations in the heart rate (Figs. 2–17 and 2–18).[2,4] Altering the pacing pattern can produce a wide range of end-diastolic volumes. An increase in end-diastolic volume, over a physiologic range of filling pressures, is associated with an increase in fetal right and left ventricular stroke volumes (see Fig. 2–16).

The left ventricle of the acutely instrumented neonatal lamb has also been shown to have a Frank-Starling relationship.[30] However, a developmental increase in the significance of the Frank-Starling relationship has been suggested to occur during neonatal life. Volume infusions have been shown to increase cardiac output by a greater percentage in the 6-week-old lamb than in the 1-week-old lamb,[50] although the 1-week-old had a greater absolute increase in output than the 6-week-old. However these findings are expressed, they indicate that a volume infusion in the neonatal lamb can result in a significant increase in cardiac output.

The Effect of Birth

Left ventricular end-diastolic volume increases with birth (see Fig. 2–13). This increase would appear to contribute to the neonatal increase in output through the Frank-Starling relationship in that in the fetus, stroke volume is related to left ventricular end-diastolic volume, and an increase in filling pressure increases stroke volume in the acutely instrumented neonate.

The neonatal increase in left ventricular end-diastolic volume, as evidenced by the increase in left ventricular end-diastolic pressure and dimensions, may result from more than one aspect of the rearrangement of the circulation with birth. The observation that in utero ventilation

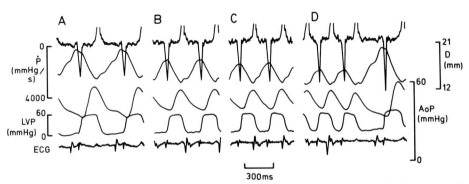

Figure 2–18. The effects of heart rate on left ventricular pressure and filling and ejection observed in a chronically instrumented fetal lamb. Heart rate was controlled by atrial pacing. With an increase in heart rate, end-diastolic volume fell while the peak first derivative of pressure increased. The group of data on the right demonstrates the effect of increasing the pacing interval and allowing pressure development to begin from the same end-diastolic dimension as that at the lowest rate. Traces from the top: first derivative of left ventricular pressure with positive deflection downward, left ventricular minor axis dimension, aortic pressure, left ventricular pressure, and electrocardiogram. AoP = aortic pressure; D = left ventricular minor axis dimension; ECG = electrocardiogram; LVP = left ventricular pressure; P = first derivative of left ventricular pressure. (Reproduced with permission from Anderson PAW, Manring A, Glick KL, Crenshaw CC Jr [1982]: Biophysics of the developing heart. III. A comparison of the left ventricular dynamics of the fetal and neonatal lamb heart. Am J Obstet Gynecol 143:195–203.)

with oxygen decreases pulmonary vascular resistance and increases pulmonary blood flow while markedly diminishing right-to-left shunting through the ductus arteriosus suggests that the neonatal fall in pulmonary vascular resistance and the increase in pulmonary venous return may be significant contributors to the neonatal increase in left ventricular end-diastolic volume.[69,91]

Left ventricular filling may be enhanced through the decrease in neonatal right ventricular afterload by way of the interaction between the right and left ventricles (see the section Passive Stress-Strain Relationship). The neonatal fall in pulmonary artery pressure would enhance left ventricular output in the following manner: A decrease in right ventricular afterload will enhance right ventricular ejection and result in a smaller right ventricular end-systolic volume. The left ventricle is then able to fill to a larger volume for a comparable filling pressure. This effect of ventricular interaction would be amplified in the fetus and the neonate because of the lower compliance of the ventricular myocardium at that age.

Afterload

The ability of the myocardium to shorten or of the ventricle to eject blood is affected by the load borne during the contraction. As contrasted to the stretch of preload that occurs prior to activation, the load borne during a contraction is termed the "afterload" and has an inverse relationship with shortening velocity or ventricular ejection (see Fig. 2–5). In all cardiac preparations, including those of the fetus, the ability of the myocardium to shorten is decreased as afterload is increased.[37] The fastest velocity of shortening is achieved at zero load, a condition not possible to obtain in the intact heart. This unloaded velocity of muscle shortening has been correlated to the rate of ATP hydrolysis by myosin ATPase, which is consistent with ATPase activity controlling the rate of cross-bridge detachment. This relationship between shortening velocity and ATPase activity is exemplified by the effects of hyperthyroidism, which changes myosin isoform expression from V_3 to V_1, the isoform with the highest ATPase activity.[61,120] The myocardium with myosin V_1 shortens more rapidly than does the myocardium expressing myosin V_3. In the presence of a load, shortening velocity also depends on the number of cross-bridge attachments.

Isolated Myocardium

When muscle shortening velocity and afterload of the fetal myocardium (corrected for cross-sectional area of the myocardium) are compared with those of the adult, the fetal myocardium shortens more slowly against the same load than does the adult myocardium.[37] This effect of afterload on the immature myocardium is not surprising in view of the developmental change in the force-generating ability of the myocardium.

When the estimated unloaded shortening velocity of the fetal sheep myocardium was compared with that of the

adult, no difference was found. In contrast, in the canine myocardium,[110] a developmental increase in muscle shortening velocity was noted from the neonate to the adult. The lack of a change in estimated unloaded shortening velocity in the sheep appears to be consistent with the absence of a change in myofibrillar ATPase in the sheep over this developmental period,[36] while the increase in muscle shortening velocity in the dog appears to be opposite of the developmental transition in myosin isoform expression (see the section Myosin).

In attempts to circumvent the complicating effects of maturational changes in the extracellular matrix on evaluating developmental changes in shortening velocity, sarcomere shortening velocity has been examined in the isolated single cardiac myocyte.[72] While no comparisons have been made among fetal and neonatal myocytes, a comparative study has been performed using neonatal and adult myocytes. The amount and velocity of sarcomere shortening were greater in the adult myocyte than in myocytes from the heart of the 3-week-old. Although these cells were externally unloaded, some internal load was present in that they reextended at the end of a contraction. This internal load has not been measured among cells from a range of development, so the presence of a developmental change in internal afterload is uncertain. However, it is clear that muscle-shortening velocity against an external afterload is enhanced with development.

Intact Heart

Arterial pressure is a major component of afterload in the intact heart and has a significant effect on ventricular ejection. For example, the higher the aortic pressure, the smaller the left ventricular stroke volume. This general relationship is true throughout development. An increase in afterload decreased fetal right ventricular output as well as that of the neonatal left ventricle.[30,90,107] In a study of the neonatal left ventricle, an increase in arterial pressure that would be well tolerated by the adult heart resulted in a fall in ventricular stroke volume.[30] Interestingly, a difference may exist in the sensitivity of the fetal right and left ventricle to afterload; that is, the fetal left ventricle may not be as sensitive as the right ventricle to an increase in afterload.[108] This apparent difference may be a reflection of the in utero differences in ventricular workload, i.e., the right ventricle performs more work than the left ventricle, and may also be due to variations in the shape and configuration of the ventricles and thus their ability to develop wall tension and to eject blood.

The Effect of Birth

With birth, aortic pressure increases (see Fig. 2–12). Given the inverse relationship between afterload and the ability of the ventricle to eject, a decrease in left ventricular ouput would be anticipated. However, the neonatal left ventricular output is markedly increased.

In contrast to the direction of change in aortic pressure, pulmonary artery pressure falls. This decrease in right ventricular afterload reduces right ventricular end-diastolic volume and thereby may enhance left ventricular filling and stroke volume, as considered earlier. Furthermore, the neonatal fall in right ventricular systolic pressure would be anticipated to enhance the ability of the left ventricle to develop pressure because of the systolic interaction of the two ventricles as well. For example, an increase in right ventricular systolic pressure decreases the ability of the neonatal left ventricle to contract, as has been demonstrated in the isolated heart.[111]

The relationship between afterload and ventricular ejection is important in considering the effects of neonatal systemic hypertension. Furthermore, the presence of this relationship in the right ventricle is important in understanding how neonatal diseases that increase right ventricular afterload affect ventricular ejection. Such diseases may impair right ventricular function and, through ventricular interaction, that of the left ventricle.

Inotropy

Inotropy can be defined simply as the strength of contraction of the myocardium. A change in inotropy reflects an increase or decrease in the ability of the myocardium to contract in the absence of a change in preload or afterload. At the cellular level, changes in inotropy can be a consequence of the isoform expression of the contractile apparatus proteins. For example, the change in myosin isoform from V_1 to V_3 would result in a decrease in ATPase activity and a fall in unloaded muscle shortening velocity,[14] while a change in thin filament regulatory protein expression could result in a shift in the force/pCa relationship[21] (see the section Developmental Changes in Protein Isoform Expression). An additional basis for a change in inotropy is an alteration in contractile protein function through posttranslational change, e.g., phosphorylation of troponin I (a result of β-agonist stimulation) decreases the sensitivity of the myofilaments to calcium.[15,117]

Another aspect of cell function that can alter inotropy is the control of cytosolic calcium. As noted in the section Contractile Properties, an alteration in sarcolemmal or sarcoplasmic reticulum function will result in a change in calcium concentration bathing the myofilaments during a contraction. Such modulation of activator calcium is a common mechanism through which inotropic agents affect the myocardium.

The Modulation of Cytosolic Calcium

In light of how cytosolic calcium is related to the ability of the thin and thick filaments to interact (see the section Contractile Properties), the control of cytosolic calcium is an important part of the process of contraction and relaxation. The increase in cytosolic calcium with activation depends on the systems that control transsarcolemmal movement of calcium. Maturational changes in some of the sarcolemmal-based systems for controlling cell calcium have been described.[33,41,48,52] If calcium concentration

is to reach levels necessary for maximum force development, release of calcium from intracellular sources appears to be necessary.[24] Consequently, the sarcoplasmic reticulum (SR) is important in the modulation of cytosolic calcium. As noted in the section Anatomy, significant changes occur in a range of SR characteristics during fetal and neonatal life. These findings suggest that maturational changes in the availability of activator calcium could be an important factor in accounting for functional differences between the immature and the adult myocardium, i.e., a lower concentration of calcium bathing the sarcomere would account for the lower sarcomere shortening and reextension velocities observed in the immature cell.[72]

A greater dependence of the immature myocardium on transsarcolemmal movement of calcium has been suggested. Force development of fetal human, cat, and rabbit myocardium as well as that of the newborn cat and rabbit is not inhibited by ryanodine, an agent that interferes with SR function, while within a few days following birth, this agent significantly decreases force development.[82] The relatively greater importance of transsarcolemmal movement of calcium in the immature myocardium is supported by a range of other findings, including the greater effect of alterations in extracellular calcium concentration on the contractile response of the immature myocardium.[52]

Maturational changes in the dependence of force development on transsarcolemmal sources of activator calcium are suggested by the maturational changes in the intracellular sites of calcium uptake and release. The SR content of the myocardium and its ability to take up calcium increase with development, including from fetal to newborn stages (see also the section Anatomy). Furthermore, when cacium release is induced from the SR, a progressive developmental increase in the sensitivity of this response to calcium is found.[34] This process is much less well developed in the fetal rat and is acquired within a few days after birth. The developmental acquisition of this aspect of SR function, calcium release, is consistent with intracellular calcium stores becoming, with maturation, more important in providing activator calcium.

Perturbations in the Pattern of Stimulation: Expression of the Developmental Changes in Membrane Function

Isolated Myocardium. The likelihood that maturational differences in the modulation of activator calcium are present is suggested by the effects of experimental perturbations such as paired pacing or the introduction of an extrasystole. These perturbations produce beat-to-beat changes in force that rapidly equilibrate following a perturbation. For example, in the adult myocardium, with the introduction of an extrasystole, the force generated in the premature extrasystole is small compared with that of a previous contraction at the basic rate, while a subsequent postextrasystole is potentiated (see Fig. 2–7). As noted previously, these differences in force are the result of differences in activator calcium, with the SR being an important contributor to postextrasystolic potentiation.

Figure 2–19. The effects of isoproterenol on postextrasystolic potentiation in a chronically instrumented
fetal lamb. A systole at the basic
pacing rate is on the left-hand side
of each panel and that following
the extrasystole is on the right.
In response to isoproterenol, a
marked enhancement in the peak
first derivative of pressure was
achieved while postextrasystolic
potentiation was markedly decreased. The groups of data were
obtained using the same heart
rates and extrasystolic intervals.
The tracings from the top: first
derivative of left ventricular pressure, left ventricular minor axis
dimension, aortic pressure, left
ventricular pressure, and electrocardiogram. AoP = aortic pressure;
D = left ventricular minor axis di-

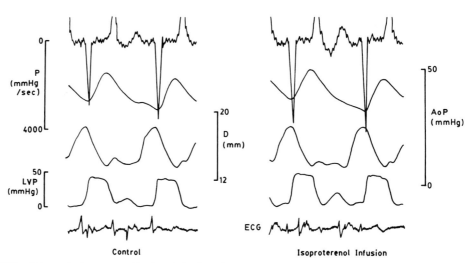

mension; ECG = electrocardiogram; LVP = left ventricular pressure; P = first derivative of left ventricular pressure. (Reproduced with permission from
Anderson PAW, Manring A, Crenshaw CC Jr [1980]: Biophysics of the developing heart. II. The interaction of the force-interval relationship with
inotropic state and muscle length [preload]. Am J Obstet Gynecol 138:44–54.)

These general physiologic properties are present across a wide range of development. For example, they have been noted in the myocardium from the human fetus. The presence of postextrasystolic potentiation in the immature myocardium demonstrates that the cellular processes that modulate activator calcium are in place. However, the extent of the enhancement in the strength of contraction with such variations in the pattern of stimulation increases with development.[3,5,7,28,66] The timing and the rate at which this increase occurs varies among species. For example, myocardium isolated from fetal sheep within 2 weeks of the end of gestation demonstrates a similar amount of postextrasystolic potentiation as that found in the lamb a month following birth, while potentiation continues to increase during neonatal life in the cat and dog. These findings demonstrate that the range over which activator calcium concentration can be modulated appears to be amplified with development.

As noted in the section Anatomy, cell growth or hypertrophy is a common maturational process. Just as postextrasystolic potentiation is enhanced with maturation, so is postextrasystolic potentiation enhanced in adult myocardium that has responded to a stimulus to hypertrophy.[6,8] Furthermore, α_1-agonist stimulation induces hypertrophy in neonatal cells,[99–101] and exposure to such an agonist enhances postextrasystolic potentiation.[62] Whether the cellular processes that bring about these similar structural and physiologic changes are coupled remains to be determined.

The restitution of contractility following a contraction (see the section Contractile Properties) is also prominently affected by development in the cat and in the rabbit (see Fig. 2–8). In the isolated kitten papillary muscle, the restitution of contractility is very rapid.[66] A maturational change in the restitution of sarcomere shortening has been found in the isolated myocyte of the 3-week-old rabbit.[72] The amount of sarcomere shortening in the most premature contraction is equal to the previous contraction at the

basic rate. This restitution of contractility in the immature myocardium is similar to that of the adult during exposure to ryanodine, suggesting that maturational changes in the sarcoplasmic reticulum (see the section Anatomy) may contribute significantly to developmental changes in the restitution of contractility.[114]

Intact Heart. Postextrasystolic potentiation is present in the intact chronically instrumented fetal lamb during the last weeks of gestation (see Figs. 2–14 and 2–19), just as it is in the isolated myocardium.[3,7] Postextrasystolic potentiation was found to be independent of ventricular volume (preload) in the developing heart. Although $[dP/dt]_{max}$ is affected by preload, the relative enhancement of $[dP/dt]_{max}$ in postextrasystole as compared with $[dP/dt]_{max}$ of the previous contraction is not affected by preload, so that a ratio of these two responses (when the two systoles begin from the same end-diastolic volume) does not vary from one ventricular volume to another.

In contrast, changes in inotropy significantly alter postextrasystolic potentiation in the immature and adult heart. For example, exposure of the heart of the intact fetus or adult to isoproterenol produces a significant decrease in postextrasystolic potentiation (Fig. 2–19).[5] The absence of an effect of preload on postextrasystolic potentiation and the sensitivity of postextrasystolic potentiation to inotropy are the bases for the use of this physiologic property as a mechanism for searching for developmental and birth-associated changes in ventricular function (see below).

The amount of postextrasystolic potentiation increases in the fetal heart in vivo during gestation (see Fig. 2–14) in a way similar to the changes in potentiation observed in the isolated myocardium. These results suggest that in the intact animal the range over which activator calcium can be modulated in the myocardium is increased prior to birth.

Effect of Birth. Neonatal left ventricular inotropy is increased from that of the fetal heart.[3,5] This conclusion is arrived at by examining the effects of birth on postextrasystolic potentiation and $[dP/dt]_{max}$ of the left ventricle (see Figs. 2–12 and 2–14). Potentiation is significantly decreased in the heart of the intact neonate as compared with postextrasystolic potentiation in the same lamb during fetal life. In addition, although $[dP/dt]_{max}$ is dependent on heart rate and end-diastolic volume, it has been possible to contrast this measure in the same lamb as a fetus and as a newborn for systoles at the same rate and end-diastolic dimension.[5] In those instances, $[dP/dt]_{max}$ was significantly higher in the newborn.

The significant fall in postextrasystolic potentiation in vivo with birth can be interpreted as a change in inotropy for the following reasons:[3,5] In the same lambs during fetal life, an isoproterenol infusion produced a significant reduction in postextrasystolic potentiation and a significant increase in $[dP/dt]_{max}$.[5] This close mimicking of the effects of an isoproterenol infusion in utero to the effects of birth on the heart in the intact lamb suggests that sympathetic stimulation is significantly enhancing ventricular function of the newborn (see the section Sympathetic Nervous System).

In the days and weeks that follow birth, $[dP/dt]_{max}$ decreases to the level found in the heart of the fetus and that of the adult, while postextrasystolic potentiation gradually increases to reattain or to exceed the fetal level of potentiation. In addition, the inotropic response to catecholamine infusion becomes greater with time following birth.[90] These maturational changes suggest that the heart is acquiring a greater functional reserve and is, in part, returning toward the reserve present in the fetal heart during late gestation.

Heart Rate

Isolated Myocardium. As noted in the sections Contractile Properties and Inotropy, alterations in the pattern of stimulation alter inotropy in the isolated myocardium. In both the adult and fetal myocardium an increase in pacing rate is associated with an increase in force development over a broad range of rates, with the characteristics of the relationship varying from species to species.

Intact Heart. The effects of heart rate on ventricular function in the intact fetus have been assessed by monitoring the ability of the left ventricle to develop pressure and by measuring right and left ventricular ejection characteristics.[2,4,5,49,90]

$[dP/dt]_{max}$ is affected positively by an increase in heart rate in the fetus, the newborn, and the adult.[5] This effect is noted even when a significant decrease in end-diastolic volume occurs, while if end-diastolic volume is maintained when rate is increased, an even greater increase in $[dP/dt]_{max}$ is observed (see Fig. 2–18).

In the fetal lamb, as in the adult animal, an increase in heart rate usually produces significant decreases in measures of ventricular ejection, e.g., stroke volume.[2,4,49] This apparently negative effect on the function of the intact heart follows from the fall in end-diastolic volume that accompanies an increase in heart rate.

The interaction between the amount of increases in heart rate (expressed as the number of beats per minute) and consequent reductions in stroke volume can lead to contradictory findings about the effect of heart rate on

ventricular output in the fetal lamb. When heart rate is increased by atrial pacing, neither right nor left ventricular output increases in the chronically instrumented fetus.[2,4] Pacing-induced increases in heart rate result in substantial decreases in end-diastolic dimension and stroke volume (Figs. 2–17, 2–18, and 2–20). If end-diastolic volume is maintained during pacing by transiently altering diastolic filling time, stroke volume increases with increases in rate, demonstrating the inotropic effect of rate and how it can be obscured by alterations in preload. These findings are consistent with those obtained from intact adult animals and humans.[89,105] In adult studies, in the absence of an increase in venous return, increases in heart rate induced by atrial pacing did not increase cardiac output.

However, a spontaneous increase in fetal heart rate has, in general, a positive effect on left and right ventricular output, although exceptions have been found.[2,4,90] The stimuli that induce spontaneous changes in heart rate also alter inotropy. Thus, in addition to the intrinsic effects of rate on inotropy, the heart of the intact fetus is responding to other endogenous inotropic stimulation. The stimuli that induce spontaneous heart rate changes can also alter venous return. For example, an increase in venous return produces a greater rate of ventricular filling, maintaining end-diastolic volume despite a decrease in diastolic filling time. Thus, the positive effect of a spontaneous increase in heart rate on fetal cardiac output may be the consequence of enhanced venous return and inotropy in addition to the increase in rate. These effects on fetal cardiac output are similar to those of rate, volume loading, and inotropic stimulation on cardiac output in the adult animal.[89,105]

Effect of Birth. With birth, heart rate increases (see Fig. 2–12).[3,5] When considered against the background of the effects of atrial pacing, the neonatal increase in heart rate might be anticipated to have no significant effect on cardiac output. However, the absence of an effect of heart rate on fetal cardiac output was due to a decrease in diastolic filling and thus a decrease in stroke volume. Following birth, pulmonary venous return is increased, and left ventricular filling may be enhanced further through the changed interaction of the right and left ventricles. Consequently, the neonatal increase in heart rate may contribute significantly to the neonatal increase in cardiac output.

Sympathetic Nervous System

Isolated Myocardium. The sympathetic nervous system and the myocardial response to various forms of sympathetic stimulation undergo a wide range of changes during development. Many aspects of the cell that are important in the response to sympathetic stimulation change; among these are changes in the adrenoceptors and the intracellular system, which transduces sympathetic stimulation into functional changes.

The intramyocardial release of norepinephrine depends on the sympathetic innervation of the myocardium. The maturation of this system varies among species and may be related to the level of the maturation of the animal at birth.[29,36,43,53,56,80] A consequence of the innervation of the myocardium is a maturational increase in the myocardial norepinephrine concentration. The timing of the increase in myocardial norepinephrine concentration varies among species. In the lamb, myocardial concentrations after 3 days of age are similar to those of the adult but are still increasing in the rabbit at the same age.

The response to exogenous catecholamines changes with development. The myocardium of the fetal lamb and of the neonate in the first few days of life is more sensitive to norepinephrine than is that of the older neonate, while no developmental difference is found in the response to isoproterenol.[36] Similar differences have been found in the rat heart.[60] In contrast, newborn pigs and dogs have a depressed contractile response to norepinephrine. A developmental increase in the response to isoproterenol and norepinephrine is found during the neonatal period in these species.[22,86]

Although these responses indicate that adrenoceptors are present in the fetal and newborn myocardium, the differences in the responses may be related to species differences in the number and proportion of α- and β-adrenoceptors between the immature and the adult hearts. The number of β-adrenoceptors has been shown to increase during fetal and newborn life in a number of species (an exception is the mouse), while the course and characteristics of the increase depend on the species studied.[13,25,27,94,115] Although the number of β-receptors has been shown to increase, the characteristics of these receptors do not appear to change with age from the fetus to the adult. Similarly, the proportion of β_1- to β_2-receptors does not differ in the rat over this developmental period.[27] In contrast to β-receptor numbers, which are high in the adult, α-adrenoceptors are found in very low levels in adult myocardium.[26,35,113,119] In several species, the number of α-adrenoceptors increases toward the end of gestation, reaches a peak in the neonatal period, and then falls. This high density of α-receptors in the neonate may be important in regard to the response of the myocardium to sympathetic stimulation during this period and, in addition, may be important in regard to the normal developmental process of hypertrophy.[99–101]

In addition to the maturational changes in innervation, catecholamine content, and adrenergic receptor density, changes have been described in the systems that transduce catecholamine stimulation; for example, basal adenylate cyclase activity is higher in the immature myocardium than in the adult, while maximally stimulated adenylate cyclase is much higher in the adult than in the immature heart.[11,84,95]

The maturational changes in the components of the cell that are affected by sympathetic stimulation, e.g., the membrane systems and the proteins that make up the contractile apparatus, are likely also to modify how changes in the sympathetic nervous system affect contractility.

Intact Heart. The ability of sympathomimetic agents to enhance ventricular function in the intact fetus depends on the measures and indices used. For example, an infusion of norepinephrine in the intact fetal lamb has been shown not to produce an increase in cardiac output.[58] In contrast, an infusion of isoproterenol in the intact fetal

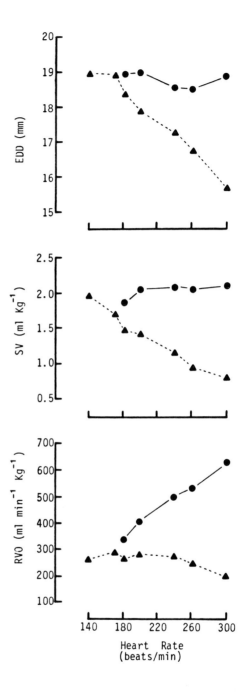

Figure 2–20. The effects of atrial pacing on right ventricular end-diastolic dimension, stroke volume (corrected for body weight), and output (corrected for body weight) during pacing over a broad range of rates. Data were obtained during pacing at a constant rate (triangle) and following an introduction of a longer pacing interval (circle). When the rate-induced fall in right ventricular dimension was circumvented by introducing the pause, stroke volume was found not to decrease with increasing heart rate. If right ventricular end-diastolic dimension and stroke volume had been maintained at the faster heart rates, right ventricular output would have increased markedly. Left atrial pacing was used to obtain these data in a fetal lamb 10 days following instrumentation. EDD = right ventricular end-diastolic dimension; RVO = output; SV = stroke volume. (Reproduced with permission from Anderson PAW, Killam AP, Mainwaring RD, Oakeley AE [1987]: In utero right ventricular output in the fetal lamb: The effect of heart rate. J Physiol 387:297–316.)

lamb results in a marked increase in $[dP/dt]_{max}$, even when heart rate and end-diastolic volume are controlled.[5] Similarly, fetal cardiac output has been shown to increase in response to an isoproterenol infusion associated with volume loading, and fetal left ventricular output is increased by an isoproterenol infusion alone.[9,39]

Isoproterenol also significantly affects postextrasystolic potentiation in the fetal lamb. As in the isolated myocardium, postextrasystolic potentiation is decreased, and on occasion postextrasystolic depression is noted (Fig. 2–19).

Effect of Birth. The importance of the sympathetic system in the neonate is suggested by the increase in circulating catecholamine concentrations that occurs with birth, as noted in humans and some other species.[31,38] Furthermore, the neonate has a blunted response to stellate ganglion stimulation in the presence of bilateral adrenalectomy,[32] while the neonatal blood pressure and heart rate are affected more by adrenalectomy than are those of the adult.[38] The markedly elevated levels of circulating catecholamines observed in the severely stressed neonate may reverse the negative inotropic effects of acidosis and thus enhance myocardial contractility.

The neonatal fall in postextrasystolic potentiation (see the section Inotropy and Fig. 2–14) also suggests the effects of sympathetic stimulation. The marked fall in postextrasystolic potentiation with birth in the intact newborn as compared with no change in postextrasystolic potentiation in isolated myocardium demonstrates that the in situ heart is subject to inotropic stimulation that is not apparent once the myocardium is removed. Studies of the effects of α- and β-antagonists on the apparently enhanced function of the intact neonatal heart during the first hours following birth remain to be performed.

DEVELOPMENTAL CHANGES IN PROTEIN ISOFORM EXPRESSION

The basis of contraction depends on the contractile proteins, e.g., myosin, actin, the troponins, and those proteins that control cell calcium such as Na^+,K^+-ATPase. In recent years it has become evident that more than one form or isoform of each of these proteins may be expressed by a cell. Of physiologic importance are the correlations of function to isoform expression that have been made in various forms of striated muscle for some of these proteins. It is likely that future studies will demonstrate such correlations in cardiac muscle.

The contractile proteins of the sarcomere have been shown to change with development. Isoforms have been shown to be expressed during development in complex temporal and chamber-specific patterns. These patterns have been used as tools for understanding differentiation and protein expression and also to suggest why the ability of the myocardium to contract changes with development.

Myosin

Myosin, a major component of the contractile apparatus, is known to change with development.[57,59,61,106,120] The myosin isozyme with the highest ATPase activity is V_1,

with V_2 having intermediate levels, and V_3 the least.[61,120] It should be recalled that the higher the ATPase activity, the faster the unloaded shortening velocity. These isozymes are composed of two heavy chains, α and β. Presently, these are the only two heavy chains that are thought to exist in cardiac myosin. The V_1 isozyme contains two α chains, V_2 contains an α and a β chain, and V_3 has two β chains.

The maturational changes in myosin heavy chain expression vary from species to species. For example, in the rat, myosin ATPase of the ventricular myocardium changes from V_3 to V_1 from the postnatal period to the adult and then returns to V_3 with senescence. In contrast, in the rabbit, V_3 is the major isoform in the fetus, with V_1 being the predominant form during the first weeks of life, and V_3 becoming the predominant isoform over the subsequent months of life. Although myosin V_1 is the common form in the ventricular myocardium of the adult mouse and rat, in general, the slower V_3 myosin is the predominant adult form in larger animals, including humans.

The developmental changes in myosin isoforms in the rabbit demonstrate the effects of the in situ environment.[57,120] Although the myosin isoform changes from V_1 to V_3 during the first months following birth, the most rapid change occurs in the left ventricle. It is of interest that the proportion of V_1 to V_3 differs between the right and the left ventricle in the same animal, from area to area within the same ventricle, and from cell to cell.

The controls of myosin isozyme expression include, besides development, the work the heart performs (e.g., the expression of V_3 in pressure-overload lesions), hormonal effects (e.g., the expression of V_1 in hyperthyroidism), and nutritional status.[59,61,106,120]

Although the control and modification of myosin isoform expression is uncertain, the change in myosin isoform from V_1 to V_3 in response to an increase in afterload is teleologically appropriate.[116] Myosin V_3 is more efficient in its consumption of ATP as compared with myosin V_1. For example, although ventricles with different proportions of V_1 and V_3 may perform similar amounts of external work, the myocardium with the higher proportion of V_3 has been shown to consume a relatively lower amount of oxygen and so demonstrates an apparently greater efficiency.

The myosin light chains vary in their expression with maturation. In the human, the fetal ventricle expresses a light chain that disappears in the postnatal ventricle and that is indistinguishable from the adult atrial light chain.[83] During the developmental changes in the myosin light chain isoforms that occur from the fetus to the infant to the adult, no differences were found between the isoforms of the right and left ventricle at any given developmental stage. Although the functional role of the light chains has yet to be delineated for cardiac muscle, the variation in isoform expression with development suggests that these proteins are important in modulating contraction.

The Thin Filament Proteins

Tropomyosin, one of the regulatory thin filament proteins, has two major isoforms, α and β.[76] The tropomyosin isoform appears to alter the interaction of troponin T and tropomyosin.[45,76] For example, troponin T binds less efficiently to β-tropomyosin. Developmental changes in the relative proportion of α and β chains have been found, with the β-isoform being predominantly expressed in the adult of large animals.[45] This maturational difference has been related to heart rate; the α-isoform is more prominent in hearts that have faster rates. In adult humans, the β-isoform is predominantly expressed.

Phosphorylation of tropomyosin also changes with development.[45,96] In the human fetal heart a greater amount of tropomyosin is phosphorylated than in adult heart. Phosphorylation has been shown with other regulatory proteins, e.g., troponin I, to alter the sensitivity of the contractile apparatus to calcium.[15,117] The developmental differences in tropomyosin isoform expression and phosphorylation may reflect the need of the fetal and newborn hearts to relax more rapidly than the adult heart because of their intrinsically faster heart rates.

The isoform expression of troponin I, C, and T has been studied in several forms of striated muscle. Isoform expression varies among muscles,[93] e.g., the troponins of slow skeletal muscle differ from those of fast skeletal muscle. Of interest, multiple troponin T isoforms have been found in fast skeletal muscle,[17] and the distribution of isoform expression appears to alter the calcium sensitivity of fast skeletal fibers.[21] Moreover, troponin T isoform expression in skeletal muscle is developmentally controlled.[98]

Adult rabbit ventricular myocardium contains at least five isoforms of troponin T.[71] This number of isoforms suggests that developmental variations in troponin T expression will be found in cardiac muscle. In light of skeletal muscle studies, such isoform variation is likely to affect the calcium sensitivity of the myofilaments.

Other Cell Constituents

Developmental studies of the cytoskeletal proteins suggest that developmental changes in isoform expression will be found in cardiac muscle.[74] Indeed, such developmental changes in isoform expression could contribute to developmental changes in the passive properties of the myocardium.

The cell systems that control cytosolic calcium also provide evidence of developmental changes in isoform expression. Recent studies suggest that developmental changes in the isoform expression of Na^+,K^+-ATPase occur from the fetus to the adult.[41] Such maturational changes in what is considered to be the digitalis receptor may be related to developmental changes in the sensitivity of the myocardium to cardiac glycosides.

Changes in isoform expression of other sarcolemmal-based systems, such as the different calcium channels, are likely. For example, electrophysiologic investigations indicate that the slow channel is insensitive to nitrendipine at younger stages of development in the chick as compared with the adult.[85] Certainly, the various effects of calcium channel antagonists during development[20] suggest that the functional characteristics of the channels are changing and can be used as evidence to imply that dif-

ferent isoforms of these channels and their associated proteins are expressed with maturation.

References

1. Allen HD, Riemenschneider TA, Epstein ML, Mason DT (1986): Hemodynamic responses of the acutely stressed neonatal right ventricle: A maturational study in lambs. Am Heart J 111:737–742.
2. Anderson PAW, Glick KL, Killam AP, Mainwaring RD (1986): The effect of heart rate on in utero left ventricular output in the fetal sheep. J Physiol (London) 372:557–573.
3. Anderson PAW, Glick KL, Manring A, Crenshaw C Jr (1984): Developmental changes in cardiac contractility in fetal and postnatal sheep: In vitro and in vivo. Am J Physiol 247:H371–H379.
4. Anderson PAW, Killam AP, Mainwaring RD, Oakeley AE (1987): In utero right ventricular output in the fetal lamb: The effect of heart rate. J Physiol (London) 387:297–316.
5. Anderson PAW, Manring A (1982): Biophysics of the developing heart. In Elkayam U, Gleicher N (eds): Cardiac Problems in Pregnancy. Diagnosis and Management of Maternal and Fetal Disease. New York, Alan R. Liss, Inc, pp 337–364.
6. Anderson PAW, Manring A, Arentzen CE, Rankin JS, Johnson EA (1977): Pressure-induced hypertrophy of cat right ventricle. An evaluation with the force-interval relationship. Circ Res 41:582–588.
7. Anderson PAW, Manring A, Nassar R (1979): Developmental changes in cardiac contractility. Pediatr Res 13:339.
8. Anderson PAW, Manring A, Serwer GA, Benson DW, Edwards SB, Armstrong BE, Sterba RJ, Floyd RD IV (1979): The force-interval relationship of the left ventricle. Circulation 60:334–348.
9. Anderson PAW, Whyte LM, Killam AP, Rosemond RL, Brown EC (1986): Fetal left ventricular output in the in utero lamb: The effect of inotropy. Circulation 74(Suppl II):491.
10. Anversa P, Olivetti G, Loud AV (1980): Morphometric study of early postnatal development in the left and right ventricular myocardium of the rat. I. Hypertrophy, hyperplasia, and binucleation of myocytes. Circ Res 46:495–502.
11. Au TLS, Collins GA, Walker MJA (1980): Rate, force and cyclic adenosine 3',5'-monophospate responses to (-)-adrenaline in neonatal rat heart tissue. Br J Pharmac 69:601–608.
12. Badke FR (1982): Left ventricular dimensions and function during right ventricular pressure overload. Am J Physiol 242:H611–H618.
13. Baker SP, Potter LT (1980): Cardiac β-adrenoceptors during normal growth of male and female rats. Br J Pharmac 68:65–70.
14. Bárány M (1967): ATPase activity of myosin correlated with speed of muscle shortening. J Gen Physiol 50:197–218.
15. Bárány M, Bárány K (1980): Phosphorylation of the myofibrillar proteins. Ann Rev Physiol 42:275–292.
16. Bassingthwaighte JB, Reuter H (1972): Calcium movements and excitation-contraction coupling in cardiac cells. In De Mello WC (ed): Electrical Phenomena in the Heart. New York, Academic Press, pp 353–395.
17. Bird IM, Dhoot G, Wilkinson JM (1985): Identification of multiple variants of fast muscle troponin T in the chicken using monoclonal antibodies. Eur J Biochem 150:517–525.
18. Borg TK, Rubin K, Lundgren E, Borg K, Obrink B (1984): Recognition of extracellular matrix components by neonatal and adult cardiac myocytes. Dev Biol 104:86–96.
19. Borg TK, Terracio L, Lundgren E, Rubin K (1985): Connective tissue of the myocardium. In Ferrans VJ, Rosenquist G, Weinstein C (eds): Cardiac Morphogenesis. New York, Elsevier Science Publishing Co., pp 69–77.
20. Boucek RJ Jr, Shelton M, Artman M, Mushlin PS, Starnes VA, Olson RD (1984): Comparative effects of verapamil, nifedipine, and diltiazem on contractile function in the isolated immature and adult rabbit heart. Pediatr Res 18:948–952.
21. Brandt PW, Diamond MS, Gluck B, Kawai M, Schachat F (1984): Molecular basis of cooperativity in vertebrate muscle thin filaments. Carlsberg Res Commun 49:155–167.

22. Buckley NM, Gootman PM, Yellin EL, Brazeau P (1979): Age-related cardiovascular effects of catecholamines in anesthetized piglets. Circ Res 45:282–292.

23. Carlsson E, Kjorell U, Thornell L-E (1982): Differentiation of the myofibrils and the intermediate filament system during postnatal development of the rat heart. Eur J Cell Biol 27:62–73.

24. Chapman RA (1983): Control of cardiac contractility at the cellular level. Am J Physiol 245:H535–H552.

25. Chen F-CM, Yamamura HI, Roeske WR (1979): Ontogeny of mammalian myocardial β-adrenergic receptors. Eur J Pharmac 58:255–264.

26. Cheng JB, Cornett LE, Goldfein A, Roberts JM (1980): α-Adrenergic receptor is present in fetal but not adult sheep myocardium. Fed Proc 39:399.

27. Cheng JB, Goldfien A, Cornett LE, Roberts JM (1981): Identification of β-adrenergic receptors using [³H] dihydroalprenolol in fetal sheep heart: Direct evidence of qualitative similarity to the receptors in adult sheep heart. Pediatr Res 15:1083–1087.

28. Davies P, Dewar J, Tynan M, Ward R (1975): Post-natal developmental changes in the length-tension relationship of cat papillary muscles. J Physiol (London) 253:95–102.

29. DeChamplain J, Malmfors T, Olson L, Sachs C (1970): Ontogenesis of peripheral adrenergic neurons in the rat: Pre- and postnatal observations. Acta Physiol Scand 80:276–288.

30. Downing SE, Talner N, Gardner TH (1965): Ventricular function in the newborn lamb. Am J Physiol 208:931–937.

31. Eliot RJ, Lam R, Leake RD, Hobel CJ, Fisher DA (1980): Plasma catecholamine concentrations in infants at birth and during the first 48 hours of life. J Pediatr 96:311–315.

32. Erath HG Jr, Boerth RC, Graham TP Jr (1982): Functional significance of reduced cardiac sympathetic innervation in the newborn dog. Am J Physiol 243:H20–H26.

33. Erman RD, Yamamura HI, Roeske WR (1983): The ontogeny of specific binding sites for the calcium channel antagonist, nitrendipine, in mouse heart and brain. Brain Res 278:327–331.

34. Fabiato A, Fabiato F (1978): Calcium-induced release of calcium from the sarcoplasmic reticulum of skinned cells from adult human, dog, cat, rabbit, rat and frog hearts and from fetal and newborn rat ventricles. Ann NY Acad Sci 307:491–522.

35. Felder RA, Calcagno PL, Eisner GM, Jose PA (1982): Ontogeny of myocardial adrenoceptors. II. Alpha adrenoceptors. Pediatr Res 16:340–342.

36. Friedman WF (1972): Neuropharmacologic studies of perinatal myocardium. Cardiovasc Clin 4:43–57.

37. Friedman WF (1972): The intrinsic physiologic properties of the developing heart. Prog Cardiovasc Dis 15:87–111.

38. Geis WP, Tatooles CJ, Priola DV, Friedman WF (1975): Factors influencing neurohumoral control of the heart in the newborn dog. Am J Physiol 228:1685–1689.

39. Gilbert RD (1982): Effects of afterload and baroreceptors on cardiac function in fetal sheep. J Dev Physiol 4:299–309.

40. Gilbert RD (1978): Venous return and control of fetal cardiac output. In Longo LD, Reneau DD (eds): Circulation in the Fetus and Newborn. New York, Garland Publishing Inc, pp 299–316.

41. Herrera VL, Ruiz-Opazo N, Schneider JW, Benz EJ, Levenson R, Medford RM, Nadal-Ginard B (1986): Two isoforms of the sodium, potassium adenosine triphosphatase: Constitutive, α-1 and brain/heart specific, α-2. Circulation 74(Suppl II):323.

42. Hilgemann DW, Delay MJ, Langer GA (1983): Activation-dependent cumulative depletions of extracellular free calcium in guinea pig atrium measured with antipyrylazo III and tetramethylmurexide. Circ Res 53:779–793.

43. Hoar RM, Hall JL (1970): The early pattern of cardiac innervation in the fetal guinea-pig. Am J Anat 128:499–508.

44. Hoerter J, Mazet F, Vassort G (1981): Perinatal growth of the rabbit cardiac cell: Possible implications for the mechanism of relaxation. J Mol Cell Cardiol 13:725–740.

45. Humphreys JE, Cummins P (1984): Regulatory proteins of the myocardium. Atrial and ventricular tropomyosin and troponin-I in the developing and adult bovine and human heart. J Mol Cell Cardiol 16:643–657.

46. Inesi G (1985): Mechanism of calcium transport. Ann Rev Physiol 47:573–601.

47. Johnson EA (1979): Force-interval relationship of cardiac muscle.

In Berne RM, Sperelakis N, Geiger SR (eds): Handbook of Physiology. Bethesda, American Physiological Society, pp 475–496.

48. Khatter JC, Hoeschen RJ (1982): Developmental increase of digitalis receptors in guinea pig heart. Cardiovasc Res 16:80–85.

49. Kirkpatrick SE, Friedman WF (1978): Myocardial determinants of fetal cardiac output. In Longo Ld, Reneau DD: Fetal and Newborn Cardiovascular Physiology. New York, Garland Press, pp 369–389.

50. Klopfenstein HS, Rudolph AM (1978): Postnatal changes in the circulation and responses to volume loading in sheep. Circ Res 42:839–845.

51. Korecky B, Rakusan K (1978): Normal and hypertrophic growth of the rat heart. Changes in cell dimensions and number. Am J Physiol 234:H123–H128.

52. Langer GA, Jarmakani JM (1984): Calcium exchange in the developing myocardium. In Legato MJ (ed): The Developing Heart. Boston, Martinus Nijhoff Publishing, pp 95–111.

53. Lebowitz EA, Novick JS, Rudolph AM (1972): Development of myocardial sympathetic innervation in the fetal lamb. Pediatr Res 6:887–893.

54. Legato MJ (1979): Cellular mechanisms of normal growth in the mammalian heart. II. A quantitative and qualitative comparison between the right and left ventricular myocytes in the dog from birth to five months of age. Circ Res 44:263–279.

55. Legato MJ (1970): Sarcomerogenesis in human myocardium. J Mol Cell Cardiol 1:425–437.

56. Lipp JM, Rudolph AM (1972): Sympathetic nerve development in the rat and guinea-pig heart. Biol Neonate 21:76–82.

57. Litten RZ, Martin BJ, Buchthal RH, Nagai R, Low RB, Alpert NR (1985): Heterogeneity of myosin isozyme content of rabbit heart. Circ Res 57:406–414.

58. Lorijn RHW, Longo LD (1980): Norepinephrine elevation in the fetal lamb: Oxygen consumption and cardiac output. Am J Physiol 239:R115–R122.

59. Lompre AM, Mercadier JJ, Wisnewsky C, Bouveret P, Pantaloni C, D'Albis A, Schwartz K (1981): Species- and age-dependent changes in the relative amounts of cardiac myosin isoenzymes in mammals. Dev Biol 84:286–290.

60. Mackenzie E, Standen NB (1980): The postnatal development of adrenoceptor responses in isolated papillary muscles from rat. Pfluegers Arch 383:185–187.

61. Mahdavi V, Matsuoka R, Nadal-Ginard B (1985): Molecular characterization and expression of the cardiac α- and β-myosin heavy chain genes. In Ferrans VJ, Rosenquist G, Weinstein C (eds): Cardiac Morphogenesis. New York, Elsevier Science Publishing Co., pp 2–9.

62. Manring A, Anderson PAW, Nassar R, Howe WR (1983): Can sympathomimetic agents be classified by their action on the force-interval relationship? Life Sci 32:329–336.

63. Markwald RR (1973): Distribution and relationship of precursor Z material to organizing myofibrillar bundles in embryonic rat and hamster ventricular myocytes. J Mol Cell Cardiol 5:341–350.

64. Martonosi AN (1984): Mechanisms of Ca²⁺ release from sarcoplasmic reticulum of skeletal muscle. Physiol Rev 64:1240–1320.

65. Martonosi A (1975): Membrane transport during development in animals. Biochim Biophys Acta 415:311–333.

66. Maylie JG (1982): Excitation-contraction coupling in neonatal and adult myocardium of cat. Am J Physiol 242:H834–H843.

67. Meissner G (1986): Ryanodine activation and inhibition of the Ca²⁺ release channel of sarcoplasmic reticulum. J Biol Chem 261:6300–6306.

68. Morad M, Goldman Y (1973): Excitation-contraction coupling in heart muscle: Membrane control of development of tension. In Butler JAV, Noble D (eds): Progress in Biophysics and Molecular Biology. Oxford, Pergamon Press, pp 257–313.

69. Morton MJ, Pinson CW, Thornburg KL (1987): In utero ventilation with oxygen augments left ventricular stroke volume in lambs. J Physiol (London) 383:413–424.

70. Nakanishi T, Jarmakani JM (1984): Developmental changes in myocardial mechanical function and subcellular organelles. Am J Physiol 246:H615–H625.

71. Nassar RN, Moore GE, Anderson PAW (1987): Troponin T isoform expression in single physiologically intact ventricular myocytes. Biophys J 51:465A.

72. Nassar R, Reedy MC, Anderson PAW (1987): Developmental changes in the ultrastructure and sarcomere shortening of the isolated rabbit ventricular myocyte. Circ Res 61:475–483.

73. Nayler WG, Fassold E (1977): Calcium accumulating and ATPase activity of cardiac sarcoplasmic reticulum before and after birth. Cardiovasc Res 11:231–237.

74. Nelson WJ, Lazarides E (1984): Assembly and establishment of membrane-cytoskeleton domains during differentiation. Spectrin as a model system. In Elson E, Frazier W, Glaser L (eds): Cell Membranes. Methods and Reviews. New York, Plenum Press, pp 219–246.

75. Nelson WJ, Lazarides E (1983): Expression of the β-subunit of spectrin in nonerythroid cells. Proc Natl Acad Sci USA 80:363–367.

76. Ohtsuki I, Nagano K (1982): Molecular arrangement of troponin-tropomyosin in the thin filament. Adv Biophys 15:93–130.

77. Olivetti G, Anversa P, Loud AV (1980): Morphometric study of early postnatal development in the left and right ventricular myocardium of the rat. II. Tissue composition, capillary growth, and sarcoplasmic alterations. Circ Res 46:503–512.

78. Page E, Buecker JL (1981): Development of dyadic junctional complexes between sarcoplasmic reticulum and plasmalemma in rabbit left ventricular myocardial cells. Morphometric analysis. Circ Res 48:519–522.

79. Page E, Surdyk-Droske M (1979): Distribution, surface density, and membrane area of dyadic junctional contacts between plasma membrane and terminal cistern in mammalian ventricle. Circ Res 45:260–267.

80. Papka RE (1981): Development of innervation to the ventricular myocardium of the rabbit. J Mol Cell Cardiol 13:217–228.

81. Pardo JV, Siliciano JD'A, Craig SW (1983): Vinculin is a component of an extensive network of myofibril-sarcolemma attachment regions in cardiac muscle fibers. J Cell Biol 97:1081–1088.

82. Penefsky ZJ (1974): Studies on mechanism of inhibition of cardiac muscle contractile tension by ryanodine: Mechanical response. Pfluegers Arch 347:173–184.

83. Price KM, Littler WA, Cummins P (1980): Human atrial and ventricular myosin light-chain subunits in the adult and during development. Biochem J 191:571–580.

84. Rabinowitz B, Parmley WW, Bonnoris G (1973): Effects of D- and DL-propranolol on myocardial adenylate cyclase activity. Proc Soc Exp Biol Med 143:1072–1076.

85. Renaud J-F, Kazazoglou T, Schmid A, Romey G, Lazdunski M (1984): Differentiator of receptor sites of [3H] nitrendipine in chick hearts and physiological relation to the slow Ca^{2+} channel and to excitation-contraction coupling. Eur J Biochem 139:673–681.

86. Rockson SG, Homcy CJ, Quinn P, Manders WT, Haber E, Vatner SF (1981): Cellular mechanisms of impaired adrenergic responsiveness in neonatal dogs. J Clin Invest 67:319–327.

87. Romero T, Covell JW, Friedman WF (1972): A comparison of pressure-volume relations of the fetal, newborn and adult heart. Am J Physiol 222:1285–1290.

88. Romero TE, Friedman WF (1979): Limited left ventricular response to volume overload in the neonatal period: A comparative study with the adult animal. Pediatr Res 13:910–915.

89. Ross J Jr, Linhart JW, Braunwald E (1965): Effects of changing heart rate in man by electrical stimulation of the right atrium: Studies at rest, during exercise, and with isoproterenol. Circulation 32:549–558.

90. Rudolph AM (1985): Distribution and regulation of blood flow in the fetal and neonatal lamb. Circ Res 57:811–821.

91. Rudolph AM, Teitel DF, Iwamoto HS, Gleason CA (1986): Ventilation is more important than oxygenation in reducing pulmonary vascular resistance at birth. Pediatr Res 20:493A.

92. Santamore WP, Lynch PR, Meier G, Heckman J, Bove AA (1976): Myocardial interaction between the ventricles. J Appl Physiol 41:362–368.

93. Schachat FH, Bronson DD, McDonald OB (1985): Heterogeneity of contractile proteins: A continuum of troponin-tropomyosin expression in mammalian skeletal muscle. J Biol Chem 260:1108–1113.

94. Schumacher W, Mirkin BL, Sheppard JR (1984): Biological maturation and β-adrenergic effectors: Development of β-adrenergic receptors in rabbit heart. Mol Cell Biochem 58:173–181.

95. Schumacher WA, Sheppard JR, Mirkin BL (1982): Biological maturation and beta-adrenergic effectors: Pre- and postnatal development of the adenylate cyclase system in the rabbit heart. J Pharmac Exp Ther 223:587–593.

96. Segura M, Palmer E, Saborio JL (1982): Phosphorylated and unphosphorylated forms of cardiac tropomyosin. Can J Biochem 60:1116–1122.

97. Sheridan DJ, Cullen MJ, Tynan MJ (1979): Qualitative and quantitative observations on ultrastructural changes during postnatal development in the cat myocardium. J Mol Cell Cardiol 11:1173–1181.

98. Shimizu N, Shimada Y (1985): Immunochemical analysis of troponin T isoforms in adult, embryonic, regenerating, and denervated chicken fast skeletal muscles. Dev Biol 111:324–334.

99. Simpson P (1985): Stimulation of hypertrophy of cultured neonatal rat heart cells through an α_1-adrenergic receptor and induction of beating through an α_1- and β_1-adrenergic receptor interaction: Evidence for independent regulation of growth and beating. Circ Res 56:884–894.

100. Simpson P, McGrath A, Savion S (1982): Myocyte hypertrophy in neonatal rat heart cultures and its regulation by serum and by catecholamines. Circ Res 51:787–801.

101. Simpson P (1983): Norepinephrine-stimulated hypertrophy of cultured rat myocardial cells is an alpha$_1$ adrenergic response. J Clin Invest 72:732–738.

102. Smith HE, Page E (1977): Ultrastructural changes in rabbit heart mitochondria during the perinatal period. Dev Biol 57:109–117.

103. Sommer JR, Johnson EA (1979): Ultrastructure of cardiac muscle. In Berne RM, Sperelakis N, Geiger SR (eds): Handbook of Physiology. Bethesda, American Physiological Society, pp 113–186.

104. Street SF (1983): Lateral transmission of tension in frog myofibers: A myofibrillar network and transverse cytoskeletal connections are possible transmitters. J Cell Physiol 114:346–364.

105. Sugimoto T, Sagawa K, Guyton AC (1966): Effect of tachycardia on cardiac output during normal and increased venous return. Am J Physiol 211:288–292.

106. Sweeney LJ, Nag AC, Eisenberg B, Manasek FJ, Zak R (1985): Developmental aspects of cardiac contractile protein. Basic Res Cardiol 80(Suppl 2):123–127.

107. Thornburg KL, Morton MJ (1983): Filling and arterial pressures as determinants of RV stroke volume in the sheep fetus. Am J Physiol 244:H656–H663.

108. Thornburg KL, Morton MJ, Anderson DF, Faber JJ (1982): Filling and arterial pressures as determinants of fetal left ventricular stroke volume. Physiologist 25:254.

109. Traub P (1985): Intermediate Filaments. A Review. Berlin, Springer-Verlag.

110. Urthaler F, Walker AA, Kawamura K, Hefner LL, James TN (1978): Canine atrial and ventricular muscle mechanics studied as a function of age. Circ Res 42:703–713.

111. Versprille A, Jansen JRC, Harinck E, Van Nie CJ, De Neef KJ (1976): Functional interaction of both ventricles at birth and the changes during the neonatal period in relation to the changes of geometry. In Longo LD, Reneau DD (eds): Fetal and Newborn Cardiovascular Physiology. New York, Garland Press, pp 399–413.

112. Warshaw JB, Terry ML (1970): Cellular energy metabolism during fetal development. II. Fatty acid oxidation by the developing heart. J Cell Biol 44:354–360.

113. Wei JW, Sulakhe PV (1979): Regional and subcellular distribution of β- and α-adrenergic receptors in the myocardium of different species. Gen Pharmac 10:263–267.

114. Weir WG, Yue DT (1986): Intracellular calcium transients underlying the short-term force-interval relationship in ferret ventricular myocardium. J Physiol (London) 376:507–530.

115. Whitsett JA, Darovec-Beckerman C (1981): Developmental aspects of β-adrenergic receptors and catecholamine-sensitive adenylate cyclase in rat myocardium. Pediatr Res 15:1363–1369.

116. Wikman-Coffelt J, Sievers R, Parmley WW (1985): Influence of myocardial isomyosins on cardiac performance and oxygen consumption. Biochem Biophys Res Commun 130:1314–1323.

117. Winegrad S (1984): Regulation of cardiac contractile proteins.

Correlations between physiology and biochemistry. Circ Res 55:565–574.

118. Wittels B, Bressler R (1965): Lipid metabolism in the newborn heart. J Clin Invest 44:1639–1646.

119. Yamada S, Yamamura HI, Roeske WR (1980): Ontogeny of mammalian cardiac α_1-adrenergic receptors. Eur J Pharmac 68:217–221.

120. Zak R, Galhotra SS (1983): Contractile and regulatory proteins. In Drake-Holland AJ, Noble MIM (eds): Cardiac Metabolism. John Wiley & Sons Ltd, New York, pp 339–364.

3 PERICARDIAL DEVELOPMENT

Thomas A. Riemenschneider

The pericardium is a unique structure that surrounds, maintains, and restricts the heart. Although the pericardium has been recognized for centuries, it has taken recent studies in the adult experimental animal and in humans to heighten our awareness of the impact of this structure on function of the heart during abnormal hemodynamic conditions.

While our knowledge of adult pericardial function has advanced dramatically in recent years, there have been few studies that have examined the effect of the pericardium on the neonatal circulation. During the transition to extrauterine life, dramatic changes of great magnitude occur in the structure, biochemistry, and function of the heart and circulation. Increased emphasis on neonatal intensive care has sparked our interest in understanding the abnormal hemodynamic alterations occurring in sick newborns, which range from premature infants with patent ductus arteriosus to term infants with persistent pulmonary hypertension of the newborn syndrome (see Chapter 51), neonatal asphyxia, or congenital heart disease.

This chapter will review recent developments in the understanding of the pericardium, present data on the impact of the pericardium on neonatal ventricular function, and speculate on the application of these data to the newborn infant.

HISTORY

The history of the pericardium is long and interesting.[10] Many prominent investigators have contributed to our understanding of the complex interactions of this organ with the heart. References to the pericardium can be found dating back to biblical times. Hippocrates provided a description of the normal pericardium. By the year 79 AD, Pliny had described a "hairy heart," a term that persisted into the sixteenth century in descriptions of pericardial adhesions. Galen described pericardial effusion in a monkey and recognized that the pericardium "protected" the heart, and that pericardial wounds could be lethal. He also probably performed the first (unsuccessful) pericardial resection.

In the seventeenth century, Rondelet described pericarditis, and Harvey reported a case of hemopericardium due to traumatic cardiac rupture. Richard Lower provided descriptions of the physiology of both pericardial tamponade and constrictive pericarditis. In the eighteenth century, Morgagni contributed important clinical observations on pericardial calcification, hemopericardium, pericardial tamponade, and pericarditis.

With Laënnec's development of the stethoscope in the nineteenth century, emphasis shifted to clinical observations of the pericardium. Pericardial rubs were described as well as other physical findings encountered in pericarditis and pericardial effusion. Laënnec described the variability of clinical findings and the difficulty in diagnosis of pericarditis. Early in the twentieth century, Barnard found that the tensile strength of the parietal pericardium was greater than that of the myocardium, while Kuno in Japan demonstrated the effect of an intact versus open pericardium on cardiac output, arterial blood pressure, heart rate, and venous pressure in the adult. All of these developments set the stage for the major advances in pericardial physiology that have been described in recent years.

ANATOMY

Toward the end of the second week of development, a cleft appears in the extraembryonic mesoderm, situated between the embryo proper and the primitive chorionic capsule. A week later, horizontal clefts also begin to form in the unsegmented embryonic mesoderm. These clefts split the mesoderm into somatic and splanchnic layers, which, in the region of the heart, are destined to become the parietal and visceral pericardium.

These isolated coelomic spaces coalesce in the head region and become continuous, connecting a space ahead of the embryo (destined to become the cardiac region) with the lateral coelomic channels in an inverted "U" shape. As the head of the embryo grows forward, separating from the underlying blastoderm, the pericardial coelom grows to lie in a ventral position relative to the embryonic head. Partitioning of the coelom into pericardial, pleural, and peritoneal cavities is completed by formation of the septum transversum, and the pleuropericardial and pleuroperitoneal membranes.

In the 4-mm embryo, the lung buds begin to develop within the medial mass of mesenchyme and bulge into the two pleural cavities. This burrowing of the lung buds into the spongy mesenchymal tissue splits off an increasingly extensive parietal pericardium from the thoracic wall. This final partitioning encloses the heart within the pericardial membranes.

The parietal pericardium consists of an outer fibrocollagenous layer together with an inner single layer of mesothelial cells, which is reflected onto the epicardial surface of the heart as the visceral pericardium. The parietal pericardium is firmly attached to the sternum and diaphragm and becomes contiguous with the adventitia of the aorta and pulmonary artery. Inferiorly, the attachment of the pericardium to the diaphragm opposes the superior attachment to the great vessels, while laterally the pericardium attaches to the roots of the lungs. These attachments limit the extent of displacement of the heart with changes in posture and respiration.

The mesothelium lining the parietal pericardium and covering the epicardial surface of the heart consists of a continuous sac, which contains 15 to 50 ml of fluid in the adult. This fluid is probably an ultrafiltrate of plasma and is eventually returned to the venous circulation through lymphatic passages.

Pressure-volume analysis of the excised intact pericardium reveals an initial flat portion of the curve wherein increasing pericardial volume causes little increase in pressure. Beyond this flat portion, there is an abrupt steep rise in the curve as increasing volume causes a rapid elevation in pressure. The difference between the volume occupied by the heart and the volume of the unstressed pericardial sac is termed the "reserve volume" of the pericardium. The reserve volume is important because it represents the volume by which the heart can increase without affecting pericardial pressure during changes in respiration, posture, hydration, and volume.

The abrupt rise in pericardial pressure that occurs with pericardial distention beyond a critical point is in part related to the high collagen content of the parietal pericardium. The collagen is arranged in bundles that spread throughout the pericardium as wavy bands and are surrounded by elastin fibers. The initial flat portion of the presssure-volume curve is associated with straightening of these wavy bands, after which the inelastic nature of the collagen results in the abrupt rise in pericardial pressure.

PHYSIOLOGY

While the pericardium has little effect on the normal circulation, numerous studies have demonstrated the impact of the intact pericardium on ventricular function under conditions of abnormal loading in the adult. Ventricular diastolic pressure and volume depend upon elasticity of the chamber, the rate and pattern of venous filling, active ventricular relaxation, and the pressure and volume of other cardiac chambers. Recent investigations have demonstrated the interaction of the two ventricles, which is manifest through the interventricular septum.[3] This interaction is greatly enhanced by the presence of an intact pericardium in the adult: If right ventricular pressure and volume are increased, the resulting elevation of left ventricular end-diastolic pressure is greater with the pericardium intact.

While pressure-volume curves have been used to examine compliance of ventricular chambers, it must be remembered that such curves may not reflect changes in compliance of the myocardium. Furthermore, pressure-volume curves may be influenced by other factors, especially the external constraints of the pericardial sac. Ventricular diastolic pressure is also altered by pleural and pericardial pressures as well as the pressure of the right ventricle. Thus, extrapolation of data from acute open-chest, open-pericardium animal preparations to the intact human must be made with caution.

Shifts of the pressure-volume curve resulting from an elevation of diastolic pressure may be due either to an increase in diastolic size or an increased stiffness of the ventricular myocardium. However, during acute volume loading, an upward shift of the entire curve is encountered, and higher end-diastolic pressures are achieved at similiar end-diastolic volumes.[1] This upward shift has been shown to be due to the impact of the intact pericardium. Ludbrook et al[5] have demonstrated that angiotensin infusion shifts the curve in an upward direction, while nitroprusside and nitroglycerin infusions shift the curve in a downward direction. In patients with congestive heart failure, the curve is also elevated.[2] In each of these circumstances, the shift in the pressure-volume curve results from the influence of the pericardium; such effects are abolished by removal of the pericardial sac. Thus, the intact pericardium has an important effect on the pressure-volume relationships under conditions of acute volume loading.

Similarly, studies in short-term chronically instrumented adult animals have revealed a similiar effect of the intact pericardium on ventricular function and filling.[9] When the pericardium is removed in these chronically instrumented volume-overloaded animals, infusion of nitroprusside does not cause the curve to return to its preinfusion level. However, longer-term chronic studies, in which the volume load was maintained for 1 month or more in instrumented adult animals, demonstrated that removal of the pericardium had no effect on pressure-volume curves,[2] suggesting that adaptation of the pericardium occurs in response to chronic volume loading of longer duration. Freeman and LeWinter demonstrated that hypertrophy of the pericardium occurs in adult animals with long-term chronic volume overload.[2]

Such studies clearly show the important impact of the pericardium on the filling and function of the left ventricle in the adult. Since most studies of the newborn circulation have been performed in animals in whom the pericardium has been removed, extrapolation of these data to the intact human newborn is difficult. Accordingly, we decided to investigate the influence of the pericardium on ventricular filling and function in the newborn lamb model.

Clinical problems such as persistent pulmonary hypertension of the newborn syndrome, neonatal asphyxia, and abnormal ventricular volume loading associated with patent ductus arteriosus and transient tricuspid insufficiency have stimulated extensive investigation of the newborn circulation and hemodynamic adaptations to extrauterine life.[4,6] These studies have described a limited ability of the neonatal ventricles to respond to acute increases in volume loading by increasing stroke volume. While there is a maturational improvement in the Starling response of the left ventricle, the right ventricle lags behind the left, with a much more limited maturation of the Starling response in the newborn lamb.[6] Most neonatal studies have been performed with the pericardium incised or partially or completely removed. Thus, extrapolation of neonatal animal data to the intact human infant is hampered by a lack of understanding of the contribution of the intact pericardium to ventricular filling and function. For this reason, I have studied the effect of the intact pericardium on left ventricular filling and function in an anesthetized neonatal lamb preparation.[7]

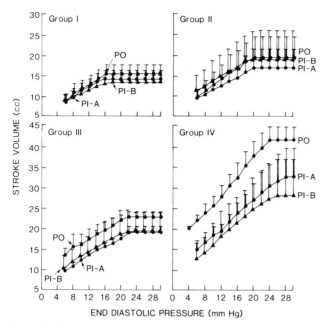

Figure 3–1. Starling curves relating mean values of stroke volume and end-diastolic pressure for lambs of groups I to IV at ages 1 to 3, 7 to 13, 17 to 21, and 34 to 49 days. Acute infusion of warmed Ringer lactate was performed with the pericardium intact (PI = A) and open (PO) in five lambs of each age group. In a second group of five lambs, fluid infusion was performed with the pericardium intact (PI = B). The lambs were then sacrificed and the heart removed with the pericardium intact; these hearts (groups I to IV, PI = B) were subjected to passive pressure volume assessment (see Fig. 3–2). Acute volume infusion demonstrated similar Starling curves for lambs of groups I, II, and III, with the pericardium intact and removed. Lambs of group IV demonstrated statistically different Starling curves, with the pericardium intact and removed. For a given end-diastolic pressure, stroke volume was significantly greater with the pericardium removed (PO).

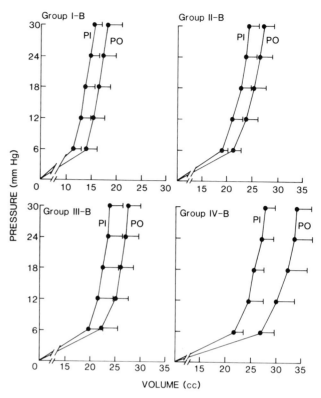

Figure 3–2. Passive pressure volume assessment of lamb hearts from groups I- to IV-B, obtained both with the pericardium intact (PI) and opened (PO). For lambs of all four groups, upright pressure volume curves were obtained, indicating that small changes in ventricular volume produced large changes in ventricular filling pressure. For lambs of groups I to II, curves obtained with the pericardium intact and removed were similar. For the oldest lambs (group IV), the curves obtained with the pericardium intact (PI) and open (PO) were statistically different. Removal of the pericardium shifted the curve such that a larger ventricular volume was required to produce a given ventricular pressure, consistent with increasing ventricular compliance.

Forty newborn lambs of ages 1 to 49 days were anesthetized and acutely instrumented for hemodynamic assessment. Ten lambs in each of four age groups were subjected to rapid infusion of warmed Ringer lactate into the left atrium, which progressively elevated left ventricular end-diastolic pressure to 30 mmHg, with the pericardium intact. Withdrawal of fluid enabled a return to resting hemodynamic conditions in all animals. The pericardium was then removed in five lambs of each age group, and the acute volume infusion was repeated to assess pump function in the absence of the pericardium. Starling curves relating ventricular end-diastolic presssure and stroke volume were constructed for each lamb, with the pericardium intact and removed (Fig. 3–1).

In the remaining five lambs of each age group, cardiac arrest was rapidly induced and the heart then removed with the pericardium intact. In these lambs, distensible balloons were introduced into both ventricular chambers in such a fashion as to allow controlled filling of the chamber and measurement of the fluid volume injected as well as the pressure within the ventricle. With the right ventricle filled to a constant pressure of 4 mmHg, left ventricular volume was determined at pressures of 6, 12, 18, 24, and 30 mmHg to assess ventricular chamber compliance with the pericardium intact.

Following removal of the fluid, the pericardium was removed, and the sequence of ventricular filling was repeated. Passive pressure-volume curves were constructed for the five lambs of each age group, demonstrating pressure-volume relationships with both the pericardium intact and following its removal (Fig. 3–2).

Starling curves for lambs in groups I and II (ages 1 to 3 and 7 to 13 days) revealed a limited response to volume loading (Fig. 3–1). Peak stroke volumes were achieved at end-diastolic pressures of 14 to 20 mmHg and were increased to levels of 50 to 70 per cent over resting stroke volume. Starling curves obtained with the pericardium removed were not statistically different in their magnitude, with similar peak stroke volumes achieved at similiar end-diastolic pressures.

In lambs of 17 to 21 days of age (group III), peak stroke volumes of 80 per cent above resting levels were achieved at end-diastolic pressures of 20 to 22 mmHg with the pericardium intact, and removal of the pericardium shifted the Starling curve to the left, so that a similiar stroke volume was achieved at lower end-diastolic pressure.

In the oldest lambs (group IV, ages 34 to 49 days), stroke volume increased approximately 100 per cent over values at resting levels, and peak stroke volume was achieved at end-diastolic pressures of 28 mmHg. When the pericardium was removed, resting stroke volume and stroke volumes at each level of end-diastolic pressure were significantly higher than corresponding values with the pericardium intact. Furthermore, peak stroke volume was achieved at 22 to 24 mmHg with the pericardium removed versus 28 mmHg with the pericardium intact. Thus, the Starling curve was significantly shifted to the left in the oldest lambs when the pericardium was removed.

Passive filling of the arrested left ventricles produced a very steep pressure-volume curve, in which even small increases in left ventricular volume produced significant elevations in ventricular pressure (Fig. 3–2). Pressure-volume curves were very similiar for lambs of groups I to III whether the pericaridium was intact or removed. In each group, the pressure-volume curve with the pericardium open was situated to the right of the curve generated with the pericardium intact. The configuration of the curve was similiar with the pericardial sac intact and removed, with a steep slope indicating that only slight changes in volume resulted in large changes in pressure. In the oldest lambs, however, the pressure-volume curve with the pericardium open was significantly shifted to the right, such that larger filling volumes could be achieved at the same pressures. In addition, the slopes of the curves were different, with the more upright slope suggesting that the intact pericardium contributes substantially to the chamber compliance in older lambs.

The results of my study demonstrate that in the newborn lamb, unlike the adult sheep, the pericardium has little impact on left ventricular filling or stroke volume. In newborn lambs chamber compliance appears to be determined primarily by the configuration, wall thickness, inherent compliance of the left ventricular wall, and the pattern of venous filling. Romero and Friedman[8] have shown that the chamber compliance of the ventricles increases with maturation. During postnatal development, as the neonatal ventricle becomes less stiff and more compliant, the inherent stiffness of the intact pericardial sac increasingly contributes to chamber compliance and eventually limits both left ventricular filling and stroke volume during acute volume loading.

While these observations demonstrate the absence of pericardial effects on the neonatal left ventricle during acute volume loading, one can only speculate about the contribution of the pericardium to ventricular interaction in the newborn. Since the interventricular septum is situated in a more midline position, and the right ventricular lateral wall thickness is as thick as that of the left ventricle at birth, it seems likely that a volume overload of the right ventricle will compromise left ventricular function to an even greater degree in the newborn than it would in the adult, with the intact pericardial sac playing an important role in ventricular interaction.

References

1. Alderman EL, Glantz SA (1976): Acute hemodynamic interventions shift the diastolic pressure-volume curve in man. Circ 54: 662–671.
2. Freeman G, LeWinter M (1984): Pericardial adaptations during chronic cardiac dilatation. Circ Res 54:294–300.
3. Hess OM, Bhargava V, Ross J Jr, Shabetai R (1983): The role of the pericardium in interactions between the cardiac chambers. Am Heart J 106:1377–1383.
4. Klopfenstein HS, Rudolph AM (1978): Postnatal changes in the circulation and response to volume loading in sheep. Circ Res 42:839–845.
5. Ludbrook PA, Byrne JD, Kurnik PB, McKnight RC (1977): Influence of reduction of preload and afterload by nitroglycerin on left ventricular diastolic pressure-volume relations and relaxation in man. Circulation 56:937–943.
6. Riemenschneider TA, Allen HD, Mason DT (1986): Maturational changes in myocardial pump performance in newborn lambs. Am Heart J 11:731–736.
7. Riemenschneider TA (1982): Role of the intact pericardium in pump function on the newborn left ventricle: Effect on ventricular filling and stroke volume (Abstr). Presented at the Cardiology Section Meeting of the American Academy of Pediatrics, 51st Annual Meeting, New York, Oct 23, 1982.
8. Romero TE, Friedman WF (1979): Limited left ventricular response to volume overload in the neonatal period. A comparative study with the adult animal. Pediatr Res 13:910–913.
9. Shirato K, Shabetai R, Bhargava V, Franklin D, Ross J Jr (1978): Alteration of the left ventricular diastolic pressure-segment length relation produced by the pericardium. Effects of cardiac distension and afterload reduction in conscious dogs. Circulation 57:1191–1198.
10. Spodick DH (1985): The hairy hearts of hoary heroes and other tales: Medical history of the pericardium from antiquity through the 20th century. In Fowler NO (ed): The Pericardium in Health and Disease. Mt. Kisco, Futura Pub, pp 1–17.

4 DEVELOPMENTAL ELECTROPHYSIOLOGY

Peter Danilo, Jr.

The need for an understanding of developmental electrophysiology has been magnified by rapid advances in the care of premature infants, which has resulted in steadily increasing survival rates for infants with lower birth weights. Many of these infants will receive drugs that affect the heart, despite the fact that our understanding of how these drugs affect the developing heart lags behind the pace at which these drugs are introduced. The pharmacologic treatment of pregnant women with cardiovascular disorders is similarly carried out without a complete understanding of how such drugs may alter fetal cardiac rate and rhythm. The etiology of the sudden infant death syndrome is still unknown. Despite the alternating hypotheses of respiratory and cardiac causes, there can be little doubt that the heart must play a key role in this syndrome whether or not apnea is the initiating event.

This chapter will summarize the changes in the cardiac transmembrane action potential that occur during development. Recent advances in the understanding of the relationship between the autonomic nervous system and the electrophysiology of the developing heart will also be reviewed. The reader is referred to recent reviews of cardiac cellular electrophysiology and of developmental aspects of the cardiac action potential for additional information.[6,14,54]

HISTORY

The developing heart has interested scientists for over 400 years. Early studies described differences in heart rate as a function of development in the chicken embryo.[22] The first pharmacologic studies of the developing heart were made in the late nineteenth century.[43] Cardioactive drugs were superfused over the hearts of chick embryos, and visual observations were made of their effects on heart rate and rhythm. With the development of more sophisticated recording and display devices, it became possible to study transmembrane action potentials.

For ease of access and cost, the chick embryo has remained the standard model for most studies of developmental electrophysiology. Additional studies have been made in mammals, including the rat, rabbit, and dog. For obvious reasons, the heart of the human embryo and fetus has been studied to a more limited extent.

The author acknowledges the expert secretarial assistance of Edda Semiday and Susan McMahon.

RESTING MEMBRANE POTENTIAL

The resting membrane potential arises as a result of an unequal distribution of potassium ions (K^+) across the cell membrane. Because the cardiac cell membrane is somewhat "leaky," K^+ tends to move out of the cell, and in association sodium ion (Na^+) moves in. This passive ion movement is countered by an energy–requiring pump that maintains ionic gradients by moving K^+ into and Na^+ out of the cell. This pump requires ATP and is crucial to the maintenance of the resting membrane potential.

In the adult, the Nernst equation predicts a 50 to 60 mV change in membrane potential with each decade change in extracellular K^+ concentration. In the embryonic chick heart near the time of hatching[55] and in fetal mammalian hearts[2,8] this relationship is equivalent to that observed for the adult heart. For the less developed chick embryo (3 to 5 days after fertilization), the relationship between extracellular K^+ and membrane potential deviates more from that of the adult, especially at lower K^+ concentrations.[55] This deviation has also been reported for the fetal rat heart[54,55] but not for the fetal dog heart.[8] These differences may be real, or they may reflect differences inherent in methods, in the animal model, and in the accessibility of the heart at different developmental stages.

Recent advances in ion selective microelectrode techniques indicate that intracellular K^+ activity increases in the chick embryo from 71 mM at the fourth incubation day to 90 mM at the eighteenth day.[15] Intracellular Na^+ activity decreases from approximately 12.5 to 7.0 mM between days 4 and 8.[15] When these values were used to calculate the equilibrium potentials, it was found that E_K increased from −73 mV at the fourth incubation day to −90 mV at the eighteenth day and that E_{Na} increased from 57.0 to 71.8 mV. This change in equilibrium potential probably arises from an increase in the activity of Na^+, K^+-ATPase.[32,53]

Resting or maximum diastolic potential increases as a function of embryonic and fetal development.[2,8,54,56] For the canine (and probably other species as well), resting potential continues to increase during neonatal life. Due in part to changes in the cell membrane and in part to changes in intracellular metabolism, during midgestation (approximately 30 to 35 days after conception), maximum diastolic potential of fetal canine Purkinje fibers is approximately −79 mV, and increases to −84 mV in late gestation.[8] Values for the neonate (0 to 10 days of age) and adult dog are −88 and −91 mV, respectively (Table 4–1).

Table 4–1. TRANSMEMBRANE ACTION POTENTIAL CHARACTERISTICS
OF FETAL, NEONATAL, AND ADULT CARDIAC PURKINJE FIBERS

	Amplitude (mV)	MDP (mV)	$\dot{V}_{max}$ (V/sec)	APD_{50} (msec)	APD_{100} (msec)
Midgestation fetus	110.0 ± 1.3	-78.6 ± 1.2	347 ± 15	104.8 ± 3.4	163.3 ± 7.8
Late gestation fetus	119.8 ± 0.8	-83.7 ± 1.2	474 ± 17	130.6 ± 4.5	214.8 ± 4.0
Neonate	122.9 ± 0.7	-88.6 ± 0.5	456 ± 12	160.0 ± 2.8	263.2 ± 3.1
Adult	127.6 ± 0.5	-90.5 ± 0.4	544 ± 10	174.7 ± 2.4	294.9 ± 2.4

Transmembrane action potentials were recorded from isolated Purkinje fibers superfused with a modified Tyrode solution (K^+ concentration = 4 mM). Fetal dog hearts were obtained from midgestation (approximately 30 to 40 days after conception) and late gestation (50 to 60 days after conception). Neonatal hearts were obtained from dogs 0 to 10 days of age and adult hearts from dogs older than 1 year. Data are presented as mean ± standard error (n = 40 to 150 for each variable) and were pooled from control data of previously published studies. MDP = maximum diastolic potential; $\dot{V}_{max}$ = maximum velocity of the action potential upstroke; APD_{50} and APD_{100} = action potential duration measured to 50 and 100 per cent polarization, respectively. (Modified after Danilo P [1984]: Electrophysiology of the fetal and neonatal heart. In Legato MJ [ed]: The Developing Heart. Boston, Martinus Nijhoff, pp 21–38.)

ACTION POTENTIAL UPSTROKE

In most normal adult cardiac cells (except those of the sinoatrial and atrioventricular nodes), depolarization during the upstroke of the action potential is rapid and brought about by inward Na^+ current through so-called fast channels. The magnitude of this current is voltage dependent. If the cell membrane is not completely polarized, then upstroke velocity may not be maximal. In this case, hyperpolarization will increase upstroke velocity by activating more fast inward Na^+ channels. A secondary current carried by Ca^{2+} is activated near the end of the rapid phase of depolarization. Inward Ca^{2+} currents during depolarization are carried through slow channels and are more important in cells of the sinoatrial (SA) and atrioventricular (AV) nodes.

During embryonic and fetal life, upstroke velocity initially is low and increases during development.[30,37,55,56] Studies of the early (≤ 6 days) embryonic chick heart indicate that the current underlying the action potential upstroke is carried primarily by Na^+ moving through a slow channel.[55,56] The low upstroke velocity does not result from the relatively low resting membrane potential because electrical hyperpolarization of the embryonic cardiac cell does not increase upstroke velocity.[55] Thus, if voltage–dependent fast channels existed, they should have been activated by an increase in resting potential.

With development, action potential amplitude and rate of rise of the upstroke both increase. Paralleling these changes may be an increase in the sensitivity of the upstroke to tetrodotoxin (TTX), a blocker of inward Na^+ current.[30,52] In embryonic myocardial cells of the chick, the action potential upstroke is reduced by the calcium blocking agents verapamil and D-600,[17,51,55] which has been interpreted to mean that these Ca^{2+} blockers also inhibit Na^+ moving through a slow inward channel.[38,51] The calcium blocking ion Mn^{2+} has no effect on action potential upstroke in the early chick embryo, whereas it does reduce contractility, thereby raising the possibility that Mn^{2+} possesses a greater activity (or specificity) for slow inward Ca^{2+} than for slow inward Na^+ channels.[55] In the fetal rat myocardium, however, at less than 10 days after conception, Mn^{2+} has been shown to reduce action potential amplitude and rate of rise at a time when TTX exerts essentially no effect.[2] By the thirteenth day these sensitivities have been reversed. TTX exerts an increasing effect on action potential upstroke and amplitude, whereas the effect of Mn^{2+} diminishes.

In contrast to an increase in sensitivity to TTX during development, other investigators demonstrated TTX–sensitive fast Na^+ channels in the chick as early as the third embryonic day.[29,35] Sensitivity (normalized with respect to age-dependent control values of $\dot{V}_{max}$) to TTX remained constant throughout development despite the fact that the rate of rise of the action potential upstroke increased. Studies of fetal canine Purkinje fibers[8] are in agreement with these data: Fibers sampled over a range of time from postimplantation to just prior to full-term had an equivalent sensitivity to TTX.

REPOLARIZATION

Repolarization of the adult cardiac cell membrane is a complex event consisting of several ionic currents, among which are two currents that display properties of a rectifier, another that apparently overlaps the slow inward current, and one that appears to be activated by Ca^{2+}. Studies of these repolarizing currents have depended on the use of isolated cardiac fibers and, more recently, single cardiac cells. The process of repolarization involves outward K^+ movement that rectifies, i.e., tends to diminish, as the membrane depolarizes. The reader is referred to current reviews of this complex subject for a more detailed description (see, for example, reference 14).

Relatively little information is available on the repolarization of the developing cardiac cell membrane. Data that are available are often difficult to compare because of differing experimental conditions. The ionic currents underlying repolarization appear to be more sensitive than those of other phases of the action potential to temperature, external ion concentration, and the rate at which action potentials are initiated. Further, the extent of the observed changes may result from differences in species or from differences in the type of tissue being studied. In the dog, the duration of the Purkinje fiber action potential increases during development (Table 4–1).

Changes in the characteristics of the transmembrane action potential by themselves do not provide sufficient insight into the effects of development on cardiac electrophysiology. At the same time that cell membranes and metabolism are developing, the autonomic nerve supply to the heart is increasing. The mature autonomic nervous system exerts complex effects on the adult heart that still are not completely understood, and our comprehension of these effects on the developing heart is even less. Not only are cardiac cell growth and differentiation occurring at a rapid rate but various receptor systems and their associated second messengers are also developing. The role of the autonomic nervous system in modulating these events is presently a subject of intense study. Data suggesting an association between innervation and electrophysiologic responsiveness of the developing heart are considered below.

ADRENERGIC EFFECTS

The effects of adrenergic stimulation of the heart are thought to be mediated by β_1-adrenergic receptors.[67] These receptors have been demonstrated in the heart by classical pharmacologic means as well as by newer techniques of receptor binding studies.

In cells of the ventricular specialized conducting system, β-adrenergic stimulation increases the rate of spontaneous diastolic depolarization,[23,47,64] an effect that increases the rate of action potential initiation. If the cell membrane is not fully polarized, beta stimulation will hyperpolarize it and increase resting membrane or maximum diastolic potential, probably through stimulation of electrogenic Na^+ pumping.[16,65] Consequent to this increase in membrane potential, the upstroke velocity of the action potential may increase. Beta stimulation generally decreases the duration of the action potential by increasing the rate of repolarization.[19,47] In addition, the plateau height (reflecting inward Ca^{2+} movement) increases, resulting in more Ca^{2+} being available to the contractile apparatus.[5]

The currents enhanced or augmented by β-adrenergic stimulation are those that function during spontaneous diastolic depolarization, during the plateau phase, and during repolarization. They are, respectively, i_f, an inward current carried by Na^+,[11] i_{si}, a slow inward current carried by Ca^{2+},[40] and an outward K^+ current, i_{x1}.[62]

Until recently, cardiac α-adrenergic receptors were thought to be lacking. However, they have now been demonstrated pharmacologically and biochemically in atrial and ventricular tissues,[44,47,50] and recent studies of isolated segments of the ventricular specialized conducting system demonstrate functional α-adrenergic receptors.[4] Electrophysiologic studies of α-adrenergic agonists demonstrate that action potential duration is increased, and resting and maximum diastolic potentials are unchanged.[19,47] In contrast to the positive chronotropic effect of β-adrenergic stimulation in isolated Purkinje fibers, α-agonists (in low concentrations) decrease the slope of spontaneous diastolic depolarization to decrease automaticity.[47] At higher concentrations, α-agonists increase automaticity. This biphasic action can be blocked by appropriate α- and β-adrenergic antagonists. The de-

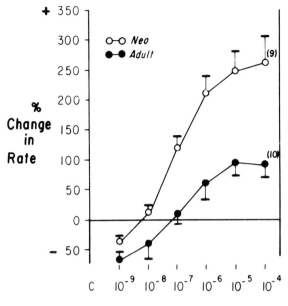

Figure 4–1. The effects of epinephrine on spontaneous rate of isolated neonatal and adult canine cardiac Purkinje fibers. Shown here are the biphasic responses of two thirds of all adult fibers and one half of all neonatal fibers. The remaining adult and neonatal fibers responded to epinephrine with a monophasic increase in spontaneous rate across the entire concentration range; these data are not shown here. Note that for the fibers in which a biphasic rate response was observed, the magnitude of the epinephrine-induced rate increase was greater in the neonate than in the adult. The control spontaneous rates were 12.2 ± 1.1 beats/min for neonates. Data are expressed as mean ± standard error. (Modified after Rosen MR, Hordorf AJ, Ilvento JP, Danilo P [1977]: Effects of adrenergic amines on electrophysiological properties and automaticity of neonatal and adult canine Purkinje fibers. Circ Res 40:340–400.)

crease in spontaneous rate is attenuated by phentolamine, and the increase in rate is reduced by propranolol. This negative chronotropic effect apparently is mediated by an α_1-adrenergic receptor in that the effects of phenylephrine on Purkinje fiber automaticity are reduced by prazosin but not by yohimbine.[48]

The effects of adrenergic stimulation on cardiac electrophysiology are modulated by growth and development. Approximately two thirds of Purkinje fibers from adult dogs show a decrease in spontaneous rate in response to epinephrine, a catecholamine with mixed α- and β-adrenergic agonist properties (Fig. 4–1). In contrast, for Purkinje fibers from neonatal dogs (0 to 10 days of age) approximately one half of all fibers respond with a negative chronotropic effect to low concentrations of epinephrine. In addition to this *qualitative* difference in the distribution of responses, a *quantitative* difference exists between adult and neonatal fibers. For fibers that respond to adrenergic stimulation with a decrease in spontaneous rate, the magnitude of the β-adrenergic receptor-mediated positive chronotropic response is greater in the neonate than in the adult—a 250 per cent increase above control compared with 75 per cent, respectively.

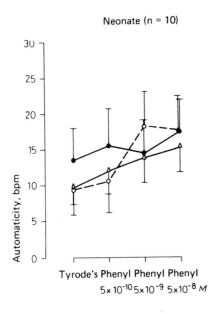

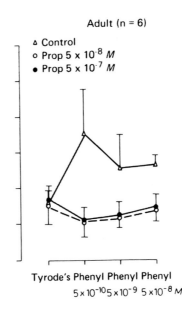

Figure 4–2. Effects of the α-agonist phenylephrine on the spontaneous rate of isolated neonatal (0- to 2-day-old) and adult canine cardiac Purkinje fibers. Control values for the spontaneous rate were obtained during superfusion with drug-free Tyrode's solution. A dose-response relationship for phenylephrine was then obtained. For both groups phenylephrine induced dose-dependent increases in the spontaneous rate. For adults, but not neonates, this rate increase was blocked by propranolol. For neonates, subsequent experiments showed that the phenylephrine-induced increase in rate could be blocked by phentolamine. (Reprinted with permission of Reder RF, Danilo P, Rosen MR [1984]: Developmental changes in alpha adrenergic effects on canine Purkinje fiber automaticity. Dev Pharmacol Ther 7:94–108, and S. Karger AG, Basel, Switzerland.)

In 0- to 2-day-old neonatal dogs, α-adrenergic stimulation by phenylephrine often induces a positive chronotropic effect of similar magnitude to that observed in adult fibers[45] (Fig. 4–2). Phenylephrine can increase spontaneous rate by causing a release of endogenous catecholamines. When propranolol was used to block this effect, adult fibers showed no phenylephrine-induced increase in rate. For neonatal fibers propranolol does not block the positive chronotropic effect of phenylephrine. Phentolamine, however, completely abolishes this effect of phenylephrine in neonatal fibers. This suggests that during development, the positive response to α-adrenergic stimulation is converted to a negative one.

The autonomic nervous system continues to develop during neonatal life. Enzymes responsible for the synthesis and degradation of catecholamines are at low levels relative to what they will be in the adult.[13,26] Similarly, the level of catecholamines and the activity of their uptake systems in the developing heart are low.[7,10,25,27,28,63] With growth, all of these parameters increase in a manner consistent with growth of the adrenergic nervous system. Thus, there is circumstantial evidence suggesting that the electrophysiologic responses of neonatal Purkinje fibers to adrenergic stimulation may be associated with innervation. The conversion of the neonatal response to alpha stimulation from excitatory to inhibitory and the increase in the proportion of the cardiac Purkinje fibers showing a negative chronotropic effect of adrenergic stimulation in adults may be associated with innervation.

In a cultured cardiac cell system, noninnervated neonatal rat myocytes respond to phenylephrine with an increase in the spontaneous rate of contraction.[12] When myocytes from neonatal rats are cocultured with sympathetic nerves, 60 per cent of them respond to phenylephrine with a decrease in rate (Fig. 4–3). Subsequent studies[58] demonstrated that the acquisition of this α-mediated negative chronotropic response occurs at the same time as the appearance of a guanosine triphosphate (GTP)–binding specific protein integral to the α-adrenergic receptor complex.

The GTP-binding proteins, called N proteins, are all chemically related and depend upon differences in a specific (α) subunit for functional specificity. This portion of the molecule has been shown to bind GTP and to be susceptible to ADP ribosylation by selective bacterial toxins, such as cholera and pertussis toxins. These N proteins appear to be crucial in the regulation of adenylate cyclase activity and phophoinositide lipid hydrolysis and in the activation of membrane ion channels.[18,31,42,57,68]

Recent studies of these N proteins led to the discovery that pertussis toxin–susceptible proteins are detectable in increasing amounts in the intact heart in association with the appearance of the α-mediated negative chronotropic effect of phenylephrine.[46,58] When neonatal rat myocytes and sympathetic neurons are cocultured, the α-induced negative chronotropic effect appears in association with this N protein.[58] When innervated myocytes are incubated in the presence of pertussis toxin, which ribosylates and inactivates the N protein, the mature–type response to alpha stimulation is converted to the immature type, in which a positive chronotropic effect is seen. These data implicate a regulatory N protein in the modulation of the α-adrenergic negative chronotropic response.

CHOLINERGIC EFFECTS

The effects of cholinergic stimulation are greatest in supraventricular tissues and least in the ventricles. The sinus and atrioventricular nodes are richly endowed with cholinergic nerves and muscarinic receptors. In the SA node, stimulation of muscarinic receptors slows the rate of action potential initiation by decreasing the slope of spontaneous diastolic depolarization and by increasing maximum diastolic potential.[23] These effects occur via an increase in outward K^+ conductance and a decrease in inward Ca^{2+} and Na^+ movement through slow channels.[60] At the AV node, muscarinic receptor stimulation decreases the rate of rise and amplitude of the action potential to decrease

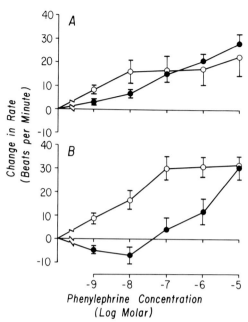

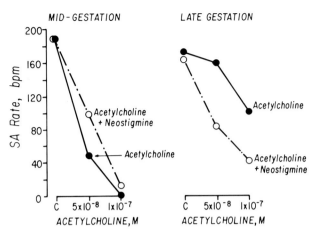

Figure 4–4. Preliminary data on the effect of acetylcholine on spontaneous sinus rate of the fetal dog heart. Hearts were obtained from fetuses during mid- (30 to 40 days after conception) and late (55 to 63 days after conception) gestation and perfused via an aortic cannula with a physiologic salt solution. Surface electrodes placed on the region of the sinus node were used to monitor sinoatrial rate. Dose-response relationships for acetylcholine were determined at two stages of gestation in the absence and presence of the cholinesterase inhibitor, neostigmine (1×10^{-7} M). In the left panel, note the greater sensitivity of the midgestation hearts to the effect of acetylcholine and the lack of effect of acetylcholinesterase inhibition on this negative chronotropic effect. In the right panel, note that the effect of acetylcholine is less in late gestation and that the effects of neostigmine now greatly enhance the negative chronotropic response to acetylcholine.

Figure 4–3. The effect of pertusssis toxin on the α_1-adrenergic mediated chronotropic response to phenylephrine in noninnervated and innervated neonatal rat myocardial cell cultures. *A*, Noninnervated myocytes. *B*, Myocytes innervated by sympathetic neurons. For both *A* and *B*, filled circles represent the control response to phenylephrine, unfilled circles represent the response to phenylephrine of myocytes exposed first to pertussis toxin, 0.5 μg/ml, for 16 to 20 hours. In *A*, note the lack of effect of pertussis toxin on the response to phenylephrine in noninnervated myocytes. In *B*, note that sympathetic innervation is associated with the appearance, at low concentrations, of a negative chronotropic effect of phenylephrine and that this event is lost after exposure to pertussis toxin. (Figure reprinted with permission from Steinberg SF et al [1985]: Acquisition by innervated cardiac myocytes of a pertussis toxin-specific regulatory protein linked to the alpha$_1$-receptor. Science 230:176–188. Copyright 1985 by the American Association for the Advancement of Science.)

the velocity of impulse conduction through the node. Increased refractoriness of the AV node also results.[23] In atrial myocardial cells, muscarinic stimulation decreases action potential duration and refractoriness. These effects result from an increase in outward K^+ conductance and a decrease in slow inward current, i_{si}, and are responsible for a negative chronotropic effect of muscarinic stimulation.[59]

Although early studies failed to demonstrate parasympathetic innervation of the ventricles, later studies demonstrated parasympathetic innervation and responsiveness to muscarinic stimulation. Relatively high concentrations of acetylcholine can shorten action potential duration of canine Purkinje fibers,[23,24] but at higher physiologic concentrations, the sole effect of acetylcholine is to suppress automaticity in a dose-dependent manner.[1,9,61]

The ontogeny of cholinergic responsiveness has been studied by a variety of methods. Anatomic and histochemical techniques have been used to establish a time course for innervation during development. Enzymes of synthesis and degradation of acetylcholine have served as markers. The presence of acetylcholinesterase in the embryonic chick heart can be detected on the first day after fertilization, at which time cholinergic innervation is not demonstrable.[70] By the tenth embryonic day, stimula-

tion of the vagus leads to the release of acetylcholine and a decrease in heart rate.[41] A similar sequence of events also occurs in mammals. In neonatal dogs[37] and in humans,[49] evidence exists indicating that vagal tone increases during pre- and postnatal life in that the ability of atropine to increase heart rate is progressive.

Acetylcholinesterase modulates the actions of acetylcholine by terminating the effect of this neurotransmitter. Indirect evidence for changes in acetylcholinesterase activity suggests that the activity of this enzyme increases during prenatal development.[33,36] In the embryonic chick heart, this enzyme was not detected until day 4.

Preliminary data from the fetal dog suggest that the sensitivity to acetylcholine of the sinus and AV nodes decreases between mid- and late gestation (Fig. 4–4). Sinoatrial rate and AV conduction are depressed by acetylcholine more at mid- than at late gestation. However, when acetylcholinesterase is inhibited by neostigmine, the sensitivity of the fetal heart during mid- and late gestation to acetylcholine is equivalent. Although direct biochemical data on the activity of cholinesterase in the fetal canine heart are lacking, studies in the fetal rat[31] and rabbit[20] indicate a developmentally related increase in the activity and quantity of this enzyme.

Recent advances in the study of acetylcholinesterase have revealed that this enzyme has a variety of molecular forms and that these forms may have different distributions within tissues.[3] In rat skeletal muscle, acetylcholinesterase may change from one molecular form to another.[66] It thus seems reasonable that developmental changes occur in the activity of acetylcholinesterase, thereby modulating the response of the heart to cholinergic stimulation.

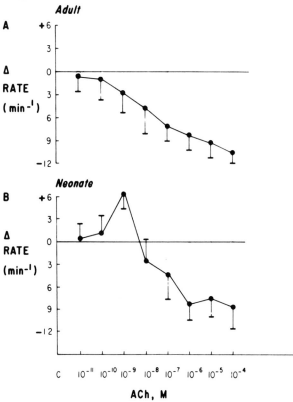

Figure 4–5. The effect of acetylcholine on the spontaneous rate of adult and neonatal cardiac Purkinje fibers. *A,* Acetylcholine produces a uniform negative chronotropic effect. *B,* Spontaneous rate is increased at low concentrations of acetylcholine ($< 1 \times 10^{-8}$ M). At higher concentrations, acetylcholine decreases the rate. For both adult and neonatal fibers, the effects of acetylcholine, including the positive chronotropic effect in neonates, were blocked by atropine. The increase in rate seen in neonates was not blocked by propranolol. (Modified after Danilo P et al [1984]: Fetal canine cardiac Purkinje fibers: Electrophysiology and ultrastructure. Am J Physiol 246:H250–H260.)

The effect of postnatal development on the cardiac response to acetylcholine has been studied. Automaticity of Purkinje fibers from neonatal dogs responds to exogenous acetylcholine with a biphasic response[9] (Fig. 4–5). At low concentrations, acetylcholine increases spontaneous rate, whereas at higher concentrations a decrease in rate occurs. This increase in spontaneous rate is not blocked by propranolol, thus ruling out the possibility that catecholamines are released secondary to muscarinic stimulation. Atropine, however, attenuates both the positive and the negative chronotropic response to acetylcholine, suggesting that both are mediated by a muscarinic receptor. In contrast to the biphasic response of the neonatal Purkinje fiber, adult fibers respond to acetylcholine with only a decrease in spontaneous rate. Although the mechanism of the neonatal response to acetylcholine remains to be determined, it suggests that innervation can influence the electrophysiologic response of the developing heart.

SUMMARY

The electrophysiologic characteristics of the normal heart undergo a gradual transition from embryonic and fetal development through neonatal and adult life. The cardiac transmembrane action potential appears to develop from one dependent on depolarization of slow channels to one in which fast channels predominate. Resting or maximum diastolic potential increases, presumably through increases in the activity of the Na^+, K^+ pump and/or changes in physiochemical properties of the cell membrane. Also developing at the same time are all the components of responsiveness to autonomic stimulation: nerves, enzymes of synthesis and degradation of neurotransmitters, neurotransmitters themselves, and receptor and effector systems. Because the sympathetic and parasympathetic nervous systems mature at different rates, it is apparent that the same balance between the two that exists in the adult is unlikely to be found in the developing heart. Mechanisms for the regulation and control of cardiac rate and rhythm are likely to be different or even lacking in the young. There is still a great need for information on how development modulates cardiac electrophysiology and responsiveness to cardioactive drugs.

References

1. Bailey JC, Greenspan K, Elizari MV, Anderson GJ, Fisch C (1973): Effects of acetylcholine on automaticity and conduction in the proximal portion of the His–Purkinje system in the dog. Circ Res 210–216.
2. Bernard C (1975): Establishment of ionic permeabilities of the myocardial membrane during embryonic development of the rat. In Lieberman M, Sano T (eds): Developmental and Physiological Correlates of Cardiac Muscle. New York, Raven Press.
3. Brimijoin S (1983): Molecular forms of acetylcholinesterase in brain, nerve and muscle: nature, localization and dynamics. Prog Neurobiol 21:291–322.
4. Buchthal SD, Bilezikian JP, Danilo P (1985): Developmental changes in beta and alpha$_1$-adrenergic receptors in cardiac Purkinje fibers. Circulation 72:III–330.
5. Carmeliet E, Vereecke J (1969): Adrenaline and the plateau of the cardiac action potential. Pflug Arch 313:300–315.
6. Danilo P (1984): Electrophysiology of the fetal and neonatal heart. In Legato MJ (ed): The Developing Heart. Boston, Martinus Nijhoff, pp 21–38.
7. Danilo P, Reder RF, Mill J, Petrie R (1979): Developmental changes in cellular electrophysiologic characteristics and catecholamine content of fetal hearts. Circulation 59:II–157.
8. Danilo P, Reder RF, Binah O, Legato MJ (1984): Fetal canine cardiac Purkinje fibers: Electrophysiology and ultrastructure. Am J Physiol 246:H250–H260.
9. Danilo P, Rosen MR, Hordof AJ (1978): Effects of acetylcholine on the ventricular specialized conducting system of the neonatal and adult dogs. Circ Res 43:777–784.
10. Dawes GS, Handler JJ, Mott JC (1957): Some cardiovascular responses in foetal, newborn and adult rabbits. J Physiol 139:123–130.
11. DiFrancesco D (1981): A new interpretation of the pacemaker current in calf Purkinje fibers. J Physiol 379:359–370.
12. Drugge E, Rosen MR, Robinson RB (1985): Neural regulation of the effects of alpha-adrenergic agonists on automaticity. Circ Res 57:415–423.
13. Enemar A, Falck B, Hakanson R (1965): Observations on the appearance of norepinephrine in sympathetic nervous system of chick embryo. Dev Biol 11:268–283.
14. Fozzard HA, Arnsdorf MF (1986): Cardiac electrophysiology. In Fozzard HA, Haber E, Jennings RB, Katz AM, Morgan HS (eds): The Heart and Cardiovascular System: Scientific Foundations. New York, Raven Press, pp 1–30.
15. Fozzard H, Sheu SS (1980): Intracellular potassium and sodium activities of chick ventricular muscle during embryonic development. J Physiol 306:579–586.

16. Gadsby DC (1983): Beta-adrenergic agonists increase membrane K+-conductance in cardiac Purkinje fibers. Nature 306:691–693.

17. Galper JB, Catterall WA (1978): Developmental changes in the sensitivity of embryonic heart cells to tetrodotoxin and D-600. Dev Biol 65:216–227.

18. Gilman AG (1984): Guanine nucleotide-binding regulatory proteins and dual control of adenylate cyclase. J Clin Invest 73:1–4.

19. Giotti A, Ledda F, Mannaioni PF (1973): Effects of noradrenaline and isoprenaline, in combination with alpha- and beta-receptor blocking substances, on the action potential of cardiac Purkinje fibers. J Physiol 229:99–113.

20. Hagopian M, Tennyson VM, Spiro D (1970): Cytochemical localization of cholinesterase in embryonic rabbit cardiac muscle. J Histochem Cytochem 18:38–43.

21. Hall EK (1957): Acetylcholine and epinephrine effects on the embryonic rat heart. J Cell Comp Physiol 49:187–200.

22. Harvey W (1653): Anatomical exercitations concerning the generation of living creatures. London, Exercitation XVII.

23. Hoffman BF, Cranefield PF (1960): Electrophysiology of the Heart. New York, McGraw-Hill, pp 104–174, pp 183–184.

24. Hoffman BF, Suckling EE (1953): Cardiac cellular potentials: Effect of vagal stimulation and acetylcholine. Am J Physiol 173:312–320.

25. Ignarro LJ, Shideman FE (1968): Appearance and concentrations of catecholamines and their biosynthesis in the embryonic and developing chick. J Pharm Exp Ther 159:38–48.

26. Ignarro LJ, Shideman FE (1968): Catechol-o-methyl transferase and monoamine oxidase activities in the heart and liver of the embryonic and developing chick. J Pharmacol Exp Ther 159:29–37.

27. Ignarro LJ, Shideman FE (1968): Norepinephrine and epinephrine in the embryo and embryonic heart of the chick: Uptake and subcellular distribution. J Pharmacol Exp Ther 159:49–58.

28. Ignarro LJ, Shideman FE (1968): The requirement of sympathetic innervation for the active transport of norephinephrine by the heart. J Pharmacol Exp Ther 159:59–65.

29. Iijima T, Pappano A (1979): Ontogenetic increase of the maximal rate of rise of the chick embryonic heart action potential. Relationship to voltage, time and tetrodotoxin. Circ Res 44:358–367.

30. Ishima Y (1968): The effect of tetrodotoxin and sodium substitution on the action potential in the cause of development of the embryonic chick heart. Proc Jap Acad 84:170–175.

31. Karazmar AG (1963): Ontogenesis of cholinesterases. In GB Koelle (ed): Handebuch der exp Pharmakol. V15. Berlin, Springer-Verlag, pp 129–186.

32. Klein RL (1963): The induction of a transfer adenosine triphosphate phosphohydrolase in embryonic chick heart. Biochem Biophys Acta 73:488–498.

33. Lelorier J, Shideman FE (1976): Acetylcholinesterase and responses to acetylcholine in the embryonic chick heart. J Pharm Pharmacol 28:196–199.

34. Mace SE, Levy MN (1983): Neural control of heart rate: A comparison between puppies and adult animals. Pediatr Res 17:491–495.

35. Marcus NC, Fozzard H (1981): Tetrodotoxin sensitivity in the developing and adult chick heart. J Mol Cell Cardiol 13:335–340.

36. McCarty LP, Lee WC, Shideman FE (1960): Measurement of the inotropic effects of drugs on the innervated and noninnervated embryonic chick heart. J Pharmacol Exp Ther 129:315–321.

37. McDonald TF, DeHaan RL (1973): Ion levels and membrane potential in chick heart tissue and cultured cells. J Gen Physiol 61:89–109.

38. McLean MJ, Shigenobu K, Sperelakis N (1976): Two pharmacological types of slow Na+ channels as distinguished by verapamil blockade. Eur J Pharmacol 26:379–382.

39. Nakamura T, Ui M (1985): Simultaneous inhibition of inosital phospholipid breakdown, arachidonic acid release and histamine secretion in most cells by islet-activating protein pertussis toxin. J Biol Chem 260:3584–3593.

40. New W, Trautwein W (1972): The ionic nature of slow inward current and its relation to contraction. Pflug Arch 334:24–38.

41. Pappano AJ, Loffelholz K (1984): Onotgenesis of adrenergic and cholinergic neuroeffector transmission in chick embryo heart. J Pharmacol Exp Ther 191:468–474.

42. Pfaffinger PJ, Martin JM, Hunter DD, Nathanson NM, Hill B (1985): GTP binding proteins couple cardiac muscarinic receptors to a K channel. Nature 317:536–538.

43. Pickering JW (1893): Observations on the physiology of the embryonic heart. J Physiol 14:383–466.

44. Posner P, Farrar E, Lambert CR (1973): Inhibitory effects of catecholamines in canine cardiac Purkinje fibers. Am J Physiol 229:99–113.

45. Reder RF, Danilo P, Rosen MR (1984): Developmental changes in adrenergic effects on canine Purkinje fiber automaticity. Dev Pharmacol Ther 7:94–108.

46. Rosen MR, Danilo P, Robinson RB, Shah A, Steinberg SF (in press): Sympathetic neural and alpha adrenergic modulation of arrhythmias. In The Sudden Infant Death Syndrome: Cardio-Respiratory Mechanisms and Intervention. New York, New York Academy of Science.

47. Rosen MR, Hordorf AJ, Ilvento JP, Danilo P (1977): Effects of adrenergic amines on electrophysiological properties and automaticity of neonatal and adult canine Purkinje fibers. Circ Res 40:340–400.

48. Rosen MR, Weiss RM, Danilo P (1984): Effect of alpha adrenergic agonists and blockers on Purkinje fiber transmembrane potentials and automaticity in the dog. J Pharm Exp Ther 231:566–571.

49. Schifferli P-Y, Caldeyro-Barcia R (1973): Effects of atropine and beta adrenergic drugs on the heart rate of the human fetus. In Boreus L (ed): Fetal Pharmacology. New York, Raven Press, pp 259–279.

50. Schumann HJ, Wagner J, Knorr A, Reidmeister JC, Sodony V, Schramm G (1978): Demonstration in human atrial preparations of alpha-adrenoceptors mediating positive inotropic effects. Naunyn-Schmied Arch Pharmacol 302:333–336.

51. Shigenobu K, Schneider JA, Sperelakis N (1974): Blockade of slow Na+ and Ca2+ currents in myocardial cells by verapamil. J Pharmacol Exp Ther 190:280–288.

52. Shigenobu K, Sperelakis N (1971): Development of sensitivity to TTX of chick embryonic hearts with age. J Mol Cell Cardiol 3:271–286.

53. Sperelakis N (1972): (Na+, K+)-ATPase activity of embryonic chick heart and skeletal muscle as a function of age. Biochem Biophys Acta 73:488–498.

54. Sperelakis N (1984): Developmental changes in membrane electrical properties of the heart. In Sperelakis N (ed): Physiology and Pathophysiology of the Heart. Boston, Martinus Nijhoff, pp 543–573.

55. Sperelakis N, Shigenobu N (1972): Changes in membrane properties of chick embryonic hearts during development. J Gen Physiol 60:430–453.

56. Sperelakis N, Shigenobu K, McLean MJ (1976): Membrane cation channels: Changes in developing hearts, in cell cultures, and in organ culture. In Lieberman M, Sano T (eds): Developmental and Physiological Correlates of Cardiac Cells. New York, Raven Press, pp 209–234.

57. Spiegel AM, Gierschik P, Levine MA, Dawns RW (1985): Clinical implications of guanine nucleotide-binding proteins as receptor-effector couplers. N Engl J Med 312:26–33.

58. Steinberg SF, Drugge ED, Bilezikian JP, Robinson RB (1985): Acquisition by innervated cardiac myocytes of a pertussis toxin-specific regulatory protein linked to the alpha₁-receptor. Science 230:176–188.

59. Ten Eick R, Nawrath H, McDonald TF, Trautwein W (1976): On the mechanism of the negative chronotropic effect of acetylcholine. Pflug Arch 361:207–213.

60. Trautwein W, Kuffler SW, Edwards C (1956): Changes in membrane characteristics of heart muscle during inhibition. J Gen Physiol 40:135–145.

61. Tse WW, Han J, Yoon MS (1976): Effect of acetylcholine on automaticity of canine Purkinje fibers. Am J Physiol 230:116–119.

62. Tsien RW, Giles W, Greengard C (1972): Cyclic AMP mediates the effects of adrenaline on cardiac Purkinje fibers. Nature New Biol 240:181–183.

63. Vapaavouri EK, Shinebourne EA, Williams RL (1973): Development of cardiovascular responses to autonomic blockage in intact fetal and neonatal lambs. Biol Neonate 22:177–188.

64. Vassalle M (1979): Electrogenesis of the plateau and pacemaker potential. Ann Rev Physiol 41:425–440.

65. Vassalle M, Barnabei O (1979): Norepinephrine and potassium fluxes in cardiac Purkinje fibers. Pflug Arch 322:287–303.

66. Vigny M, Koenig J, Rieger F (1976): The motor end plate specific of acetylcholinesterase: Appearance during embryo-genesis and reinnervation of rat muscle. J Neurochem 27:1347–1353.

67. Watanabe AM, Jones LR, Manalan AS, Besch HR (1982): Cardiac autonomic receptors. Recent concepts from radiolabeled ligand-binding studies. Circ Res 50:161–174.

68. Watanabe AM, Lindemann JP (1984): Mechanisms of adrenergic and cholinergic regulation of myocardial contractility. In Sperelakis N (ed): Physiology and Pathophysiology of the Heart. Boston, Martinus Nijhoff, pp 377–404.

69. Wildenthal K (1973): Maturation of responsiveness to cardioactive drugs: Differential effects of acetylcholine, norepinephrine, theophylline, tyramine, glucagon, and dibutyryl cyclic AMP on atrial rate in hearts of fetal mice. J Clin Invest 52:2250–2258.

70. Zachs SI (1954): Esterases in the early chick embryo. Anat Rec 118:509–537.

5 PULMONARY VASCULAR DEVELOPMENT

Sheila G. Haworth

The state of the pulmonary vascular bed frequently determines the outcome of palliative and corrective surgery in newborn infants with congenital heart disease. Dramatic structural and functional changes occur in the pulmonary circulation at birth, but babies with congenital heart disease may be subjected to anesthesia, mechanical ventilation, and even cardiopulmonary bypass before the lungs have had time to adapt completely to extrauterine life. Also, certain types of congenital heart disease compromise pulmonary vascular development before birth, producing abnormalities that complicate clinical management. An increase in pulmonary arterial smooth muscle in children with hypoplastic left heart syndrome or obstructed total anomalous pulmonary venous return, for example, can lead to a delay in adaptation, an excessive lability of the pulmonary vasculature, and the abrupt increases in pulmonary arterial pressure known as pulmonary hypertensive crises. The majority of children with congenital heart disease do not need an operation in the neonatal period, but in planning the future management of these children the effect of the hemodynamic abnormalities on pulmonary vascular development will influence the timing and sometimes the choice of operation. It is essential to understand the normal development of the pulmonary circulation in order to understand how abnormalities in structure and function can influence the practice of pediatric cardiology.

HISTORICAL PERSPECTIVE

Harvey first described the fetal circulation correctly. "In the embryo, whilst the lungs are yet in a state of inaction... nature uses two ventricles of the heart as if they formed but one, for the transmission of the blood."[31] The fetal circulation was first visualized in vivo in 1939 when Barclay et al performed cineangiographic studies on the exteriorized fetal lamb.[3] The first direct physiologic measurements on the pulmonary vascular bed of the fetus and newborn were made by Born and his colleagues at Oxford in the 1950s.[5] They showed that the high pulmonary arterial pressure and vascular resistance of the fetal lamb fell abruptly upon gaseous expansion of the lung, a change accompanied by a six- to tenfold increase in pulmonary blood flow.[11,21] The reduction in pulmonary vascular resistance was attributed to both the mechanical effect of gaseous expansion and to a direct effect of oxygen on the lung. Ten years later, Rudolph and Heymann[55–57] used radioactive microspheres to show that the lung of the fetal lamb receives 3.7 per cent of the combined ventricular output at 0.4 to 0.7 gestation, increasing to 7 per cent near term.

The fetal and neonatal pulmonary vasculature was shown to be exquisitely sensitive to small changes in arterial oxygen tension, with the pulmonary vascular resistance increasing in a curvilinear manner as oxygen tension fell.[5,58] Hypercarbia and acidosis were shown to augment the vasoconstrictor response to hypoxia.[11,17,59] Conversely, an increase in arterial oxygen tension achieved by keeping the mother in a state of hyperbaric oxygen reduced pulmonary vascular resistance and increased the pulmonary blood flow.[55] Chronic changes in the oxygen environment of the pregnant rat were associated with changes in the thickness of the fetal pulmonary arteries,[26] attributed by some to an increase in the amount of vascular smooth muscle and by others to vasoconstriction.[24,26]

The fetal and newborn pulmonary vasculature is more reactive than the mature pulmonary vasculature, responding briskly to many drugs as well as to changes in the concentration of oxygen, carbon dioxide, and hydrogen ion. For example, in the fetal lamb, acetylcholine lowers pulmonary vascular resistance and extends the period of time during which blood flows forward into the pulmonary vascular bed during each cardiac cycle.[58] Instead of flowing forward only during early systole, when velocity is high, blood flows forward throughout systole, as occurs in the normal lung after birth.

In 1887 His described the early anatomic development of the human fetal lung, finding a right and left stem bronchus passing into a primary lung sac at an early stage.[43] Congdon[16] used wax plate reconstructions to show that the lungs are perfused by paired segmental arteries arising from the dorsal aortae until the 18-mm stage, when the lungs became connected to the right ventricle by the definitive pulmonary arteries. Hislop and Reid showed that the pulmonary arterial and venous branching patterns are complete by midgestation, except for the vessels at the lung periphery, which form as the alveoli form during late gestation and after birth.[44,45] The high pulmonary arterial wall thickness characteristic of fetal life was described by Civin in 1950.[14] Subsequently, quantitative morphometric techniques were used to describe pre- and postnatal pulmonary vascular development and to correlate the postnatal fall in pulmonary vascular resistance with the reduction in pulmonary arterial wall thickness.[34,35,44,45] Early studies indicated a reduction in pulmonary arterial muscle mass after birth.[53] Recent ultrastructural work, however, has shown that the pulmonary arteries adapt to extrauterine life not by reducing the amount of muscle but by reorganizing the components of the arterial wall to reduce wall thickness and increase lumen diameter.[29,30,33]

In the immediate future we shall learn about the innervation of the developing pulmonary vasculature by classical and peptidergic neurotransmitters and about the

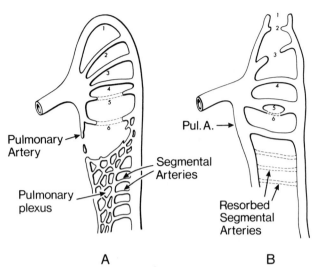

Figure 5–1. Development of the aortic arches and pulmonary artery. In (A) the pulmonary plexus is connected to the segmental arteries, which have atrophied in (B), where the pulmonary plexus is connected solely to the pulmonary artery. Pul. A = pulmonary artery. (Redrawn with permission from Hungington GS [1919–1920]: The morphology of the pulmonary artery in the mammalia. Anat Rec 17:165–201.)

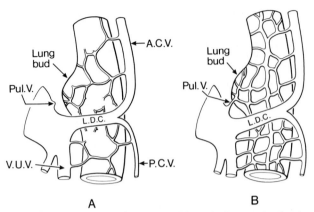

Figure 5–2. Development of the lung bud from the foregut, showing the pulmonary venous outgrowth from the atrial sinus in (A) connecting with the foregut plexus in (B). A.C.V. = anterior cardinal vein; P.C.V. = posterior cardinal vein; L.D.C. = left duct of Cuvier; Pul. V. = pulmonary vein; V.U.V. = vitello-umbilical vein. (Redrawn with permission from Butler H [1952]: Some derivatives of the foregut venous plexus of the albino rat, with reference to man. J Anat 86:95–109, Cambridge University Press.)

pharmacology of the immature pulmonary circulation. These studies should help optimize the management of newborn infants with pulmonary hypertension. The current literature on adults abounds with studies on the metabolism and functional properties of the pulmonary endothelial cell and on the interaction between endothelium and vascular smooth muscle. Extension of these investigations to the immature pulmonary circulation offers an exciting challenge.

EMBRYONIC DEVELOPMENT

The heart tube is formed by the end of the third week of gestation, and about 5 days later the lung bud develops at the caudal end of the laryngotracheal sulcus. The lung bud expands laterally and divides into two lung sacs, each of which elongates and divides into lobes and then into bronchopulmonary segments. The lobar bronchi to each lung are present by 5 weeks gestation (8 mm stage) and all subsegmental bronchi are present by 6 weeks gestation (13.4 mm stage).[61] As the lung buds push out from the laryngeal floor, they become invested by the surrounding mesenchyme of the splanchic mesoderm of the ventral surface of the foregut. The intrapulmonary blood vessels develop from this mesenchyme as the pulmonary plexus and become connected to paired segmental arteries that arise from the dorsal aortae cranial to the celiac arteries (Fig. 5–1A).

At about 32 days of gestation (5 mm stage) the sixth branchial arches appear, which give off branches to the lungs and the pulmonary arteries (Fig. 5–1A).[16] By 50 days after ovulation (18 mm stage) the segmental arteries cease to supply the lung, and the adult pattern of blood supply is achieved (Fig. 5–1B). All the bronchopulmonary segments are connected exclusively to the central pulmonary arteries derived from the sixth branchial arches, and these vessels provide the intrapulmonary arteries with their only source of blood supply. Occasionally, one or more of the early segmental arteries persists, permanently capturing a lobe or segment of lung.[41]

The intrapulmonary veins, like the arteries, are derived from the splanchnic plexus associated with the lung buds (Fig. 5–2). They drain into the systemic venous system until day 28 to 30 of gestation, when the proximal pulmonary vein develops as an outgrowth from the left atrium and connects with the intrapulmonary veins.[9] In the human lung some connections remain between esophageal and pulmonary veins at the hilus of the lung[9] and offer an alternative pathway for pulmonary venous outflow. They assume considerable importance in babies born with absent extrapulmonary veins or obstructed pulmonary venous return.

The bronchial arteries appear relatively late in fetal life, between the ninth and twelfth week of gestation, as a secondary arterial system implanted on the walls of the bronchi and large pulmonary vessels that extends down the bronchial tree as the cartilage develops.[6] The bronchial arteries arise from the aorta itself or from the right or left posterior intercostal rami of the aorta. Anastomoses between pulmonary and bronchial arteries are frequent in the fetal and newborn lung but decrease in size and number during the first years of life.[60]

FETAL DEVELOPMENT: PHYSIOLOGIC AND MORPHOLOGIC CHANGES

Physiologic Development

Studies on the fetal circulation of the lamb have shown that the right ventricle ejects 66 per cent of the combined ventricular output.[56] Consequently, the main pulmonary trunk is large and continues as the ductus arteriosus into

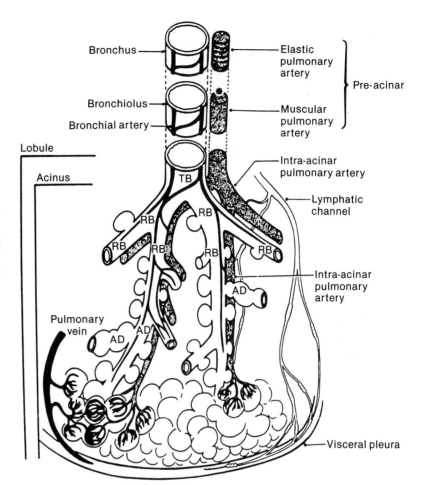

Figure 5–3. Diagram of the branching pattern of airways and pulmonary artery (stippled). TB = terminal bronchiolus; RB = respiratory bronchiolus; AD = alveolar duct. (Reproduced by permission of Anderson RH, Macartney FJ, Shineboune EA, Tynan M [1987]: Paediatric Cardiology. Edinburgh, Churchill Livingstone.)

the descending thoracic aorta. The mean pressure in the pulmonary trunk is similar to that in the aorta throughout gestation but during the last third of gestation the systolic pressure may be 5 to 8 mmHg higher.[55] Reflecting the similarity in distending pressures, the media of the pulmonary trunk has a similar thickness to that of the aorta and is composed of parallel elastic fibers of uniform thickness arranged in a compact fashion.[40] The pulmonary arteries convey only 4 to 10 per cent of the combined ventricular output to the lungs.[57] This blood is mainly superior vena caval blood and has an oxygen tension of 16 to 18 mmHg, and an oxygen saturation of 50 to 55 per cent. As gestation advances, the amount of blood perfusing the lungs increases from approximately 20 to 40 ml/min/kg fetal body weight, and the proportion of the combined ventricular output increases from 4 per cent to 8 to 10 per cent.[55,57] The increase in pulmonary blood flow is accompanied by a slight fall in pulmonary vascular resistance from approximately 2 to 1.6 mmHg/ml/min/kg. The increase in flow is matched by an increase in cross-sectional area of the pulmonary vascular bed as new arteries form and as existing ones increase in size.

Morphologic Development

In the mature lung the arteries accompany the airways (Fig. 5–3) and these structures develop together during fetal life.[44,45] The preacinar arteries and airways are those structures extending down to, but not including, the respiratory (acinar) region of the lung. The majority of the preacinar arteries and bronchi, 65 to 75 per cent, are formed between the tenth and fourteenth week of gestation, and the entire preacinar branching pattern is complete by the sixteenth week[7,44] (Fig. 5–4). By contrast, the intra-acinar arteries develop relatively late in fetal life and continue to form after birth as the alveolar ducts and alveoli develop[44,45] (Fig. 5–4). The pre- and postnatal development of the intrapulmonary veins parallels that of the arteries.[46] The preacinar branching pattern is complete by 20 weeks of gestation, and veins continue to develop in the intra-acinar region of the lung after birth. The veins do not accompany the arteries and airways but lie in the intersegmental plane (Fig. 5–3).

In the adult lung the proximal half of the preacinar arterial pathway down to the seventh generation has an elastic wall structure, and beyond this it is muscular (Fig. 5–3). In fetal life the adult distribution of elastic structure is achieved by the nineteenth week of gestation.[44] In the smaller preacinar and intra-acinar arteries, wall structure is related to the diameter of an artery, the muscle giving way to a partially muscular structure and this to a nonmuscular structure that is the same diameter in the fetus as in the adult lung but is located at a more proximal level along the arterial

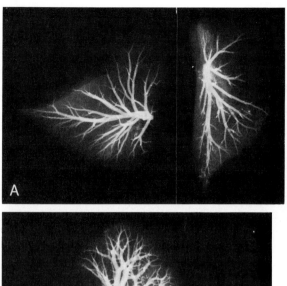

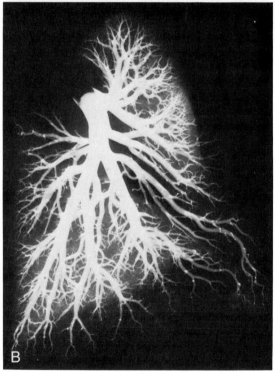

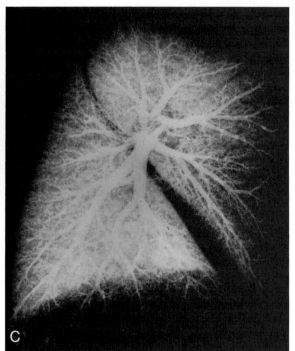

Figure 5–4. Postmortem arteriograms. *A,* Normal fetus of 19 weeks' gestation. The preacinar arteries are all present. (Reproduced by permission of Dr. A. Hislop.) *B,* Normal fetus of 40 weeks' gestation. (Reproduced by permission of Davis JA, Dobbing J [eds] [1981]: Scientific Foundations of Paediatrics. London, Heinemann Professional Publishing.) *C,* Normal 18-month-old child. A dense background haze has appeared since birth due to filling of newly formed intra-acinar arteries and growth of existing vessels (Magnification: *A, B,* and *C* × 95).

pathway (Fig. 5–5). At birth, therefore, relatively few intra-acinar arteries contain muscle; muscle cells gradually differentiate in progressively more peripheral arteries as the child grows.[45] During fetal life, the wall thickness of the muscular and partially muscular pulmonary arteries is high, and the lumen is small[14,44] (Fig. 5–6A). As new arteries are formed, they acquire a muscle coat whose thickness is commensurate with their size.[44] Thus, as gestation advances, the number of muscularized arteries rises, increasing the amount of smooth muscle per unit area of lung tissue. The thickness of the muscle coat of each individual artery, however, does not change. Premature infants are born with arteries that are slightly smaller than normal and therefore have less muscle than is normal at term.

The vein wall is thin throughout fetal and postnatal life. Muscle cells are rarely found in the wall before 28 weeks of gestation.[46]

ADAPTATION TO EXTRAUTERINE LIFE AND EARLY POSTNATAL GROWTH

Physiologic Changes

Immediately after birth, the pulmonary vascular resistance falls rapidly as the lungs are ventilated, and pulmonary blood flow increases. In the lamb, resistance decreases from approximately 1.6 to 0.3 mmHg/ml/min/kg, flow increases from 35 to 150 to 200 ml/kg/min,[11,21,55] and pulmonary arterial pressure falls. The pressure is determined mainly by pulmonary vascular resistance but is also related to closure of the ductus arteriosus and does not become independent of the systemic arterial pressure until the ductus has closed. While the ductus arteriosus remains patent, a transient change in the

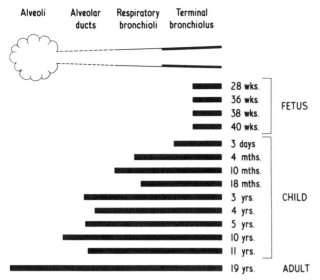

Figure 5–5. Diagram illustrating the appearance of muscle in the wall of intra-acinar arteries. (Reproduced by permission of Hislop A et al [1973]: Pulmonary arterial development during childhood. Thorax 28:129–135.)

resistance of either pulmonary or systemic circulation leads to bidirectional shunting—the circulation is transitional. In humans the pulmonary arterial pressure falls abruptly from a mean of approximately 60 to 30 mmHg during the first 10 hours of life[20] and gradually achieves a normal mature level during the first month. The reduction in resistance is accompanied by a reduction in the work of the right ventricle, which in the pig is halved during the first 2 weeks of life.[28] The postnatal reduction in pulmonary vascular resistance is associated with a dramatic increase in the cross-sectional area of the pulmonary vascular bed.

Morphologic Development

In the normal human lung, pulmonary arterial wall thickness decreases rapidly during the first days of life, particularly in arteries less than 250 μm in diameter and reaches a mature adult level in all arteries during the first 3 months of life[35,45] (Figs. 5–6 and 5–7). Ultrastructural studies on the normal pig lung have shown that the thick-walled fetal pulmonary arteries are composed of thick endothelial and smooth muscle cells, with both cell types having a low surface-volume ratio[29,30,33] (Figs. 5–8 to 5–11). The endothelial cells have deep, interdigitating cell contacts, and the smooth muscle cells overlap each other.[29] Smooth muscle cells are immature, and even at birth contain a relatively small proportion of contractile filaments. Thus, the high pulmonary vascular resistance of fetal life appears to be due to the shape and organization of the cells within the vessel wall rather than to marked contraction of well-differentiated smooth muscle cells (Fig. 5–12). Adaptation to extrauterine life can be divided into three overlapping stages, which will be described in the following sections.

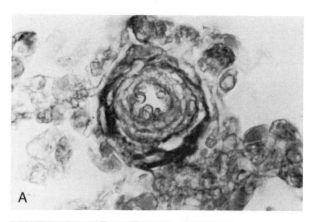
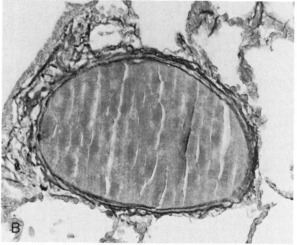

Figure 5–6. Photomicrographs of arteries accompanying a respiratory bronchiolus in a fetus (A) (magnification × 500) and an adult (B) (magnification × 300).

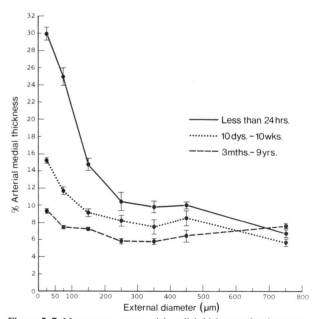

Figure 5–7. Mean percentage arterial medial thickness related to external diameter in peripheral pulmonary arteries. Bars indicate standard error of the mean. (Reproduced by permission of Haworth SG, Hislop AA [1983]: Pulmonary vascular development: normal values of peripheral vascular structure. Am J Cardiol 52:578–583.)

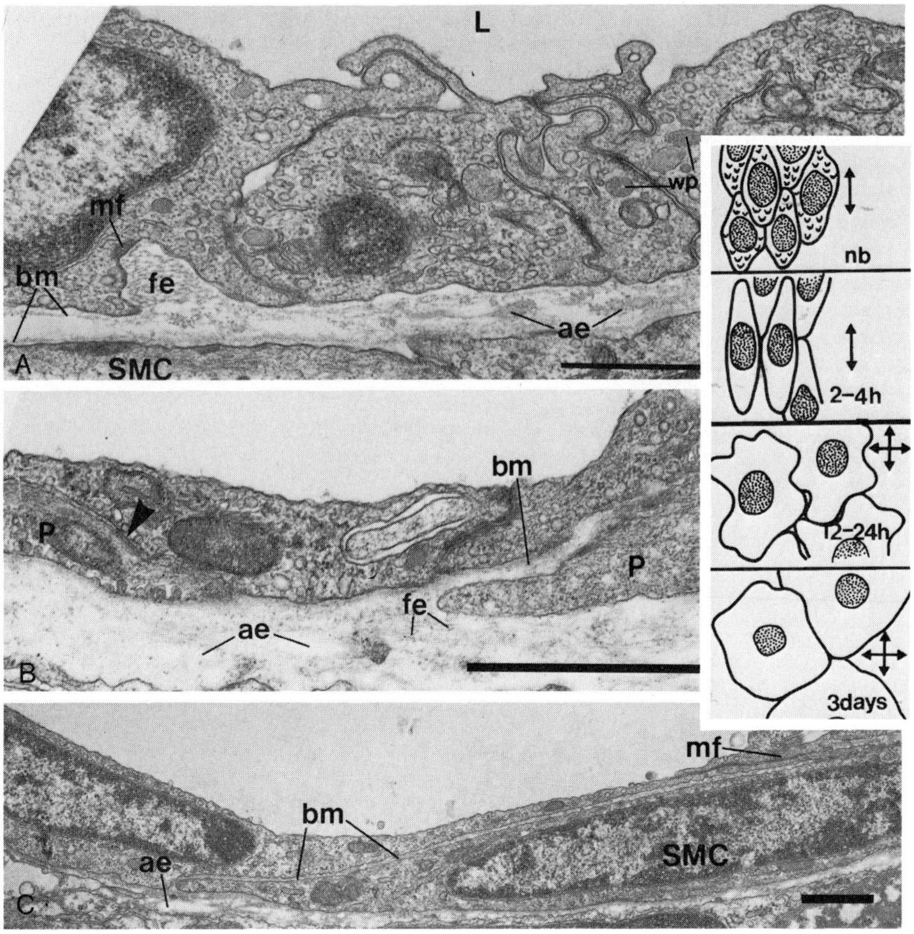

Figure 5–8. Electron micrographs of small intra-acinar vessels. *A*, Partially muscular artery from stillborn pig, transverse section. *B*, Nonmuscular artery from a pig age 8 hours, transverse section. *C*, Partially muscular artery from pig age 3 days, transverse section. Arrow = endothelial/pericyte close contact; ae = amorphous elastin; bm = basement membrane; fe = microfibrillar elastin; L = lumen; mf = microfilaments; P = pericyte; SMC = smooth muscle cell; wp = Weibel-Palade bodies; scale bar = 1 μm. (From Haworth SG [1986]: Pulmonary arterial adaptation to extra-uterine life. J Pathol 149:57. Copyright 1986. Reprinted by permission of John Wiley & Sons, Ltd.) *Inset*, Illustration of en face shape changes in endothelial cells. nb = newborn; h = hours.

Stage 1: Rapid Adaptation

During the first minutes after birth, the first structural changes are seen in the endothelial cells lining the nonmuscular arteries of the alveolar walls (Fig. 5–13). These cells become thinner, and the cell contacts become reduced in depth and complexity (Fig. 5–8). The cells appear to be stretched in a longitudinal direction, which are changes consistent with the vessels' being stretched as the lung is expanded at birth[29] (Fig. 5–8). Within the first 30 minutes the wall thickness of the slightly larger muscular respiratory unit arteries also decreases as both endothelial and smooth muscle cells become thinner, show less overlap between adjacent cells, and appear to spread within the vessel wall (Figs. 5–9 and 5–10). These changes continue rapidly during the first 24 hours (Fig. 5–10) and then more slowly in order to increase both lumen and external diameter (the arteries dilate). During the first 12 hours, many small muscular arteries with a slitlike lumen become recruited into the circulation (Figs. 5–11 and 5–13).

At this time the vessels contain relatively little "fixed" connective tissue, collagen, and amorphous elastin, which might restrict changes in cell shape and position. The intra-acinar arteries do not even contain a definitive elastic lamina that might limit expansion; only small profiles of elastin are present.

The morphologic findings are consistent with several physiologic studies that indicate that physical expansion of the fetal lung with gas lowers pulmonary vascular resistance, presumably by stretching and reducing the wall thickness of the nonmuscular alveolar wall vessels.[5,11] Expansion of the fetal lung can generate a negative intrapleural pressure of −42 mmHg, which would exert considerable traction on these thin-walled vessels.[47] The vasodilator effect of oxygen might facilitate these changes and be crucial to the dilation of slightly larger muscularized arteries. The mechanisms involved in oxygen-dependent vasodilation are unknown. Lloyd suggested that oxygen stimulates the release of a vasodilator substance from the lung tissue surrounding the vessel.[51] Oxygen may also stimulate the release of bradykinin from kininogen at birth. Bradykinin is a potent vasodilator of fetal pulmonary arteries;[10,42] the levels of circulating bradykinin are elevated transiently at birth, and the deactivator of bradykinin, bradykinase, appears relatively late in gestation.[23] Bradykinin is also a potent stimulator of arachidonic acid metabolites, which can produce the vasodilator prostaglandins prostacyclin and prostaglandin E_2, both of which dilate the fetal and newborn pulmonary circulation.[12,13] When animals are exposed to a hypoxic environment from birth, adaptation fails to occur because the endothelial and smooth muscle cells are prevented from thinning and spreading within the vessel wall.[33] In

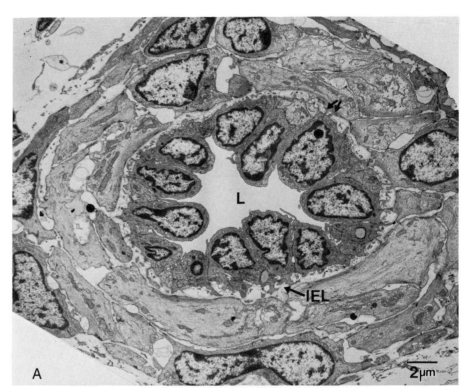

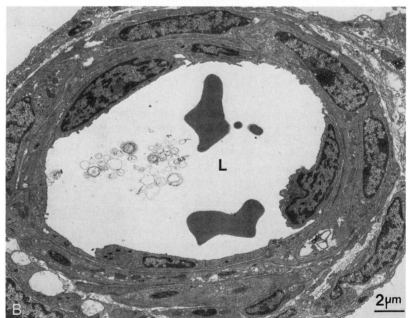

Figure 5–9. Electron micrographs of small muscular pulmonary arteries from animals. *A*, Stillborn. *B*, Aged 5 minutes. IEL = internal elastic lamina; L = lumen; arrows = narrow processes making contact with adjacent smooth muscle cells.

addition, the density of contractile myofilaments increases significantly within 3 days.

Although the most dramatic changes occur in the peripheral pulmonary arteries at birth, the walls of the conducting pulmonary arteries (elastic vessels) are also remodeled during the first days of life.[30] Wall thickness decreases as the interlamellar distance and smooth muscle cell diameter decrease. Remodeling occurs more slowly in these vessels than in the more peripheral vessels and takes days rather than hours to complete.

At birth, adaptive changes in the pulmonary circulation are accompanied by adaptive changes in the heart. The ability to increase cardiac output by increasing stroke volume improves, the myocardium develops greater active tension with age, and, at the molecular level, the ratio of the different cardiac myosin isoenzymes alters.[52,55] The entire cardiopulmonary system adapts rapidly to extrauterine life so that it may function efficiently as an integrated whole.

Stage 2: Structural Stabilization

After a phase of rapid adaptation, the remodeling of the arterial wall continues more gradually during the first

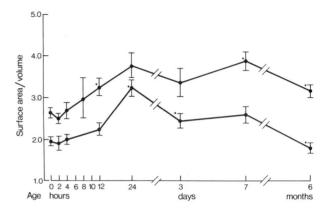

Figure 5–10. Mean surface/volume ratio of smooth muscle cells in terminal bronchiolar (top line) and small preacinar muscular (bottom line) arteries from birth to 6 months. * = significant difference from newborn and then from each subsequent significantly different value (p = < 0.05 to 0.005); ⌡ = standard error.

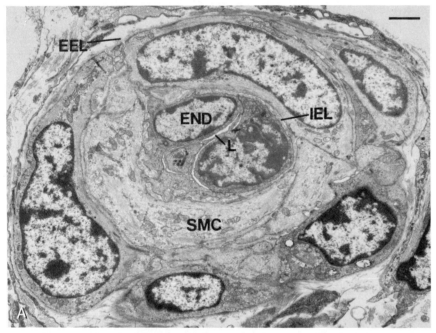

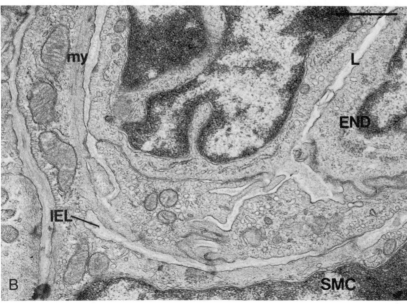

Figure 5–11. Electron micrographs of transverse sections of undilated arteries from two stillborn pigs. *A*, Low power magnification shows endothelium surrounded by a single layer of overlapping smooth muscle cells; the lumen is minute. Scale bar line = 2 μm. *B*, Detail of another artery showing interdigitating junctions between endothelial cells. Scale bar line = 1 μm. L = lumen; END = endothelial cell; SMC = smooth muscle cell; IEL = internal elastic lamina; EEL = external elastic lamina; my = myofilaments.

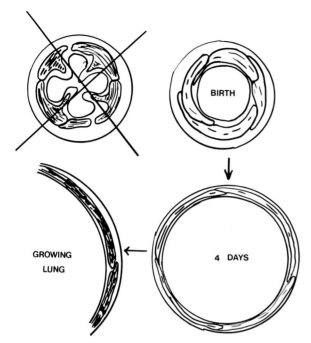

Figure 5–12. Diagram illustrating fetal luminal obstruction prior to birth, overlapping smooth muscle cells containing few myofilaments at birth, thin muscle cells with little overlap at 4 days, and muscle cells containing more myofilaments in the older lung. At birth, arteries do not have a constricted appearance.

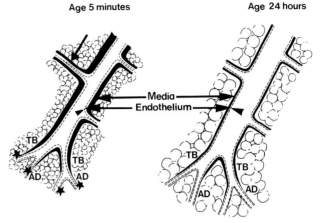

Figure 5–13. Diagram illustrating peripheral arterial pathway. At age 5 minutes arteries have a thick media and endothelium (interrupted line between arrow heads). Both these structures are thinner at 24 hours. Arteries that have a minute lumen at 5 minutes are dilated at 24 hours (arrow). * = arteries in which structural changes are noted in the first minutes of life; AD = alveolar duct; TB = terminal bronchiolus.

weeks of life. The wall thickness of the respiratory unit arteries reaches an adult level by 3 months of age.[35] In all arteries, from the hilar to the precapillary vessels, remodeling is characterized by deposition of connective tissue and maturation of the smooth muscle cells.[30] There are fewer contractile myofilaments in the smooth muscle cells of the newborn than in those of the mature lung. The cells of the human infant take 6 months to achieve maturity.

In the newborn the smooth muscle cells contain predominantly synthetic rather than contractile organelles, and, having assumed a more definitive position within the vessel wall after birth, the smooth muscle cells appear to deposit connective tissue around themselves and so stabilize the new wall structure.[30] In the conducting arteries the sheets of amorphous elastin become thicker, and the fine fibrils of collagen present at birth are replaced by thick bundles of striated collagen (Fig. 5–14). Collagen is the major stress-bearing component. In the pulmonary circulation, as in other developing blood vessels, more collagen than elastin is formed after birth. These structural changes are mirrored by changes in the mechanical properties of the vessel wall.[27] During the first weeks of life the structural stiffness of the vessel wall increases (Fig. 5–15), although the pressure-strain elastic modulus (functional distensibility) is unchanged at the low pressure to which the pulmonary arteries are exposed after birth.

Deposition of connective tissue separates the cells from each other and probably reduces the ease with which they can communicate.[29] In the large arteries the increase in thickness and integrity of the internal elastic lamina separates endothelial from smooth muscle cells, with there being relatively few gaps in the lamina. At the entrance to the respiratory unit, however, the internal elastic lamina of the terminal bronchilar arteries remains thin and patchy throughout life. It is in these arteries that intimal proliferation first develops in young children with pulmonary hypertensive congenital heart disease.[32] There is no physical barrier to communication and interaction between smooth muscle and endothelial cells nor to the migration of smooth muscle cells from the media to the intima to produce intimal proliferation.

Stage 3: Growth

Within the respiratory unit the medial thickness of the pulmonary arteries remains low once adaptation has occurred,[35] but with growth the conducting arteries show an increase in wall thickness, interlamellar distance, and smooth muscle cell diameter as lumen diameter increases.[30]

The progressive growth and remodeling of the vascular bed ensures that as the cardiac output increases with growth, pulmonary vascular resistance does not rise. Proximal to the arterial pathways of the microcirculation, resistance is mainly determined by lumen diameter, and total pulmonary vascular resistance is determined by the number of resistance pathways arranged in parallel. With growth, not only does vessel size increase, but the number of peripheral intra-acinar arterial and venous pathways also increases, thus ensuring a progressive rise in the capacity of the peripheral pulmonary vascular bed during childhood. The majority of these vessels form during the first year of life as new alveoli form.[35,45] As in fetal life, the intra-acinar arteries acquire a muscle coat as they increase in size, but the development of smooth muscle usually lags behind the increase in size; and therefore, throughout childhood the intra-acinar arterial bed contains fewer muscular arteries than are seen in adult life.[45] To the cardiologist, this structural difference has important practical implications. In a lung biopsy, the presence of

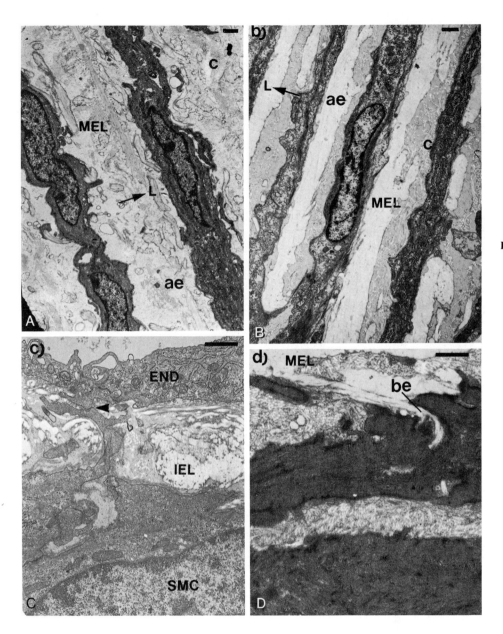

Figure 5-14. Electron micrographs of transverse sections of walls of elastic arteries in pigs aged (*A*) 12 hours, (*B*) 3 weeks, (*C*) 24 hours, and (*D*) from an adult. ae = amorphous elastin; be = branch elastin; c = collagen; END = endothlium; IEL = internal elastic lamina; L = lumen orientation; MEL = medial elastic lamina; SMC = smooth muscle cells; arrows = endothelial smooth muscle cell contact. Scale bar line = 1 μm.

muscle in more peripheral arteries instead of in those in which it is normally seen with respect to age is an early indication of the structural response of the pulmonary circulation to pulmonary hypertension.

POSTNATAL CHANGES IN THE STRUCTURE OF THE PULMONARY TRUNK

At birth the right and left pulmonary arteries have a smaller diameter than the main pulmonary artery and arise from the main vessel at a more acute angle than is seen in postnatal life. This appearance can persist for several weeks after birth and accounts for a small pressure gradient of 5 to 8 mm between the main pulmonary artery and the right and left pulmonary arteries.[19] The structure of the pulmonary trunk changes more gradually. The ratio of the thickness of the media of the pulmonary trunk to that of the aorta decreases from 1 to a mean value of 0.6 at about 8 months of age, and this ratio is maintained throughout life.[40] The elastic fibers of the pulmonary trunk become fragmented and consist of short thick rods, with some having clubbed ends. The pulmonary trunk has an adult appearance by the end of the second year of life.

EFFECT OF ALTITUDE ON ADAPTATION TO EXTRAUTERINE LIFE

In babies born at high altitude, at birth the weight of the right ventricle and the muscularity of the pulmonary arterial circulation are similar to those found in babies born at sea level.[1] After birth, however, pulmonary arterial muscularity does not decrease at the same rate nor reach the same low level.[2,54] From the age of 1 month the peripheral pulmonary arteries show medial hypertrophy as compared with the normal at sea level. This difference represents an adaptive phenomenon, not disease. There is evidence, however, to suggest that the incidence of "primary" pulmonary hypertension in childhood is greater at high altitude.[4,50]

DEVELOPMENT OF THE INNERVATION OF THE PULMONARY VASCULATURE

Oxygen has a direct effect on the pulmonary vasculature, but even during fetal life the autonomic nervous system contributes to the vasoconstrictor response to asphyxia. Stimulation of the sympathetic nerves to the lung of the fetal lamb causes vasoconstriction, as does injection of adrenaline and noradrenaline, while sympathectomy and administration of β-receptor drugs causes pulmonary vasodilation.[15,20] Some of these responses can be elicited at only 0.6 gestation. Vasoactive peptides, such as bradykinin, and the prostaglandins I_2 and E_2 produce vasodilation and modify the vasoconstrictor response to hypoxia.[12,25,42,49]

Surprisingly, despite the physiologic evidence of autonomic activity, there has been no systematic study of the development of nerves, neurotransmitters, and regulatory peptides in the pulmonary vasculature. Studies on the systemic arteries of different animal species indicate that nerve growth begins with outgrowth of axons and is followed by an increase in nerve fiber density and formation of varicosities.[18] Elastic arteries are innervated earlier and more densely than peripheral muscular vessels.[18] There are considerable differences in the timing of innervation of perivascular adrenergic nerves of systemic arteries in different organs during development, and noradrenergic and peptidergic nerves show differences in nerve density and in the age at which peak nerve density is reached in the same blood vessel.[22] A trophic role has been postulated for perivascular peptide-containing nerves.[8]

WITH REFERENCE TO CONGENITAL HEART DISEASE

Structural abnormalities of the pulmonary circulation may arise during early fetal development in association with an intracardiac abnormality or occur in late fetal or postnatal life as a result of the hemodynamic consequences of the cardiac defect. In pulmonary atresia with ventricular septal defect, for example, lobar or segmental pulmonary arteries usually remain permanently connected to the segmental arteries while acquiring, in addition, a normal connection to a central pulmonary artery.[36] A prenatal increase in pulmonary arterial pressure or flow, as in hypoplastic left heart syndrome or obstructed total

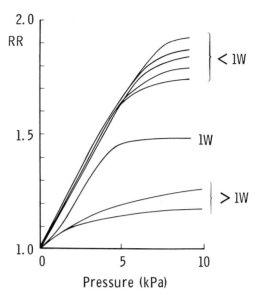

Figure 5–15. Changes in relative radius (RR) of elastic and muscular pulmonary arteries related to distending pressure in groups of pigs of different ages. Relative radius at any pressure is defined by the ratio of the radius at that pressure to the radius at a positive pressure close to zero (0.5 kPa). (Reproduced by permission of Haworth SG [1982]: Changes in distensibility of intrapulmonary arteries. Cardiovasc Res 16:725.)

anomalous pulmonary venous return, leads to a prenatal increase in pulmonary vascular smooth muscle and sometimes also to an increase in number of intra-acinar pulmonary arteries.[37,39] The converse is true of children with pulmonary atresia and an intact ventricular septum.[38] Adaptation to extrauterine life may be impaired immediately after birth by the association of thick-walled pulmonary arteries, hypoxia, and acidosis, and occur more gradually in the presence of a large left-to-right shunt. The clinical evidence suggests that the postnatal reduction in peripheral pulmonary arterial wall thickness occurs more slowly in infants with left-to-right shunts than in normal infants.

References

1. Arias-Stella J, Recavarren S (1962): Right ventricular hypertrophy in native children living at high altitude. Am J Pathol 41:55–64.
2. Arias-Stella J, Saldãna M (1962): The muscular pulmonary arteries in people native to high altitude. Med Thorac 19:484–493.
3. Barclay AE, Barcroft J, Barron DH, Franklin KJ (1939): A radiographic demonstration of the circulation through the heart in the adult and in the foetus and the identification of the ductus arteriosus. Br J Radiol 12:505–517.
4. Berthrong M, Cochran TH (1955): Pathological findings in nine children with "primary" pulmonary hypertension. Bull Johns Hopk Hosp 97:69–111.
5. Born GVR, Dawes GS, Mott JC, Widdicombe JG (1954): Changes in the heart and lungs at birth. Cold Spring Harbor Symp Quant Biol 19:102–108.
6. Boyden EA (1970): The developing bronchial arteries in a fetus of the twelfth week. Am J Anat 129:357–368.
7. Bucher U, Reid L (1961): Development of the intrasegmental bronchial tree: The pattern of branching and development of cartilage at various stages of intra-uterine life. Thorax 16:207–218.

8. Burnstock G (1982): Neuropeptides as trophic factors. In Bloom SR, Polak JM, Lindenlaub E (eds): Systemic Role of Regulatory Peptides. Stuttgart, F.K. Schattauer, pp 423–441.

9. Butler H (1952): Some derivatives of the foregut venous plexus of the albino rat, with reference to man. J Anat 86:95–109.

10. Campbell AGM, Dawes GS, Fishman AP, Hyman AI (1966): Bradykinin and pulmonary blood flow in the foetal lung. J Physiol 184:80P.

11. Cassin S, Dawes GS, Mott JC, Ross BB, Strang LB (1964): The vascular resistance of the foetal and newly ventilated lung of the lamb. J Physiol 171:61–79.

12. Cassin S, Tyler T, Leffler C, Wallis R (1979): Pulmonary and systemic vascular responses of perinatal goats to protaglandins E_1 and E_2. Am J Physiol 236:H828–H832.

13. Cassin S, Winikor I, Tod M, Philips J, Frisinger J, Jordan J, Gibbs C (1981): Effects of prostacyclin on fetal pulmonary circulation. Pediatr Pharmacol 1:197–207.

14. Civin WH (1950): The postnatal changes in the intrapulmonary arteries, arterioles and the changes in these vessels in isolated ventricular septal defects and the Eisenmenger complex. Thesis, University of Minnesota.

15. Colebatch HJH, Dawes GS, Goodwin JW, Nadeau RA (1965): The nervous control of the circulation in the foetal and newly expanded lungs of the lamb. J Physiol 178:544–562.

16. Congdon ED (1922): Transformation of the aortic-arch system during the development of the human embryo. Contrib Embryol 14:47–110.

17. Cook CD, Drinker PA, Jacobson HN, Levison M, Strang LB (1963): Control of pulmonary blood flow in the foetal and newly born lamb. J Physiol 169:10–29.

18. Cowen T, Haven AJ, Wen-Qin C, Gallen DD, Franc F, Burnstock G (1982): Development of the aging of perivascular adrenergic nerves in the rabbit. A quantitative fluorescence histochemical study using image analysis. J Auto Nerv Syst 5:317–336.

19. Danilowicz D, Rudolph AM, Hoffman JIE (1965): Vascular resistance in the large pulmonary arteries in infancy. Circulation 32 (Suppl II):74.

20. Dawes GS (1968): Foetal and Neonatal Physiology. Chicago, Year Book Medical Publishers, Inc, pp 167–188.

21. Dawes GS, Mott JC, Widdicombe JG, Wyatt DG (1953): Changes in the lungs of the newborn lamb. J Physiol 121:141–162.

22. Dhall U, Cowen T, Haven AJ, Burnstockl G (1986): Perivascular noradrenergic and peptide-containing nerves show different patterns of change during development and aging in the guinea pig. J Auto Nerv Syst 16:109–126.

23. Friedli B, Kent G, Olley PM (1973): Inactivation of bradykinin in the pulmonary vascular bed of newborn and fetal lambs. Circ Res 33:421.

24. Geggel RL, Aronovitz MJ, Reid LM (1986): Effects of chronic in utero hypoxemia on rat neonatal pulmonary arterial structure. J Pediatr 108:756–759.

25. Gerber JG, Voelkel N, Nies AS, McMurty IF, Reeves JT (1980): Moderation of hypoxic vasoconstriction by infusion of arachidonic acid: Role of PGI_2. J Appl Physiol 49:107–112.

26. Goldberg SJ, Levy RA, Siassi B, Betten J (1971): The effects of maternal hypoxia and hyperoxia upon the neonatal pulmonary vasculature. Pediatrics 48:528–533.

27. Greenwald SE, Berry CL, Haworth SG (1982): Changes in the distensibility of the intrapulmonary arteries in the normal newborn and growing pig. Cardiovasc Res 16:716–725.

28. Greenwald SE, Johnson RJ, Haworth SG (1985): Pulmonary vascular input impedance in the newborn and infant pig. Cardiovasc Res 19:44–50.

29. Hall SM, Haworth SG (1986): Normal adaptation of pulmonary arterial intima to extrauterine life in the pig: Ultrastructural studies. J Pathol 149:55–66.

30. Hall SM, Haworth SG (1987): Conducting pulmonary arteries: Structural adaptation to extrauterine life in the pig. Cardiovasc Res 21:208–216.

31. Harvey W (1847): The works of William Harvey, MD. London, Sydenham Society.

32. Haworth SG (1984): Pulmonary vascular disease in different types of congenital heart disease. Implications for interpretation of lung biopsy findings in early childhood. Br Heart J 52:557–571.

33. Haworth SG (1985): Structural adaptation to extrauterine life in the normal and in neonates with pulmonary hypertension. In Doyle EF, Engle MA, Gersony WM, Rashkind WJ, Talner NS (eds): New York, Springer-Verlag.

34. Haworth SG, Hislop AA (1981): Adaptation of the pulmonary circulation to extrauterine life in the pig and its relevance to the human infant. Cardiovasc Res 15:108–119.

35. Haworth SG, Hislop AA (1983): Pulmonary vascular development: Normal values of peripheral vascular structure. Am J Cardiol 52:578–583.

36. Haworth SG, Macartney FJ (1980): Growth and development of pulmonary circulation in pulmonary atresia with ventricular septal defect and major aortopulmonary collateral arteries. Br Heart J 44:14–24.

37. Haworth SG, Reid L (1977): A quantitative structural study of the pulmonary circulation in the newborn with aortic atresia, stenosis or coarctation. Thorax 32:121–128.

38. Haworth SG, Reid L (1977): Quantitative structural study of pulmonary circulation in the newborn with pulmonary atresia. Thorax 32:129–133.

39. Haworth SG, Reid L (1977): Structural study of pulmonary circulation and of heart in total anomalous pulmonary venous return in early infancy. Br Heart J 39:80–92.

40. Heath D, DuShane JW, Wood EH, Edwards JE (1959): The structure of the pulmonary trunk at different ages and in cases of pulmonary hypertension and pulmonary stenosis. J Pathol Bacteriol 77:443–456.

41. Hessel EA, Boyden EA, Stamm SJ, Sauvage LR (1970): High systemic origin of the sole artery to the basal segments of the left lung: Findings, surgical treatment and embryologic interpretation. Surgery 67:624–632.

42. Heymann MA, Rudolph AM, Nies AS, Melmon KL (1969): Bradykinin production associated with oxygenation of the fetal lamb. Circ Res 25:521.

43. His W (1887): Zur bildungsgeschichte der lungen beim menschlichen embryo. Arch Anat Entwick, pp 89–106.

44. Hislop A, Reid L (1972): Intrapulmonary arterial development during fetal life—branching pattern and structure. J Anat 113:35–48.

45. Hislop A, Reid L (1973): Pulmonary arterial development during childhood: Branching pattern and structure. Thorax 28:129–135.

46. Hislop A, Reid L (1973): Fetal and childhood development of the intrapulmonary veins in man—branching pattern and structure. Thorax 28:313–319.

47. Howatt WF, Humphreys PW, Normand ICS, Strang LB (1965): Ventilation of liquid by the fetal lamb during asphyxia. J Appl Physiol 20:496–502.

48. Huntingdon GS (1919–1920): The morphology of the pulmonary artery in the mammalia. Anat Rec 17:165–201.

49. Kadowitz PJ et al (1981): Pulmonary responses to prostaglandins. Fed Proc 40:1991–1996.

50. Khoury GH, Hawes CR (1963): Primary pulmonary hypertension in children living at high altitude. J Pediatr 62:177–185.

51. Lloyd TC (1968): Hypoxic pulmonary vasoconstriction: Role of perivascular tissue. J Appl Physiol 25:560–565.

52. Lompre A-M, Mercadier J-J, Wisnewsky C, Bouveret P, Pantaloni C, D'Albis A, Schwartz K (1981): Species and age-dependent changes in the relative amounts of cardiac myosin isoenzymes in mammals. Dev Biol 84:286–290.

53. Naeye RL (1961): Arterial changes during the perinatal period. Arch Pathol 71:121–128.

54. Naeye RL (1965): Children at high altitude: Pulmonary and renal abnormalities. Circ Res 16:33–38.

55. Rudolph AM (1974): Congenital diseases of the heart. Clinical-physiologic considerations in diagnosis and management. Chicago, Year Book Medical Publishers Inc, pp 30–40.

56. Rudolph AM, Heymann MA (1967): The circulation of the fetus in utero. Methods for studying distribution of blood flow, cardiac output and organ blood flow. Circ Res 21:163–184.

57. Rudolph AM, Heymann MA (1970): Circulatory changes during growth in the fetal lamb. Circ Res 26:289–299.

58. Rudolph AM, Heymann MA, Lewis AB (1977): Physiology, pharmacology of the pulmonary circulation in the fetus and newborn.

In Hodson WA (ed): Lung Biology in Health and Disease. Vol 6. Development of the Lung. New York, Marcel Dekker Inc, pp 503–505.

59. Rudolph AM, Yuan S (1966): Response of the pulmonary vasculature to hypoxia and H+ ion concentration changes. J Clin Invest 45:399–411.

60. Wagenvoort CA, Wagenvoort N (1967): Arterial anastomoses bronchopulmonary arteries and pulmobronchial arteries in perinatal lungs. Lab Invest 16:13–24.

61. Wells LJ, Boyden EA (1954): The development of the bronchopulmonary segments in human embryos of horizons XVII to XIX. Am J Anat 95:163–201.

6 DEVELOPMENTAL PHYSIOLOGY OF THE DUCTUS ARTERIOSUS

Ronald I. Clyman

HISTORICAL PERSPECTIVE

In 200 AD Galen identified the ductus arteriosus in the fetus as a vessel that formed a junction between the aorta and pulmonary artery. He also described its postnatal obliteration.[66] Some 1300 years later, in 1564, Botallus (for whom the vessel is named) described a new way for blood to enter the left ventricle. It is interesting that the ductus should be named after Botallus as he came onto the scene so late and never mentioned the vessel in his treatise. Apparently, what he rediscovered was the foramen ovale![60] Not until William Harvey wrote his *Exercitatio anatomica de motu Cordis et Sanguinis in animalibus* in 1628 was it appreciated that in the fetus the ductus arteriosus was not a nutrient artery that brought blood from the aorta to the lungs but rather allowed right ventricular blood to bypass the lungs, enabling the fetus to have a common ventricular ejection into the aorta.[76] Three hundred years later, the angiographic studies of Barclay, Franklin, and Pritchard[8] in the lamb and of Lind and Wegelius[103] in the human showed Harvey's description to be correct.

Sciacca and Condorelli have reviewed the various theories proposed to account for ductus closure.[134] One group of theories proposes external forces that compress the ductus after birth: a large bronchus filled with air, bending of the aortic arch by increased pressure after birth, respiration altering the position of the thoracic viscera, fibrous bands connected to the diaphragm that occlude the ductus with respiration, and tension by the recurrent laryngeal nerve. Another group of theories proposes obliteration of the ductus from within: a thickened valve at the aortic end, thrombosis within the lumen, inflammation of the vessel wall, fibrous growth within the intima, and active contraction of the vessel wall. Gérard[67] clearly distinguished two phases of ductus closure: primary functional closure of the vessel by some mechanical process within a few minutes of birth, followed by a secondary anatomic obliteration of the lumen. This chapter will examine the factors and events that influence each of these two phases of ductus closure.

EMBRYOLOGY

The ductus arteriosus is the terminal aortic portion of the pulmonary or sixth branchial arch. The arch system goes through two phases: the branchial phase, during which the vessels are in a pattern resembling a primitive gill system, and the postbranchial phase, during which the vessels are in a pattern resembling the adult mammalian arterial system.[29] When the right pulmonary arch separates from the right aortic arch, the formation of separate systemic and pulmonary circulations begins. In the human fetus, the completion of both branchial phases occurs by about day 26.[29]

The aortic arches connect the central aortic sac (a vascular bulge above the heart) with the paired dorsal aortae. The pulmonary arch begins to be formed by independent extensions from the dorsal aorta and the aortic sac. The primitive left subclavian artery originates at a point below the fusion of the paired dorsal aortae and subsequently migrates upward on the dorsal aorta beyond the insertion of the left pulmonary arch; this may explain why the ductus occasionally anomalously joins the aorta above the left subclavian artery. The postbranchial phase begins when the right pulmonary arch separates from the right dorsal aorta; the proximal portion of the right pulmonary arch persists as the origin of the right pulmonary artery. On the left, the pulmonary arch persists as the primitive pulmonary artery and its continuation into the aorta, the ductus arteriosus.

REGULATION OF DUCTUS PATENCY AND CLOSURE

In the full-term animal or human, the ductus arteriosus begins to constrict rapidly once the neonate is delivered and initiates air breathing. The rate at which this functional closure occurs varies from a few minutes in guinea pigs and rabbits to 10 to 15 hours in humans.[55,81,92,114,133] In 1942, based on studies performed in guinea pigs, Kennedy and Clark concluded that oxygen was responsible for constricting the ductus arteriosus after birth.[92] Experiments performed both in vitro and in vivo have substantiated these initial findings.[5,16,58,97,120,159] In addition, ductus closure is delayed or absent in human neonates exposed to low oxygen environments, either experimentally or when born at high altitudes.[3,115,124]

The biochemical basis for the oxygen response is not fully explained. Fay and colleagues have hypothesized that the contractile response to oxygen begins with an interaction between oxygen and cytochrome a_3.[58-59a] They have suggested that oxidation of cytochrome a_3 results in generation of ATP, which causes the ductus to contract through alteration in intracellular calcium. Coceani et al

I wish to thank Mr. Richard Truelove and Mr. Paul Sagan for their skillful preparation of this manuscript.

have suggested that oxygen works through an unidentified cytochrome P_{450}-catalyzed enzymatic process, which can be inhibited by carbon monoxide.[48] They hypothesize that an epoxide metabolite of an arachidonic acid monooxygenase pathway in the ductus has contractile properties, but no active metabolites have been identified to date.

Another theory of ductal closure at birth postulates that thromboxane A_2 (TxA_2) is the mediator,[62] a hypothesis that assumes that TxA_2 is carried to the ductus from the lungs by the circulation because it is not synthesized in the ductus tissue.[122,127] Consistent with this idea is the finding that TxA_2 production by the lung increases during the perinatal period.[126,145] However, it is unlikely that TxA_2 is a mediator of ductus constriction at birth because the compound is inactive on the ductus arteriosus and is exceedingly labile in blood.[46]

It has been hypothesized that direct innervation of the ductus could play a role in ductus closure. Sympathetic innervation of the ductus arises chiefly from the thoracic trunk and from the inferior cervical sympathetic nerve.[1] Some innervation also is derived from the vagus.[1] Although Aronson et al[4] were able to find only scattered bundles of acetylcholinesterase-containing nerve fibers in the adventitia of 10- to 20-week-old human fetuses, Silva and Ikeda[139] have shown extensive fibers and ganglia in the adventitia and outer one third of the medial muscle layer in lamb fetuses. In addition, the ductus does constrict well when exposed to acetylcholine.[14,58,97,119] Several groups have found norepinephrine-containing nerve terminals throughout the media of both human and lamb fetal ductuses.[4,14,139] Although only a few specimens in younger fetuses were studied, the nerves appeared not to penetrate as deeply into the media in the younger fetuses as in the older fetuses.[14] It is interesting that sections of the ductus arteriosus obtained from children (2 months to 6 years) who had a patent ductus arteriosus (PDA) requiring surgical ligation showed no adrenergic innervation of the media,[21,28] suggesting that lack of innervation could play a role in persistent ductal patency. On the other hand, catecholamines produce ductus constriction only at concentrations well above physiologic levels.[4,97,108] In addition, the catecholamine-induced constriction is not as potent as the acetylcholine-produced constriction.

Other vasoactive factors (such as histamine, 5-hydroxytryptamine, and bradykinin) produce dose-dependent contractile responses of the ductus arteriosus in vitro.[4,97,108,109,140] Although these neural and hormonal factors possibly contribute to the closure of the ductus under physiologic conditions, they do not mediate oxygen-induced vessel closure. In fact, a recent investigation suggests that none of these factors (except acetylcholine) has any contractile effect on the fetal lamb ductus in vivo.[62]

Until the early 1970s it was commonly believed that the ductus arteriosus was a relatively passive structure in the fetus and that regulation of blood flow to the pulmonary and systemic circulations was largely regulated by the relative vascular resistances within those circulations. It is now obvious that the relative patency of the ductus, even during fetal life, is regulated by both contracting and dilating factors. Recent studies have suggested that circulating concentrations of adenosine may play a role in maintaining ductus patency during fetal life.[111] Adenosine causes ductus relaxation during oxygen-induced vasoconstriction, and plasma adenosine concentrations fall when oxygen tension rises after delivery.

Evidence that prostaglandins participate in maintaining patency of the ductus began to accumulate with observations that prostaglandin E_1 (PGE_1) and E_2 (PGE_2) would relax isolated strips of ductus arteriosus in vitro.[50,143] Parallel studies demonstrated that the ductus arteriosus could be closed in vivo and in vitro by administration of agents known to inhibit the synthesis of prostaglandins.[136,137] These same effects were demonstrated in humans when it was shown that PGE_1 could maintain the patency of the ductus in infants with congenital heart disease, and that indomethacin could induce ductus constriction in premature infants with PDA.[61,77,121]

Several groups have shown that tissue homogenates or intact rings of ductus arteriosus produce prostaglandin E_2, I_2 (PGI_2), and $F_{2\alpha}$ ($PGF_{2\alpha}$) as well as 11-, 12-, and 15-monohydroxy metabolites from arachidonic acid.[40,65,122,127] The lipoxygenase products as well as the leukotrienes C_4 and D_4 have no effect on ductal patency and are unlikely to have a role in its closure at birth.[49] $PGF_{2\alpha}$ in physiologic or pharmacologic doses has no effect on the ductus arteriosus. PGI_2 has been shown to be a potent vasodilator in several vascular tissues; however, in the ductus arteriosus the ability of PGI_2 to dilate the vessel was two to three orders of magnitude less potent than that of PGE_2.[45,47] Therefore, even though PGE_2 is a minor product of arachidonic acid metabolism and prostaglandin production (the ratio of PGE_2:PGI_2 formation is 1:10), the marked sensitivity of the tissue to PGE_2 makes it the most important endogenous prostaglandin in the regulation of patency of the vessel. In fact, what makes the ductus arteriosus such a unique vessel, compared with other blood vessels, is its extraordinary sensitivity to PGE_2.

DEVELOPMENTAL DIFFERENCES IN DUCTUS ARTERIOSUS BEHAVIOR

The delayed closure of the ductus arteriosus in premature infants may be related to an ineffective contractile response of the ductus to the increasing oxygen tension that occurs after birth.[45,109,119,120] Oxygen has a greater constrictor effect in ductuses from older fetuses than in those from younger fetuses, but this is not due to differences in the ability of the vessel to achieve maximal contraction in younger versus older ductuses. There are comparable contractile responses at all gestational ages tested when the agonists are potassium, acetylcholine, or indomethacin plus oxygen.[45,109,119]

The diminished contractile response to oxygen of the immature ductus arteriosus appears to be due to a developmental alteration in the sensitivity of the vessel to locally produced prostaglandins. In the presence of inhibitors of prostaglandin synthesis, such as indomethacin, immature and near-term ductuses exhibit no difference in their ability to contract in response to oxygen.[45] We have found that the ductus arteriosus from immature lambs is much more sensitive to the dilating effects of PGE_2 than is the ductus from near-term animals.[45] While fetal blood vessels synthesize greater amounts of cyclooxygenase products than do adult vessels,[65] we have found no change in the rate of PGE_2 formation by the ductus arteriosus with advancing gestation. Therefore, we have hypothesized that the increased sensitivity of the immature ductus to vasodilation induced by PGE_2 may be the major factor responsible for the immature vessel's diminished response to oxygen. In other words, it is not the lack of contractile force that explains the oxygen insensitivity of the very immature ductus but rather the greater sensitivity of the ductus smooth muscle in younger fetuses to the dilating action of PGE_2.

SOURCE OF PGE_2

The exact production site of the PGE_2 responsible for the regulation of the ductus arteriosus in vivo currently is unknown. It has been shown from in vitro studies that the ductus is capable of synthesizing and catabolizing PGE_2 itself.[45,122,123]

However, isolated rings of lamb ductus arteriosus produce very little PGE_2 at the low ambient oxygen tensions found in the fetus; much more PGE_2 is produced at high oxygen tensions.[38] Thus, it is likely that circulating PGE_2 controls the ductus arteriosus in utero; after birth, when arterial oxygen tension rises, the ductus is capable of producing increased quantities of PGE_2, which, in some circumstances, may maintain the ductus in a dilated state.

When compared with term lambs, fetal and preterm newborn lambs have decreased plasma clearance rates and decreased pulmonary metabolism of PGE_2,[30,39,42] resulting in elevated concentrations of PGE_2 in fetal and preterm newborn lamb plasma.[30,42] By 2 hours after birth, full-term lambs have circulating PGE_2 concentrations well below the in vivo threshold concentrations required to produce ductus dilation. In contrast, circulating PGE_2 concentrations in premature lambs are two times greater than the in vivo threshold concentration required to produce ductal dilation. Therefore, circulating PGE_2 concentrations probably play a significant role in the patency of the ductus arteriosus in premature animals during the first hours after birth.[43]

HORMONAL REGULATION OF DUCTUS CONTRACTILITY

The factors that alter the sensitivity of the ductus to locally produced PGE_2 are unknown. Ever since Burnard's original description,[24] the association has been recognized between lung immaturity (as manifested by the respiratory distress syndrome) and a patent ductus arteriosus. The relationship between lung immaturity and patent duc-

tus arteriosus is supported by the observation that ductus closure occurs early in premature infants with no respiratory distress;[117,138,149] ductus closure also occurs early in premature infants who have been exposed to chronic intrauterine stress, which is known to accelerate lung maturation.[94,150] Because intrauterine stress is associated with increased production of fetal glucocorticoids, glucocorticoids may accelerate ductus closure in preterm infants. Cortisol normally is found in low concentrations in the fetus until it rises rapidly near term.[112]

We studied the effects of a 48-hour intravenous infusion of hydrocortisone on the ductus arteriosus of premature fetal lambs. The concentrations of circulating cortisol produced by the hydrocortisone infusions approximated the concentrations found in the fetal lambs near term. After the 48-hour infusions, the fetuses were delivered by cesarean section, and estimations of ductus patency were made in the premature newborn lambs at 1 hour of age using radioactive microsphere injections into the left ventricle.[41] The ductus was more widely patent in the untreated control animals than in the hydrocortisone-treated animals. There were no significant differences in circulating concentrations of PGE_2, PaO_2, cardiac output, pulmonary vascular resistance, systemic vascular resistance, or ductus arteriosus PGE_2 production in the two groups of animals. These findings are similar to those reported by Thibeault et al[151] for fetal lambs and by Momma et al[113] for fetal rats. Forty-eight hours of prenatal exposure to hydrocortisone decreased the sensitivity of the preterm ductus to PGE_2 and made it more like that of the full-term ductus.[41] In the undisturbed fetus, the normal increase in endogenous cortisol, which occurs near the end of gestation, probably influences ductus development in the same manner as exogenously administered steroids. As one might anticipate from the data collected from studies in lambs, prenatal administration of dexamethasone or betamethasone in human pregnancies causes a significant reduction in the incidence of PDA in premature infants.[33,51,155]

That the effect of glucocorticoids on ductal patency is a function of biochemical effects on the ductus itself, rather than of glucocorticoid-induced improvements in lung function secondary to increased surfactant release, is supported by studies of surfactant replacement therapy. Preterm infants treated with artificial surfactant for respiratory distress syndrome have a high incidence of patent ductus arteriosus.[64] In premature lambs with respiratory distress syndrome,[37] ductus reactivity was not altered by artificial surfactant administration; however, left-to-right shunt through the ductus was larger after surfactant administration because pulmonary vascular resistance was reduced.

LOSS OF DUCTUS REACTIVITY

In the full-term guinea pig and human neonate, the relaxing effects of PGE_2 and hypoxia are lost shortly after birth, and the ductus remains "irreversibly" closed thereafter.[16,59,115] In the guinea pig there was a correlation between irreversible closure and the cellular necrosis that occurs during the first days after delivery.[59] Fay and Cook[59] suggested that the ductus loses its ability to reopen as a result of the central plug of cells that fills the lumen; they hypothesized that this central mass must be cohesive and adhere to the inner walls of the ductus. However, in both the human and in the lamb, loss of ductus relaxation in response to PGE_2 and hypoxia takes place before there are obvious signs of cellular necrosis. The ability of the ductus arteriosus to dilate and to contract decreases within the first hours after postnatal ductus constriction in full-term lambs and humans.[16,44,115] Loss of ductus responsiveness is directly related to the degree of prior ductus constriction and consequent reduction in ductus luminal blood flow,[44] which appears to be the major source of ductus smooth muscle nutrition. There are small vessels on the surface of the ductus that provide vasa vasorum to its wall.[32,56,92,139] The vasa vasorum of the ductus originate both from terminal branches of the internal mammary artery and from branches of the vasa vasorum that lie in the adventitia of the pulmonary artery and thoracic aorta.[32,56] Until 28 weeks of intrauterine life in the human fetus, no vessels can be seen in the wall of the ductus; between 28 weeks and term, the vasa vasorum are distributed to the ductus wall in the adventitia.[32] Vasa vasorum extend only into the outer one third to one half of the muscle media.[139] Because luminal blood flow is the major source of ductus smooth muscle nutrition, the generalized loss of vessel responsiveness may be due to the ischemic damage that occurs when the ductus constricts.

How does the ductus remain closed once it has suffered ischemic damage? One may infer from Laplace's law that as a vessel constricts, greater transmural pressures will be required to cause any subsequent increase in vessel diameter. Mathematical considerations suggest that there is a critical closing pressure below which the lumen of a vessel will be obliterated.[25,107,118] It would therefore follow that once the ductus is constricted, it may be kept constricted by very little muscular effort.[107]

In normal full-term animals, loss of responsiveness to PGE_2 shortly after birth prevents the ductus arteriosus from reopening once it has constricted. In premature infants, it recently has become apparent that once the ductus has closed (either spontaneously or as a result of indomethacin administration), it may reopen at a later date, with recurrence of the left-to-right shunt.[110] The incidence of ductus reopening is inversely related to the birthweight: 33 per cent of infants with birth weights less than 1000 g reopened their ductus after initial closure, while only 8 per cent of infants with birth weights greater than 1500 g reopened their ductus.[35]

We have found that in contrast to more mature lambs the immature neonatal lamb is likely to have a ductus that continues to dilate in response to PGE_2 after its postnatal constriction. The propensity of the immature lamb to reopen the ductus in response to PGE_2 probably has several explanations: (1) Immature lambs do not constrict their ductus as tightly as more mature lambs, probably as a result both of increased sensitivity of the immature ductus to PGE_2 and of higher circulating concentrations of

PGE_2 (see above). (2) Even in those premature lambs in which the ductus constricts tightly in vivo, the ductus does not lose its sensitivity to the dilating action of PGE_2 (as it does in the full-term animal).[35] Such persistence of ductus responsiveness after ductus constriction may account for the high rate of ductus reopening observed in preterm infants after successful indomethacin-induced closure. It is noteworthy that 80 per cent of infants whose ductus reopened after initial closure still appeared to be responsive to indomethacin.[35]

The factors that maintain the persistence of ductus responsiveness to PGE_2 in immature lambs after ductus constriction are unknown. We hypothesized that the ductus smooth muscle in premature lambs may have a lower rate of oxygen consumption than in lambs near term. We would anticipate a lower rate of oxygen consumption in preterm ductus smooth muscle because of the low circulating concentrations of thyroid hormones in immature fetuses and neonates. If oxygen consumption were less in the preterm ductus, then the ductus from immature fetuses would be more resistant to ischemic damage during ductus constriction. Consistent with this hypothesis, we have found that premature infants with low levels of circulating thyroid hormones have an increased incidence of PDA compared with those with normal thyroid hormone levels.[34] To test this hypothesis, we infused premature lamb fetuses with triiodothyronine for 4 days to elevate circulating thyroid hormone concentrations to levels similar to those found in full-term newborn lambs.[34] Prior to delivery, there were no differences between the T_3-infused and control fetuses, either in the contractile response of their ductus to oxygen and indomethacin or in the relaxation response to PGE_2. Following the thyroid hormone infusions, some premature fetuses were delivered by cesarean section and were studied as newborns. In the preterm newborn lambs infused with T_3 in utero, there was a generalized loss of ductus responsiveness as the ductus constricted after birth. The loss of ductus responsiveness during postnatal constriction in the T_3-infused premature lambs was similar to that found in full-term lambs. In contrast, the ductus arteriosus in the premature control lambs was still responsive to vasoactive agonists after postnatal constriction.[34] Although increases in thyroid hormone concentrations, which occur with advancing gestation, may not alter the balance between the vasoactive effects of oxygen and PGE_2 on the ductus (as do glucocorticoids[41]), they may play a role in preventing a ductus' reopening once it has constricted after birth.

ANATOMIC CLOSURE OF THE DUCTUS ARTERIOSUS

In addition to the functional closure of the ductus arteriosus that occurs after birth, there is an anatomic closure that leads to the ultimate obliteration of the ductus lumen. Histologic studies of the ductus arteriosus may be found as far back as Billard in 1828,[12] but Langer[98] is credited with first describing the main histologic differences between the ductus and the aorta and pulmonary artery. The ductus is a more muscular artery compared with the elastic vessels at either end; it has a looser structure, with increased amounts of acid mucopolysaccharide in the muscle media; and there is less elastic tissue and no external elastic lamina.[19,54,86,93] While other species such as the lamb, rat, and rabbit[79,90,158] have been found to have longitudinally oriented smooth muscle in the inner part of the media and circularly oriented smooth muscle in the outer media, the orientation of muscle cells in the human ductus has varied.[54,57,86] The different muscle fiber orientations in the media of the human ductus may be a result of studies done in different states of contraction or relaxation. Von Hayck[154] sectioned the human ductus in different planes and observed two coats of smooth muscle: Both were helical spirals going in opposite directions. In the outer layer, the spiraling was more acute, making the fibers appear circular in cross-sectional views. In the inner layer, the spiraling was more gradual, and therefore the appearance was more longitudinal.

Prior to delivery, the ductus undergoes changes in the architecture of its wall. In the human fetus at 15 to 22 weeks' gestation, there is a single continuous internal elastic lamina with a single layer of flattened endothelial cells lining the lumen of the vessel.[153] The endothelial cells have abundant rough endoplasmic reticulum and ribosomes. The subendothelial space contains rod-shaped elastic fibers. Smooth muscle cells are not found in the intima and are restricted to the media. These smooth muscle cells are noted to have rich glycogen deposits, abundant rough endoplasmic reticulum, and dilated cisternae.[153]

The extracellular space of the media contains mucopolysaccharides and only scanty elastic fibers. The adventitia and surrounding connective tissue contain smooth muscle cells, fibroblasts, and myelinated nerve fibers. The prominence of the intracytoplasmic synthetic organelles is not seen in the adjacent aorta and pulmonary artery. These findings are similar to those observed in the immature fetal rabbit ductus.[158] With advancing gestation, there is decreasing evidence of mitotic cells among the endothelial and smooth muscle cells.[158] Increases in the number of myofilaments and rough endoplasmic reticulum, apparent reductions in smooth muscle cell glycogen, and increases in extracellular mucopolysaccharides also occur with advancing gestation.[153,158] The smooth muscle cells become less tightly packed as the amount of amorphous extracellular material increases.[153]

In addition to the increased synthetic capacity of the ductus, suggested by increases in smooth muscle endoplastic reticulum, several studies indicate both intimal thickening and fragmentation of the internal elastic lamina[90,153,158] with advancing gestation. This intimal thickening appears to be due to migration of smooth muscle cells from the media[106,153] and not due to cellular proliferation.[106] Several investigators have addressed the question of whether this intimal thickening occurs prior to delivery or is an artifact of postmortem contraction.[23,81] Bunce[23] found that the intima is compressed in the distended vessel but may be greatly thickened in collapsed vessels, with reductions in vessel lumen. Hornblad[81] used whole body freezing in five species of animals and found

that at birth the ductus had a smooth inner surface lined by a single layer of flat endothelial cells. During the last part of intrauterine life, Hornblad found that there was an increase in the ductal lumen in the guinea pig, rabbit, rat, and mouse, but that an increase in wall thickness could be demonstrated only in the guinea pig and the rabbit.[81] The subendothelial zone of the fetal ductus "was of inappreciable extent in the rat and mouse, whereas in the pig, guinea pig and rabbit, fibroblasts and elastic and collagen fibers were visible, being most prominent in the rabbit."[80] Yoder has suggested that these intimal "fibroblasts" really are smooth muscle cells that have migrated from the media.[158] It is worth noting that at no time has intimal thickening been observed without fragmentation of the underlying internal elastic lamina.[54,57,74,153,158] Whether this means that intimal thickening is a result of medial constriction,[54] or whether intimal thickening occurs without contraction is still a subject of speculation.

Obliteration of the ductus takes place after birth. During postnatal closure of the ductus in the human, the media indentates into the lumen, and the intima increases in size and forms intimal mounds or cushions that partially occlude the lumen. These intimal changes are probably secondary to extensive shortening of the ductus as well as to reductions in ductal radius. Fragmentation of the internal elastic membrane, first noted with advancing gestation, continues. Shortly after birth, cells in the inner part of the media appear to disintegrate.[59,74,82,90,158] Mucoid lakes appear in the media as the muscle cells become more densely packed.[54,74] Thrombosis within the lumen of the ductus only rarely is observed on postmortem examination. It may be that after muscular closure of the ductus lumen, the central part no longer is able to obtain a supply of blood through either vasa vasorum or through the lumen and degenerates as a result. If this hypothesis is true, the precipitating cause of the histologic changes would be a lack of blood supply brought on by muscular contraction of the wall.[92]

From 1 to 3 months after birth, the obliteration is caused by the increasing size of the intimal mounds with overlying caps of connective tissue.[86] The connective tissue caps are subendothelial and are differentiated from the mounds themselves by the absence of elastic fibers.[73,86] The intimal mounds contain more elastic tissue and increasing amounts of collagen. Hemorrhages appear in the wall of 20 per cent of the vessels studied.[57] The muscle fibers of the media atrophy and are replaced by elastic and connective tissue; only a remnant of the outer circular muscular layer remains.

The closure of the ductus in other species follows a pattern similar to the human one. However, in contrast to the human ductus, which has no elastic lamellae in the media, the ductus of the guinea pig, lamb, calf, rabbit, rat, and mouse all have concentric elastic lamellae.[19,81] The media of the ductus contain fewer elastic lamellae than the aorta, although the mouse has as much elastic tissue in its ductus as in its aorta.[82] During closure, all species, except for the rat and mouse (the two smallest species studied), develop medial indentations into the lumen;[19,79,82] intimal cells pile up during ductal closure in all species, but only the human develops thick intimal mounds or cushions. The tissue eventually obliterating the ductus also varies between species: In the guinea pig and rabbit connective tissue rich in collagen and mucopolysaccharide, with sparse elastic fibers, initially fills the lumen; ultimately, only collagen containing little mucopolysaccharide or elastin is left. In the calf, the tissue that obliterates the ductus is composed of mucopolysaccharides and elastic fibers.[19]

Starting at the end of the first week of postnatal life, the wall of the ductus arteriosus becomes progressively vascularized; the wall and luminal tissue reach maximal vascularity by the third week.[32] The vasa vasorum then start to regress; by the end of the first year, the vasa vasorum are confined to the adventitial layer.

In the human, anatomic closure has been reported to be complete from one to several months after birth;[86] similar periods have been given for the pig and calf.[81] Complete obliteration in the dog, cat, guinea pig, and rat occurs between 1 and 4 weeks after birth.[81]

There have been only a limited number of studies of the histology of the persistently patent ductus arteriosus. Dogs, especially poodles, have a hereditary persistent ductus arteriosus.[22] When the ductus remains patent in the dog, the medial architecture is much more elastic and compact than normal[72] and resembles the aortic media. In contrast to the findings of intimal thickening and fragmentation of the internal elastic lamina observed in the normally closing ductus, dogs with a persistently patent ductus show no intimal edema, and their endothelial cells adhere to the underlying internal elastic lamina.[72] Such canine "aortification" of the persistently patent ductus is seen only in a minority of human ductus with permanent patency;[74] usually in the human, only a normal amount of smooth muscle is present in the patent ductus. Gittenberger-de-Groot studied patent ductus from infants who were full term when they were delivered and who were more than 3 months old when they died.[74] She found no obvious increase in the amount of elastic material. Mucoid lakes were present, but cytolytic necrosis was rarely encountered.[74] In general, the intimal cushions were not very pronounced, and the internal elastic lamina underneath them was often not fragmented.[74] The most striking feature she noted was a wavy, unfragmented subendothelial elastic lamina.[74] When she reviewed the histology of ductus taken from preterm infants, Gittenberger-de-Groot noted that intimal cushions of various sizes, with or without connective tissue caps, were associated with functional ductus closure.[73] In those infants with a functionally patent ductus at the time of death, the ductus appeared like that in a fetus or like that in a term infant with a permanently patent ductus (i.e., intact subendothelial elastic lamina and absence of cytolytic necrosis).[73] One wonders whether the different histologic picture in the preterm infants with patent ductus is due to a lack of ischemic damage of the ductus during the postnatal period. Therefore, the question still remains whether the transient physiologic contraction of the ductus that occurs with air breathing is a necessary step in the orderly process of histologic closure.

SIGNIFICANCE

The exact consequences of a left-to-right shunt through a patent ductus arteriosus (PDA) have not been elucidated clearly for the preterm infant. The pathophysiologic features of a PDA depend on the magnitude of the left-to-right shunt and the cardiac and pulmonary responses to the shunt.

Cardiovascular Responses

There are important differences between the hearts of immature and mature infants and their ability to handle a volume load. Before term, the myocardium has more water and less contractile mass. Therefore, the ventricles in the immature fetus are less distensible than at term and generate less force per gram of myocardium (even though they have the same ability to generate force per sarcomere as those in more mature infants).[63] The relative lack of distensibility of the left ventricle in immature infants is more a function of tissue constituents than of poor muscle function. As a result, left ventricular distention secondary to a large left-to-right PDA shunt may produce a higher left ventricular end-diastolic pressure at smaller ventricular volumes in the immature than in the mature infant. Elevations in left ventricular end-diastolic pressures, which increase pulmonary venous pressures and cause pulmonary congestion, occur with smaller left-to-right shunts in the immature than mature infant. Several studies have also demonstrated the poorer cardiac sympathetic innervation in immature infants.[63,99]

Several investigators have reported that fetal lambs respond poorly to acute volume loading as compared with adults.[70,96] In newborn lambs, the effects of rapid acute volume loading depend on postnatal age.[96] In 1-week-old lambs, volume loading increased cardiac output by only 35 per cent; by 6 weeks after delivery, volume loading increased cardiac output by 75 per cent above control values. Since cardiac output normally is much higher in the newborn period and falls over the next several weeks, it has been postulated that the limited ability of the neonatal heart to increase its cardiac output with volume loading is due not to reduced myocardial performance but rather to limited reserve.[96] Teitel et al recently have examined the resting contractility, inotropic reserve, and maximal inotropic state in newborn lambs over the first month after birth, by examining the end-systolic pressure-volume relationship.[148] Resting contractility was maximal in the first weeks after birth and fell by 4 weeks. Contractility was not affected by isoproterenol in the first weeks but increased by 50 per cent at 4 weeks; maximal contractility was similar at all ages studied.[148] These studies and others[10] demonstrate that the preterm and full-term newborn myocardium is operating at maximal performance with little inotropic reserve and may adapt to acute volume loads primarily through the Frank-Starling mechanism by increasing its left ventricular preload.[11]

On the other hand, several investigators have shown that the fetal and neonatal myocardial response to an acute volume load is dependent on afterload resistance.[70,71,131,152] When the ductus is widely patent and pulmonary vascular resistance is low, aortic runoff into the pulmonary bed can markedly reduce afterload resistance; as a result, the neonatal myocardium can better accommodate to the substantial increases in stroke volume required to maintain effective systemic blood flow when the ductus is patent.

The effects of a PDA on cardiovascular performance have been studied mostly in adult animals or infants beyond the newborn period. Children with long-standing PDA shunts have been found to have increased left ventricular end-diastolic pressures, heart rate, pulse pressure, pulse pressure with exercise, blood volume, and cardiac work.[26,142] In addition, large ductal flow increases forward flow in the ascending aorta and forearm and retrograde flow in the descending aorta below the ductus.[27,141] Increases in oxygen consumption and metabolism have been observed in older infants with PDA[100] and may contribute to the poor weight gain observed in premature infants with PDA.[104]

In studies of adult dogs with a prosthetic aortopulmonary shunt, Rudolph et al found that opening the shunt caused immediate decreases in aortic and left ventricular systolic pressure and increases in pulmonary arterial pressure, left atrial pressure, left ventricular end-diastolic pressure, stroke volume, and heart rate.[133] Other changes Rudolph et al observed included a doubling of pulmonary blood flow, a moderate decrease in systemic blood flow, and a marked increase in pulmonary diastolic blood flow; as a result, peripheral pulmonary blood flow became much more continuous. In other cardiac lesions with increased pulmonary blood flow (e.g., atrial or ventricular septal defects), a similar increase in pulmonary diastolic flow is not evident. Continuous distention of the pulmonary vessels in PDA may be particularly important in the production of pulmonary vascular disease.

Decreases in systemic arterial oxygen saturation have been observed after PDA closure in adult dogs with a prosthetic shunt,[133] in older children during PDA ligation,[26] and in newborn lambs following PDA occlusion.[55] In preterm lambs with an occluder around the ductus arteriosus, we have observed that temporary occlusion of the ductus after birth reduces the volume of blood flowing through the lungs and causes a fall in arterial oxygen saturation with no change in the minute ventilation.[36] Dawes et al demonstrated that recirculation of arterial blood through lungs that were only partially expanded could account for this phenomenon and suggested that the continued patency of the ductus arteriosus after birth may serve a useful function in preterm infants whose lungs were not fully expanded.[15,55] Unrecognized changes in ductal patency (or pulmonary vascular resistance, when ductal patency is constant) in premature infants with respiratory distress syndrome thus will confound interpretation of arterial PO_2 values, which are commonly, but mistakenly, assumed to reflect only pulmonary pathology. Closure of a PDA (or elevation in pulmonary vascular resistance with no change in PDA) will cause a drop in PaO_2 that may be mistaken for increasing atelectasis with increased venous admixture.[18]

Whether or not a PDA causes redistribution of cardiac output and a "steal" of systemic organ blood flow into the lower resistance pulmonary vascular bed is a question that recently has been approached experimentally. The results, as published so far, unfortunately are equivocal. In an initial series of experiments using premature lambs with a PDA, Baylen and coworkers observed a reduced "effective" systemic blood flow and organ (carcass, heart, gastrointestinal tract, brain, kidney, and liver) hypoperfusion.[9] They found that the preterm lamb was unable to increase left ventricular output and "effective" systemic blood flow sufficiently to compensate for the left-to-right shunt. However, using the same experimental protocol, the same researchers reported results a year later[11] that contradicted their earlier observation. In their follow-up study, they found that preterm lambs, with the same size left-to-right shunt (44 per cent of left ventricular output) as observed in the initial study, were able to increase their left ventricular output to compensate for the ductus shunt.[11] We recently concluded a series of experiments in preterm lambs to examine the effects of left-to-right shunts on cardiac output and its distribution. Several days prior to delivery, the fetal lambs had an inflatable occluder placed around the ductus arteriosus. Subsequently, the lambs were delivered (at 131 days' gestation, with 150 days being term), and the ductus was intermittently obstructed with the occluder while measurements of cardiac output and its distribution were made using radioactive microspheres. We found that the preterm lamb could increase its left ventricular output and maintain "effective" systemic blood flow without altering organ perfusion with ductal shunt less than 40 to 50 per cent of left ventricular output. With shunts greater than 50 per cent of left ventricular output, "effective" systemic blood flow fell, and organ perfusion decreased. Blood flow to the carcass was most likely to be affected by left-to-right ductal shunts; the next most likely organs to be affected were the gastrointestinal tract and the kidneys.[36]

A PDA may affect myocardial blood flow and metabolism by means of the coronary "steal" (due to forward flow from the aortic arch to the pulmonary vessels during diastole instead of retrograde flow to the coronary arteries); other factors may interfere with coronary blood flow as well. One striking feature of a large PDA is the low aortic diastolic blood pressure (frequently 20 to 25 mmHg). Because coronary flow to the subendocardial muscle occurs entirely during diastole, such reductions in aortic diastolic pressure may produce subendocardial ischemia and inhibit myocardial function.[78] In fact, electrocardiographic findings of myocardial strain in neonates with a PDA have been reported.[27,157]

At this time, we can only guess what importance the magnitude and duration of left-to-right shunt and the changes in pulmonary arterial and venous pressures caused by PDA may have in preterm human infants. Unlike older infants, the preterm infant with respiratory distress syndrome appears to have a diminished capacity to increase cardiac output in response to volume loading. Alverson et al[2] observed that the left ventricular output was increased in the presence of a left-to-right ductus shunt and fell significantly after closure of the ductus. The increase in left ventricular output seen in the presence of PDA did not provide an increase in effective systemic blood flow; femoral blood flow velocity was low prior to closure of the PDA and returned to normal after closure.[2]

Very low birthweight infants with a PDA have been found to have increased flow in the ascending aorta (with increased forearm blood flow) and decreased flow in the descending aorta, with an associated metabolic acidosis.[89] Such alterations in cardiac output distribution have been implicated in the high incidence of intracranial hemorrhage[105,125] and necrotizing enterocolitis[52,95] associated with PDA. Significant aortic backflow has been observed over large distances in some infants with PDA, consistent with a "diastolic steal" of blood from the abdominal organs to the pulmonary artery.[141] The continuous distention of the pulmonary vessels during diastole may be important in the production of pulmonary vascular disease and bronchopulmonary dysplasia.[20,133,141]

The decreased ability of the preterm infant to maintain active pulmonary vasoconstriction[102] may be responsible in part for the earlier presentation of a "large" left-to-right PDA shunt in the most immature infants.[69,85] Therapeutic maneuvers (e.g., surfactant replacement) that lead to decreased pulmonary vascular resistance can exacerbate the amount of left-to-right shunt in preterm infants with respiratory distress syndrome.[37,64]

Pulmonary Responses

The factors responsible for preventing fluid and proteins from moving from the plasma to the lung interstitium (microvascular barrier) and from the interstitium to the air spaces (alveolar barrier) have been described previously in detail.[144] The lymphatic system is essential for both "barriers," draining off excessive fluid filtrate and protein that enters the interstitium and preventing the build-up of pressure that would lead to alveolar flooding. A low microvascular barrier conductance to fluid and small molecules prevents excessive leakage of plasma into the lung's interstitium. It has been hypothesized that the alveolar barrier has an even lower conductance for fluid and small molecules.[144] The interstitial hydrostatic pressure opposes the pressure driving fluid from the microvasculature. Increased alveolar gas pressure and a low alveolar air-liquid surface tension, produced by alveolar surfactant, decrease the effective driving pressure from the interstitium into the alveolar space.

A very low microvascular barrier conductance to protein transport provides the osmotic pressure difference between the plasma and the interstitium. This safety factor plays an essential role in protecting patients with elevated pulmonary vascular hydraulic pressures (as in PDA) from developing gross pulmonary edema. Increases in pulmonary microvascular perfusion pressure seen in association with PDA (which predispose the patient to pulmonary edema) are partially offset by simultaneous decreases in interstitial osmotic pressure caused by protein washout from the interstitial compartment as a result of increased fluid filtration. Such reductions in interstitial osmotic pressure reduce the force driving fluid across the alveolar barrier into the air spaces, and thus protect the patient from pulmonary edema.

Patients with low plasma protein concentrations, such as preterm infants with respiratory distress syndrome, are at higher risk for developing clinical pulmonary edema at lower levels of left atrial pressure than are patients with normal plasma protein concentrations.[53] The protective effect of plasma proteins depends on a normal microvascular barrier. Experimental work in 1-week-old, full-term lambs suggests that there is no increased microvascular permeability to plasma proteins when compared with adult sheep.[13] However, more recent studies have shown that premature newborn lambs requiring artificial ventilation have an increased protein leak across the microvascular barrier, which is independent of peak inspiratory airway pressure; this increased protein leak increases with decreasing gestational age.[88] In addition, premature newborn lambs with respiratory distress syndrome appear to have increased lung microvascular protein permeability compared with preterm lambs without respiratory distress syndrome.[146] Studies in human infants with respiratory distress syndrome have suggested that there is an increased permeability to small solutes, which diminishes toward normal adult levels as the respiratory distress resolves.[87]

Leakage of plasma proteins into the alveolar space may inhibit surfactant function and increase the air-liquid surface tension, as has been observed in patients with pulmonary edema.[91] Newborn infants with respiratory distress syndrome have been found to have specific proteins in their airways that inhibit the surface tension–lowering properties of surfactant.[84] These protein inhibitors diminish as the respiratory distress improves.

Clinical and animal studies of the effects of PDA and increased pulmonary blood flow on respiratory symptoms have been conducted mainly after the newborn period. In studies of older infants with congenital heart disease and increased pulmonary blood flow and without pneumonia, pulmonary edema, or airway disease,[101] Lees et al found that alveolar ventilation, dead space, and the alveolar ventilation-oxygen consumption ratio were normal. Respiratory rate was slightly increased, and tidal volume was diminished.[101] Alveolar diffusing capacity has been found to be increased in cardiac lesions with left-to-right shunts.[27]

Griffin et al studied the pulmonary compliance of infants with heart disease.[75] Infants with an isolated PDA had decreased pulmonary compliance, which improved after surgical ligation. Diminution of compliance was related to peak pulmonary systolic pressure. Lesions associated with increased flow but normal pulmonary artery pressure (atrial septal defect, small ventricular septal defect) had normal compliance.[75]

Bancalari et al studied infants between 2 weeks and 9 months of age who had no evidence of "pulmonary complications nor a clinical diagnosis of congestive heart failure."[7] These infants had shunt ratios ($\dot{Q}_p/\dot{Q}_s$) between 1.3 and 6.3. There was no change in tidal volume or functional residual capacity. Respiratory rate and pulmonary resistance were higher in infants with left-to-right shunts. Dynamic compliance was decreased significantly in infants with an increased pulmonary blood flow,[7] but the mechanism remains unclear. Increases in left atrial and pulmonary venous pressure have been shown to decrease lung compliance in experimental animals,[17] but this was not the explanation in the patients studied by Bancalari et al.[7] Premature infants with PDA and obvious pulmonary edema sometimes may have low left atrial pressures at cardiac catheterization.[132] In fact, Bancalari et al observed no correlation between specific compliance and the magnitude of the left-to-right shunt in their study of older infants with left-to-right shunt;[7] however, Bancalari et al did observe a significant correlation between specific compliance and mean pulmonary pressure.[7] The association between increased mean pulmonary pressure and decreased compliance in infants with left-to-right shunts has been observed by others as well.[75,83,156]

Several groups have observed an improvement in lung compliance in preterm infants following PDA ligation.[68,89,116] With a wide-open PDA, the pulmonary vasculature is exposed to systemic blood pressure and increased pulmonary blood flow. Because the premature infant with respiratory distress syndrome frequently has a low plasma oncotic pressure and may have increased capillary permeability, increases in microvascular perfusion pressure that result from PDA may increase interstitial and alveolar lung fluid. Leakage of plasma proteins into the alveolar space may inhibit surfactant function and increase surface tension in the immature air sacs, which are already compromised by surfactant deficiency. The increased FiO_2 and mean airway pressures required to overcome these early changes in compliance caused by PDA may be important factors in the association of PDA with chronic lung disease.[20,52]

We have not observed decreased pulmonary compliance in preterm lambs with PDA during the first 6 hours after delivery.[36] Acute relaxation and occlusion of the ductus arteriosus produced no changes in functional residual capacity or dynamic compliance in paralyzed and mechanically ventilated lambs, despite increases in pulmonary artery blood pressure to systemic levels and increases in pulmonary blood flow to systemic blood flow ratio ($\dot{Q}_p/\dot{Q}_s$) to greater than 2:1.[36] Even 12-hour exposures of the pulmonary vascular bed to systemic pressures and high blood flows had no effect on pulmonary mechanics. Only future studies can determine whether these animals would require several days of an increased PDA shunt before showing changes in compliance. However, at this time it appears that acute increases in pulmonary blood flow and mean pulmonary pressure do not interfere with pulmonary expansion and do not decrease pulmonary compliance.

Another mechanism by which the patent ductus arteriosus might produce respiratory distress in the preterm newborn is through respiratory muscle fatigue. The ability of striated respiratory muscles to obtain adequate energy supplies to sustain rhythmic contraction at high work rates depends on muscle blood flow.[6] Studies in dogs have shown that to sustain high levels of contractile effort the respiratory muscles, and especially the diaphragm, increase their blood flow significantly.[128,129] Respiratory

muscle fatigue is an important component of ventilatory limitation in patients with airway obstruction.[130,135] Teague et al have observed power spectral patterns in the diaphragmatic muscle electromyograms of preterm infants consistent with diaphragmatic fatigue.[147] These changes exist even before infants are challenged with increasing respiratory loads or chemoreceptor stimulation.[147] Because of both reduction and redistribution of effective systemic perfusion, blood flow to respiratory muscles in infants with a large left-to-right PDA shunt may be reduced; as a result, respiratory muscle blood flow may be limited to levels less than those required by the work of breathing (work that may be increased by PDA, as considered above), and respiratory failure may result.

Alternatively, the redistribution of cardiac output in infants with a large PDA shunt may reduce brain blood flow and thereby affect the central control of respiration. In goats, a 50 per cent reduction in cerebral blood flow causes ventilatory depression, and a further decrease leads to respiratory arrest.[31]

References

1. Allan FD (1955): The innervation of the human ductus arteriosus. Anat Rec 122:611–631.
2. Alverson DC, Eldridge MW, Johnson JD, Burstein R, Papille LA, Dillon T, Yabek, Berman W Jr (1983): Effect of patent ductus arteriosus on left ventricular output in premature infants. J Pediatr 102:754–757.
3. Alzamora-Castro V, Battilana G, Abugattas R, Sialer R (1960): Patent ductus arteriosus and high altitude. Am J Cardiol 5:761–763.
4. Aronson SG, Gennser G, Owman C, Sjoberg NO (1970): Innervation and contractile response of the human ductus arteriosus. Eur J Pharmacol 11:178–186.
5. Assali MS, Morris JA, Smith RW, Manson WA (1963): Studies on ductus arteriosus circulation. Circ Res 13:478–489.
6. Aubier M, Trippenbach T, Roussos C (1981): Respiratory muscle fatigue during cardiogenic shock. J Appl Physiol 51:499–508.
7. Bancalari E, Jesse MJ, Gelband H, Garcia O (1977): Lung mechanics in congenital heart disease with increased and decreased pulmonary blood flow. J Pediatr 90:192–195.
8. Barclay AE, Franklin KJ, Pritchard MML (1944): The Foetal Circulation. Oxford, Blackwell Scientific Publications.
9. Baylen BG, Ogata H, Ikegami M, Jacobs HC, Jobe AH, Emmanouildes G (1983): Left ventricular performance and regional blood flows before and after ductus arteriosus occlusion in premature lambs treated with surfactant. Circulation 67:837–843.
10. Baylen BG, Ogata H, Jacobs H, Ikegami M, Jobe A, Emmanouilides G (1983): Frank-Starling performance and "contractile state" of the preterm and term left ventricle. Pediatr Res 17:108A.
11. Baylen BG, Ogata H, Oguchi K, Ikegami M, Jacobs H, Jobe A, Emmanouilides GC (1985): The contractility and performance of the preterm left ventricle before and after early patent ductus occlusion in surfactant treated lambs. Pediatr Res 19:1053–1058.
12. Billard CM (1828): Traité des maladies des enfants nouveau-nés et á la mamelle fondée sur de nouvelles observations cliniques et d'anatomie pathologique, faites á l'hopital des enfants trouvés de Paris. Paris.
13. Bland RD, McMillan DD (1977): Lung fluid dynamics in awake newborn lambs. J Clin Invest 60:1107–1115.
14. Boreus LO, Malmfors T, McMurphy DM, Olson L (1969): Demonstration of adrenergic receptor function and innervation in the ductus arteriosus of the human fetus. Acta Physiol Scand 77:316–321.

15. Born GVR, Dawes GS, Mott JC, Rennick BR (1955): The relief of central cyanosis caused by pulmonary arterio-venous shunts by constriction of an artificial ductus arteriosus. J Physiol 130:167–190.

16. Born GVR, Dawes GS, Mott JC, et al (1956): Constriction of the ductus arteriosus caused by oxygen and asphyxia in newborn lambs. J Physiol 132:304–342.

17. Borst HG, Berglund E, Whittenberger JL, Mead J, McGregor M, Collier C (1957): The effect of pulmonary vascular pressures on the mechanical properties of the lungs of anesthetized dogs. J Clin Invest 36:1708–1714.

18. Bratton DL, Mellander M, Krueger ED, Stahlman MT, Cotton RB (1984): Influence of early indomethacin on venous admixture in infants with HMD. Pediatr Res 18:150A.

19. Broccoli F, Carinci P (1973): Histological and histochemical analysis of the obliteration processes of ductus arteriosus. Botalli Acta Anat 85:69–83.

20. Brown E (1979): Increased risk of bronchopulmonary dysplasia in infants with patent ductus arteriosus. J Pediatr 95:865–866.

21. Brundin T, Norberg KA, Soderlund S (1971): Lack of adrenergic nerves in the circular smooth muscles of ductus arteriosus persistens. Scand J Thorac Cardiovasc Surg 5:16–18.

22. Buchanan JW, Patterson DF, Pyle RL (1971): Morphologic studies in dogs with hereditary patent ductus arteriosus. Circulation 44 (Suppl II):131–147.

23. Bunce DFM (1965): Structural differences between distended and collapsed arteries. Angiology 16:53–56.

24. Burnard ED (1959): Discussion on the significance of continuous murmurs in the first few days of life. Proc R Soc Med 52:77–78.

25. Burton AC (1951): On the physical equilibrium of small blood vessels. Am J Physiol 164:319–329.

26. Cassels DE, Morse M, Adams WE (1950): Effect of the patent ductus arteriosus on the pulmonary blood flow, blood volume, heart rate, blood pressure, arterial blood gases and pH. Pediatrics 6:557–571.

27. Cassels DE (1973): The Ductus Arteriosus. Springfield, Charles C Thomas, pp 143–160.

28. Cassels DE (1973): The Ductus Arteriosus. Springfield, Charles C Thomas, pp 67–69.

29. Cassels DE (1973): The Ductus Arteriosus. Springfield, Charles C Thomas, pp 25–36.

30. Challis JRG, Dilley SR, Robinson JS, et al (1976): Prostaglandins in the circulation of the fetal lamb. Prostaglandins 11:1041–1052.

31. Chapman RW, Santiago TV, Edelman NH (1979): Effects of graded reduction of brain blood flow in ventilation in unanesthetized goats. J Appl Physiol 47:104–111.

32. Clarke JA (1965): An x-ray microscopic study of the vasa vasorum of the human ductus arteriosus. J Anat 99:527–537.

33. Clyman RI, Ballard PL, Sniderman S, Ballard RA, Roth R, Heymann MA, Granberg JP (1981): Prenatal administration of betamethasone for prevention of patent ductus arteriosus. J Pediatr 98:123–126.

34. Clyman RI, Breall J, Maher P, Campbell D, Mauray F (1985): Thyroid hormones and the ductus arteriosus. Pediatr Res 19:338A.

35. Clyman RI, Campbell D, Heymann MA, Mauray F (1985): Persistent responsiveness of the neonatal ductus arteriosus in immature lambs: A possible cause for reopening of patent ductus arteriosus after indomethacin-induced closure. Circulation 71:141–145.

36. Clyman RI, Heymann MA, Mauray F (1985): Cardiopulmonary effects of a patent ductus arteriosus. Pediatr Res 19:92A.

37. Clyman RI, Jobe A, Heymann MA, Ikegami M, Roman C, Payne B, Mauray F (1982): Increased shunt through the patent ductus arteriosus after surfactant replacement therapy. J Pediatr 100:101–107.

38. Clyman RI, Mauray F, Demers LM, Rudolph AM, Roman C (1980): Does oxygen regulate prostaglandin induced relaxation in the lamb ductus arteriosus? Prostaglandins 19:489–498.

39. Clyman RI, Mauray F, Heymann MA, Roman C (1981): Effect of gestational age on pulmonary metabolism of prostaglandin E_1 and E_2. Prostaglandins 21:505–513.

40. Clyman RI, Mauray F, Koerper MA et al (1978): Formation of prostacyclin (PGI_2) by the ductus arteriosus of fetal lambs at different stages of gestation. Prostaglandins 16:633–642.

41. Clyman RI, Mauray F, Roman C, Heymann MA, Ballard PL, Rudolph AM, Payne B (1981): Effects of antenatal glucocorticoid administration on ductus arteriosus of preterm lambs. Am J Physiol 241:H415–H420.

42. Clyman RI, Mauray F, Roman C, Rudolph AM, Heymann MA (1980): Circulating prostaglandin E_2 concentrations and patent ductus arteriosus in fetal and neonatal lambs. J Pediatr 97:455–461.

43. Clyman RI, Mauray F, Roman C, Heymann MA, Payne B (1983): Effect of gestational age on ductus arteriosus response to circulating prostaglandin E_2. J Pediatr 102:907–911.

44. Clyman RI, Mauray F, Roman C, Heymann MA, Payne B (1983): Factors determining the loss of ductus arteriosus responsiveness to prostaglandin E. Circulation 68:433–436.

45. Clyman RI (1980): Ontogeny of the ductus arteriosus response to prostaglandins and inhibitors of their synthesis. Semin Perinatol 4:115–124.

46. Coceani F, Bishai I, White E, et al (1978): Action of prostaglandins, endoperoxides and thromboxanes on the lamb ductus arteriosus. Am J Physiol 234:H117–H122.

47. Coceani F, Bodach E, White E, et al (1978): Prostaglandin I_2 is less relaxant than prostaglandin E_2 on the lamb ductus arteriosus. Prostaglandins 15:551–556.

48. Coceani F, Hamilton NC, Labuc J, Olley PM (1984): Cytochrome P 450-linked monooxygenase: Involvement in the lamb ductus arteriosus. Am J Physiol 246:H640–H643.

49. Coceani F, Jhamandas VM, Bodach E, Labuc J, Olley PM (1982): Evidence against a role for lipoxygenase derived products of arachidonic acid in the lamb ductus arteriosus. Can J Physiol Pharmacol 60:345–349.

50. Coceani F, Olley PM (1973): The response of the ductus arteriosus to prostaglandins. Can J Physiol Pharmacol 51:220–225.

51. Collaborative Group on Antenatal Steroid Therapy (1985): Prevention of Respiratory Distress Syndrome: Effect of Antenatal Dexamethasone Administration. NIH Publication No 85-2695, p 44.

52. Cotton RB, Stahlman MT, Berder HW, Graham TP, Catterton WZ, Kover I (1978): Randomized trial of early closure of symptomatic patent ductus arteriosus in small preterm infants. J Pediatr 93:647–651.

53. DaLuz PL, Shubin H, Weil MH, Jacobsen E, Stein L (1975): Pulmonary edema related to changes in colloid osmotic and pulmonary artery wedge pressure in patients after acute myocardial infarction. Circulation 51:350–357.

54. Danesino VL, Reynolds SRM, Rehman IH (1955): Comparative histological structure of the human ductus arteriosus according to topography, age and degree of constriction. Anat Rec 121:801–829.

55. Dawes GS, Mott JC, Widdicombe JG (1955): The patency of the ductus arteriosus in newborn lambs and its physiological consequences. J Physiol 128:361–383.

56. Dawes GS (1968): Foetal and Neonatal Physiology. Chicago, Year Book Medical Publishers, p 165.

57. Deslignerves S, Larroche JC (1970): Ductus arteriosus. Biol Neonate 16:278–296.

58. Fay FS (1971): Guinea pig ductus arteriosus. I. Cellular and metabolic basis for oxygen sensitivity. Am J Physiol 221:470–479.

59. Fay FS, Cooke PH (1972): Guinea pig ductus arteriosus. II. Irreversible closure after birth. Am J Physiol 222:841–849.

59a. Fay FS, Jobsis FF (1972): Guinea pig ductus arteriosus. III. Light absorption changes during response to O_2. Am J Physiol 223:588–595.

60. Franklin KJ (1949): A Short History of Physiology. London, Staples Press, p 47.

61. Friedman WF, Hirschklau MJ, Printz MP, Pitlick PT, Kirkpatrick SE (1976): Pharmacologic closure of patent ductus arteriosus in the premature infant. N Engl J Med 295:526–529.

62. Friedman WF, Printz MP, Kirkpatrick SE, Haskins EJ (1983): The vasoactivity of the fetal lamb ductus arteriosus studied in utero. Pediatr Res 17:331–337.

63. Friedman WF (1972): The intrinsic physiologic properties of the developing heart. In Friedman WF, Lesch M, Sonnenblick EH (eds): Neonatal Heart Disease. New York, Grune & Stratton, pp 21–49.

64. Fujiwara T, Maeta H, Morita T, Watamabe V, Chida S, Abe T (1980): Artificial surfactant therapy in hyaline membrane disease. Lancet 1:55–59.

65. Funk CD, Powell WS (1985): Release of prostaglandins and monohydroxy and trihydroxy metabolites of linoleic and arachidonic acids by adult and fetal aortae and ductus arteriosus. J Biol Chem 260:7481–7488.

66. Galen (1884): Opera Omnia IV:243. Kuhn edition. Translation from Dalton JC: Doctrines of the Circulation. Philadelphia, Lea's Son and Co, p 64.

67. Gérard G (1900): De l'oblitération du canal artériel, les théories et les faits. J Anat (Paris) 36:323–357.

68. Gerhardt T, Bancalari E (1980): Lung compliance in newborns with patent ductus arteriosus before and after surgical ligation. Biol Neonate 38:96–105.

69. Gersony WM, Peckham GJ, Ellison RC, Miettinen OS, Nadas AS (1983): Effects of indomethacin in premature infants with patent ductus arteriosus. Results of a national collaborative study. J Pediatr 102:895–906.

70. Gilbert RD (1982): Effects of afterload and baroreceptors on cardiac function in fetal sheep. J Dev Physiol 4:299–309.

71. Gilbert RD (1980): Control of fetal cardiac output during changes in blood volume. Am J Physiol 238:H80–H86.

72. Gittenberger-de-Groot AC, Strengers JLM, Mentink M, Poelmann RE, Patterson DF (1985): Histologic studies on normal and persistent ductus arteriosus in the dog. J Am Coll Cardiol 6:394–404.

73. Gittenberger-de-Groot AC, Van Ertbruggen I, Moulaert AJMG, Harinck E (1980): The ductus arteriosus in the preterm infant: Histologic and clinical observations. J Pediatr 96:88–93.

74. Gittenberger-de-Groot AC (1977): Persistent ductus arteriosus: Most probably a primary congenital malformation. Br Heart J 39:610–618.

75. Griffin AJ, Ferrara JD, Lax JO, Cassels DE (1972): Pulmonary compliance. An index of cardiovascular status in infancy. Am J Dis Child 123:89–95.

76. Harvey W (translated by Chauncey Leake) (1941): Anatomical Studies on the Motion of the Heart and Blood. 3rd ed. Springfield, Charles C Thomas.

77. Heymann MA, Rudolph AM, Silverman NH (1976): Closure of the ductus arteriosus in premature infants by inhibition of prostaglandin synthesis. N Engl J Med 295:530–533.

78. Hoffman JIE, Buckberg GD (1976): Transmural variations in myocardial perfusion. Prog Cardiol 5:37–89.

79. Hornblad PY, Larsson KS, Marsk L (1969): Studies on closure of the ductus arteriosus. VII. Closure rate and morphology of the ductus arteriosus in the lamb. Cardiologia 54:336–342.

80. Hornblad PY (1969): Embryological observations of the ductus arteriosus in the guinea pig, rabbit, rat, and mouse: Studies on closure of the ductus. IV. Acta Physiol Scand 76:49–57.

81. Hornblad PY (1969): Experimental studies on closure of the ductus arteriosus utilizing whole-body freezing. Acta Paediatr Scand (Suppl) 190:6–21.

82. Hornblad PY (1967): Studies on closure of the ductus arteriosus. III. Species differences in closure rate and morphology. Cardiologia 51:262–282.

83. Howlett G (1972): Lung mechanics in normal infants and infants with congenital heart disease. Arch Dis Child 47:707–715.

84. Ikegami M, Jacobs H, Jobe A (1983): Surfactant function in respiratory distress syndrome. J Pediatr 102:443–447.

85. Jacob J, Gluck L, DiSessa T, Edwards D, Kulovich M, Kurlinski J, Merritt TA, Friedman WF (1980): The contribution of PDA in the neonate with severe RDS. J Pediatr 96:79–87.

86. Jager BV, Wollenman J Jr (1942): Anatomic study of closure of the ductus arteriosus. Am J Pathol 18:595–613.

87. Jefferies AL, Coates G, O'Brodorich HM (1984): Pulmonary epithelial permeability in hyaline membrane disease. N Engl J Med 311:1075–1080.

88. Jobe AH, Ikegami M, Jacobs HC, Berry D (1984): Increased lung protein permeability of prematurely delivered and ventilated lambs. Pediatr Res 18:394A.

89. Johnson DS, Rogers JH, Null DM, DeLemos RA (1978): The physiologic consequences of the ductus arteriosus in the extremely immature newborn. Clin Res 26:826A.

90. Jones M, Barrow MV, Wheat MW Jr (1969): An ultrastructural evaluation of the closure of the ductus arteriosus in rats. Surgery 66:891–898.

91. Kahana LM, Thurlbeck WM (1972): Surface tension and static volume-pressure hysteresis in pulmonary emphysema and other conditions. Am Rev Respir Dis 105:217–228.

92. Kennedy JA, Clark SL (1942): Observations on the physiological reactions of the ductus arteriosus. Am J Physiol 136:140–147.

93. Kennedy JA, Clark SL (1941): Observations on the ductus arteriosus of the guinea pig in relation to its method of closure. Anat Rec 79:349–371.

94. King DT, Emmanouilides GC, Andrews JC, Hirose FM (1980): Morphologic evidence of accelerated closure of the ductus arteriosus in preterm infants. Pediatrics 65:872–880.

95. Kitterman JA (1975): Effects of intestinal ischemia in necrotizing enterocolitis in the newborn infant. In Moore TD (ed): Report of the 68th Ross Conference of Pediatric Research. Columbus, Ross Laboratories, p 38.

96. Klopfenstein HS, Rudolph AM (1978): Postnatal changes in the circulation, and responses to volume loading in sheep. Circ Res 42:839–845.

97. Kovalcik V (1963): The response of the isolated ductus arteriosus to oxygen and anoxia. J Physiol (Lond) 169:185–197.

98. Langer C (1857): Zur Anatomie der fotalen Kreislanfsorgane. Z Ges Aerzte Wien 36:329–339.

99. Lebowitz EA, Novick JS, Rudolph AM (1972): Development of myocardial sympathetic innervation in the fetal lamb. Pediatr Res 6:887–893.

100. Lees MH, Bristow JD, Griswold HE, Olmsted RW (1965): Relative hypermetabolism in infants with congenital heart disease. Pediatrics 36:183–191.

101. Lees MH, Way RC, Ross BB (1967): Ventilation and respiratory gas transfer of infants with increased pulmonary blood flow. Pediatrics 40:259–271.

102. Lewis AB, Heymann MA, Rudolph AM (1976): Gestational changes in pulmonary vascular responses in fetal lambs in utero. Circ Res 39:536–541.

103. Lind K, Wegelius C (1949): Angiocardiographic studies on the human foetal circulation. Pediatrics 4:391–400.

104. Mahony L, Carnero V, Brett C, Heymann MA, Clyman RI (1982): Prophylactic indomethacin therapy for patent ductus arteriosus in very low-birthweight infants. N Engl J Med 306:506–510.

105. Martin CG, Snider AR, Katz SM, Peabody JL, Brady JP (1982): Abnormal cerebral blood flow patterns in preterm infants with a large patent ductus arteriosus. J Pediatr 101:587–593.

106. Mato M, Aikawa E, Uchiyama Y (1970): Radioangiographic study on the obliteration of the ductus arteriosus Botalli. Virchows Arch (Pathol Anat) 349:10–20.

107. McIntyre TW (1969): An analysis of critical closure in the isolated ductus arteriosus. Biophys J 9:685–699.

108. McMurphy DM, Boreus L (1971): Studies on the pharmacology of the perfused human fetal ductus arteriosus. Am J Obstet Gynecol 109:937–942.

109. McMurphy DM, Heymann MA, Rudolph AM et al (1972): Developmental changes in constriction of the ductus arteriosus: Responses to oxygen and vasoactive substances in the isolated ductus arteriosus of the fetal lamb. Pediatr Res 6:231–238.

110. Mellander M, Leheup B, Lindstrom DB, Palme C, Graham TP Jr, Stahlman MT, Cotton RB (1984): Recurrence of symptomatic patent ductus arteriosus in extremely premature infants treated with indomethacin. J Pediatr 105:138–143.

111. Mentzer RM, Ely SW, Lasley RD, Mainwaring RD, Wright EM, Berne RM (1985): Hormonal role of adenosine in maintaining patency of the ductus arteriosus in fetal lambs. Ann Surg 202:223–230.

112. Mescher EJ, Platzker ACG, Ballard PL, Kitterman JA, Clements JA, Tooley WH (1975): Ontogeny of tracheal fluid, pulmonary surfactant, and plasma corticoids in the fetal lamb. J Appl Physiol 39:1017–1021.

113. Momma K, Mishihara S, Ota Y (1981): Constriction of the fetal ductus arteriosus by glucocorticoid hormones. Pediatr Res 15:19–21.

114. Moss AJ, Emmanouilides GC, Rettori O, Higashino SM, Adams

FH (1966): Postnatal circulatory and metabolic adjustments in normal and distressed premature infants. Biol Neonate 8:177–197.

115. Moss AJ, Emmanouilides GC, Adams FH, Chuang K (1964): Response of ductus arteriosus and pulmonary and systemic arterial pressure to changes in oxygen environment in newborn infants. Pediatrics 33:937–944.

116. Naulty CM, Horn S, Conry J, Avery GB (1978): Improved lung compliance after ligation of patent ductus arteriosus in hyaline membrane disease. J Pediatr 93:682–684.

117. Neal WA, Bessinger FB, Hunt CE, Lucas RV (1975): Patent ductus arteriosus complicating respiratory distress syndrome. J Pediatr 86:127–131.

118. Nichol J, Girling F, Jerrard W, Claxton EB, Burton AC: Fundamental instability of the small blood vessels and critical closing pressures in vascular beds. Am J Physiol 164:330–344.

119. Noel S, Cassin S (1976): Maturation of contracile response of ductus arteriosus to oxygen and drugs. Am J Physiol 231:240–243.

120. Oberhansli-Weiss I, Heymann MA, Rudolph AM, Melmon KL (1972): The pattern and mechanisms of response to oxygen by the ductus arteriosus and umbilical artery. Pediatr Res 6:693–700.

121. Olley PM, Coceani F, Bodach E (1976): E-type prostaglandins: A new emergency therapy for certain cyanotic heart malformations. Circulation 53:728–731.

122. Pace-Asciak CR, Rangaraj G (1977): The 6 keto-prostaglandin $F_{1\ alpha}$ pathway in the lamb ductus arteriosus. Biochim Biophys Acta 486:583–585.

123. Pace-Asciak CR, Rangaraj G (1978): Prostaglandin biosynthesis and catabolism in the lamb ductus arteriosus, aorta and pulmonary artery. Biochim Biophys Acta 529:13–20.

124. Penaloza D, Arias-Stella J, Sime F, Recavarren S, Marticorena E (1964): The heart and pulmonary circulation in children at high altitudes. Pediatrics 34:568–582.

125. Perlman JM, Hill A, Volpe JJ (1981): The effect of patent ductus arteriosus on flow velocity in the anterior cerebral arteries: Ductal steal in the premature newborn infant. J Pediatr 99:767–771.

126. Powell WS, Solomon S (1978): Biosynthesis of prostaglandins and thromboxane B_2 by fetal lung homogenates. Prostaglandins 15:351–364.

127. Powell WS, Solomon S (1977): Formation of 6 oxoprostaglandin $F_{1\ alpha}$ by arteries of the fetal calf. Biochem Biophys Res Commun 75:815–822.

128. Robertson CH Jr, Foster CH, Hohnson RL Jr (1977): The relationship of repiratory failure to the oxygen consumption of, lactate production by, and distribution of blood flow among respiratory muscles during increasing inspiratory resistance. J Clin Invest 59:31–42.

129. Rochester DF, Bettini G (1976): Diaphragmatic blood flow and energy expenditure in the dog. Effects of inspiratory airflow resistance in hypercapnia. J Clin Invest 57:661–672.

130. Rochester DF (1980): Respiratory disease. Attention turns to the air pumps. Am J Med 68:803–805.

131. Romero TE, Friedman WF (1979): Limited left ventricular response to volume overload in the neonatal period: A comparative study with the adult animal. Pediatr Res 13:910–915.

132. Rudolph AM, Drorbaugh JE, Auld PAM, Rudolph AJ, Nadas AS, Smith CA, Hubbell JP (1961): Studies on the circulation in the neonatal period. Pediatrics 27:551–566.

133. Rudolph AM, Scarpelli EM, Golinko RJ, Gootman NL (1964): Hemodynamic basis for clinical manifestations of patent ductus arteriosus. Am Heart J 68:447–458.

134. Sciacca A, Condorelli M (1960): Involution of the ductus arteriosus. Bibl Cardiol 10:1–52.

135. Sharp JT (1980): Respiratory muscles. A review of old and new concepts. Lung 157:185–199.

136. Sharpe GL, Larsson KS, Thalme B (1975): Studies on closure of the ductus arteriosus. XII. In utero effect of indomethacin and sodium salicylate in rats and rabbits. Prostaglandins 9:585–596.

137. Sharpe GL, Thalme B, Larsson KS (1974): Studies on closure of the ductus arteriosus. XI. Ductal closure in utero by a prostaglandin synthetase inhibitor. Prostaglandins 8:363–368.

138. Siassi B, Blanco C, Cabal LA, Goran AG (1976): Incidence and clinical features of patent ductus arteriosus in low-birthweight infants: A prospective analysis of 150 consecutively born infants. Pediatrics 57:347–351.

139. Silva DG, Ikeda M (1971): Ultrastructural and acetylcholinesterase studies on the innervation of the ductus arteriosus, pulmonary trunk, and aorta of the fetal lamb. J Ultrastruct Res 34:358–374.

140. Smith RW, Morris JA, Assali NS, Beck R (1964): Effects of chemical mediators on the pulmonary and ductus arteriosus circulation in the fetal lamb. Am J Obstet Gynecol 89:252–260.

141. Spach MS, Serwer GA, Anderson PAW, Canent RV Jr, Levin AR (1980): Pulsatile aortopulmonary pressure flow dynamics of patent ductus arteriosus in patients with various hemodynamic states. Circulation 61:110–122.

142. Spann JF Jr, Mason DT, Zelis R, Braunwald E (1968): Differences in left ventricular performance and myocardial mechanics in patent ductus arteriosus and ventricular septal defect. Circulation 37 (Suppl 4):187.

143. Starling MB, Elliot RB (1974): The effects of prostaglandins, prostaglandin inhibitors and oxygen on the closure of the ductus arteriosus, pulmonary arteries and umbilical vessels in vitro. Prostaglandins 8:187–203.

144. Staub NC (1980): Pathogenesis of pulmonary edema. Prog Cardiovasc Dis 23:53–80.

145. Sun FF, McGuire JC (1978): Metabolism of prostaglandins and prostaglandin endoperoxides in rabbit tissues during pregnancy: Differences in enzyme activities between mother and fetus. In Coceani F, Olley PM (eds): Advances in Prostaglandin and Thromboxane Research 4. New York, Raven Press, pp 75–85.

146. Sundell HW, Rojas J, Grogaard J, Mohan P, Brigham KL (1984): Lung lymph studies in newborn lambs with hyaline membrane disease. Pediatr Res 18:351A.

147. Teague WG, Targett RC, Heldt G (1985): Do hypoxia and hypercapnia contribute to diaphragmatic fatigue in preterm infants. Pediatr Res 19:418A.

148. Teitel D, Sidi D, Chin T, Brett C, Heymann MA, Rudolph AM (1985): Developmental changes in myocardial contractile reserve in the lamb. Pediatr Res 19:948–955.

149. Thibeault DW, Emmanouilides GC, Dodge ME, Lachman RS (1977): Early functional closure of the ductus arteriosus associated with decreased severity of respiratory distress syndrome in preterm infants. Am J Dis Child 131:741–745.

150. Thibeault DW, Emmanouilides GC (1977): Prolonged rupture of fetal membranes and decreased frequency of respiratory distress syndrome and patent ductus arteriosus in preterm infants. Am J Obstet Gynecol 123:43–46.

151. Thibeault DW, Emmanouilides GC, Dodge ME (1978): Pulmonary and circulatory function in preterm lambs treated with hydrocortisone in utero. Biol Neonate 34:238–247.

152. Thornburg KL, Morton MJ (1983): Filling and arterial pressures as determinants of RV stroke volume in the sheep fetus. Am J Physiol 244:H656–H663.

153. Toda T, Tsuda N, Takagi T, Nishimori I, Leszczynski D, Kummerow F (1980): Ultrastructure of developing human ductus arteriosus. J Anat 131:25–37.

154. Von Hayck H (1935): Der funktionelle Bau der Nabelarterien und des Ductus Botalli. Z Anat Entwicklungsgesch 105:15–24.

155. Waffarn F, Siassi B, Cabal L Schmidt PL (1983): Effect of antenatal glucocorticoids on clinical closure of the ductus arteriosus. Am J Dis Child 137:336–338.

156. Wallgren G, Geubelle F, Koch G (1960): Studies of the mechanics of breathing in children with congenital heart lesions. Acta Paediatr Scand 49:415–425.

157. Way GL, Pierce JR, Wolfe RR, McGrath R, Wiggins J, Merenstein GB (1979): ST depression suggesting subendocardial ischemia in neonates with respiratory distress syndrome and patent ductus arteriosus. J Pediatr 95:609–611.

158. Yoder MJ, Banmann FG, Grover-Johnson NM, Brick I, Imparato AM (1978): A morphological study of early cellular changes in the closure of the rabbit ductus arteriosus. Anat Rec 192:19–40.

159. Zapol WM, Kolobow T, Doppman J, Pierce JE (1971): Response of ductus arteriosus and pulmonary blood flow to blood oxygen tension in immersed lamb fetuses perfused through an artificial placenta. J Thorac Cardiovasc Surg 61:891–903.

7 DEVELOPMENTAL PULMONARY CIRCULATORY PHYSIOLOGY

Walker A. Long

Yet nature desiring that the blood should be strained through the lungs, was forc'd to add the right ventricle, by whose pulse the blood should be forc'd through the very lungs out of the vena cava *into the receptacle of the left ventricle.*

William Harvey, 1628

The neonatal pulmonary circulation is an ephemeral phase in the dramatic metamorphosis of the pulmonary circulation that takes place during the passage from fetal to adult life. During fetal life, which is really a water-breathing phase of existence analogous to the tadpole stage of a frog's life, the pulmonary circulation is a low flow, high resistance parallel circuit that receives only a small proportion of cardiac output and that appears to serve very little purpose other than providing some practice at traversing the pathways through which the entire circulation must course after birth (presumably most nutritive requirements of the developing fetal lung could be supplied by the bronchial circulation). In contrast, during adult life the pulmonary circulation is a high flow, low resistance series circuit that receives the entire cardiac output and that permits delivery of carbon dioxide to and retrieval of oxygen from the lungs. In between lies the neonatal pulmonary circulation, an insufficiently explored, rapidly changing form of the pulmonary circulation, which certainly plays an important role in the successful adaptation of newborn animals to extrauterine life and which may hold the key to understanding many forms of unexplained pulmonary hypertension.

Since the neonatal pulmonary circulation serves the same function as the adult pulmonary circulation (i.e., the neonatal pulmonary circulation serves as the carrier system for pulmonary gas exchange), it would seem likely that physiologic regulation of the neonatal pulmonary circulation would be more similar to the physiologic regulation of adult life rather than fetal life. Paradoxically, however, the neonatal pulmonary circulation's function is that of adult life but its regulation remains closer to that of fetal life.

The purposes of this chapter are to review what is known about physiologic regulation of the neonatal pulmonary circulation and to compare and to contrast these observations with what is known about the physiologic regulation of the fetal and adult pulmonary circulations. This chapter is written with two hopes. First, it is hoped that clinicians caring for newborn infants at risk of developing or already having persistent pulmonary hypertension of the newborn syndrome (PPHNS) (see Chapter 51) may be influenced to think carefully about many aspects of routine care that can unwittingly influence the pulmonary circulation. Second, it is hoped that researchers interested in the pulmonary circulation will be stimulated to explore new areas and that their discoveries will eventually lead to new explanations and new therapies for pulmonary hypertension in both newborn infants and adults.

HISTORICAL PERSPECTIVE

Three hundred and fifty years ago Sir William Harvey brilliantly deduced the pathways of the systemic and pulmonary circulations during both fetal and adult life.[115] Many great physicians and scientists have studied the pulmonary circulation since the time of Harvey, but none have come close to matching Harvey's contribution.

In the nineteenth century many physiologists observed that vascular pressures were much lower in the pulmonary circulation than in the systemic circulation, and several noted that asphyxia caused marked increases in pulmonary arterial pressure. Some very sophisticated experiments on the regulation of the pulmonary circulation were being conducted by the end of the nineteenth century.[28,29] In 1904 Plumier demonstrated that simply reducing the oxygen tension of inspired air in the dog also caused pulmonary hypertension.[196] However, physiologic studies of the pulmonary circulation did not become commonplace until after the rediscovery of cardiac catheterization in the 1930s (see Chapter 27). Cardiac catheterization accelerated investigations of the pulmonary circulation for two reasons. First, cardiac catheterization made access to the pulmonary circulation much easier. Second, it provided the first direct physiologic confirmation of the fact that pulmonary hypertension accompanied many clinical disorders, and thereby stimulated investigative interest in the pulmonary circulation.

In 1942 Beyne confirmed Plumier's observations of 1904 that reducing inspired oxygen tension in the dog increased pulmonary arterial pressure, but left atrial pressure was not measured.[23] In 1946 von Euler and Liljestrand published what proved to be a landmark paper in the physiologic investigation of the pulmonary circulation when they demonstrated that 10 to 11 per cent oxygen caused considerable increases in pulmonary arterial pressure in cats without increasing left atrial pressure.[84] In that same paper, von Euler and Liljestrand also showed that increasing alveolar

CO_2 tension caused a similar but smaller rise in pulmonary arterial pressure.[84] In the ensuing 40 years the phenomenon of hypoxia-induced pulmonary vasoconstriction has attracted much attention, but its mechanisms remain unexplained. Carbon dioxide–induced pulmonary vasoconstriction has also attracted much attention, and changes in pH have been shown to be responsible for the carbon dioxide effects, but the mechanisms by which changes in hydrogen ion concentration alter pulmonary vascular tone also remain unexplained. Some investigators have expended not inconsiderable thought in wondering what the purposes of hypoxia- and carbon dioxide–induced pulmonary vasoconstriction might be, but the obvious answer was clearly suggested by von Euler and Liljestrand themselves in their original paper— to match perfusion and ventilation. However, in the enthusiastic investigation of the mechanisms of hypoxia– induced and carbon dioxide–induced pulmonary hypertension, many other important physiologic mechanisms for regulation of the pulmonary circulation have long been overlooked. Indeed, it may turn out that explanations for many forms of unexplained pulmonary hypertension lie in these other, long-neglected physiologic pathways.

PHYSIOLOGIC FACTORS ALTERING NEONATAL PULMONARY VASCULAR TONE

Studies of the regulation of the neonatal pulmonary circulation are in their infancy, but it is already quite clear that it is unsafe to simply extrapolate forward from the fetus or backward from the adult. Observations from fetal or adult regulation of the pulmonary circulation must be specifically confirmed or denied in neonatal animals, for the newborn animal is neither a delivered fetus nor a small adult. Unfortunately, many of the physiologic factors known to influence pulmonary vascular tone in the adult or fetal animal have not been tested in newborn animals. In such cases, one cannot say whether the same, opposite, or no effects are present in newborn animals, but one can say that the experiments are worth repeating in newborn animals to find out.

Certainly oxygen levels and pH are well established as important and powerful determinants of pulmonary vascular tone during all stages of development. However, many other influences also have important roles in regulation of the pulmonary circulation. In the following discussion most of the factors that have been described to influence pulmonary vascular tone in either fetal, neonatal, or adult life are considered; when direct neonatal observations are not available, a guess as to how the newborn animal may respond has been offered, but the reader's intuition as to whether the newborn animal responds similarly or not may differ from the author's. However, as suggested above, it is far more important that the experiments be done to find out the truth of the matter rather than whether the reader or author is right.

Four other caveats should be offered. First, species differences must always be kept in mind in comparing the results of physiologic experiments. For example, alveolar hypoxia is a potent pulmonary vasoconstrictor in the adult sheep but a very modest pulmonary vasoconstrictor in the adult cat. Such species differences, whether recognized or unrecognized, may play a large role in the outcome of a given series of experiments. Thus, inability to document that the autonomic nervous system contributes substantially to hypoxic pulmonary vasoconstriction in the newborn calf[209] and adult dog[173,230] does not invalidate observations that sectioning of the autonomic nervous system in the fetal[54] and newborn sheep[62] and that alpha blockade in the adult cat[197] greatly reduce hypoxic pulmonary vasoconstriction in those species.

Second, any factor or mechanism that appears to have a relatively small effect in the normal animal or human may have a much more dramatic effect in the sick patient. It must be recalled that resistance to blood flow in a given vessel is inversely proportional to the fourth power of that vessel's radius; therefore, any additional small increment or decrement in pulmonary vasoconstriction in already constricted vessels can have a major influence on pulmonary vascular resistance. These observations are particularly pertinent to the newborn infant, whose pulmonary vessels are small to begin with.

Third, for obvious ethical or technical reasons, very few data are available on regulation of the pulmonary circulation in healthy premature infants, sick premature infants, or healthy premature animals (the latter are particularly difficult to come by). In fact, except for a number of observations in premature lambs and premature primates ill with hyaline membrane disease, and a few observations in premature infants with hyaline membrane disease[70,207a,220a] or bronchopulmonary dysplasia (see Chapter 31), the premature pulmonary circulation remains largely unexplored. Virtually no animal data are available on the premature pulmonary circulation after the third postnatal day, and the few clinical observations recorded have usually been made in ill, not healthy, premature infants. Fetal observations would suggest that pulmonary vasoconstriction would be less powerful in preterm infants than in term infants. Indeed, rapid postnatal reductions in pulmonary vascular resistance in extremely preterm infants with respiratory distress syndrome have been postulated to increase left-to-right ductal shunt markedly and thereby account for the worse outcome among younger babies.[133a] Nevertheless, how the pulmonary circulation of the premature infant may react to most of the phenomena discussed below is totally unknown.

Fourth, this chapter will perforce focus on pulmonary vasoconstriction because much more information is available on physiologic factors that cause pulmonary vasoconstriction than on physiologic factors that cause pulmonary vasodilation.[168] However, in the long run, identification of the normal vasodilatory mechanisms in the pulmonary circulation, which must exist to counterbalance the many vasoconstricting mechanisms already identified, may lead to the new forms of therapy clinicians working with pulmonary hypertension patients so desperately seek.

Oxygen

Oxygen is an important determinant of pulmonary vascular tone during fetal, neonatal, and adult life. Alveolar oxygen tension, mixed venous oxygen tension, and systemic arterial oxygen tension have all been demonstrated to influence pulmonary vascular tone at one stage of development or another, as considered further in the sections to follow.

Alveolar Hypoxia

During fetal life, the lungs are not collapsed; instead, the alveoli are expanded by endogenously produced pulmonary fluid.[1] Ventilation of fetal lungs with pure nitrogen reduces pulmonary vascular resistance[40,54,58,72,73] because mechanical expansion of fetal lungs with gas reduces resistance to pulmonary blood flow and because the lungs are already hypoxic during fetal life and do not become any more so during nitrogen ventilation. (The effects of lung inflation on pulmonary vascular resistance during fetal, neonatal, and adult life are considered fully in a later section.)

In contrast, alveolar hypoxia has been demonstrated to cause substantial pulmonary vasoconstriction in newborn calves,[199,209] lambs,[31,62,63,128] newborn piglets,[166,202] and newborn humans,[2,18,19,79,134] and of course the same phenomenon is well demonstrated in most adult species.[84,111,116,160,172,197,201,230] Because resting pulmonary arterial pressures are higher in the newborn animal than in the adult animal, the magnitude of increase in pulmonary artery pressure during alveolar hypoxia in newborn animals is greater than in adult animals exposed to equivalent levels of alveolar hypoxia. However, the percentage increase in pulmonary arterial pressure during alveolar hypoxia appears to be the same for the newborn and adult cow[199] and pig,[202] but in the sheep the newborn lamb exhibits more vigorous alveolar hypoxia-induced pulmonary vasoconstriction than the adult does.[62,63] The explanation for this developmental difference in sheep remains uncertain, but recent experiments implicate the autonomic nervous system.[62]

Mixed Venous PO_2

Pulmonary arterial (mixed venous) blood oxygen tension has been demonstrated to have an effect on pulmonary vascular tone in fetal sheep[36,40,41,58,72,122,153a] and in adult cats[127] but not in the newborn lamb[128] or adult rat.[116] In the adult dog, conflicting observations have been reported.[201,205a] Increases in pulmonary vascular tone caused by reductions in mixed venous PO_2 are more easily demonstrable in the fetus than in the adult (because the alveoli do not contain oxygen in the fetus). The normally low mixed venous PO_2 (18 to 22 mmHg) of fetal life apparently plays a major role in maintaining high fetal pulmonary vascular resistance in utero.[36,40,58,72,153a] Further, reductions in mixed venous PO_2 cause greater increases in pulmonary vascular resistance in the fetal sheep as gestation progresses,[206] indicating a developmental increase in the fetal pulmonary vascular bed's response to reductions in mixed venous PO_2. Increases in mixed venous PO_2 cause pulmonary vasodilation in fetal sheep[122] and adult cats,[127] indicating that normal mixed venous PO_2 contributes to pulmonary vascular tone in the fetal sheep and adult cat. However, factors counterbalancing the increasing pulmonary vasoconstricting effects of mixed venous fetal PO_2 during fetal development must exist because sheep fetal pulmonary vascular resistance actually drops as gestation progresses;[206,207] otherwise, a progressive increase in fetal pulmonary vascular resistance would be expected during gestation (as a result of expected developmental increases in the pulmonary vasoconstrictor response to fetal hypoxia). Most likely the 20-fold increase in the cross-sectional area of the pulmonary vascular bed during the last half of gestation permits a progressive drop in fetal pulmonary vascular resistance during gestation[206,207] in the face of increasing pulmonary vascular responsiveness to hypoxia. In the adult cat, alveolar oxygen tension is a much more powerful influence than mixed venous PO_2.[127]

The effect of mixed venous PO_2 on pulmonary vascular tone in humans is largely unstudied, but most likely the human pulmonary circulation responds to mixed venous PO_2 at all stages of development. Mixed venous PO_2 is likely to be important in two clinical situations. First, if diffuse alveolar hypoxia is present, reductions in mixed venous PO_2 are likely to exacerbate alveolar hypoxia-induced pulmonary hypertension because any small increment in pulmonary vascular tone in already constricted vessels can markedly increase pulmonary vascular resistance. Second, marked reductions in mixed venous PO_2 are likely to compromise systemic arterial PO_2 when right-to-left intrapulmonary shunt (venous admixture) is present, and, as considered in the following discussion, systemic arterial PO_2 is an important determinant of pulmonary vascular tone at all stages of development. In newborn animals, marked reductions in mixed venous PO_2 can also compromise systemic arterial PO_2 when extrapulmonary right-to-left shunts across the foramen ovale and arterial duct are present, as in persistent pulmonary hypertension of the newborn syndrome (PPHNS).

Systemic Arterial PO_2

Reductions in systemic arterial PO_2 cause reflex pulmonary vasoconstriction in fetal sheep[36] and adult dogs;[11,66] the afferent loop of the reflex arc is via the peripheral chemoreceptors (carotid and aortic bodies), and in at least the fetal sheep the efferent loop is the sympathetic nervous system.[36] The reflex effects of reductions in systemic arterial PO_2 on pulmonary vascular tone may well contribute to the physiology observed in infants with PPHNS (see Chapter 51). Reflex pulmonary hypertension induced by systemic hypoxemia could also account for the long recognized but heretofore unexplained phenomenon of early and severe pulmonary vascular disease seen in infants with transposition of the great vessels.

In infants with transposition of the great vessels, alveolar oxygen tension is normal, blood pH is normal, pulmonary arterial (i.e., mixed venous) oxygen tension is high (which vasodilates the lung circulation in adult cats[127]), and the pulmonary circulation receives a volume load from excess pulmonary blood flow. However, infants with atrial septal defects often have equal or greater pulmonary blood flows and yet do not develop pulmonary vascular disease for at least 20 years. In contrast, untreated infants with transposition of the great vessels frequently develop irreversible pulmonary vascular disease before the end of their second year of life. Further, although polycythemia is usually present in infants with transposition of the great vessels, and polycythemia increases pulmonary vascular tone (see the following), neither the magnitude nor time course of polycythemia in infants with transposition suggests that the polycythemia is responsible for the early and severe pulmonary vascular disease seen in infants with transposition. It is possible that the obligatory profound systemic arterial hypoxemia found in infants with transposition causes sustained chemoreceptor discharge and results in persistent reflex pulmonary vasoconstriction, which accounts for the early and severe pulmonary vascular disease often observed.

The peripheral chemoreceptors' reflex role in regulation of pulmonary vascular tone is considered in a subsequent section.

Carbon Dioxide

The addition of carbon dioxide to alveolar gas has been known to increase pulmonary arterial pressure in the adult lung since at least the 1920s[164] and in the fetal[40,58] and neonatal[209] lung since the 1960s. However, only relatively recently have the arguments been conclusively settled in both the adult and newborn animal about whether the effects of carbon dioxide on pulmonary arterial pressure are direct effects or are due to carbon dioxide–induced changes in pH. All effects of alveolar and pulmonary arterial CO_2 tension on pulmonary vascular tone in adult[21] and newborn[128,211] animals are due to changes in pH; this relationship does not appear to have been studied in the fetus but presumably the same holds true at that stage of development as well.

pH

The hydrogen ion concentration in the pulmonary capillaries is an important determinant of pulmonary vascular tone during neonatal,[128,171,209,211] and adult life,[21] and certainly fetal life as well, since fetal alveolar CO_2 has been shown to influence fetal pulmonary vascular tone.[40,58] Hydrogen ion concentration is of course influenced by many different physiologic processes, but in general the lung is responsible for acute adjustments, and the kidneys are responsible for chronic adjustments. Both elevations and reductions in hydrogen ion concentration alter pulmonary vascular tone.

Acidosis

Nisell[184] was probably the first to suggest that changes in pH accounted for the effects of inhaled carbon dioxide (and of hypoxia) on the pulmonary circulation. Liljestrand[154] studied the mechanisms by which increasing carbon dioxide tension in isolated, perfused cat lungs caused pulmonary vasoconstriction and showed that increasing alveolar carbon dioxide and administering acid intravenously both increased pulmonary vascular resistance; Liljestrand correctly concluded that changes in blood pH were responsible for the pulmonary vasoconstricting effects of inhaled carbon dioxide. Bergofsky et al[21] demonstrated that comparable decreases in pH increased pulmonary vascular tone similarly regardless of whether respiratory or metabolic acidosis was responsible. Subsequently, a number of investigators have confirmed that acidosis causes pulmonary vasoconstriction in neonatal[128,171,209,211] and adult[21,83,109,114a,154] life. Whether the acidosis is metabolic or respiratory is totally irrelevant; only the magnitude of the acidosis is important in determining the effects on the pulmonary circulation. However, whether there are developmental differences in the magnitude of response to a given level of acidosis during fetal, neonatal, and adult life does not appear to have been explored.

Alkalosis

Just as acidosis is a pulmonary vasoconstrictor at all stages of development, so too is alkalosis a potent pulmonary vasodilator at all stages of development.[48,77a,171,178,211] As for acidosis, whether the alkalosis is metabolic or respiratory is totally irrelevant in determining its effects on the pulmonary circulation; only the magnitude of the alkalosis is important. Also, as in acidosis, whether there are developmental differences in the magnitude of response to a given level of alkalosis during fetal, neonatal, and adult life remains largely unexplored.

Temperature

Hypothermia has been demonstrated to cause pulmonary vasoconstriction in adult animals,[74,92,142,225] largely by constricting pulmonary veins.[225] Hyperthermia appears to have opposite effects.[74] Since adrenergic blockade can abolish hypothermia-induced pulmonary vasoconstriction,[225] it would seem likely that reflex effects from the hypothalamic nuclei responsible for temperature control play a role in the pulmonary vascular bed's responses to changes in temperature. Whether fetal and newborn animals exhibit pulmonary vascular responses to changes in temperature similar to those of adult animals remains unknown, but intuition would suggest that similar pulmonary vascular responses to hypothermia are likely to be present in at least the newborn animal.

The deleterious effects of hypothermia on other aspects of perinatal adaptation are well known to neonatologists, but the probable pulmonary vascular effects of hypothermia in newborn infants remain largely unrecognized. The neonatal pulmonary vascular response to hypothermia probably has substantial importance in outcome in the perioperative period, particularly after the performance of cardiac surgery for congenital heart disease under hypothermic arrest. Given the recent advances in neonatal heart surgery (see Chapters 57 to 67), investigation of the neonatal pulmonary vascular response to hypothermia is certainly warranted.

Blood

Hematocrit, hemoglobin oxygen affinity, and blood viscosity have important influences on pulmonary vascular tone during fetal, neonatal, and adult life. Such hematologic influences on the pulmonary circulation are often overlooked.

Hematocrit

The fact that the fetus compensates for its hypoxic environment in part by increasing red cell mass has been recognized since at least the 1930s.[77] However, the influence of hematocrit on pulmonary vascular resistance has been recognized only relatively recently in adult[2a,138a,178a] and newborn animals.[88] In isolated adult dog lungs, resistance to pulmonary perfusate flow increased gradually as hematocrit was increased from 0 to 40 per cent, but at hematocrits above 40 per cent, pulmonary vascular resistance increased steeply with further increases in hematocrit.[2a,178a] In 1973, Fouron and Hebert demonstrated that increasing hematocrit in neonatal lambs also caused pulmonary vascular resistance to rise more than systemic vascular resistance.[88] In 1982 Lister et al[158] confirmed these observations in humans by demonstrating that increasing hemoglobin concentration in children with ventricular septal defects reduced left-to-right shunt by increasing pulmonary vascular resistance more than systemic vascular resistance.

These observations have important implications for newborn infants. First, neonatal patients with symptomatic pulmonary hypertension should be transfused quite cautiously and only when absolutely necessary. Rote replacement of "blood out" in such patients is not a good idea. Second, phlebotomy (with crystalloid replacement) should certainly be performed in newborn infants with polycythemia (hematocrit > 65 per cent) and symptomatic pulmonary hypertension. Third, phlebotomy should also be considered in newborn infants with symptomatic pulmonary hypertension and relatively high hematocrits (> 50 per cent) who prove refractory to simple supportive measures such as oxygen, alkali, and warming. However, as Fouron et al[89] have recently pointed out, further reducing circulating blood volume in infants with polycythemia when hypovolemia is present reduces oxygen transport; for this reason, all blood removed from neonates with high hematocrits and symptomatic pulmonary hypertension should be replaced with crystalloid, and volume expansion with crystalloid should be undertaken if blood volume is low. Indeed, one of several possible mechanisms for the putative success of extracorporeal membrane oxygenator (ECMO) therapy in managing refractory PPHNS, if in fact ECMO is more beneficial than standard therapy, may be reduction in hematocrit.

Hemoglobin Oxygen Affinity

The fact that the fetus compensates for a hypoxic environment in part by making a form of hemoglobin with a greater oxygen affinity than that of adult hemoglobin has also been recognized since at least the 1930s.[77] In 1984, Lister[157] showed that isovolemic substitution of adult blood for fetal blood in the newborn lamb increased P_{50} 8 ± 3 mm Hg and permitted better maintenance of cardiac output and systemic oxygen transport during inhalation of 10 per cent oxygen. During those experiments, Lister did insert pulmonary artery catheters for sampling of mixed venous blood, but the effects of increasing P_{50} on pulmonary vascular resistance and pulmonary artery pressures were not reported. In 1985 Fouron et al[89] showed that isovolemic substitution of adult blood for fetal blood in the newborn lamb increased pulmonary vascular resistance. Whether replacing normal blood in the adult with fetal blood alters pulmonary vascular tone has not been studied. Neither does it appear that pulmonary vascular resistance has been measured in the fetus after replacement of fetal blood with adult blood. On the other hand, the observations of Fouron and colleagues in newborn lambs[89] do suggest that P_{50} may be an important determinant of pulmonary vascular tone; if so, alterations in oxygen availability in the pulmonary capillary bed oxygen-sensing sites are probably responsible.

However, in replacing blood from one stage of development with that from another, more is changed than just the concentration of fetal hemoglobin and the P_{50}.[89] Whether shifting P_{50} alone without other changes truly alters pulmonary vascular tone has not been established at any age. Experiments to study the question of whether P_{50} truly affects pulmonary vascular tone should be performed using recently discovered pharamacologic agents capable of altering P_{50} directly.[17,87]

Viscosity

Blood viscosity is an important determinant of resistance to blood flow, and for unknown reasons the pulmonary vascular bed appears to be more sensitive to changes in viscosity than the systemic vascular bed. Also for unknown reasons, fetal red cells are less viscous than adult red cells at the same hematocrit.[203,204] Whether there are developmental differences in the pulmonary vascular bed's response to changes in viscosity has apparently not been studied.

High Altitude

In infants born at high altitude the normal postnatal drop in pulmonary vascular resistance occurs more slowly and is smaller than in infants born at sea level.[9,10,179,215] Similarly, pulmonary vascular resistance is higher in adults living at high altitude than in adults living at sea level.[106,107,192] Whether pulmonary vascular resistance is different in the fetus living at high altitude remains unproven, but most likely fetal pulmonary vascular resistance is higher at high altitude as well. Reductions in oxygen tensions are likely to account for the higher pulmonary vascular resistance observed at high altitude, but the effects of normoxic hypobaria on pulmonary vascular tone do not appear to have been studied in fetal, neonatal, or adult life. It is possible that barometric pressure itself affects pulmonary vascular tone.

Gestational Age

Pulmonary vascular resistance is progressively reduced during fetal life,[153a,206,207] and birth accelerates the decline. How postmaturity affects fetal pulmonary vascular tone has not been studied. Postnatally, pulmonary vascular resistance drops dramatically within 24 hours of birth in calves,[199] puppies,[208] goats,[208] humans,[2,8,18,19,81,134,155,156] and presumably other species. Pulmonary vascular resistance continues a more gradual decline in the first several postnatal weeks in the piglet[198,202] and human[205] and presumably other species, after which a nadir is reached that appears to remain relatively constant throughout youth and adult life. Whether gestational age at birth (i.e., degree of prematurity or postmaturity) has any influence on ultimate pulmonary vascular tone in the adult is not known. Further, the question of whether age-related changes in pulmonary vascular tone occur normally in adult life does not appear to have been studied rigorously.

Another important question that does not appear to have been studied is whether prematurity affects the normal postnatal drop in pulmonary vascular resistance. Conventional wisdom says that premature infants go into heart failure from left-to-right patent ductus arteriosus (PDA) shunt within a few days of birth, and term infants with left-to-right ventricular septal defect (VSD) shunt do not go into heart failure for 4 to 6 weeks because pulmonary vascular resistance drops much more rapidly postnatally in preterm infants. However, it is possible that pulmonary vascular resistance is normally low from birth in the healthy premature infant.

Labor

One echocardiographic study in newborn infants has suggested that labor prior to delivery reduces pulmonary vascular resistance.[136] Altered circulating prostaglandin levels in infants who experienced labor have been documented,[25] and such differences could account for labor-associated reductions in pulmonary vascular resistance.[38] Whether such labor-induced differences in pulmonary vascular resistance, if they exist, persist into adult life is unknown, but this possibility seems unlikely.

Lung Influences

Local pulmonary factors other than oxygen tension and pH also influence resistance to pulmonary blood flow. For example, as considered further in the following sections, lung inflation, pulmonary surfactant, mechanical ventilation, positive end-expiratory pressure (PEEP), atelectasis, and patent ductus arteriosus all affect pulmonary vascular resistance.

Inflation

The lungs are expanded during all stages of development, but during fetal life the lungs are normally expanded with fluid[1] rather than gas. Inflation of the lungs with saline during fetal life has no effect on pulmonary vascular resistance,[58,73] but inflation of the lungs with nitrogen during fetal life causes pulmonary vasodilation;[40,54,58,72,73] these latter effects may be mechanical. Once gas breathing is established in the fetus, reductions in tidal volume increase pulmonary vascular resistance,[58] as do deflations of fetal lungs to a state of collapse.[58]

Lung inflation has similar effects in adult animals. The relationship between lung inflation and pulmonary vascular resistance can be examined in terms of both lung volumes and lung pressures. When lung volumes are low, pulmonary inflation reduces pulmonary vascular resistance.[34,125,241] When lung volumes are high, pulmonary inflation increases pulmonary vascular resistance.[34,125,241] In excised lungs of adult dogs, lung inflation has been shown to increase the volume of large vessels and to decrease the volume of small vessels;[125] the latter effect accounts for the increase in pulmonary vascular resistance seen when the lungs are expanded beyond moderate inflation.[34]

At low levels of transpulmonary pressure, state of inflation has little effect on pulmonary vascular resistance in excised adult canine lungs, but at high levels of transpulmonary pressure, state of inflation markedly affects pulmonary vascular resistance.[241] At low blood flow and the same transpulmonary pressure, there is a hysteresis between the inflation and deflation limbs of the pulmonary vascular resistance–inflation curve such that pulmonary vascular resistance is lower during inflation than deflation.[241]

Inflation of fetal lungs with oxygen rather than nitrogen causes immediate and dramatic pulmonary vasodilation by a bradykinin-dependent mechanism;[37,122] some indirect evidence suggests that bradykinin's vascular effects are mediated through prostacyclin release.[179a]

The pulmonary vasodilation induced by oxygen inflation of fetal lungs has two phases, the first an immediate phase that is not cyclooxygenase dependent and the second a slower phase that can be inhibited by indomethacin[152] and that is probably a result of prostacyclin production.[149a,150,152] In fetal goats, indomethacin causes greater reductions in pulmonary vasodilation induced by oxygen inflation of the lungs in younger fetuses,[152] indicative that the pulmonary vasodilating effects of lung inflation are more prostacyclin-dependent at younger gestational ages. In any case it would appear that maternal indomethacin administration can predispose to PPHNS by more than one mechanism (see Chapter 51 for additional mechanisms). Lung inflation promotes pulmonary vasodilation by prompting release of prostacyclin in adult life as well,[77a,107a] for prostacyclin is a potent pulmonary vasodilator at all stages of development.[39,46,80,169,221,223] Lung inflation with gas also causes release of pulmonary surfactant during both neonatal[148] and adult[48] life, and, as considered in the following section, pulmonary surfactant also reduces pulmonary vascular resistance.

Pulmonary Surfactant

Administration of pulmonary surfactant reduces pulmonary vascular resistance in premature lambs.[16,50] In adult dogs, pulmonary vascular resistance increases in lung areas from which surfactant is washed out.[182] Whether the presence or absence of pulmonary surfactant influences pulmonary vascular resistance only on a mechanical basis or also provokes active pulmonary vasoconstriction or active pulmonary vasodilation remains unknown.

Mechanical Ventilation: Positive Versus Negative Pressure Ventilation

Positive pressure ventilation mechanically impedes pulmonary blood flow during inspiration, particularly at high inflation pressures, high lung volumes, or high transpulmonary pressures;[34,125,241] presumably, physical compression of the pulmonary vascular channels is involved. Whether positive pressure mechanical ventilation, like PEEP (see later discussion), also provokes active pulmonary vasoconstriction remains unknown.

Controversy exists over whether negative pressure mechanical ventilation also increases pulmonary vascular resistance. Some observations would suggest that negative pressure mechanical ventilation has little mechanical impact on resistance to pulmonary blood flow,[109,125] which may at least partially explain why negative pressure mechanical ventilation can be useful in infants with refractory PPHNS. Others remain skeptical that negative pressure mechanical ventilation has different effects because ostensibly transpulmonary pressure should be the same in the two modes of ventilation.[34] However, the only safe assertion is that the issue should be settled experimentally in the intact organism, particularly in the newborn period.

Positive End-Expiratory Pressure

Distention of the lungs with positive end-expiratory pressure (PEEP) increases pulmonary vascular resistance by mechanically impeding pulmonary capillary blood flow as a result of physical compression of the pulmonary vascular channels in term newborn lambs,[238] adult dogs,[231] and adult humans,[114] but distension also causes calcium-dependent pulmonary vasoconstriction in term newborn lambs.[238] In premature newborn lambs with hyaline membrane disease, PEEP at 5 to 8 cm H_2O had no effect on pulmonary vascular resistance,[59] presumably because lung overdistension did not take place.

Atelectasis

By the same token, collapse of large lung segments also physically compresses enclosed pulmonary vascular channels and causes regional elevation in pulmonary vascular resistance.[22] However, other factors such as local hypoxia and local acidosis also contribute to elevations of pulmonary vascular tone in areas of atelectasis.

Patent Ductus Arteriosus

Recent evidence demonstrates that elevations in pulmonary arterial pressure reduce the resistance of the arterial duct in the newborn lamb and preserve its responsiveness to the ductal vasodilator prostaglandin E_2 (PGE_2).[52] As yet, there is no evidence that the converse is true, i.e., that patency of the arterial duct directly influences pulmonary vascular tone. However, there are several mechanisms by which the arterial duct can influence pulmonary arterial pressure and by which, at least indirectly, pulmonary arterial pressure can influence pulmonary vascular tone.

First, when pulmonary vascular tone is high (as in most forms of PPHNS [see Chapter 51]), patency of the arterial duct permits at least part of the antegrade flow through the pulmonary valve to avoid the pulmonary vascular bed and thereby limits elevations in pulmonary artery pressure. Pressure is a function of resistance and flow (pressure = resistance/flow), and any reductions in pulmonary blood flow unaccompanied by an increase in resistance (i.e., unaccompanied by pulmonary vasoconstriction) will reduce pulmonary artery pressure. At least in infants, elevations in pulmonary artery pressure (but not elevations in pulmonary artery flow) decrease lung compliance;[12,102] certainly infants with PPHNS frequently exhibit marked reductions in lung compliance.[213] (In contrast, pulmonary hypertension does not appear to affect lung compliance in the lamb.[35,50]) Whether airway compliance directly influences pulmonary vascular resistance in either species is unclear. However, if pulmonary hypertension–induced reductions in pulmonary compliance are lessened by right-to-left ductal shunt and either impairments in gas exchange or applications of PEEP or mechanical ventilation are thereby reduced, pulmonary vascular resistance will be reduced.

Second, when pulmonary vascular tone is low (as is presumably the case in most premature infants), patency of the arterial duct permits increased pulmonary blood flow as a result of left-to-right ductal shunt, and left-to-right shunts predispose to pulmonary hypertension. As noted previously, pulmonary hypertension reduces pulmonary compliance in infants,[12,102] and changes in pulmonary compliance can indirectly affect pulmonary vascular tone by altering gas exchange or by altering applications of PEEP or mechanical ventilation. Indeed, closure of patent ductus arteriosus in the human neonate has been shown repeatedly to improve lung compliance.[102,180,243] Thus, it seems likely that pulmonary hypertension caused by left-to-right shunts such as patent ductus arteriosus can reduce lung compliance in infants, and thereby indirectly influence pulmonary vascular tone.

Central Neural Influences

In the classical view, the pulmonary circulation is held to be regulated solely by local factors such as oxygen and pH. If this concept were accurate, one would have to wonder at nature's lack of economy in richly innervating both the arterial and venous sides of the pulmonary circulation in most mammalian species.[117] On the contrary, and despite skepticism,[76,121] a substantial body of evidence indicates that neural mechanisms can influence the pulmonary circulation at all stages of development.[168] What remains less clear is how important neural influences are in the regulation of the normal pulmonary circulation and what role neural mechanisms play in various forms of pulmonary hypertension.

The central nervous system has been demonstrated to influence the pulmonary circulation in at least three ways: by way of reflex mechanisms, by way of direct autonomic influences, and by way of direct brain influences. Important developmental differences in central neural regulation of the pulmonary circulation may exist; for example, the brain may be particularly important in the neonatal regulation of the pulmonary circulation.[168]

Reflex Mechanisms

Several reflex mechanisms have been proved to influence pulmonary vascular tone, including reflexes initiated by baroreceptors, peripheral chemoreceptors, and the upper airway. Most likely the efferent arm of each of these reflex mechanisms is the sympathetic nervous system, but alternative possibilities exist.[29,168]

Baroreceptors. Baroreceptors are well known to play an important role in regulation of systemic arterial pressure and systemic vascular resistance. However, the fact that baroreceptors may also play a role in regulation of the pulmonary circulation is not widely recognized.

Carotid Baroreceptors. In a constantly perfused isolated left lower lobe model, Daly and Daly demonstrated in 1957 that stimulation of the carotid baroreceptors caused substantial reflex increases in pulmonary arterial pressures.[65] They were unable to demonstrate conclusively the efferent limb of carotid baroreceptor–induced pulmonary vasoconstriction, but in at least one animal it appeared that the lung sympathetic nerve supply was responsible. Later, Pace could not confirm Daly and Daly's findings,[191] but more recently Shoukas and colleagues presented convincing evidence that carotid baroreceptor stimulation increases pulmonary vascular tone.[212]

Pulmonary Baroreceptors. Several studies have identified pulmonary artery baroreceptors,[24,32,55a,56,183,190] but their function remains unknown. Some investigators have described what appears to be pulmonary artery distention–induced reflex pulmonary hypertension,[15,138,145] but more recent observations suggest artifact may be responsible.

Chemoreceptors. Chemoreceptors sense carbon dioxide and oxygen tensions in the blood. In the adult, the central chemoreceptor is in the brain stem, and senses carbon dioxide alone. The peripheral chemoreceptors in the adult are located in the carotid and aortic bodies and sense both carbon dioxide and oxygen tensions. During fetal life, additional chemoreceptors are located in the adrenal glands in some species, but these disappear with postnatal development. The function of the adrenal che-

moreceptors during fetal life is largely unknown. The increase in breathing caused by reduction in systemic arterial oxygen tension (and consequent stimulation of the peripheral chemoreceptors) is now well recognized during fetal, neonatal, and adult life, but the reflex pulmonary hypertension that also results is often overlooked.

Peripheral Chemoreceptors. The aortic chemoreceptors were demonstrated in 1927 by Heymans and Heymans,[123] who also demonstrated the carotid chemoreceptors 4 years later, thereby proving Castro's 1928 hypothesis[47] that the carotid body was also a chemosensory organ. Heymans used a cross-perfusion technique to supply hypoxic blood from one animal to the isolated aorta or carotid artery of another animal (which was otherwise well oxygenated) and demonstrated that breathing was stimulated in the recipient animal. Heymans was awarded the Nobel Prize for these discoveries. Using derivations of the Heymans' elegant experimental model, others subsequently demonstrated that hypoxia restricted to the peripheral chemoreceptors not only stimulated breathing but also caused reflex pulmonary hypertension in fetal lambs[36] and adult dogs.[11,66] Other studies in simpler preparations have confirmed that the peripheral chemoreceptors cause reflex pulmonary vasoconstriction in adult cats[224,226] and adult dogs.[227] However, in the adult animal it appears that the peripheral chemoreceptors have a much larger influence on pulmonary vascular compliance than resistance.[227,229] Since isolated systemic hypoxia (with normal alveolar PO_2) causes reflex pulmonary vasoconstriction in adult dogs,[242] but isolated brain hypoxia does not,[189] it appears that the peripheral chemoreceptors are the afferents for hypoxia-induced reflex central neural pulmonary vasoconstriction.

The efferent pathway for peripheral chemoreceptor–induced pulmonary vasoconstriction has been shown to be the sympathetic nervous system in the fetal lamb[36] and adult dog.[66,227]

The aortic and carotid chemoreceptors appear to have different physiologic effects. In the adult dog, aortic chemoreceptors have modest effects on ventilation but increase systemic vascular resistance, whereas carotid chemoreceptors markedly stimulate breathing and have little effect on systemic vascular resistance.[57,69] In the adult dog, carotid chemoreceptors slow the heart,[68] while apparently aortic chemoreceptors do not. Further, aortic chemoreceptors predominantly constrict pulmonary veins in the adult dog,[224] whereas presumably carotid chemoreceptors predominantly constrict pulmonary arterioles. Explanations for these differences are obscure but probably have something to do with defense of the fetus against hypoxia. Developmental differences in the relative contributions of the aortic and carotid chemoreceptors to hypoxic pulmonary vasoconstriction are not well studied, but they may exist.[168] Custer and Hales have shown that chemical sympathectomy markedly inhibits hypoxic pulmonary vasoconstriction in newborn sheep but has little effect in adult sheep;[62] chemical sympathectomy may eliminate the efferent arm of the chemoreceptor-induced reflex pulmonary hypertension. As illustrated in Figure 7–1, surgical extirpation of the peripheral chemoreceptors in newborn piglets also markedly reduces the magnitude

PART A   **PART B**

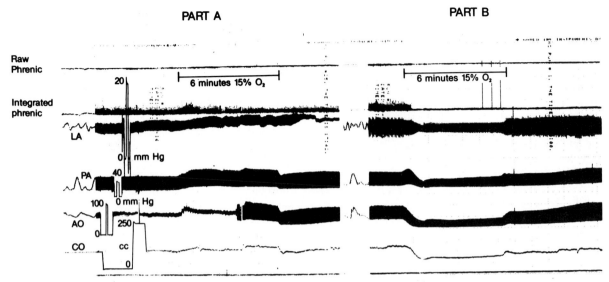

Figure 7–1. The effects of chemodenervation on the pulmonary circulation's response to alveolar hypoxia in a 3-day-old anesthetized, paralyzed, mechanically ventilated, ductus-ligated, otherwise intact piglet are shown. In *part A*, the chemoreceptors were intact; in *part B*, the carotid sinus nerves and vagal nerves were severed (the aortic chemoreceptor fibers run in the vagus). On the top line, amplified phrenic activity (Raw Phrenic) did not reproduce well. On the second line, full-wave rectified phrenic neural activity (Integrated phrenic) is recorded; each deflection is a breath, and the height of each deflection is proportional to tidal volume. On the third, fourth, fifth, and sixth lines, left atrial pressure (LA), pulmonary arterial pressure (PA), aortic pressure (AO), and cardiac output (CO), respectively, are shown. In *part A* before chemodenervation, 15 per cent oxygen increased phrenic neural activity, pulmonary artery pressure, and aortic pressure. Left atrial pressure increased slightly, and cardiac output was largely unaffected. In the middle of the hypoxia exposure it was realized that the pulmonary artery pressure tracing was damped, and the catheter was flushed. In *part B* after chemodenervation, phrenic neural activity decreased rather than increased during repeat exposure to 15 per cent oxygen (indicating successful chemodenervation), and left atrial pressure, pulmonary artery pressure, aortic pressure, and cardiac output fell. These observations indicate that the peripheral chemoreceptors contribute substantially to hypoxic pulmonary hypertension in newborn piglets.

of pulmonary vasoconstriction induced by alveolar hypoxia, and in fact can result in death during the hypoxia exposure.[166] Similarly, in neonatal rats, exposure to hypoxia after chemodenervation was fatal,[124] but in adult rats chemodenervation simply reduced the magnitude of alveolar hypoxia-induced pulmonary hypertension.[144] These observations demonstrate that the peripheral chemoreceptors contribute significantly to the pulmonary hypertension induced by alveolar hypoxia in both adult and newborn animals and that the chemoreceptor contribution to alveolar hypoxia-induced pulmonary vasoconstriction (and to survival of hypoxia) may be particularly important in the neonatal period.

Central Chemoreceptor. The central chemoreceptor responds to carbon dioxide, not oxygen. Whether the central chemoreceptor, like the peripheral chemoreceptors, has a role in the regulation of the pulmonary circulation remains unexplored. However, it seems probable that the central chemoreceptor can initiate both vasodilatory and vasoconstricting pulmonary vascular reflexes, depending on the level of brain stem carbon dioxide. Experiments to explore this possibility should be conducted because identifying and taking advantage of such central neural vasodilatory pathways may eventually prove more important in treating pulmonary hypertension than blocking vasoconstricting pathways.

Upper Airway. Several lines of evidence suggest that upper airway reflexes may play a role in regulation of pulmonary vascular tone. In adult dogs[55,113] and newborn sheep,[104] intratracheal injections of small volumes of fresh- or saltwater cause apnea and pulmonary hypertension. In at least the adult dog, pulmonary arterial pres-

sures seemed to increase more than would be expected for the magnitude of apnea and respiratory acidosis observed.[55] Supplemental oxygen in the adult dog[55] lessened but did not abolish the increases in pulmonary arterial pressure observed during the tracheal injections. In newborn sheep experiments,[104] oxygen and mechanical ventilation did counteract the hypoxia and respiratory acidosis accompanying laryngeal water-induced apnea and did reduce the systemic effects observed, but whether oxygen and mechanical ventilation also reduced the increases in pulmonary artery pressure caused by laryngeal installations of water was not reported.[104] Tracheal installation of tetracaine and intravenous administration of hexamethonium in adult dogs lessened tracheal water-induced increases in pulmonary artery pressure, and atropine prevented the response.[55] Vagotomy had no effect on freshwater-induced pulmonary hypertension in adult dogs, but the site of vagal sectioning was not mentioned.[55] A local pulmonary reflex was concluded to be responsible for tracheal freshwater-induced pulmonary hypertension.[55] Similarly, pharmacologic blocking experiments with alpha antagonists and atropine in neonatal sheep[104] altered systemic responses to laryngeal water installation, but pulmonary artery pressures during the latter experiments were not reported.

One possible explanation for tracheal fluid-induced pulmonary hypertension lies in stimulation of the laryngeal chemoreceptors, which fire in response to low or high chloride concentrations.[26] The larynx also contains mechanoreceptors; both types of fibers travel to the central nervous system via the superior laryngeal nerve, which is a branch of the vagus nerve. As illustrated in

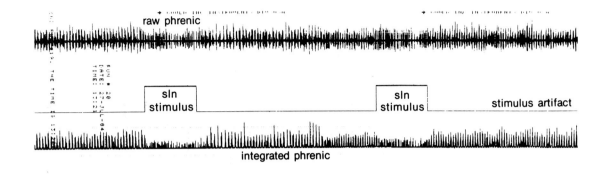

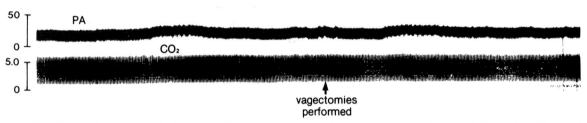

Figure 7–2. The effects of electrically stimulating the superior laryngeal nerve on pulmonary artery pressure before and after cutting of the vagal nerves distal to the point of entry of the superior laryngeal nerves into the vagal nerves are demonstrated in a 3-day-old anesthetized, paralyzed, mechanically ventilated piglet. On the top line, the amplified phrenic neural activity is recorded (raw phrenic). On the second line, full-wave rectified phrenic neural activity (integrated phrenic) is recorded; each deflection is a breath, and the height of each deflection is proportional to tidal volume. On the third line, two 3-minute electrical superior laryngeal nerve stimulations are indicated (sln stimulus), between which at the arrow the vagal nerves were severed in the low cervical area. On the fourth and fifth lines, pulmonary arterial pressure (PA) and end-tidal carbon dioxide (CO_2), respectively, are shown. Note that superior laryngeal nerve stimulation caused inhibition of phrenic neural activity and increased pulmonary artery pressure both before and after low cervical sectioning of the vagal nerves. By design, end-tidal CO_2 was held constant.

Figures 7–2 and 7–3, electrical stimulation of the superior laryngeal nerve has recently been shown to cause pulmonary vasoconstriction in newborn piglets in whom blood gases were held constant.[165,168] Sectioning of the vagal nerves distal to the superior laryngeal nerve had no effect on superior laryngeal nerve–induced pulmonary vasoconstriction (Fig. 7–2).[165,168] These observations demonstrate that afferent input from the upper airway can cause pulmonary hypertension in newborn piglets and that the central nervous system is responsible. The efferent limb of this reflex is as yet unproven but is probably the sympathetic nervous system. Possible developmental aspects of this reflex also deserve study.

These observations suggest that particular care should be taken to avoid laryngeal irritation in newborn infants with PPHNS. Dumping 0.9 per cent saline down the airway, tracheal suctioning, and endotracheal tube manipulations quite possibly could worsen pulmonary hypertension. Further, therapeutic approaches in PPHNS such as negative pressure ventilation may work not only because removal of positive airway pressure decreases pulmonary vascular resistance but also because the endotracheal tube is removed from the larynx. In addition, it is possible that application of local anesthetics to the upper airway could be of value in intubated infants with PPHNS.

Direct Autonomic Influences

The autonomic nervous system is well known to influence the systemic circulation, but only recently has the role of the autonomic nervous system in regulation of the pulmonary circulation received much attention.

Fetal Life. Rudolph has expressed skepticism that the autonomic nervous system plays a role in the regulation of the fetal pulmonary circulation in utero[206,207] despite observations in the exteriorized fetus consistent with modest tonic sympathetic-mediated pulmonary vasoconstriction, vagal-induced pulmonary vasodilation, and reflex pulmonary vasoconstriction in response to hypoxia.[41,54] Rudolph's skepticism is largely due to the fact that he and his colleagues were unable to document any effect of the alpha blockers phentolamine and Dibenzyline, the beta blocker propranolol, or the parasympathetic blocker atropine on either resting pulmonary blood flows or pressures[206] or on the pulmonary vascular response to hypoxia in chronically instrumented fetal sheep.[153a] Rudolph implied that something about exteriorizing the fetal sheep causes the autonomic nervous system to assume a more active role in the regulation of the pulmonary circulation.[206] On the other hand, Rudolph himself found that isoproterenol,[206] acetylcholine,[153a] and tolazoline[206] produced marked decreases in pulmonary vascular resistance in chronically instrumented fetal sheep and that the fall in fetal pulmonary vascular resistance caused by acetylcholine increased with advancing gestation.[153a] Similarly, Campbell et al[36] found that reflex-induced pulmonary vasoconstriction from systemic hypoxia was detectable only in late gestation fetuses, and Colebatch et al[54] found that thoracic sympathectomy reduced pulmonary vascular resistance only in late gestation fetuses. Thus, available data suggest that the autonomic nervous system *can* influence the

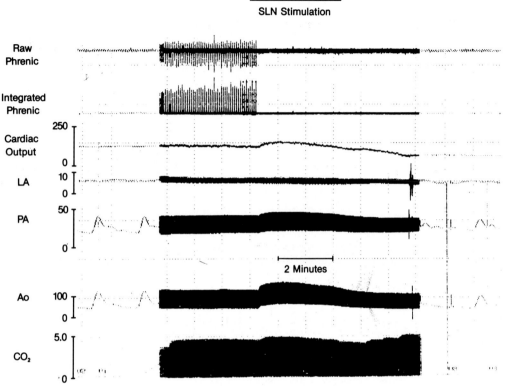

Figure 7–3. The respiratory and hemodynamic effects of electrically stimulating the superior laryngeal nerve in a 5-day-old anesthetized, paralyzed, mechanically ventilated (with 100 per cent oxygen) piglet are shown. On the top line, the amplified phrenic neural activity is recorded (Raw Phrenic). On the second line, full-wave rectified phrenic neural activity (Integrated Phrenic) is recorded; each deflection is a breath, and the height of each deflection is proportional to tidal volume. On the third line, cardiac output is recorded. On the fourth, fifth, sixth, and seventh lines, left atrial pressure (LA), pulmonary arterial pressure (PA), aortic pressure (Ao) and end-tidal carbon dioxide (CO_2), respectively, are shown. The 3-minute electrical superior laryngeal nerve stimulus (10 hertz, 1 volt) is indicated by the solid bar. Note that superior laryngeal nerve stimulation caused total apnea (which persisted after stimulus cessation), decreased left atrial pressure slightly, increased cardiac output briefly, and caused sustained increases in pulmonary artery pressure and systemic arterial pressure. In other experiments, increases in pulmonary artery pressure occurred during superior laryngeal nerve stimulations without any even transient increases in cardiac output. These observations indicate that the superior laryngeal nerve can increase pulmonary vascular tone.

pulmonary circulation during fetal life and that the capacity of the autonomic nervous system to influence the fetal pulmonary circulation increases with development. What remains unknown is whether the autonomic nervous system actually *does* play an important role in the regulation of the fetal pulmonary circulation, either in the basal state or during times of stress. It would certainly appear that the sympathetic nerve and vagal nerve stimulation experiments of Colebatch et al in exteriorized fetal sheep[54] should be repeated in utero in chronically instrumented fetal sheep. In view of the neonatal and adult data to be considered in the following sections, it seems likely that important autonomic influences on the fetal pulmonary circulation would be found.

Neonatal and Adult Life. During neonatal and adult life, the evidence documenting that the autonomic nervous system can influence the pulmonary circulation is substantial. Most studies have shown that the sympathetic nervous system can influence the tone of the pulmonary circulation;[64,67,80,110,133,197,225–229,236,237] a few studies, depending on species and experimental model, have not found adrenergic effects.[172,174,175,230] However, recent work by Hyman and colleagues has pointed out that

underlying pulmonary vascular tone has very important effects on the results observed with autonomic intervention.[130,131]

Sympathetic Stimulation. Depending on the existing tone of the pulmonary bed and whether alpha or beta stimulation predominates, stimulation of the pulmonary sympathetic nerves electrically can cause either elevations or reductions in pulmonary vascular tone.[130,131] Szidon and Fishman found that electrical stimulation of the left stellate ganglion in a pulsatile but constantly perfused canine isolated left lower lobe model caused elevations in systolic pulmonary artery pressure but not in diastolic or mean pulmonary artery pressures without changing calculated pulmonary vascular resistance.[227] Szidon and Fishman concluded that the small resistance vessels were largely unaffected but that the distensibility and tension of the large pulmonary vessels were altered by sympathetic stimulation.[227] In contrast, Hyman, Kadowitz, and Lippton have found that electrical stellate ganglion stimulation elevates pulmonary vascular resistance in a similar cat model with continuous rather than pulsatile constant left lower lobe flow.[130,131] Hyman, Kadowitz, and Lippton also noted that electrical stellate ganglion stimulation predominantly stimulates pulmonary vascular alpha receptors, but beta receptors were also stimulated.[130,131] Pulmonary vasoconstriction caused by electrical stellate ganglion stimulation was enhanced by beta blockade with propanolol and reversed by alpha blockade with phenoxybenzamine.[131] Enhanced prostacyclin production could contribute to sympathetic nerve–induced pulmonary vasodilation.[80] In the adult dog, both pulmonary arteries and pulmonary veins are constricted by sympathetic stimulation.[139]

Efferent Vagal Stimulation. The effects of vagal stimulation on pulmonary vascular tone in the exteriorized fetal lamb[54] and in the adult cat[131] have been studied using electrical stimulation of the left cervical vagosympathetic nerve. However, the vagosympathetic nerves carry both vagal and sympathetic fibers. Hyman, Lippton, and Kadowitz have found that under basal conditions in their cat model with continuous rather than pulsatile constant left lower lobe flow, left cervical vagosympathetic nerve stimulation causes modest elevations in pulmonary vascular resistance that are blockable by phenoxybenzamine.[131] After elevation of pulmonary vascular tone with the alpha agonist U-46619 or with PGF_{2a} in that same model, left cervical vagosympathetic nerve stimulation causes pulmonary vasodilation.[131] Atropine but not propanolol blocked cervical vagosympathetic-mediated pulmonary vasodilation, indicating that cholinergic nerves were responsible.[131] Parasympathetic nerve-induced pulmonary vasodilation could be a result of increased prostacyclin production,[30] as may be the case with sympathetic nerve-induced pulmonary vasodilation.[80]

Afferent Vagal Stimulation. Electrical stimulation of the cut *central* end of the vagus was demonstrated to cause increases in pulmonary arterial pressure by Bradford and Dean in 1894.[29] Although Weber confirmed the existence of this phenomenon in 1910 (cited by Daly and von Euler[67]), the fact that afferent stimulation of the central end of the cut vagus can cause brain-mediated reflex pulmonary vasoconstriction has received very little subsequent attention.

Direct Brain Influences

Hypothalamus. Pulmonary vasomotor tone is also influenced by direct brain stimulation. Anderson and Brown[6] reported in 1967 that electrically stimulating the hypothalamus in cats caused marked increases in pulmonary arterial pressure and modest (6 to 8 per cent) increases in pulmonary vascular resistance. Although cardiac output also increased in Anderson and Brown's experiments, increases in pulmonary arterial pressure began before blood flow changed.[6] Hypothalamic-induced pulmonary vasoconstriction was blocked by hexamethonium and by sectioning of the stellate ganglion but not by vagotomy.[6] Hypothalamic-induced increases in pulmonary arterial pressure were exacerbated by atropine.[6] These observations indicate that the sympathetic nervous system mediates hypothalamic-induced pulmonary vasoconstriction.

Similar increases in pulmonary arterial pressure and cardiac output were observed by Szidon and Fishman in intact dogs during electrical stimulation of the hypothalamus.[227] However, Szidon and Fishman also stimulated the hypothalamus electrically in an isolated canine left lower lobe preparation designed to permit constant pulsatile blood flow.[227] In that model as well considerable increases in pulmonary systolic pressure were observed, but pulmonary diastolic pressures either remained unchanged or only increased slightly.[227] However, the distribution of pulmonary blood flow improved during hypothalamic stimulation,[227] which was a role predicted for pulmonary vasomotor nerves 38 years earlier by Daly and von Euler.[67] Hypothalamic-induced increases in pulmonary artery pressure were blocked by phenoxybenzamine.[227] From these experiments, one can conclude that in the adult dog hypothalamic stimulation alters the distensibility of large pulmonary vessels more than the resistance of small pulmonary blood vessels, that the hypothalamus might have a role in maintaining homogenous pulmonary perfusion, and that hypothalamic influences on the pulmonary circulation are mediated by the sympathetic nervous system.[227]

Brain Stem. In 1894 Bradford and Dean reported that electrical stimulation of the high medulla in an area they termed a "vasomotor center" increased pulmonary arterial pressure.[28] Bradford and Dean found that sectioning of the spinal cord at C_7 prior to electrical stimulation of the high medulla largely abolished accompanying increases in systemic artery pressure but had no effect on increases in pulmonary artery pressure. Bradford and Dean also found that sectioning of the spinal cord at C_2 prior to medullary electrical stimulation abolished increases in pulmonary artery pressure. Bradford and Dean further noted that pulmonary artery pressure also increased during electrical stimulation of the spinal roots of C_2, C_3, and C_4 and that sectioning of the splanchnic nerves did not alter the increases in pulmonary artery pressure caused by electrical stimulation of the C_2, C_3, and C_4 spinal roots but did prevent accompanying changes in the systemic artery pressure.

Unaware of Bradford and Dean's discoveries, Dr. D. L. Brown and I recently began to investigate the effects of electrical brain stem stimulations on the pulmonary circulation.[168] Our experiments were based on recent developments in identifying the brain stem vasomotor center,[33] which is a 0.5 mm³ (in rats) area located in the rostral brain stem in the area of the nucleus paragigantocellularis (Fig. 7–4). The brain stem vasomotor center is the hub of sympathetic circulatory control and is capable of causing tremendous changes in the systemic circulation, but its effects on the pulmonary circulation are unexplored. The preparation (Fig. 7–5) consisted of anesthetized newborn piglets who were tracheotomized, ventilated with 100 per cent O_2 at constant end-tidal carbon dioxide and constant body temperature, and then paralyzed with gallamine. Pulmonary, femoral, and left atrial pressures as well as cardiac output were measured continuously. The ventral brain stem was exposed. Brief (10 to 30 seconds) electrical stimulations (10 to 50 hertz, 50 to 100 milliamps)

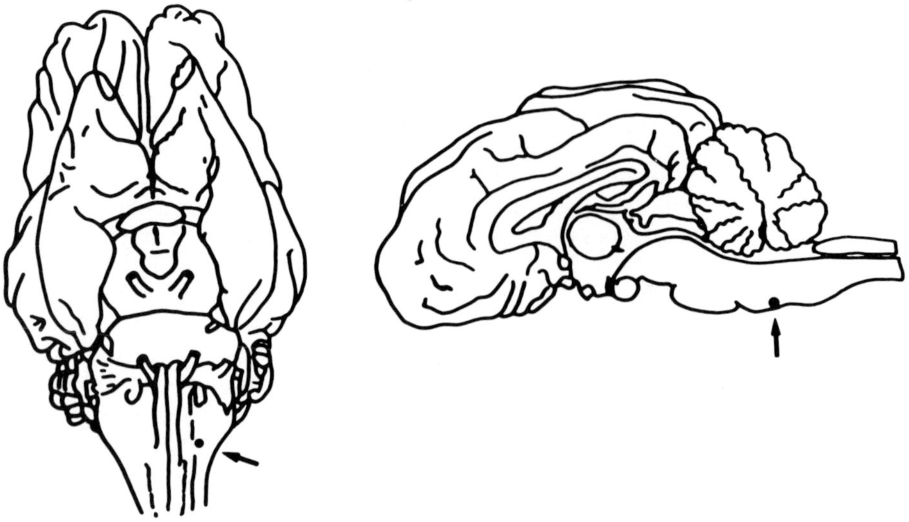

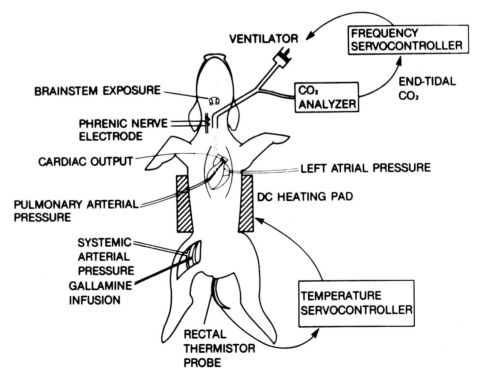

Figure 7–4. The location of the brain stem vasomotor center is illustrated by the arrows.

were applied to various parts of the brain stem vasomotor center with a fine monopolar stimulating electrode, and hemodynamic changes were noted. Areas of the brainstem vasomotor center causing hemodynamic changes of interest were marked by direct current destruction and subsequently identified histologically.

Slight shifts in electrode position within the brain stem vasomotor center caused substantial variations in responses to electrical stimulation. Both immediate and

delayed effects on systemic arterial pressure, cardiac output, and pulmonary arterial pressure have been observed. In some younger piglets (2 to 3 days of age), we have found what appears to be significant pulmonary vasoconstriction (Fig. 7–6) with no changes in cardiac output and relatively small changes in the systemic resistance.[168] Although these observations are preliminary, they do suggest that a specific pulmonary vasoconstrictor area does exist within the brain stem vasomotor center.

Figure 7–5. The preparation for determining pulmonary vascular resistance during electrical stimulation of the brain stem in newborn piglets is illustrated. Note that both temperature and end-tidal CO_2 are held constant by electronic servocontrolled mechanisms. The inspired gas is 100 per cent oxygen throughout the preparation.

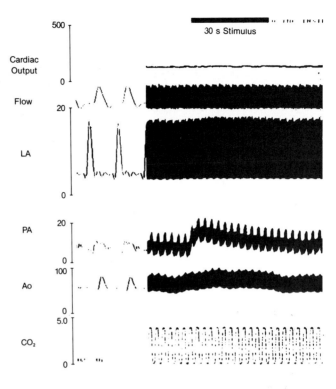

Figure 7–6. The effects of electrically stimulating the brain stem vasomotor center in an anesthetized, paralyzed, mechanically ventilated newborn piglet are shown. The 10 hertz, 50 milliampere electrical stimulus is indicated by the bar; the stimulation lasted 30 seconds. On the top line, mean cardiac output measured at the pulmonary artery is recorded. On the second line, instantaneous cardiac output measured at the main pulmonary artery (Flow) is recorded. On the third, fourth, fifth, and sixth lines, left atrial presssure (LA), pulmonary artery pressure (PA), aortic pressure (Ao), and end-tidal CO_2 (CO_2) are recorded. Note that electrical stimulation of the brain stem vasomotor center caused substantial increases in pulmonary artery pressure and modest increases in aortic pressure without changing cardiac output, instantaneous pulmonary flow, or left atrial pressure. These observations indicate that neurally mediated pulmonary and systemic vasoconstriction occurred.

CHEMICAL MEDIATORS AND MESSENGERS

Cells read very little if any extracellular information directly; at a minimum, second messengers such as cyclic AMP transmit information from receptor binding at the cell surface to the cell interior. It is doubtful that even hypoxia or hydrogen ion, which stimulate contraction of isolated pulmonary vascular smooth muscle cells in vitro, actually act directly; instead, chemical mediators probably are responsible for resulting pulmonary vascular smooth muscle contraction. However, the chemical mediators for even these two relatively straightforward phenomena still elude definition; the chemical mediators and messengers for the many other influences on pulmonary vascular tone considered above remain even more obscure.

On the other hand, a great many endogenous agents have been found to alter pulmonary vascular tone, and in some cases second messengers for these agents are well described. Administration or inhibition of agents affecting pulmonary vascular tone may eventually prove useful clinically in treating pulmonary hypertension long before their true roles, if any, in normal regulation of the pulmonary circulation are known. Prostacyclin is a case in point.[169] Below are reviewed a number of neurochemicals, eicosanoids, peptides, and other substances that have been shown to influence pulmonary vascular tone at various stages of development.

Neurochemicals

As considered in the preceding discussion, evidence is substantial that the autonomic and central nervous systems can have important influences on the lung circulation during fetal, neonatal, and adult life. It seems likely that eventually successful new therapies for pulmonary hypertension will consist of altering central or peripheral neural transmission rather than administering direct smooth muscle dilators. The following sections consider some of the neurochemicals known to affect the pulmonary circulation.

Catecholamines

Many investigators have looked at the roles of various catecholamines in regulation of pulmonary vascular tone.[82,86,91,101,112,118,119,163,181,197,236,237] In general, alpha adrenergic agonists constrict the pulmonary circulation at all stages of development, and alpha adrenergic antagonists dilate the pulmonary circulation.[31,100,161,223] Similarly, beta adrenergic agonists generally dilate the pulmonary circulation at all stages of development, and beta adrenergic antagonists constrict the pulmonary circulation.

Serotonin

Serotonin is a potent pulmonary vasoconstrictor in most species, including the adult dog,[202a] but serotonin is not the mediator of hypoxic pulmonary vasoconstriction.[86] Serotonin antagonists can reduce pulmonary vascular tone in some models.

Acetylcholine

Acetylcholine is a pulmonary vasodilator in adult humans[90,113a] and fetal sheep,[153a,206,207] but is a pulmonary vasoconstrictor in newborn puppies.[209] Explanations

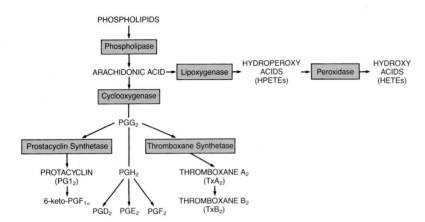

Figure 7–7. The prostaglandin cascade is illustrated. Products of the lipoxygenase pathway are pulmonary vasoconstrictors at all stages of development. In the fetal lamb, all products of the cylooxygenase pathway except $PGF_{2\alpha}$ and thromboxane are pulmonary vasodilators. In contrast, in the adult sheep the only product of the entire prostaglandin cascade that is a pulmonary vasodilator is prostacyclin. These developmental differences appear to hold true in other species as well. For discussion of eicosanoid effects in neonatal lambs, see text.

for these developmental or species differences remain obscure.

Eicosanoids

Eicosanoids are biologically active 20-carbon compounds usually derived from arachidonic acid (Fig. 7–7); prostaglandins, leukotrienes, and thromboxane are all eicosanoids derived from arachidonic acid. Like thromboxane, leukotrienes are potent pulmonary vasoconstrictors at all stages of development,[129,132,140,151,177,185,216] as is PGF_{2a}.[126,153,220] In contrast, prostacyclin is a potent pulmonary vasodilator at all stages of development[42,46,169,187,188,214,221,223] and may have clinical utility in many forms of pulmonary hypertension,[169] including PPHNS (see Chapters 51 and 55). PGE_1 is also a pulmonary vasodilator at all stages of development;[5,44,45,126,169,223] PGE_1, however, is not a product of arachidonic acid, but instead of gamma linolenic acid, and appears to cause pulmonary vasodilation by binding to the prostacyclin receptor.[169]

For unexplained reasons, the effects of three other arachidonic acid–derived prostaglandins (PGH_2, PGD_2, and PGE_2) vary markedly with development. PGH_2 is a pulmonary vasodilator in unventilated fetal sheep,[234] but is a pulmonary vasoconstrictor in ventilated fetal sheep[234] and adult sheep.[141] PGD_2 and PGE_2 are pulmonary vasodilators during fetal life and immediately after birth,[42,43,195,214,217,218] but within a short period after birth, PGD_2 becomes a pulmonary vasoconstrictor,[7,39,187,194,218] and remains so throughout adult life. PGE_2[5,220] is also a pulmonary vasoconstrictor during adult life, but the timing of PGE_2's postnatal metamorphosis from pulmonary vasodilator to pulmonary vasoconstrictor has not been studied.

Thus, during fetal life, all products of cyclooxygenase except PGF_{2a} and thromboxane are pulmonary vasodilators. At birth PGH_2 joins the pulmonary vasoconstrictor

ranks; during neonatal life, PGD_2 also joins the pulmonary vasoconstrictor ranks; and at some later point PGE_2 as well becomes a pulmonary vasoconstrictor. As a result, the only product of the cyclooxygenase pathway that continues to dilate the pulmonary circulation in adult life is prostacyclin. The fact that three cyclooxygenase products (PGI_2, PGD_2, and PGE_2) are pulmonary vasodilators at birth but that two of the three (PGD_2 and PGE_2) become pulmonary vasoconstrictors during postnatal development may account for meclofenamate's causing less pulmonary vasoconstriction with increasing postnatal age.[198]

In addition to their direct effects, it is also possible that prostaglandins influence the pulmonary circulation indirectly by modulating the autonomic nervous system.[181,237,240]

Peptides

Peptides are increasingly recognized as playing an important role in the regulation of the systemic circulation;[93] there is little doubt that future investigations will reveal that the peptidergic nervous system also plays an important role in the regulation of the pulmonary circulation. For example, vasoactive intestinal peptide dramatically decreases pulmonary vascular resistance in neonatal lambs,[162] and in adult rabbit lungs neuroepithelial bodies containing opiates and other peptides release their contents in response to alveolar hypoxia.[147] Similar neuroepithelial bodies have been described in several species, including humans, and at all stages of development. In addition, the opiate leu-enkephalin causes dose-dependent pulmonary vasoconstriction in rat lungs,[97,98] and naloxone can diminish hypoxic pulmonary vasoconstriction in adult dogs.[14]

Endogenous opiates are increasingly recognized to have roles as co-neurotransmitters in the autonomic nervous system,[239] and can either enhance or diminish the response to a given level of neurotransmitter by altering the neurotransmitter's receptor. Such endogenous opiate-induced neurotransmitter receptor alterations are not induced by direct binding to the neurotransmitter receptors but by distant bindings that nevertheless cause conformational changes in the neurotransmitter receptors.

Other peptides could also play important roles in regulation of the pulmonary circulation. If the brain stem vasomotor center proves to have an important role in pulmonary vascular tone (as is clearly the case for the systemic circulation), peptides such as substance P[99] and amino acids such as glutamate[108] may provide keys to new therapeutic avenues in treatment of pulmonary hypertension. Because adults with essential systemic hypertension also exhibit elevations in pulmonary artery pressure[4,85] and because newborns with PPHNS also exhibit elevations in systemic vascular resistance,[176] it would appear that the regulations of the two circulations are far from independent.

References

1. Adams FH, Latta H, El-Salawy A, Nozaki M (1969): The expanded lung of the term fetus. J Pediatr 75:59–66.
2. Adams FH, Lind J (1957): Physiologic studies on the cardiovascular status of newborn infants (with special reference to the ductus arteriosus): Pediatrics 19:431–437.
2a. Agarwal JB, Paltoo R, Palmer WH (1970): Relative viscosity of blood at varying hematocrits in pulmonary circulation. J Appl Physiol 29:866–871.
3. Alexander JM, Nyby MD, Jasberg KA (1977): Prostaglandin synthesis inhibition restores hypoxic pulmonary vasoconstriction. J Appl Physiol 42:903–908.
4. Alpert MA, Bauer JH, Parker BM, Sanfelippo JF, Brooks CS (1985): Pulmonary hemodynamics in systemic hypertension. South Med J 78:784–789.
5. Altura BM, Chand N (1981): Differential effects of prostaglandins on canine intrapulmonary arteries and veins. Br J Pharmacol 73:819–827.
6. Anderson FL, Brown AM (1967): Pulmonary vasoconstriction elicited by stimulation of the hypothalamic integrative area for defense reactions. Circ Res 21:747–756.
7. Angerio AD, Ramwell PW, Kot PA, Rose JC (1977): Cardiovascular responses to PGD$_2$ in the dog. Proc Soc Exp Biol Med 156:393–395.
8. Arcilla RA, Oh W, Lind J (1966): Pulmonary artery pressure of newborn infants with early and late clamping of the cord. Acta Pediatr Scand 55:305–315.
9. Arias-Stella J, Recavarren S (1962): Right ventricular hypertrophy in native children living at high altitude. Am J Pathol 41:55–64.
10. Arias-Stella J, Saldana M (1962): The muscular pulmonary arteries in people native to high altitude. Med Thorac 19:484–493.
11. Aviado DM Jr, Ling JS, Schmidt CF (1957): Effects of anoxia on pulmonary circulation: reflex pulmonary vasoconstriction. Am J Physiol 189:253–262.
12. Bancalari E, Jesse MJ, Gelband H, Garcia O (1977): Lung mechanics in congenital heart disease with increased and decreased pulmonary blood flow. J Pediatr 90:192–195.
13. Bard H, Fouron JC (1987): Neonatal circulatory changes in polycythemia. Comparison between fetal and adult type blood. In Stern W, Oh W, Friis-Hansen B (eds): Physiologic Foundations of Perinatal Care, Vol 2. New York, Elsevier, pp 50–62.
14. Bar-Or, D, Good JT, Marx JA, Moore EE, Winkler JV (1984): Naloxone: Effects on hypoxic pulmonary vasoconstriction. Ann Emerg Med 13:495–498.
15. Baylen BG, Emmanouilides GC, Jurastch CE, Yoshida Y, French WJ, Criley JM (1980): Main pulmonary artery distention: A potential mechanism for acute pulmonary hypertension in the newborn infant. J Pediatr 96:540–544.
16. Baylen BG, Ogata H, Ikegami M, Jacobs HC, Jobe AH, Emmanouilides GC (1983): Left ventricular performance and regional blood flows before and after ductus arteriosus occlusion in premature lambs treated with surfactant. Circulation 67:837–843.
17. Beddell CR, Goodford PJ, Kneen G, White RD, Wilkinson S, Wootton R (1984): Substituted benzaldehydes designed to increase the oxygen affinity of human haemoglobin and inhibit the sickling of erythrocytes. Br J Pharmacol 82:397–407.
18. Berglund G (1955): Studies of circulation in the neonatal period. Acta Pediatr 103:138–139.
19. Berglund G, Korlberg P, Lind J (1955): Studies of the respiration and circulation during the neonatal period. Acta Pediatr 44:136–137.
20. Bergofsky EH (1974): Mechanisms underlying vasomotor regulation of regional pulmonary blood flow in normal and disease states. Am J Med 57:378–394.
21. Bergofsky EH, Lehr DE, Fishman AP (1962): The effects of changes in hydrogen ion concentration on the pulmonary circulation. J Clin Invest 41:1492–1501.
22. Berry D, Jobe A, Jacobs H, Ikegami M (1985): Distribution of pulmonary blood flow in relation to atelectasis in premature ventilated lambs. Am Rev Resp Dis 132:500–503.
23. Beyne J (1942): Influence de l'anoxemie sur la grande circulation et sur la circulation pulmonaire. C R Soc Biol (Paris) 136:399–400.
24. Bianconi R, Green JH (1959): Pulmonary baroreceptors in the cat. Arch Ital Biol 97:305–315.
25. Bibby JG, Brunt JD, Hodgson H, Mitchell MD, Anderson ABM, Turnbull AC (1979): Prostaglandins in umbilical plasma at elective C-section. Br J Obstet Gynaecol 86:282–284.
26. Boggs DF, Bartlett D Jr (1982): Chemical specificity of a laryngeal apneic reflex in puppies. J Appl Physiol 53:455–462.
27. Born GVR, Dawes GS, Mott JC, Widdicombe JG (1954): Changes in the heart and lungs at birth. Cold Spring Harbor Symp Quant Biol 19:102–108.
28. Bradford JR, Dean HP (1889): On the innervation of the pulmonary vessels. J Physiol (Lond) 10:Pi–iv.
29. Bradford JR, Dean HP (1894): The pulmonary circulation. J Physiol (Lond) 16:34–96.
30. Brandt R, Dembinska-Kiec A, Korbut R, Gryglewski RJ, Nowak J (1984): Release of prostacyclin from the human pulmonary vascular bed in response to cholinergic stimulation. Naun-Schemid Arch Pharmacol 325:69–75.
31. Bressack MA, Bland RA (1981): Intravenous infusion of tolazoline reduces pulmonary vascular resistance and net fluid filtration in the lungs of awake, hypoxic newborn lambs. Am Rev Resp Dis 123:217–221.
32. Bronfman BL, Charms BL, Kohn PM, Elder J, Newman R, Rizika M (1959): Unilateral pulmonary artery occlusion in man. J Thorac Surg 34:206–227.
33. Brown DL, Guyenet PG (1985): Electrophysiological study of cardiovascular neurons in the rostral venterolateral medulla of the cat. Circ Res 56:359–369.
34. Burton AC, Patel DJ (1958): Effect on pulmonary vascular resistance of inflation of the rabbit lungs. J Appl Physiol 12:239–246.
35. Caeton AJ, Goetzman BW, Bennett SH, Millstein JM (1987): Effect of pulmonary hypertension on lung compliance in newborn lambs. Pediatr Pulmonol 3:324–327.
36. Campbell AGM, Cockburn F, Dawes GS, Milligan JE (1967): Pulmonary vasoconstriction in asphyxia during cross-circulation between twin foetal lambs. J Physiol (Lond) 192:111–121.
37. Campbell AGM, Dawes GS, Fishman AP, Hyman AI, Perks AM (1968): The release of bradykinin-like pulmonary vasodilator substance in foetal and newborn lambs. J Physiol (Lond) 195:83–96.
38. Casaba IF, Sulyok E, Hadnagy J (1977): Caesarean section and respiratory distress syndrome. Br Med J 1:977.
39. Cassin S (1983): Arachidonic acid metabolites and the pulmonary circulation of fetus and newborn. In MacLeod SM, Okey AB, Spielberg SP (eds): Developmental Pharmacology. New York, Alan R Liss Inc, pp 227–250.
40. Cassin S, Dawes GS, Mott JC, Ross BB, Strang LB (1964): The vascular resistance of the foetal and newly ventilated lung of the lamb. J Physiol (Lond) 171:61–79.

41. Cassin S, Dawes GS, Ross BB (1964): Pulmonary blood flow and vascular resistance in immature foetal lambs. J Physiol 171:80–89.

42. Cassin S, Tod M (1985): Arachidonic acid and the pressor response to hypoxia in perinatal and adult sheep. In Jones CT, Nathanielsz PW (eds): The Physiologic Development of the Fetus and Newborn. New York, Academic Press, pp 299–303.

43. Cassin S, Tod M, Philips J, Frisinger J, Jordan J, Gibbs C (1981): Effects of prostaglandin D_2 on perinatal circulation. Am J Physiol 240:H755–H760.

44. Cassin S, Tyler T, Leffler C, Wallis R (1979): Pulmonary and systemic vascular responses of perinatal goats to prostaglandins E_1 and E_2. Am J Physiol 236:H828–H832.

45. Cassin S, Tyler T, Wallis R (1975): The effects of prostaglandin E_1 on fetal pulmonary vascular resistance. Proc Soc Exp Biol Med 148:584–587.

46. Cassin S, Winikor I, Tod M, Philips J, Frisinger J, Jordan J, Gibbs C (1981): Effects of prostacyclin on the fetal pulmonary circulation. Pediatr Pharmacol 1:197–207.

47. Castro F de (1928): Sur la structure et l'innervation du sinus carotidien de l'homme et des mammiferes. Nouveaux faits sur l'innervation et la fonction du glomus caroticum. Trabajos Lab Invest Biol Univ Madrid 25:331–384.

48. Chander A, Dodia CR, Fisher AB (1988): Respiratory alkalosis and β-adrenergic agonist mediated increases in lung surfactant are additive. Am Rev Resp Dis 37:278A.

49. Clyman RI, Heymann MA, Mauray F (1985): Cardiopulmonary effects of a patent ductus arteriosus. Pediatr Res 19:92A.

50. Clyman RI, Jobe A, Heymann MA, Ikegami M, Roman C, Payne B, Mauray F (1982): Increased shunt through patent ductus arteriosus after surfactant replacement therapy. J Pediatr 100:101–107.

51. Clyman RI, Mauray F, Rudolph AM, Heymann MA (1980): Age-dependent sensitivity of the lamb ductus arteriosus to indomethacin and prostaglandins. J Pediatr 96:94–98.

52. Clyman RI, Mauray F, Heymann MA, Roman C (1988): PDA and pulmonary blood pressure. Pediatr Res 23:432A.

53. Coceani F, Olley PM, Lock JE (1980): Prostaglandins, ductus arteriosus, pulmonary circulation: Current concepts and clinical potential. Eur J Clin Pharmacol 18:75–81.

54. Colebatch HJH, Dawes GS, Goodwin JW, Nadeau RA (1965): The nervous control of the circulation in the foetal and newly expanded lungs of the lamb. J Physiol (Lond) 178:544–562.

55. Colebatch HJH, Halmagyi DFJ (1963): Reflex pulmonary hypertension of fresh-water aspiration. J Appl Physiol 18:179–185.

55a. Coleridge JCG, Kidd C (1960): Electrophysiological evidence of baroceptors in the pulmonary artery of the dog. J Physiol 150:319–326.

56. Coleridge JCG, Kidd C (1963): Reflex effects of stimulating baroreceptors in the pulmonary artery. J Physiol 166:197–210.

57. Comroe JH (1939): The location and function of the chemoreceptors of the aorta. Am J Physiol 27:176–191.

58. Cook CD, Drinker PA, Jacobson HN, Levison H, Strang LB (1963): Control of pulmonary blood flow in the fetal and newly born lamb. J Physiol 169:10–29.

59. Cotton RB, Lindstrom DP, Kanarek KS, Sundell H, Stahlman MJ (1980): Effect of positive end expiratory pressure on right ventricular output in lambs with hyaline membrane disease. Acta Pediatr Scand 69:603–606.

60. Cox RH, Peterson LH, Detweiler DK (1976): Hemodynamic responses to stellate ganglion stimulation in mongrels and greyhounds. Am J Physiol 231:1062–1067.

61. Crone RK (1984): The cardiovascular effects of isoproterenol in the preterm rabbit pup. Crit Care Med 12:33–35.

62. Custer JR, Hales CA (1986): Chemical sympathectomy decreases alveolar hypoxic vasoconstriction in lambs but not sheep. J Appl Physiol 60:32–37.

63. Custer JR, Hales CA (1985): Influence of alveolar oxygen on pulmonary vasoconstriction in newborn lambs versus sheep. Am Rev Resp Dis 132:326–331.

64. Daly IdB (1961): An analysis of active and passive effects on the pulmonary vascular bed in response to pulmonary nerve stimulation. Quart J Exp Physiol 46:257–271.

65. Daly IdB, Daly MdB (1957): Observations on the changes in resistance of the pulmonary vascular bed in response to stimula-

tion of the carotid sinus baroreceptors in the dog. J Physiol 137:427–435.

66. Daly IdB, Daly MdB (1959): The effects of stimulation of the carotid body chemoreceptors on the pulmonary vascular bed in the dog: The "vasosensory controlled perfused living animal" preparation. J Physiol 148:201–219.

67. Daly IdB, von Euler V (1931): The functional activity of the vasomotor nerves to the lungs in the dog. Proc R Soc Lond 60B:92–111.

68. Daly MdB, Scott MJ (1958): Effects of stimulation of the carotid body chemoreceptors on heart rate in the dog. J Physiol 144:148–166.

69. Daly MdB, Ungar A (1966): Comparison of the reflex responses elicited by stimulation of the separately perfused carotid and aortic body chemoreceptors in the dog. J Physiol 182:379–403.

70. Danilowicz D, Rudolph AM, Hoffman JIE (1966): Delayed closure of the ductus arteriosus in premature infants. Pediatrics 37:74–78.

71. Dauber IM, Weil JV (1983): Lung injury edema in dogs: Influence of sympathetic ablation. J Clin Invest 72:1977–1986.

72. Dawes GS, Mott JC (1962): The vascular tone of the foetal lung. J Physiol 164:465–477.

73. Dawes GS, Mott JC, Widdicombe JG, Wyatt DG (1953): Changes in the lungs of the newborn lamb. J Physiol 121:141–162.

74. Despasquale MP, Burch GE, Hyman AL (1965): Pulmonary venous response to immersion hypothermia and hyperthermia. Am Heart J 70:486–493.

75. Dickstein PJ, Trindad O, Goldberg RN, Bancalari E (1984): The effect of calcium antagonists on hypoxic pulmonary hypertension in the piglet. Pediatr Res 18:1252–1265.

76. Downing SE, Lee JC (1980): Nervous control of the pulmonary circulation. Ann Rev Physiol 42:199–210.

77. Eastman NJ (1930): Foetal blood studies. I. The oxygen relationships of umbilical cord blood at birth. Bull Johns Hopkins Hosp 47:221–230.

77a. Edwards JF, Berry E, Wyllie JH (1969): Release of prostaglandin caused by distention of the lungs. Br J Surg 56:622–623.

78. Eldridge FL, Hultgren HN, Wigmore ME (1954): The physiologic closure of the ductus arteriosus in newborn infants: A preliminary report. Science 119:731–732.

79. Eldridge FL, Hultgren HN, Wigmore ME (1955): The physiologic closure of the ductus arteriosus in the newborn infant. J Clin Invest 34:987–996.

80. Ellsworth ML, Gregory TJ, Newell JC (1983): Pulmonary prostacyclin production with increased flow and sympathetic stimulation. J Appl Physiol 55:1225–1231.

81. Emmanoulides GC, Moss AJ, Duffie ER Jr, Adams FH (1964): Pulmonary arterial pressure changes in human newborn infants from birth to 3 days of age. J Pediatr 65:327–333.

82. Engel G (1981): Subclasses of beta-adrenoreceptors—a quantitative estimation of $beta_1$- and $beta_2$-adrenoreceptors in guinea pig and human lung. Postgrad Med J 57S:77–83.

83. Enson Y, Giuntini C, Lewis ML, Morris TQ, Ferrer MI, Harvey RM (1964): The influence of hydrogen ion concentration and hypoxia on the pulmonary circulation. J Clin Invest 43:1146–1162.

84. von Euler US, Liljestrand G (1946): Observations on the pulmonary arterial blood pressure in the cat. Acta Physiol Scand 12:301–320.

85. Fiorentini C, Barbier P, Galli C, Loaldi A, Tamoborini G, Tosi E, Guazzi MD (1985): Pulmonary vascular overreactivity in systemic hypertension: A pathophysiological link between the greater and lesser circulation. Hypertension 7:885–1002.

86. Fishman AP (1986): Hypoxia on the pulmonary circulation: How and where it acts. Circ Res 38:221–231.

87. Fitzharris P, McLean AEM, Sparks RG, Weatherley BC, White RD, Wootton R (1985): The effects of BW 12C, a compound designed to left-shift the blood-oxygen saturation curve. Br J Clin Pharmacol 19:471–481.

88. Fouron J-C, Hebert F (1973): The circulatory effects of hematocrit variations in normovolemic newborn lambs. J Pediatr 82:995–1003.

89. Fouron J-C, Bard H, Riopel L, De Muylder X, Van Ameringen MR, Urfer F (1985): Circulatory changes in newborn lambs with experimental polycythemia. Comparison between fetal and adult type blood. Pediatr 75:1054–1060.

90. Fritts HW Jr, Harris P, Clauss RH, Odell JE, Cournand A (1958):

The effect of acetylcholine on the human pulmonary circulation under normal and hypoxic conditions. J Clin Inv 37:99–110.

91. Gabriel M, Hunneman DH, Gahr M (1983): Plasma levels of catecholamine metabolites in the newborn period. Biol Neonate 44:203–209.

92. Galleti PM, Salisbury PF, Rieben A (1958): Influence of blood temperature on the pulmonary circulation. Circ Res 6:275–282.

93. Ganten D, Land RE, Archelos J, Unger T (1984): Peptidergic systems: Effects on blood vessels. J Cardiovasc Pharmacol 6:S598–S607.

94. Gatto C, Johnson MG, Seybold V, Kulik TJ, Lock JE, Johnson DE (1984): Distribution and quantitative developmental change in guinea pig pulmonary beta receptors. J Appl Physiol 57:1901–1907.

95. Gessner I, Krovetz LJ, Benson RW, Prytowsky H, Stenger V, Eitzman V (1965): Hemodynamic alterations in the newborn infant. Pediatrics 36:752–762.

96. Gilbert RD, Hessler JR, Eitzman DV, Cassin S (1972): Site of pulmonary vascular resistance in fetal goats. J Appl Physiol 32:47–53.

97. Gillespie MN, Bowdy BD, Renisel CN, Iwamoto ET, Crooks PA (1964): Leu-enkephalin provokes naloxone-insensitive pulmonary vasoconstriction. Life Sci 34:1177–1183.

98. Gillespie MN, Renisel CN, Bowdy BD (1984): Pulmonary vasoactivity of endocrine cell-related peptides. Life Sci 34:1177–1183.

99. Gillis RA, Helke CJ, Hamilton BL, Norman WP, Jacobwitz DM (1980): Evidence that substance P is a neurotransmitter of baro- and chemoreceptor afferents in nucleus tractus solitarius. Brain Res 181:476–481.

100. Goetzman BW, Milstein JM (1979): Pulmonary vasodilator action of tolazoline. Pediatr Res 13:942–944.

101. Goldring RM, Turino GM, Cohen G, Jameson G, Bass BG, Fishman AP (1962): The catecholamines in the pulmonary arterial pressor response to acute hypoxia. J Clin Invest 41:1211–1212.

102. Griffin AJ, Ferrara JD, Lax JO, Cassels DE (1972): Pulmonary compliance. An index of cardiovascular status in infancy. Am J Dis Child 123:89–95.

103. Grimm DJ, Dawson CA, Hakim TS, Linehan JH (1978): Pulmonary vasomotion and the distribution of vascular resistance in a dog lung lobe. J Appl Physiol 45:545–550.

104. Grogaard J, Lindstrom DP, Marchal F, Stahlman MT, Sundell H (1982): The cardiovascular responses to laryngeal water administration in young lambs. J Dev Physiol 4:353–370.

105. Grogaard J, Sundell H (1983): Effect of beta adrenergic agonists on apnea reflexes in newborn lambs. Pediatr Res 17:213–219.

106. Grover RF, Okin JT, Overy HR, Treger A, Spracklen FHN (1965): Natural history of pulmonary hypertension in normal adult residents of high altitude (abstr). Circulation 32(Suppl II):102.

107. Grover RF, Vogel JHK, Voight GC, Blount SG (1966): Reversal of high altitude pulmonary hypertension. Am J Cardiol 18:928–932.

107a. Gryglewski RJ, Korbut R, Ocetkiewskiez A (1978): Generation of prostacyclin by lungs "in vivo" and its release into the arterial circulation. Nature 273:765–767.

108. Guyenet PG, Miao-Kun S, Brown DL (1987): Role of GABA and excitatory amino acids in medullary baroreflex pathways. In Organization of the Autonomic Nervous System: Central and Peripheral Mechanisms. New York, Alan R Liss Inc, pp 215–225.

109. Haas F, Bergofsky EH (1968): Effect of pulmonary vasoconstriction on balance between alveolar ventilation and perfusion. J Appl Physiol 24:491–497.

110. Hakim TS, Dawson CA (1979): Sympathetic nerve stimulation and vascular resistance in a pump-perfused dog lung lobe. Proc Soc Exp Biol Med 160:38–41.

111. Hales CA, Rouse E, Buchwald IA, Kazemi H (1977): Role of prostaglandins in alveolar hypoxic vasoconstriction. Res Physiol 29:151–162.

112. Halmagyi DFJ (1959): Role of the autonomous nervous system in the genesis of pulmonary hypertension in heart disease. J Chronic Dis 9:525–535.

113. Halmagyi DFJ, Colebatch HJH (1961): Ventilation and circulation after fluid aspiration. J Appl Physiol 16:35–40.

113a. Harris P (1957): Influence of acetylcholine on the pulmonary arterial pressure. Br Heart J 19:272–278.

114. Harris P, Segel N, Green I, Housley E (1968): The influence of the airways resistance and alveolar pressure on the pulmonary vascular resistance in chronic bronchitis. Cardiovasc Res 2:84–92.

114a. Harvey RM, Enson Y, Betti R, Lewis ML, Rochester DF, Ferrer MI (1967): Further observations on the effect of hydrogen ion on the pulmonary circulation. Circulation 35:1019–1027.

115. Harvey W (1628): Exercitatio Anatomica De Motu Cordis et Sanguinis In Animalibus. The Keynes Translation of 1928. Birmingham, The Classics of Medicine Library, 1978.

116. Hauge A (1969): Hypoxia and pulmonary vascular resistance: The relative effects of pulmonary arterial and alveolar pO_2. Acta Physiol Scand 76:121–130.

117. Hebb C (1969): Motor innervation of the pulmonary blood vessels of mammals. In Fishman AP, Hecht HH (eds): The Pulmonary Circulation and Interstitial Space. Chicago, The University of Chicago Press, pp 195–222.

118. Hedquist P (1976): Further evidence that prostaglandins inhibit the release of noradrenaline from adrenergic nerve terminals by restriction of available calcium. Br J Pharmacol 58:599–603.

119. Hedquist P (1977): Basic mechanisms of prostaglandin action on autonomic neurotransmission. Am Rev Pharmacol Toxicol 17:259–279.

120. Herman AG, Verburuen TJ, Moncada S, Vanhoutte PM (1978): Effect of prostacyclin on myogenic activity and adrenergic neuroeffector interaction in canine isolated veins. Prostaglandins 16:911–921.

121. Heymann MA (1984): Control of the pulmonary circulation in the perinatal period. J Devel Physiol 6:281–290.

122. Heymann MA, Rudolph AM, Nies AS, Melmon KL (1969): Bradykinin production associated with oxygenation of the fetal lamb. Circ Res 25:521–534.

123. Heymans J-F, Heymans C (1927): Sur les modifications directes et sur la regulation reflexe de l'activite du centre respiratoire de la tête isolée du chien. Arch Int Pharmacodynam 33:272–370.

124. Hofer MA (1984): Lethal respiratory disturbance in neonatal rats after arterial chemoreceptor denervation. Life Sci 34:489–496.

125. Howell JBL, Permutt S, Proctor DF, Riley RL (1961): Effect of inflation of the lung on different parts of pulmonary vascular bed. J Appl Physiol 16:71–76.

126. Hyman AL (1969): The active responses of pulmonary veins in intact dogs to prostaglandins F_2-alpha and E_1. J Pharmacol Exp Ther 165:267–273.

127. Hyman AL, Higashi RT, Spannhake EW, Kadowitz PJ (1981): Pulmonary vasoconstrictor responses to graded decreases in precapillary blood PO_2 in intact chest cats. J Appl Physiol 51:1009–1016.

128. Hyman AL, Kadowitz PJ (1975): Effects of alveolar and perfusion hypoxia and hypercapnia on pulmonary vascular resistance in the lamb. Am J Physiol 228:397–403.

129. Hyman AL, Kadowitz PJ (1984): Analysis of responses to leukotriene D4 in the pulmonary vascular bed. Circ Res 55:707–717.

130. Hyman AL, Kadowitz PJ (1986): Enhancement of α- and β-adrenoreceptor responses by elevations in vascular tone in pulmonary circulation. Am J Physiol 250:H1109–H1116.

131. Hyman AL, Lippton HL, Kadowitz PJ (1985): Autonomic regulation of the pulmonary circulation. J Cardiovas Pharmacol 7S:S80–S95.

132. Iacopino VJ, Compton S, Fitzpatrick T, Ramwell P, Rose J, Kot P (1984): Responses to leukotriene C4 in the perfused rat lung. J Exp Pharmacol Ther 229:654–657.

133. Ingram RH, Szidon JP, Skalak R, Fishman AP (1968): Effects of sympathetic nerve stimulation on the pulmonary arterial tree of the isolated lobe perfused in situ. Circ Res 22:801–815.

133a. Jacobs J, Gluck L, Disessa J, Edwards D, Kulovich M, Kurlinski J, Merritt TA, Friedman WF (1980): The contribution of PDA in the neonate with severe RDS. J Pediatr 96:79–87.

134. James LS, Rowe RD (1957): The pattern of response of pulmonary and systemic arterial pressures in newborn and older infants to short periods of hypoxia. J Pediatr 51:5–11.

135. Janicki JS, Weber KT, Likoff MJ, Fishman AP (1985): The pressure-flow response of the pulmonary circulation in patients with heart failure and pulmonary vascular disease. Circulation 72:1270–1278.

136. Jacobstein MD, Hirschfield SS, Flinn C, Riggs T, Fanaroff A (1982): Neonatal circulatory changes following elective cesarean section: An echocardiographic study. Pediatrics 69:374–376.

137. Johansson B (1974): Determinants of vascular reactivity. Fed Proc 33:121–126.

138a. Julien M, Hakim TS, Vahi R, Chang HK (1985): Effect of hematocrit on vascular pressure profile in dog lungs. J Appl Physiol 58:743–748.

138. Juratsch CE, Jengo JA, Laks MM (1977): Role of the autonomic nervous system and pulmonary artery receptors in production of experimental pulmonary hypertension. Chest 71S:265–269.

139. Kadowitz PJ, Joiner PD, Hyman AL (1975): Influence of sympathetic stimulation and vasoactive substances on the canine pulmonary veins. J Clin Invest 56:354–365.

140. Kadowitz PJ, Hyman AL (1984): Analysis of responses to leukotriene D4 in the pulmonary vascular bed. Circ Res 55:707–717.

141. Kadowitz PJ, Spannhake EW, Levin JL, Hyman AL (1980): Differential actions of the prostaglandins on the pulmonary vascular bed. Adv Prostaglandin Thrombox Res 7:731–743.

142. Kuhn LH, Turner J (1959): Alteration in pulmonary and peripheral vascular resistance in immersion hypothermia. Circ Res 7:366–374.

143. Kulik TJ, Johnson DE, Elde RP, Locke JE (1984): Pulmonary vascular effects of vasoactive intestinal peptide in conscious newborn lambs. Am J Physiol 246:H716–H719.

144. Lagneaux D (1986): Relation between peripheral chemoreceptors stimulation and pulmonary arterial pressure in rats. Arch Int Physiol Biochim 94:127–134.

145. Laks MM, Jurastch CE, Garner D, Beazell J, Criley JM (1975): Acute pulmonary artery hypertension produced by distention of the main pulmonary artery of the conscious dog. Chest 68:807–813.

146. Lauer RM, Evans JA, Aoki M, Kittle CF (1965): Factors controlling pulmonary vascular resistance in fetal lambs. J Pediatr 67:568–577.

147. Lauweryns JM, De Bock V, Guelinckx P, Decramer M (1983): Effects of unilateral hypoxia on neuroepithelial bodies in rabbit lungs. J Appl Physiol 55:1665–1668.

148. Lawson EE, Birdwell RL, Huang PS, Taeusch HW Jr (1979): Augmentation of pulmonary surfactant secretion by lung expansion at birth. Pediatr Res 13:611–614.

149. Lees MH, Way C, Ross BB (1967): Ventilation and respiratory gas transfer of infants with increased pulmonary blood flow. Pediatr 40:259–271.

149a. Leffler CW, Hessler JR (1981): Prostacyclin is synthesized by fetal lung in response to ventilation with air. Fed Proc 40:591A.

150. Leffler CW, Hessler JR, Terrango NA (1980): Ventilation-induced release of prostaglandin-like material from fetal lungs. Am J Physiol 238:H282–H286.

151. Leffler CW, Mitchell JA, Green RS (1984): Cardiovascular effects of leukotrienes in neonatal piglets. Circ Res 66:780–787.

152. Leffler CW, Tyler TL, Cassin S (1978): Effect of indomethacin on pulmonary vascular response to ventilation in fetal goats. Am J Physiol 234:H346–H351.

153. Leffler CW, Tyler TL, Cassin S (1979): Responses of pulmonary and systemic circulations of perinatal goats to prostaglandin F2alpha. Can J Physiol Pharm 57:167–173.

153a. Lewis AB, Heymann MA, Rudolph AM (1976): Gestational changes in pulmonary vascular responses in fetal lambs in utero. Circ Res 39:536–541.

154. Liljestrand G (1958): Chemical control of the distribution of the pulmonary blood flow. Acta Physiol Scand 44:216–240.

155. Lind J (1977): Eleventh Edgar Mannheimer Lecture. Human fetal and neonatal circulation. Some structural and functional aspects. Eur J Cardiol 5:265–281.

156. Lind J, Wegelius C (1954): Human fetal circulation: Changes in the cardiovascular system at birth and disturbance of postnatal closure of the foramen ovale and ductus arteriosus. Quant Biol 19:109–125.

157. Lister G (1984): Oxygen transport in the intact hypoxic newborn lamb: Acute effects of increasing P50. Pediatr Res 18:172–177.

158. Lister G, Hellenbrand WE, Kleiman CS, Talner NS (1982): Physiologic effects of increasing hemoglobin concentration in left-to-right shunting in infants with ventricular septal defects. N Eng J Med 306:502–506.

159. Lister G, Moreau G, Moss M, Talner NS (1984): Effects of alterations of oxygen transport on the neonate. Semin Perinatol 8:192–204.

160. Lloyd T (1964): Effect of alveolar hypoxia on pulmonary vascular resistance. J Appl Physiol 19:1086–1094.

161. Locke JE, Coceani F, Olley PM (1979): Direct and indirect effects of tolazoline in the newborn lamb. J Pediatr 96:600–605.

162. Locke JE, Hamilton F, Luide H, Coceani F, Olley P (1980): Direct pulmonary vascular responses in the conscious newborn lamb. J Appl Physiol 48:188–196.

163. Locke JE, Olley PM, Coceani F (1981): Enhanced beta-adrenergic function in fetal sheep. Am J Obstet Gynecol 112:1114–1121.

164. Lohr H (1924): Untersuchungen zur physiologie und pharmakologie der lunge. Z Ges Exp Med 32:67–130.

165. Long WA (1987): Superior laryngeal nerve–induced reflex pulmonary hypertension in neonatal piglets. Am Rev Resp Dis 135:A299.

166. Long WA (1987): Effects of chemoreceptor sectioning on hypoxia induced pulmonary hypertension. Am Rev Resp Dis 135:A520.

167. Long WA (1989): Persistent pulmonary hypertension of the newborn syndrome. In Long WA (ed): Fetal and Neonatal Cardiology. Philadelphia, WB Saunders Co.

168. Long WA, Brown DL (in press): Central neural regulation of the pulmonary circulation. In Fishman AP (ed): Pulmonary Circulation. Normal and Abnormal. Philadelphia, University of Pennsylvania Press.

169. Long WA, Rubin LJ (1987): Prostacyclin and PGE1 treatment of pulmonary hypertension. Am Rev Resp Dis 136:773–776.

170. Lovick TA, Hilton SM (1986): Vasodilator and vasoconstrictor neurones of the ventrolateral medulla in the cat. Brain Res 331:353–357.

171. Lyrene RK, Welch KA, Godoy G, Philips JB III (1985): Alkalosis attenuates hypoxic pulmonary vasoconstriction in neonatal lambs. Pediatr Res 19:1268–1271.

172. Malik AB, Kidd BSL (1973): Adrenergic blockade and the pulmonary vascular response to hypoxia. Res Physiol 19:96–106.

173. Malik AB (1985): Mechanisms of neurogenic pulmonary edema. Circ Res 57:1–18.

174. McKenzie JC, Klein RM (1984): The effect of neonatal guanethidine administration on hemodynamic and physical alterations in the adult rat pulmonary artery during the development of hypoxia-induced pulmonary hypertension. J Auton Nerv Syst 10:199–203.

175. McLean JR, Twarog BM, Bergofsky EH (1985): The adrenergic innervation of pulmonary vasculature in the normal and pulmonary hypertensive rat. J Auton Nerv Syst 14:111–123.

176. Milstein JM, Goetzman BW, Riemenschneider TA, Wennberg RP (1979): Increased systemic vascular resistance in neonates with pulmonary hypertension. Am J Cardiol 44:1159–1162.

177. Morganroth ML, Reeves JT, Murphy RC, Voelkel NF (1984): Leukotriene synthesis and receptor blockers block hypoxic pulmonary vasoconstriction. J Appl Physiol 56:1340–1346.

178. Morin FC III (1986): Hyperventilation, alkalosis, prostaglandins, and pulmonary circulation of the newborn. J Appl Physiol 61:2088–2094.

178a. Murray JF, Karp RB, Nadel JA (1969): Viscosity effects on pressure-flow relations and vascular resistance in dogs' lungs. J Appl Physiol 27:336–341.

179. Naeye RL (1965): Children at high altitude: Pulmonary and renal abnormalities. Circ Res 16:33–38.

179a. Nasjletti A, Malik KU (1979): Relationships between the kallikrein-kinin and prostaglandin systems. Life Sci 25:99–110.

180. Naulty CM, Horn S, Conry J, Avery GB (1978): Improved lung compliance after ligation of patent ductus arteriosus in hyaline membrane disease. J Pediatr 93:682–684.

181. Neri Serneri GG, Masotti G, Castellani S, Scarti L, Trotta F, Mannelli M (1983): Role of PGE2 in the modulation of the adrenergic response in man. Cardiovasc Res 17:662–670.

182. Nieman GF, Hakim TS, Bredenberg CE (1988): Effect of increased alveolar surface tension on segmental pulmonary vascular resistance. J Appl Physiol 64:154–161.

183. Nishi K, Sakanashi M, Takenaka F (1974): Afferent fibres from pulmonary arterial baroreceptors in the left cardiac sympathetic nerve of the cat. J Physiol (Lond) 240:53–66.

184. Nisell O (1948): The action of oxygen and carbon dioxide on the circulation of isolated and perfused lungs of the cat. Acta Physiol Scand 16:121–127.

185. Noonan TC, Malik AB (1986): Pulmonary vascular responses to leukotriene D4 in unanesthetized sheep: Role of thromboxane. J Appl Physiol 60:765–769.

186. Nowak J (1984): Eicosanoids and the lungs. Ann Clin Res 16:269–286.

187. Olley PM, Coceani F (1980): Use of prostaglandins in cardiopulmonary diseases of the newborn. Semin Perinatol 4:131–141.

188. Olley PM, Coceani F (1984): The biochemistry and characteristics of the prostaglandins: Possible therapeutic implications in persistent fetal circulation. In Sandor GS, McNab AJ, Rastogi RB (eds): Persistent Fetal Circulation: Etiology, Clinical Aspects, and Therapy. Mt. Kisco, Futura Media Services, pp 127–140.

189. Olson NC, Robinson NE, Scott JB (1983): Effects of brain hypoxia on pulmonary hemodynamics. J Surg Res 35:21–27.

190. Osorio J, Russek M (1962): Reflex changes on the pulmonary and systemic pressures elicited by stimulation of the baroreceptors of the pulmonary artery. Circ Res 10:664–667.

191. Pace JB (1978): Influence of carotid occlusion on pulmonary vascular resistance in anesthetized dog. Proc Soc Exp Biol Med 158:215–219.

192. Penaloza D, Sime F, Banchero N, Gamboa R (1963): Pulmonary hypertension in healthy men born and living at high altitudes. In Grover RF (ed): Normal and Abnormal Pulmonary Circulation. Basel, S Karger, p 257.

193. Peterson MB, Huttemeuerm PC, Zapol WM, Martin EG, Watkins DW (1982): Thromboxane mediates acute pulmonary hypertension in sheep extracorporeal perfusion. Am J Physiol 243:H471–H479.

194. Philips JB (1984): Prostaglandins and related compounds in the perinatal pulmonary circulation. Pediatr Pharmacol 4:129–142.

195. Philips JB III, Lyrene RK, McDevitt M, Perlis W, Satterwhite C, Cassady G (1983): Prostaglandin D$_2$ inhibits hypoxic pulmonary vasoconstriction in neonatal lambs. J Appl Physiol 54:1585–1589.

196. Plumier L (1904): La circulation pulmonaire chez la chien. Arch Int Physiol 1:176–213.

197. Porcelli RJ, Bergofsky EH (1973): Adrenergic receptors in pulmonary vasoconstrictor responses to gaseous and humoral agents. J Appl Physiol 34:483–488.

198. Redding GJ, McMurtry I, Reeves JT (1984): Effects of meclofenamate on pulmonary vascular resistance correlate with postnatal age in young piglets. Pediatr Res 18:579–583.

199. Reeves JT, Leathers JE (1964): Circulatory changes following birth of the calf and the effect of hypoxia. Circ Res 15:343–354.

201. Reeves JT, Leathers JE, Eisman B, Spencer FC (1962): Alveolar hypoxia versus hypoxemia in the development of pulmonary hypertension. Med Thorac 19: 561–572.

202. Rendas A, Brathwaite M, Reid L (1978): Growth of pulmonary circulation in normal pig—structural analysis and cardiopulmonary function. J Appl Physiol 45:806–817.

202a. Ricaby DA, Dawson CA, Marion MB (1980): Pulmonary inactivation of serotonin and site of serotonin pulmonary vasoconstriction. J Appl Physiol 48:606–612.

203. Riopel L, Fouron JC, Bard H (1982): Blood viscosity during the neonatal period: The role of plasma and red blood cell type. J Pediatr 100:449–453.

204. Riopel L, Fouron JC, Bard H (1983): A comparison of blood viscosity between the adult sheep and newborn lamb: The role of plasma and red blood cell type. Pediatr Res 17:452–455.

205. Rowe RD, James LS (1957): The normal pulmonary arterial pressure during the first year of life. J Pediatr 51:1–4.

205a. Rubin LJ, Hughes JD (1984): Relation between mixed venous oxygen tension and pulmonary vascular tone during normoxic, hyperoxic, and hypoxic ventilation in dogs. Am J Cardiol 54:1118–1123.

206. Rudolph AM (1977): Fetal and neonatal pulmonary circulation. Am Rev Resp Dis 115:11–18.

207. Rudolph AM (1979): Fetal and neonatal pulmonary circulation. Ann Rev Physiol 41:383–395.

207a. Rudolph AM, Drorbaugh JE, Auld PAM, Rudolph AJ, Nadas AS, Smith CA, Hubbell JP (1961): Studies on the circulation in the newborn period. The circulation in the respiratory distress syndrome. Pediatr 27:551–556.

208. Rudolph AM, Auld PAM, Golinko RJ, Paul MH (1964): Pulmonary vascular adjustments in the neonatal period. Pediatr 28:28–34.

209. Rudolph AM, Yuan A (1966): Response of the pulmonary vasculature to hypoxia and H$^+$ ion concentration changes. J Clin Invest 45:399–411.

210. Said SI (1982): Pulmonary metabolism of prostaglandins and vasoactive peptides. Ann Rev Physiol 44:257–268.

211. Schreiber MD, Heymann MA, Soifer SJ (1986): Increased arterial pH, not decreased PaCO$_2$, attenuates hypoxia-induced pulmonary vasoconstriction in newborn lambs. Pediatr Res 20:113–117.

212. Shoukas AA, Brunner MJ, Frankle AE, Greene, AS, Kallman CH (1984): Carotid sinus baroreceptor reflex control and the role of autoregulation in the systemic and pulmonary arterial pressure-flow relationships of the dog. Circ Res 54:674–682.

213. Shutack JG, Moomian AS, Wagner HR, Peckham GJ, Fox WW (1979): Severe obstructive airway disease associated with pulmonary artery hypertension in the neonate. Pediatr Res 13:541A.

214. Sideris EB, Yokochi K, Van Helder T, Coceani F, Olley PM (1983): Effects of indomethacin, and prostaglandins E$_2$, I$_2$, and D$_2$ on the fetal circulation. Adv Prostaglandin Thromboxane Leukotriene Res 12:477–482.

215. Sime F, Banchero N, Penaloza D, Gambia R, Cruz J, Marticorena E (1963): Pulmonary hypertension in children born and living at high altitudes. Am J Cardiol 11:143–149.

216. Soifer SJ, Loitz RD, Roman C, Heymann MA (1985): Leukotriene end organ antagonists increase pulmonary blood flow in fetal lambs. Am J Physiol 249:H570–H576.

217. Soifer SJ, Morin FC III, Heymann MA (1982): Prostaglandin D$_2$ reverses hypoxia-induced pulmonary hypertension in the newborn lamb. J Pediatr 100:458–463.

218. Soifer SJ, Morin FC III, Kaslow DC, Heymann MA (1983): The developmental effects of PGD$_2$ on the pulmonary and systemic circulations in the newborn lamb. J Develop Physiol 5:237–250.

219. Spannhake EW, Lemen RJ, Wegmann MJ, Hyman AL, Kadowitz PJ (1978): Effects of arachidonic acid and prostaglandins on lung function in the intact dog. J Appl Physiol 44:397–405.

220. Sprague RS, Stephenson AH, Heitmann LJ, Lonigro AJ (1984): Differential response of the pulmonary circulation to prostaglandins E$_2$ and F$_{2\alpha}$ in the presence of unilateral alveolar hypoxia. J Pharmacol Exp Ther 229:38–43.

220a. Stahlman M, Blakenship WJ, Shepard FM, Gray J, Young WC, Malon AF (1973): Circulatory studies in clinical hyaline membrane disease. Biol Neonate 20:300–320.

221. Starling MB, Neutze JM, Elliott RL (1979): Control of elevated pulmonary vascular resistance in neonatal swine with prostacyclin (PGI$_2$): Prostaglandins Med 3:105–117.

222. Starling MB, Neutze JM, Elliott RL, Elliott RB (1976): Studies of the effects of prostglandins E$_1$, E$_2$, A$_1$, and A$_2$ on the ductus arteriosus of swine in vivo using cineangiography. Prostaglandins 12:355–367.

223. Starling MB, Neutze JM, Elliott RL, Elliott RB (1981): Comparative studies of the hemodynamic effects of prostaglandin E$_1$, prostacyclin, and tolazoline upon elevated pulmonary vascular resistance in neonatal swine. Prostaglandins Med 7:349–361.

224. Stern S, Braun K (1965): Effect of chemoreceptor stimulation on the pulmonary veins. Am J Physiol 210:535–539.

225. Stern S, Braun K (1970): Pulmonary arterial and venous response to cooling: Role of alpha adrenergic receptors. Am J Physiol 219:982–985.

226. Stern S, Ferguson RE, Rappaport E (1964): Reflex pulmonary vasoconstriction due to stimulation of the aortic body by nicotine. Am J Physiol 206:1189–1195.

227. Szidon JP, Fishman AP (1969): Autonomic control of the pulmonary circulation. In Fishman AP, Hecht HH (eds): The Pulmonary Circulation and Interstitial Space. Chicago, The University of Chicago Press, pp 239–268.

228. Szidon JP, Fishman AP (1971): Participation of pulmonary circulation in the defense reaction. Am J Physiol 220:364–370.

229. Szidon JP, Flint JF (1977): Significance of sympathetic innervation of pulmonary vessels in response to acute hypoxia. J Appl Physiol 43:65–71.

230. Thilenius OG, Candiolo BM, Beug JL (1967): Effect of adrenergic blockade on hypoxia-induced pulmonary vasoconstriction in awake dogs. Am J Physiol 213:990–998.

231. Thoraldson J, Ilebekk A, Kiil F (1985): Determinants of pulmonary blood volume. Effects of acute changes in airway pressure. Acta Physiol Scand 125:471–479.
232. Tod ML, Cassin S (1984): Perinatal pulmonary responses to arachidonic acid during normoxia and hypoxia. J Appl Physiol 57:977–983.
233. Tod ML, Cassin S (1985): Thromboxane synthase inhibition and perinatal pulmonary response to arachidonic acid. J Appl Physiol 58:710–716.
234. Tod ML, Cassin S, McNamara DB, Kadowitz PJ (1986): Effects of prostaglandin H_2 on perinatal pulmonary circulation. Pediatr Res 20:565–569.
235. Tolins M, Weir K, Chesler E, Nelson DP, From AHL (1986): Pulmonary vascular tone is increased by a voltage-dependent calcium channel potentiator. J Appl Physiol 60:942–948.
236. Tong EY, Mathe' AA, Tusher PW (1978): Release of norepinephrine by sympathetic nerve stimulation from rabbit lungs. Am J Physiol 235:H803–H808.
237. Torok TL, Bunyevac Z, Nguyen TT, Hadhazy P, Magyar K, Vizi ES (1984): The inhibitory action of $PGF_{2\alpha}$ on release of [H3]noradrenaline enhanced by α_2-adrenergic blockade, sodium pump inhibition and 4-aminopyridine in the main pulmonary artery of the rabbit. Neuropharmacology 23:37–41.
238. Venkataraman ST, Fuhrman BP, Howland DF (1988): Air trapping during mechanical ventilation raises pulmonary vascular tone in neonatal lungs. Pediatr Res 23:529A.
239. Viveros OH, Diliberto EJ Jr, Hazum E, Chang KJ (1979): Opiate-like material in the adrenal medulla: Evidence for storage and secretion with catecholamines. Mol Pharmacol 16:1101–1108.
240. Weitzell R, Steppeler A, Starke K (1978): Effects of prostaglandin E_2, I_2, and 6-keto prostaglandin $F_{1\alpha}$ on adrenergic neurotransmission in the pulmonary artery of the rabbit. Eur J Pharmacol 52:137–141.
241. Whittenberger JL, McGregor M, Berglund EW, Borst HG (1960): Influence of the state of inflation of the lung on pulmonary vascular resistance. J Appl Physiol 15:878–882.
242. Wilcox BR, Autin WG, Bender HW (1964): Effect of hypoxia on pulmonary artery pressure in dogs. Am J Physiol 207:1314–1318.
243. Yeh TF, Thalji A, Luken L, Lilien L, Carr I, Pildes RS (1981): Improved lung compliance following indomethacin therapy in premature infants with persistent ductus arteriosus. Chest 80:698–700.

8 NEONATAL GAS EXCHANGE AND OXYGEN TRANSPORT

Enid R. Kafer

Delivery of adequate oxygen to the tissues and removal of metabolic products are critical at all stages of development. The respiratory, cardiovascular, and endocrine systems must interact efficiently but quite differently during fetal, neonatal, and adult life to supply adequate oxygen and to remove metabolic products, particularly during times of stress. At birth, major changes occur in these systems as well as in metabolism. Further, following birth, changes in these systems and in the erythrocyte and hemoglobin structure continue.[17,33,40,75,94,107,108,109,142] Impairments in the maturation of any components of the systems responsible for oxygen transport and metabolic removal necessitate compensary changes by other organ systems. The ability to compensate for impaired function is a test of the biologic characteristics of the organism as well as its maturation.[33,37,75,94]

This chapter will discuss metabolism, gas exchange, hemodynamic functions, and the red cell, focusing on the end product, oxygen delivery, and the ability of the supporting systems to compensate for individual and multisystem impairment. A list of abbreviations is provided at the end of the chapter.

METABOLIC RATE AND OXYGEN TRANSPORT

Metabolism and Oxygen Consumption

Metabolic rate, which is measured as oxygen consumption ($\dot{V}O_2$) is high in the neonate compared with the adult. In sheep, in which accurate data are available, neonatal metabolic rate is also higher than the fetal rate (Table 8–1).[2,23,34,75,76] The components of energy expenditure and therefore oxygen consumption are basal metabolic rate, specific dynamic energy of food, physical activity, and heat production. The basal metabolic rate of the newborn includes a relatively large expenditure for growth.[52] In the lamb, which is an animal that grows rapidly, estimates of the growth component of the basal metabolic rate are as high as 30 to 35 per cent.[112] In comparison, in neonates with slower growth rates, only 2 to 3 per cent of the $\dot{V}O_2$ is attributed to growth, except in the premature neonate, in which the percentage is higher.[16,52] However, the variability of measured $\dot{V}O_2$ within and between subjects in the neonate is large,[114] particularly when the duration of measurements is brief.[1,141] The $\dot{V}O_2$ of the neonate rapidly increases with activity (Table 8–2),[16,141] place-

I gratefully acknowledge the secretarial support of Diena Burton and the artistic excellence of Ann Jennings, Medical Illustration.

ment in a nonthermoneutral environment,[112] therapeutic and diagnostic procedures (Table 8–2),[141] and increased work of breathing. The $\dot{V}O_2$ for respiratory work is normally a small fraction of the metabolic rate. However, when mechanical abnormalities or ventilatory compensation for ventilation–blood flow maldistribution increases the work of breathing, the work of breathing may constitute more than 20 per cent of the metabolic rate.[22] In experimental studies in normothermic lambs placed in a cool environment ($17.4 \pm 1.1°C$), the $\dot{V}O_2$ increased by 40 per cent from 14.9 to 20.8 $ml \cdot kg^{-1} \cdot min^{-1}$.[112] In addition there were increases in arteriovenous oxygen content difference ($a\bar{v}O_2D$) of 19 per cent, cardiac output (CO) of 18 per cent and heart rate (HR) of 14 per cent. However, severe hypoxemia or hypothermia or both depress the responses to cold exposure and result in a decrease in the metabolic rate. During experimental exposure of normothermic lambs to both cool environment and hypoxemia, the $\dot{V}O_2$ decreased, and the increases in the cardiac output and heart rate were reduced.[112] Therefore, as a result of hypoxemic impairment of the thermogenic response to a cool environment, the core temperature decreases during hypoxemia. Both severe cyanotic congenital heart disease and exposure to hypoxic gas mixtures are also associated with a reduced $\dot{V}O_2$.[25,60,73] In infants with severe cyanotic congenital heart disease ($PaO_2 = 21$ mmHg), the $\dot{V}O_2$ was 3.14 $ml \cdot min^{-1} \cdot kg^{-1}$, whereas with less severe cyanotic congenital heart disease ($PaO_2 = 27$ mmHg), the $\dot{V}O_2$ was 7.70 $ml \cdot min^{-1} \cdot kg^{-1}$. The thermogenic response was also reduced in some infants with cyanotic congenital heart disease.[60]

Oxygen Transport

The oxygen availability (AVO_2), which is the product of the cardiac output and the arterial oxygen content, is also elevated in the neonate (Table 8–1). The estimated oxygen delivery in the resting neonate (33 $ml \cdot min^{-1} \cdot kg^{-1}$) is 75 per cent higher than in the adult (Table 8–1).[75] However, because of the limits of invasive monitoring in normal human neonates, more comprehensive information on the normal and compensatory responses to impaired oxygen transport is available from animal models such as the lamb. Therefore, this review of the effects of and compensatory cardiovascular responses to impaired oxygen transport will be based on experimental studies in the lamb. The neonatal lamb, however, differs from the human neonate, and those differences include a lower hematocrit.[75] Therefore, data obtained from experimental studies in the lamb should be applied to the human neonate with caution.

Table 8–1. THE RELATIONSHIP AMONG BODY WEIGHT, FRC, OXYGEN CONSUMPTION, AND OXYGEN AVAILABILITY IN THE NEAR-TERM FETUS, NEONATE, AND ADULT

Species (Age)	Weight (kg)	FRC (ml)	Cardiac Output ($ml \cdot min^{-1} \cdot kg^{-1}$)	Oxygen Consumption ($ml \cdot min^{-1} \cdot kg^{-1}$)	Oxygen Availability ($ml \cdot min^{-1} \cdot kg^{-1}$)
Human					
Near-term fetus	3.2		500	8 ± 1.4	–
Neonate	3.0	80 (26.7)	400	6 ± 1.1	33
Adult	75.0	3000 (40.0)	100	3 ± 0.6	19
Sheep					
Near-term fetus	3.5		400	7.3	22
Lamb (1 month)	4.0		250	15.0	50
Adult sheep	70.0		100	4.5	10

Notes: Mean $\pm$ SD. The FRC values in parenthesis are expressed as $ml \cdot kg^{-1}$. Sources: Adams and Lind, 1957;[2] Crone, 1983;[23] Emmanoulides et al, 1970;[34] and Lister et al, 1979, 1984.[75,76]

Impaired Oxygen Availability and Increased Demand

Three major processes impair oxygen availability. They are (1) hypoxemia resulting from ventilation–blood flow maldistribution or shunt or both, or experimentally, hypoxemia is induced by administration of a hypoxic gas mixture; (2) reduced oxygen binding capacity as a result of reduced hemoglobin (THB) or increased dyshemoglobins, e.g., carboxyhemoglobin (COHb); and (3) reduced cardiac output. In addition, the inability of the oxygen transport system to compensate for an increased metabolic rate and the resulting reduced mixed venous oxyhemoglobin saturation ($S\bar{v}O_2$) and increased alveolar-arterial oxygen pressure difference (AaO_2P) become self-perpetuating when pulmonary or intracardiac right-to-left shunts are present, and further hypoxemia and impaired oxygen transport result.[59,129,130]

Qualitatively, the cardiovascular, endocrine, and respiratory responses to impaired oxygen transport in the neonate are similar to those in the adult.[17,32,33,37,40,55,75,118] For example, a reduction in cardiac output results in a redistribution of blood flow, with preservation of flow to the heart and brain and reduction in blood flow to the kidneys and the splanchnic areas. In addition, whole body oxygen extraction increases, and the $a\bar{v}O_2D$ widens; as a result, $S\bar{v}O_2$ decreases and AaO_2P increases. Eventually, $\dot{V}O_2$ decreases and becomes dependent on oxygen transport. However, it is argued that the high values of cardiac output, $\dot{V}O_2$, and AVO_2 in the neonate indicate that the

neonate is physiologically near the maxima of those variables, and thus the neonate has limited reserve.[107,108] Therefore, when the compensation for impaired oxygen transport involves an increase in cardiac output, the maximum is rapidly reached, and further oxygen demands are associated with an increase in oxygen extraction ratio, $a\bar{v}O_2D$, and a decrease in the $S\bar{v}O_2$, with the ensuing events as described above.[59,129,130]

Hypoxemia

In normal awake lambs (1 to 7 days old), hypoxemia induced by breathing an F_IO_2 of 0.1 ($PaO_2 = 31 \pm 4$ mmHg) resulted in *decreases* in $\dot{V}O_2$, $a\bar{v}O_2D$, AVO_2 and system vascular resistance (SVR) and an *increase* in oxygen extraction from 44 per cent to 65 per cent (Table 8–3).[74] Although there were increases in both the CO and the HR, the increase in the CO was not statistically significant. The decrease in $a\bar{v}O_2D$ was therefore the result of the decrease in $\dot{V}O_2$. The critical PO_2, or oxygen availability at which the $\dot{V}O_2$ becomes dependent on oxygen delivery, was not examined. However, following exchange transfusion that resulted in an increase in the P_{50}, CO, stroke volume (SV) and oxygen extraction were increased, and the $\dot{V}O_2$ was not significantly different from normoxia (Table 8–3). Return to normoxia was associated with normalization of the $\dot{V}O_2$, CO, SV, AVO_2, and $P\bar{v}O_2$, and an increase in the $a\bar{v}O_2D$ (5.60 ± 0.92 versus pretransfusion normoxia of 4.91 $ml \cdot dl^{-1}$). Therefore, the P_{50} and the associated oxygen release in the myocar-

Table 8–2. EFFECT OF DIAGNOSTIC AND THERAPEUTIC PROCEDURES ON THE METABOLIC RATE IN PREMATURE NEONATES

Physical State (Procedure)	Oxygen Consumption Average ($ml \cdot min^{-1} \cdot kg^{-1}$)	Oxygen Consumption Peak ($ml \cdot min^{-1} \cdot kg^{-1}$)
Resting	6.2 ± 1.5	–
Chest therapy	8.0 ± 2.0	14.8 ± 1.6
Heel stick	9.4 ± 1.5	16.8 ± 3.2
IV insertion	9.8 ± 1.6	18.6 ± 4.3

Notes: Mean $\pm$ SD, n = 10; age = 32 weeks' gestation; body weight = 1.32 ± 0.37 kg. (Adapted with permission from S Karger AG, Basel. From Yeh TF et al [1984]: Increased O_2 consumption and energy loss in premature infants following medical care procedures. Biol Neonate 46:157–162.)

Table 8–3. OXYGEN TRANSPORT: COMPARISON OF THE EFFECTS OF HYPOXEMIA AND NORMOXIA AT DIFFERENT P_{50} VALUES ON OXYGEN TRANSPORT

Physiologic Variable	Normoxia	Hypoxemia	Hypoxemia and Exchange Transfusion	Normoxia and Exchange Transfusion
Hematocrit (%)	28 ± 3	29 ± 2	31 ± 3	31 ± 4
P_{50} (mmHg)	27 ± 3.9	27 ± 3.9	35.5 ± 3.0	35.5 ± 3.0
PaO_2 (mmHg)	81 ± 12	31 ± 4*	31 ± 5	94 ± 13
SaO_2 (%)	95 ± 2	47 ± 8*	39 ± 11*	94 ± 2
CaO_2 (ml·dl^{-1})	11.23 ± 1.32	6.07 ± 1.17*	5.31 ± 1.06*	12.48 ± 1.70
$P\bar{v}O_2$ (mmHg)	36 ± 5	19 ± 6*	17 ± 3	38 ± 5
$a\bar{v}O_2D$ (ml·dl^{-1})	4.91 ± 0.78	3.90 ± 0.77*	3.74 ± 0.88	5.60 ± 0.92*
CO	361 ± 55	390 ± 66	506 ± 166*	338 ± 39
AVO_2	40.7 ± 9.5	23.2 ± 5.0*	26.5 ± 4.5*	41.5 ± 7.4
O_2 ER	0.438 ± 0.071	0.647 ± 0.121*	0.686 ± 0.080	0.459 ± 0.100
$\dot{V}O_2$ (ml·min^{-1}·kg^{-1})	17.5 ± 3.1	14.6 ± 2.0*	17.8 ± 3.2*	18.5 ± 3.8
HR (beats·min^{-1})	227 ± 51	260 ± 52*	260 ± 54	239 ± 55
LVSV (ml)	1.66 ± 0.47	1.64 ± 0.54	2.03 ± 0.67*	1.52 ± 0.49
Ao (mmHg)	75 ± 9	73 ± 11	74 ± 15	78 ± 12
SVR	230 ± 55	202 ± 45*	163 ± 62*	238 ± 63

Notes: Mean ± SD, n = 10; AVO_2 = oxygen availability, ml O_2 min^{-1}·kg^{-1}; CO = ml·min^{-1}·kg^{-1}; SVR = mmHg liter^{-1} min^{-1}·kg^{-1}; $a\bar{v}O_2D$ = ml·dl^{-1}; $\dot{V}O_2$ = ml·min^{-1}·kg^{-1}; O_2ER:O_2 extraction ratio = $\dot{V}O_2/AVO_2$. * = statistically significant difference from normoxia, $p < 0.05$. (Adapted with permission from Lister G [1984]: Oxygen transport in the intact hypoxic newborn lamb: Acute effects of increasing P_{50}. Pediatr Res 18:172–177.)

dium appear to have a critical effect on the ability of the neonatal myocardium to respond reflexly to hypoxemia in order to compensate for impaired O_2 transport.[37] Further evidence that changes in P_{50} in the neonate (unanesthetized lamb) are of critical importance in tissue oxygenation is shown by the reduced increase in cerebral blood flow in response to hypoxemia following blood transfusion and an increase in P_{50}.[67]

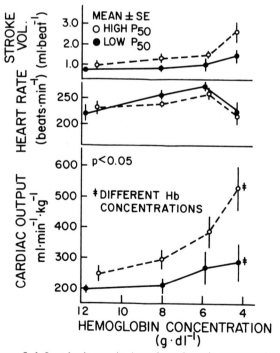

Figure 8–1. Isovolemic anemia. Acute hemodynamic responses (stroke volume, heart rate, and cardiac output) to graded isovolemic anemia in newborn normal lambs and the effects of high and low oxygen affinity hemoglobin. (Redrawn with permission from Van Amerigan MR et al [1981]: Oxygenation in anemic newborn lambs with high or low oxygen affinity red cells. Pediatr Res 15:1500–1503.)

Isovolemic Anemia

In lambs with high affinity hemoglobin (P_{50} = 19.4 mmHg) and graded isovolemic anemia (4, 6, 8, and 10 g·dl^{-1}), in addition to the direct relationship between the hemoglobin concentration and both arterial (CaO_2) and mixed venous oxygen contents ($C\bar{v}O_2$), $P\bar{v}O_2$, mean aortic pressure (Ao), and SVR decreased significantly with isovolemic anemia (Fig. 8–1). The CO and SV increased at all levels of hemoglobin, and the HR increased down to a hemoglobin of 6 g·dl^{-1}. The increase in CO and SV was greater where the hemoglobin oxygen affinity was reduced (high P_{50}) (Fig. 8–1).[125] The $\dot{V}O_2$ decreased with high affinity hemoglobin concentrations of less than 8 g·dl^{-1} (Fig. 8–2). These observations are again consistent with the concept that the maintenance of adequate myocardial function and oxygen delivery during stress in the

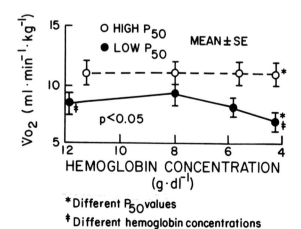

Figure 8–2. Isovolemic anemia. Effect of graded isovolemic anemia and hemoglobin with high and low oxygen affinity on oxygen consumption ($\dot{V}O_2$, ml·min^{-1}·kg^{-1}) in normal newborn lambs. (Redrawn with permission from Van Amerigan MR et al [1981]: Oxygenation in anemic newborn lambs with high or low oxygen affinity red cells. Pediatr Res 15:1500–1503.)

Table 8–4. OXYGEN TRANSPORT: LONGITUDINAL STUDY EXAMINING THE CONCOMITANT CHANGES IN HEMOGLOBIN CONCENTRATION, O_2 CONSUMPTION, CARDIAC OUTPUT, AND OXYGEN TRANSPORT IN NEWBORN LAMBS

	1 to 2 Days	3 to 5 Days	1 Week	2 Weeks	4 Weeks	6 Weeks	8 Weeks
Weight (kg)	4.13 ± 0.78	4.95 ± 1.11	5.98 ± 1.40	7.86 ± 2.15	11.43 ± 2.25	11.59 ± 3.55	14.53 ± 4.62
PaO_2 (mmHg)	85 ± 18	81 ± 7	83 ± 7	84 ± 10	80 ± 12	79 ± 9	78 ± 11
$a\bar{v}O_2D$ (ml·dl^{-1})	3.99 ± 0.68	4.30 ± 0.79	4.12 ± 1.09	3.85 ± 0.87	3.92 ± 1.01	4.21 ± 1.16	4.24 ± 1.02
AVO_2	49.8 ± 9.2	45.4 ± 11.1	43.6 ± 15.0	35.1 ± 14.2	24.9 ± 11.3	27.1 ± 12.4	28.4 ± 10.5
O_2ER	0.339 ± 0.102	0.358 ± 0.073	0.350 ± 0.094	0.389 ± 0.113	0.427 ± 0.188	0.359 ± 0.119	0.331 ± 0.088

Notes: Mean ± SD, n = 9 to 14; AVO_2 = ml O_2 min^{-1}·kg^{-1}. (Adapted with permission from Lister G et al [1979]: Oxygen delivery in lambs: Cardiovascular and hematologic development. Am J Physiol (Heart Circ Physiol) 237:H668–H675.)

neonate is dependent on the release of oxygen to the myocardium and other organ systems.

Impaired Cardiac Output

In order to examine the responses to impaired oxygen transport resulting from reduced cardiac output, experimental studies on cord compression in fetal lambs will be described.[54] With a 50 per cent reduction in umbilical blood flow, the fraction of fetal cardiac output distributed to the brain, heart, carcass, kidneys, and gastrointestinal tract increased, whereas the pulmonary blood flow decreased. In addition, graded decreases in umbilical blood flow resulted in proportionate decreases in the combined ventricular output, such that with a 50 per cent decrease in umbilical blood flow, the decrease in combined ventricular output was 20 per cent. The proportion of umbilical venous blood passing through the ductus venosus increased, and the proportion of this blood preferentially distributed through the foramen ovale also increased. Similarly, the inferior vena caval blood flow increased, and it was also preferentially distributed through the foramen ovale. These responses were associated with an increase in the vascular resistance of the lower body (73 per cent), whereas the resistance of the upper body was unchanged, as was total body fetal vascular resistance. As a consequence of these changes, O_2 delivery to the brain and myocardium was preferentially maintained, and O_2 delivery was reduced to the periphery, to the kidneys, and to the gastrointestinal tract. In essence, fetal umbilical compression to 50 per cent reduction in flow causes a redistribution of (but no increase in) fetal vascular resistance and an increase in placental vascular resistance; in contrast, maternal hypoxemia causes an increase in total fetal vascular resistance and has no effect on placental vascular resistance. The explanation for this difference may lie in differences in myocardial preload and neural reflex responses from baro- and chemoreceptors as well as circulating hormones such as catecholamines, vasopressin, and angiotension. In addition, after birth, circulatory

(including pulmonary vascular) and other changes will alter the pattern of response to impaired oxygen transport from reduced cardiac output.

Increased Metabolic Demands

Using the resting lamb as a model of the neonate, Lister and associates examined the concomitant changes in $\dot{V}O_2$, CO, and oxygen transport during the first 8 weeks of life (Table 8–4).[76] During the first 2 months of life there is a fall in hemoglobin concentration (THb) and a rightward shift in the oxyhemoglobin dissociation curve (ODC), which enables more O_2 to be released from the hemoglobin molecule at the same capillary O_2 tension (Fig. 8–3).[76] However, if tissue oxygenation is to remain adequate for the metabolic demands of extrauterine life including motor activity, then the increase in P_{50} must compensate for the reduced THb. The other alternatives include increased O_2 extraction or an increase in cardiac output or both. The pattern of changes observed included a decline in THb to a nadir at 3 to 4 weeks and a subsequent rise to adult hemoglobin values, a progressive shift in P_{50} to the right, and an early increase in 2,3-diphosphoglycerate (2,3-DPG) with a decline after 2 weeks (Fig. 8–3). From the high values at birth there was a progressive decline in both the $\dot{V}O_2$ and CO to near-adult, lower levels at 2 months (Fig. 8–3). Therefore, AVO_2 (CO × CaO_2) decreased from very high values at birth (49.80 ± SD 9.18 ml O_2·kg^{-1}·min^{-1}) to significantly reduced values at 2 months (28.35 ± 10.45 ml O_2·kg^{-1}·min^{-1}), with, however, considerable interindividual variation. The oxygen extraction ratio ($\dot{V}O_2$/CO × CaO_2) did vary throughout the 8-week period, but the variation was not statistically significant (Table 8–4). The $P\bar{v}O_2$ increased rapidly during the first week and then slowly thereafter. Further analysis of this longitudinal study demonstrated parallel changes in $\dot{V}O_2$ and CO, and therefore the $a\bar{v}O_2D$ remained constant. Thus, the cardiac output was adjusted to compensate for changing $\dot{V}O_2$, THb, and P_{50}. However, below a critical THb, failure of the cardiac output to com-

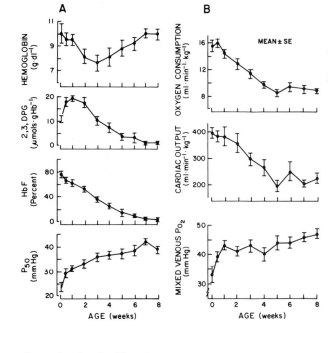

Figure 8–3. Chronologic adaptations to changes in oxygen consumption and transport in neonatal lambs. Chronologic changes in (*A*) hemoglobin concentration, 2,3-DPG (μ moles$\cdot$g Hb^{-1}), HbF (%), P_{50} (mmHg) and (*B*) oxygen consumption (ml$\cdot$min$^{-1}\cdot$kg^{-1}), cardiac output (ml$\cdot$min$^{-1}\cdot$kg^{-1}), and the P$\bar{v}O_2$ during the first 8 weeks of life. (Redrawn with permission from Lister G et al [1979]: Oxygen delivery in lambs: Cardiovascular and hematologic development. Am J Physiol 237:H668–H675.)

pensate for the reduced CaO_2 necessitated a redistribution of cardiac output; otherwise, it is argued, tissue hypoxia would ensue. As reviewed elsewhere, the neonatal cardiovascular system has limited reserve[107] and has reduced ability to respond to volume (preload)[62,94,105] or to an increase in SVR (afterload).

PULMONARY FUNCTION

Development of the Bronchoalveolar and Pulmonary Vasculature

The epithelial structure of the human lung arises from the foregut (seventh pair of pharyngeal pouches) and can be recognized in the third week of embryologic development (3-mm embryo). By the sixth or seventh week (14-mm embryo), through a combination of monopodal and irregular dichotomous branching of the bronchial system, 10 principal branches may be discerned on the right and 8 on the left. These are the basis of the adult bronchopulmonary segments. Although the bronchial tree is developed by the sixteenth week of intrauterine life, the number of alveoli continues to increase and the alveolar volume increases in a parallel fashion with the increase in volume of the chest wall until completion of adolescence. At approximately 48 days of intrauterine life the bronchopulmonary tree becomes ensheathed in a vascular plexus. As growth continues, variations in both the bronchial and vascular pattern occur. As a result of these variations, the mature lung may have many bronchial and vascular pattern variations.[84,99] In addition, during development, the gas exchange and airway structures are innervated by elements of the autonomic nervous system, including the vagi. These neural elements provide the basis for the lung inflation reflexes.[24,90]

Bronchoalveolar Development

The postembryonic development of the lung may be divided into three periods: (1) *pseudoglandular*, in which the bronchial divisions are established; (2) the *canalicular* period, which extends from week 16 to 17 to week 24, a potentially viable stage in which the respiratory areas become delineated and vascularized; and (3) the *terminal sac* period, which is from 24 weeks to term and in which the definitive alveoli are differentiated.[119] During the canalicular period, the bronchioles are vascularized, and the alveolar type I and II cells, with the intracellular organelles in the latter, can be identified. The maturation of these structures parallels the synthesis of surface active lipoprotein and the viability of the preterm neonate. During the terminal sac period, the duct system becomes more extensive, and the surface area increases as a result of the formation of saccules. The histologic features of the saccules consist of a capillarized epithelium on one side and a ciliated cuboidal epithelium on the other. Gradually, the connective tissue between the saccules thins, and the air spaces enlarge.

Postnatal Development. Lung growth should be considered in relation to the growth of the rest of the organism, and although not always recognized, the growth rate in the immediate postnatal period is the most rapid.[119] During the postnatal period, considerable alveolar multiplication occurs and continues until 8 to 10 years of age. There is, however, considerable dispute as to the age at which multiplication ceases.[119] In addition, throughout childhood and into adolescence there is an increase in the volume of the alveoli. However, the general consensus is that the majority of alveoli appear in the postnatal period, with the peak alveolar multiplication phase occurring between birth and 3 months and maximum growth in volume and surface area occurring during the first year of life.[119] Distortion and impaired development of the rib cage in infancy, e.g., infantile kyphoscoliosis, not only distorts the shape of the lung but also impairs alveolar development.[27] Other factors that modify lung growth include hypoxia (e.g., altitude), hyperoxia, and possibly certain endocrine functions.[119]

Pulmonary Vasculature

The sixth, or pulmonary, arches appear at 32 days (5-mm stage) and give off branches to the existing lung bud. The left sixth arch will develop into the main pulmonary artery. At this stage the lung bud is also supplied by paired segmental branches arising from the dorsal aorta. These are later lost and the bronchial arteries develop from the aorta much later. By the 18-mm stage (50 days) the adult pattern of blood supply to the lung is complete, the right sixth arch has disappeared, and the left arch gives rise to the main as well as the left and right pulmonary arterial branches. The main pulmonary vein develops later than the pulmonary arteries. Before the lung is linked to the heart by the pulmonary veins, the pulmonary vessels drain into the systemic system of the foregut and trachea. The systemic and pulmonary vessels are both derived from the same splanchnic plexus. These connections are subsequently lost except for persistent connections at the lung roots between the esophageal and pulmonary venous systems.

Fetal Development of Pulmonary Vasculature. Within the lung the endothelial canals differentiate, and in the 8-mm embryo they are interconnected. The branches of the pulmonary arterial system assume a position next to the bronchial system and maintain this relationship as both the bronchial and vascular structures ramify during the pseudoglandular and canalicular periods. Thus, by 16 weeks there is a full complement of vessels leading to the respiratory bronchioles, alveolar ducts, and saccules. The arteries within the structure comprising the terminal units continue to proliferate up to and for several years following birth. In addition, at 35 days (8-mm embryo) a new outgrowth appears from the left side of the atrial chamber, which is the primitive pulmonary vein. This primitive pulmonary vein starts as a blind capillary that grows posteriorly and bifurcates several times to contact the lung buds. After connections are made within the lung, the first two branches are reabsorbed to form the left atrial chamber. Therefore, by the seventh week the adult pattern of vessels connecting the heart to the lung is developing.

During fetal life pulmonary artery pressure is high, and the histologic structure of the pulmonary artery resembles the structure of the aorta. These features include the thickness and configuration of the elastic fibrils, which are mostly parallel, compact, and uniform in thickness, and the medial muscle layer. After birth, changes occur that are obvious at 6 months; at 2 years the wall of the main pulmonary artery is only 40 to 70 per cent as thick as the aorta. The structure of the large fetal pulmonary arteries is similar to that of the main pulmonary artery, and they have a media of elastic and muscle fibers (elastic arteries). Progressing peripherally, the number of elastic layers

decreases to a transitional stage. The muscle layers also become thinner. This pattern of change from proximal to distal pulmonary arteries is similar to that of the adult, in whom vessel structure is also related to the diameter of the vessel.

Postnatal Development of the Pulmonary Vasculature. The immediate major hemodynamic changes with the first breath are characterized by a decrease in the pulmonary vascular resistance and an increase in the systemic vascular resistance. In addition there is a functional closure of both the foramen ovale and the patent ductus arteriosus. As a result of these hemodynamic changes, the neonatal pulmonary vasculature assumes the functions of the adult vasculature, which include absorption of alveolar and perivascular fluid (together with the lymphatic system); filtration of particulates; absorption, release, and/or biotransformation of vasoactive and other bioactive substances;[72,98] and maintenance of a vascular volume reservoir. The "effective" pulmonary blood flow continues to increase during the early days of life. The "effective" blood flow is, however, less than the total blood flow, which is consistent with the concept that perfusion to unventilated or poorly ventilated regions contributes to the increased AaO_2P observed in neonates.[65]

At birth, although the arteries to the terminal respiratory units are completely formed, there are few arteries within the terminal respiratory units. Therefore, during the first decade of life, the number of arteries with their capillaries within the gas exchange areas increases enormously, and their development parallels the formation of new respiratory bronchioles, alveolar ducts, and alveoli.

Bronchial Vasculature

In the human fetus the bronchial arteries are a secondary system and connect relatively late to the lung to supply the walls of the bronchial tree and larger pulmonary vessels. The bronchial arteries appear only in the ninth and twelfth weeks of gestation and the number in each lung varies substantially. The bronchial arteries grow along the airways as the cartilage develops. The more peripheral lung regions are supplied by branches of the pulmonary arteries rather than by bronchial arteries. The veins draining the bronchi (bronchial veins) empty into the systemic venous system (e.g., azygous vein) and the right atrium, whereas veins draining the bronchiolar capillaries drain into the pulmonary veins (bronchopulmonary veins) and therefore may contribute to the pulmonary arteriovenous shunt. The respective proportions are 25 to 33 per cent and 67 to 75 per cent.

Structural and Functional Requisites for Gas Exchange

Development of the bronchoalveolar and pulmonary vascular structures together with maturation of the respiratory neuromotor and mechanical systems provides an adequate and stable gas exchange system. The dependence of adequate and stable gas exchange on the maturation of respiratory control, the neuromotor system, and

Table 8–5. NORMAL ARTERIAL BLOOD GASES, ACID BASE VARIABLES, AND HEMATOCRIT IN FULL-TERM NEONATES BREATHING AIR

Age	PaO_2 (mmHg)	$PaCO_2$ (mmHg)	pHa	Standard Bicarbonate Concentration (mequiv·liter^{-1})	Hematocrit (%)
Birth, 5 to 10 minutes	49.6 ± 9.9	46.1 ± 7.0	7.207 ± 0.051	16.7 ± 1.6	53.0 ± 5.0
1 hour	63.3 ± 11.3	36.1 ± 4.2	7.332 ± 0.031	19.2 ± 1.2	54.1 ± 4.9
5 hours	73.7 ± 12.0	35.2 ± 3.6	7.339 ± 0.028	19.4 ± 1.2	52.4 ± 5.9
24 hours	72.7 ± 9.5	33.4 ± 3.1	7.369 ± 0.032	20.2 ± 1.3	54.8 ± 7.2
5 days	72.1 ± 10.5	34.8 ± 3.5	7.371 ± 0.031	20.6 ± 1.7	50.1 ± 6.9
7 days	73.1 ± 9.7	35.9 ± 3.1	7.371 ± 0.026	21.8 ± 1.3	51.0 ± 7.8

Notes: Mean ± SD, n = 30 to 42. (Adapted with permission from S Karger AG, Basel. From Koch G, Wendel H [1968]: Adjustment of arterial blood gases and acid base balance in the newborn infant. Biol Neonate 12:136–161.)

the mechanical properties of the respiratory system will be discussed in the following sections.

Gas Exchange and Arterial Blood Gases

Gas exchange and the arterial blood gases are products of (1) the neural control of ventilation and respiratory timing, (2) the mechanical properties of the respiratory system, (3) the stability of the end-expiratory lung volume, (4) ventilation–blood flow relationships and shunt, (5) the oxyhemoglobin dissociation curve, (6) the adequacy of the cardiac output in relation to the $\dot{V}O_2$, and, (7) the ensuing mixed venous oxygen content. The adaptive processes that occur at birth and in the subsequent hours and days may be described in three phases. Those three adaptive phases are (1) first breath, (2) rapid adaptive processes of the first few hours, and (3) relative "steady state" conditions during the succeeding days. However, even in phase 3 the neonate has structural constraints because of the relatively small alveolar surface area resulting from the incomplete development of the alveoli and pulmonary vasculature[119] and the high chest wall–lung compliance ratio.[80]

Arterial Blood Gases

In both normal full-term infants (Table 8–5)[66] and in "uncomplicated" premature infants (Table 8–6)[91] following an initial low PaO_2 and an elevated $PaCO_2$ there is a significant increase in the PaO_2 and a decrease in the $PaCO_2$ during the early hours of life.[42,66,91] In the full-term infant at 1 hour after birth the $PaCO_2$ reaches a plateau, and within 5 hours the PaO_2 reaches a plateau,[66] whereas in the premature infant up to 6 hours elapse before the PaO_2 reaches a plateau.[91] In addition, in the premature infant the coefficients of variation of the PaO_2

were high and ranged from 13 per cent at birth to 29 per cent, with the maximum value at the 24- to 48-hour period (Table 8–6). In "uncomplicated" premature infants the $PaCO_2$ values from 6 to 24 hours were below the normal range and less than those observed in normal full-term infants. Orzalesi and associates[91] subdivided these premature infants into three groups, which were characterized as normal (n = 21), tachypneic (n = 11), and having mild respiratory distress syndrome (MRDS) (n = 4). They demonstrated that the PaO_2 was less and the calculated venous admixture (VA) was higher in the tachypneic and MRDS groups than in the normal group. In the normal group at age 6 to 24 hours the PaO_2 was 68.2 ± 13.4, and the VA was 15.6 ± 5.7%; whereas PaO_2 in the tachypneic and MRDS groups was 58.7 ± 10.2 (P < 0.05) and 52.5 ± 12.4 (P < 0.05), respectively, and the VA was 21.4 ± 9.3% (P > 0.05) and 28.7 ± 8.3% (P < 0.01), respectively. The hypocapnia was unrelated to the magnitude of hypoxemia. The elevated VA returned to within the "normal" range of 10 per cent within 5 days.[91]

Analysis of Blood Gas Abnormalities

Conventional theoretical analysis of the factors that contribute to an increase in the AaO_2P difference are (1) ventilation–blood flow maldistribution (distribution effect), (2) pulmonary or intracardiac right-to-left shunts, and (3) impaired diffusion.[35] In addition, there are two contributing factors: (1) reduced mixed venous oxygen content in the presence of shunt[59,129] and (2) position of the oxygen dissociation curve (ODC) in the presence of ventilation–blood flow maldistribution.[129] It is now well recognized and has been quantitatively demonstrated that an inadequate cardiac output for $\dot{V}O_2$ and which results in a reduced $C\bar{v}O_2$, increases the AaO_2P and may therefore result in hypoxemia.[59,129] Although it was thought that the alinearity of the ODC contributes to the AaO_2P, it has

Table 8–6. ARTERIAL BLOOD GASES CALCULATED VENOUS ADMIXTURE AND ACID BASE VARIABLES IN UNCOMPLICATED AND PRETERM INFANTS BREATHING AIR

Age	n	PaO$_2$ (mmHg)	SaO$_2$ (%)	VA (%)	PaCO$_2$ (mmHg)	pHa	BE (mequiv·liter^{-1})
3 to 5 hours	4	59.5‡ ±7.7	91.3‡ ±1.7	19.5 ± ±4.5	47.0* ±8.5	7.329* ±0.038	-3.7‡ ±1.5
6 to 12 hours	9	69.7‡ ±11.8	95.2‡ ±1.2	14.5 ± ±4.8	28.2† ±6.9	7.425 ±0.072	-4.7‡ ±3.1
13 to 24 hours	2	67.0‡ ±15.2	95.3* ±2.1	16.3 ± ±6.3	27.2† ±8.4	7.464 ±0.064	-3.0‡ ±3.3
25 to 48 hours	22	72.5‡ ±20.9	95.0‡ ±2.0	13.8† ±8.7	31.3* ±6.7	7.434 ±0.054	-2.3‡ ±3.0
3 to 4 days	13	77.8* ±16.4	95.7‡ ±1.5	9.8* ±5.5	31.7* ±6.7	7.425 ±0.044	-2.9‡ ±2.3
5 to 10 days	12	80.3* ±12.0	95.1† ±1.3	8.2 ±4.2	36.4 ±4.2	7.378 ±0.043	-3.5† ±2.3
11 to 40 days	8	77.8† ±9.6	96.0† ±0.6	8.4 ±2.9	32.9 ±4.0	7.425 ±0.033	-2.1† ±2.2
Adult	13	91.8 ±12.4	97.1 ±1.1	5.5 ±5.1	37.9 ±6.4	7.443 ±0.044	+1.4 ±1.5

Notes: Mean ± SD. Statistical significance of difference from adult values: * = P < 0.05; † = P < 0.01; ‡ = P < 0.001. VA = calculated venous admixture. (Adapted with permission from Orzalesi MM et al [1967]: Arterial oxygen studies in premature newborns with and without mild respiratory disorders. Arch Dis Child 42:174–180.)

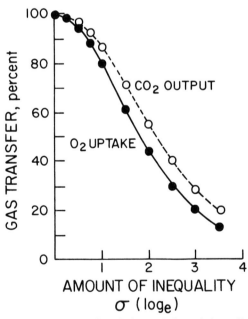

Figure 8–4. Acute effects of ventilation-perfusion ratio inequality on the oxygen uptake and carbon dioxide output of a lung model. In this figure, the composition of the mixed venous blood is held constant, and the gas transfer is shown as a percentage of its value for steady state conditions with no inequality (300 ml·min^{-1} and 240 ml·min^{-1}, for oxygen and carbon dioxide, respectively). The abscissa shows the log SD of ventilation or blood flow; both give identical results. Note that the interference with carbon dioxide transfer is almost as great as oxygen. (Reproduced with permission from West JB [1969]: Ventilation-perfusion inequality and overall gas exchange in computer models of the lung. Respir Physiol 7:88–110.)

now been demonstrated theoretically that the *position* of the ODC has a major impact on oxygen exchange in the presence of the ventilation–blood flow maldistribution.[122,123,129,130,136] In a theoretical study, Wagner demonstrated that the alveolar PO$_2$ (PAO$_2$) is most sensitive to the P$_{50}$ where the $\dot{V}_A/\dot{Q}$ ratios are within the normal range. As an example, a spread of 10 mmHg in the P$_{50}$ value results in a 30 mmHg difference in PAO$_2$ when the $\dot{V}_A/\dot{Q}$ ratio is 0.5. The higher affinity curve (P$_{50}$ = 22 mmHg) results in a PAO$_2$ of 96, whereas the lower affinity curve (P$_{50}$ = 32 mmHg) results in a PAO$_2$ of 66 mmHg. Therefore, pulmonary oxygenation (defined by Wagner as the difference between CaO$_2$ and C$\bar{v}$O$_2$) is increased with the lower P$_{50}$. However, the relationships for a nonhomogeneous whole lung are complex. Although the foregoing quantitative analysis shows the effects of changes in the position of the ODC, maldistribution of ventilation–blood flow and major shunt are the major factors causing an increased AaO$_2$P in pulmonary or cyanotic congenital heart disease. Further, the effects of changes in P$_{50}$ on oxygenation also depend on the severity of hypoxemia.[122,123]

Ventilation–blood flow maldistribution also impairs the exchange of CO$_2$.[135,137] Theoretical studies using digital computer analysis with multicompartment lung models and algorithms for the nonlinear and interdependent dissociation curves for oxygen and carbon dioxide have compared the exchange of O$_2$ and CO$_2$. These studies have demonstrated that $\dot{V}_A/\dot{Q}$ maldistribution similarly impairs O$_2$ and CO$_2$ exchange, resulting in fairly comparable decreases in PaO$_2$ and increases in PaCO$_2$ (Figs. 8–4 and 8–5). In this model, increasing $\dot{V}_A/\dot{Q}$ maldistribution resulted in a precipitous fall in the PaO$_2$ and a somewhat less rapid rise in the PaCO$_2$ (Fig. 8–5). In addition, there was an increase in the venous admixture and the dead space–tidal volume ratio (V_D/V_T). Increasing the minute ventilation ($\dot{V}_E$) reduced the $PaCO_2$, which could be returned to normal values. However, even though increases in $\dot{V}_E$ increased the PaO_2, normal values could not be regained.

Indices of $\dot{V}_A/\dot{Q}$ Maldistribution and Shunt in the Neonate

The conventional indices of $\dot{V}_A/\dot{Q}$ maldistribution and shunt, i.e., V_D/V_T ratio, AaO_2P and venous admixture after breathing air, and AaO_2P and shunt fraction after breathing 100 per cent oxygen, are consistent with the concept that pulmonary or intracardiac right-to-left shunt is the major contributor to AaO_2P.[86] However, as demonstrated by Wagner and associates using the inert gas excretion technique,[131,132] breathing 100 per cent O_2 results in an increase in shunt fraction. While breathing 100 per cent oxygen, regions with low $\dot{V}_A/\dot{Q}$ ratios are converted to areas of shunt ($\dot{V}_A/\dot{Q} = O$). Unfortunately, there are no definitive data in the neonate using the inert gas excretion technique to address this problem. Measurements of nitrogen washout are consistent with a uniform distribution of ventilation.[86] Lees and associates also reported normal V_D/V_T ratios in the neonate.[71] In addition, measurements of the "anatomic" dead space using the single breath nitrogen expirate method show that the relationship between dead space and body size in the neonate is similar to that of the adult.[44]

Therefore, as a result of the data on shunt fraction after breathing 100 per cent oxygen, most attention has been directed to an examination of the anatomic basis for the presumed increase in pulmonary arteriovenous shunt in the neonate.[51] However, there is inadequate anatomic explanation to support the concept of pulmonary arteriovenous shunts. Therefore, there remains the possibility that the shunt is in fact primarily the result of areas of low $\dot{V}_A/\dot{Q}$ ratio, which are converted to areas of $\dot{V}_A/\dot{Q} = O$.

Pulmonary Diffusion Capacity

Only a few studies have measured diffusion capacity in the neonate.[65,87,115] Koch, using the steady state method in full-term infants at 1 and 7 days of age, obtained values that when normalized for $\dot{V}O_2$ or $\dot{V}_A$ were in close agreement with normal adult values.[65] In addition, recent studies using inert gas techniques to measure the relative contributions of impaired diffusion, $\dot{V}_A/\dot{Q}$ maldistribution, and shunt in pulmonary disease, including adult respiratory distress syndrome, have confirmed the concept that impaired diffusion of oxygen is not a major contributor to the AaO_2P.[133]

Mechanical Properties of the Respiratory System

The maturation of the mechanical properties of the neonatal respiratory system plays an essential role in optimizing ventilation–blood flow distribution in the lung

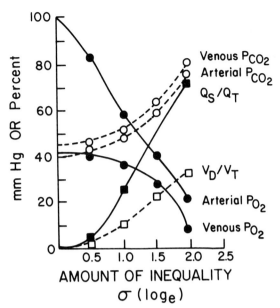

Figure 8–5. Effect of increasing ventilation-perfusion ratio inequality on gas exchange in a lung model in which oxygen uptake and carbon dioxide output are maintained at 300 and 240 ml·min⁻¹, respectively (steady state conditions). Note the rapid fall in arterial and mixed venous PO_2 and the corresponding rise in arterial and mixed venous PCO_2. (Reproduced with permission from West JB [1969]: Ventilation-perfusion inequality and overall gas exchange in computer models of the lung. Respir Physiol 7:88–110.)

and in stabilizing the end-expiratory lung volume (EELV) and therefore also the alveolar gas exchange units. In addition, the ability of the respiratory system to compensate for increased mechanical and ventilatory loads is dependent on the stability of the chest wall. The high chest wall–lung compliance ratio, particularly in the premature infant, impairs and limits the efficacy of an increase in neural drive in compensating for increased ventilation–blood flow maldistribution, increased metabolic rate ($\dot{V}O_2$ and $\dot{V}CO_2$), and increased mechanical load to breathing.[80]

Mechanical Aspects of the Onset of Breathing and Maintenance of Lung Volume

Prior to birth the lungs are distended with fluid of their own production, and the fetal breathing movements are irregular.[19] Therefore, at birth the essential changes in mechanical and neural function are fluid reabsorption, onset and maintenance of regular respiratory neural drive, and establishment of end-expiratory lung volume (EELV). During prenatal development, the lungs contribute to the production of amniotic fluid, and at term the fluid in the lung is estimated to be 30 ml·kg⁻¹.[89] This volume is similar to the volume of the EELV at birth (Table 8–1). The term fetus has lungs that are filled with fluid (thereby eliminating surface tension) and has a compliant chest wall; as a result the lungs are close to their relaxation volume, and elastic recoil (pleural pressure, Ppl) is close to zero. During labor, pulmonary filtration ceases and absorption begins. After birth one third of the remaining fluid is absorbed by the lymphatics and the remainder by the pulmonary vasculature.

Table 8-7. MECHANICAL PROPERTIES OF THE RESPIRATORY
SYSTEM, LUNG VOLUMES, AND RESPIRATORY PATTERN

Physiologic Variables	Newborn	6 Months	12 Months	Adult
Respiratory frequency (breaths·min^{-1})	50 ± 10	30 ± 5	24 ± 6	12 ± 3
Tidal volume (ml, BTPS)	21	45	78	575
Minute ventilation (liter·min^{-1}, BTPS)	1.05	1.35	1.78	6.4
Alveolar ventilation (ml·min^{-1}, BTPS)	665	–	1248	3100
VC (ml, BTPS)	120			4000
FRC (ml, BTPS)	80			3000
TLC (ml, BTPS)	160			6000

Notes: Reprinted by permission of Crone RK [1983]: The respiratory system. In Gregory GA (ed): Pediatric Anesthesia. New York, Churchill Livingstone, p 54.

The characteristics of the first breath include parallel changes in pleural pressure (Ppl) and volume (V_T), a peak Ppl of -30 to -100 cmH$_2$O (higher than the spontaneous breathing swings of -5 to -7 cmH$_2$O), a V_T of 35 to 45 ml, which is less than a crying vital capacity (VC) but more than the resting V_T (Table 8–7),[23] and retention during the next exhalation of 15 ml or 40 per cent of the inhaled breath.[80] The major forces that oppose the inspiratory muscle force during the first breath are elasticity of lung tissue, surface forces and frictional resistance to the movement of air, and fluid in the tracheobronchial tree. The frictional resistance of the column of fluid is much higher during the first breath than during subsequent air breathing because of the high viscosity of the pulmonary fluid. Additional forces opposing the first breath include distortion of the rib cage and inertial resistance of the chest wall and the pulmonary fluid. The expiration following the first inspiration is often slow and prolonged. The esophageal pressures recorded are often larger than passive recoil would predict and are therefore consistent with active expiration. This positive airway pressure during expiration promotes clearing of the fluid from the airway. There is a large intersubject variation in the amount of air retained in the lungs after the first expiration (10 to 20 ml), and the volume represents 10 to 20 per cent of the EELV established in the several-day-old infant. This volume of air may in part be explained by air bubble formation in the peripheral airways. Therefore, lung surfactants play an essential role in maintaining the stability of peripheral air spaces and allow the retention of air in the lung at end expiration. In addition, surfactants also reduce the inspiratory muscle force required for expansion and facilitate clearance of fluid from the lung.

First Hours After Birth

The breathing pattern and mechanical characteristics of the respiratory system during successive hours include the following:

1. A breathing frequency that increases to 70 to 90 breaths·min^{-1} for the first few days; periods of apnea can also occur. Early postnatal tachypnea is prolonged when fluid absorption is slow, and is probably mediated by the pulmonary J receptors.[40] Tachypnea also correlates with the hypocapnia observed in the preterm infant (Table 8–6).

2. A shortening of expiratory time (T_E), which maintains the EELV above the relaxation volume (dynamic control of EELV).

3. Low compliance of the total respiratory system (Crs) and a high total respiratory resistance (Rrs). The Crs increases by 80 per cent, lung compliance increases, chest wall compliance (Ccw) decreases, and the Rrs decreases by 20 per cent over several days; while the relaxation volume (Vr) increases, and the Ppl at Vr becomes more negative but remains less negative than in the adult (-1.9 cmH$_2$O). Within a few hours, therefore, the EELV is established, and ventilation–blood flow distribution and arterial blood gases in the infant are stabilized (Table 8–5).[66,91]

4. Absorption of most pulmonary fluid in the term infant within 2 to 6 hours of birth.

5. Incomplete aeration of alveoli, despite increases in lung compliance and stabilization of EELV. Therefore, $\dot{V}_A/\dot{Q}$ maldistribution continues, as does the potential for pulmonary shunt.

Mechanical Properties of the Respiratory System of the Neonate

The mechanical properties of the respiratory system of the neonate are described as the following:

1. *Static compliance of the lung* (Clstat) is characterized by an S-shaped inflation limb of the static pressure-volume curve of the lung, with evidence consistent with "airways opening" or recruitment and/or complex changes in the shape of the surface tension area in the region of the EELV.[38] Thus, based on the above description, only a portion of the alveoli are aerated, and the features of the P-V inflation limb are consistent with retention of some fluid in the alveoli or the interstitial spaces. Therefore, in the region of the EELV the change in volume in response to a change in Ppl is small; as volumes increase, the slope of the pressure-volume (P-V)

curve increases initially but eventually decreases at higher volumes when pleural pressures are above −15 to −20 cmH$_2$O. In addition, the neonatal deflation P-V curve of the lung differs from that of the adult, in that it is concave toward the pressure axis. Interspecies comparisons have shown that static pulmonary compliance is directly proportional to body mass, 3.3 ml·cmH$_2$O^{-1}·kg^{-1}.[80]

2. *Dynamic compliance of the lung* (Cldyn) in children and in the newborn, in contrast to adults, is less than the Clstat and the difference is greater at younger ages.[80] The difference in Clstat and Cldyn, which is also present in isolated lungs, is frequency dependent and increases with increasing breathing frequencies. This phenomenon is considered to be the result of asynchronous behavior of peripheral lung units and the viscoelastic properties of the lung tissue. Complementary evidence includes stress relaxation, which is greater in the newborn (decay in Ppl after a step inflation); lung tissue resistance, which is three times higher in children than in adults; and other factors, which include distortion of the chest wall, causing inequalities of the mechanical behavior of peripheral units.

3. *Resistance of the total respiratory system* (Rrs) in the newborn infant is about 55 per cent of the adult value. Despite technical difficulties, in the newborn infant the time constant of decay for Rrs (including upper airways) has been estimated to be 0.21 s (seconds), and total resistance per kilogram body weight has been estimated to be 0.20 cmH$_2$O ml^{-1}·s^{-1}·kg^{-1}.[80] No study has specifically addressed the relative contribution of various components of Rrs in neonates; hence, the information comes from pooling different sources and therefore must be interpreted with caution.[80] Estimates indicate that the airway resistance (Raw) and lung resistance (Rl) constitute 75 per cent of Rrs, and that Rl contributes 40 per cent of the combined Raw plus Rl; this latter fraction is larger than that in adults. The high contribution of lung resistance to Rrs could reflect the larger proportion of lung tissue to airspace in the neonate. Direct measurement of the peripheral airways resistance in infants and children shows that these airways also contribute a greater fraction of Rrs than in the adult.

Mechanical Properties and Dynamic Characteristics of the Chest Wall

The chest wall comprises all those structures that are external to the lung and move with passive changes in lung volume. The chest wall is considered to have two compartments, the diaphragm-abdominal system and the rib cage. The dynamic performance of these two components depends not only on their individual performance but also on coordination (timing and direction of force), configuration, and elastic and resistance properties. In neonates the compliance of the chest wall is very high (the P-V curve is almost vertical), and therefore there is a large volume change per pressure increment. However, as in the adult, below EELV, chest wall compliance is reduced. On the other hand, the ribs are disposed more horizontally in neonates,[3] and the differences between the

major and the minor diameters are smaller than in the adult.[117] The most striking dynamic characteristic of neonatal breathing is the paradoxical movement of the rib cage with inspiration. Although this paradoxical motion is largely the result of the high compliance of the chest wall, it is also a function of the pattern of activation of the diaphragm and the intercostal muscles (neural coordination). Indeed, during rapid eye movement (REM) sleep in infants the intercostal muscles are inactive. In addition, effective intercostal counteraction of distortion requires a functional gamma loop. Experimental studies in kittens indicate that, as in skeletal muscles, the intercostal gamma loop is not mature. However, activation of intercostal muscles in infants has been observed with large breaths and when there is electroneurographic evidence of diaphragmatic fatigue.[121]

Control of End-Expiratory Lung Volume

During resting, breathing infants normally keep their EELV above the relaxation volume (functional residual capacity, FRC) (dynamic control). Several different or even combined mechanisms contribute to the dynamic control of the EELV in the neonate. These mechanisms are (1) shortening of T$_E$ so that there is insufficient T$_E$ for the volume to reach the relaxation volume; (2) prolongation of inspiratory muscle activity into the expiratory phase (the slow decay of inspiratory muscle activity is frequently observed in the diaphragmatic electromyogram or in the phrenic electroneurogram); and (3) an increase in expiratory resistance primarily from laryngeal and pharyngeal closure. The advantages of the dynamic maintenance of the EELV include a more uniform distribution of the alveolar volume and elastic properties, and therefore a more uniform distribution of ventilation. The dynamic control of EELV therefore supplements the role of surfactants in maintaining the stability of the gas exchange units. In addition it should be noted that in adult mammals, including primates, both the control of diaphragmatic–rib cage coordination[110] and of the upper airway caliber[58] are sensitive to the effects of sedation and general anesthesia.

Effect of Position on the Ventilation–Blood Flow Distribution

Bronchospirometric and radioisotopic studies of regional ventilation in spontaneously breathing adults have demonstrated that both blood flow and ventilation are preferentially distributed to the *dependent* regions of the lung. In addition, in the lateral position in the unanesthetized spontaneously breathing adult, the dependent lung again receives preferential distribution of both ventilation and blood flow. When this observation was extended to clinical practice, it was demonstrated in adults with unilateral pulmonary disease that oxygenation was improved when the good lung was dependent.[101] However, several recent studies in infants with unilateral pulmonary disease have shown that oxygenation was improved when the normal lung was nondependent.[21,46] A more recent

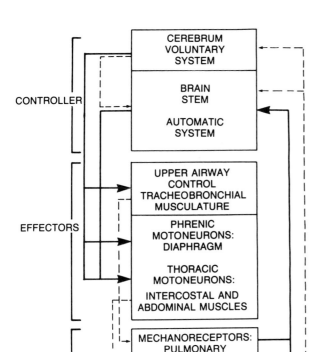

Figure 8–6. Schematic of the respiratory control system showing the controller, afferents from chemoreceptors, mechanoreceptors, pain receptors and higher centers, and the efferent pathways. Major pathways are shown as continuous line and minor pathways are shown as dashed lines. (Reproduced with permission from Kafer ER [1987]: Neurophysiology of respiration and the effects of anesthesia. Appl Cardiopul Pathophysiol 2:183–202.)

study using radioisotopic techniques has confirmed that in infants with and without unilateral pulmonary disease there is a reversal of the adult pattern of distribution of ventilation in the lateral position.[26] The difference from the adult may be the result of a Ppl in the newborn infant that is closer to atmospheric pressure, and therefore the infant breathes at a relatively lower EELV. When Ppl is close to atmospheric pressure in adults, ventilation in the lateral position is indeed preferentially distributed to the nondependent lung.[82] These observations have important clinical implications in optimizing oxygenation in the neonate. Furthermore, the usual effects of lateral positioning in the newborn infant may be modified by positive end-expiratory pressure during conventional mechanical ventilation, by continuous positive airway pressure, or by high frequency ventilation.

RESPIRATORY CONTROL

The respiratory control system comprises a controller, sensors, and the effector systems (Fig. 8–6).[58] In the adult, the controller and the pathways to the effector system are composed of two anatomically and functionally different neural systems: a metabolic, or automatic, system and a behavioral, or voluntary, system. Successful development of the automatic respiratory control system is essential for gas exchange, and for compensatory responses to (1) increased metabolism, (2) ventilation–blood flow maldistribution and shunt, (3) metabolic disturbances in acid-base balance, and (4) sustained mechanical loads. The function of this automatic respiratory control system is, of course, dependent on several factors, including central nervous system development, peripheral responses to increased neural drive, integrity of the diaphragm and associated respiratory musculature, and maturation of the mechanical properties of the respiratory system.

Respiratory Rhythm and Drive

In the absence of chemoreceptor stimulation, the appearance and maintenance of respiratory rhythm in the fetus is dependent on behavioral status. In the fetal lamb, respiratory movements are often observed during a state comparable to REM or active sleep.[28] However, with increasing chemoreceptor input, particularly during hypoxemia, respiratory movements are also observed during non-REM sleep.[19,20]

Following birth, major changes in somatic afferent stimuli (temperature, touch, hearing, and sight) occur, and a relatively regular respiratory rhythm develops.[70] However, in preterm infants, recurrent apneic episodes represent a major clinical problem.[39,69,79] Although it is assumed that immaturity of the central neural control of respiratory rhythm underlies the apnea of prematurity, the neurophysiologic and neurochemical mechanisms responsible have not been defined. Studies using brain stem auditory-evoked responses have shown increased latencies in preterm infants that parallel the immaturity of the respiratory control system.[47] These data support the general concept of the immaturity or impaired development of the brain stem as an associated phenomenon with the apnea of prematurity. Further considerations include the role of neurochemical transmitters and modulators in the maturation of respiratory control. In contrast to normal adults, naloxone increases respiratory drive in newborn animals, and therefore it is concluded that during the first few postnatal days endorphins may depress central respiratory drive.[45,77]

In addition, there is neurophysiologic evidence that in the absence of somatic stimuli or in the presence of impaired afferent transmission, chemoreceptor stimuli are essential to the maintenance of the respiratory rhythm.[111,134] Similarly, with minimal input from higher centers, the chemoreceptor stimuli are important in maintenance of respiratory rhythm and drive.[43,134] Further, considerations have also been given to afferent stimuli, such as from the upper airway, that may inhibit respiratory rhythm and drive.[14] In addition, it has also been demonstrated that as in adult animals, intercostal-phrenic reflexes are inhibitory to respiratory drive in newborn infants[64] and may be activated by changes in lung volume.[48]

Chemical Regulation of Respiratory Rhythm and Drive

The chemical regulation of ventilation is usually measured as the minute ventilation ($\dot{V}_E$), tidal volume (V_T), frequency (f), and airway occlusion pressure responses to CO_2 and/or hypoxemia. The stimulus patterns used for evaluating chemical regulation of ventilation in newborn infants differ for single breath, rebreathing, and steady state methods, and therefore so do the physiologic responses and their interpretations. Obviously, only an overview may be described in this chapter. Both uncomplicated preterm and full-term neonates increase their V_T in response to CO_2.[102,103] As in adults, the increase in f in response to CO_2 in newborn infants is variable. The increase in $\dot{V}_E$ in response to CO_2 observed in newborn infants is normalized for body size, and is regarded as a "normal" response to central chemoreceptor stimulation.[102] However, two features of the CO_2 response in preterm infants have been noted. First, in preterm infants exposed to CO_2, f increases only transiently.[78] Second, measurement of the steady state responses to CO_2 in preterm infants has shown a lower response in apneic infants than in nonapneic infants.[39]

In neonates an important feature of the ventilatory response to hypoxemia is the failure of sustained response.[79] After an increase in $\dot{V}_E$ for approximately a minute, there is a decrease in ventilation within 2 to 3 minutes. The phenomenon is more consistently observed during active sleep. By 2 to 3 weeks the increase in $\dot{V}_E$ in response to hypoxemia is sustained. Hypotheses advanced to explain the late hypoxic depression of ventilation in neonates include increases in cerebral blood flow, exhaustion of neurotransmitters and/or neuromodulators, and suprapontine inhibition. Respiratory depression from hypoxemia is, however, not unique to the neonate. Anesthetic drugs such as halothane—even in subanesthetic doses—depress the ventilatory response to hypoxemia.[56,57] Further, reexamination of the effects of most central nervous system drugs on the chemical regulation of ventilation demonstrates a greater depression of the ventilatory response to hypoxemia than to CO_2.[57] In addition, postanesthesia apnea is well documented in preterm infants.[69]

Compensatory Responses to Mechanical Loads

The compensatory responses to an increase in the mechanical loads to breathing are complex. In summary, they may be divided into the following:

1. Nonneural or "intrinsic" load adjustment responses, which include the elastic and resistance properties of the respiratory system, the force-length and force-velocity relationships of the diaphragm, and also the Laplace relationships of the diaphragm. In the unanesthetized adult or the vagotomized anesthetized animal these are major contributors to the first breath load adjustment.[95,100]

2. A neurally mediated increase in intercostal muscle activity (via the gamma loop) that is probably minor.

3. Neurally mediated (probably via pulmonary vagal stretch receptors) prolongation in inspiratory time (T_I) and therefore peak inspiratory force during the first loaded breath.[24,90] However, during active sleep in infants, load compensation is disorganized, possibly as a result of inhibition of the intercostal muscles.[48,63]

4. Progressive increase in neural drive resulting from an increase in chemoreceptor stimuli during sustained mechanical loads.

Therefore, in neonates the ability to compensate for an increase in mechanical load is influenced by behavioral state, integrity of neural reflexes, including responses to chemoreceptor stimuli, and mechanical properties (particularly of the rib cage). Further, drugs that impair neural control may depress the normally sustained response to an increase in mechanical load. Finally, the development of neuromuscular fatigue, evidenced by changes in the diaphragmatic electromyogram, may further impair the maintenance of gas exchange.[83]

Reflex Cardiorespiratory Responses to Hypoxemia

In the normal unanesthetized adult, the cardiorespiratory reflex responses to hypoxemia are the result of a complex interaction of direct responses to peripheral chemoreceptor stimuli and secondary reflex circulatory responses to the respiratory response (Fig. 8–7).[56,57] In addition to the increase in $\dot{V}_E$, V_T, and f, during hypoxemia, HR and CO increase and peripheral vascular resistance decreases.[56,57,113] However, when the respiratory response is inhibited, the direct cardiovascular reflex responses to peripheral chemoreceptor stimuli are characterized by a decreased heart rate and an increase in peripheral vascular resistance. Therefore, the cardiovascular reflex responses to hypoxemia are dependent on the integrity of the respiratory responses to hypoxemia. Other variables include the magnitude of hypoxemia,[36] gestational age,[113] and environmental temperature,[15] as well as drugs that impair the neural reflex responses to hypoxemia. In neonates, as in adults, specific organ vascular responses to hypoxemia depend on the balance of direct vasodilation (e.g., cerebral blood flow)[55] and vasoconstriction mediated by the sympathetic nervous system (e.g., renal blood flow).[17,40,56,57]

RED CELL AND HEMOGLOBIN FUNCTION IN THE NEWBORN

Several aspects of the red cell and hemoglobin molecule have profound effects on oxygen transport and tissue uptake. Those aspects include (1) the oxygen dissociation curve (ODC) and the affinity for oxygen, which is measured as the P_{50};[8] (2) the red cell concentration and structure and the plasma constituents, which determine the viscosity of the blood and the deformity of the erythrocyte;[68,104] and (3) extracellular fluid plasma and blood volumes and the fetal and maternal osmolality together with the neural reflex and humoral responses to volume and osmolality changes in the newborn.[140] In this discussion attention is focused on hemoglobin and the erythrocyte function.

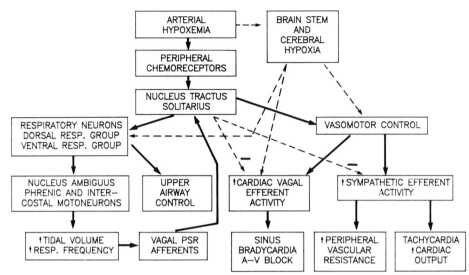

Figure 8–7. Schematic of the acute reflex respiratory and cardiovascular responses to hypoxemia. Arrows with heavy lines = major pathways; arrows with dashed lines = minor pathways; − = inhibition. (Reproduced with permission from Kafer ER [1985]: Cardiorespiratory effects of hypoxemia. Anaesthesiol Inten Care Med 180:33–52.)

Erythrocyte and Hemoglobin O_2 Affinity

The major function of the erythrocyte is to serve as a vehicle to transport oxygen to the organs and carbon dioxide to the lungs. The transport of oxygen is performed primarily by hemoglobin, which is present in high concentration in the erythrocyte. The mature erythrocyte is a "specialized" organ whose metabolic activities are those of the cytoplasm. Nevertheless, the mature erythrocyte modulates the affinity of hemoglobin by production of 2,3-diphosphoglycerate (2,3-DPG) and other organic phosphates.[12,13,18,93]

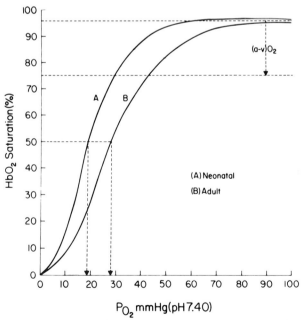

Figure 8–8. The oxyhemoglobin dissociation curves in adult (B) and neonatal (A) hemoglobin and their respective P_{50} values. (Reproduced with permission from Sachs LM, Delivoria-Papadopoulos M [1984]: Hemoglobin-oxygen interactions. Semin Perinatol 8:168–183.)

The affinity of hemoglobin for oxygen is described by the ODC[120] and may be expressed as the P_{50}.[8] The P_{50} is the partial pressure in mmHg of oxygen at which the hemoglobin is 50 per cent saturated with oxygen under standard conditions of temperature and pH. An *increase* in the P_{50} results in a *decrease* in affinity (shift to the right), whereas a *decrease* in P_{50} results in an *increase* in affinity (shift to the left) for oxygen (Fig. 8–8).[109] In addition, hemoglobin is an allosteric protein, i.e., interaction with one substance at one or more sites influences the interaction with other substances at other (noncontiguous) sites. The allosteric behavior of hemoglobin enables the complex interactions between oxygen and 2,3-DPG, and also between CO_2 and hydrogen ions and gives hemoglobin its biologic behavior.[106,109]

Structure of Hemoglobin and the ODC

Hemoglobin is a nearly spherical molecule with a diameter of 55 Å and is made up of four subunits (globin), each with an oxygen binding group, the prosthetic heme group or moiety. In adult hemoglobin (HbA), the globin units comprise two pairs of amino acid chains, a pair of α-chains (141 amino acids) and a pair of β-chains (146 amino acids). The amino acid composition (primary structure) of the chains is genetically determined and is pertinent to the oxygen transport function of hemoglobin. Fetal hemoglobin (HbF) differs from HbA by having two α- and two γ-chains (146 amino acids) ($α_2 γ_2$:HbF). The β- and γ-chains differ from each other: in position 143, histidine in the β-chain is replaced by serine in the γ-chain.[4] This amino acid difference is critical for the binding of 2,3-DPG to the HbA molecule and the reduced binding of 2,3-DPG to HbF and therefore their differences in P_{50}. The secondary structures of each subunit are composed of largely α-helices of the individual chains, and the tertiary folding of the secondary structures results in a similar globular structure of both chains.[106] The spatial relationship of the subunit globin chains to each other constitutes the quarternary structure. Within the secondary structure, the E and F helices form a hydrophobic cleft in which the heme group is inserted. The hydrophobic characteristics protect the heme group from oxidation, and therefore the iron remains in the ferrous state.[106] Each heme group contains a porphyrin ring and a ferrous iron with five (RHb) or six (O_2Hb) coordinated groups. Four of these are nitrogen atoms of the porphyrin ring, the fifth is an imidazole group of the histidine residue in the F helix of the globin chain, and the sixth coordinated group of O_2Hb is oxygen or another ligand, e.g., CO_2. The distance between the heme groups is considerable, and therefore their interaction to form the sigmoid dissociation curve is indirect and the result of conformational changes. X-ray crystallographic studies have shown that O_2Hb and RHb differ markedly from each other in their quarternary structure, and the O_2Hb is the more compact form (tense T-form).[97] In addition, there is evidence that there are two contact regions between the α- and the β-chains, termed $α_1$, $β_1$, (also $α_2$, $β_2$) and $α_2$ $β_1$ (also $α_1$ $β_2$) contacts. In the transition from O_2Hb to RHb, the atoms at the $α_2$, $β_1$ site shift by 6 Å and are stabilized by hydrogen bonding. Thus, structural changes such as amino acid substitutions in the $α_2$, $β_1$ region affect the heme-heme interaction.[109]

From a teleologic point of view the interaction between the heme groups to form the sigmoid-shaped ODC is advantageous. The shape of the curve ensures optimal binding of oxygen in the pulmonary capillaries and release in the peripheral tissues. Similarly, shifts in the position of the ODC occur as a result of changes in temperature, partial pressure of CO_2, and pH (Bohr effect). Further, the effects of oxygen on the binding of CO_2 and hydrogen ions (CDH effect) are also advantageous for CO_2 transport and release as well as hydrogen ion homeostasis. The molecular groups involved and the mechanism proposed for the Bohr effect are the C terminal histidine of the β-chain (HC3 [146] his), N terminal amino groups of the α-chains (NA1 [1] val), and possibly the α-chain, histidine 122.[106] As a result of the Bohr effect, an increase in PCO_2 and/or H^+ ion shifts the ODC to the right in both adult and fetal blood.[49,50] The Bohr effect expressed as log P_{50} per change in pH ($\Delta - log P_{50}/\Delta - pH$) is −0.48 and −0.44 for adult and fetal red cells, respectively.[109] However, there is also evidence that the Bohr effect is also influenced by the presence of 2,3-DPG.[4] It should be noted that the effect of varying the PCO_2 at the same pH exceeds that of varying the pH at the constant PCO_2.[49] In addition, the effect of prolonged changes in pH (2 to 3 hours) is dependent on the red cell organic phosphates. Further, the slope of the log P_{50} per change in pH relationship is increased at low oxygen tensions when 2,3-DPG is depleted.[49,109]

Control and Effects of Erythrocyte Organic Phosphates

2,3-DPG and other organic phosphates (adenosine triphosphate [ATP], diphosphate [ADP], and monophosphate [AMP] in descending order of affinity) bind to hemoglobin and modulate hemoglobin affinity for oxygen.[12,13,18] 2,3-DPG is produced by intracellular erythrocyte metabolism and forms salt bridges with valine 1 and histidine 2 and 143 of both β-chains and to the lysine[82] of one β-chain.[4] A single molecule of 2,3-DPG is therefore linked by salt bridges to cations at the entrance of the central cavity. As a result of the conformational changes of the hemoglobin molecule, in its reduced form (RHb) the hemoglobin cavity accommodates the 2,3-DPG molecule, but in its oxygenated form (compact or tense [T] form of O_2Hb), the 2,3-DPG molecule is extruded.[4] In the normal adult erythrocyte the concentration of 2,3-DPG is 4 to 5 $\mu mol \cdot ml^{-1}$ RBC and the remaining organic phosphates constitute a small concentration (e.g., ATP 0.8 to 1.4 $\mu mol \cdot ml^{-1}$ RBC). Through a wide range of 2,3-DPG concentrations in adult erythrocytes there is a linear change in P_{50}; as the concentration of 2,3-DPG increases, the affinity for oxygen decreases.[92,93] The slope of the relationship is such that a change of 430 nmol of 2,3-DPG per ml erythrocyte results in a shift of 1 mmHg in the P_{50}.[92] These features are not shared by the erythrocyte of the newborn.[92,93,127]

Multiple biochemical and physiologic factors control the erythrocyte concentration of 2,3-DPG[92,93,127] as well as the affinity of hemoglobin for 2,3-DPG. Factors that influence the binding of 2,3-DPG to hemoglobin are pH, temperature, other anions (e.g., chloride), PCO_2, and the hemoglobin concentration.[106] The concentration of 2,3-DPG is also influenced by those variables as well as pathophysiologic processes, including cardiac failure, shock, and hypoxemia.[92] Pregnancy increases 2,3-DPG, which shifts the maternal ODC further to the right and thereby facilitates O_2 unloading to the fetal HbF.[9] In addition, the concentration of 2,3-DPG falls in stored blood, resulting in a reduction in P_{50}, but several hours after transfusion the P_{50} of the transfused cells returns to normal.[124] Therefore, it has been proposed that the reduced P_{50} with increased affinity for O_2 might impair the ability of stored blood to release oxygen in the tissues in patients receiving major stored blood transfusions. However, oxygen delivery in the periphery is also limited by organ perfusion and capillary density, and therefore it is difficult to quantitate the clinical significance of changes in 2,3-DPG and P_{50} at any age.

Fetal Hemoglobin and Postnatal Changes

Fetal hemoglobin is uniquely suited to advantageously take up oxygen at the placenta, because its increased affinity for oxygen (reduced P_{50}) situates the fetal ODC to the left of maternal ODC.[53] The increased affinity of HbF for oxygen is the result of its reduced affinity for 2,3-DPG and other organic phosphates. The effect of 2,3-DPG on the affinity of HbF for oxygen is only 40 per cent that of HbA. The molecular basis of HbF's reduced affinity for 2,3-DPG is the substitution of serine in the γ-chain for histidine in the β-chain (His 143).[4] During fetal life and the first few months of postnatal life, as the concentrations of HbA and 2,3-DPG increase, the P_{50} and oxygen affinity

Table 8–8. HEMOGLOBIN CONCENTRATION, P_{50}, HbF, AND 2,3-DPG
CONCENTRATION IN INFANT AND ADULT BLOOD

Age	Hemoglobin Concentration ($g \cdot dl^{-1}$)	HbF (%)	P_{50} (mmHg)	2,3-DPG ($\mu mol \cdot ml\ RBC^{-1}$)
Premature	16.26	74.8 ± 3.8	19.91 ± 1.44	4.00 ± 1.26
Full term	17.65	59.1 ± 7.9	21.50 ± 1.57	3.94 ± 1.09
5 to 10 days	16.89	53.7 ± 6.6	22.87 ± 1.40	4.93 ± 0.71
11 to 20 days	15.87	50.3 ± 4.5	23.60 ± 1.33	4.80 ± 0.94
21 to 30 days	13.54	42.8 ± 6.2	24.60 ± 1.45	4.59 ± 1.11
60 to 120 days	11.00	19.4 ± 6.2	26.74 ± 2.64	4.73 ± 1.19
6 months	11.12	4.1 ± 2.1	27.47 ± 2.43	4.41 ± 0.86
6 years	13.10	1.2 ± 0.8	27.15 ± 1.59	3.99 ± 0.55
Adult	14.28	0	25.87 ± 1.28	4.11 ± 0.76

Notes: Mean ± SD, n = 6 to 12 infants. The hemoglobin concentrations were estimated from the blood oxygen concentrations and the hemoglobin oxygen capacity ($1.34\ ml \cdot g^{-1}$ hemoglobin). The values were not corrected for dissolved oxygen. (Adapted with permission from Versmold HT et al [1973]: Blood oxygen affinity in infancy. The interaction of fetal and adult hemoglobin, oxygen capacity, and red cell hydrogen ion and 2,3-diphosphoglycerate concentration. Respir Physiol 18:14–25.)

correlate with the concept of "functioning DPG fraction," i.e., the product of HbA per cent × DPG $nmol \cdot ml^{-1}$ RBC (Table 8–5) (Figs. 8–9 and 8–10).[30,31,81,126,128] In addition, ATP does not bind to HbF as well as to HbA, and this difference may prevent depletion of membrane ATP by HbF, a condition that may predispose to red cell rigidity. Reduced HbF binding of ATP may be particularly advantageous during fetal life because hypoxemia increases cell rigidity. Fetal red cell rigidity in combination with the already high fetal hematocrit would markedly increase the blood viscosity and resistance to flow.

As the embryo develops, multiple allelic genes give rise to different types of fetal hemoglobin.[88] In humans at least seven different hemoglobin subunits develop, and their appearance is precisely scheduled. The embryonic hemoglobins, Gower 1 and 2 and Portland, usually disappear by 10 weeks' gestation. HbF is the predominant hemoglobin from 8 weeks to approximately 40 weeks after conception.[88] Formation of HbA begins as early as the tenth week of gestation. However, at 30 weeks it constitutes only 5 to 10 per cent and at term, is only 20 to 30 per cent of the total hemoglobin.[5-7] The switchover from almost exclusively HbF (90 to 95 per cent) to increasing HbA synthesis, which occurs at 30 weeks, is determined by gestational age and is not altered by premature birth.[5-7] HbF synthesis rapidly declines after birth and is negligible at 16 to 20 weeks of age (Table 8–8).[7,128] Recently, a number of environmental factors have been

shown to alter the timing of HbA synthesis, including maternal diabetes[96] and hypoxemia.[11] Changes in the fetal erythrocyte metabolism parallel the declining synthesis in HbF and probably represent a maturation to the adult form of erythropoiesis.[81]

The postnatal decrease in HbF and increase in HbA result in a progressive right shift in the ODC; by 6 to 8 months of age the infant's ODC and P_{50} are similar to the adult's. In the term infant, the P_{50} increases from 19.4 ± 1.8 to 20.6 ± 1.7 mmHg in the first 5 postnatal days (Figs. 8–9 and 8–10, Table 8–8).[10,31,126,128] The shift in the ODC over the succeeding 6- to 8-month period is gradual. Again, the postnatal changes in erythrocyte metabolism and enzyme activity parallel the decline in HbF and represent maturation of erythropoiesis.

Physiologic Implications of the ODC in Neonatal O_2 Transport

Although HbF is uniquely suited to optimize O_2 exchange at the placenta and to carry out oxygen transport in the fetus, it has been speculated that in the neonate, particularly when oxygen transport is compromised, HbF with its high O_2 affinity may be disadvantageous to tissue O_2 release. In the presence of fetal hemoglobin, the myocardium, which normally has a large $a\bar{v}O_2D$, may receive insufficient O_2 to ensure an adequate compen-

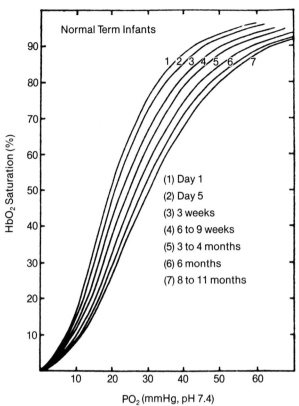

Figure 8–9. Progressive shift in the oxyhemoglobin dissociation curve from day 1 to 8 to 11 months of life in normal term infants. (Reproduced with permission from Delivoria-Papadopoulos M et al [1971]: Postnatal changes in oxygen transport of term, premature, and sick infants: The role of red cell 2,3-diphosphoglycerate and adult hemoglobin. Pediatr Res 5:235–245.)

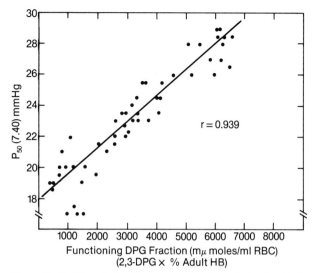

Figure 8–10. The relationship between the P_{50} and the functioning 2,3-DPG fraction (m µ moles/ml RBC) in full-term infants at normal pH. (Reproduced with permission from Delivoria-Papadopoulos M et al [1971]: Exchange transfusion in the newborn infant with fresh and "old" blood: The role of storage on 2,3-diphosphoglycerate hemoglobin-oxygen affinity, and oxygen release. J Pediatr 79:898–903.)

satory response to compromised O_2 delivery. Although a number of clinical studies, particularly in premature neonates with respiratory distress, have shown clinical improvement with exchange transfusion (and the improvement has been associated with a rightward shift in the ODC),[29,30,41,139] it is argued that there have been no major clinical controlled trials of its efficacy.[61] Multiple factors, which include administration of vasoactive substances and/or improved volume loading, may have contributed to improved tissue perfusion, O_2 delivery, and neonatal outcome after exchange transfusion. However, a number of physiologic studies in lambs in which O_2 transport has been compromised have demonstrated improvement in O_2 delivery and tissue oxygenation following transfusion with low affinity hemoglobin. Therefore, although the results of experimental studies in lambs should be interpreted with caution, the evidence from these experimental studies is supportive of the concept that tissue O_2 delivery may be improved with low affinity hemoglobin.

Control of Erythropoiesis

Erythropoietin is considered to be the primary hormone controlling erythropoiesis in both the adult and the fetus.[85]

In the fetus, as in the adult, the level of erythropoietin is dependent on O_2 delivery. An example of this is the demonstration that fetal hypoxemia results in an immediate increase in erythropoietin.[138] Because erythropoietin does not cross the placenta, it is assumed that fetal levels represent fetal synthesis. The early postnatal level of erythropoietin was closely correlated with an index of tissue oxygen release.[116] The interaction of hemoglobin concentration (O_2 capacity) with shifting P_{50} and the changing O_2 tissue release that results account for the "physiologic" anemia of prematurity. This anemia is maximum at 2 to 3 months of age.[116]

SUMMARY

In comparison to the adult, the neonate has an increased tendency to develop hypoxemia and a reduced ability to compensate for impaired O_2 transport. The factors that lead to hypoxemia include (1) reduced FRC relative to the $\dot{V}O_2$ and therefore reduced O_2 stores even when 100 per cent oxygen is being breathed; (2) increased ventilation–blood flow maldistribution and shunt, which increases the AaO_2P; (3) reduced ability to increase ventilation in response to mechanical and/or chemical loads, together with hypoventilation in response to sustained hypoxemia; and (4) relatively high metabolic rate. The limited ability to compensate for impaired O_2 transport is the result of the reduced ability of the myocardium to respond to volume and pressure loads; high hemoglobin O_2 affinity, which impairs tissue oxygen delivery and which is critical to the myocardial function because of its high $a\bar{v}O_2D$; high blood viscosity; and possible limitations in redistributing CO to facilitate oxygenation of critical organs.

ABBREVIATIONS

Gas Exchange and O_2 Transport

AaO_2P	=	alveolar-arterial oxygen pressure gradient, mmHg
$a\bar{v}O_2D$	=	arterial-mixed venous oxygen content difference, $ml \cdot dl^{-1}$
AVO_2	=	oxygen availability or delivery, $ml \cdot min^{-1}$ or $ml \cdot min^{-1} \cdot kg^{-1} = \dot{Q}_t \times CaO_2 \times 10$
CaO_2	=	arterial oxygen content, $ml \cdot dl^{-1}$
$C\acute{c}O_2$	=	end pulmonary capillary oxygen content, $ml \cdot dl^{-1}$
$C\bar{v}O_2$	=	mixed venous oxygen content, $ml \cdot dl^{-1}$
CO	=	cardiac output, $ml \cdot min^{-1}$ or $ml \cdot min^{-1} \cdot kg^{-1}$
2,3-DPG	=	2,3-diphosphoglycerate
O_2ER	=	oxygen extraction, ratio, or percentage, $\dot{V}O_2/CO \times CaO_2$
PaO_2	=	arterial oxygen tension, mmHg
PAO_2	=	alveolar oxygen tension, mmHg
$PaCO_2$	=	arterial carbon dioxide tension, mmHg
pHa	=	arterial pH
$P\bar{v}O_2$	=	mixed venous oxygen tension, mmHg
$\dot{Q}_{sh}$	=	amount of shunted cardiac output, $ml \cdot min^{-1}$
$\dot{Q}_t$	=	total cardiac output, $ml \cdot min^{-1}$
$\dot{Q}_{sh}/\dot{Q}_t$	=	shunt fraction, %
SaO_2	=	arterial oxygen hemoglobin saturation, %
$S\bar{v}O_2$	=	mixed venous oxyhemoglobin saturation, %
VA	=	calculated venous admixture, %
$\dot{V}_A$	=	alveolar ventilation, ml or $liter \cdot min^{-1}$, BTPS
V_T	=	tidal volume, ml, BTPS
V_D	=	dead space, ml, BTPS
V_D/V_T	=	dead space/tidal volume ratio
$\dot{V}O_2$	=	oxygen consumption, $ml \cdot min^{-1}$ or $ml \cdot min^{-1} \cdot kg^{-1}$, STPD
$\dot{V}CO_2$	=	carbon dioxide production, $ml \cdot min^{-1} \cdot kg^{-1}$, STPD

Hemodynamic Function

Ao	=	mean aortic pressure, mmHg
CO	=	cardiac output, $ml \cdot min^{-1}$ or $ml \cdot min^{-1} \cdot kg^{-1}$
HR	=	heart rate, $beats \cdot min^{-1}$
SVR	=	systemic vascular resistance

Hemoglobin Species and Status

HbA	=	adult hemoglobin
HbF	=	fetal hemoglobin
RHb %	=	reduced hemoglobin, %
O_2Hb	=	oxyhemoglobin, % (SO_2 %)
COHb %	=	carboxyhemoglobin, %
MetHb %	=	methemoglobin, %
THb	=	total hemoglobin concentration, $g \cdot dl^{-1}$
ODC	=	oxyhemoglobin dissociation curve
P_{50}	=	partial pressure of oxygen at which hemoglobin is 50% saturated with oxygen, pH 7.40, and 37°C

Respiratory Mechanics and Timing

Cldyn	=	dynamic compliance of the lung, $ml \cdot cm\ H_2O^{-1}$
Clst	=	static compliance of the lung, $ml \cdot cm\ H_2O^{-1}$
Ccw	=	compliance of the chest wall, $ml \cdot cm\ H_2O^{-1}$
Crs	=	compliance of the respiratory system, $ml \cdot cm\ H_2O^{-1}$
EELV	=	end-expiratory lung volume, liter or ml, BTPS
FRC	=	functional residual capacity, ml, BTPS
f	=	respiratory frequency, $breaths \cdot min^{-1}$
Ppl	=	pleural pressure, cm H_2O
Raw	=	airway resistance, cm $H_2O \cdot liter^{-1} \cdot s^{-1}$
Rl	=	lung resistance, cm $H_2O \cdot liter^{-1} \cdot s^{-1}$
Rrs	=	total respiratory resistance, cm $H_2O \cdot liter^{-1} \cdot s^{-1}$
T_E	=	expiratory time, s
T_I	=	inspiratory time, s
T_T	=	total respiratory time, s
TLC	=	total lung capacity, liter or ml, BTPS
V	=	volume, liter or ml
$\dot{V}_I$ or $\dot{V}_E$	=	minute ventilation or flow, liter or $ml \cdot min^{-1}$, BTPS
VC	=	vital capacity, liter or ml, BTPS
Vr	=	static relaxation volume of the respiratory system, liter or ml, BTPS
V_T	=	tidal volume, liter or ml, BTPS

References

1. Abdulrazzaq YM, Brooke OG (1984): Respiratory metabolism in preterm infants: The measurement of oxygen consumption during prolonged periods. Pediatrics Res 18:928–931.
2. Adams FH, Lind J (1957): Physiologic studies on the cardiovascular status of normal newborn infants (with special reference to the ductus arteriosus). Pediatrics 19:431–437.
3. Agostoni E, Kinematics (1970): In Campbell, EJM, Agostoni E, Davis JN (eds): The Respiratory Muscles: Mechanics and Neural Control. Philadelphia, WB Saunders Co, pp 23–47.
4. Arnone A (1972): X-ray diffraction study of binding of 2,3-diphosphoglycerate in human erythrocytes to human deoxyhemoglobin. Nature 237:146–149.
5. Bard H (1973): Postnatal fetal and adult hemoglobin synthesis in early preterm newborn infants. J. Clin Invest 52:1789–1795.
6. Bard H (1975): Postnatal decline of hemoglobin F synthesis in normal infants. J Clin Invest 55:395–398.
7. Bard H, Prosmanne J (1982): Postnatal fetal and adult hemoglobin synthesis in preterm infants whose birth weight was less than 1000 grams. J Clin Invest 70:50–52.
8. Bartels H, Harms H (1959): Sauerstoffdissoziationskurven de Blutes von Saugertieren. Pflugers Arch Ges Physiol 268:334–365.
9. Bauer CH, Ludwig M, Ludwig I, Bartels H (1969): Factors governing the oxygen affinity of human adult and fetal blood. Respir Physiol 7:271–277.
10. Baumann R, Bauer CH, Rathschlag-Schaefer AM (1972): Causes of the postnatal decrease of blood oxygen affinity in lambs. Respir Physiol 15:151–158.
11. Baumann R, Padeken S, Haller E-A, Brilmayer T (1983): Effects of hypoxia on oxygen affinity, hemoglobin pattern, and blood volume of early chicken embryos. Am J Physiol 244:R733–R741.
12. Benesch R, Benesch RE (1969): Intracellular organic phosphates as regulation of oxygen release by hemoglobin. Nature 221:618–622.
13. Benesch RE, Benesch R (1970): The reaction between diphosphoglycerate and hemoglobin. Fed Proc 29:1101–1104.
14. Boggs DF, Bartlett D (1982): Chemical specificity of a laryngeal apneic reflex in puppies. J Appl Physiol Respirat Environ Exercise Physiol 53:455–462.
15. Brady JP, Ceruti E (1966): Chemoreceptor reflexes in the newborn infant: Effects of varying degrees of hypoxia on heart rate and ventilation in a warm environment. J Physiol (London) 184:634–645.
16. Brooke OG, Alvear J, Arnold M (1979): Energy retention, energy expenditure and growth in healthy immature infants. Pediatr Res 13:215–220.
17. Buckley NM (1983): Regional circulatory function in the perinatal period. In Gootman I, Gootman RM (eds): Perinatal Cardiovascular Function. New York, Marcel Dekker, Inc, pp 227–264.
18. Chanutin A, Curnish RR (1967): Effect of organic and inorganic phosphates on the oxygen equilibrium of human erythrocytes. Arch Biochem Biophys 121:96–102.
19. Chernick V (1978): Fetal breathing movements and the onset of breathing at birth. Clin Perinatol 5:257–268.
20. Chernick V, Faridy EE, Pagtakhan, RD (1975): Role of peripheral chemoreceptors in the initiation of fetal respiration. J Appl Physiol 38:407–410.
21. Cohen RS, Smith DW, Stevenson DK, Moskowitz PS, Graham CB (1984): Lateral decubitus position as therapy for persistent focal pulmonary interstitial emphysema in neonates: A preliminary report. J Pediatr 104:441–443.
22. Cogswell JJ, Hatch DJ, Kerr AA, Taylor B (1975): Effects of continuous positive pressure airway on lung mechanics of babies after operation for congenital heart disease. Arch Dis Child 50:799–804.
23. Crone RK (1983): The respiratory system. In Gregory GA (ed): Pediatric Anesthesia. New York, Churchill Livingstone, pp 35–62.
24. Cross KW, Klaus M, Tooley WH, Weisser K (1960): The response of the newborn baby to inflation of the lungs. J Physiol (London): 151:551–565.
25. Cross KW, Tizard JPM, Trythall DAH (1958): The gaseous metabolism of the newborn infant breathing 15% oxygen. Acta Paediatr Scand 47:217–237.
26. Davies H, Kitchman R, Gordon I, Helms P (1985): Regional ventilation in infancy. Reversal of adult pattern. N Engl J Med 313:1626–1628.
27. Davies G, Reid L (1970): Growth of the alveoli and pulmonary arteries in childhood. Thorax 23:669–681.
28. Dawes GS, Fox HE, Leduc BM, Liggins GG, Richards RT (1972): Respiratory movements and rapid eye movement sleep in the foetal lamb. J Physiol (London) 220:119–143.
29. Delivoria-Papadopoulos M, Miller LD, Forster RE et al (1976): The role of exchange transfusion in the management of low birth weight infants with and without severe respiratory distress syndrome. I. Initial observations. J Pediatr 89:273–278.
30. Delivoria-Papadopoulos M, Morrow G, Oski FA (1971): Exchange transfusion in the newborn infant with fresh and "old" blood: The role of storage on 2,3-diphosphoglycerate hemoglobin–oxygen affinity and oxygen release. J Pediatr 79:898–903.
31. Delivoria-Papadopoulos M, Roncevic NP, Oski FA (1971): Postnatal changes in oxygen transport of term, premature and sick infants: The role of red cell 2,3-diphosphoglycerate and adult hemoglobin. Pediatric Res 5:235–245.
32. Downing SE, Talner NS, Gardner TH (1965): Ventricular function in the newborn lamb. Am J Physiol 208:931–937.
33. Edelstone DI (1984): Fetal compensatory responses to reduced oxygen delivery. Semin Perinatol 8:184–191.
34. Emmanouilides GC, Moss AJ, Monset-Couchard M, Marcano BA, Rzeznic B (1970): Cardiac output in newborn infants. Biol Neonate 15:186–197.
35. Farhi LE, Rahn H (1955): A theoretical analysis of the alveolar-arterial O_2 difference with special reference to the distribution effect. J Appl Physiol 7:669–703.
36. Finley JP, Kelly C (1986): Heart rate and respiratory patterns in mild hypoxia in unanesthetized newborn mammals. Can J Physiol Pharmacol 64:122–124.
37. Fisher DJ (1984): Oxygenation and metabolism in the developing heart. Semin Perinatol 8:217–225.
38. Fisher JJ, Mortola JP (1980): Status of the respiratory system in newborn mammals. Respir Physiol 41:155–172.
39. Gerhadt T, Bancalari E (1984): Apnea of prematurity. I. Lung function and regulation of breathing. Pediatrics 74:58–62.
40. Gootman PM (1983): Neural regulation of cardiovascular function in the perinatal period. In Gootman N, Gootman PM (eds): Perinatal Cardiovascular Function. New York, Marcel Dekker, Inc, pp 265–328.
41. Gottuso MA, William ML, Oski FA (1976): The role of exchange transfusions in the management of low-birth weight infants with and without severe respiratory distress syndrome. II. Further observations and studies of mechanisms of action. J Pediatrics 89:279–285.
42. Gregory GA (1983): Anesthesia for premature infants. In Gregory GA (ed): Pediatric Anesthesia. New York, Churchill Livingstone, pp 579–606.
43. Haddad GG, Leisterner HL, Epstein RA (1980): CO_2 induced changes in ventilation and ventilatory pattern in normal sleep infants. J Appl Physiol Respirat Environ Exercise Physiol 48:684–688.
44. Hart MC, Orzalesi MM, Cook CS (1963): Relationship between anatomic respiratory dead space and body size and lung volume. J Appl Physiol 18:519–522.
45. Hazinski TA, Grunstein MM, Schlueter MA, Tooley WH (1981): Effect of naloxone on ventilation in newborn rabbits. J Appl Physiol 50:713–718.
46. Heaf DP, Helms P, Gordon I, Turner HM (1983): Postural effects on gas exchange in infants. N Engl J Med 308:1505–1508.
47. Henderson-Smart DJ, Pettigrew G, Campbell DJ (1983): Clinical apnea and brain stem neural function in preterm infants. N Engl J Med 308:353–357.
48. Henderson-Smart DJ, Read DJC (1979): Reduced lung volume during behavioral active sleep in the newborn. J Appl Physiol Respirat Environ Exercise Physiol 46:1081–1085.
49. Hlastala MP, Woodson RD (1975): Saturation dependency of the Bohr effect interactions among H^+, CO_2 and DPG. J Appl Physiol 38:1126–1131.

50. Hlastala MP, Standaert TA, Franada RL, McKenna HP (1978): Hemoglobin-ligand interaction in fetal and maternal sheep blood. Respir Physiol 34:185–194.

51. Hodson WA, Alden ER, Woodrum DE (1977): Gas exchange in the developing lung. In Hodson WA (ed): Development of the Lung. New York, Marcel Dekker, Inc, pp 469–496.

52. Hommes FA, Drost YM, Geraets WXM, Reijenga MAA (1975): The energy requirement for growth: An application of Atkinson's metabolic price system. Pediatr Res 9:51–55.

53. Itskovitz J, Goetzman BW, Roman C, Rudolph AM (1984): Effects of fetal-maternal exchange transfusion on fetal oxygenation and blood flow distribution. Am J Physiol (Heart Circ Physiol): 247:H655–H660.

54. Itskovitz J, LaGamma EF, Rudolph AM (1987): Effects of cord compression of fetal blood flow distribution and O_2 delivery. Am J Physiol (Heart Circ Physiol) 252:H100–H109.

55. Jones MD Jr, Traystam RJ (1984): Cerebral oxygenation in the fetus, newborn and adult. Semin Perinatol 8:205–216.

56. Kafer ER (1985): Cardiorespiratory effects of hypoxemia. Anaesthesiol Inten Care Med 180:33–52.

57. Kafer ER (1987): Effects of anesthesia on the cardiovascular and respiratory reflex response to hypoxemia. Appl Cardiopul Pathophysiol 1:143–160.

58. Kafer ER (1987): Neurophysiology of respiration and the effects of anesthesia. Appl Cardiopul Pathophysiol 2:183–202.

59. Kelman GR, Nunn JR, Prys-Roberts C, Greenbaum R (1967): The influence of cardiac output on arterial oxygenation: theoretical study. Br J Anaesth 39:450–458.

60. Kennaird DL (1976): Oxygen consumption and evaporation loss in infants with congenital heart disease. Arch Dis 51:34–41.

61. Kim HC (1983): Red blood cell transfusion in the neonates. Semin Perinatol 7:159–174.

62. Klopfenstein HS, Rudolph AM (1978): Postnatal changes in circulation and responses to volume loading in sheep. Circ Res 42:839–845.

63. Knill R, Andrews W, Bryan DC, Bryan MH (1976): Respiratory load compensation in infants. J Appl Physiol 40:357–361.

64. Knill R, Bryan AC (1976): An intercostal-phrenic inhibition reflex in human newborn infants. J Appl Physiol 40:352–356.

65. Koch G (1968): Alveolar ventilation, diffusion capacity and the $AaPO_2$ difference in the newborn infant. Respir Physiol 4:168–192.

66. Koch G, Wendel H (1968): Adjustment of arterial blood gases and acid base balance in the normal newborn infant during the first week of life. Biol Neonate 12:136–161.

67. Koehler RC, Traystam RJ, Jones MD, Jr (1986): Influence of reduced oxyhemoglobin affinity on cerebrovascular response to hypoxia. Am J Physiol (Heart Circ Physiol) 251:H756–H763.

68. Kon K, Maeda N, Shiga T (1983): The influence of deformation of transformed erythrocytes during flow on the rate of oxygen release. J Physiol (London) 339:573–584.

69. Kurth CD, Spitzer AR, Broennie AM, Downes, JJ (1987): Postoperative apnea in preterm infants. Anesthesiology 66:483–488.

70. LaFramboise WA, Tuck RE, Woodrum DE, Guthrie RD (1984): Maturation of eupneic respiration in the neonatal monkey. Pediatric Res 18:943–948.

71. Lees MH, Way RC, Ross BB (1967): Ventilation and respiratory gas transfer of infants with increased pulmonary flow. Pediatrics 43:259–271.

72. Leffler CW, Hessler JR, Green RS (1984): The onset of breathing at birth stimulates pulmonary vascular prostacyclin synthesis. Pediatric Res 18:938–942.

73. Levison H, Delivoria-Papadopoulos M, Swyer PR (1965): Variations in oxygen consumption in the infant with hyoxaemia due to cardiopulmonary disease. Acta Paediat Scand 54:369–374.

74. Lister G (1984): Oxygen transport in the intact hypoxic newborn lamb: Acute effects of increasing P_{50}. Pediatr Res 18:172–177.

75. Lister G, Moreau G, Ross N, Talner NS (1984): Effects of alterations of oxygen transport on the neonate. Semin Perinatol 8:192–204.

76. Lister G, Walter TK, Versmold HT, Dallman PR, Rudolph AM (1979): Oxygen delivery in lambs: Cardiovascular and hematologic development. Am J Physiol (Heart Circ Physiol) 237:H668–H675.

77. Long WA, Lawson EE (1983): Developmental aspects of the effect of naloxone on control of breathing in piglets. Respir Physiol 51:119–129.

78. Martin RJ, Carlo WA, Robertson SS, Day WR, Bruce EN (1985): Biphasic response of respiratory frequency to hypercapnia in preterm infants. Pediatr Res 19:791–796.

79. Martin RJ, Miller MJ, Carlo WA (1986): Pathogenesis of apnea in preterm infants. J Pediatric 109:733–741.

80. Mortola JP (1987): Dynamics of breathing in newborn mammals. Physiol Rev 67:187–243.

81. Mueggler PA, Carpenter S, Black JA (1983): Postnatal regulation of 2,3-DPG in sheep erythrocytes. Am J Physiol (Heart Circ Physiol) 245:H506–H512.

82. Milic-Emili J, Henderson JAM, Dolovich MB, Trop D, Kaneko K (1966): Regional distribution of gas in the lung. J Appl Physiol 21:749–759.

83. Muller N, Gulston G, Cade D, Bryan AC, Bryan MH (1979): Diaphragmatic muscle fatigue in the newborn. J Appl Physiol Respir Environ Exercise Physiol 46:688–695.

84. Murray JF (1976): The Normal Lung. The Basis for Diagnosis and Treatment of Pulmonary Disease. Philadelphia, WB Saunders Co.

85. Nathan DG, Sytkowski A (1983): Erythropoietin and the regulation of erythropoiesis. (Editorial) N Engl J Med 308:520–523.

86. Nelson NM, Prod'hom LS, Cherry RB, Lipsitz PH, Smith CA (1963): Pulmonary function in the newborn infant: The alveolar-arterial oxygen gradient. J Appl Physiol 18:534–538.

87. Nelson NM, Prod'hom LS, Cheng RB, Smith CA (1964): Contribution of the diffusion component to the alveolar-arterial oxygen tension difference in the newborn infants (Abstract). J Pediatr 65:110.

88. Nienhuis AW, Benz EJ (1977): Regulation of hemoglobin synthesis during the development of the red cell. N Engl J Med 297:1318–1328; 1371–1381; 1430–1436.

89. Normand ICS, Oliver RE, Reynolds EOR, Strang LB (1971): Permeability of lung capillaries and alveoli to non-electrolyte in the foetal lamb. J Physiol (London) 219:303–330.

90. Olinsky A, Bryan MH, Bryan AC (1974): Influence of lung inflation on respiratory control in neonates. J Appl Physiol 36:426–429.

91. Orzalesi MM, Mendicini M, Bucci G, Sacalamandre A, Savignoni PG (1967): Arterial oxygen studies in premature newborns with and without mild respiratory disorders. Arch Dis Child 42:174–180.

92. Oski FA, Gottlieb AJ, Miller WW, Delivoria-Papadopoulos M (1970): The effect of deoxygenation of adult and fetal hemoglobin on the synthesis of red cell 2,3-diphosphoglycerate and its in-vivo consequences. J Clin Invest 49:405–407.

93. Oski FA, Delivoria-Papadopoulos M (1970): The red cell 2,3-diphosphoglycerate and tissue oxygen release. J Pediatr 77:941–956.

94. Penefesky ZJ (1983): Perinatal development of cardiac contractile mechanisms. In Gootman N, Gootman PM (eds): Perinatal Cardiovascular Function. New York, Marcel Dekker, Inc, pp 109–199.

95. Pengelly LD, Alderson AM, Mulic-Emili J (1971): Mechanics of the diaphragm. J Appl Physiol 30:797–805.

96. Perrine SP, Greene MF, Faller DV (1985): Delay in fetal globin switch in infants of diabetic mothers. N Engl J Med 312:334–338.

97. Perutz MF (1976): Structure and mechanism of hemoglobin. Br Med Bull 32:195–208.

98. Pitt BR, Lister G (1983): Pulmonary metabolic function in the awake lamb: Effect of development and hypoxia. J Appl Physiol Respirat Environ Exercise Physiol 55:383–391.

99. Polgar G, Weng TR (1979): The functional development of the respiratory system. From the period of gestation to adulthood. Am Rev Respir Dis 120:625–695.

100. Read DJC, Freedman S, Kafer ER (1974): Pressures developed by loaded inspiratory muscles in conscious and anesthetized man. J Appl Physiol 37:207–218.

101. Remolina C, Khan AU, Santiago TV, Edelman NH (1981): Positional hypoxemia in unilateral lung disease. N Engl J Med 304:523–525.

102. Rigatto H, Brady JP, dela Torre-Verdezeo R (1975): Chemoreceptor reflexes in the preterm infants. II. The effect of gestation and

postnatal age on the ventilatory response to inhaled carbon dioxide. Pediatric 55:614–620.

103. Rigatto H, Kalapesi Z, Leahy FN, Durand M, Maccallum M, Cates D (1980): Chemical control of respiratory frequency and tidal volume during sleep in preterm infants. Respir Physiol 41:117–125.

104. Riopel L, Fouron JC, Bard H (1983): A comparison of blood viscosity between the adult sheep and newborn lamb. The role of plasma and red blood cell type. Pediatr Res 17:452–455.

105. Romero TE, Friedman WF (1979): Limited left ventricular response to volume overload in the neonatal period: Comparative study with the adult animal. Periatr Res 13:910–915.

106. Rorth M (1972): Hemoglobin interactions and red cell metabolism. Series Hematologia 5:7–102.

107. Rudolph AM (1984): Oxygenation in the fetus and neonate—a perspective. Semin Perinatol 8:158–167.

108. Rudolph AM (1985): Distribution and regulation of blood flow in the foetal and neonatal lamb. Circ Res 57:811–821.

109. Sachs LM, Delivoria-Papadopoulos M (1984): Hemoglobin-oxygen interactions. Semin Perinatol 8:168–183.

110. Schmid ER, Rehder K (1981): General anesthesia and the chest wall. Anesthesiology 55:668–675.

111. See WR, Schalefke ME, Loesheke HH (1983): Role of chemical afferents in the maintenance of rhythmic respiratory movements. J Appl Physiol Respirat Environ Exercise Physiol 54:453–459.

112. Sidi D, Kuipers JRG, Heymann MA, Rudolph AM (1983): Effects of ambient temperature on oxygen consumption and the circulation in newborn lambs at rest and during hypoxemia. Pediatr Res 12:254–258.

113. Sidi D, Kuipers JRG, Teitel D, Hyman MA, Rudolph AM (1983): Developmental changes in oxygenation and circulatory responses to hypoxemia in lambs. Am J Physiol (Heart Circ Physiol) 245:H674–H682.

114. Smales ORC, Hull D (1978): Metabolic response to cold in the newborn. Arch Dis Child 53:407–410.

115. Stahlman MT (1957): Pulmonary ventilation and diffusion in the human newborn infant. J Clin Invest 36:1081–1091.

116. Stockman JA III, Garcia JF, Oski FA (1977): The anemia of prematurity. N Engl J Med 296:647–650.

117. Takashimi E, Atsumi H (1955): Age differences in thoracic form as indicated by thoracic index. Hum Biol 27:65–74.

118. Teitel D, Sidi D, Bernstein D, Heyman MA, Rudolph AM (1985): Chronic hypoxia in the newborn lamb: Cardiovascular, hematopoietic, and growth adaptators. Pediatric Res 19:1004–1010.

119. Thurlbeck WM (1975): Postnatal growth and development of the lung. Am Rev Resp Dis 111:803–844.

120. Torrance JS, Lenfant C (1969/1970): Methods for determination of O_2 dissociation curves including Bohr effect. Respir Physiol 8:172–136.

121. Trippenbach T, Kelly G (1983): Phrenic activity and intercostal muscle EMG during inspiratory loading in newborn kittens. J Appl Physiol 54:496–501.

122. Turek Z, Kreuzer F (1981): Effect of shifts of the O_2 dissociation curve upon alveolar-arterial O_2 gradients in comparison models of the lung with ventilation-perfusion mismatching. Respir Physiol 45:133–139.

123. Turek Z, Kreuzer F, Ringnalda BEM (1978): Blood gases of several levels of oxygenation in rats with a left-shifted blood oxygen dissociation curve. Pflugers Arch 376:7–13.

124. Valeri CR, Collins FB (1971): Physiologic effects of 2,3- DPG-depletion red cells with high affinity for oxygen. J Appl Physiol 31:823–827.

125. Van Amerigan MR, Fouron JC, Bard H, Guennec LC, Prosmanne J (1981): Oxygenation in anemic newborn lambs with high or low oxygen affinity red cells. Pediatr Res 15:1500–1503.

126. Versmold H, Horn K, Windthorst H, Riegel KP (1973): The rapid postnatal increase of red cell 2,3 diphosphoglycerate: Its relation to plasma thyroxine. Respir Physiol 18:26–33.

127. Versmold HT, Linderkamp O, Donlemann C, Riegel KP (1976): Oxygen transport in congenital heart disease: Influence of fetal hemoglobin, red cell pH and 2,3-diphosphoglycerate. Pediatr Res 10:566–570.

128. Versmold HT, Seifert G, Riegel KP (1973): Blood oxygen affinity in infancy. The interaction of fetal and adult hemoglobin, oxygen capacity, and red cell hydrogen ion and 2,3-diphosphoglycerate concentration. Respir Physiol 18:14–25.

129. Wagner PD (1974): The oxyhemoglobin dissociation curve and pulmonary gas exchange. Semin Hematol 11:405–421.

130. Wagner PD (1977): Recent advances in pulmonary gas exchange. Inter Anesthesiol Clin 15:81–111.

131. Wagner PD, Saltzman HA, West JB (1974): Measurement of continuous distributions of ventilation perfusion ratios: Theory. J Appl Physiol 36:588–599.

132. Wagner PD, Laravuso RB, Uhl RR, West JB (1974): Continuous distributions of ventilation-perfusion ratios in normal subjects breathing air and 100 percent O_2. J Clin Invest 54:54–68.

133. Wagner PD, Dantsker DR, Dueck R, Clausen JL, West JB (1977): Ventilation-perfusion inequality in chronic obstructive pulmonary disease. J Clin Invest 59:203–216.

134. Wennergren G, Wennergren M (1983): Neonatal breathing control mediated via the central chemoreceptors. Acta Physiol Scand 119:139–146.

135. West JB (1969): Ventilation-perfusion inequality and overall gas exchange in computer models of the lung. Respir Physiol 7:88–110.

136. West JB (1969/1970): Effect of slope and shape of dissociation curve on pulmonary gas exchange. Respir Physiol 8:66–85.

137. West JB (1971): Causes of carbon dioxide retention in lung disease. N Engl J Med 284:1232–1236.

138. Widness JA, Teramo KA, Clemons GK, Garcia JF (1986): Temporal response of immunoreactive erythropoietin to acute hypoxemia in fetal sheep. Pediatric Res 20:15–19.

139. Wilkinson AR, Phibbs RH, Heilbron DC, Gregory GA, Versmold HT (1980): In-vivo oxygen dissociation curves in transfused and untransfused newborns with cardiopulmonary disease. Am Rev Respir Dis 122:629–634.

140. Woods LL, Brace RA (1986): Fetal blood volume, vascular pressure, and heart rate responses to fetal and maternal hyperosmolality. Am J Physiol (Heart Circ Physiol) 251:H716–H721.

141. Yeh TF, Ulien LD, Leu St, Pildes RS (1984): Increased O_2 consumption and energy loss in premature infants following medical care procedures. Biol Neonate 46:157–162.

142. Yao AC (1983): Cardiovascular changes during the transition from fetal to neonatal life. In Gootman N, Gootman PM (eds): Perinatal Cardiovascular Function. New York, Marcel Dekker, Inc, pp 1–41.

9 BLOOD GAS AND ACID-BASE ALTERATIONS IN NEONATAL CONGESTIVE HEART FAILURE

Norman S. Talner
George Lister

The changes in blood gas composition and acid-base equilibrium that occur in neonatal congestive heart failure are a result of the interplay of several factors. Myocardial loading conditions and decreases in organ blood flow (particularly to the kidneys and liver) as well as the adaptive responses of the respiratory, renal, and hematologic systems all influence metabolism and gas exchange. This chapter will consider the fundamental pathophysiologic effects of congestive heart failure on cardiopulmonary performance and regional organ function and will show the effects of such disturbances on neonatal blood gas composition and acid-base equilibrium.

VOLUME LOADING

The commonest cause of congestive heart failure in premature neonates is the large volume left-to-right patent ductus arteriosus (PDA) shunt. In term neonates ventricular septal defects (VSD) complicated by PDA, atrial septal defects (ASD), or atrioventricular valve (AV) regurgitation also commonly cause congestive heart failure. In addition, large systemic AV fistulas (vein of Galen malformation, hepatic AV fistula), and isolated left-sided atrioventricular valve regurgitation can cause volume-induced cardiac failure in neonates, but they are much rarer.

Volume loading alters ventilatory performance by increasing pulmonary blood flow and fluid transudation. Significant aberrations in blood gas tensions and pH as well as reductions in systemic perfusion can occur during volume overload despite preservation of ventricular function. Increases in pulmonary perfusion, pulmonary hypertension, and left atrial distention initiate a chain of events that results in the production of many of the classical signs of congestive heart failure in the infant. These signs include tachypnea (rapid shallow respirations), wheezing, tachycardia, cardiac enlargement, and hepatic enlargement. The respiratory signs initially reflect the accumulation of water in the pulmonary interstitial space, followed by peribronchiolar edema. Lung water clearance follows the same pathway.[7] When interstitial pulmonary edema develops, breathing becomes rapid and shallow secondary to decreases in lung compliance and possible stimulation of receptors in the interstitial space.[4] Tachypnea is the bedside correlate of increased lung water and decreased compliance. As long as edema does not accumulate in

alveolar spaces, gas exchange may be near normal, and only a respiratory alkalosis might be observed.[9] However, with increasing fluid transudation and development of alveolar edema, gas exchange is compromised, and hypoxemia occurs. Hypoxemia (which will further stimulate ventilation) results from perfusion of nonventilated areas and decrements in mixed venous oxygenation. As congestive heart failure worsens and fluid moves into peribronchiolar spaces (small airway edema), small airway resistance increases, and wheezing may become evident. In addition, the large conducting airways can be compressed by pulmonary artery dilatation or left atrial distention or both.[6] Obstructive emphysema and/or lobar collapse can result and further impair ventilatory function and oxygenation. Progressive reductions in pulmonary compliance can cause fatigue of the respiratory muscles, particularly the diaphragm, and respiratory failure can develop.[1] Severe mismatches in ventilation-perfusion, marked increases in the work of breathing (increased airway resistance, decreased lung compliance), and poor nutrition all likely contribute to the development of respiratory failure in congestive heart failure.

As mentioned previously, myocardial function seems to be preserved in the face of a large left-to-right shunt. Ventricular function is maintained by increased adrenergic tone. Enhanced sympathetic discharge is manifested clinically by tachycardia, pallor, and sweating. This augmented adrenergic tone results in a redistribution of cardiac output; blood flow is decreased not only to the skin (pallor) but also to the kidneys (decreased urine formation). Serum catecholamine levels as well as the urinary excretion of catecholamine metabolites are increased in the presence of large volume left-to-right shunts with congestive heart failure.[5]

Increased work of breathing and elevated serum catecholamine levels both increase oxygen consumption. Failure to thrive may develop, since caloric requirements are elevated at the same time that nutritional intake is limited by tachypnea and fatigue. Feeding is the infant's equivalent of climbing a flight of stairs; if the infant cannot feed without resting, it has little cardiopulmonary reserve. With more advanced congestive heart failure, oxygen consumption may fall if systemic perfusion is inadequate; metabolic acidosis follows. Thus, in the late stages of congestive heart failure there is a combined metabolic and respiratory acidosis.

When organ systemic perfusion, particularly that of the kidneys, becomes diminished, the renin-angiotension-aldosterone system is stimulated. Renin is released, which initiates a cascade involving activation of angiotensinogen and the conversion of angiotensin I to angiotensin II. The latter is a potent vasoconstrictor and the principal regulator of adrenal aldosterone production. Aldosterone causes renal sodium retention leading to volume expansion. Increased serum aldosterone and elevated urinary levels have been observed in newborn infants with congestive heart failure.

When systemic transport of oxygen is impaired by volume loading, tissue oxygenation can be improved by shifting the oxyhemoglobin dissociation curve to the right. Both increased production of 2,3-diphosphoglycerate in the red blood cells[10] and acidosis produce a rightward shift of the oxyhemoglobin dissociation curve (i.e., increase P_{50}); this right shift permits more oxygen to be released for a given arterial oxygen tension. Maximum oxygen extraction, evident from wide arteriovenous oxygen content differences, serves to preserve tissue oxygenation.

Hemoglobin concentration is an important determinant of the magnitude of left-to-right shunt[3] and thus influences blood gas and acid-base alterations observed in volume-induced congestive heart failure. Blood viscosity decreases during the normal postnatal fall in hemoglobin concentration and thereby contributes to increased left-to-right shunt during postnatal development despite constant cardiac anatomy.

Cyanotic congenital cardiac lesions characterized by volume loading may cause an early and severe decrease in arterial pH because of the combination of metabolic acidosis secondary to arterial hypoxemia and respiratory acidosis secondary to increased lung water and decreased lung compliance. Examples include lesions such as transposition of the great arteries with a large ventricular septal defect, total anomalous pulmonary venous connection, and truncus arteriosus.

Figure 9–1 depicts the pathophysiology of volume loading conditions as illustrated by a large ventricular septal defect. Shown in the diagram are the pulmonary sites at which lung water accumulation may take place and interfere with gas exchange. The effects on the myocardium and systemic circulation are also depicted, as are the various adaptive mechanisms that may modify regional blood flows and tissue oxygen delivery.

LOW PERFUSION STATES

The commonest causes of congestive heart failure in term neonates are pressure overloads and asphyxia, but there are also many other causes of low output congestive heart failure in neonates. Severe obstructive lesions of the left side of the heart (coarctation, aortic stenosis, hypoplastic left heart syndrome), impaired filling (diabetic cardiomyopathy), tachyarrhythmias, and impaired contractility (asphyxia, myocarditis, endocardial fibroelastosis, glycogen storage disease, carnitine deficiency) can all result in similar impairment of systemic perfusion.

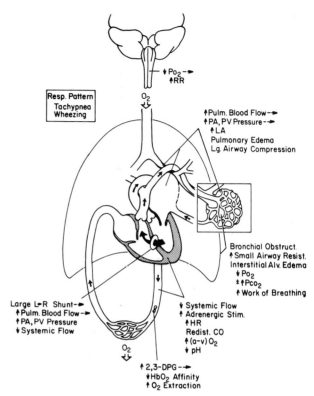

Figure 9–1. The effect of large volume left-to-right shunts on acid-base equilibrium and blood gas tensions as illustrated by an infant with a large ventricular septal defect. As a consequence of increased pulmonary blood flow (PBF), pulmonary artery and left atrial pressures are increased. Interstitial, alveolar, and peribronchial edema may impair gas exchange and increase small airway resistance. Large airways may be compressed by left atrial enlargement and pulmonary artery distention. As a result of gas trapping and pulmonary edema, PaO_2 may fall and $PaCO_2$ may rise. Interstitial pulmonary and small airway edema cause tachypnea and wheezing. Systemic perfusion may be diminished secondary to the large run-off into the pulmonary circulation (although total cardiac output is high); heart rate is increased, and cardiac output is redistributed (adrenergic effects). Oxygen extraction may be improved by the synthesis of 2,3-diphosphoglycerate.

Reductions in cardiac output compromise tissue oxygen delivery and thereby cause metabolic acidemia.[8] Typically, serum acidosis causes rapid deep respirations (hyperpnea), as encountered in diarrheal states, ketoacidosis, and hypovolemia. However, in low output congestive heart failure, pulmonary edema is often present, and the breathing pattern is that of rapid and shallow respirations, as with left-to-right shunts. In an attempt to compensate for serum acidosis, marked hyperventilation can result in dramatic reductions in arterial carbon dioxide tension. In situations in which pulmonary flow exceeds the diminished systemic flow, a left-to-right atrial shunt (as a result of left atrial distention, stretching of the foramen ovale, and poor left ventricular filling) can produce a high pulmonary arterial oxygen tension. As a result, the blood shunted right-to-left via the ductus in lesions such as hypoplastic left heart syndrome can maintain relatively normal systemic arterial oxygen tensions.

Patency of the ductus arteriosus is an important determinant of physiology and symptoms in many of the lesions associated with decreased systemic perfusion. As

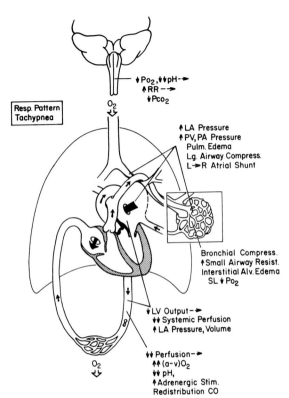

Figure 9–2. The effects of acutely curtailed systemic perfusion on acid-base equilibrium and blood gas tensions as illustrated by critical aortic valve stenosis. With obstruction to LV outflow, LV filling pressures rise along with LV systolic pressures. As a result of the increased filling pressures, pulmonary venous and pulmonary arterial pressures rise. Pulmonary edema, both interstitial and alveolar, may develop. Small airways may be compromised by peribronchiolar edema; large airways may be compromised by left atrial enlargement and pulmonary artery distention. Although tachypnea and arterial hypoxemia occur, the major effect is impairment of systemic perfusion. Diminished arterial pulsations, cool extremities, poor capillary refill, and severe metabolic acidemia are the clinical results. Oxygen extraction is increased, and arteriovenous oxygen content differences are markedly widened.

the ductus arteriosus undergoes postnatal constriction, systemic blood flow may be curtailed at the same time that pulmonary flow may be augmented (by left-to-right atrial shunting and the normal postnatal decrease in pulmonary vascular resistance). Systemic blood flow can be further compromised in ductal-dependent lesions by administration of high oxygen concentrations; administration of high oxygen concentrations may increase arterial PaO_2, but at the same time pH and $PaCO_2$ may fall dramatically. This phenomenon occurs because the rise in oxygen tension constricts the ductus arteriosus, which then decreases systemic blood flow while maintaining a high pulmonary flow. The large volume of oxygenated pulmonary venous return mixes with the small volume of systemic venous return at the atrial level. The net effect is an increase in arterial oxygen tension and a fall in systemic perfusion; the latter effect results in metabolic acidosis. Administration of prostaglandin E_1 to patients with ductal-dependent systemic blood flow dilates the ductus arteriosus, improves systemic perfusion, and reduces metabolic acidosis;[2] pH rises despite the decline in

systemic arterial oxygen content. This phenomenon illustrates the importance of systemic blood flow for oxygen transport and acid-base equilibrium. Since oxygen transport is the product of cardiac output and arterial oxygen content, improvements in systemic perfusion may easily offset small decreases in arterial oxygen content.

As a result of limitations in oxygen supply, oxygen consumption is often diminished in patients with reduced cardiac output, even though demands may be elevated. In contrast, infants with large volume left-to-right shunts tend to be hypermetabolic.

Congestive heart failure often develops rapidly in the patient with low systemic perfusion; as a result, there is little opportunity for renal compensation. The capacity of the kidneys to excrete acid may be impaired by reductions in renal plasma flow. Hepatic blood flow is also reduced; as a result, further elevations in blood lactate concentration, or hypoglycemia, may occur.

Neonates with congestive heart failure and impaired systemic perfusion challenge the clinician to improve systemic blood flow rapidly. Prompt initiation of prostaglandin E_1 infusion (to dilate the ductus arteriosus) or inotropic agents (to improve myocardial contractility) or immediate termination of life-threatening tachyarrhythmia may be essential if vital organ function is to be preserved.

Figure 9–2 depicts the pathophysiology of acutely curtailed systemic perfusion as illustrated by critical aortic stenosis. Blood gas and acid-base alterations induced by critical aortic stenosis, and various adaptive mechanisms are illustrated.

SUMMARY

This chapter has reviewed the pathophysiology responsible for alterations in blood gas composition and acid-base equilibrium in neonates with congestive heart failure. Neonatal congestive heart failure may result from either volume loading or lesions that impair systemic perfusion. Both types of neonatal congestive heart failure cause changes in pH, PaO_2, and $PaCO_2$. For neonates with congestive heart failure secondary to a large volume left-to-right shunt, interventions that limit pulmonary blood flow and its deleterious effects on lung function are needed. For neonates with congestive heart failure secondary to lesions that impair systemic perfusion, therapy to improve systemic blood flow is required.

References

1. Auber M, Trippenbach T, Roussos C (1981): Respiratory muscle fatigue during cardiogenic shock. J Appl Physiol 51:499–508.
2. Freed MD, Heymann MA, Lewis AB, Roehl SL, Kensey RC (1981): Prostaglandin E_1 in infants with ductus-dependent congenital heart disease. Circ 64:899–905.
3. Lister G, Hellenbrand WE, Kleinman CS, Talner NS (1982): Physiologic effects of increasing hemoglobin concentration in left-to-right shunting in infants with ventricular septal defects. N Engl J Med 306:502–506.
4. Paintal AS (1970): The mechanism of excitation of type J receptors and the J reflex. In Porter R (ed): Breathing: Hering-Breuer Centenary Symposium. London, J and A Churchill, pp 59–76.

5. Ross RD, Daniels SR, Schwartz DC, Hannon DW, Skukla R, Kaplan S (1987): Plasma norepinephrine levels in infants and children with congestive heart failure. Am J Cardiol 59:911–914.
6. Stanger P, Lucas R, Edwards J (1969): Anatomic factors causing respiratory distress in acyanotic congenital cardiac disease. Special reference to bronchial obstruction. Pediatrics 47:760–769.
7. Staub NC (1974): State of the art review—pathogenesis of pulmonary edema. Am Rev Resp Dis 109:358–372.
8. Talner NS, Campbell AGM (1972): Recognition and management of cardiologic problems in the newborn infant. Prog Cardiov Dis 15:153–188.
9. Talner NS, Lister G (1980): Oxygen transport in congenital heart disease. In Engle MA (ed): Pediatric Cardiovascular Disease, Vol 11. Philadelphia, FA Davis, pp 129–148.
10. Versmold HT, Linderkamp O, Dohlemann C, Riegel KP (1976): Oxygen transport in congenital heart disease: Influence of fetal hemoglobin, red cell pH, and 2,3-diphosphoglycerate. Ped Res 10:566–570.

PART 2

Prenatal (Fetal) Cardiology

10 GENETICS AND RECURRENCE RISKS OF CONGENITAL HEART DISEASE

Catherine A. Neill

Several etiologic and pathogenetic questions confront the physician caring for the newborn infant with congenital heart disease. First, what genetic factors or environmental teratogens may be involved? Second, what are the risks of recurrence in a subsequent pregnancy? Recently, because of the improved survival rate of children born with congenital cardiovascular malformations (CCVM) and because many of these children are reaching reproductive age, a third question arises: Namely, what are the risks of recurrence in the offspring? Several new areas are receiving increased attention: Is this a defect isolated to the heart or are other systems involved? If other systems are involved, is this a defined syndrome[53] or a collection of anomalies awaiting further analysis? The proportion of neonates with CCVM who have other noncardiac defects is higher than that in a referral clinic in part because of increased mortality of those neonates with multisystem defects and in part because cardiac consultation is now sought early for any infant with a noncardiac anomaly (such as omphalocele or fetal alcohol syndrome) which is known to be associated with CCVM.[16,59] Doppler echocardiographic techniques now allow for early and accurate cardiac diagnosis.

Knowledge and understanding of genetic factors and recurrence risk are in a phase of rapid growth.[7,25,56] In this chapter I will use the pathogenetic classification of CCVM proposed by Clark,[13] which has been used in analysis of familial risks of congenital heart defect assessed in a population-based epidemiologic study,[7] and also in an extensive literature review on recurrences in specific CCVM.[60] The chapter will focus attention on how new studies are addressing the questions of genetic factors, recurrence risk, and syndrome identification.

The overall risk of CCVM is approximately 8 per 1000 live births,[35,47] with one quarter to one third recognized in the first year of life.[29] In a regional case control study of the Baltimore-Washington area (Baltimore-Washington Infant Study, BWIS), Ferencz[25] investigated the resident birth cohort and obtained complete ascertainment of all live-born infants with structural cardiac abnormalities less than 1 year old, in whom the diagnosis was confirmed by echocardiography, cardiac catheterization, surgery, or autopsy. The sole defect excluded was patent ductus arteriosus in infants of gestational age less than 38 weeks. In the first 3 years of the study the prevalence of CCVM was 3.7 per 1000, a figure very compatible with prior studies using confirmed cardiac diagnosis.[7,25]

If either a parent or sibling had an isolated congenital cardiovascular malformation (ICCVM), earlier studies reported a *recurrence risk* of 3 to 5 per cent,[2,55,64] a figure compatible with multifactorial inheritance. However, recent studies have shown a much higher risk among the offspring of affected parents, particularly affected mothers.[61,77] This apparent discrepancy between first degree relatives, i.e., between siblings and offspring, is now under intensive investigation and will be discussed further later. Boughman et al,[7] using families with ICCVM in the population-based epidemiologic BWIS, recently described a *precurrence risk* of 12 per cent in first degree relatives of infants with abnormalities of left heart flow, a risk that is much higher than that in other types of defect. This study strongly suggests that precurrence (and probably recurrence) risks may vary among different developmental subsets or pathogenetic groupings.[12,13,14]

Certain *mendelian syndromes* or genetic disorders are known to have a high incidence of associated CCVM, ranging from 90 per cent in trisomy 13 to around 13 per cent in the recessive disorder of Ellis-van Creveld syndrome. Although associated anomalies have been known to occur in 20 to 25 per cent of individuals with CCVM,[32] it has proved difficult to compare recurrence risks between different reported series because of uncertainty as to whether syndromes with a cardiac component were being included. For example, inadvertent inclusion of patients with Noonan syndrome[53,74] into a family study of pulmonic stenosis will greatly increase the apparent "recurrence risk." Ferencz et al[28] have shown that of all infants presenting with confirmed CCVM under 1 year of age, only 73 per cent have isolated cardiac malformations, and the remaining 27 per cent have defects involving other systems.

Although in this chapter we will focus on the genetic information and recurrence risks in ICCVM, we will also discuss the role of the cardiologist and neonatologist in syndrome recognition and in adding further to our knowledge in this rapidly expanding field. An excellent review by Copel et al[16] has analyzed the extracardiac malformations that are often associated with major cardiac defects.

I am grateful to Dr. Edward B. Clark for his ideas and continuing encouragement, to Dr. Charlotte Ferencz for her leadership of the Baltimore-Washington Infant Study, and to Mrs. R. M. Cherry for her secretarial skills and long enjoyable working partnership.

125

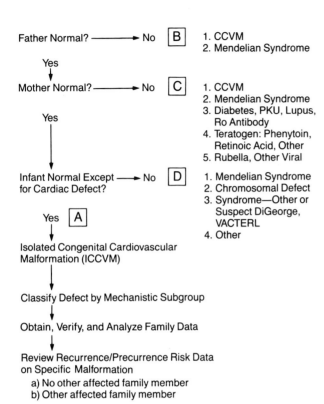

Figure 10–1. Analytical approach to congenital cardiovascular malformation (CCVM) recurrence risk.

Maternal disorders and metabolic defects, sometimes clinically silent, may also affect the developing heart. Maternal diabetes and maternal phenylketonuria are associated with an increased risk of CCVM, with the incidence probably varying with the severity of the metabolic disorder.[16,44] The presence of Ro antibodies in the mother is associated with heart block with or without endocardial fibroelastosis in the fetus. Infections and certain drugs ingested by the mother may lead to embryopathy with varying cardiac involvement.[59] These various risk factors need to be analyzed before calculating recurrence risks in an individual family.[51,55]

The major role of genetic mechanisms in CCVM is suggested by the relative constancy of the incidence and types of these defects in various nationalities and at different times. Animal studies have shown species predilection for certain CCVM in inbred strains.[58] Taussig[70] has suggested the importance of both evolutionary and genetic factors.

The subject of genetic predisposition and recurrence risks, always one of passionate interest to patients and their families, is now being advanced by contributions from geneticists and experimental embryologists and through new approaches to pathogenetic classification.[14] Data from the BWIS of Ferencz et al[25] provide an epidemologic basis for detailed analysis of genetic and environmental risk factors. Fetal echocardiography[1] and echocardiographic studies of family members[21,23] provide new tools for accurate cardiac diagnosis and genetic

studies. There is now enough information to allow tentative construction of a decision tree for considering genetic factors and recurrence risks in an individual family (Fig. 10–1).

Clearly, with the use of modern technology this analytic approach, or decision tree, may be used at different times and levels. For example, fetal echocardiography was performed at 30 weeks on Mrs. W., a 35-year-old healthy multiparous mother, with the indication being fetal non-immune hydrops fetalis. She had previously refused amniocentesis. The recognition of complete AV canal and cardiac arrhythmia led to an in utero diagnosis of Down syndrome, which was confirmed by chromosomal studies after birth. This infant could thus be placed in group D even prior to delivery, and recurrence risks and genetic counseling would be as for other Down syndrome families. (There may be interesting differences between families with Down syndrome and CCVM and those with Down syndrome without CCVM, but this subject is beyond the scope of this chapter.)

Similarly, in utero diagnosis of fetal congenital heart block in the second pregnancy of a healthy 21-year-old black woman led to detection of a high Ro antibody titer.[71] Recurrence risks and genetic counseling appropriate for her are completely different, despite her clinically normal health to date, from that suitable for a mother of an infant with a small ventricular septal defect.

In the following sections, some of the background for this decision tree will be given, with particular reference to the new information on recurrence risks in ICCVM and on certain syndromes with specific cardiac defects. The dramatic advances in cardiac diagnosis and therapy of the past 2 decades have tended to overshadow recognition of the major importance of associated extracardiac defects and their clinical and etiologic implications.

HISTORICAL PERSPECTIVE

The earliest family studies were those of Campbell.[11] Numerous subsequent analyses of "recurrence risks" in siblings have been undertaken since that time.[55,64] In some studies, precurrence and recurrence risks were not clearly separated. More recently, "precurrence risks," i.e., the incidence of congenital heart disease in the previously born siblings and parents of affected and control infants, have become available[7] and suggest a much higher precurrence risk in first degree relatives of infants with abnormalities of left heart flow, including coarctation, hypoplastic left heart syndromes, and aortic stenosis, as compared with first degree relatives of infants with lesions falling into other pathogenetic groupings.

Recurrence risks in the *offspring* of surviving patients with cardiac defects have been studied by a number of authors[18,19] and are reviewed later under the various pathogenetic groupings. In our own early study of patients reaching adult life,[50] we found a recurrence risk of 1.8 per cent in live-born offspring. At that time, however, most of the mothers with tetralogy of Fallot had not had total repair, and their arterial unsaturation led to a high incidence of fetal loss; the incidence of cardiac defects in these spontaneous abortuses was not known. Taussig et al[69] reported in their long-term tetralogy of Fallot follow-up study that 3 of 96 infants born to affected mothers had CCVM, but none of 100 infants born to affected fathers had CCVM. Whittemore et al[77] showed a high overall risk of 16.1 per cent in the offspring of 233 mothers with varying cardiac defects who had a total of 482 pregnancies. Rose[61] found that 8.8 per cent of offspring of 219 propositi (100 male and 119 female) had cardiac defects. Ferencz[27] found no affected offspring among 52 children of 78 fathers with varying CCVM interviewed in 1972. Czeizel[18] reported 4.9 per cent affected offspring among the 246 live-born children of 166 propositi. Nora and Nora[56] recently reviewed the literature and some of their own unpublished data and concluded that there is a maternal effect in that the offspring of affected mothers are at higher risk than the offspring of affected fathers.

Mendelian syndromes involving CCVM have been increasingly recognized since Cockayne[15] suggested that dextrocardia and situs inversus were inherited by an autosomal recessive mechanism. In Table 10–1 some of the mendelian syndromes with CCVM and the date of their recognition are listed. This list omits cardiomyopathies and also the Williams-Beuren, DiGeorge, and other syndromes discussed elsewhere. Inheritance patterns in the prolonged QT syndrome[37] are now the subject of a major cooperative study.

Chromosomal defects and their cardiac manifestations have an interesting history in that the high frequency of cardiac anomalies and the preponderance of atrioventricular septal type defects in Down syndrome were recognized many years before definition of the specific disorder of chromosome 21. Rowe and Uchida[62] clearly established the high (approximately 45 per cent) incidence of cardiac septation defect in Down syndrome, and later studies have emphasized the preponderance of atrioventricular septal defects. In a study of aborted fetuses with CCVM Ursell et al[75] found 57 per cent had chromosomal anomalies.

Chromosomal disorders, including Down syndrome, are reviewed in Chapter 47. Burn and associates[10] have emphasized the importance of chromosomal analysis, including chromosome banding techniques, in dysmorphic infants with CCVM who may have some phenotypic features simulating Noonan syndrome but with atypical cardiac anomalies. When the cardiac defect is associated with parental translocation, they state that there is a one in five recurrence risk of chromosomal abnormalities in subsequent pregnancies.

Varying percentages have been quoted for the proportion of live-born patients with CCVM who have chromosomal defects. The figure of 12 per cent in the population-based BWIS[28] establishes definitively the extreme importance of chromosomal anomalies in infants presenting with cardiac defects in the first year of life.

Other named syndromes with CCVM are reviewed elsewhere in this book. Those of major clinical significance in the neonatal period include DiGeorge,[31,41,76] the Pierre-Robin anomalad, and the VATER association.[4]

"Suspect syndromes," in which CCVM were associated with one or more significant defects in other systems, were recognized in 1.1 per cent of infants in the BWIS.[28] Copel et al[16] give an excellent review of associated anomalies in CCVM, with particular emphasis on the implications for fetal echocardiography. Many prior studies of such associations have not separated affected infants clearly into those with mendelian, chromosomal, or other known syndromes. Elucidation of the recurrence risks of these suspect syndromes (for example, omphalocele associated with CCVM) must await further detailed analysis of population-based studies. A historic review of this group will not be attempted here.

Isolated CCVM was the major focus of study by Campbell[11] and other early reviews of recurrence risks. It is clear that referral patterns, including age at first diagnosis,

Table 10–1. MENDELIAN SYNDROMES WITH CCVM

	Partial List of Major Contributors		
Year	**Syndrome (Author)**	**Cardiac**	**Extracardiac**
1938	R (Cockayne)[15]	Dextrocardia	Situs inversus
1940	R Ellis-van Creveld[20]	Single atrium	Ectodermal chondrodystrophy: polydactyly
1955	D Marfan[45]	MVP Aortic dilatation	Connective tissue disorder
1960	D Holt-Oram[36]	ASD	Radial anomalies
1968	D Noonan[54]	Dysplastic pulmonary valve	"Turner phenotype"
1969	R Thrombocytopenia[34] Absent radius	ASD TOF	Skeletal Hematologic
1978	D Shprintzen[67]	VSD R aortic arch TOF	Face and palate

Notes: D = dominant; R = recessive; ASD = atrial septal defect; MVP = mitral valve prolapse; VSD = ventricular septal defect; TOF = tetralogy of Fallot.

were different in past years, accounting to a significant degree for the discrepancy between Campbell's reported incidence of 3 per cent of major chromosomal anomalies and the 12 per cent found in the BWIS. The concept that in only 73 per cent of infants with CCVM is the cardiac defect *isolated* has major clinical and genetic implications, which are not yet fully recognized and accepted. Syndrome recognition will be discussed further in the following section.

CLINICAL APPROACH AND CLASSIFICATION

Classification of cardiac defects has not been standardized in the past, which has led to problems in deciding whether defects in family members were "concordant" or "discordant."[17] In this chapter, Clark's pathogenetic classification, which integrates some of the recent embryologic and clinical advances, will be used.[12,13]

Because the neonatologist is the first to see infants with multiple handicaps, his or her awareness of the cardiac problems in various syndromes is particularly important. The fetus or neonate is at high risk (greater than 25 per cent) of CCVM if there is a major chromosomal defect present or if the family history is positive for known mendelian syndromes with cardiac involvement. Thus, fetal or neonatal echocardiography in addition to clinical evaluation is warranted in all infants with Down syndrome, even if no cardiac murmurs are present. Similarly, a search for subtle evidence of coarctation or bicuspid aortic valve is warranted in Turner syndrome. Later in this chapter I will consider the converse of this principle, namely, the types of cardiac malformation that frequently are not isolated and that should lead to a careful search for associated anomalies of other systems.

The classification below is a brief review of what is known of the genetics of anomalies of cardiac looping, conotruncal defects, defects involving extracellular matrix (or cardiac jelly), defects related to hemodynamic molding, and others.

Looping Anomalies

This is a useful term embracing visceral heterotaxia, dextrocardia with or without situs inversus, and situs inversus with levocardia. Family data on dextrocardia with abnormal cardiac anatomy are still incomplete, but our center favors inclusion of dextrocardia in this group. Many authors also include corrected or levotransposition with ventricular inversion. These disorders are rare, but there is a growing consensus favoring recessive mendelian inheritance with incomplete penetrance.[9,48,78] Animal models have provided useful insight. Layton[42] hypothesized that the normal allele at the iv locus controls normal visceral asymmetry: Absence of this control allows situs to be determined in a random fashion. Families with some members showing isomerism and others showing disorders of ciliary motility[65] suggest that continuing research will reveal further overlap between these syndromes. Opitz[57] comments on the powerful role of the midline in the mammalian morphogenesis and suggests that "polyasplenia" should be considered as a complex developmental field defect (Table 10–2).

Disorders of Mesenchymal Tissue Migration (Conotruncal Anomalies)

Recent experimental work by Kirby et al[39,40] has emphasized the importance of migration of neural crest cells in the formation of the developing conotruncal area. The clinical implications of these data still await clarification, but there are some specific *syndromes* with neurologic, branchial arch, and conotruncal involvement that are of great importance to the neonatologist, cardiologist, and family. These include DiGeorge syndrome,[41,76] a disorder of the third and fourth branchial arches associated with thymic hypoplasia and hypocalcemia, and with cardiac lesions, including truncus arteriosus, interrupted aortic arch, and extreme tetralogy of Fallot with pulmonary outflow atresia. The genetic mechanisms of this syndrome remain controversial, with dominant and recessive mech-

Table 10–2. LOOPING ANOMALIES

	Empiric Recurrence Risk (Siblings)	Inheritance
Atrial isomerism Right atrial (asplenia syndrome) Left atrial (polysplenia syndrome)	15 per cent	R
Kartagener Ciliary dyskinesis syndrome		R
Dextrocardia Situs inversus Normal heart	20 per cent	R
Corrected (levo) Transposition (Ventricular inversion)	NA	

Note: R = recessive.

anisms being invoked and partial deletion of chromosome 22 having been reported.[31] In Shprintzen syndrome[67] (velocardiofacial syndrome), tetralogy of Fallot or ventricular septal defect with right aortic arch is combined with facial and palatal abnormalities. This syndrome appears to be inherited as an autosomal dominant. In Goldenhar syndrome involving the first and second pharyngeal pouch, ocular, auricular, and vertebral anomalies may be accompanied by severe tetralogy of Fallot. Some evidence suggests that Goldenhar syndrome may be inherited by an autosomal dominant mode of inheritance.[63] Tetralogy of Fallot has also been described in other familial dysmorphic syndromes.[38]

When tetralogy of Fallot, the most frequent conotruncal defect, presents as an isolated defect, it has a low *recurrence risk* in siblings, between 2 and 3 per cent in most previous studies and 0/150 in the BWIS to date.[7] Isolated arterial transposition also recurs very infrequently and has a remarkably low incidence of associated anomalies,[28] strongly suggesting a different underlying pathogenesis from other conotruncal defects.

If the mother has tetralogy of Fallot, the *offspring's* risk is as yet uncertain, but until new data are available, we believe it must be considered to be at least 10 per cent, a figure intermediate between that in Whittemore's studies[77] and previous data.[56] If the father has tetralogy of Fallot, the previously quoted recurrence risk of 5 per cent or less appears well founded. No data are yet available on the offspring of individuals born with transposed great arteries, so in the absence of any additional risk factors or teratogens, a recurrence risk of 10 per cent or less may be quoted reasonably.

Anomalies Involving Extracellular Cardiac Matrix (Atrioventricular Septal Defects)

Defects involving the formation of cardiac cushions from the cardiac jelly are often referred to as endocardial cushion or atrioventricular septal defects. Although they may occur in otherwise normal subjects, the overwhelming preponderance of atrioventricular (AV) septal defects in trisomy 21 syndrome (Down syndrome) has long been recognized.

The *recurrence risk* in siblings of children with isolated AV septal defects has shown considerable variation in different series, ranging from 1.5 to 8.7 per cent.[64] The AV septal defect is concordant about two thirds of the time. Few studies are available on the *offspring* of affected individuals. However, Emanuel et al[24] have published data on the 56 offspring of 90 individuals mostly with the complete form of AV septal defect. None of the propositi had Down syndrome. The recurrence risk in offspring was 9.6 per cent overall, and 14.3 per cent if only female propositi were included. In three of five of the affected children, the AV septal defect was concordant in type to that of the parent.

Defects of Hemodynamic Molding (Flow Defects)

In utero disorders of *left heart flow* may lead to a spectrum of disorders, including bicuspid aortic valve,

aortic stenosis, aortic coarctation, and left heart hypoplasia.[13] It is possible that in some cases left heart flow is diminished because of an in utero restrictive cardiomyopathy.[52] Boughman et al[7] found that first degree relatives of infants with left heart flow disorders had a 12 per cent incidence of cardiac malformations, mostly also disorders of left heart flow, though of varying severity. This observation is extremely important and is being further pursued. Previous studies of hypoplastic left heart syndrome have shown variable recurrence risks in siblings, and sibling clusters have been reported.[8]

The *offspring* of adults with aortic stenosis were found by Rose et al[61] to have an 11.5 per cent incidence of cardiac defects (N = 96). The offspring of those with coarctation had a 4.4 per cent risk of cardiac defect, with the risk being higher if the affected parent was a mother. In an interesting clinical and echocardiographic study of 41 families with bicuspid aortic valves, Emanuel et al[23] found that 14.7 per cent of families had more than one affected member.

Right heart flow defects include secundum atrial septal defect (ASD) and pulmonic stenosis. In uncomplicated ASD of the secundum type, the recurrence risk in both siblings and offspring has been reported at around 5 per cent in many previous studies. Rose et al[61] found 10 per cent of 194 offspring to have defects and noted that the child was 3.5 times more likely to be affected if the mother, rather than the father, had an atrial defect. When ASD is seen complicating the hand-arm syndrome of Holt-Oram,[36] recurrence risk in both siblings and offspring is around 40 per cent. When major conduction anomalies are present in addition to the atrial defect, the recurrence risk seems to be higher, and some families with defects occurring in three generations have been reported.[5] A large familial constellation without extracardiac or conduction defects has been described by Thomas et al.[73]

Pulmonic stenosis as an isolated lesion has a recurrence risk of between 2 and 5 per cent[60,64] in both siblings and offspring. However, when the pulmonary valve is dysplastic, a high suspicion should be entertained of Noonan syndrome, which has autosomal dominant recurrence risks.

Other flow defects include perimembranous (type II) ventricular septal defect (VSD). Definition of the true VSD recurrence risk is complicated because of the possibility of overdiagnosis without echocardiography confirmation, the risk of underdiagnosis if only echocardiographic criteria are used, and the variable rate of spontaneous closure. However, at the present time the VSD recurrence risk in both siblings and offspring appears to be 5 per cent or less unless additional maternal problems of teratogenic significance such as the fetal alcohol syndrome are present.

Sherman et al[66] describe a remarkable family, with 11 of 13 direct descendants of one female member having either atrial or ventricular septal defects. They postulate a cytoplasmic, possibly mitochondrial, mechanism of inheritance.

VSD is the most common cardiac anomaly in the VATER association,[4,72] or "axial mesodermal dysplasia spectrum," as it is in a number of multisystem disorders. Among 393 infants with VSD enrolled in the BWIS, 80 per cent had VSD as an isolated defect, 9 per cent had a chromosomal disorder, 3 per cent had a recognized mendelian syndrome, and 8 per cent had other "non-syndromic" extracardiac malformations.[28] This high incidence of associated abnormalities will probably decrease as more infants with small defects are referred for Doppler echocardiographic assessment of hemodynamically insignificant lesions. However, these data serve as a reminder that in about 20 per cent of infants with confirmed VSD, the heart is not the only organ affected.

Now that precise anatomic definition of even small ventricular septal defects is possible with Doppler echocardiographic techniques, it will be possible to construct family pedigrees and see whether there are family differences between the different pathogenetic groupings of VSD.[14]

Anomalies of Targeted Growth

These include total anomalous pulmonary venous return, atrial septal defect of the sinus venosus type, and cor triatriatum. Familial recurrences have been described in all of these disorders[3,6] and in the cardiopulmonary anomaly known as the scimitar syndrome.[30,49] Recurrence risk in first degree relatives is not clearly established.

Abnormalities Related to Cell Death

These include defects in the muscular part of the ventricular septum and possibly Ebstein's anomaly of the tricuspid valve. Recurrence risks do not appear to be higher than 3 to 5 per cent, although family constellations have been observed.[22,60] Malcolm[43] has reviewed possible associations between Ebstein's anomaly and mitral valve prolapse (MVP).

Other Disorders

Cardiomyopathies are reviewed elsewhere in this book (Chapter 39) and will not be discussed further. *Supravalvar aortic stenosis*[53] has been the subject of numerous family studies since an early description in a maternal grandmother and grandson raised the possibility of an autosomal dominant mode of inheritance.[68] The Williams-Beuren syndrome involving supravalvar aortic stenosis and facial anomalies was originally thought to be sporadic and the recurrence risk in siblings was thought to be low, but recent analysis of an extensive series by Grimm and Wesselhoeft[33] suggests an autosomal dominant mode of inheritance. McKusick[46] has reviewed the complex literature and emphasized the value of the characteristic "stellate" or "lacy" appearance of the iris in Williams-Beuren syndrome diagnosis in the neonate.

Mitral valve prolapse (MVP) is rarely recognized in the newborn unless associated with Marfan or Ehlers-Danlos syndrome. However, MVP occurs in 4 to 8 per cent of otherwise normal young adults, and family studies have supported an autosomal dominant mode of inheritance. Malcolm[43] has provided a valuable analytic review on the association of MVP with cardiac and other anomalies. In the BWIS, MVP was self-reported in 7 of 1020 mothers of infants with CCVM (0.69 per cent), and 4 of 1339 control mothers (0.30 per cent).[26] Four of the seven affected infants (57 per cent) had major multisystem defects. At present, parents with isolated MVP should be made aware of the familial nature of this usually extremely benign valve anomaly but should not be quoted an increased risk of other types of CCVM. Prospective studies of pregnancy outcome in MVP may soon be forthcoming.

SUMMARY

Syndrome Recognition

The cooperative efforts of cardiologists, neonatologists, and geneticists are needed to allow clear separation of ICCVM from syndromic associations. In Table 10–3, CCVM is listed according to the probability of associated defects or syndromes. For example, pulmonary atresia with intact septum usually occurs in isolation, while pulmonary atresia with ventricular septal defect (extreme tetralogy of Fallot) has at least a 25 per cent risk of associated extracardiac anomalies. Pulmonary atresia with abnormal cardiac looping indicates an isomerism disorder, and extracardiac anomalies are present in 50 per cent or more of the infants. This table will need further revision as knowledge advances but may be useful to the physician confronted with a newborn with heart disease.

Recurrence Risks

CCVM forms a heterogeneous group of defects. By using the algorithm in Figure 10–1 and Clark's pathogenetic classification as outlined in this chapter, it is possible to define subsets, probably with varying recurrence risk. Present data suggest that abnormalities of left heart flow may carry a higher recurrence risk (around 10 to 15 per cent) than those of other groups, although there is a great variation in phenotypic expression. The multifactorial model may not apply to all pathogenetic groups. However, with the exception of left heart flow defects, recurrence risks in siblings are 5 per cent or less.

The offspring of mothers with ICCVM appear to have a recurrence risk of approximately 10 per cent, higher than previously recognized and greater than that of affected fathers. These observations and others will provide a major stimulus to future embryologic, fetal, genetic, echocardiographic, and population-based studies.

Table 10–3. SPECIFIC CCVM DEFECTS
PROBABILITY OF ASSOCIATED DEFECTS OR SYNDROMES[28,32]

Cardiac Diagnosis	Syndrome	Probability of Some Extracardiac Defect
Truncus arteriosus Pulmonary atresia + VSD Interrupted aortic arch type B	DiGeorge	50 per cent or more
Supravalvar aortic stenosis	Williams	
AV septal defect	Down	
Dysplastic pulmonary valve	Noonan	
Interrupted inferior vena cava Discordance cardiac, abdominal situs "looping anomalies"	Isomerism syndromes (asplenia, polysplenia)	↓
Tetralogy of Fallot	Neural crest or branchial arch defects	20 to 30 per cent (in approximate order of decreasing frequency)
Complex cyanotic defects		
Coarctation of aorta	Pierre-Robin anomalad, other	
Aortic stenosis		
Pulmonary stenosis		
Atrial septal defect	Holt-Oram	
VSD (type II perimembranous)	Renal, skeletal	↓
Total anomalous pulmonary venous return		10 per cent or less
Hypoplastic left heart		
Tricuspid atresia		
D-transposition of great arteries		
Pulmonary atresia with intact ventricular septum		↓

Note: VSD = ventricular septal defect.

References

1. Allan LD, Crawford DC, Sunder KC, Anderson RH, Tynan M (1986): Familial recurrence of congenital heart disease in a prospective series of mothers referred for fetal echocardiography. Am J Cardiol 58:333–337.
2. Anderson RC (1976): Fetal and infant death, twinning and cardiac malformations in families of 2000 children with and 500 without cardiac defects. Am J Cardiol 38:218–224.
3. Arensman FW, Boineau JP, Balfour IC, Flannery DB, Moore HV (1986): Sinus venosus atrial septal defect and pacemaker requirement in a family. Am J Cardiol 57:368–369.
4. Auchterlonie IA, White MP (1982): Recurrence of the VATER association within a sibship. Clin Genet 21:122–124.
5. Bizarro RO, Callahan JA, Feldt RH, Kurland LT, Gordon H, Brandenburg RO (1970): Familial atrial septal defect with prolonged atrioventricular conduction: A syndrome showing the autosomal dominant pattern of inheritance. Circulation 41:677–684.
6. Baron P, Gutgesell H, Hawkins E, McNamara D (1982): Infradiaphragmatic total anomalous pulmonary venous connection in siblings. Am Heart J 104:1107–1109.
7. Boughman JA, Berg KA, Astemborski JA, Clark EB, McCarter RJ, Rubin JD, Ferencz C (1987): Familial risks of congenital heart disease in a population based epidemiologic study. Am J Med Genet 26:839–850.
8. Brownell LG, Shokeir MHK (1976): Inheritance of hypoplastic left heart syndrome (HLHS): Further observations. Clin Genet 9:245–249.
9. Burn J, Colley R, Allan LD, Pembrey ME, Robinson P, Macartney FJ (1984): Isomerism—A family study. (abstr) J Med Genet 21:301.
10. Burn J, Baraitser M, Hughes DT, Saldano-Garcia P, Taylor JFN

(1984): Absent right atrioventricular connection and double-inlet left ventricle due to an unbalanced familial 8:13 chromosome translocation: A cautionary tale. Pediatr Cardiol 5:55–60.
11. Campbell M (1965): Causes of malformations of the heart. Br Med J 2:895.
12. Clark EB (1986): Cardiac embryology. Its relevance to congenital heart disease. Am J Dis Child 140:41–44.
13. Clark EB (1987): Mechanisms in the pathogenesis of congenital cardiac malformations. In Pierpont MEM, Moller JH (eds): The Genetics of Cardiovascular Disease. Boston, Martinus Nijhoff Publishing, pp 3–11.
14. Clark EB (1987): Growth morphogenesis and function: The dynamics of heart development. In Moller JH, Neal WA, Lock JE (eds): Fetal Neonatal and Infant Heart Disease. New York, Appleton-Century-Crofts.
15. Cockayne EA (1938): The genetics of transposition of the viscera. Quart J Med 7:479–493.
16. Copel JA, Gianluigi P, Kleinman CS (1986): Congenital heart disease and extracardiac anomalies: Association and indications for fetal echocardiography. Am J Obstet Gynecol 154:1121–1132.
17. Corone P, Bonati C, Feingold J, Fromond S, Berthet-Bondet D (1983): Familial congenital heart disease: How are the various types related? Am J Cardiol 51:941–945.
18. Czeizel A, Pornoi A, Peterffy E, Tarcal E (1982): Study of children of parents operated on for congenital cardiovascular malformations. Br Heart J 47:290–293.
19. Dennis NR, Warren J (1981): Risks of the offspring of patients with some common congenital heart defects. J Med Genet 18:8.
20. Ellis RWB, van Creveld S (1940): A syndrome characterized by ectodermal dysplasia, polydactyly, chondrodysplasia, and congenital morbus cordis. Report of 3 cases. Arch Dis Child 15:85.

21. DiSegni E, Pierpont MEM, Bass JL, Kaplinsky E (1985): Two-dimensional echocardiography in detection of endocardial cushion defects in families. Am J Cardiol 55:1649–1652.

22. Emanuel R, O'Brian K, Ng R (1976): Ebstein's anomaly. Genetic study of 26 families. Br Heart J 38:5–7.

23. Emanuel R, Withers R, O'Brian K, Ross P, Feizi O (1978): Congenitally bicuspid aortic valves: Clinico-genetic study of 41 families. Br Heart J 40:1402–1407.

24. Emanuel R, Somerville J, Inns A, Withers R (1983): Evidence of congenital heart disease in the offspring of parents with atrioventricular defects. Br Heart J 49:144–147.

25. Ferencz C, Rubin JD, McCarter RJ, Brenner JI, Neill CA, Perry LW, Hepner SI, Downing JW (1985): Congenital heart disease: Prevalence at livebirth. The Baltimore-Washington Infant Study. Am J Epidemiol 121:31–36.

26. Ferencz C, Rubin JD, McCarter RJ, Brenner JI, Neill CA, Perry LW, Hepner SI, Downing JW (1985): Maternal mitral valve prolapse and congenital heart disease in the offspring. Am Heart J 110:899–900.

27. Ferencz C (1986): Offspring of fathers with cardiovascular malformations. Am Heart J 111:1212–1213.

28. Ferencz C, Rubin JD, McCarter RJ, Boughman JA, Wilson PD, Brenner JI, Neill CA, Perry LW, Hepner SI, Downing JW (1987): Cardiac and noncardiac malformations: Observations in a population-based study. Teratology 141:1281–1220.

29. Fyler DC, Buckley LP, Hellenbrand WE, Cohen HE (1980): Report of the New England Regional Infant Cardiac Program. Pediatrics 65:376–461.

30. Gikonyo DK, Tandon R, Lucas RV Jr, Edwards JE (1986): Scimitar syndrome in neonates: Report of four cases and review of the literature. Pediatr Cardiol 6:193–197.

31. Greenberg F, Crowder WE, Paschall V, Colon-Linares J, Lubianski B, Ledbetter DH (1984): Familial DiGeorge syndrome and associated partial monosomy of chromosome 22. Hum Genet 65:317–319.

32. Greenwood RD, Rosenthal A, Parisi L, Fyler DC, Nadas AS (1975): Extracardiac abnormalities in infants with congenital heart disease. Pediatrics 55:485.

33. Grimm T, Wesselhoeft H (1980): Genetics of the Williams-Beuren syndrome and of the isolated form of supravalvar aortic stenosis (Study of 128 families). Z Kardiol 69:168–172.

34. Hall JG, Levin J. Juhn JP, Ottenheimer EJ, Berkum KAP, McKusick VA (1969): Thrombocytopenia with absent radius (TAR) Medicine 48:411–439.

35. Hoffman JIE, Christianson R (1978): Congenital heart disease in a cohort of 10,502 births with long-term follow-up. Am J Cardiol 42:641–647.

36. Holt M, Oram S (1960): Familial heart disease with skeletal anomalies. Br Heart J 22:236–242.

37. Itoh S, Munemura S, Satoh H (1982): A study of the inheritance pattern of Romano-Ward syndrome: Prolonged Q-T interval, syncope and sudden death. Clin Pediatr 21:20–24.

38. Jones MC, Waldman JD (1985): Tetralogy of Fallot—Autosomal dominant syndrome of characteristic facial appearance, preauricular pits, fifth finger clinodactyly and tetralogy of Fallot. Am J Med Genet 22:135–141.

39. Kirby ML, Gale TF, Stewart DE (1983): Neural crest cells contribute to normal aorticopulmonary septation. Science 220:1059–1061.

40. Kirby ML (1987): Cardiac morphogenesis—Recent research advances. Ped Res 21:219–224.

41. Lammer EJ, Opitz JM (1986): The DiGeorge anomaly as a developmental field defect. Am J Med Genet Suppl 2:113–127, Developmental Field Concept 323–337.

42. Layton WM (1978): Heart malformations in mice homozygous for a gene causing situs inversus. Birth Defects 14:277–293.

43. Malcolm AD (1985): Mitral valve prolapse associated with other disorders. Casual coincidence, common link or fundamental genetic disturbance? Br Heart J 53:353–362.

44. McCarter RJ, Kessler II, Comstock GW (1987): Is diabetes mellitus a teratogen or a coteratogen? Am J Epidemiol 125:195–205.

45. McKusick VA (1955): The cardiovascular aspects of Marfan's syndrome: A heritable disorder of connective tissue. Circulation 11:321–342.

46. McKusick VA (1986): Mendelian Inheritance in Man. Catalogues of Autosomal Dominant, Autosomal Recessive and X-linked Phenotypes. 7th ed. Baltimore, Johns Hopkins University Press, p 766.

47. Mitchell SC, Korones SB, Berendes HW (1971): Congenital heart disease in 56,109 births. Incidence and natural history. Circulation 43:323–332.

48. Moreno A, Murphy EA (1981): Inheritance of Kartagener syndrome. Am J Med Genet 8:305–313.

49. Neill CA, Ferencz C, Sabiston DC, Sheldon H (1960): The familial occurrence of hypoplastic right lung with systemic arterial supply and venous drainage "Scimitar Syndrome." Bull Johns Hopkins Hospital 107:1–21.

50. Neill CA, Swanson S (1961): Outcome of pregnancy in congenital heart disease. (abstr) Circulation 24:1003.

51. Neill CA (1973): Genetics of congenital heart disease. In Cregar WP (ed): Annual Review of Medicine. Palo Alto, Annual Reviews, Inc.

52. Neill CA, Ursell P (1984): Endocardial fibroelastosis and left heart hypoplasia revisited. Inter J Cardiol 5:547–550.

53. Neill CA (1987): Congenital heart disease and syndromes. In Pierpont MEM, Moller JH (eds): The Genetics of Cardiovascular Disease. Boston, Martinus Nijhoff Publishing, pp 95–112.

54. Noonan JA (1968): Hypertelorism with Turner phenotype: A new syndrome associated congenital heart disease. Am J Dis Child 116:373–380.

55. Nora JJ, Nora AH (1978): The evolution of specific genetic and environmental counseling in congenital heart diseases. Circulation 57:205–213.

56. Nora JJ, Nora AH (1987): Maternal transmission of congenital heart disease: New recurrence risk figures and the questions of cytoplasmic inheritance and vulnerability to teratogens. Am J Cardiol 59:459–463.

57. Opitz JM (1985): Editorial comment on the paper by de la Monte and Hutchins on familial polyasplenia. Am J Med Genet 21:175–176.

58. Patterson DF, Pyle RI, Van Mierop LHS, Melbin J, Olson M (1974): Hereditary defects of the conotruncal septum in Keeshond dogs: Pathologic and genetic studies. Am J Cardiol 34:187–205.

59. Pexieder T (1987): Teratogens. In Pierpont MEM, Moller JH (eds): The Genetics of Cardiovascular Disease. Boston, Martinus-Nijhoff Publishing, pp 25–68.

60. Pierpont MEM, Moller JH (1987): Congenital cardiac malformations. In Pierpont MEM, Moller JH (eds): The Genetics of Cardiovascular Disease. Boston, Martinus-Nijhoff Publishing, pp 13–24.

61. Rose V, Gold RJM, Lindsay G, Allen M (1985): A possible increase in the incidence of congenital heart defects among the offspring of affected patients. J Am Coll Cardiol 6:376–382.

62. Rowe RD, Uchida IA (1961): Cardiac malformation in mongolism. A prospective study of 184 mongoloid children. Am J Med 31:726.

63. Regenbogen L, Godel V, Goya V, Goodman RM (1982): Further evidence for an autosomal dominant form of oculoauriculovertebral dysplasia. Clin Genet 21:161–167.

64. Sanchez-Cascos A (1978): The recurrence risk in congenital heart disease. Eur J Cardiol 7:197–210.

65. Schidlow DV, Katz SM, Turtz MG, Donner RM, Capasso S (1982): Polysplenia and Kartagener syndrome in a sibship: Association with abnormal respiratory cilia. J Pediatr 100:401–403.

66. Sherman J, Angulo M, Boxer RA, Gluck R (1985): Possible mitochondrial inheritance of congenital cardiac septal defects. N Engl J Med 313:186–187.

67. Shprintzen RJ, Goldberg RB, Lewin ML, Sidoti EJ, Berkman MD, Argamaso RV, Young D (1978): A new syndrome involving cleft palate, cardiac anomalies, typical facies and learning disabilities: Velo-cardio-facial syndrome. Cleft Palate J 15:56–62.

68. Sissman NJ, Neill CA, Spencer FC, Taussig HB (1959): Congenital aortic stenosis. Circulation 19:458–468.

69. Taussig HB, Crocetti A, Eshaghpour E, Keinonen R, Yap KN, Bachman D, Momberger N, Kirk H (1971): Long-time observations on the Blalock-Taussig operation. I. Results of first operation. Johns Hopkins Med J 129:243–257.

70. Taussig HB (1982): World survey of the common cardiac malformations: Developmental error or genetic variant? Am J Cardiol 50:544–559.

71. Taylor PV, Scott JS, Gerlis LM, Esscher E, Scott O (1986): Maternal antibodies against fetal cardiac antigens in congenital complete heart block. N Engl J Med 315:667–673.

72. Texeira OHP, Malhotra K, Sellers J, Mercer S (1983): Cardiovascular anomalies with imperforate anus. Arch Dis Child 58:747–749.

73. Thomas D, Lassault G, Caille B, Drobinski G, Huberman JP, Shqueir A, Grosgogeat Y (1985): Familial forms of ostium secundum atrial septal defect. Arch mal Coeur 78:1205–1209.

74. Traisman ES, Traisman HS (1982): Noonan syndrome. A report of male-to-male transmission. Clin Pediatr 21:51–53.

75. Ursell P, Byrne JM, Strobino BA (1985): Significance of cardiac defects in the developing fetus: A study of spontaneous abortions. Circulation 72:1232–1236.

76. van Mierop LHS, Kutsche L (1986): Cardiovascular anomalies in DiGeorge syndrome and importance of neural crest as a possible pathogenetic factor. Am J Cardiol 58:133–137.

77. Whittemore R, Hobbins JC, Engle MA (1983): Pregnancy and its outcome in women with and without surgical treatment of congenital heart disease. Am J Cardiol 50:641–650.

78. Zlotogora J, Elian E (1981): Asplenia and polysplenia syndromes with abnormalities of lateralization in a sibship. J Med Genet 18:301–302.

11 MATERNAL DISEASES AFFECTING THE FETAL CARDIOVASCULAR SYSTEM

Vern L. Katz
Watson A. Bowes, Jr.

INTRODUCTION

Many maternal diseases cause infertility. Disease may inhibit ovulation or cause spontaneous abortion through interference with embryogenesis and/or the formation of a normal placenta. When maternal diseases occur after embryogenesis and placental formation, the pattern of fetal response is frequently not lethal. This chapter will concentrate primarily on the fetal cardiovascular response to maternal diseases after embryogenesis is finished, although reference will be made to significant teratogenic effects of maternal diseases. Chapter 12 will concentrate on the fetal cardiovascular response to treatments of various disease states. This chapter will not attempt to discuss the pathophysiology of maternal diseases in pregnancy. For such discussions the reader is referred to a number of excellent obstetric and medical textbooks.[26,53,116]

The Patterns of Fetal Cardiovascular Response

The fetal cardiovascular system may respond to maternal diseases either directly or indirectly (Table 11–1). Maternal diseases that affect the fetus directly do so by a variety of mechanisms such as immunoglobulins, hormones, or metabolites that cross the placenta. Examples of such direct-acting maternal diseases are hyperthyroidism, diabetes mellitus, and systemic lupus erythematosus. The fetal cardiac response to direct-acting maternal diseases ranges from asymptomatic fetal cardiac arrhythmias to fetal or neonatal cardiac failure and death. Maternal diseases that indirectly affect the fetus do so by disrupting uteroplacental function. Severe maternal renal disease and maternal cardiac disease are examples of maternal diseases that can indirectly affect fetal cardiovascular function. The fetal cardiovascular response to abnormalities of uteroplacental function includes a wide spectrum of fetal disorders, from mild asymmetric intrauterine growth retardation to intrauterine fetal death.

Fetal Response to Maternal Diseases That Affect the Fetus Directly

Maternal diseases affect the fetal cardiovascular system directly through several mechanisms. Most important quantitatively are maternal diseases that specifically affect the fetal heart. Diseases such as rubella and diabetes mellitus lead to developmental cardiac abnormalities. The SSA-Ro (Ro) antibody found in patients with connective tissue diseases may destroy the fetal cardiac conducting system. Maternal disease may lead to decreased oxygen-carrying capacity of fetal blood. This situation may be found in inherited fetal hemoglobinopathies and maternal-fetal blood incompatabilities. Maternal disease may lead to vascular disease in the fetus as with congenital syphilis. The end stage fetal cardiac response to a maternal disease that attacks the fetus directly is similar to that of an infant or an adult—heart failure.

Cardiac failure (hydrops fetalis) in the fetus is not manifested by pulmonary edema because the fetal pulmonary vascular bed has a relatively high resistance and receives less than 10 per cent of cardiac output.[63,121] When fetal cardiac failure occurs, it is essentially a right heart failure. The fetal ventricles beat in series, and the first sign of failure is right atrial dilation. The next sign is increased cardiac size, which may be seen ultrasonographically as a predominantly right-sided dilation. Liver enlargement, ascites, umbilical vein dilation, pericardial and pleural effusions, and placental enlargement secondary to edema are further manifestations of fetal cardiac failure.[6] Clinically, such fetuses are hydropic or swollen. However, not all cases of hydrops fetalis are cardiogenic; for example, the generalized edema of Turner syndrome is a noncardiogenic hydrops. The evaluation, pathogenesis, and differential diagnosis of hydrops is discussed in Chapters 18 and 19. The picture of cardiogenic failure in the fetus is dynamic, and in early states of fetal cardiac compromise, mild cardiac dilation may be present prior to the formation of full-blown failure.

The diagnosis and management of hydrops fetalis is dependent on the cause of the insult.[63,143] Since the first manifestation of the disease will often be polyhydramnios (presumably caused by decreased swallowing of amniotic fluid by the ailing fetus), the diagnosis of hydrops fetalis is often made when an ultrasonographic examination for maternal size greater than normal for gestational dates detects fetal ascites or cardiomegaly. Retrospective evaluation may then uncover the subtle maternal abnormality responsible for the fetal cardiac compromise. This situation is different from fetal cardiac compromise secondary to uteroplacental insufficiency, in which the maternal disease state is usually quite pronounced. In the latter situation, fetal evaluation is ongoing during the pregnancy.

Many cardiac lesions may cause only mild difficulty in utero but cause severe problems after delivery because of the changes in fetal circulation that occur at birth. An example is diabetic hypertrophic cardiomyopathy. This lesion rarely inhibits fetal cardiac function because it primarily affects the left ventricle, which is of much less importance prior to birth.

Uteroplacental Insufficiency and Its Relation to the Fetal Cardiovascular System

When a maternal disease or condition alters utero-placental function, the fetus attempts to compensate. To understand the maternal-fetal interaction we must first look directly at uteroplacental function and then review the fetal response.

The normal term placenta is discoid and weighs between 400 and 500 g.[52] It averages 20 mm in thickness. The maternal surface appears as 15 to 20 lobules, which are not specifically functional units. The lobules are composed of two to three fetal cotyledons. Each cotyledon is a functional unit composed of an arborized fetal main stem villus unit or tertiary villus supplied by one of the maternal spiral arterioles.[110] As will be discussed below, if maternal disease, such as lupus, leads to vascular occlusion of the spiral arteriole, then the whole cotyledon unit is functionally lost, appearing histologically as a partial placental infarction.

The cotyledon may be thought of as a blood-filled cavity, with multiple branching capillaries of fetal origin floating free in a pool of maternal blood (a giant upside-down bowl sitting on top of several closely packed trees). Thus, the human placenta is classified as hemochorial, i.e., maternal blood in direct continuity with fetal tissue. The villi are composed of three layers: an outermost trophoblastic layer, next a supporting connective tissue layer, and an innermost layer of fetal capillary wall. The villi are lined by a trophoblastic layer that decreases in thickness as pregnancy progresses. At term, the trophoblastic layer is very thin and hardly recognizable. In disease states, however, fibrin may accumulate between the trophoblastic layers and the capillaries and inhibit nutrient and oxygen exchange.[52,110] Blood enters the villi through perpendicularly placed spiral arterioles.[15] Blood spurts into the cotyledons under the back pressure of the spiral arterioles and is driven toward the chorionic plate. The blood then percolates back toward the maternal surface, entering a large plexus of veins that run parallel to the placental surface.[15]

The maternal component of this system is the uterus, which grows to accept a volume over 500 times that of the nonpregnant state, with a blood flow of nearly a liter per minute, 85 per cent of which goes to the placenta.[47,120] The functional components of the uteroplacental exchange are the radial arteries that branch off from the uterine arteries and traverse perpendicularly through the myometrial fibers. Contraction of the myometrium leads to occlusion of these vessels.[46] The radial arteries then branch into the spiral arterioles, which supply each of the fetal mainstem villi.

Table 11–1. CLASSIFICATION OF MATERNAL DISEASES AFFECTING THE FETAL CARDIOVASCULAR SYSTEM

Category I: **Maternal diseases that directly affect the fetal cardiovascular system (excluding teratogenic effects)**

Pheochromocytoma
Hyperthyroidism
Diabetes mellitus
Collagen vascular disease (e.g., Ro antibody)
Smoking
Rubella
Cytomegalovirus
Enterovirus infection
Toxoplasmosis
Listeriosis
Maternal group B streptococcal colonization with fetal invasion
Syphilis
Inherited metabolic diseases

Category II: **Maternal diseases that may indirectly affect the fetal cardiovascular system as a result of abnormalities of uteroplacental function**

Neoplastic diseases
Diabetes mellitus
Maternal cardiac disease
Anemia (including the hemoglobinopathies)
Hypertensive disorders
Collagen vascular disease (e.g., lupus anticoagulant and SLE)
Renal disease (associated with hypertension)
Smoking
Asthma
Cholestatic jaundice of pregnancy
Cytomegalovirus
Bacterial infections

The trophoblast cells of the developing placenta invade the spiral arterioles within the endometrium and myometrium and eliminate the muscular layer of these vessels.[119] Consequently, in the normal state, blood supply to the placenta is directly dependent on maternal cardiac output, there being no autoregulation of blood flow. Disease states may inhibit trophoblastic growth into the myometrium, resulting in persistent vasoactive arterioles and potential reduction of uteroplacental blood flow.

Uteroplacental function may be adversely affected in several ways by maternal disease (Table 11–2). The first type of dysfunction is caused by decreased uterine blood flow; examples of maternal diseases or conditions that induce this phenomenon are supine hypotension, maternal exercise, hypertensive states of pregnancy, and maternal dehydration. After 20 weeks of pregnancy, the uterus has risen in the abdomen to the level of the abdominal aorta and inferior vena cava. When a woman lies in a supine position the uterus may cause aortocaval compression. As a result, there is inadequate venous return and a decreased cardiac output. The decreased cardiac output then leads to decreased uterine blood flow. During exercise a physiologic redistribution of blood flow away from the abdominal viscera to the exercising muscles may occur; and consequent decreases in uterine blood flow may lead to uteroplacental dysfunction.[96] The hypertensive disorders of pregnancy may decrease uterine blood flow through a

Table 11–2. MECHANISMS OF
ABNORMAL UTEROPLACENTAL FUNCTION

I. Decreased uteroplacental blood flow
   A. Decreased flow to the uterus
      Exercise
      Postural changes in cardiac output
      Dehydration
      Plasma volume reduction—hypertensive disorders
   B. Decreased blood flow to the placenta
      Uterine vascular spasm—hypertensive
        disease
      Placental abruption
      Vascular endarteritis

II. Decreased oxygen content in maternal blood
      Hemoglobinopathies
      Cyanotic heart disease
      Severe asthma

III. Decreased transplacental diffusion or transport
      Placental villitis from infection or nonspecific
        inflammation
      Placental edema
      Smoking
      Senescent changes in postmature placentas

variety of mechanisms. The volume contraction of pre-eclampsia may lead to a generalized decrease in uterine blood flow.[118] Uterine arterial atherosclerotic changes that are found in the chronic hypertensive disorders may also lead to a decreased uteroplacental blood flow.[13] If the functional area between the placenta and the uterus is diminished by a blood clot, as in the condition of abruptio placentae, uteroplacental exchange is also diminished.

A second category of uteroplacental dysfunction includes maternal disorders that lead to decreased oxygen content in the maternal blood. This situation is found, for example, in women with cyanotic heart disease, severe asthma, or maternal hemoglobinopathies.[27] A third category of decreased uteroplacental function is one in which there is a decrease in diffusion of oxygen across the placenta. This situation may be due to a variety of factors, including villitis, which could be secondary to infection from a variety of organisms.[12] The normal senescent placental changes that accompany prolonged pregnancies may lead to increased fibrin deposition in the placenta, which may also inhibit oxygen diffusion.[14] Placental diffusion capacity is also diminished by maternal smoking.[82]

The Fetal Response to Decreased Uteroplacental Function

The physiology of the uteroplacental unit leaves the fetus with little control over uterine blood flow and placental oxygen exchange. However, several compensatory mechanisms assist the fetus in adapting to vagaries in uteroplacental exchange. The higher oxygen-carrying capacity of fetal hemoglobin facilitates oxygen transport to the fetal side of the placenta. Serum protein levels are higher in the fetus, and fetal protein binding of a variety of nutrients and metabolites is enhanced. The trophoblast secretes hormones that not only affect maternal fuel metabolism but also affect maternal fluid balance and vascular function. However, the most important fetal adaptive mechanisms are cardiovascular.

When a maternal disease compromises uteroplacental function, the fetal cardiovascular system responds by a redistribution of fetal blood flow. Since increases in fetal cardiac output will not increase uteroplacental exchange, when faced with oxygen shortage, the fetus must ration the available resources. The fetal cardiovascular system shunts away blood from less vital areas such as the liver, intestines, and extremities and shunts toward the more vital areas, specifically the adrenal glands, the brain, and the heart. The result over time is decreased growth of the fetus in length, weight, and abdominal girth but a sparing of the head size.[134,135,136] This chronic intrauterine oxygen stress is appreciated clinically as asymmetric growth retardation. The degree of blood redistribution is dependent on the degree of deprivation of oxygen. As the insult becomes more severe, head growth is also impaired.[123] Further deprivation leads to a large enough reduction in renal blood flow that amniotic fluid production is decreased and oligohydramnios results.[136] The end result, as oxygen supply continues to decrease in relation to fetal needs, is intrauterine fetal death.[135] If the fetus is stressed during the period of uteroplacental dysfunction, such as with labor and uterine contractions, the manifestation may be the "fetal distress" seen clinically as heart rate decelerations, bradycardias, or tachycardias. Fetal asphyxia is further discussed in Chapter 17.

Recent research using pulsed Doppler ultrasonography has substantiated the theory of fetal cardiovascular redistribution in response to decreased uteroplacental flow leading to subsequent intrauterine growth retardation. With the use of linear array real time ultrasonography, pulsed Doppler examinations have been made of blood flow through the descending aorta. Normal pregnancies were compared with growth retarded pregnancies. In a study of infants at varying gestational ages by Tong et al, an increase in peripheral vascular resistance was found in fetuses with growth retardation.[141] Increased peripheral vascular resistance leads to redistribution of flow, as has been documented in animal studies.[136] The conclusion that peripheral vascular resistance is increased in the growth-retarded fetus is supported by the findings of decreased peak velocity and decreased end-diastolic velocity in the descending aorta. Another report by Joupila and Kirkinen that compared waveforms in growth-retarded versus normal fetuses, both of hypertensive mothers, further confirmed the study of Tong et al.[72] The study of Joupila and Kirkinen showed that although both groups of fetuses came from pregnancies in which maternal hypertension was approximately equal, the growth-retarded fetuses had significantly decreased end-diastolic velocities in the descending aorta (implying an increased peripheral vascular resistance).

The remaining sections of this chapter will focus on various maternal disease states known to affect the fetal cardiovascular system and the typical fetal effects of those diseases.

DISEASES OF THE MATERNAL ENDOCRINE SYSTEM

The function of the reproductive tract is closely related to and often dependent upon the normal functioning of the other endocrine organs, specifically the pituitary, thyroid, and adrenal glands. Untreated severe endocrinopathies are therefore rare in pregnancy.

Pheochromocytoma

Fewer than 200 cases of pheochromocytoma in pregnancy have been reported to date; these have been reviewed recently.[130] The intrauterine fetal death rate from this disease is over 50 per cent; fetal demise is thought to be due to decreased perfusion of the placental bed caused by high levels of circulating catecholamines. Higher than normal umbilical cord blood levels of catecholamines have been found in fetuses and in infants of mothers with pheochromocytoma.[130]

Thyroid Disease

Maternal hypothyroidism, though associated with infertility, does not appear to affect the fetal cardiovascular system.[19] Hyperthyroidism due to Graves disease, however, may lead to fetal and neonatal thyrotoxicosis. Thyrotoxicosis is found in the offspring of 1 per cent of women with a history of autoimmune thyroid disease.[20,22,75] The woman need not have active hyperthyroidism at the time of the pregnancy. Transplacental passage of thyroid-stimulating immunoglobulins may cause effects directly on the fetal cardiovascular system. Tachycardia is the most common symptom.[75] The mortality from neonatal and fetal thyrotoxicosis has been reported to be as high as 25 per cent, with heart failure being the most common cause of death.[20,22,75]

Diabetes

Diabetes is the most common medical problem seen in pregnancy.[131] As many as 10 per cent of pregnant women have disorders of glucose intolerance. The disease affects the fetal cardiovascular system in multiple ways, both directly and indirectly (Table 11–3).

Indirect effects on the fetal cardiovascular system caused by maternal diabetes may result from associated conditions, such as small vessel disease or renal disease, or from placental abnormalities associated with diabetes. The placentas of diabetic women are larger than normal because of increased glycogen.[38] Though no specific "diabetic lesion" exists, associated vasculopathies are common. Approximately one quarter of placentas from

Table 11–3. EFFECTS OF MATERNAL DIABETES ON THE FETAL CARDIOVASCULAR SYSTEM

1. Increased risk of developmental cardiac lesions
2. Diabetic cardiomyopathy
3. Increased risk of respiratory distress syndrome
4. Increased risk of stillbirth
5. Increased placental pathology
6. Increased maternal vascular disease, leading to decreased uterine blood flow

diabetic pregnancies have endarteritis. Edema and abnormal maturation, both advanced and retarded on the cellular level, are also common features.[37] Abnormally thick basement membranes are found in the capillaries.[7] If a diabetic woman has severe vascular disease, her placenta may be small, with decreased uteroplacental flow. Babies of these women tend to be growth retarded. Fetuses of diabetic mothers are at twice the normal risk of sudden in utero death,[18] most probably secondary to a combination of decreased uteroplacental perfusion and an increased metabolic rate induced by fetal hyperinsulinism.

Infants of diabetics have a congenital anomaly rate that is quoted to be as high as 20 per cent.[18] Cardiovascular abnormalities make up a prominent fraction of that anomaly rate, although cardiovascular defects are not as common as skeletal or neural tube defects.[104] The level of maternal glucose during embryogenesis has been correlated directly with the incidence of anomalies.[105] Elevated glucose levels not only lead to abnormal cellular organization and cellular divisions but also adversely affect oxygen transport.[48] Common cardiovascular anomalies seen in infants of diabetic mothers are transposition of the great vessels, ventricular septal defect, single ventricle, and hypoplastic left heart. In one series of 116 diabetics followed prospectively, nine of the 15 anomalies observed were severe cardiovascular lesions.[105] The risk of having a structural cardiovascular anomaly in an infant of a diabetic mother is five times that of the general population.[127]

Maternal diabetes also affects the fetal cardiovascular system after embryogenesis is complete. During pregnancy the fetus is exposed to increased levels of maternal blood sugar, which lead to increased levels of fetal glucose and result in increased fetal insulin levels. Higher levels of insulin, which acts like a growth hormone in the fetus, lead to fetal enlargement and a macrosomic morphology.

Fetuses of diabetic mothers are also likely to develop hypertrophic cardiomyopathy. Beginning in the late 1930s, a large percentage of infants of diabetic mothers were noted to have cardiomegaly on chest radiographic examination and at autopsy.[66] Initially, the hypertrophy of the ventricles was thought to be due to hyperglycemia and increased glycogen deposition.[55,56] Recently, the hypertrophy has been attributed to a more complex mechanism. Fetal hyperinsulinemia coupled with a normally increased level of insulin receptors in the fetal heart causes myocardial cell hyperplasia and hypertrophy from increased fat and protein synthesis. The increases in myocardial cell fat and protein synthesis are in addition to increased glycogen deposition.[17,140] The cardiac hypertrophy, which is greatest in the intraventricular septum, may or may not be symptomatic.[152] The heart silhouette is enlarged, although ventricular function is usually adequate. Hypertrophy of both ventricles occurs, but more hypertrophy occurs in the left ventricle than in the right. Most of the time, the cardiac hypertrophy is asymmetric, and the interventricular septum is more profoundly affected. Diabetic hypertrophic cardiomyopathy is primarily a third trimester phenomenon (although it has been documented as early as 24 weeks' gestation). Resolution of diabetic hypertrophic cardiomyopathy ranges from 2 to 20 months but usually occurs within 6 months of birth.[17,55,56,92,152] Unlike other hypertrophic cardiomyopathies, diabetic cardiomyopathy is not familial, spontaneously resolves, and does not have myocardial fiber disarray when examined histologically.[17,55,56,74,92,152] While up to 30 per cent of term infants of diabetic mothers have diabetic cardiomyopathy, less than 1 in 10 infants of diabetic mothers actually develop cardiac dysfunction.[92,152]

The risk for respiratory distress syndrome in infants of diabetic mothers is increased five to six times compared with infants of nondiabetic mothers of similar gestational ages.[35] The high incidence of respiratory dysfunction (thought to be due to the effect of hyperinsulinemia altering lipid and surfactant production[74]) and the high incidence of cardiac structural abnormalities obscure accurate assessment of the incidence of diabetic hypertrophic cardiomyopathy. Furthermore, the degree of cardiac hypertrophy and clinical disease in the infant does not correlate with the severity of the maternal disease.[17,55,56,92,152] While long-standing maternal diabetes does not always produce severe infant disease, there does seem to be a correlation with maternal glucose control during the pregnancy.[17,92,152] The work-up and treatment of the symptoms of diabetic hypertrophic cardiomyopathy will be discussed in detail in Chapter 40.

NEOPLASTIC DISEASE

Transplacental passage of metastatic cancer is extremely rare. Placental metastases, although reported, are also uncommon. When they occur, they may lead to uteroplacental insufficiency. Melanoma, breast cancer, and leukemia and lymphomas are the main types of cancers that may involve the placenta. However, case reports exist of many other types of malignancies involving the placenta.[32]

MATERNAL CARDIAC DISEASE

Severe maternal cardiac disease may lead to compromised uteroplacental exchange and intrauterine growth retardation. The mechanism by which maternal cardiac disease affects the fetus is thought to be the mother's inability to increase cardiac output, which is a normal physiologic change during pregnancy. This deficiency may occur in various valvular lesions, both inherited and acquired, such as mitral valve or aortic valve disease.[114,146] The severity of maternal compromise is directly correlated with a relative reduction in uterine blood flow and hence uteroplacental insufficiency.[114,147] Patients with tachyarrhythmias may also have uteroplacental insufficiency and fetal distress secondary to decreased cardiac output.[77] Congenital diseases associated with right-to-left shunting also have an increased incidence of fetal compromise.[101] In conditions of maternal cyanotic heart disease (right-to-left shunting) the fetus is affected in direct proportion to the degree of maternal compromise.[145]

In addition, as considered in Chapter 10, offspring of patients with congenital heart disease are themselves at increased risk of congenital heart disease; the recurrence risk varies by lesion.

HEMATOLOGIC DISEASES

Anemias produce detrimental fetal effects when they are severe (hemoglobin less than 6.5).[103] The placenta may be enlarged and slightly edematous, which is thought to be a compensatory change.[41] Fetuses of mothers with hemoglobin SS have a significantly higher rate of intrauterine growth retardation and stillbirth, which is related to the severity of maternal symptoms during pregnancy.[102,106,108] One explanation for these observations in the offspring of pregnant sickle cell patients is that placental infarction is increased, perhaps due to sludging of maternal blood.[41] Results of some studies suggest that increasing maternal hemoglobin A through transfusions may decrease fetal morbidity and mortality.[5,102,117]

Thalassemia in the mother does not affect the fetus unless the fetus inherits the homozygous state. α-Thalassemia in utero usually leads to cardiovascular failure and hydrops fetalis, with intrauterine fetal demise or perinatal demise.[67,98,143] G6PD deficiency is an x-linked disease, and male fetuses of mothers with this disease have been reported to develop severe anemia, and rarely hydrops fetalis, after exposure to drugs that precipitate hemolysis, such as nitrofurantoin or sulfa.[5,113]

Idiopathic or immune thrombocytic purpura is not uncommon in pregnant women. The IgG antiplatelet antibody does cross the placenta and may lead to neonatal thrombocytopenia. However, a specific cardiovascular effect has not been seen.[5,34,65,80,99] Isoimmune thrombocytopenia, in which the mother has an antibody to the baby's platelets, may also affect fetal hemostasis but is much more rare.[5,24,139]

HYPERTENSIVE DISORDERS

The hypertensive disorders in pregnancy affect 5 per cent to 10 per cent of all gestations and include chronic hypertension, preeclampsia/eclampsia, preeclampsia superimposed on chronic hypertension, and transient gestational hypertension.[24,115] These disorders have been known and described since the time of Hippocrates.[23] These diseases affect the fetal cardiovascular system by causing uteroplacental insufficiency.

Preeclampsia, the etiology of which is obscure, is characterized by generalized vasospasm and increased capillary permeability; plasma and blood volumes decrease as a result.[23,24,115,122,124,159] The vasculature of the myometrium and placental bed undergoes constrictive atherosis and a necrotizing arteriopathy.[24,124,155] These changes begin early in pregnancy.[94] The placenta of women with hypertensive disorders may demonstrate decreased vascularity, decreased size, and endarteritis. There are often findings of cytotrophoblastic hyperplasia, increased fibrinoid necrosis in the cotyledons, and increased fibrin deposition in the basement membranes of placental vessels. The trophoblastic membrane may also be thickened. These changes are most often proportional to the severity of the disease.[42] The consequences of these changes are smaller placentas, intrauterine growth retardation, higher incidence of placental infarction, and increased incidence of premature placental separation. Fetal-maternal bleeding is also increased. As a result of placental insufficiency, stillbirth and neonatal asphyxia are not infrequent.[23,24,42,94,115,122,124,159]

The treatment of pregnant patients with hypertensive disorders is beyond the scope of this discussion; however, the assurance of fetal well-being by means of real time ultrasound and fetal cardiac monitoring both antepartum and intrapartum is essential in any management plan. As described above, Doppler analysis of the fetal cardiovascular system may aid in determining the effects of hypertensive disorders on the baby.

CONGENITAL METABOLIC DISEASE

Advances in the treatment of congenital metabolic disorders now permit affected women to reach childbearing age. As a result it is now recognized that fetal disease may result from deficiencies or surpluses of substrates in the maternal circulation.[21] Women with homocystinuria have a higher than expected rate of fetal loss, the mechanism of which is unclear.[148] Infants of mothers with phenylketonuria have an increased incidence of congenital heart defects.[90,91] The maternal PKU syndrome appears to be related to maternal phenylalanine levels (greater than or equal to 10 mg/dl).[91] Among 123 mothers with PKU and with phenylalanine levels greater than 20 mg/dl, the rate of congenital heart disease in the offspring was 17 per cent. In mothers with phenylalanine levels below 10 mg/dl no structural heart lesions were found. The lesions observed in maternal PKU syndrome include tetralogy of Fallot, ventricular septal defect, coarctation of the aorta, single ventricle, and atrial septal defects.[91]

CONNECTIVE TISSUE DISORDERS

Disorders variably classified as connective tissue disorders, collagen vascular diseases, or nonendocrine autoimmune diseases have a wide range of clinical manifestations. Many such diseases are common in women in their childbearing years. As a general rule, collagen vascular diseases that cause vasculopathies (such as lupus) may affect the fetal cardiovascular system by causing uteroplacental insufficiency, as described above. Although nonspecific, the common vascular findings in the placentas of mothers with connective tissue disorders and vasculopathies (excluding mothers with the lupus anticoagulant) include fibrinoid necrosis of the vessels, "variable vascular architecture disruption, subintimal edema in the small vessels, and marked necrotic dissolution of the vascular wall."[1] An increased incidence of placental infarction and abruption and preeclampsia are also seen.[36,39,60,100,154] This placental pathology leads to uteroplacental insufficiency, and intrauterine growth retardation, stillbirth, or fetal distress during labor can result, particularly when maternal hypertension or renal disease is present.[36,39,60,100,154] Such placental lesions are infrequently seen in rheumatoid arthritis and scleroderma, but are often present in periarteritis nodosa.[154]

Two autoimmune-related phenomena associated with the connective tissue disorders significantly affect the fetal cardiovascular system in a direct manner. The first is the Ro antibody. The second is the lupus anticoagulant.

The Ro antibody, so called for its first description in a Mrs. Robair,[132] causes the congenital heart block found in neonatal lupus syndrome. This antibody reacts to the SSA-Ro antigen, which is a soluble ribonucleoprotein. The antibody is found in 25 to 30 per cent of women with systemic lupus erythematosus (SLE), and as an IgG antibody, it crosses the placenta. Approximately 40 per cent of patients with Sjögren syndrome and 5 per cent of patients with rheumatoid arthritis also possess the antibody.[84,93,132,133] Twenty-five per cent of the infants with congenital heart block due to this abnormality will be born to mothers who are asymptomatic and previously undiagnosed.[84,132] Using immunofluorescent histology, Letsey et al[93] have shown antibody attached to the epicardium and the myocardium of the right atrium in an infant with congenital heart block whose mother had Ro antibodies.[93] The result was inflammation and destruction. The right atrium and interventricular septum of the infant demonstrated destruction and calcification in the area of the AV node and bundle of His. Fetuses of mothers with the Ro antibodies may present with a variety of problems, including stillbirth, bradycardia and cardiac failure, incomplete block without cardiac failure, or minor sinus node dysfunction.[84,132,133] Some fetuses are unaffected. The outcome of affected infants is dependent on the degree of destruction in the conducting system; severely affected infants with irreversible changes who survive may need permanent pacing.[36,84,132,133]

The "lupus anticoagulant" is an immunoglobulin, usually of the IgG class but occasionally of the IgM class, which is nearly always lethal to the fetus.[16,28,29,36,62,97] The lupus anticoagulant became widely recognized in the late 1970s,[62] and at that time acquired its name, which is misleading. The lupus anticoagulant is found in only 5 to 15 per cent of patients with SLE, although 40 per cent of patients with the antibody have SLE.[16,62,28] The antibody is associated with many diseases, including neoplastic disease, myeloproliferative diseases, rheumatoid arthritis, and polyarteritis nodosa.[62] In vitro the antibody inhibits coagulation by interfering in phospholipid-dependent clotting. In vivo the antibody causes thrombosis, and women who are pregnant often present with venous and occasional arterial thrombosis.[1,29,62,97,154] The increased clotting is due to alterations in the vascular endothelium, which lead to an increased thromboxane to prostacyclin ratio. The accompanying interference with platelet function leads to a thrombocytopenia due to consumption of platelets. The patient usually has an elevated aPTT, which will not correct when diluted in equal amounts with normal plasma. The aPTT will correct when mixed with phospholipid substrate to bind the antibody. Within the placenta the antibody causes multiple infarctions as a result of clotting of uterine vessels. The spiral arterioles may be obliterated by thrombosis.[28,150] The continued loss of functioning placenta leads to intrauterine growth retardation and fetal death, usually in the second or early third trimester. If the fetus survives, it may suffer from severe growth retardation.[16,28,62,97,150] These patients frequently develop preeclampsia, which further compromises the fetus.[1,16,28,60,62,97,150,154] Some patients have been successfully treated with a regimen of high dose prednisone and low dose aspirin, preferably for several months prior to conception.[16,62] Unfortunately, this regimen is not invariably successful.[16] In 162 untreated patients reviewed by Branch et al, only two live infants were delivered, and both had severe growth retardation.[16]

RENAL DISEASE

For the most part, maternal renal disease affects the fetus to the extent that it is associated with hypertension and a reduction in uteroplacental perfusion. In these cases the fetus is at risk for uteroplacental insufficiency, growth retardation, and stillbirth.[11,31,59,76] In all types of renal disease, the presence of hypertension in addition to the patient's preexisting lesion is the most significant factor influencing fetal health and viability.[11,30,31,59,73,76] Chronic renal failure is frequently complicated by superimposed preeclampsia, which further compromises uteroplacental blood flow.[11,59,76]

PULMONARY DISEASE

The most common noninfectious pulmonary disease occurring in pregnancy is asthma, affecting nearly 1 per cent of pregnant women.[33] The effect of asthma on the fetal cardiovascular system is minimal. However, chronic mild hypoxia may lead to a slightly increased incidence of growth retardation owing to mechanisms described above.[5,15,54,153] Most studies have not found maternal asthma to have a detrimental effect on the fetus. Other primary pulmonary diseases such as sarcoid do not tend to affect the fetal cardiovascular system.[33,54,153,155] Smoking

and nicotine (reviewed in Chapter 49) do affect the fetal cardiovascular system, and can cause significant uteroplacental insufficiency.

LIVER DISEASES

In general, liver diseases have minimal effects on the fetal cardiovascular system except when the liver disease is a manifestation of another systemic disorder.[50] The rare syndrome of acute fatty liver of pregnancy, which may be part of the spectrum of hypertensive disorders, is associated with stillbirth.[50,157] Cholestatic jaundice of pregnancy is a poorly understood disease manifested by pruritus, jaundice, and slightly elevated liver enzymes.[25,70,83,137,156,176] Although cholestatic jaundice of pregnancy causes only mild maternal discomfort, it is associated with chronic and acute compromise of the fetus. The fetal effects include intrauterine growth retardation, fetal distress, stillbirth, and a relatively increased rate of meconium passage.[25,83,156,176] Intravillous edema in the placenta is often found with this condition.[156] Other investigators have noted a variety of placental abnormalities.[40] A correlation does exist between fetal distress and the level of maternal bile acids.[70,156]

INFECTIOUS DISEASES

Infections in the mother significantly affect the fetal cardiovascular system in both indirect and direct manners. It is impossible to list every infecting agent in this review, so only the most common and most important will be reviewed. Table 11–4 summarizes the major infecting agents that influence the fetal cardiovascular system.

VIRAL DISEASES

Most viral infections do not affect the fetal cardiovascular system. These include herpes simplex and herpes varicella, rhinovirus, parainfluenza virus, respiratory syncytial virus, and adenovirus.[3,45,85] Maternal influenza infection, although associated with increased stillbirth,[86] does not seem to cause increased structural cardiac defects.[86,149] Maternal hepatitis and rubeola also do not affect the fetal cardiovascular system.[51,151] Maternal infection with mumps in the first trimester has been associated with fetal endocardial fibroelastosis.[9,51,128,149] However, currently most authors feel that endocardial fibroelastosis is not related to maternal mumps.

Rubella

Maternal rubella is covered in detail in Chapter 47. The incidence of rubella infection has declined in the past 20 years since the last major epidemic in 1964. However, because of the reservoir of susceptible women in the population, rubella is an everpresent threat.[4] Rubella infection affects growth in all organ systems, and the extent of the damage to the cardiovascular system is related to the timing of infection.[3,51,64] If the maternal infection occurs in the first trimester, up to 85 per cent of fetuses are affected.[3,51] Approximately one half of affected infants will have serious cardiovascular disorders.[149] The most common lesions include patent ductus arteriosus, pulmonary valvular stenosis, both central and peripheral pulmonary artery stenosis, aortic valvular stenosis, coarctation, and endomyocardial disease.[64,149] In addition to its teratogenic effects, rubella has been reported to cause fetal myocarditis leading to in utero death and to neonatal morbidity and mortality.[2,149]

Cytomegalovirus

Maternal infection with cytomegalovirus (CMV) is currently the most common in utero viral infection. CMV tends not to cause structural anomalies of the heart, although such anomalies are occasionally reported.[64,138,142,149] Mitral and pulmonary valvular stenosis and tetrology of Fallot are the lesions most commonly noted. Cases of fatal neonatal myocarditis have also been reported[86,129,149] as well as in utero cardiac failure, hydrops fetalis, and stillbirth.[63,143] In utero CMV infection can cause placental villitis with necrosis,[43] which may lead to intrauterine growth retardation. Because CMV infection affects fetal cellular growth, other reasons besides uteroplacental insufficiency exist for growth retardation.[43,64,138,142,149]

The Enterovirus Group

In contrast to many agents, the enteroviruses do cause myocarditis. ECHO virus, Coxsackie virus, and poliovirus are enteroviruses. The first two viruses are especially dangerous to the fetus and neonate,[58,69,85,129,149] and may cause myocarditis manifested by either fetal or neonatal cardiac failure. The inner myocardium tends to be most affected, with lymphocytic infiltrates, interstitial edema, and areas of necrosis.[10,58,69,128,129,149] Cases occur from sporadic maternal infections as well as from epidemics.[68,85] In cases of severe fetal disease, the outcome is often fatal, but recovery has been reported.[149] Case reports suggest that enteroviruses may infect the fetus at any time in gestation, since nonimmune hydrops fetalis from cardiac failure has been seen early in pregnancy. It is not known if enteroviruses cause structural cardiac lesions in human fetuses.

TOXOPLASMOSIS

A primary maternal infection with *Toxoplasma gondii* may produce discernible lesions of congenital toxoplasmosis in 10 to 15 per cent of infants. The fetal cardiovascular system is only rarely involved in congenital toxoplasmosis.[51,88,89,149] The earlier in pregnancy the disease is acquired by the mother, the more severe the effect on the fetus. Myocarditis with lymphocytic infiltrates and focal

Table 11–4. MAJOR INFECTIOUS AGENTS THAT AFFECT THE FETAL CARDIOVASCULAR SYSTEM

I. Viral
Rubella
Cytomegalovirus
ECHO virus
Coxsackie virus
II. Parasitic
Toxoplasmosis
III. Bacterial
Listeria
Syphilis
Group B streptococcus

necrosis has been reported in the neonate[89]; in utero heart failure and hydrops may also occur.[63,143]

BACTERIAL INFECTIONS

In general, bacteremias that occur in the mother often lead to labor, whether gestation is preterm or term. The placentitis and chorioamnionitis resulting from bacterial invasion lead to prostaglandin release, which may initiate uterine contractions. The fetus is usually affected indirectly by maternal signs of infection, specifically uteroplacental insufficiency from maternal dehydration or shock. Maternal fever in the first trimester may increase the risk of congenital structural defects, but these anomalies are rarely cardiovascular and tend to involve the neural tube if they occur. Two important bacterial agents that may directly affect the fetal cardiovascular system but not cause labor are syphilis and *Listeria*. Maternal bacteremia from *Listeria monocytogenes* may lead to a transplacental passage of the bacteria. The mother may experience only mild, flulike symptoms with slight fever. The fetus may develop septicemia and die. All fetal organ systems are affected, and the fetal disease has been termed granulomatosis infantiseptica.[79,158]

Maternal infection with *Treponema pallidum* may cause congenital disease of the fetal heart, in utero cardiac failure, stillbirth, and placental disease.[87,95] The longer the duration of maternal disease with syphilis prior to pregnancy, the less severe the fetal manifestations. For example, primary syphilis in the first trimester is associated with up to a 50 per cent perinatal mortality.[126] Structurally affected areas include the aorta and pulmonary arteries as well as systemic vessels. However, cardiovascular lesions are much less common than anomalies in other organ systems. Hemolytic anemia is common with congenital syphilis.[51,87,95,149] Stillbirth is also common in untreated primary syphilis and may be preceded by hydrops fetalis.[143] The placental involvement may be part of the pathogenesis of the fetal heart failure. The placenta may be infiltrated with inflammatory cells. Perivasculitis and endarteritis may also occur.[44,57] Syphilitic placentas in general are pale, enlarged, and edematous.[44,57,95]

Maternal colonization of the urorectogenital tract with group B β-hemolytic streptococci is a condition that is potentially lethal to the fetus. In the United States three perinatal deaths per thousand are caused by this agent, and the rate has not decreased in frequency in the past 20 years.[8,126] The infection may be ascending after ruptured membranes, but in over 40 per cent of cases infection may occur through intact membranes.[8,78] The organism has been shown to cross membranes in vitro and has been found in amniotic fluid in women with intact membranes.[49,107] The organism's effect on the fetal cardiovascular system contributes to its lethal nature. When introduced into the fetal circulation, the exotoxin of group B streptococci has been shown in animal models to induce a rapid response of marked pulmonary hypertension with a large pulmonary vascular leak. An initial phase of this reaction is then followed by a period of increased pulmonary vascular permeability with pulmonary sequestration of neutrophils. Lung parenchymal and lung vascular destruction leads to shock.[8,111,125,126] The exotoxin may also initiate a prostaglandin-mediated myocardial depression.[112] Unlike most bacterial infections that ascend through the vagina, group B streptococci may lead to stillbirth without labor.

SUMMARY

Maternal diseases may affect the fetal cardiovascular system both directly and indirectly. The placenta serves as a sea wall resisting the invasion of the tides of maternal diseases. However, when a maternal disease compromises the uteroplacental unit, the fetus can only respond by redistributing its limited resources to the most vital areas. This redistribution leads to resultant intrauterine growth retardation; if uteroplacental compromise is severe enough, stillbirth can occur. If the maternal disease breaches the placental barrier, the fetal cardiovascular system may be affected directly. Agents such as immunoglobulins or viruses can cause congenital heart lesions, abnormal fetal cardiac rates, or myocardial disease. In general, if the maternal disease affecting the baby causes only uteroplacental insufficiency, the neonatal prognosis is relatively good if labor is delayed until the fetus reaches viability. However, if the maternal disease causes the fetus to be affected directly (with the exception of diabetes and thyroid disease), the effects on the fetal cardiovascular system tend to be long lasting. In diseases that affect the fetus indirectly through uteroplacental insufficiency, often the severity of the disease is directly correlated with the severity of uteroplacental insufficiency. However, in diseases in which the fetal cardiovascular system is affected directly, the mother may be asymptomatic and the fetus severely affected.

References

1. Abramowsky CR, Vegas ME, Swineheart G, et al (1980): Decidual vasculopathy of the placenta in lupus erythematosus. N Engl J Med 303:668–672.

2. Ainger LE, Lawyer NG, Fitch CW (1966): Neonatal-rubella myocarditis. Br Heart J 28:691–697.

3. Amstey MS (1985): Chickenpox and herpes zoster. In Gleicher N (ed): Principles of Medical Therapy in Pregnancy. New York, Plenum Medical Book Co, p 566.

4. Amstey MS (1985): Rubella. In Gleicher N (ed): Principles of Medical Therapy in Pregnancy. New York, Plenum Medical Book Co, p 563.

5. Anderson HM (1984): Maternal hematologic disorders. In Creasy RK, Resnick R (eds): Maternal-Fetal Medicine: Principles and Practice. Philadelphia, WB Saunders, p 795.

6. Arcilla RA, Thilenius OG, Ranniger K (1969): Congestive heart failure from suspected ductal closure in utero. J Pediatr 75:74–78.

7. Asmussen I (1982): Vascular morphology in diabetic placentas. Contrib Gynecol Obstet 7:76–85.

8. Baker CJ, Edwards MS (1983): Group B streptococcal infection. In Remington JS, Klein JO (eds): Infectious Diseases of the Fetus and Newborn Infant, 2nd ed. Philadelphia, WB Saunders, p 520.

9. Baker DA (1985): Mumps. In Gleicher N (ed): Principles of Medical Therapy in Pregnancy. New York, Plenum Medical Book Co, p 589.

10. Bose CL, Goosh WM, Sanders GO, et al (1983): Dissimilar manifestations of intrauterine infection with echo virus 11 in premature twins. Arch Pathol Lab Med 197:361.

11. Becker GJ, Ihle BU, Fairley KF, et al (1986): Effect of pregnancy on moderate renal failure in reflux nephropathy. Br Med J 292:796–798.

12. Bjøro K Jr, Myhre E (1984): The role of chronic non-specific inflammatory lesions of the placenta in intrauterine growth retardation. Acta Pathol Microbiol Immunol Scand Sect A 92:133–137.

13. Blaustein A (1977): Pathology of the Female Genital Tract. New York, Springer-Verlag, p 684.

14. Ibid, p 689.

15. Bonnar J, Sheppard BL (1977): The vascular supply of the placenta in normal and abnormal pregnancy. In Blaustein A (ed): Pathology of the Female Genital Tract. New York, Springer-Verlag, p 626.

16. Branch SW, Scott JR, Kockenour NC (1985): Obstetric complications associated with lupus anticoagulant. N Engl J Med 313:1322–1326.

17. Breitweser JA, Meyer RA, Sperling MA, et al (1980): Cardiac septal hypertrophy in hyperinsulinemic infants. J Pediatr 96:535–539.

18. Burrow GN, Ferris TF (1982): Medical Complications during Pregnancy. 2nd ed. Philadelphia, WB Saunders, p 48.

19. Burrow GN (1982): Thyroid disease. In Burrow GN, Ferris TF (eds): Medical Complications during Pregnancy. 2nd ed. Philadelphia, WB Saunders, p 196.

20. Burrow GN (1982): Thyroid disease. In Burrow GN, Ferris TF (eds): Medical Complications during Pregnancy. 2nd ed. Philadelphia, WB Saunders, p 208.

21. Caufin E, Gleicher N (1985): Metabolism during pregnancy. In Gleicher N (ed): Principles of Medical Therapy in Pregnancy. New York, Plenum Medical Book Co, p 281.

22. Check JH, Rezvani I, Goodner D, et al (1982): Prenatal treatment of thyrotoxicosis to prevent intrauterine growth retardation. Obstet Gynecol 60:122–124.

23. Chesley LC (1984): History and epidemiology of pre-eclampsia and eclampsia. Clin Obstet Gynecol 27:801–820.

24. Chesley LC (1985): Hypertensive disease in pregnancy. In Gleicher N (ed): Principles of Medical Therapy in Pregnancy. New York, Plenum Medical Book Co, p 751.

25. Costoya AL, Leontic EA, Rosenberg HG, et al (1980): Morphological study of placental terminal villi intrahepatic cholestasis of pregnancy: Histochemistry, light and electron microscopy. Placenta 1:361–368.

26. Creasy RK, Resnick R (eds) (1984): Maternal-Fetal Medicine: Principles and Practice. Philadelphia, WB Saunders.

27. Creasy RK, Resnick R (1984): Intrauterine growth retardation. In Creasy RK, Resnick R (eds): Maternal-Fetal Medicine: Principles and Practice. Philadelphia, WB Saunders, p 498.

28. Carreras LO, Defreyn G, Machin SJ, Vermylen J (1981): Arterial thrombosis, intrauterine death and lupus anticoagulant. Lancet 1:244.

29. Carreras LO, Vermylen J, Spitz B, et al (1981): Lupus anti-coagulant and inhibition of prostacyclin formation in patients with repeated abortion, intrauterine growth retardation and intra-uterine death. Br J Obstet Gynecol 88:890–894.
30. Davison JM, Lindheimer MD (1985): Pregnancy in women with chronic renal disease. In Gleicher N (ed): Principles of Medical Therapy in Pregnancy. New York, Plenum Medical Book Co, p 791.
31. Davison JM, Katz AI, Lindheimer MD (1985): Kidney disease and pregnancy: Obstetric outcome and long-term renal prognosis. Clin Perinatol 12:497–519.
32. Deppe G, Smith PE (1985): Neoplasia and pregnancy. In Gleicher N (ed): Principles of Medical Therapy in Pregnancy. New York, Plenum Medical Book Co, p 1057.
33. de Swiet M (1984): Maternal pulmonary diseases. In Creasy RK, Resnick R (eds): Maternal-Fetal Medicine: Principles and Prac-tice. Philadelphia, WB Saunders, p 786.
34. Eden RF (1985): Platelet disorders. In Gleicher N (ed): Principles of Medical Therapy in Pregnancy. New York, Plenum Medical Book Co, p 1193.
35. Felig P, Coustan D (1982): Diabetes mellitus. In Burrow GN, Ferris TF (eds): Medical Complications During Pregnancy, 2nd ed. Philadelphia, WB Saunders, p 49.
36. Fine LG, Barnett EV, Danovitch GM, et al (1981): Systemic lupus erythematosus in pregnancy. Ann Intern Med 94:667–677.
37. Fox H (1978): Pathology of the Placenta. Philadelphia, WB Saunders, p 226.
38. Ibid, p 223.
39. Ibid, p 233.
40. Ibid, p 232.
41. Ibid, p 231.
42. Ibid, p 214.
43. Ibid, p 310.
44. Ibid, p 304.
45. Trofatter KE (1985): Herpes simplex virus. In Gleicher N (ed): Principles of Medical Therapy in Pregnancy. New York, Plenum Medical Book Co, p 569.
46. Freeman RK, Garite TJ (1981): Fetal Heart Rate Monitoring. Baltimore, Williams & Wilkins, p 7.
47. Ibid, p 8.
48. Freinkel N, Dooley SL, Metzger BE (1985): Care of the pregnant woman with insulin dependent diabetes mellitus. N Engl J Med 313:96–101.
49. Galask RP, Varner MW, Petzold CR (1984): Bacterial attachment to the chorioamniotic membranes. Am J Obstet Gynecol 148:915–926.
50. Galbraith RM (1985): Liver disease: General considerations. In Gleicher N (ed): Principles of Medical Therapy in Pregnancy. New York, Plenum Medical Book Co, p 829.
51. Gileles RS, Sweet RC (1984): Maternal and fetal infections. In Creasy RK, Resnick R (eds): Maternal-Fetal Medicine: Principles and Practice. Philadelphia, WB Saunders, p 603.
52. Glass RH (1984): Sperm and egg transport, fertilization, and implan-tation. In Creasy RK, Resnick R (eds): Maternal-Fetal Medicine: Principles and Practice. Philadelphia, WB Saunders, pp 115–122.
53. Gleicher N (1985): Principles of Medical Therapy in Pregnancy. New York, Plenum Medical Book Co.
54. Greenberger PA (1985): Asthma in pregnancy. Clin Perinatol 12:571–584.
55. Gutgesell HP, Speer ME, Rosenberg HS (1980): Characterization of the cardiomyopathy in infants of diabetic mothers. Circulation 61:441–450.
56. Gutgesell HP, Mullins CE, Gillette PC (1976): Transient hyper-trophic subaortic stenosis in infants of diabetic mothers. J Perinatol 89:120–125.
57. Manif GRG (1974): Infectious Diseases in Obstetrics and Gynecology. Hagerstown, MD, Harper & Row, p 182.
58. Hall CB, Miller DG (1969): Detection of a silent Coxsackie B-5 virus perinatal infection. J Pediatr 75:124–127.
59. Hou SH, Grossman SD, Madias NE (1985): Pregnancy in women with renal disease and moderate renal insufficiency. Am J Med 78:185–194.
60. Hayslett JP, Reece EA (1985): Systemic lupus erythematosus in pregnancy. Clin Perinatol 12:539–550.
61. Heymann MA (1984): Fetal cardiovascular physiology. In Creasy RK, Resnick R (eds): Maternal-Fetal Medicine: Principles and Practice. Philadelphia, WB Saunders, p 263.
62. Lubbe WF, Liggins GC (1985): Lupus anticoagulant and preg-nancy. Am J Obstet Gynecol 153:322–327.
63. Holzgreve W, Curry CJR, Golbus MS, et al (1984): Investigation of nonimmune hydrops fetalis. Am J Obstet Gynecol 150:805–812.
64. Houtsman DM (1982): Viral infections. In Burrow GN, Ferris TF (eds): Medical Complications during Pregnancy. 2nd ed. Philadelphia, WB Saunders, p 333.
65. Huffman PC (1985): ITP in pregnancy. Clin Perinatol 12:599.
66. Hurwitz D, Irving FC (1937): Diabetes and pregnancy. Am J Med Sci 194:85–92.
67. Hutchison AA, Drew JH, Yu VYH, et al (1982): Nonimmunologic hydrops fetalis: A review of 61 cases. Obstet Gynecol 59:347–352.
68. Javett SN, Heymann S, Mundel B, et al (1956): Myocarditis in the newborn infant; a study of an outbreak associated with Coxsackie group B virus infection in a maternity home in Johannesburg. J Pediatr 48:1–22.
69. Jennings RC (1966): Coxsackie Group B fatal neonatal myocar-ditis associated with cardiomegaly. J Clin Pathol 19:325–327.
70. Johnston WG, Baskett TF (1979): Obstetric cholestasis: A 14 year review. Am J Obstet Gynecol 133:299–301.
71. Jones P, McNay A, Walker W (1969): Association between foeto-maternal bleeding and hypertension in pregnancy. Br Med J 3:738.
72. Jouppila P, Kirkinen P (1986): Blood velocity waveforms of the fetal aorta in normal and hypertensive pregnancies. Obstet Gynecol 67:856–860.
73. Jungers P, Forget D, Henry-Amor M (1986): Chronic kidney dis-ease and pregnancy. In Grunfeld P, Maxwell MH (eds): Advances in Nephrology. Vol 15. Chicago, Year Book Medical Publishers, Inc, p 103.
74. Kalhan SC, Heed RH (1985): Diabetics in pregnancy. In Gleicher N (ed): Principles of Medical Therapy in Pregnancy. New York, Plenum Medical Book Co, p 251.
75. Kaplan MM (1985): Thyroid disease in pregnancy. In Gleicher N (ed): Principles of Medical Therapy in Pregnancy. New York, Plenum Medical Book Co, p 204.
76. Katz AL, Davison JM, Hayslett JP, et al (1980): Pregnancy in women with kidney disease. Kidney Int 18:192–206.
77. Katz VL (1985): Unpublished observations.
78. Katz VL, Bowes WAB Jr: Perinatal GBS infections across intact amniotic membranes. J Reprod Med (in press).
79. Katz VL, Weinstein L (1982): Antepartum treatment of Listeria monocytogenes septicemia. South Med J 75:1353–1354.
80. Kelton JG (1983): Management of the pregnant patient with idiopathic thrombocytopenic purpura. Ann Intern Med 99:796–800.
81. Kibrick S, Benirschke K (1954): Acute aseptic myocarditis in the newborn child infected with Coxsackie virus group B type 3. N Engl J Med 233:883.
82. Killam AP (1985): Tobacco smoking. In Gleicher N (ed): Prin-ciples of Medical Therapy in Pregnancy. New York, Plenum Medical Book Co, p 115.
83. Latham PS (1985): Liver diseases of pregnancy. In Gleicher N (ed): Principles of Medical Therapy in Pregnancy. New York, Plenum Medical Book Co, p 832.
84. Lee LA, Bias WB, Arnett FC, et al (1983): Immunogenetics of the neonatal lupus syndrome. Ann Intern Med 99:592–596.
85. Lebrman SN (1985): Common viral respiratory illnesses. In Gleicher N (ed): Principles of Medical Therapy in Pregnancy. New York, Plenum Medical Book Co, p 547.
86. Lebrman SN (1985): Influenza. In Gleicher N (ed): Principles of Medical Therapy in Pregnancy. New York, Plenum Medical Book Co, p 556.
87. Lee RN (1982): Sexually transmitted diseases. In Burrow GN, Ferris TF (eds): Medical Complications during Pregnancy. 2nd ed. Philadelphia, WB Saunders, p 351.
88. Lee RV (1982): Parasitic infections. In Burrow GN, Ferris TF (eds): Medical Complications during Pregnancy. 2nd ed. Philadelphia, WB Saunders, p 387.

89. Lee RV (1985): Protozoan infections in pregnancy. In Gleicher N (ed): Principles of Medical Therapy in Pregnancy. New York, Plenum Medical Book Co.

90. Lenke RR (1985): Maternal hyperphenylalinemia. In Gleicher N (ed): Principles of Medical Therapy in Pregnancy. New York, Plenum Medical Book Co, p 286.

91. Lenke RR, Levy HL (1980): Maternal phenoketonuria and hyperphenylalaninemia. N Engl J Med 303:1202–1208.

92. Leslie J, Shen SC, Strauss L (1982): Hypertrophic cardiomyopathy in a midtrimester fetus born to a diabetic mother. J Pediatr 100:631–632.

93. Litsey SE, Noonan JA, O'Connor WN, et al (1984): Maternal connective tissues disease and congenital heart block. N Engl J Med 312:98–100.

94. Lichtig C, Deutch M, Brandes J (1984): Vascular changes of endometrium in early pregnancy. Am J Clin Pathol 81:702.

95. Livengaad CH (1985): Syphilis. In Gleicher N (ed): Principles of Medical Therapy in Pregnancy. New York, Plenum Medical Book Co, p 504.

96. Lotgering FK, Gilbert RD, Longo LD (1985): Maternal and fetal responses to exercise during pregnancy. Phys Rev 65:1–36.

97. Lubbe WF, Butler WS, Palmare SJ, Liggins GC (1984): Lupus anticoagulant in pregnancy. Br J Obstet Gynaecol 91:357–363.

98. Morrison JC, Harris JB (1985): Disorders of structure and function of hemoglobin synthesis. In Gleicher N (ed): Principles of Medical Therapy in Pregnancy. New York, Plenum Medical Book Co, p 1186.

99. Martin JN, Morrison JC, Files JC (1984): Autoimmune thrombocytopenic purpura: Current concepts and recommended practices. Am J Obstet Gynecol 150:86–96.

100. Mathias CG (1984): Skin and pregnancy. In Creasy RK, Resnick R (eds): Maternal-Fetal Medicine: Principles and Practice. Philadelphia, WB Saunders, p 1058.

101. McAnulty JA, Metcalfe J, Leland K (1982): Cardiovascular disease. In Burrow GN, Ferris TF (eds): Medical Complications during Pregnancy. 2nd ed. Philadelphia, WB Saunders, p 145.

102. McLaughlin BN, Martin RW, Morrison JC (1985): Clinical management of sickle cell hemoglobinopathies during pregnancy. Clin Perinatol 12:585–597.

103. Meeks GR, Goakin KS, Marrison JC (1985): Iron deficiency anemia. In Gleicher N (ed): Principles of Medical Therapy in Pregnancy. New York, Plenum Medical Book Co, p 1177.

104. Mennuti MT (1985): Teratology and genetic counseling in the diabetic pregnancy. Clin Obstet Gynecol 28:486–495.

105. Miller E, Hare JW, Cloherty JP (1981): Elevated maternal hemoglobin A1c in early pregnancy and major congenital anomalies in infants of diabetic mothers. N Engl J Med 304:1331–1334.

106. Miller JM, Horger EO, Key TC (1981): Management of sickle hemoglobinopathies in pregnant patients. Am J Obstet Gynecol 141:237–241.

107. Miller JM, Pupkin MJ, Hill GB (1980): Bacterial colonization of amniotic fluid from intact fetal membranes. Am J Obstet Gynecol 136:796–804.

108. Milner PF, Jones BR, Döbler J (1980): Outcome of pregnancy in sickle cell anemia and sickle cell hemoglobin c disease. Am J Obstet Gynecol 138:239–245.

109. Naeye R (1978): Cause and consequences of placental gravata retardation. J Am Med Assoc 239:1145–1147.

110. Novak ER, Woodruff JD (1979): Gynecologic and Obstetric Pathology. 8th ed. Philadelphia, WB Saunders.

111. O'Brien WF, Golden SM, Bibro MC et al (1985): Short-term responses in neonatal lambs after infusion of Group B streptococca extract. Obstet Gynecol 65:802–806.

112. Peevy KJ, Chartrand SA, Wiseman HJ et al (1985): Myocardial dysfunction in Group B streptococcal shock. Pediatr Res 19:511–513.

113. Perkins RP (1971): Hydrops fetalis and stillbirth in a male with glucose-6-phosphate dehydrogenase-deficient fetus possibly due to maternal ingestion of sulfisoxazole: A case report. Am J Obstet Gynecol 111:379–381.

114. Perloff JK (1985): Congenital heart disease and pregnancy. In Gleicher N (ed): Principles of Medical Therapy in Pregnancy. New York, Plenum Medical Book Co, p 668.

115. Placin PF, Chatellier C, Breant C et al (1986): Frequent perinatal consequences of hypertensive disease of pregnancy. Advances Nephrol 15:57.

116. Pritchard JA, MacDonald PC, Gant NF (1985): Williams Obstetrics. 17th ed. Norwalk, CT, Appleton-Century-Crofts.

117. Ibid, p 371.

118. Ibid, p 533.

119. Ibid, p 108.

120. Ibid, p 181.

121. Ibid, p 150.

122. Ibid, p 539.

123. Queenan JT (1980): Intrauterine growth retardation. In Queenan JT (ed.): Management of High Risk Pregnancy. Oradell, NJ, Medical Economics Book Co, p 459.

124. Roberts JM (1984): Pregnancy related hypertension. In Creasy RK, Resnick R (eds): Maternal-Fetal Medicine: Principles and Practice. Philadelphia, WB Saunders, p 703.

125. Rojas J, Green RS, Hellerqvist CG et al (1981): Studies on Group B beta-hemolytic streptococcus. II. Effects on pulmonary hemodynamics and vascular permeability in unanesthetized sheep. Pediatr Res 15:899–904.

126. Rojas J, Stahlman M (1984): Effects of group B streptococcus and other organisms on the pulmonary vasculature. Clin Perinatol 11:591–599.

127. Rowe RD, Freedom RM, Mehviz A (1982): The Neonate with Congenital Heart Disease. Philadelphia, WB Saunders, p 116.

128. Ibid, p 117.

129. Rowe RO, Izukawa T, Mulholland HC et al (1978): Nonstructural heart disease in the newborn: Observations during one year in a perinatal service. Arch Dis Child 53:726–730.

130. Schenker JG, Granat M (1982): Phaeochromocytoma and pregnancy—an updated appraisal. Austr NZ J Obstet Gynecol 22:1–10.

131. Schneider JM, Curet LB (1983): Obstetrical management of the pregnant diabetic. In Sciarra JJ (ed): Gynecology and Obstetrics. Vol 3. New York, Harper & Row.

132. Scott JS (1985): Connective tissue disease antibodies and pregnancy. In Gleicher N (ed): Principles of Medical Therapy in Pregnancy. New York, Plenum Medical Book Co, p 994.

133. Scott JS, Maddison PJ, Taylore PV, et al (1983): Connective tissue disease, antibodies to ribonucleoprotein, and congenital heart block. N Engl J Med 309:209–212.

134. Seeds JW (1984): Impaired fetal growth: Definitions and clinical diagnosis. Obstet Gynecol 64:303–310.

135. Seeds JW (1984): Impaired fetal growth: Ultrasound evaluation and clinical management. Obstet Gynecol 64:577–584.

136. Seeds JW, Cefalo RC (1986): Practical Obstetrical Ultrasound. Rockville, MD, Aspen Publishing Co, p 73.

137. Shaw D, Frohlich J, Wittmann BA, et al (1982): A prospective study of 18 patients with cholestasis of pregnancy. Am J Obstet Gynecol 142:621–625.

138. Stagno S, Whitley RJ (1985): Herpes virus infections of pregnancy. Pt. I: Cytomegalovirus and Epstein-Barr virus infections. N Engl J Med 313:1270–1274.

139. Surainder SY, Bellur B, Choudhry A, et al (1981): Isoimmune thrombocytopenia: Coordinated management of mother and infant. Obstet Gynecol 57:124.

140. Susa JB, Schwartz R (1985): Effects of hyperinsulinemia in the primate fetus. Diabetes 34: Suppl. 2:36–41.

141. Tonge HM, Wladimiroff JW, Noordam J, et al (1986): Blood flow velocity waveforms in the descending fetal aorta: Comparison between normal and growth-retarded pregnancies. Obstet Gynecol 56:851–855.

142. Trofatter KF (1985): CMV infection. In Gleicher N (ed): Principles of Medical Therapy in Pregnancy. New York, Plenum Medical Book Co, p 575.

143. Turkel SB (1982): Conditions associated with nonimmune hydrops fetalis. Clin Perinatol 9:613–625.

145. Ueland K (1984): Cardiac disease. In Creasy RK, Resnick R (eds): Maternal-Fetal Medicine: Principles and Practice. Philadelphia, WB Saunders, p 691.

146. Ueland K (1985): Rheumatic heart disease. In Gleicher N (ed): Principles of Medical Therapy in Pregnancy. New York, Plenum Medical Book Co, p 660.

147. Ueland K (1980): The pregnant cardiac patient in management of

high risk pregnancy. In Queenan JT (ed): Management of High Risk Pregnancy. Oradell, NJ, Medical Economics Book Co, p 225.

148. Vermesh M, Gleicher N (1985): Disorders of amino acid metabolism. In Gleicher N (ed): Principles of Medical Therapy in Pregnancy. New York, Plenum Medical Book Co, p 283.

149. Wagner HR (1981): Cardiac disease in congenital infections. Clin Perinatol 8:481–497.

150. DeWolf F, Carreras LO, Moerman P, et al (1982): Decidual vasculopathy and extensive placental infarction in a patient with repeated thromboembolic accidents, recurrent fetal loss, and a lupus anticoagulant. Am J Obstet Gynecol 142:829–834.

151. Wands JR (1979): Viral hepatitis and its effects on pregnancy. Clin Obstet Gynecol 22:301–311.

152. Way GL, Wolfe RR, Eshaghpour E, et al (1979): The natural history of hypertrophic cardiomyopathy in infants of diabetic mothers. J Pediatr 95:1020–1025.

153. Weinberger SE, Weiss ST (1982): Pulmonary diseases. In Burrow GN, Ferris TF (eds): Medical Complications during Pregnancy. 2nd ed. Philadelphia, WB Saunders, p 405.

154. Weinstein A, Parke AL (1985): Pregnancy and the rheumatic diseases: The connective tissue diseases. In Gleicher N (ed): Principles of Medical Therapy in Pregnancy. New York, Plenum Medical Book Co, p 1013.

155. Wilson AF (1985): Pulmonary physiology and pulmonary disorders in pregnancy. In Gleicher N (ed): Principles of Medical Therapy in Pregnancy. New York, Plenum Medical Book Co, p 739.

156. Wilson BR, Haverkamp HD (1979): Cholestatic jaundice of pregnancy: New perspectives. Obstet Gynecol 54:650–652.

157. Yip DM, Baker AL (1985): Liver diseases in pregnancy. Clin Perinatol 12:683–694.

158. Zervoudakis IA, Cederqvist LL (1972): Effect of *Listeria monocytogenes* septicemia during pregnancy on the offspring. Am J Obstet Gynecol 129:465–467.

159. Zuspan FP (1984): Chronic hypertension in pregnancy. Clin Obstet Gynecol 27:854–873.

12 MATERNAL THERAPY AFFECTING THE FETAL CARDIOVASCULAR SYSTEM

Vern L. Katz

Watson A. Bowes, Jr.

Both prescribed and illicit drugs may affect the fetal cardiovascular system. Some drugs, such as nicotine and digitalis, may directly alter fetal cardiac function. Others, like furosemide, may affect the fetal cardiovascular system in an indirect fashion by affecting uteroplacental function. This chapter will review both direct and indirect responses of the fetal cardiovascular system to drugs. For indepth reviews of fetal-maternal drug interactions, the reader is directed to the detailed reviews of medications in pregnancy listed in the bibliography.[7,95] Because new drugs are continually being developed and new experiences with these agents are continually being reported, this chapter can only serve as a guide and an outline. Specific teratogenic effects leading to structural changes in the heart are covered in Chapter 49. The reader is also directed to Chapter 16, which describes the in utero pharmacologic therapy of fetal cardiac arrhythmias. In this chapter, drugs and medications are discussed by therapeutic classification, i.e., antimicrobial agents, anti-inflammatory agents, and so on. Often, drugs are used for more than one indication; in such instances, this chapter will consider the drug under its most common usage during pregnancy. Drugs will be referred to by their generic nomenclature.

FETAL CARDIAC RESPONSES

The fetal cardiac response to maternal drugs may be direct or indirect. Direct responses are caused by specific pharmacologic effects on the fetal cardiovascular system. The tachycardia caused by the drug terbutaline, used for tocolysis, is an example of a direct effect. The fetal cardiovascular system is under central (CNS), sympathetic, and parasympathetic neural control. Agents such as narcotics, which depress both central and sympathetic fetal cardiovascular control, will decrease short-term beat-to-beat fetal heart rate variability. The sinus arrhythmia known as fetal heart rate variability (discussed in Chapter 13) is extremely important for the evaluation of fetuses in utero. Variability in fetal heart rates may be both short-term or beat-to-beat (defined as rate changes from second to second) and long-term (defined as changes in rate over 20 to 30 seconds to a few minutes). The acceleration in heart rate with fetal movement is an established measure of fetal well-being. The fetal heart rate response to contractions during labor is often mediated by the parasympathetic nervous sys-

tem. Drugs that are vagolytic may abolish the normal fetal cardiac responses during labor.

Indirect responses of the fetal cardiovascular system to maternal drug therapy include the redistribution of blood flow away from the extremities and viscera to the heart, brain, and adrenals, usually in response to placental hypoxia and/or nutritional deprivation. Such deprivation, known as uteroplacental insufficiency, may be caused by a variety of problems, including abnormalities in the umbilical circulation, such as a knot in the cord; problems in the placenta leading to fibrosis and poor oxygen exchange; separation of the placenta from the uterine wall (abruptio placentae); and problems involving poor uterine blood flow either from spasm in the uterine vessels or relative hypovolemia in the mother. Maternal drugs may create and affect many of these problems. Cardiac responses to acute uteroplacental insufficiency include fetal bradycardia, fetal tachycardia, or, during labor, late decelerations in response to contractions. Chronic uteroplacental insufficiency is often manifested by reductions in amniotic fluid volume (a sign of decreased blood flow to the fetal kidneys) as well as intrauterine growth retardation (a sign of decreased blood flow to the fetal liver and extremities).

ANTIMICROBIAL AGENTS

The antimicrobial agents have been fairly well studied in pregnancy. With but a few exceptions, these drugs do not seem to have an effect on the fetal cardiovascular system.[38,55] Of the commonly used agents, the penicillins, cephalosporins, aminoglycosides, clindamycin, and erythromycin (the nonestolate preparations) are safe. Tetracyclines are rarely used during pregnancy because of noncardiac toxicity. Sulfonamides may be prescribed but are usually not used in the late third trimester because of potential bilirubin displacement. Sulfonamides may cause hemolytic anemia in infants with a G6PD deficiency.[115] Because of theoretic teratogenic risks, metronidazole is rarely used during the first trimester; however, it does not affect the cardiovascular system. The nitrofurantoins have been linked in rare cases to hemolysis in G6PD deficient infants;[115] however, nitrofurantoin is used frequently for treatment of urinary tract infections. Chloramphenicol is associated with gray baby syndrome, manifested by palid cyanosis, vascular collapse, and death. This syndrome was described in preterm infants treated with chloramphenicol postnatally who were incapable of metabolizing and excreting the drug. Gray baby syndrome has not been reported in infants or fetuses born to mothers who received chloramphenicol. Nevertheless, chloramphenicol is rarely used in the United States, especially in the third trimester.[10,38,55,124]

Isoniazid has no fetal cardiotoxicity and may be used in pregnancy with pyridoxine supplementation.[55] Topical antifungal agents have no fetal cardiovascular effects. The systemic antifungal agent ketoconazole is not known to have fetal cardiovascular effects.[38] Amphotericin has not been known to have fetal cardiovascular effects, either.[61,120]

Acyclovir has not been shown to be embryotoxic in animals and does not appear to have fetal cardiotoxic effects. However, acyclovir is incompletely studied at this time.[38,114]

Of the antiparasitic agents, chloroquine and quinine may be used with caution. Neither of these drugs seems to have fetal cardiovascular toxicity. Pyrimethamine and primaquine are contraindicated in pregnancy.[61] Metronidazole, as mentioned above, does not appear to have fetal cardiotoxic effects but is not used in the first trimester.

ANTI-INFLAMMATORY AGENTS

Corticosteroids have been well evaluated in pregnancy. They are used both chronically in varying doses as anti-inflammatory agents and acutely in bolus form to induce fetal lung maturation. The fetal cardiovascular system seems unaffected either directly or indirectly by glucocorticoids.[73,125] In mothers receiving large doses, babies may theoretically be born with suppressed adrenal glands and need tapering doses of steroids.[7] Azathioprine does not have fetal cardiotoxic effects.[73,91,121]

The nonsteroidal anti-inflammatory agents include the large group of prostaglandin synthetase inhibitors, such as indomethacin, ibuprofen, and naproxen. This group of drugs is discussed under the section Tocolytics. Acetaminophen does not affect the fetal cardiovascular system and is considered safe in pregnancy.[8] Acetylsalicylic acid (aspirin) is one of the most frequently used medications in pregnancy. The deleterious effects of aspirin on the fetus are based primarily to its effect on clotting. Increased clotting times, increased incidence of intraventricular hemorrhage in premature infants, cephalohematomas, and a higher stillbirth incidence in an Australian study have all been related to maternal aspirin ingestion. Hemostatic effects appear to be dose related.[9,103,110] Maternal aspirin therapy can also cause fetal ductal constriction (see the following section). Large amounts and chronic use of aspirin are thus contraindicated in pregnancy.

ANTICOAGULANTS

Heparin does not cross the placenta and thus does not affect the fetal cardiovascular system directly. Heparin has no indirect cardiovascular effects, either.[11] Sodium warfarin (Coumadin) and related drugs do cross the placenta. During the first trimester, these drugs are associated with the fetal warfarin syndrome—a multiple embryopathy that can affect the heart (Chapter 49); use during the second and third trimesters has led to central nervous system abnormalities as well as severe fetal and neonatal hemorrhage and stillbirth.[12,58] Coumadin is contraindicated in pregnancy.

ANESTHETICS

All *inhalation agents*, if given in large enough concentrations, can lead to maternal cardiac depression, which may cause indirect but potentially lethal fetal compromise.[71] In the usual concentrations, NO_2 is unlikely to affect the fetal cardiovascular system; NO_2 does not seem to decrease uterine blood flow or affect fetal heart rate.[40] During administration in routine concentrations, methoxyflurane, isoflurane, enflurane, and halothane do not usually affect the fetal cardiovascular system.[40,105] In studies of the effect of halogenated agents upon fetal sheep, large anesthetic concentrations caused mild decreases in fetal blood pressure and decreases in fetal cardiac index.[101] Inhalation agents cause a potentially beneficial decrease in circulating maternal catecholamines, which can increase uterine blood flow and improve fetal oxygenation.[105]

The local anesthetics, used in spinal, epidural, paracervical, and pudendal injections as well as in perineal analgesia, are subdivided into the esters and the amides. Both readily cross the placenta.[71] These agents affect the fetal cardiovascular system not only directly but also indirectly. The esters, chloroprocaine being the most popular in obstetrics, are rapidly metabolized.[71] The amides have longer half-lives but longer time for onset of action. Bupivacaine and lidocaine are the most popular amide local anesthetics.[71,106] The local anesthetics are weak acids and are not ionized in the maternal circulation. Local anesthetics readily cross the placenta and may become ionized in the more acidic fetal circulation, especially during labor. Once ionized, local anesthetics remain trapped in the fetal circulation, and large concentrations may accumulate. Amide local anesthetics are metabolized in the liver and accumulate more readily than esters (since fetal metabolism is immature), thus predisposing to fetal cardiac toxicity.[71,75,92] Local anesthetics had few direct fetal cardiovascular effects in acidotic, nonlaboring fetal lambs.[53] Increased cerebral blood flow and tachycardia were seen in acidotic, nonlaboring sheep.[53] In women in labor, direct fetal effects of local anesthetics include decreased heart rate variability (both short term and long term), bradycardia, fetal acidosis, and stillbirth.[72,92,105,106] Similarly, the indirect effects of local anesthetics on the fetal cardiovascular system include decreased beat-to-beat fetal heart rate variability, bradycardia, acidosis, and stillbirth.[71,75,92,94] Thus, it is often difficult to ascertain which is a direct effect from the local anesthetic and which is an indirect effect.

Local anesthetics may affect the fetus indirectly through three mechanisms. Peripherally, local anesthetics may lead to a relative maternal sympathetic blockade, thereby causing vasodilation, maternal hypotension, and uterine hypoperfusion.[105,106,122] Such maternal sympathetic blockade may also lead to uterine hyperstimulation, thereby causing uteroplacental insufficiency and fetal cardiovascular distress; when uterine tone is greater than 20 mmHg, uteroplacental blood flow is effectively stopped.[45,92,94] One of the most devastating potential effects of local anesthetics is uterine vascular spasm, which can lead to acute and profound fetal bradycardia.[71,92,94,106] Uterine hyperstimulation and uterine vascular spasm only occur with high maternal blood levels of the local anesthetics. Serious adverse effects are seen more commonly with the amide agents because of the rapid metabolism of the ester type local anesthetics.[72]

Bupivacaine, in the concentration of 0.75 per cent, causes maternal cardiovascular toxicity and has been removed from obstetric use.[76] When spinal or epidural anesthesia causes hypotension, the most commonly used medication to reverse the hypotension is ephedrine. In this setting, ephedrine has been noted to increase fetal heart rate and increase beat-to-beat variability.[123]

Paracervical injections, currently out of vogue in obstetrics, were quite common during the past 2 decades. More recently, paracervical injections have fallen into disuse because of significant fetal cardiac effects. Paracervical injections produced decreased fetal heart rate variability, bradycardia, acidosis, and occasionally intrauterine demise due to their anesthetic effects. The fetal bradycardia ensued approximately 2 minutes after paracervical injection and lasted for up to 30 minutes with lidocaine and up to 2 hours with bupivacaine.[71,92,94,106] The fetal cardiovascular changes from paracervical injections were postulated to be caused by the passage of the local anesthetic into the uterine arteries and then into the placental and fetal circulations. Uterine artery spasm and umbilical artery spasm were the result of high uterine levels of the local anesthetics. Fetal cardiac effects were so frequent (25 to 35 per cent of the time) that paracervical local anesthetic injections have largely given way to other forms of obstetric analgesia.[71,92,94,106,118]

TOCOLYTIC AGENTS

Prematurity is the most frequent cause of neonatal mortality. Mechanisms responsible for and agents designed to stop preterm labor are well studied. Modern agents, though, have profound effects on the fetal heart. Uterine contractility is controlled in part by the release of calcium ions from the sarcoplasmic reticulum of the myometrial cells. Calcium activates the actin-myosin filaments through phosphorylation of a myosin light chain kinase. Intracellular calcium may be regulated by several factors, including prostaglandins and oxytocin. The myosin kinase is also regulated by cyclic AMP levels, which are under β_2-adrenergic control. Thus, several pharmacologic approaches may be used to decrease contractility.[63] Almost all pharmacologic approaches not only affect contractions but also affect the fetal cardiovascular system.

Calcium Channel Blockers

Tocolytic therapy with calcium channel blockers is largely experimental in the United States. Three agents that have been studied include nocardipine, nifedipine, and verapamil. Calcium channel blockers decrease uterine contractility by inhibiting the influx of calcium ions through cell membranes, thus decreasing intracellular calcium and decreasing myosin activation.[50] Although tocolytic therapy with calcium channel blockers is currently only investigational, preliminary reports have shown few fetal cardiovascular effects in animals at doses sufficient to stop labor. An early report on treatment of premature labor with nifedipine found no fetal heart changes during drug therapy, which successfully stopped labor.[116] In animal studies, nifedipine caused no significant changes in uterine blood flow in the pregnant pygmy goat.[119] In pregnant ewes, nifedipine tocolysis led to a significant increase in fetal heart rate.[57] In a study of pregnant rhesus monkeys, fetal acidosis was reported with tocolytic doses of nifedipine.[13] Mean fetal arterial pressure declined slightly also. When used to treat hypertension in pregnancy, calcium channel blockers have not been found to have significant fetal cardiovascular effects.[13,49] Verapamil crosses the placenta but not freely. However, nifedipine and nocardipine are thought to cross the placenta easily. With the use of these agents for maternal arrhythmias, no fetal cardiovascular effects have been seen.

Nonsteroidal Anti-Inflammatory Agents

Nonsteroidal anti-inflammatory agents (NSAI) decrease uterine contractions by inhibiting prostaglandin synthetase, which reduces prostaglandin-mediated calcium influx into the cells.[87] Indomethacin is the NSAI agent most frequently used for tocolysis. An important complication of maternal indomethacin and other nonsteroidal therapy is premature closure of the ductus arteriosus; patency of the fetal ductus is prostaglandin-dependent.[33,87] Fetal ductal closure may be partial or total. When the ductus closes in utero, cardiomegaly, right heart failure, pulmonary hypertension, edema, and hydrops fetalis ensue. Case reports have been published documenting premature closure of the ductus in utero with hydrops fetalis and intrauterine cardiac failure.[15] Dudley and Hardie reviewed 167 patients receiving indomethacin therapy and found no fetal cardiovascular side effects.[46] Neibyl reported on another 46 infants and found no abnormal fetal cardiovascular effects.[87] However, animal studies have shown indomethacin to have mild to severe effects on the fetal ductus and the fetal vasculature.[102] The consensus in the U.S. literature at this time is that NSAIs have the greatest effect on the fetal ductus after 34 weeks' gestation and that the ductal effects are dose dependent.[33,46,87,88] Since tocolysis is rarely initiated beyond 33 weeks' gestation, premature closure of the ductus does not tend to be a complication of tocolytic therapy. Studies to evaluate the effects of indomethacin in utero on the fetal vascular system are ongoing. Neonatal effects from maternal non-steroidal anti-inflammatory use are discussed in detail in Chapter 51. Obviously, inadvertent use of NSAI agents late in pregnancy may be catastrophic. These agents are now sold as over-the-counter preparations and can be expected to cause increasing perinatal problems, since their hazards are not yet well recognized.

β_2-Adrenergic Agonists

The most commonly used tocolytic medications in the United States are the beta sympathicomimetic agents. Currently, intravenous ritodrine is the most popular form of tocolytic therapy. Alternatively, some medical centers use intravenous terbutaline. Isoxsuprine had been used in the late 1970s and early 1980s but is not used currently. After premature labor has been stopped, mothers are often given oral ritodrine or terbutaline for a period of 4 to 6 weeks. Europeans have used fenoterol and salbutamol (albuterol) since the mid-1970s for tocolysis. Myometrial cells have β_2-adrenergic receptors, activation of which inhibits intracellular calcium release[63,95] by increasing intracellular levels of cyclic AMP.

The most common fetal cardiovascular effects of beta sympathicomimetics are direct. β_2-mimetics pass into the fetal circulation, and tachycardia and tachyarrhythmias are the most frequent fetal affects. Although ritodrine, terbutaline, and fenoterol are primarily β_2-agents, they also have crossover effects on cardiac β_1-receptors.[95] Indirect fetal effects due to maternal cardiovascular changes from beta sympathicomimetic therapy are caused by an increased systolic and decreased diastolic maternal blood pressure.[95] Some mothers have experienced EKG changes, ischemia, and myocardial infarction during tocolytic therapy with beta mimetics.[5] These effects tend to be dose related, and clinicians currently discontinue beta sympathicomimetic therapy when any maternal cardiovascular signs or symptoms appear. Guinea pigs given ritodrine may have a decrease in uteroplacental blood flow.[117] However, other animal studies have shown ritodrine to have little or no effect on uteroplacental flow.[95] Further, Doppler ultrasonographic studies in normotensive women between 31 and 36 weeks' gestation have found no evidence of changes in fetal umbilical blood flow after maternal ritodrine administration.[65]

The beta sympathicomimetics cross the placenta and do cause tachycardia in the fetus. If drug levels are present at birth, the incidences of hypotension and respiratory distress may be increased.[34,97,111] Thus, if labor progresses despite the use of beta sympathicomimetic tocolytic therapy, the drug should be stopped.

Large numbers of infants have been treated with beta mimetics without apparent problems. However, over the past 15 years investigators have noted permanent deleterious effects on the fetal heart from beta mimetic use. Just as cardiac changes of ischemia and infarction can occur in the mother, such changes have been documented in fetuses of mothers receiving beta mimetics. Focal subendocardial necrosis, fatty degeneration in myocardial cells, and nuclear polyploidization of subendocardial areas were found in a study of 28 newborns whose mothers had been treated with beta mimetics and who died of noncardiac causes.[32] Another study found parenchymal necrosis in the hearts of 21 newborns born after maternal beta sympathicomimetic therapy. Using M-mode ultrasonography, Nuchpuckdee et al found significantly greater interventricular septal hypertrophy in infants exposed to ritodrine compared with control infants delivered at the same gestational age.[89] From these studies, and several case reports in the literature, it is clear that beta mimetics may have long-lasting effects upon the fetal heart. These effects are thought to be due to increased calcium in the myocardial cells. The myocardial damage is similar to the adrenergic cardiomyopathy of pheochromocytoma. Although long-term follow-up studies have demonstrated that beta mimetics may be used safely in the great majority of fetuses,[97] benefits should clearly outweigh the potential risks before these drugs are used.

Magnesium Sulfate

The use of magnesium sulfate as a tocolytic agent is increasing in popularity throughout the United States. $MgSO_4$ crosses the placenta freely to the infant. Direct fetal cardiac effects of $MgSO_4$ include decreases, increases, and no change in heart rate variability;[92–94,97,108] indirect effects do not appear to occur. Magnesium sulfate does not seem to affect uterine blood flow. Indeed, animal studies suggest an increase in uterine blood flow with magnesium sulfate use.[3,93,113] However, maternal serum magnesium levels greater than 15 mg/dl are associated with respiratory depression, and higher levels may cause cardiac dysfunction and arrest. Maternal hypothermia and decreased maternal serum calcium levels are important side effects of $MgSO_4$ therapy.[93] Hypertensive patients are often treated with magnesium sulfate to prevent seizures during labor. Hemodynamic studies in these patients suggest that $MgSO_4$ transiently decreases peripheral resistance; pressures return to baseline levels within 1 hour of initiation of magnesium administration.[42] Overall, magnesium sulfate seems much safer than beta mimetic agents for the fetus. However, postnatal respiratory depression and lethargy are observed with high fetal levels of $MgSO_4$. Serum calcium levels appear to be lower in infants of mothers treated with magnesium sulfate compared with those of control infants but remain within normal limits.[43] In another study, fetal calcium levels after maternal $MgSO_4$ administration were the same as those of control infants.[83]

OXYTOTIC DRUGS

Two types of drugs are used to stimulate labor in the United States: oxytocin and prostaglandins. Oxytocin, the posterior pituitary hormone, does not cross the placenta and thus has no direct fetal effects. However, large doses of oxytocin may lead to uterine hyperstimulation, which may in turn cause uteroplacental insufficiency and indirect fetal cardiovascular effects.[97] Late decelerations, fetal tachycardia, and fetal bradycardia may result from uterine hyperstimulation with oxytocin.

The main prostaglandins used to stimulate labor are PGF_2 and PGE_2. These agents are currently not approved by the FDA for induction of labor in term pregnancies.[97] Little is known about their fetal effects. Although PGE suppositories are often used to cause cervical changes prior to delivery and can cause uterine hyperstimulation, direct fetal effects have not been noted.[97]

Maternal hypotension may occur during the use of prostaglandin agents; therefore, in volume-depleted or intravascularly depleted women, caution must be used. Maternal hyperthermia may also be caused by prostaglandins, and fetal tachycardia can result.[97]

Ergot alkaloids are used postpartum to constrict uterine arteries and increase uterine contractility. Ergot alkaloids are powerful agents that cause sustained uterine contractions and are therefore contraindicated during pregnancy; their use can produce fetal anoxia.

NARCOTICS AND BARBITURATES

Both prescribed and illicit narcotics cross the placenta and depress the fetal central nervous system; as a result, beat-to-beat heart rate variability is decreased.[71] Meperidine is used quite often during labor, and in the United States it may be the most commonly used medication for relief of labor pain. Meperidine crosses freely into the fetal circulation.[16] Postnatal respiratory depression may be seen in the fetus if excessive amounts of meperidine are given to the mother. Decreased beat-to-beat fetal heart rate variability also occurs as a direct fetal cardiac effect of meperidine.[71] Meperidine and promethazine together have been reported to cause a sinusoidal fetal heart rate pattern during labor in 11 of 350 patients.[36] Freeman and Garite define a sinusoidal pattern as a "sine wave above and below the baseline fetal heart rate with a cyclicity of approximately up to 8 per minute."[51] In this pattern, increased long-term fetal heart rate variability is accompanied by decreased short-term fetal heart rate variability.[51] In some situations, a sinusoidal fetal heart rate pattern is associated with anemia or severe hypoxia but may also indicate abnormal fetal central nervous system (CNS) input into heart rate regulation.[52] Not uncommonly, alphaprodine (Nisentil) has also been associated with a sinusoidal fetal heart rate pattern during labor.[52,71] Morphine and heroin also depress the fetal central nervous system and decrease fetal heart rate variability, but they are not commonly used during labor.[71]

The barbiturates also cross freely to the fetus[71] and cause fetal CNS depression. As a result, barbiturates decrease fetal heart rate variability, both long-term and short-term.[71,92] Other problems associated with barbiturates include an absence or decrease in the normal fetal heart rate acceleration seen with fetal movements and neonatal hemorrhage secondary to suppression of vitamin K–dependent factors.[17] Maternal thiopental injection for induction of general anesthesia reaches the umbilical circulation within 30 seconds.[105] During anesthetic induction, barbiturates have been found to decrease uterine and specifically placental blood flow, although in healthy fetuses these effects are thought to be minimal.[90] Other than fetal CNS depression and consequent changes in fetal heart rate variability, the effects of barbiturates on the fetal cardiovascular system are minimal.

PSYCHIATRIC DRUGS

Generally, the phenothiazines do not affect the fetal cardiovascular system directly. However, phenothiazines can affect the fetal cardiac system through their CNS effects, with rhythm disturbances being a potential problem.[71] Chlorpromazine has been found to cause maternal hypotension during labor, thus indirectly affecting fetal cardiovascular function.[18] Haloperidol, which also crosses to the fetus, has not been shown to have fetal cardiovascular effects.[19] These agents are used not only as antipsychotics during pregnancy but also as antiemetics and narcotic adjuvants during labor;[71] their effects on fetal cardiovascular systems are minimal. Promazine and promethazine are used most commonly during the first trimester as antiemetics and also to potentiate narcotics during labor. The anticholinergic and CNS effects of promazine and promethazine can potentially affect the fetal cardiac rate and rhythm. Meperidine and promethazine used together are associated with a sinusoidal fetal heart rate pattern.[36] Promethazine in labor has been associated with maternal tachycardia and hypotension.[22,71,76] Potential indirect fetal effects such as decreased beat-to-beat fetal heart rate variability have also been noted with these agents.[18,71,75,94]

Tricyclic antidepressants cross readily to the fetus,[20,56] but usually do not affect the fetal cardiovascular system. However, cases of fetal distress at birth have been noted after maternal tricyclic therapy, including a case of transient heart failure unrelated to structural defects and another case of unexplained transient tachycardia.[56] Lithium, besides causing the anomalies discussed in Chapter 49, may significantly affect fetal cardiac function. Lithium crosses readily to the fetus and may cause bradycardia, atrial flutter, cardiomegaly, and ECG abnormalities in the newborn.[21] Because of these effects, maternal ingestion of lithium should be avoided if at all possible.

Benzodiazepines cross readily to the fetus, which has limited ability to metabolize these agents.[76] The primary fetal cardiovascular effect of benzodiazepines is a marked decrease in short-term fetal heart rate variability;[76] the direct and indirect fetal cardiovascular effects are otherwise minimal. On occasion benzodiazepines may lead to significant fetal depression after delivery if they are used in large quantities.[76]

ANTICHOLINERGIC AGENTS

Anticholinergic agents, such as atropine and glycopyrrolate, are used in obstetrics primarily to inhibit oral, pharyngeal, and gastric secretions prior to induction of anesthesia. Glycopyrrolate does not cross the placenta, and thus does not affect the fetal heart rate. Glycopyrrolate may increase maternal heart rate slightly without changes in maternal blood pressure.[1] Atropine does cross the placenta and induces fetal vagal blockade and elevation in basal fetal heart rate. Atropine abolishes vagal-dependent fetal heart rate decelerations induced by head and cord compressions during labor. The effect of atropine on heart rate increases as gestation advances, suggesting an increased parasympathetic control of the heart as pregnancy continues.[52] Decreased beat-to-beat fetal heart rate variability may also be seen with atropine administration.[52,64]

ANTIHISTAMINES AND DECONGESTANTS (CHLOROPHENIRAMINE, PHENIRAMINE, DIPHENHYDRAMINE)

These over-the-counter agents, often formulated in combination with other drugs, are widely used in pregnancy. In small amounts for short periods, the antihistamines and decongestants considered here do not affect the fetal cardiovascular system.[23,59] The decongestants pseudoephedrine and ephedrine are also popular over-the-counter medications prepared in combination with antihistamines. Pseudoephedrine and ephedrine can lead to fetal tachycardia. (The use of parenteral ephedrine to reverse hypotension has been described above under the section Anesthesia.) The adrenergic activity of decongestants may influence uterine blood flow and thus indirectly affect fetal cardiac function.[104] Very large oral doses of ephedrine and pseudoephedrine would be required to reduce uterine blood flow in normal pregnancies; however, in cases of preexisting uteroplacental insufficiency, caution is warranted in the use of sympathomimetic agents of any amount.[24]

ANTIEPILEPTICS

Trimethadione and valproic acid are not recommended in pregnancy, owing to their severe teratogenic effects (see Chapter 49). Phenytoin may cause hemorrhage in the infant, hypocalcemia, and folate deficiency.[25,109] Other than cardiac structural effects (see Chapter 49), phenytoin does not appear to affect the fetal heart directly. The barbiturates are discussed above.

ANTITHYROID MEDICATIONS

Both propylthiouracil (PTU) and methimazole cross the placenta. PTU is preferred in pregnancy because methimazole is teratogenic. Both PTU and methimazole may cause transient hypothyroid effects in the fetus in approximately 1 per cent of treated women.[35,96]

MEDICATION FOR MYASTHENIA GRAVIS

Neostigmine, pyridostigmine, and less commonly ambenonium act as cholinergic agonists, but none of them seem to cross the placenta, since they are ionized at physiologic pH.[44]

SMOKING, CARBON MONOXIDE, AND NICOTINE

The fetal cardiovascular effects of tobacco smoking are both acute and chronic and are a combination of responses to carbon monoxide, nicotine, and hypoxia. Tobacco smoking affects fetal heart rate acutely and retards intrauterine growth chronically. Tobacco smoking causes placental and uterine artery damage and has an indirect chronic fetal cardiovascular effect.[84] Placental abruption, placental infarction, stillbirth, subchorionic fibrin deposition, and calcification are more common in smokers than nonsmokers.[39,85] Elevated fetal hemoglobin levels may be found in infants of mothers who smoked during pregnancy.[86]

Nicotine is transferred across the placenta and may be found in higher concentrations in the fetus than in the mother. Nicotine is also found in higher concentrations in fetal amnionic fluid than in maternal serum.[78] Nicotine decreases beat-to-beat fetal heart rate variability, and in the second trimester it elevates fetal heart rate.[74] Smoking cigarettes containing nicotine does increase fetal aortic and umbilical blood flows (as measured by Doppler ultrasonography). Presumably, nicotine-induced increases in fetal peripheral vasoconstriction raise fetal blood pressure.[47,120] Long-term and short-term fetal heart rate variability are decreased with as little as one cigarette.[47] Nicotine also indirectly affects fetal cardiovascular function by decreasing uterine blood flow.[104]

Carbon monoxide passes freely across the placenta in proportion to the maternal and fetal partial pressure difference.[77] Carbon monoxide exposure is much more lethal to the fetus than to the mother because of fetal oxygenation kinetics. Smoking increases maternal carbon monoxide levels; the resultant increase in maternal carboxyhemoglobin shifts the maternal oxygen dissociation curve to the left; therefore, less oxygen is transferred to the fetus. As fetal carboxyhemoglobin levels also rise, the availability of fetal blood to accept oxygen decreases at a time when less oxygen is available from maternal hemoglobin.[77] Maternal and fetal carbon monoxide poisoning may result in acidosis and stillbirth, which is often preceded by fetal distress. During labor, high carbon monoxide levels may cause late decelerations and fetal tachycardia. The high carbon monoxide levels may also result from exposure to exhaust gases or from exposure to poorly ventilated barbecues. With lower concentrations of carbon monoxide and with chronic exposure (such as with smoking or poorly vented indoor cooking or heating), growth retardation may occur. The loss of oxygen from smoking two packs of cigarettes per day is equivalent to decreasing uterine blood flow by 60 per cent.[120]

CAFFEINE

Approximately 80 per cent of pregnant women are exposed to caffeine during pregnancy.[100] Caffeine does pass the placenta freely; in normal human doses (fewer than 10 cups of coffee per day) chronic caffeine ingestion does not affect the fetal cardiovascular system.[81] Maternal caffeine ingestion can cause premature atrial beats in the fetus as well as sinus tachycardia.[98]

COCAINE

Cocaine is being used with increasing frequency. Unfortunately, little information is available on its use during pregnancy. However, intravenous cocaine appears to be potentially lethal to the fetus. In animals, cocaine has been shown to reduce uterine blood flow by markedly increasing uterine vascular resistance. As a result, fetal hypoxemia occurs, fetal catecholamines rise, and fetal heart rate and mean arterial pressures increase. Spontaneous abortions and placental abruptions among cocaine users are most likely the result of sudden uterine artery vasoconstriction.[37] Such cocaine-induced fetal losses may not be necessarily related to dose or chronicity of use.

Narcotics, both illicit and prescribed, cause decreased beat-to-beat fetal heart rate variability through central nervous system depression but otherwise do not directly affect the fetal cardiovascular system. Withdrawal of narcotics from pregnant narcotic addicts may lead to fetal demise in utero. The fetus, like the mother, may become addicted to narcotics, and as withdrawal occurs, fetal tachycardia and some increase in beat-to-beat fetal heart rate variability may result from increased levels of circulating fetal catecholamines.[41,126] Intrauterine meconium aspiration may occur during narcotic withdrawal as well as intrauterine death. Therefore, addicts must be managed very carefully if the fetus is to survive.

Marijuana and lysergic acid diethylamide–25 (LSD) do not appear to affect the fetal cardiovascular system,[41,126] but both do cross the placenta.

ETHANOL

Ethanol crosses the placenta freely.[54] At one time ethanol was used therapeutically to inhibit labor. However, today in the United States ethanol is rarely used in obstetrics. Ethanol passes the placenta and causes depression of fetal left ventricular function and depressed fetal myocardial contractility.[69] Initially, ethanol elevates fetal heart rate as fetal ethanol levels rise, but fetal heart rate returns to basal levels within 15 minutes of ethanol exposure.[69] In one study, fetal arterial pressure decreased after ethanol infusion.[2] In human studies fetal heart rate seems to be unchanged or elevated during third trimester ethanol exposure.[54,82] High alcohol levels may cause severe fetal metabolic acidosis[54,66] or neonatal hypotension and shock.[66] Neonatal metabolism of ethanol lags behind that of the adult, and infants whose mothers have been intoxicated may have severe CNS depression at birth.[54]

Ethanol consumption in early pregnancy can also cause structural cardiac defects (Chapter 49).

ANTIHYPERTENSIVES

Diuretic Agents

Furosemide crosses the placenta, as does hydrochlorothiazide.[5,6] Diuretics reduce maternal plasma volume, which can decrease uteroplacental blood flow and indirectly affect the fetal cardiovascular system.[127] However, diuretic-induced adverse effects on the fetus are rare. Diuretic-induced maternal and fetal hypocalcemia can cause fetal cardiac rhythm irregularities, stillbirths, and bradycardias.[26,127] Thiazides have induced thrombocytopenia (rarely) in the neonate as well as rebound hypertension after delivery.[26,127]

Beta Blocking Agents

During pregnancy, beta blockers are useful for a variety of disorders. One of the most common usages in pregnant women is for the control of hypertension. After moderate beta blocker doses, both maternal and fetal levels are equal.[27] Because the uterus is under an anticontractile influence from the β_2-adrenergic receptors, in high doses, beta blockers may lead to increased uterine activity.[27] Fetal bradycardia, lower baseline fetal heart rate, and decreased beat-to-beat fetal heart rate variability may also be seen with the use of beta blockers. Long-term beta blocker use has been questionably linked to fetal growth retardation, but separating the influence of beta blockers on fetal growth versus the influence of the maternal disease for which the beta blockers were prescribed is difficult. However, it does appear that beta blockers may decrease fetal movement in utero; short umbilical cords have been seen in animals exposed to these agents prenatally.[67] Further, the stresses of labor and delivery may not be tolerated as well by the fetus if beta blockade is present.[27,79,127] Propranolol (Inderal) has been used successfully for in utero treatment of fetal supraventricular tachycardia.[70,112]

Hydralazine

Hydralazine is widely used in obstetrics because it increases uterine blood flow. Hydralazine is a vasodilator, and although most vasodilators cause relative hypotension and reductions in uterine blood flow, hydralazine does not.[99] Hydralazine crosses the placenta freely and does not seem to have direct effects on the fetal cardiovascular system.[28] In women with decreased intravascular volume, intravenous hydralazine has been shown to cause hypotension, which may lead to uteroplacental insufficiency.[99] Diazoxide is less frequently used in pregnancy than hydralazine. Diazoxide is a potent vasodilator that may significantly decrease uterine blood flow secondary to maternal hypotension.[28,99] However, diazoxide does not tend to affect either fetal heart rate variability or fetal responses to movement or contractions.[4]

Nitroprusside is a rapid-acting and potent vasodilator, which, like most other vasodilators, may decrease uterine blood flow by reducing maternal blood pressure. Nitroprusside may cause high cyanide levels in the fetus.[90,99] This effect has been seen in animal studies but not in human studies; however, nitroprusside use is recommended only immediately prior to delivery.

CARDIAC DRUGS

The treatment of maternal and fetal arrhythmias is often similar. Therapy for fetal arrhythmias is covered in Chapter 16. Agents used for treatment of fetal arrhythmias include digitalis, propranolol, verapamil, procainamide, and quinidine. Digoxin crosses moderately well from the maternal to the fetal circulation, but usually high maternal levels are needed to obtain adequate fetal levels.[29] However, fetal toxicity and neonatal death from maternal digoxin overdoses have been reported.[29,90] Digitalis has mild oxytotic effects on the uterus. Quinidine may also have an oxytotic effect on the uterus;[30,107] it is used alone or in combination with digitalis to treat fetal arrhythmias, but its use may be associated with neonatal thrombocytopenia.[30] The effect of bretylium on the fetus is not known.[31] Dopamine is rarely used outside of life-threatening situations. Animal studies have suggested that dopamine decreases uterine blood flow by increasing uterine vascular resistance.[79,90] Use of dopamine for spinal hypotension at cesarean delivery may reduce fetal PO_2.[79] Ephedrine is a better agent for spinal hypotension, as discussed above.

CONCLUSION

Overall, most agents in the pharmacologic armamentarium do not affect the fetal cardiovascular system directly. However, any drug that affects maternal blood volume or causes uterine vasospasm will indirectly affect the fetal cardiovascular system, which must compensate for the loss of oxygen and nutrients. Drugs that affect the maternal cardiac system usually cross the placenta and cause similar changes in the fetal cardiac system. Drugs that a patient may take unwittingly and that directly affect the fetal cardiovascular system include the NSAIs, which may cause premature closure of the ductus and fetal embarrassment. Other drugs that cause direct fetal cardiac problems include beta sympathomimetics, which overstimulate the fetal myocardium and lead to myocardial damage.

One of the main principles of obstetrics is that the fetus tolerates maternal cardiovascular compromises less well than the mother. Therefore, in any emergency, maintaining maternal cardiovascular homeostasis takes precedence over the theoretic untoward effects of medications on the fetal cardiovascular system. However, if delivery is imperative, it is important to recall that many drugs are relatively less well metabolized by the newborn infant than by the adult. Drug effects that are transient in the mother may linger in the newborn and lead to cardiovascular changes. Therefore, a careful maternal drug history is necessary for the evaluation of any neonatal cardiac problems.

References

1. Abboud TK, Read J, Miller F, Chen T (1981): Use of glycopyrrolate in the parturient. Obstet Gynecol 57:224–227.
2. Abel EC (1981): A critical evaluation of the obstetric use of alcohol in preterm labor. Drug Alcohol Depend 7:367–378.
3. Ayromlooi J, Desiderio D, Tobias M, Berg P (1982): Effect of $MgSO_4$ on maternal and fetal hemodynamics and fetal brain function. Ped Pharm 2:305–312.
4. Barr PA, Gallery DM (1982): Effect of diazoxide on the antepartum cardiotocograph in severe pregnancy associated hypertension. Aust NZ J Obstet Gynaecol 21:11–15.
5. Beerman B, Fahraeus L, Groschinsky GM, Lindstrom B (1980): Placental transfer of hydrochlorothiazide. Gynecol Obstet Invest 11:45–48.
6. Beerman B, Groschinsky GM, Fahraeus L, Lindstrom B (1978): Placental transfer of furosesmide. Clin Pharm Ther 24:560–562.
7. Briggs GG, Freeman RK, Yaffe SJ (1986): Drugs in Pregnancy and Lactation. 2nd ed. Baltimore, Williams & Wilkins, p 105.
8. Ibid, p 2.
9. Ibid, p 26.
10. Ibid, p 76.
11. Ibid, p 204.
12. Ibid, p 106.
13. Ibid, p 309.
14. Ibid, p 468.
15. Ibid, p 221.
16. Ibid, p 267.
17. Ibid, p 343.
18. Ibid, p 85.
19. Ibid, p 203.
20. Ibid, p 218.
21. Ibid, pp 251–253.
22. Ibid, pp 374–376.
23. Ibid, pp 147–148.
24. Ibid, p 348.
25. Ibid, pp 350–356.
26. Ibid, pp 80–83.
27. Ibid, pp 378–382.
28. Ibid, pp 132–134.
29. Ibid, p 142.
30. Ibid, pp 398–399.
31. Ibid, p 44.
32. Bohm N, Adler CP (1981): Focal necroses, fatty degeneration and subendocardial nuclear polyploidization of the myocardium in newborns after beta-sympathomimetic suppression of premature labor. Eur J Ped 163:149–157.
33. Brash AR, Hickey DE, Graham TP, Stuhlman MT, Oates JA, Cotton RB (1981): Pharmacokinetics of indomethacin in the neonate. N Engl J Med 305:67–72.
34. Brazy JE, Little V, Grimm J (1981): Isoxuprine in the perinatal period. II. Relationships between neonatal symptoms, drug exposure, and drug concentration at the time of birth. J Ped 98:164–151.
35. Burrow GN (1982): Thyroid diseases. In Burrow GN, Ferris TF (eds): Medical Complications during Pregnancy, 2nd ed. Philadelphia, WB Saunders, pp 187–214.
36. Busacca M, Gementi P, Ciralli I, Vignali M (1982): Sinusoidal fetal heart rate associated with maternal administration of meperidine and promethazine in labor. J Perinat Med 10:215–218.

37. Chasnoff IJ, Burns WJ, Schnale SH, Burns KA (1985): Cocaine use in pregnancy. N Engl J Med 313:666–669.

38. Chow AW, Jewesson P (1985): Pharmacokinetics and safety of antimicrobial agents during pregnancy. Rev Infect Dis 7:287–313.

39. Christianson RA (1979): Gross differences observed in the placenta of smokers and nonsmokers. Am J Epidem 110:178–187.

40. Cohen SE (1987): Inhalation analgesia and anaesthesia for vaginal delivery. In Shnider SM, Levinson G (eds): Anaesthesia for Obstetrics. Baltimore, Williams & Wilkins, pp 142–156.

41. Confino E, Gleicher N (1985): Drug abuse in pregnancy. In Gleicher N (ed): Principles of Medical Therapy in Pregnancy. New York, Plenum Medical Book Co, pp 90–102.

42. Cotton DB, Gonik B, Dorman KF (1984): Cardiovascular alterations in severe pregnancy induced hypertension: Acute effects of intravenous $MgSO_4$. Am J Obstet Gynecol 148:162–166.

43. Cruikshank DP, Pitkin RM, Reynolds WA, Williams GA (1979): Effects of $MgSO_4$ treatment on perinatal Ca^{++} metabolism. Am J Obstet Gynecol 134:243–249.

44. Dajessio DJ (1986): Neurologic diseases. In Burrow GN, Ferris TF (eds): Medical Complications during Pregnancy, 2nd ed. Philadelphia, WB Saunders, 1986, pp 435–473.

45. DeVore JS, Eisler EA (1987): Effects of anesthesia in uterine activity and labor. In Shnider SM, Levinson G (eds): Anaesthesia for Obstetrics. Baltimore, Williams & Wilkins, 1987, pp 41–49.

46. Dudley DK, Hardie MI (1985): Fetal and neonatal effects of indomethacin used as a tocolytic agent. Am J Obstet Gynecol 151:180–184.

47. Eriksen PS, Gennser G, Lindvall R, Nilsson K (1985): Acute effects of maternal smoking on fetal heart beat intervals. Acta Obstet Gynecol Scand 63:385–390.

48. Finn S, Schoenbaum SC, Morison RE, Rosner G (1982): No association between coffee consumption and adverse outcomes of pregnancy. N Engl J Med 306:141–145.

49. Ferris TF (1988): Toxemia and hypertension. In Burrow GN, Ferris TN (eds): Medical Complications During Pregnancy. 3rd ed. Philadelphia, WB Saunders, pp 1–34.

50. Forman A, Andersson KE, Ulmsten A (1981): Inhibition of myometrial activity by calcium antagonists. Semin Perinatol 5:288–294.

51. Freeman RK, Garite TJ (1981): Fetal Heart Rate Monitoring. Baltimore, Williams & Wilkins, p 83.

52. Ibid, pp 10–11.

53. Friesen C, Yarnell R, Bachman C, Meatheral K, Biehl D (1986): Effect of lidocaine on regional blood flow and cardiac output in the nonstressed and stressed fetal lamb. Can Anaesth Soc J 33:130–151.

54. Fuchs AR, Fuchs F (1981): Ethanol for prevention of preterm birth. Semin Perinatol 5:236–251.

55. Gibbs RS, Sweet RC (1984): Maternal and fetal infections. In Creasy RK, Resnik R (eds): Maternal Fetal Medicine. Philadelphia, WB Saunders, pp 653–678.

56. Goldberg HL, DiMascio A (1978): Psychotropic drugs in pregnancy. In Lipton MA, DeMascio A, Killam KF (eds): Psychopharmacology: A Generation of Progress. New York, Raven Press, pp 1047–1055.

57. Golichowski AM, Hathoway DR, Frieberg N, Peleg D (1985): Tocolytic and hemodynamic effects of nifedipine in the ewe. Am J Obstet Gynecol 151:1134–1140.

58. Green D (1985): Management of thrombotic disorders in pregnancy. In Gleicher N (ed): Principles of Medical Therapeutics in Pregnancy. New York, Plenum Medical Book Co, pp 731–736.

59. Greenberger P, Patterson R (1978): Safety of therapy for allergic symptoms during pregnancy. Ann Intern Med 89:234–239.

60. Guntheroth WG, Dal RC, Mack LA, Benedetti T (1985): Hydrops from reciprocating tachycardia in a 27-week fetus requiring quinidine for conversion. Obstet Gynecol (3 Suppl) 66:295–335.

61. Ho JL, Barza M (1985): Chemotherapy of infection. In Gleicher M (ed): Principles of Medical Therapy in Pregnancy. New York, Plenum Medical Book Co, pp 406–419.

62. Hofmann W, Scheich A, Schroeter D, Weidinger H, Wiest W (1977): Herzmuskelnekrosen durch β-sympathomimetika. Virchow Arch 373:85–95.

63. Huszar G (1984): Physiology of the myometrium. In Creasy RK, Resnik R (eds): Maternal Fetal Medicine. Philadelphia, WB Saunders, pp 146–154.

64. James FM (1987): Anesthesia for nonobstetric surgery during pregnancy. Clin Obstet Gynecol 30:621–628.

65. Jouppila P, Kirkinen P, Kowula A, Yeikorkala O (1985): Ritodrine infusion during late pregnancy: Effects on fetal and placental blood flow, prostacyclin and thromboxane. Am J Obstet Gynecol 151:1028–1032.

66. Jung AI, Roan VR (1980): Neonatal death associated with acute transplacental ethanol intoxication. Am J Dis Child 134:419–420.

67. Katz V, Blanchard G, Dingman C, Bowes WA (1987): Atenolol and short umbilical cords. Am J Obstet Gynecol 156:1271–1272.

68. Keegan KA, Paul RH, Broussard PM, McCort D (1979): Antepartum fetal heart rate testing. Am J Obstet Gynecol 133:519–580.

69. Kirkpatrick SE, Pitlick PT, Hirschklan MJ, Friedman WF (1976): Acute effects of maternal ethanol infusion on cardiac performance. Am J Obstet Gynecol 126:1034–1037.

70. Klein AM, Holzman IR, Austin EM (1979): Fetal tachycardia prior to development of hydrops. Am J Obstet Gynecol 134:347–348.

71. Kryc JJ (1986): Management of pain during labor. In Rayburn WF, Zuspan FP (eds): Drug Therapy in Obstetrics and Gynecology. 2nd ed. Norwalk, Appleton-Century-Crofts, pp 205–224.

72. Lavin JP, Samuels SL, Miodvnik M, Halroyde J (1981): Effects of bupivicane and chloroprocaine as local anesthetics for epidural anesthesia. Am J Obstet Gynecol 141:717–722.

73. Lavin JP (1986): Pharmacologic therapy for chronic medical disorders during pregnancy. In Rayburn WF, Zuspan FP (eds): Drug Therapy in Obstetrics and Gynecology. 2nd ed. Norwalk, Appleton-Century-Crofts, pp 129–146.

74. Lehtovirta P, Farss M, Rauvamoro I, Kariniemi V (1983): Acute effects of nicotine on fetal heart rate variability. Br J Obstet Gynaecol 90:710–715.

75. Levinson G, Schnider SM (1987): Controversies in selecting a drug. In Schnider SM, Levinson G (eds): Anesthesia for Obstetrics, 2nd ed. Baltimore, Williams & Wilkins, pp 69–78.

76. Levinson G, Shnider SM (1987): Systemic medication for labor and delivery. In Shnider SM, Levinson G (eds): Anesthesia for Obstetrics, 2nd ed. Baltimore, Williams & Wilkins, pp 89–108.

77. Longo LD (1977): Biological effects of carbon monoxide on the pregnant woman, fetus and newborn. Am J Obstet Gynecol 129:69–102.

78. Luck W, Nan H, Hansen R, Steldinger R (1985): Extent of nicotine transfer to the human fetus. Dev Pharmacol Ther 8:384–395.

79. Mangano DT (1987): Anesthesia for the pregnant cardiac patient. In Shnider SM, Levinson G (eds): Anesthesia for Obstetrics, 2nd ed. Baltimore, Williams & Wilkins, pp 345–381.

80. Marsal K (1984): Acute effects of maternal smoking on fetal blood flow after smoking. Acta Obstet Gynecol Scand 63:391–395.

81. Martin JC (1982): An overview: Maternal nicotine and caffeine consumption. Toxic Terat 4:421–427.

82. McLeod W, Brien J, Loomis C, Carmichael L (1983): Effect of maternal ethanol ingestion on fetal breathing movements and heart rate at 37–40 weeks' gestation. Am J Obstet Gynecol 145:251–256.

83. McGuinness GA, Weinstein MM, Cruikshank DP, Pitkin RM (1980): Effects of $MgSO_4$ treatment on perinatal Ca metabolism. Obstet Gynecol 56:595–604.

84. Naeye RL (1981): Influence of maternal cigarette smoking during pregnancy on fetal growth. Obstet Gynecol 57:18–21.

85. Naeye RL, Harkness WL, Utts J (1977): Abruptio placenta and perinatal death, a prospective study. Am J Obstet Gynecol 128:740–746.

86. Naeye RL, Peters EC (1984): Mental development of children whose mothers smoked. Obstet Gynecol 64:601–608.

87. Niebyl JR (1981): Prostaglandin synthetase inhibitors. Semin Perinatol 5:274–287

88. Niebyl JR, Witten FR (1987): Neonatal outcome after indomethacin treatment for preterm labor. Am J Obstet Gynecol 155:747.

89. Nuchpuckdee P, Grodsky N, Porat R, Hurt H (1986): Ventricular septal thickness and cardiac function in neonates after in utero ritodrine exposure. J Pediatr 109:687–691.

90. Cosmi EV, Shnider SM (1979): Obstetric anesthesia and uterine

blood flow. In Shnider SM, Levinson G (eds): Anesthesia for Obstetrics. 2nd ed. Baltimore, Williams & Wilkins, pp 22–70.

91. Parke AL (1985): Pregnancy and the rheumatic diseases. In Gleicher N (ed): Principles of Medical Therapy in Pregnancy. New York, Plenum Medical Book Co, pp 1003–1013.

92. Petrie RH (1978): Effects of drugs and anesthetics on the fetal heart rate. Semin Perinatol 2:147–153.

93. Petrie RH (1981): Tocolysis using MgSO$_4$. Sem Perinat 5:266–273.

94. Petrie RH, Yen SY, Murata Y, Paul RH (1978): The effect of drugs on fetal heart rate variability. Am J Obstet Gynecol 130:294–299.

95. Rayburn WF, DeDonato DM, Rand WK III (1986): Drugs to inhibit premature labor. In Rayburn WF, Zuspan FP (eds): Drug Therapy in Obstetrics and Gynecology. 2nd ed. Norwalk, Appleton-Century-Crofts, pp 172–190.

96. Rayburn WF, McNulty RM, O'Shaughnessy RW (1986): Endocrine disorders during pregnancy. In Rayburn WF, Zuspan FP (eds): Drug Therapy in Obstetrics and Gynecology. 2nd ed. Norwalk, Appleton-Century-Crofts, pp 93–111.

97. Rayburn WF, Russ JS (1986): Uterine stimulation. In Rayburn WF, Zuspan FP (eds): Drug Therapy in Obstetrics and Gynecology. 2nd ed. Norwalk, Appleton-Century-Crofts, pp 191–204.

98. Resch BA, Lapp JG (1985): Effects of caffeine on the fetal heart. Am J Obstet Gynecol 146:231–232.

99. Roberts JM (1984): Pregnancy related hypertension. In Creasy RK, Resnik R (eds): Maternal Fetal Medicine. Philadelphia, WB Saunders, pp 653–678.

100. Rodgers BD, Lee RV (1988): Drug abuse. In Burrow GN, Ferris TF (eds): Medical Complications during Pregnancy. 3rd ed. Philadelphia, WB Saunders, pp 570–582.

101. Rosen MA (1987): Anesthesia for fetal surgery. In Shnider SM, Levinson G (eds): Anesthesia for Obstetrics. 2nd ed. Baltimore, Williams & Wilkins, pp 206–216a.

102. Rudolph AM (1981): Effect of nonsteroidal antiinflammatory compounds on fetal circulation and pulmonary function. Obstet Gynecol 58:635–675.

103. Rumack CM, Guggenheim MA, Rumack BH, Peterson RC (1981): Neonatal intracranial hemorrhage and maternal use of aspirin. Obstet Gynecol 58:525–275.

104. Shad RF, Rayburn WF (1987): Antiemetics, iron preparations, OTC drugs. In Rayburn WF, Zuspan FP (eds): Drug Therapy in Obstetrics and Gynecology. 2nd ed. Norwalk, Appleton-Century-Crofts, pp 24–36.

105. Shnider SM, Levinson G (1987): Anesthesia for cesarean section. In Shnider SM, Levinson G (eds): Anesthesia for Obstetrics. 2nd ed. Baltimore, Williams & Wilkins, pp 159–178.

106. Shnider SM, Levinson G, Ralston GH (1987): Regional anesthesia for labor and delivery. In Shnider SM, Levinson G (eds): Anesthesia for Obstetrics. 2nd ed. Baltimore, Williams & Wilkins, pp 109–122.

107. Spinnato JA, Shaver DC, Flims GS, Sibai BM (1984): Fetal supraventricular tachycardia: in utero therapy with digoxin and quinidine. Obstet Gynecol 64:730–735.

108. Stallworth JC, Yen SY, Petrie RH (1981): The effect of MgSO$_4$ on fetal heart rate variability. Am J Obstet Gynecol 140:702.

109. Stengal LE, Rayburn WF (1987): Anticonvulsant therapy in pregnancy. In Rayburn WF, Zuspan FP (eds): Drug Therapy in Obstetrics and Gynecology. 2nd ed. Norwalk, Appleton-Century-Crofts, pp 53–71.

110. Stuart MJ, Gross SO, Elrod H, Graeber JE (1982): Effects of acetylsalicylic acid ingestion on maternal and neonatal hemostasis. N Engl J Med 307:909–912.

111. Svenningsen NW (1982): Follow-up studies on preterm infants after maternal β-receptor agonist treatment. Acta Obstet Gynecol Scand Suppl 108:67–70.

112. Teuscher A, Bossi E, Imhof P, Erb E (1978): Effect of propranolol on fetal tachycardia. Am J Card 42:304–307.

113. Thiagarajah S, Harbert GM, Burgeios FJ (1985): MgSO$_4$ and ritodrine: Systemic and uterine effects. Am J Obstet Gynecol 153:666–674.

114. Trofatter KF (1985): Herpes simplex virus. In Gleichner N (ed): Principles of Medical Therapy in Pregnancy. New York, Plenum Medical Book Co, pp 569–575.

115. Turkel SB (1982): Conditions associated with nonimmune hydrops fetalis. Clin Perinatol 9:613–625.

116. Ulmsten U, Andersson KE, Wengerup L (1980): Treatment of premature labor with the Ca^{++} antagonist nifedipine. Arch Gynecol 229:1–5.

117. Van der Walle AFGM, Martin CB (1986): Effect of ritodrine on uteroplacental blood flow and cardiac output distribution in unanesthetized guinea pigs. Am J Obstet Gynecol 154:189–194.

118. Van Dorsten JP, Miller FC (1981): Fetal heart rate changes after accidental intrauterine lidocaine. Obstet Gynecol 57:257–259.

119. Veille JC, Bissonette JM, Hohimer AR (1986): Effect of calcium channel blocker on uterine blood flow in the pregnant goat. Am J Obstet Gynecol 154:1160–1166.

120. Weinberger SE, Weiss ST (1988): Pulmonary diseases. In Burrow GN, Ferris TF (eds): Medical Complications of Pregnancy. 3rd ed. Philadelphia, WB Saunders, pp 448–484.

121. Williamson RA, Karp LE (1981): Azathioprine teratogenicity: Review of the literature and case report. Obstet Gynecol 58:247–250.

122. Wright RG, Shnider SM (1987): Hypotension and regional anesthesia in obstetrics. In Shnider SM, Levinson G (eds): Anesthesia for Obstetrics. 2nd ed. Baltimore, Williams & Wilkins, pp 293–299.

123. Wright RG, Shnider SM, Levinson G, Rollins SH (1981): The effect of maternal administration of ephedrine on fetal heart rate and variability. Obstet Gynecol 57:734–739.

124. Yaffe SJ (1981): Antimicrobial therapy and the neonate. Obstet Gynecol 58:855–945.

125. Zuspan FP, Cardero L (1986): Glucocorticoids and fetal pulmonary maturity. In Rayburn WF, Zuspan FP (eds): Drug Therapy in Obstetrics and Gynecology. 2nd ed. Norwalk, Appleton-Century-Crofts, pp 162–171.

126. Zuspan FP, Rayburn WF (1987): Drug abuse during pregnancy. In Rayburn WF, Zuspan FP (eds): Drug Therapy in Obstetrics and Gynecology. 2nd ed. Norwalk, Appleton-Century-Crofts, pp 37–52.

127. Zuspan FP, Zuspan KJ (1986): Acute and chronic hypertension during pregnancy. In Rayburn WF, Zuspan FP (eds): Drug Therapy in Obstetrics and Gynecology. 2nd ed. Norwalk, Appleton-Century-Crofts, pp 73–92.

13 FETAL ELECTROCARDIOGRAPHY

Ron Auslender

Julian T. Parer

The original description of the adult electrocardiogram was published in 1903 by Einthoven. Three years later in 1906 Cremer published the first fetal electrocardiogram (FECG). The record was obtained using two maternal leads, with one being intravaginal and the other abdominal.[6]

For the next 30 years there were few reports, probably because of the low success rate in recording FECG. With further improvement of the recording equipment and increased ability to amplify the ECG signal, new interest arose in FECG. The technique was evaluated for the diagnosis of twins, fetal position, fetal life, congenital heart disease, and asphyxia.[2,15,20,21,22,26,34,36] Despite this renewed promise, the difficulty of recording abdominal FECG and its questionable yield limited the clinical utility of this technique, and it was used primarily for research purposes.

In 1953 Smyth[35] made direct intrauterine recordings of FECG by passing a silver wire electrode into the amniotic sac. Further development of the direct technique gave a better signal than that recorded by abdominal leads and again raised hopes that FECG could be used as a diagnostic tool for the detection of intrapartum asphyxia. Subsequently, direct recording of FECG became the basis for continuous fetal heart rate monitoring, and the classification and interpretation of different heart rate patterns became widespread.[14] Despite the general loss of interest in the actual FECG, there is still an active interest in seeking clinically applicable results from both human and experimental animal studies.

THE TECHNIQUE OF RECORDING FECG

There are two distinct methods of detecting the FECG signal: indirect recording, in which the signal is picked up from maternal electrodes, and direct recording, in which the signal is obtained by direct attachment of electrodes to the fetus.

Indirect Recording

With this technique one can obtain QRS signals during pregnancy in a noninvasive manner. Such FECGs have been recorded as early as the second trimester of pregnancy.[4,20]

Possible Pathways Through Which FECG Is Propagated to the Maternal Surface

Electrodes on the maternal surface pick up the maternal ECG and, at a lower voltage, the FECG. The volume conduction theory, which is applicable to adult electrocardiography, presumes that the whole body is a heterogeneous conductor from the point of view of transmission of electrical signals. In contrast to this theory, electrical potentials created by the fetal heart are thought to be transmitted to the maternal surface mainly through the umbilical vessel–placental pathway and the mucus-lined areas of the fetus, such as the nasopharynx and oropharynx.[18,31]

These low resistance transmission pathways appear to be favored because of the high impedance of the fetal skin (which is aproximately 100 times greater than that of the amniotic fluid and the uterine muscle). Fetal skin attenuates the electrical signal to such an extent that conduction by this pathway (i.e., the skin) cannot be measured at the maternal surface. This high impedance may result from the vernix that covers the fetal skin.[18,31]

Conventional leads have been established in adult electrocardiography: The body is considered as a volume conductor, and the electrical vector can be examined along most of the cardiac axes by using the correct pairs of electrodes. Because of the above noted peculiarity of fetal signal transmissions, the recording of FECG through maternal leads creates a waveform that is not affected by changing electrode placement, as would be expected if the volume conductor theory applied.[31]

Although the FECG wave configuration does not change when the position of the recording electrodes is changed on the surface of the mother's body, the amplitude of the electrical signal may change. Therefore, when recording from the maternal surface, the electrodes are moved about until the strongest signal is obtained.

Amplitude of the FECG Recorded from the Maternal Surface

The amplitude of the QRS complex recorded through abdominal leads varies between 0 and 121 microvolts (μV) (with a mean of 27 μV), and is higher in pregnancies with occiput posterior fetal presentation.[41] The amount of vernix and amniotic fluid and the degree of maternal obesity do not affect the amplitude of the FECG complex because of the voltage transmission pathway. The location of the placenta does not influence the FECG amplitude significantly.[31] The duration of the QRS complex varies from a mean of 29 ± 2 (SD) msec at 17 weeks' gestation to 53 ± 4 (SD) msec at 41 weeks' gestation.[5] This developmental increase in QRS duration correlates with increasing heart size.

The main limitation of indirect FECG recording is the low amplitude signal coming from the fetal heart and the relatively high background noise created by the maternal ECG complex, skin potentials, electromyograms, and electrical equipment. This low signal-to-noise ratio usually results in the fetal P and T waves being undetectable. At times a filter is used to remove the background noise, which further interferes with detection of fetal P and T waves. The best location of maternal leads for FECG recording is generally along the linea alba. Maternal leads located in other places, such as the limbs, rectum, vagina, and lower back, give less satisfactory results, probably because of the increased distance from the fetal heart and increased background noise due to the higher likelihood of muscular activity.

Direct Recording

In contrast to maternal abdominal FECG recordings, in which generally only the R waves are seen, direct FECG allows for detection of the entire ECG complex, including P, QRS, and T waves produced by the electrical activity of the fetal heart.

Electrodes are usually applied transvaginally to the presenting fetal part, although transabdominally placed electrodes have also been used in the past.[7,19] Currently, direct recording is restricted to the intrapartum period after rupture of membranes. As noted previously, the main advantage of direct FECG recording is the accuracy achieved because of the relatively high signal-to-noise ratio.[7,19] The use of bipolar electrodes for direct FECG recording gives better results, with less fluctuation of the baseline and a clearer ECG signal than that obtained with unipolar electrodes.

CHARACTERISTICS OF NORMAL FECG

It is difficult to set up normal standards for the FECG because there are no conventional leads as exist for recording ECG's in newborns and adults. In experimental animals, standardized leads would be feasible, but it is not possible to achieve this clinically in the human fetus.

Three main characteristics can be measured in the normal FECG:
1. Fetal heart rate
2. Amplitudes of the different waves
3. The durations of waves, segments, and intervals.

The normal range for fetal heart rate is conventionally stated as between 120 and 160 beats per minute (bpm), with an average of 140 bpm. There is a tendency for this rate to decrease linearly during gestation. Thus, the mean

value at 20 weeks' gestation is 155 bpm, and at term it is 140 bpm.[16]

In a comprehensive study, Figueroa-Longo and co-workers[7] measured fetal ECGs on nine fetuses. They measured the fetal ECG with three different electrode placements: the fetal head and buttocks, the fetal buttocks and maternal abdomen, and the fetal head and maternal abdomen. It is of interest that the voltages obtained with two electrodes directly attached to the fetus are similar to those obtained in the newborn infant.

Table 13–1 shows the values obtained for the amplitudes of the P, R, and T waves. Note that the highest voltages are obtained when two electrodes are placed on the fetus, the next highest with one breech electrode, and the lowest with one electrode attached to the vertex. This is of potential clinical importance because most monitored babies are in the vertex presentation. The breech electrodes were placed transabdominally onto fetuses in the vertex presentation, and it is not known whether the breech presentation with the breech electrode has similar voltages.

The durations of wave segments and intervals were measured in the same study noted above.[7] The mean values obtained in this study are shown in Figure 13–1. As in the case of the amplitudes noted above, no important differences in these intervals and segments were found between the fetus and the newborn immediately after delivery.

Some data have been obtained in early pregnancy with indirect (maternal abdominal) recording using averaging techniques.[5] The QRS duration at 17 to 18 weeks' gestation was 28.7 ± 4.1 (SD) msec, and this increased to 53.0 ± 4.3 (SD) msec at 41 weeks' gestation. There was also a linear correlation between fetal weight and the QRS duration.[5]

Table 13–1. AMPLITUDE OF THE FECG WAVES IN MILLIVOLTS USING THREE DIFFERENT ELECTRODE PLACEMENTS

Electrodes	Mean	Standard Deviation
Vertex-Breech		
P wave	0.064	0.019
R wave	0.529	0.102
T wave	0.071	0.017
Breech-Maternal		
P wave	0.036	0.011
R wave	0.404	0.162
T wave	0.040	0.012
Vertex-Maternal		
P wave	0.023	0.007
R wave	0.158	0.051
T wave	0.025	0.008

Notes: Modified from Figueroa-Longo JG et al (1966): Fetal electrocardiogram at term labor obtained with subcutaneous fetal electrodes. Am J Obstet Gynecol 96:556–564.

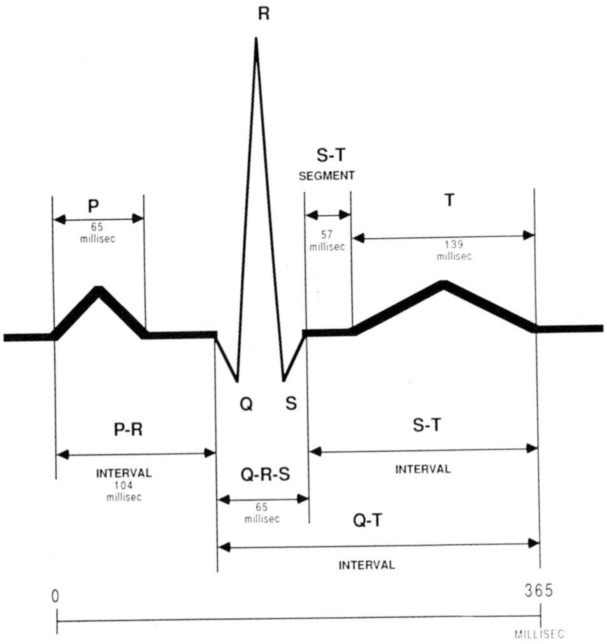

Figure 13–1. Mean values of waves, intervals, and segments of the human FECG, determined by bipolar electrodes, one on the scalp and the other on the buttock. (Modified from Figueroa-Longo JG et al [1966]: Fetal electrocardiogram at term labor obtained with subcutaneous fetal electrodes. Am J Obstet Gynecol 96:556–561.)

Marvell and coworkers[24] have carried out a comprehensive study of the fetal electrocardiogram during labor using computerized techniques. The labors studied were all normal by clinical and biochemical outcome, and fetal ECG was determined by direct means. Trends through labor were normalized to the time of delivery as zero time. Trends over the preceding 140 minutes were noted. They concluded that certain changes in the fetal ECG, previously thought to be characteristic of fetal distress, occurred in normal patients. PR interval was up to 10 per cent shorter during contractions at the end of labor, and there was a long-term trend toward the end of labor for the PR interval to fall by 7 per cent. The P wave amplitude fell by 30 per cent over the last hour. The QRS complex was found to lengthen slightly toward the end of labor, but the RT interval and the ST segment displacement displayed no significant changes. It is against these normal events that changes due to asphyxia must be measured.

INFLUENCE OF ASPHYXIA AND HYPOXIA ON FECG

Waveform Changes

The main interest in fetal ECG in recent years has been for the detection of fetal asphyxia. Studies have been done in both humans and experimental animals, but most of the manipulative experimental work in this field

has been carried out on animals. There are a number of reasons for believing that findings in other species may not apply exactly to humans. There are differences of anatomy, size, and gestational age that may contribute to variations in results. Individual species vary in their physiologic maturity at different gestational ages, and the fetal vectors may also be different. Some animals are studied under acutely operated conditions with anesthesia, while other experiments are done under chronically instrumented conditions. In addition, experimental asphyxia has been induced either by having the mother breathe low oxygen gas mixtures or by decreasing uterine or umbilical blood flow. In some studies fetal asphyxia is induced gradually while in other cases, abruptly.

The most obvious ECG changes are found in the ST waveform of the hypoxic fetus.[9] The ST waveform includes the T wave, which represents repolarization of the ventricles. The QRS deflection represents depolarization of the ventricles. Repolarization is an active process, which consumes energy. Thus, T wave changes may be expected to reflect more accurately metabolic and electrolyte changes within the myocardium. Variations in T waves may also be a consequence of changes in the sequence of ventricular depolarization.

Three features of the ST waveform have been used to indicate abnormalities: (1) T wave amplitude expressed as T/QRS ratio, (2) ST segment elevation or depression, and (3) existence of negative T waves.

The T/QRS ratio is used so that comparative changes in the T wave can be detected even under conditions when the whole complex is changing in amplitude. ST segment elevation or depression represents changes in the relationship between depolarization and repolarization (i.e., repolarization occurs earlier than expected). Negative T waves represent changes in the direction of repolarization.

Rosen et al[33] used a grading system for determining the severity of FECG changes with deliberately imposed hypoxia in fetal sheep.

1. Grade 1. The appearance of inverted T waves, the amplitude of which exceeds that of the P waves.

2. Grade 2. Maximally negative T wave changes.

3. Grade 3. A gradual decrease in the amplitude of the negative T wave changes.

4. Grade 4. Elevation of the ST segments and T wave, with the amplitude of the T wave higher than that of the P wave.

5. Grade 5. A maximal increase in the amplitude of the T wave.

6. Grade 6. A decrease in the amplitude of the T wave during continuous hypoxia.

Our own work[1] shows an increase in T wave amplitude in lead 2, which is expressed as a T/QRS ratio from a mean of 0.30 in controls to 0.53 during fetal asphyxia in fetal sheep. These changes were not related to the degree of asphyxia. The QRS axis varies between animals, which limits use of absolute numbers for the normal amplitude of the T wave from a given lead.

Waveform Changes in Relation to Blood Changes

As a convenient measure of the degree of hypoxia or asphyxia, many workers have used changes in blood acid-base state or oxygenation. There are ST changes within the first few minutes of hypoxia that correlate with a decrease in blood oxygen saturation; however, during prolonged (though relatively mild) hypoxia, the ST changes correlate better with the lactic acid blood level than with decreased pH and oxygen saturation levels.[23] It is presumed that fetal blood lactate levels increase as a result of local anaerobic metabolism in organs that undergo vasoconstriction during fetal hypoxia.

Initial changes in the T/QRS ratio are correlated with blood oxygen saturation via activation of adrenoreceptors.[12,13] Further changes in the T/QRS ratio occur in metabolic acidosis with lactate accumulation.[13,33]

Biochemical Changes within the Myocardium

Myocardial biopsy has been used to study tissue changes in the heart under conditions of fetal asphyxia, which permits analysis of various biochemical and enzymatic changes in relationship to FECG alterations. A linear correlation was found between the decrease in myocardial glycogen content and the increase in T/QRS ratios during fetal hypoxia.[12] The decrease in glycogen content is presumed to be due to an increase in glycogenolysis as a result of catacholamine secretion during asphyxia or hypoxia. Similar FECG changes can be found after injection of B-adrenergic agonists.[12,32]

Levels of ATP in the myocardium have been studied as a measure of dependence on anaerobic metabolism. In the fetal guinea pig it was shown that ATP levels were maintained until glycogen was almost depleted. However, studies on the fetal lamb showed that there was a parallel decrease in ATP level and myocardial glycogen concentration.[12]

Myocardial metabolism has been studied by catheterizing the descending aorta and coronary sinus in the sheep fetus in order to determine changes occurring with induced hypoxia.[8] When blood arterial oxygen content was reduced by 50 per cent, oxygen consumption was maintained by an increase in myocardial blood flow, which compensated for the decrease in oxygen content. Maintenance of myocardial oxygen uptake during fetal hypoxia contradicts the presumption that changes in FECG in moderate hypoxia result from myocardial anaerobic metabolism.

Control Mechanisms

There are thought to be two phases in the hypoxic changes in fetal T waves. The first is seen in mild hypoxia, in which the FECG changes are mainly the result of activation of B-adrenoreceptors. These changes in FECG can be reversed after injection of the B-adrenergic receptor blocking agent propranolol.[12,32] FECG changes similar to those of mild hypoxia have been produced by injection of the B-adrenergic agonist isoprenalin. These latter changes were also subsequently blocked by propranolol,[12] suggesting that FECG changes in mild hypoxia are due to B-adrenergic stimulus of hypoxia on the myocardium.

The second phase of FECG change is seen during severe hypoxia when ECG changes are thought to be a direct result of myocardial hypoxia.

Factors Associated with Changes in Conduction Time

The main FECG changes with respect to the conduction system are (1) sinus bradycardia, (2) changes in P-R interval, and (3) wandering pacemaker.

Bradycardia occurs early during experimental fetal asphyxia or hypoxia as a result of vagal stimulation. The initial bradycardic response is chemoreceptor mediated, but the baroreflex plays a role shortly thereafter.[17] If the asphyxia is prolonged, a sinus tachycardia may intervene, owing to either catecholamine secretion or carbon dioxide accumulation.[10] Vagal stimulation may also delay atrioventricular node conduction, which results in a prolongation of the P-R interval. In addition, in response to vagal stimulation, sinoatrial node activity decreases and may be replaced by alternative atrial foci. We have frequently noted this phenomenon, known as wandering atrial pacemaker, in association with fetal bradycardia induced by asphyxia.

Nonvagal fetal bradycardia is a sign of severe myocardial hypoxia and probably results when hypoxia is of such a degree that myocardial oxygen consumption falls. There is a high concentration of glycogen within the conduction system, which probably makes it less vulnerable (and the last to fail) during asphyxia or hypoxia.

In our work with asphyxiated fetal sheep[1] we found a significant increase in S-T interval measured from lead 2 from a mean of 0.15 sec control time to 0.18 sec during asphyxia. The corrected Q-T interval in the same lead was not changed, which suggests that the increase in S-T interval was not the result of myocardial damage but probably vagally induced.

CLINICAL APPLICATIONS

Fetal Heart Rate Monitoring

The electrical activity of the fetal heart is used clinically almost exclusively to trigger cardiotachometers for intrapartum fetal heart rate monitoring. The direct mode using a fetal electrode gives the most accurate detection of R-R intervals. External maternal electrodes, though reasonably accurate, have largely been discarded in favor of the more convenient Doppler ultrasonography for noninvasive monitoring.

Fetal heart rate monitoring depends on the visual interpretation of patterns of fetal heart rate as traced on a cardiotachometer. There are standardized scales for fetal heart rate and paper speed, and specific heart rate patterns are recognized. Most of the changes seen in heart rate patterns are transient decreases in heart rate, which are termed decelerations; the majority of decelerations are seen in association with uterine contractions. The decelerations have been ascribed to various causes, although not necessarily on a rigid experimental basis. We will describe the patterns, their presumed etiology, and associated FECG changes.

Early Decelerations

Early decelerations are transient decreases in heart rate of gradual onset and recovery occurring over the same time period as the uterine contraction. The nadir of heart rate is less than 20 bpm below baseline. Early decelerations are not associated with compromised fetuses, and there are no associated FECG changes.

Late Decelerations

Late decelerations, like the early decelerations described above, are smooth in contour, but the onset and nadir are delayed for periods of up to 1 minute from the contraction. They are thought to include a fetal chemoreceptor response to reduced fetal oxygen transfer secondary to relative insufficiency of uterine blood flow during the uterine contraction. The severity of late decelerations is generally indicated by an increase in depth or absence of beat-to-beat heart rate variability.[29] Absence of fetal heart rate variability in the presence of late decelerations is considered to represent severe asphyxia, which warrants emergency delivery.

FECG changes using the group averaging technique have been described during late decelerations. With relatively mild decelerations (less than 20 bpm), the P-R interval was prolonged. With increasing severity of decelerations, the P-R interval was shortened. With further severity, the P wave became biphasic or disappeared.[28]

In approximately 50 per cent of cases there are also ST segment and T wave changes. These usually consist of ST segment depression and an increase in the amplitude of the T wave. The incidence of these changes was not well correlated with changes in fetal blood pH.

The P-R interval and P wave changes suggest vagal stimulation as a cause, in accordance with other physiologic information.[30] It has been suggested that the ventricular repolarization changes may be due to generalized myocardial depression.[28]

Variable Decelerations

Variable decelerations are decreases in fetal heart rate that are abrupt in onset and recovery and generally differ in appearance from contraction to contraction. These decelerations vary in their duration and depth and are described as "severe" when below 70 bpm for more than 60 seconds. This latter pattern, if persistent, has been associated with fetal acidosis and depression, particularly when unaccompanied by beat-to-beat fetal heart rate variability. Their etiology in most clinical settings is unknown, although they can be reproduced by compression of the umbilical cord or severe head compression.[29]

With variable decelerations of moderate intensity, the P-R interval became progressively shorter, and the P wave became biphasic or disappeared. These changes reversed when the heart rate recovered. Only with severe variable decelerations (heart rate below 70 bpm for 60 seconds) was there sometimes ST segment depression or an increase in T wave amplitude.[28]

As noted above, in changes with late decelerations, the P wave and P-R interval changes are indications of vagal influences on the sinus node and on conduction; at times a nodal rhythm can occur.[28]

Arrhythmias

In recent years there has been an increasing number of reports on fetal arrhythmias, including extrasystoles, tachyarrhythmias, and bradyarrhythmias.[37] The majority of reported fetal arrhythmias are either supraventricular or ventricular arrhythmias. Most morbidity is confined to fetuses or newborns with the tachy- or bradyarrhythmias.[3,25]

Major abnormalities in fetal cardiac rate are generally detected by auscultation of the fetal heart. Antepartum FECGs with maternal abdominal electrodes have been generally unrewarding in the diagnosis of either the arrhythmias themselves or associated heart defects, and fetal echocardiography is the standard diagnostic technique. Fetal arrhythmias and fetal echocardiography are covered in Chapters 10, 14, and 15, respectively.

Fetal Systolic Interval Measurements

A number of investigators have examined the fetal systolic interval in the hope that it would be useful as an index of myocardial health, as it is in the adult. The interval that has gained the most popularity for study in the fetus is the preejection period (PEP). PEP is defined as the interval from the onset of ventricular depolarization (the Q wave onset in the fetal ECG) to the onset of aortic valve opening, generally measured by Doppler ultrasonography. Several modifications of this definition have been proposed, mainly for convenience of processing.[11]

PEP increases with gestational age and decreases as mean heart rate decreases. Like the beat-to-beat heart rate, PEP tends to be characteristic for each fetus. Hence, in a given fetus, trends over time rather than absolute values are important; variations in preload, afterload, myocardial contractility, and heart rate all affect PEP.

There has been controversy in the literature regarding the importance of PEP measurements in clinical obstetrics, and varying results have been obtained during clinical and experimentally induced asphyxia and hypoxia. Much of the disagreement can be resolved by recognizing the complex fetal events during progressive asphyxia, i.e., the stages from the cardiorespiratory compensations during mild and moderate asphyxia to the decompensation occurring with severe or prolonged asphyxia. During the initial stages of acute asphyxia (the "stress" phases), the fetus responds with neurohumoral activity, which includes sympathetic nervous and adrenal medullary responses. During this time, the PEP shortens, and there is main tenance of myocardial oxygenation. As the asphyxia continues, the myocardial function is depressed because of decreased myocardial oxygenation and acidosis, and the PEP is prolonged.[27] This pattern probably corresponds to the decompensation phase of severe fetal asphyxia.

The PEP may ultimately be shown to reflect central tissue oxygen adequacy like fetal heart rate variability. An important difference is that whereas certain changes in the PEP may reflect myocardial oxygenation, fetal heart rate variability is thought to reflect oxygenation of the central nervous system.[29]

Measurement of fetal PEP is unlikely to become clinically applicable for awhile because the equipment and technique are quite complex, computer processing is required, and interpretation is not yet clarified.

References

1. Auslender RA, Field DR, Parer JT, Ross B, Johnson J (1987): The fetal ECG during asphyxial decompensation. Abstracts of Scientific Papers, 34th annual meeting, Society for Gynecologic Investigation, Atlanta, Georgia.
2. Bell GH (1938): The human foetal electrocardiogram. Br J Obstet Gynaecol 45:802–809.
3. Bergmans MGM, Jonker GJ, Kock HCLV (1985): Fetal supraventricular tachycardia. Review of the Literature. Obstet Gynecol Survey 40:61–68.
4. Bernstein P, Mann H (1942): A clinical evaluation of fetal electrocardiography. Am J Obstet Gynecol 43:21–31.
5. Brambati B, Pardi G (l980): The intraventricular conduction time of fetal heart in uncomplicated pregnancies. Br J Obstet Gynaecol 87:941–948.
6. Cremer MV (l906): Ueber die direkte ableitung der akionsstrome des menschlichen herzens vom oesophagus und uber das elektrokardiogramm des fotus. Muenchener Medizinische Wochenschrift 53:811–813.
7. Figueroa-Longo JG, Poseiro JJ, Alvarez LO, Caldeyro-Barcia R (l966): Fetal electrocardiogram at term labor obtained with subcutaneous fetal electrodes. Am J Obstet Gynecol 96:556–564.
8. Fisher DJ, Heymann MA, Rudolph AM (l982): Fetal myocardial oxygen and carbohydrate consumption during acutely induced hypoxemia. Am J Physiol 242:H657–H661.
9. Greene KR, Dawes GS, Lilja H, Rosen KG (1982): Changes in the ST waveform of the fetal lamb electrocardiogram with hypoxemia. Am J Obstet Gynecol 144:950–958.
10. Gu W, Jones CT, Parer JT (1985): Metabolic and cardiovascular effects on fetal sheep of sustained reduction of uterine blood flow. J Physiol 368:109–129.
11. Hawrylyshyn PA, Organ LW, Bernstein A (1980): A new computer technique for continuous measurements of the pre-ejection period in the human fetus. Physiologic significance of pre-ejection period patterns. Am J Obstet Gynecol 137:801.
12. Hokegard K-H (1979): Fetal and neonatal electrocardiographic changes in relation to fetal hypoxia. Thesis, University of Goteborg, Sweden.
13. Hokegard K-H, Karlsson K, Kjellmer I, Rosen KG (1979): ECG changes in the fetal lamb during asphyxia in relation to beta-adrenoreceptor stimulation and blockade. Acta Physiol Scand 105:195–203.
14. Hon EH, Quilligan EJ (1967): The classification of fetal heart rate. Connecticut Med 31:779.
15. Hon EH, Hess OW (1960): The clinical value of fetal electrocardiography. Am J Obstet Gynecol 79:1012–1023.
16. Ibarra-Polo AA, Guiloff E, Gomez-Rogers C (1972): Fetal heart rate throughout pregnancy. Am J Obstet Gynecol 113:814–818.
17. Itskovitz J, Goetzman BW, Rudolph AM (1982): The mechanism of late deceleration of the heart rate and its relationship to oxygenation in normoxemic and chronically hypoxemic fetal lambs. Am J Obstet Gynecol 142:66.
18. Kahn AR (1963): Transmission characteristics in fetal electrocardiography. l6th Annual Conference on Engineering in Medicine and Biology. Baltimore, Maryland, Vol V, p 134.
19. Kaplan S, Toyama S (1958): Fetal electrocardiography: Utilizing abdominal and intrauterine leads. Obstet Gynecol 11:391–397.
20. Larks SD (1959): The fetal electrocardiogram in multiple pregnancy. Am J Obstet Gynecol 77:1109–1115.
21. Larks SD, Faust R, Longo L, Anderson G (1960): Experiences in the diagnosis of fetal life with fetal electrocardiogram. Am J Obstet Gynecol 80:1143–1150.
22. Lee ST, Hon EH (1965): The fetal electrocardiogram. IV. Unusual variations in the QRS complex during labor. Am J Obstet Gynecol 92:1140–1147.
23. Lilja H, Greene KR, Karlsson K, Rosen KG (1985): ST waveform changes of the fetal electrocardiogram during labour—a clinical study. Br J Obstet Gynaecol 92:611–617.
24. Marvell CJ, Kirk DL, Jenkins HM, Symonds EM (1980): The normal condition of the fetal electrocardiogram during labour. Br J Obstet Gynaecol 87:786–796.
25. Michaelsson M, Engle MA (1972): Congenital complete heart block: An international study of the natural history. Cardiovasc Clin 4:86–101.
26. Miller ML, Werch SC, Milton JD, Ferguson JH (1958): Determination of fetal life by electrocardiography. Obstet Gynecol 11:398–402.
27. Organ LW, Bernstein A, Hawrylyshyn PA (1980): The pre-ejection period as an antepartum indicator of fetal well-being. Am J Obstet Gynecol 137:810.
28. Pardi G, Tucci E, Uderzo A, Zanini D (1974): Fetal electrocardiogram changes in relation to fetal heart rate patterns during labor. Am J Obstet Gynecol 118:243–250.
29. Parer JT (1983): Handbook of fetal heart rate monitoring. Philadephia, WB Saunders.
30. Parer JT, Krueger TR, Harris JL (1980): Fetal oxygen consumption and mechanisms of heart rate response during artificially produced late decelerations of fetal heart rate in sheep. Am J Obstet Gynecol 136:478–482.
31. Roche JB, Hon EH (1965): The fetal electrocardiogram. V. Comparison of lead systems. Am J Obstet Gynecol 92:1149–1159.
32. Rosen KG, Dagbjartsson A, Henriksson BA, Lagercrantz H, Kjellmer I (1984): The relationship between circulating catecholamines and ST waveform in the fetal lamb electrocardiogram during hypoxia. Am J Obstet Gynecol 149:190–194.
33. Rosen KG, Hokegard KH, Kjellmer I (1976): A study of the relationship between the electrocardiogram and hemodynamics in the fetal lamb during asphyxia. Acta Physiol Scand 98:275–284.
34. Southern EM (1957): Fetal anoxia and its possible relation to changes in the prenatal fetal electrocardiogram. Am J Obstet Gynecol 73:233–247.
35. Smyth CN (1953): Experimental electrocardiography of the foetus. Lancet 1:1124–1126.
36. Vara P, Halminen E (1951): On foetal electrocardiography. II. Acta Obstet Gynecol Scand 39:179–185.
37. Voigt HJ, Singer H (1985): Fetale Arrhythmien: Differential diagnostik, klinische bedeutung und prognose. Geburtsh u Frauenheilk 45:251–359.

14 FETAL ECHODOPPLER AND COLOR FLOW MAPPING

David J. Sahn

Continuous wave Doppler detectors have been used to detect and to record fetal heart rate (a gross index of fetal cardiac function) since the late 1960s. However, it was not until high resolution real time cardiac imaging of the fetus became available[1,7,8] that accurate prenatal diagnosis of heart disease became possible. Using M-mode echocardiography, Kleinman and coworkers[6] were able to diagnose Ebstein anomaly prenatally and to perform elegant studies on the detection and treatment of fetal arrhythmias, but it was only as recently as 1977–78 that gross cardiac malformations (such as single ventricle, hydrops fetalis, and hypoplastic left heart) could be recognized prenatally with echocardiography. By 1982[10] prenatal echocardiographic diagnosis of a large number of fetal heart disorders had been reported.

The application of range-gated pulsed Doppler echocardiography to fetal diagnosis was probably first reported by Redel and Hansmann,[11] who used it to detect premature obstruction of the foramen ovale in a hydropic fetus.

Several subsequent technologic advances have significantly enhanced the utility of Doppler technologies in delineation of both normal and abnormal prenatal cardiac physiology. Accurate quantitation of flow velocity in cm/sec and calculation of volume flow appear feasible when fast Fourier transform spectral analysis Doppler velocity is combined with a real time echocardiographic device, which is a duplex concept developed by Griffith and Henry.[3] Most recently, the development by Kasai and Namekawa[4] of real time color flow mapping, which displays the spatial orientation of flows within the heart, has substantially improved noninvasive characterization of blood flow within the fetal heart.

INSTRUMENTATION FOR FETAL DOPPLER ECHOCARDIOGRAPHIC STUDIES

Instruments designed to perform high quality fetal Doppler echocardiography need several features: (1) high frequency and high resolution front end image acquisition systems, (2) flexible scan converters for display, (3) digital memory for review, (4) good Doppler sensitivity with small and tightly focused sample volumes (single gate or multigate for flow mapping), and (5) adequate frame rates for flow mapping. Combining these capabilities in a single machine is not simple, and presently it is fair to say that few Doppler systems and practically no

flow imaging systems are optimized for fetal cardiac studies. In a brief discussion of these requirements, only pulsed Doppler technology will be discussed, but continuous wave Doppler is of importance for studying and quantifying valvular insufficiency.

Resolution requirements are, in fact, similar for imaging and for Doppler echocardiography. In imaging, transducer configurations that permit short pulse bursts, transducer damping, and use of high frequencies provide the best axial resolution. Lateral resolution at depth (resolution of structures side by side) is best with phased or linear array systems with flexible electronic transmit focus and dynamic receive focus algorithms. Slice thickness or azimuthal resolution remains a problem.

In fetal echocardiography, high resolution and high sensitivity in all three planes combined with tight Doppler beam profile focusing at depth would be ideal. Dynamic focus algorithms increase the depth of the tightly focused field, but for most phased or linear array technologies, focus in azimuth is achieved by an acoustic lens that focuses at mainly one preselected depth. Either a family of these elevational focuses will be required to deal with fetal hearts at different depths from the transducer, or variable elevational focus will be required in biplanar arrays. In mechanically swept systems, annular arrays can achieve a cylindrical three-dimensional focus both in azimuth and within the plane for lateral resolution (see Color Figure 1). The same factors that determine the discreteness of image lines and image resolution also determine the discreteness of Doppler sampling loci. Sampling sensitivity, pulse burst duration, and receiver gate time period determine the axial length of the pulsed Doppler sample volume, i.e., the axial length of single gate as well as the length of individual gates for multigate flow mapping. Providing adequate elevational and azimuthal focus for Doppler sampling to separate fetal heart flows, which are located millimeters apart and yet may be 6 to 10 cm from the interrogating transducer, is more difficult. Doppler beam antennae patterns are often wider than the equivalent imaging antennae patterns, both in width and azimuth. (Doppler is processing signals from scatterers [the red cells] which are not usually imaged, and the sensitivity required to accomplish this determines a wider beam profile). Hence, it is common to pick up Doppler signals from structures to the side or even above or below the plane of the structures being imaged (i.e., coronary flow in the right ventricular outflow tract or left ventricular outflow tract flow near the mitral valve). Thus, tight and flexible beam focusing is important for Doppler and for flow imaging, especially in the fetus.

In adults, Doppler studies are performed at lower transducer frequencies to improve sensitivity, but significant beam degradation occurs at lower frequencies during fetal echocardiographic studies. Tight and discrete sampling yields clear signals from a single location and improves sensitivity. The best Doppler signals are attained with very high resolution imaging systems built with excellent flexibility in optimizing scan sequence and focusing. In linear array systems, this flexibility should include the capacity to obtain Doppler samples from different directions. For processing the Doppler shift and achieving display, the spectral processors need high sampling rates, high dynamic range for weak signals, and good signal-to-noise characteristics. Display flexibility and digital memory requirements will be discussed after a brief review of flow mapping concepts.

DISPLAY MAGNIFICATION AND DIGITAL MEMORY

Magnification modes that recalculate and sample data only in the region of interest can produce not only larger but also enhanced (rather than degraded) images, Doppler studies, and color flow maps, all of which are of obvious importance in fetal echocardiography. Additional requirements in color flow mapping are optimization of pulse repetition frequency (PRF) and data collection over only a specific region. Mixed imaging modes in which real time images share screen space (either in true real time or as a frozen locator image of either tissue or tissue and flow map) with waveform velocity traces, M-mode, or color velocity–coded M-mode must not only allocate display space to any of the three types of traces but also must provide flexibility within the scan converter and magnification modes, or zoom modes, for any of the windows in the display. Real time Doppler imaging and flow mapping systems process and display large quantities of information at very fast rates; thus, the capacity for redisplay and review of primary quality digitally recorded and stored information in slow motion with reallocation of display space, color assignment, or zero shift is of significant importance. Digital storage capability already exists, for instance, to store up to 8 seconds of real time digital image and flow map information for review and measurement. When the information is played back through the system itself, the data can be measured, magnified, and/or manipulated in a number of ways. Lastly, it is of considerable importance that tissue information be stored in memory locations separate from flow information, so that the flow information can be looked at separately or superimposed on the tissue and so that the tissue can be looked at separately or with the flow superimposed. As a result of these combinations, the relationships between anatomy and flow can be accurately studied (see Color Figure 2).

REAL TIME COLOR-ENCODED FLOW MAPPING DOPPLER SYSTEMS

In single gate spectral Doppler systems, a single gate is sampled through time along a single direction for the Doppler frequency shift. In real time color-coded flow mapping, many gates (perhaps 120) along each line are sampled. Gate length has often been chosen at around 0.4 mm, since very short gates contain progressively smaller volumes of moving red cells and can compromise sensitivity. Further, while the moving scan sequence is sampling different directions to make up the image, multiple lines are also being sampled for Doppler, and each of those lines is being sampled along multiple gates to assemble a real time spatial matrix of flow. The density of the flow matrix is a function of the number of gates and the number of lines sampled. Unfortunately, sampling is limited by the time required for the ultrasound signal to return from the tissue being examined. Thus, travel time determines how much time has to be spent receiving before the next pulse is sent out, and thereby determines PRF. While certain parallel processing algorithms have been applied in attempts to sample simultaneously along several adjacent lines, PRF remains a fundamental limitation in the assembly of Doppler flow maps. A given PRF has to provide simultaneously all lines of sight sampled for imaging and all lines of sight sampled for Doppler and to determine the sampling density within a given sector (or scan raster). The more lines of sight sampled (whether over a narrow angle with a high sample line density or over a wider angle with a lower sample line density), the lower the frame rate. Obviously, rapid frame rates are desirable when heart rates are high, as in the fetus. Limiting the number of sample lines (for example, using a narrow focus) and placing the transducer near the structures being imaged can provide faster frame rates. However, the fetal heart not only beats rapidly, but is also a long distance from the transducer. Further, the accuracy of Doppler velocity determinations is a function of the number of times one line of sight is sampled sequentially (a number called N); usually, each line of sight is sampled 5 to 8 times. In essence, the scanner sends out one sound wave pulse for image and then another 5 to 8 pulses along that same one line of sight for Doppler, thus sharing PRF. Since these devices are designed for postnatal cardiac imaging, sampling begins near the transducer.

Fetal echocardiography and Doppler could be greatly improved by designing equipment with the capacity to sample small tissue volumes at substantial depths from the transducer with both high information density and high frame rates (or by "windowing" and implementing Doppler sampling only when the information received is returning and using the other time to sample other directions or other depths). Despite the obvious usefulness of current systems in supplying information about fetal flow, much room for improvement remains (see Color Figure 1).

Just as in pulse spectral Doppler studies, axial gate length and lateral and azimuthal resolution also determine the resolution of flow mapping scans. The resolution of flow mapping is poor when flow signals spread onto tissue areas and above and below the plane of the imaged structures, a common problem in fetal flow mapping with present instruments. Flow mapping resolution can be improved by use of intelligent scan converter algorithms, which do not superimpose flow signals onto pixels that contain tissue information.

Flow mapping display systems should provide flexibility in color allocation and an adjustable zero (no color) point. These features are important in accurately identifying both low velocities (such as the foramen ovale flow [see Color Figure 2], identification of which requires good sensitivity at depth and flexible wall filtering) and high velocities exceeding the Nyquist limit (and causing color aliasing). In the flow map systems currently in existence, velocity is estimated at the individual loci by statistical autocorrelations that compare the Doppler shift in any one location with model curves in memory; tremendous memory and speed are required to calculate velocity in each gate and to assign color to each pixel in real time. Usually, flow velocities moving toward the transducer are shown as increasingly bright shades of red, and those moving away from the transducer as increasingly bright shades of blue. Significant variance in velocities within a given locus results in a turbulence allocation, to which the color green has been assigned. The variance technique provides unique highlighting of the disorganized turbulent flows resulting from valvular insufficiency and other abnormalities. If, instead of calculating the mean frequency within a locus, one calculates the amplitude or power of the Doppler shift over all frequencies within the locus, the signal-to-noise ratio can be improved, and low flow velocities can be detected. Such calculations, independent of velocity, are called power mode. These displays will probably be quite important in fetal flow mapping in determining whether flow is toward or away from the transducer, especially for low flow velocity areas.

THE QUESTION OF BIOHAZARD FOR FETAL DOPPLER ECHOCARDIOGRAPHIC STUDIES

The safety of routine Doppler ultrasonographic investigations of fetal hearts has been questioned because there is some evidence that growth retardation, behaviorial changes in newborn animals, or chromsomal breaks can be observed after exposure to ultrasound during early gestation.[9] Most fetal Doppler investigations of the heart involve at most 60 to 90 minutes of exposure to pulsed ultrasound at relatively low pulse repetition frequencies (because of distance); energy exposures invariably fall below 100 mW/cm^2 (spatial peak temporal average) with instruments recently redesigned to meet the new standards for pediatric echocardiographic examinations. There is not any convincing evidence that fetal Doppler echocardiography performed after 10 weeks' gestation (long after completion of organogenesis)[9] poses a significant biohazard. Indeed, in the first days of postnatal life, the average fetus born at 26 to 27 weeks' gestation would have several cranial echo imaging and Doppler studies to detect intracranial hemorrhage and assess cerebral blood flow as well as several echocardiographic Doppler examinations to assess ductal patency. Instrumentation used in performing these postnatal studies typically functions at higher PRF and shorter interrogation distances than instrumentation used in fetal Doppler echocardiography. There is little doubt that information gained from medically indicated fetal Doppler echocardiographic studies performed and interpreted with appropriate expertise justifies the minimal risk of the energy exposure. Even with those considerations, it behooves the examiner to complete the examination as quickly as possible using the lowest possible PRF and power output setting on each instrument. Further, it behooves the manufacturer to design the equipment so that all fetal Doppler systems, although adjustable, are preset at low PRFs and power outputs when initially turned on and provide a continuous, cumulative total of energy delivered during that examination. Exceeding energy doses of 100 mW/cm^2 should be done only under the direction of a physician supervising the imaging laboratory or with his knowledge and specific order.

APPLICATIONS OF SPECTRAL DOPPLER FOR FETAL CARDIAC EVALUATION

Among the fetal applications of spectral Doppler velocimetry are assessments of systolic fetal cardiac function, volume flows, diastolic function, and valvular insufficiency. Since the orientation of the fetal heart may vary and is not under the examiner's control, angle correction often has to be used for quantitative Doppler velocimetry. Nonetheless, efforts should be made to decrease the incident angle to less than 30 degrees whenever possible, since the accuracy of angle correction decreases as the cosine function gets steeper. Reed et al[12] published normal flow velocity values for aortic, pulmonary, tricuspid, and mitral flow for the human fetus. These observations established the right heart dominance of the fetus with higher tricuspid than mitral velocities (Fig. 14–1). Such velocities can provide indices of cardiac performance as well as information on the distribution of intracardiac flows and cardiac output. As an example, Berman et al[2] suggest that cardiac acceleration time for the aorta as well as peak aortic velocity is an indice of left ventricular performance. The maintenance of forward flow in the descending aorta throughout diastole (i.e., a relatively high descending aorta velocity at end-diastole in comparison to peak systolic aortic or umbilical artery velocities) is

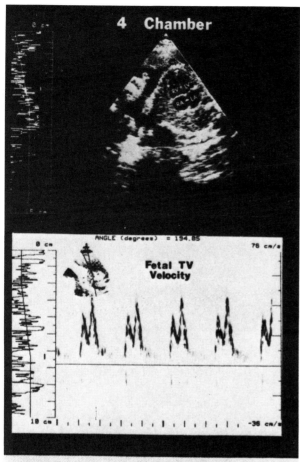

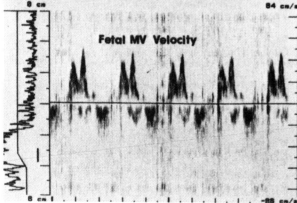

Figure 14–1. Normal right (middle panel) and left (lower panel) atrioventricular valve Doppler velocities for the human fetus obtained from the four-chamber view (upper panel). The right-sided velocities are almost always higher. LA = left atrium; LV = left ventricle; MV = mitral valve; RA = right atrium; RV = right ventricular; TV = tricuspid valve. (Reprinted by permission of the American Heart Association, from Reed KL et al [1986]: Cardiac Doppler flow velocities in human fetuses. Circ 73:41.)

also believed to be an indicator of low placental resistance. Loss of end-diastolic forward flow in the aorta has been associated with maternal hypertension and intrauterine growth retardation. Cardiac output and the length of diastole (heart rate) also undoubtedly influence the

relationships of systolic and diastolic aortic and umbilical artery flow. The velocity time integral (the area under a systolic aortic or pulmonary flow curve or under a diastolic atrioventricular valve flow curve) can be easily measured through planimetery to provide estimates of volume flow. For example, aortic and pulmonary velocity time intervals were decreased (consistent with low cardiac output) in two fetuses we studied with hydrops fetalis and intrauterine myocarditis. In contrast, flow velocity integrals were increased during systole across semilunar valves and in diastole across atrioventricular valves in fetuses we studied with intrauterine anemia and increased cardiac output. We have also observed increases in mitral and tricuspid flow velocity integrals after conversion of fetal tachycardia to sinus rhythm, indicating that cardiac output improved despite the lower heart rate after conversion. Using flow velocity integrals, we have demonstrated that the fetus exhibits postextrasystolic potentiation after ectopic beats (Fig. 14–2), a capability that has been questioned in view of the fetus's reduced cardiac compliance and reduced tolerance of volume loading. Doppler

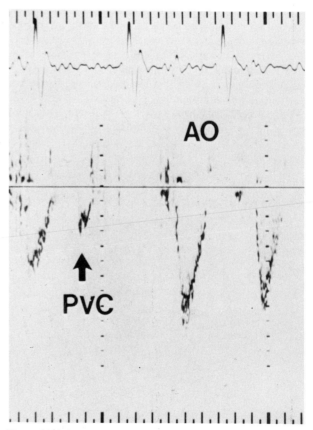

Figure 14–2. Fetal descending aortic flow is shown during a fetal premature ventricular contraction. Unlike the normal fetal QRS complexes, the QRS complex of the premature ventricular contraction was not recorded on the fetal ECG. The postextrasystolic beat shows a larger velocity time integral and a higher peak velocity. AO = aortic velocity time integral; PVC = premature ventricular contraction. (Courtesy of Kathy Reed, Department of Obstetrics, University of Arizona, Tucson.)

studies may also be used to look at flow deflections resulting from atrial as well as ventricular mechanical activity. Huhta (personal communication) has demonstrated a combined ventricular inflow and outflow view with a large sample volume, which provides a beat-by-beat demonstration of the relationship between atrial and ventricular activity. Such Doppler recordings complement M-mode traces in the diagnostic analysis and treatment of fetal arrhythmias.

Accurate estimates of volume flow can be calculated from the area or diameter of the flow and the flow velocity integral if the diameter measurements are made from axially directed fetal echocardiographic images or flow maps. Using this approach, Reed et al[12] showed right ventricular flows of around 307 ml/kg/min in human fetuses in midgestation and left ventricular flows of 232 ml, suggesting a right-to-left ventricular output ratio close to 1:3/1. Berman et al[2] showed descending aortic volume flows close to 180 to 200 ml/kg/min; these measurements are relatively similar to observations in fetal lambs[14,15] if one considers the increased flow to the head in human fetuses compared with sheep.

In studies on the sequence of diastolic filling in the human fetus, Reed et al[13] have shown that late atrial diastolic filling velocities across both mitral and tricuspid valves exceed the early diastolic filling velocities, especially in earlier gestation (Fig. 14–3). The ratio of late to early diastolic filling velocities in the ventricle (A/E) was found to be approximately 1.5 at 17 to 20 weeks' gestation.[13] Such diastolic filling patterns have been associated with abnormally decreased myocardial compliance (increased stiffness)[5] and are concordant with experimental studies, demonstrating gradual maturation

of diastolic function and increasing diastolic compliance with advancing gestation.[14]

Doppler studies in abnormal hearts not only provide functional data but also flow patterns that sometimes have prognostic significance. Silverman et al[19] have suggested that the presence of tricuspid insufficiency or atrioventricular valve insufficiency in fetuses with hydrops fetalis and structural heart disease is a sign of impending fetal demise; our experience has been the same. Further, image-guided continuous wave Doppler echocardiography (Fig. 14–4) can provide estimates of intracardiac pressures and/or gradients[20] when valvular insufficiencies or stenoses are present. The demonstration and characterization of valvular insufficiency and abnormal intracardiac flows in fetal examinations is greatly facilitated by real time Doppler color flow mapping studies.

DOPPLER COLOR FLOW MAPPING STUDIES IN HUMAN FETUSES

In clinical adult and pediatric cardiology, the recent flow mapping technologies appear to provide new insights into both normal and abnormal cardiac physiology. The spatial distribution and velocity profiles of normal flows are well characterized by color flow mapping. Color flow mapping also provides new information on the direction and extension of abnormal flows from stenotic valve jets and regurgitant and shunt flows and may have a role in quantitation.[8,16] Color flow mapping appears to carry equal promise in fetal cardiology. The flow map can show ventricular inlet and great artery flows (see Color

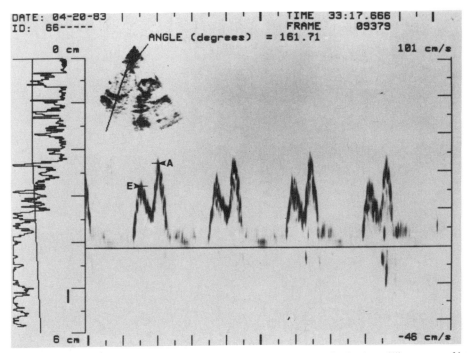

Figure 14–3. Early and late diastolic flow velocity peaks from a 26-week-old human fetus show the dominant filling pattern of late diastole. E = early ventricular filling; A = late ventricular filling.

Figures 1, 3, and 4) and can provide complete flow visualization of the ductal arch and aortic arch. Information on the normal flow profiles present at various points in the fetal circulation can be useful in evaluating fetal cardiovascular well-being. In view of documented cases of hydrops fetalis secondary to intrauterine foramen ovale obstruction[11] and concern over possible premature ductal constrictions in utero, we recently studied the flow diameters and velocity characteristics of both the foramen ovale (see Color Figure 2) and ductus arteriosus (see Color Figure 4) in the human fetus. Flow dimensions were expressed as a percentage of the diameter of the aortic root measured in short axis.[17] The foramen ovale flow diameter was 74 per cent of the diameter of the aortic root, and the mean A wave dominant diastolic velocity was 42 cm/sec. At its insertion into the descending aorta, the ductus flow diameter was 85 per cent of the aortic root, and the mean velocity was 86 cm/sec. The highest systolic velocity occurs in the fetal ductus, which appears to be constricted at its insertion. In contrast, we recently observed a foramenal flow diameter of 19 per cent and a turbulent A wave dominant foramenal velocity of 120 cm/sec in a hydropic fetus with premature closure of the foramen ovale, suggesting a transatrial gradient of up to 5 or 6 mmHg. At autopsy after intrauterine fetal demise, the foramen was 1.5 × 1.5 mm in size. We have also shown that the turbulent flows when imaged permit characterization of AV valve regurgitation in AV septal defects as well as characterization of transventricular flows and left ventricular–to–right atrial shunts. In fetal AV septal defect and in fetal Ebstein or other tricuspid dysplasias, a qualitative relationship exists between the degree of flow map turbulent regurgitant flow and the severity of valve insufficiency (see Color Figure 5); reverse inferior caval and umbilical vein flows can be detected on spectral waveform Doppler. Our preliminary experience suggests that these techniques will be quite useful in volume flow calculations, in quantitation of valvular insufficiency, and in characterization of the direction and orientation of intraventricular shunts (which are of low velocity in the fetus).

SUMMARY

While imaging systems and Doppler interrogation systems have not as yet been optimized for fetal studies, it is clear that high resolution echocardiographic imaging and flow velocity determinations already provide important information about fetal cardiovascular well-being. Currently available mapping systems have even greater limitations in imaging the very small fetal heart from the maternal abdomen wall, but the potential value of fetal color flow mapping is already obvious. The physics of sound wave imaging cannot be altered, but technical advances in equipment design will provide important improvements in the resolution, recording, and display of fetal flow mapping images.

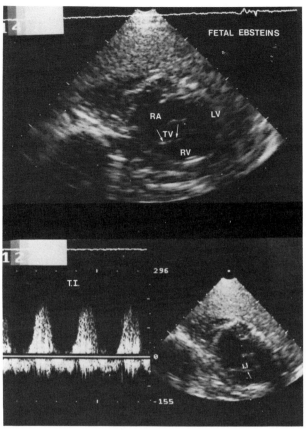

Figure 14–4. This fetal echo showed a large right ventricle and very enlarged right atrium (upper panel) and 2.2 m/sec of right ventricular–to–right atrial tricuspid insufficiency flow (lower panel) in a 26-week-old hydropic fetus who was later stillborn. The arrows identify the tricuspid valve. LV = left ventricle; RA = right atrium; RV = right ventricle; TI = tricuspid insufficiency; TV = tricuspid valve.

References

1. Allan LD, Joseph MC, Boyd EGCA, Campbell S, Tynan M (1982): M-mode echocardiography in the developing human fetus. Br Heart J 47:573–583.
2. Berman W, Alverson DC, Eldridge M, Dillon T (1985): Pulsed Doppler evaluation of the fetal circulation. In Altobelli SA, Voyles WF, Greene ER (eds): Cardiovascular Ultrasonic Flowmetry. New York, Elsevier, pp 411–430.
3. Griffith JM, Henry, WL (1978): An ultrasound system for combined cardiac imaging and Doppler blood flow measurement in man. Circulation 57:925–930.
4. Kasai C, Namekawa, K (1984): Principle and equipment. In Omoto R (ed): Color Atlas of Real-time Two-dimensional Doppler Echocardiography. Tokyo, Shindan-To-Chiryo Co., pp 5–13.
5. Kitabatake A, Inoue M, Asao M, Tanouchi J, Masuyama T, Abe H, Morita H, Senda S, Matsuo H (1982): Transmitral blood flow reflecting diastolic behavior of the left ventricle in health and disease—a study by pulsed Doppler technique. Jap Circ J 46:92–102.
6. Kleinman CS, Hobbins JC, Jaffe CC, Lynch DC, Talner NS (1980): Echocardiographic studies of the human fetus: Prenatal diagnosis of congenital heart disease and cardiac dysrhythmias. Pediatrics 65:1059–1067.
7. Lange LW, Sahn DJ, Allen HD, Goldberg SJ, Anderson C, Giles H (1980): Qualitative real-time cross-sectional echocardiographic imaging of the human fetus during the second half of pregnancy. Circulation 62:799–806.
8. Miyatake K, Okamoto M, Kinoshita N, Izumi S, Owa M, Takao S,

Sakakibara H, Nimura Y (1984): Clinical applications of a new type of real-time two-dimensional flow Doppler imaging system. Am J Cardiol 54:857–868.

9. Obrien WD (1986): Biological effects of ultrasound: Rationale for the measurement of selected ultrasonic output quantities. Echocardiography 3:165–180.

10. Dellenbach P, ed (1982): Proceedings of the 1er Symposium International D'echocardiologie Foetale. Strasbourg, Roche Bioelectronics and Milupa Dietetique.

11. Redel DA, Hansmann M (1981): Fetal obstruction of the foramen ovale detected by two-dimensional Doppler echocardiography. In Rijsterborgh H (ed): Echocardiology. Boston, Martinus Nijhoff Publishers, pp 425–429.

12. Reed KL, Meijboom EJ, Sahn DJ, Scagnelli, SA, Valdes-Cruz LM, Shenker L (1986): Cardiac Doppler flow velocities in human fetuses. Circulation 73:41–46.

13. Reed KL, Sahn DJ, Scagnelli S, Anderson CA, Shenker, L (1986): Doppler echocardiographic studies of diastolic function in the human fetal heart: Changes during gestation. J Am Coll Cardiol 8:391–395.

14. Romero T, Covell J, Friedman WF (1972): A comparison of pressure-volume relations of the fetal, newborn and adult heart. Am J Physiol 222:1285–1290.

15. Rudolph AM, Heymann MA (1974): Fetal and neonatal circulation and respiration. Ann Rev Physiol 36:187–207.

16. Sahn DJ (1985): Real-time two-dimensional Doppler echocardiographic flow mapping. Circulation 71:849–853.

17. Sahn DJ, Hagen-Ansert S (1986): Echo Doppler color flow mapping studies for elucidation of cardiovascular anatomy and physiology in the human fetus. (Abstr) J Am Coll Cardiol 7:37A.

18. Sahn DJ, Lange LW, Allen HD, Goldberg SJ, Anderson C, Giles H, Haber K (1980): Quantitative real-time cross-sectional echocardiography in the developing normal human fetus and newborn. Circulation 62:588–597.

19. Silverman NH, Kleinman CS, Rudolph AM, Copel JA, Weinstein EM, Enderlein MA, Golbus M (1985): Fetal atrioventricular valve insufficiency associated with nonimmune hydrops: A two-dimensional echocardiographic and pulsed Doppler ultrasound study. Circulation 72:825–832.

20. Yock PG, Popp RL (1984): Noninvasive estimation of right ventricular systolic pressures by Doppler ultrasound in patients with tricuspid regurgitation. Circulation 70:657–662.

15 FETAL DIAGNOSIS OF CONGENITAL HEART DISEASE

James C. Huhta

The effort and cooperation necessary for accurate diagnosis of congenital defects prior to birth demand that the question be asked, why is it important? If accurate prenatal diagnosis of congenital heart disease is possible, what are the options for its application?

Knowledge of a congenital heart defect in utero requires prenatal counseling of the parents regarding the likely outcome prior to and after birth, with and without any intervention, as well as increased surveillance of the pregnancy. The latter is required both to detect the presence of other noncardiac lesions (such as genetic abnormalities or potentially treatable defects) and to determine whether the lesions identified become more severe with increasing gestational age. When the heart defect identified prenatally is one that causes fetal compromise or a potentially shortened pregnancy, obstetric management may be altered. Whether the detection of congenital heart disease results from a state-sponsored screening system, an incidental ultrasonographic study, a positive family history, or an examination as a result of a complication of pregnancy, the overriding issue is the *accuracy of the diagnosis and the prognosis* for delivery and later palliation or correction of the congenital heart defect. Early experience with fetal echocardiographic predictions of cardiac anatomy has yielded a large degree of success.[1,2,11,16] However, technical considerations in fetal imaging[9] give the fetal diagnosis of congenital heart disease no more and possibly less accuracy than is currently being achieved in newborn infants. The possibility of fetal surgery[15] for congenital defects makes the issue of diagnostic accuracy very important.

Prenatal screening for congenital heart disease by a perinatologist or pediatrician means a new physician-patient relationship—namely that between the doctor and the fetus. The recognition of the human qualities and personal attributes of the patient is the physician's first step in the relationship. Regardless of the gestational age or state or federal laws, it should be obvious to all that once the fetus is identified as a person in need of medical care, then the need for a "personal physician" exists. A pediatrician is well-suited to involvement at this point, since pediatric training allows the physician to surmise the likely outcome of a given heart defect. The participation of neonatologists, pediatric cardiac surgeons, and pediatric cardiologists in decisions about management of the pregnancy is mandatory from the time of fetal diagnosis of congenital heart disease.

INDICATIONS

The pediatric cardiologist should be viewed as a consultant in the area of prenatal screening and evaluation of congenital defects.[11] Optimally, he or she should be consulted after an abnormality has been detected—either of the heart or of a system associated with the heart, which would include nearly every life-threatening congenital defect. For example, a fetus with esophageal atresia will be more likely to have a congenital cardiac defect, which could dramatically alter the prognosis of the defect that first came to attention. Genetic syndromes are strongly associated with severe congenital heart disease, as is diabetes mellitus in the mother that is poorly controlled in early gestation. Drug exposures are associated with relatively few heart defects today (e.g., Ebstein anomaly with lithium exposure); however, a careful history will almost certainly add to the list of known cardiac teratogens, especially as more fetal cardiac lesions that are fatal prior to birth become identified. Maternal exposure to medications suspected of causing harm to the fetus, such as prostaglandin inhibitors, is reason to perform Doppler studies for the evaluation of fetal ductal constriction. The increasing experience with fetal arrhythmias reveals that a wide spectrum of rhythm disorders can begin in utero; many fetal arrhythmias that are benign, such as premature atrial contractions, may not persist until term. A positive family history for congenital heart disease is also reason for a careful prenatal examination, particularly with certain lesions that have a high recurrence rate (Chapter 10).

HISTORICAL PERSPECTIVE

Congenital heart disease has a natural and unnatural history. The natural history of various lesions was determined before treatment became a possibility. The first successful operation for congenital heart disease was ligation of a patent ductus arteriosus in 1938. The first successful open heart operation was achieved in 1957 using cardiopulmonary bypass for artificial support of the circulation. The first interventional treatment catheterization was the Rashkind balloon atrial septostomy which was performed in 1966; Portsmann first reported successful closure of a patent ductus arteriosus with a catheter system in 1967.

As these advances in treatment occurred, the need for a better understanding of each lesion's natural history and accurate diagnosis became urgent. A similar situation exists today in the prenatal evaluation of congenital defects. Eventually, the availability of effective antenatal treatments will stimulate collection of adequate information about the natural history of fetal congenital heart disease. Early experience in the surgical closure of ventricular septal defects in which there was well-advanced pulmonary vascular disease (Eisenmenger syndrome) was a case in point; only by proper patient selection can effective management strategies be devised. Therefore, the prognosis of a defect detected in utero is the key factor in deciding on management. Prognosis depends not only upon the type of lesion but also on its severity; unfortunately, the natural histories of many fetal cardiac defects are as yet incompletely known. In a lesion with what appears to be a poor prognosis, often little is to be gained by artificial termination of pregnancy, considering the emotional impact on the family. Confident prognosis is not possible with current technology prior to 16 to 20 weeks' gestation.

Factors that affect the mother's health should be considered.[1] As technological advances permit earlier fetal cardiac diagnosis, it will be possible to study the fetal natural history of various congenital cardiac defects. Such studies will be necessary to learn when in utero surgery will be beneficial, when early spontaneous uterine death will occur regardless of therapy, and when the fetus should await term delivery for postnatal cardiac surgery.

SURVIVAL WITH CONGENITAL HEART DISEASE

The situation regarding survival with currently available treatment of children born with congenital heart disease has changed in the last 20 years. Since the advent of surgical and interventional catheterization treatment of congenital heart defects, there has been a changing spectrum, increasing prevalance, and improving outcome for those so afflicted. One example is the infant with tricuspid atresia. The mortality for this lesion was quoted in 1970 as 85 per cent in the first year of life. Recent studies of surgical outcome have shown that nearly 75 per cent of children with tricuspid atresia will be alive at age 15.

It is evident that the prognosis for congenital heart disease patients is far from dim and continues to improve; nearly every category of defect has a large spectrum of lesions for which there is a well-defined treatment. The rehabilitation of the majority of children born with congenital heart defects and treated successfully with surgery is far ahead of that for any other type of congenital abnormality. Two persistent areas of difficulty are the neonate with multiple congenital defects, including heart disease, and the premature infant with a heart defect (see Chapter 32). In cases of multiple congenital defects, the noncardiac congenital defects usually determine the early outcome; for this reason, the fetal echocardiographer must work with a sonographer experienced in the intrauterine detection and accurate diagnosis of noncardiac congenital defects.

CLASSIFICATION—PASSIVE VERSUS ACTIVE CONGENITAL DEFECTS

It is now becoming clear that congenital defects may be divided into those that are passive or "active" in utero. So-called "active" lesions are those in which congestive heart failure develops prior to birth owing to either myocardial disease or valvular regurgitation (e.g., Ebstein malformation of the tricuspid valve, atrioventricular septal defect, or hypoplastic left heart syndrome with valvular regurgitation)[12] (see below). In such situations, polyhydramnios or hydrops fetalis can result,[10] and the fetal heart disease may well affect the pregnancy and determine its outcome. In many cases the fetus with a severe active cardiac defect does not come to medical attention until its condition deteriorates to a poor level or a spontaneous terminal event is imminent. Sometimes such complex defects are associated with a rhythm disturbance such as complete heart block.

ULTRASONIC TECHNOLOGY

Improved noninvasive imaging techniques have made ultrasonic imaging of fetal intra- and extracardiac anatomy feasible after 20 weeks' gestation. Fetal imaging requires high resolution at depth. The rapid development of real time, gray scale imaging allows imaging of the cardiovascular system of the fetus as never before possible.[9] Phased-array technology, computerization of imaging techniques, advanced digital scan converters, dynamic focusing, and annular array imaging now allow for improved azimuthal resolution and image quality not believed possible just a few years ago. Newer techniques give current equipment the cabability to image cardiac anatomy even at very fast heart rates of over 200 beats per minute. Gradually, experience is being gained with pre- and postprocessing of the images to optimize them for each application; the previous superiority of mechanical and B scan modalities over phased-array techniques has been largely eliminated, though some exceptions still exist in near-field imaging after birth (see Chapter 25).

Doppler techniques can aid in obtaining functional information about the cardiovascular system in the fetus. Concerns about energy hazards in the fetus[8] can be reduced by improvement in receiver sensitivity and better energy focusing. Color Doppler techniques are being applied to supplement other modes of ultrasonographic scanning (see the following section). Color Doppler provides information about the flow of blood in the structures being visualized (see Chapter 14). New techniques for tissue characterization may improve the prognostic capabilities for ultrasonography in myocardial assessment.

TECHNIQUE

The segmental approach to the diagnosis of congenital heart disease with a step-by-step methodology is very applicable to the fetus. The process consists of sequential identification of the side of the cardiac apex, the atrial situs, the connection of the atria and ventricles, the great artery connections, and the extracardiac anatomy of the arteries and veins. For purposes of screening, it has been stated that a normal four-chamber view of the fetal heart (Fig. 15–1) effectively excludes most congenital heart disease; this is true. Lacking in such a method is the detection of anomalies of the pulmonary and systemic veins; abnormalities of ventriculoarterial connection when there are two normal-sized ventricles, such as with transposition of the great arteries; obstruction of the left ventricular outflow tract, such as aortic stenosis (although right ventricular enlargement may be recognized in such a case); and septal defects. As a result, most of the early series of defects detected in utero were heavily weighted by very complex lesions[1,2] and do not effectively mirror the spectrum of heart disease seen after birth.

The atrial situs can be identified indirectly by the position of the descending aorta with respect to the inferior vena cava at the level of the liver.[11] When the aorta is on the left of the spine in the normal position and the inferior vena cava is normal, the atrial situs is nearly always situs solitus (normal). In situs ambiguous, the aorta may run with the vena cava on the right or left of the spine (in cases of right atrial isomerism), or the vena cava may be interrupted with azygous continuation located behind the aorta on the right or left (left atrial isomerism). Occasionally, the morphology of the atrial appendages aids in the diagnosis of situs (Fig. 15–2). In cases of dextrocardia and situs solitus with a normal arch, the cardiac apex is on the side opposite the descending aorta (Fig. 15–3).

Abnormal atrioventricular connection such as tricuspid atresia or double inlet ventricle is readily identified by fetal examination after 16 weeks' gestation in most pa-

tients.[1] A common and complex abnormality is atrioventricular septal defect, which is often associated with situs ambiguous. Instead of two separate atrioventricular valves, there is a common valve and a common atrioventricular valve orifice (Fig. 15–3). The presence of atrioventricular valve regurgitation (Fig. 15–4) may indicate a poor prognosis.[12]

Semilunar (aortic and pulmonary) valve abnormalities may be difficult to diagnose in the fetus because of limited imaging of these very small structures and their movement. However, the presence of obstruction to one ventricle induces enlargement in the other. For example, aortic valve stenosis often leads to hypoplasia of the left ventricle and relative enlargement of the right ventricle (Fig. 15–5). Fetal Doppler ultrasonography may not show a marked increase in the velocity across the stenotic aortic valve before birth.

M-mode and Doppler ultrasound techniques can be used in the fetus to assess cardiac function[7] and to diagnose rhythm disorders.[6] Typical Doppler velocity patterns may aid imaging in the identification of some extracardiac structures. Although the aortic and ductal arches appear similar, they can be differentiated by the origin of the brachiocephalic arteries from the aorta. The pattern of blood velocity is similar, but velocity is consistently higher in the ductus (Fig. 15–6). As another example, the Doppler velocity pattern in the fetal pulmonary arteries is quite different from that in the ductus arteriosus, but the two could be mistaken by imaging alone (Fig. 15–7).

Fetal rhythm abnormalities can be the cause of fetal demise, particularly in the case of supraventricular tachycardia. One of the premier successes of the application of ultrasonography to the fetus has been the ability to diagnose rhythm disturbances and to treat the fetus transplacentally by administering antiarrhythmics to the

Text continued on page 176

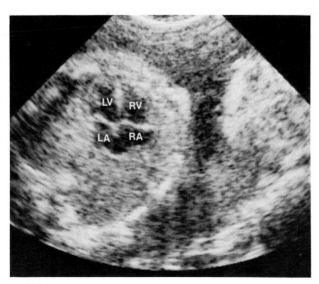

Figure 15–1. Normal four-chamber view of a fetal heart showing the left ventricle (LV), right ventricle (RV), left atrium (LA), and right atrium (RA).

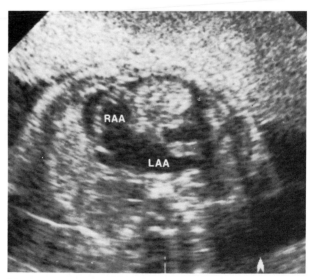

Figure 15–2. Fetal echocardiographic imaging of the atrial appendages. The right appendage has a broad base (RAA) and the left appendage has a narrower base (LAA). Such imaging of the morphology of the atrial appendages may aid the diagnosis of atrial situs.

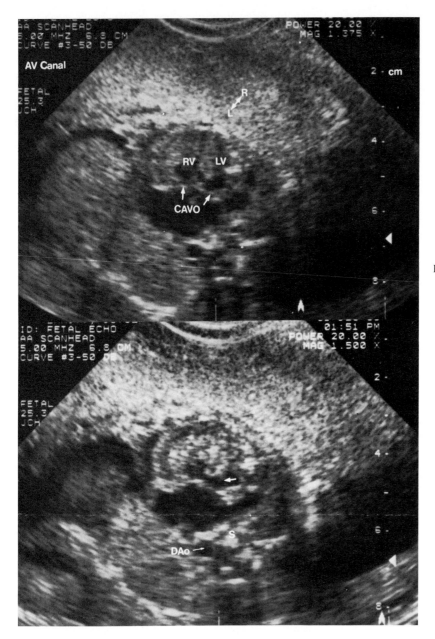

Figure 15–3. Complex congenital heart disease at 25 weeks' gestation. There is complete atrioventricular septal defect with a common AV orifice (CAVO) and a free-floating anterior bridging leaflet (arrow in upper panel) with a common atrium. The descending aorta (DAo) (lower panel) is to the left of the spine (S) and there is dextrocardia. LV = left ventricle; RV = right ventricle; L = left; R = right.

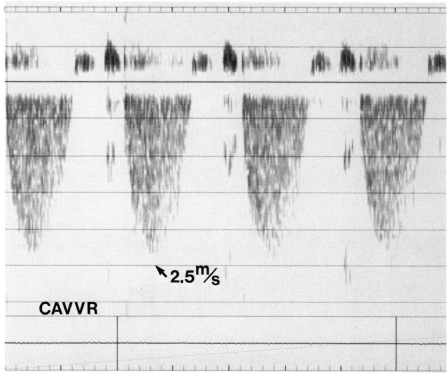

Figure 15–4. Fetal continuous wave Doppler showing common atrioventricular valve regurgitation (CAVVR) in an 18-week-old fetus with a single ventricle. The holosystolic nature of the velocity jet and the high velocity (2.5 meters per second) indicate significant valve leak in the fetus using current techniques.

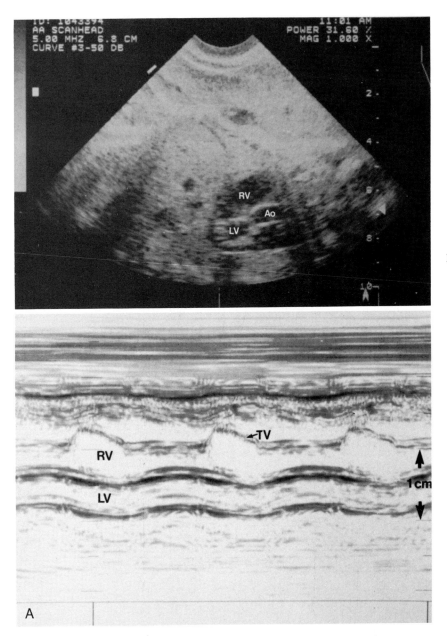

Figure 15–5. *A,* Fetal echocardiography at 33 weeks' gestation in a fetus with critical aortic valve stenosis and hypoplasia of the left ventricle (LV). In the imaging portion of the study the marked enlargement of the right ventricle (RV) is noted with echogenicity of the left ventricular walls. The M-mode shows the hypoplasia of the left ventricle. There is enlargement of the ascending aorta with respect to the aortic valve anulus, which is hypoplastic.

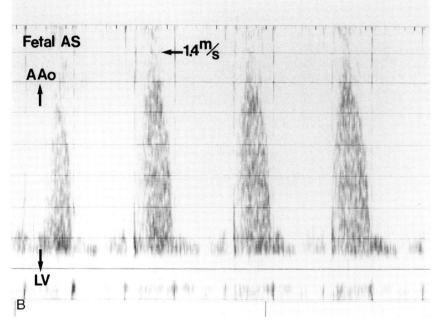

Figure 15–5 *Continued. B*, Fetal pulsed Doppler in the ascending aorta shows a slightly increased velocity of 1.4 meters per second due to fetal aortic stenosis (AS). This velocity pattern confirms the presence of a pressure gradient between the left ventricle (LV) and the ascending aorta (AAo).

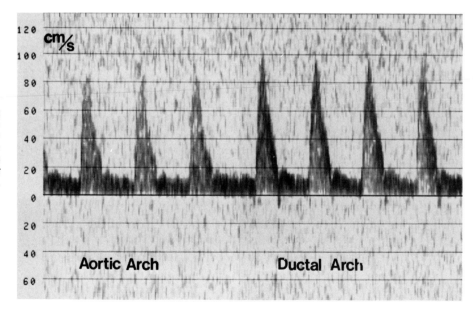

Figure 15–6. Fetal Doppler comparing aortic arch (left) and the ductus arteriosus (right). Note that the velocity in the ductus arteriosus is normally higher than that in the aortic arch (100 versus 80 cm/sec), but diastolic runoff in the two vessels is similar. cm = centimeter; s = second.

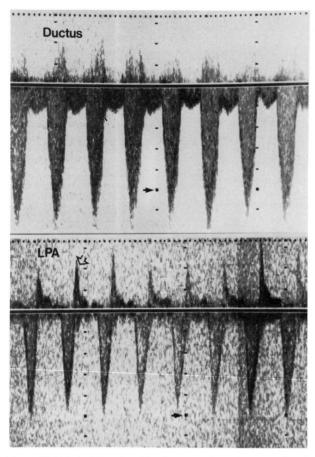

Figure 15–7. Pulsed Doppler of the ductus arteriosus (upper panel) and left pulmonary artery (LPA) (lower panel) velocity patterns. The ductal pattern is a higher systolic peak (upper limits of normal at 1.4 meters per second in this normal fetus), with a lower velocity directed toward the descending aorta in diastole. In contrast, the LPA has a high peak systolic velocity but reversal of flow in early diastole (open black arrow), confirming that the pulmonary bed in the human fetus has relatively high resistance. Solid black arrows indicate 1 meter per second velocity.

mother. Doppler ultrasonography may aid in the rhythm diagnosis (Fig. 15–8).[13] It is also important to differentiate between cardiac and noncardiac causes of hydrops fetalis, which, for example, could be due to Rh disease with some fetal tachycardia. However, in such situations the anemia is responsible for fetal tachycardia. In a recent case of severe hydrops fetalis the atrial rate appeared to be fast owing to a large pleural effusion and rapid movement of the collapsed fetal lung. The fluttering movement near the heart was not the atrial appendages but the prominent pulsations of the superior vena cava (Fig. 15–9).

PRENATAL CONGENITAL HEART DEFECTS—CLINICAL EXPERIENCE AND DIAGNOSTIC ACCURACY

Diagnostic Errors

In a series of 30 consecutive fetuses, two fetuses with moderate or large ventricular defects were not diagnosed.

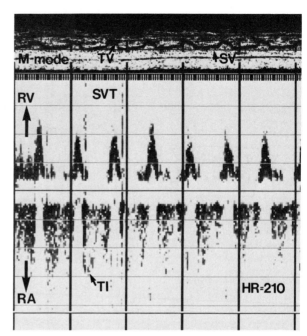

Figure 15–8. Fetal Doppler of the tricuspid valve during supraventricular tachycardia at a rate of 210 per minute. Tricuspid insufficiency (TI) was present. RA = right atrium; RV = right ventricle.

In a fetus with left atrial isomerism and atrioventricular septal defect, most of the intracardiac diagnosis was correct; however, the most important anomaly, interrupted aortic arch, was missed. In a patient with tricuspid atresia, the diagnosis of mitral atresia was made erroneously.

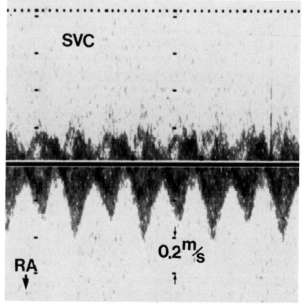

Figure 15–9. Fetal Doppler velocity in the superior vena cava (SVC) in a fetus with severe hydrops fetalis of unknown cause and a normal heart rate. The prominent biphasic pattern of blood velocity toward the right atrium (RA) in the superior cava was transmitted to the pleural effusion, making the heart rate appear to be approximately 300 beats per minute. Time marks = 1 second between depth markers.

Prognosis

In a recent review of imaging combined with Doppler techniques in the evaluation of intrauterine congenital heart defects at Baylor College of Medicine, my department found that significant atrioventricular valve regurgitation in association with structural congenital heart disease correlated with a poor prognosis for the pregnancy and survival of the child. In that study, the characteristics of "significant" regurgitation were defined by occurrence throughout systole and by high peak velocity (greater than 2 meters per second), indicating a signal of more than trivial intensity (Fig. 15–4).

At times, the prognosis of one defect is altered by the presence of another. For example, pulmonary stenosis will improve the survival of a child with many types of interventricular defect.[4]

Impact

From the preceding discussion it is clear that most types of cardiac abnormalities detected in utero are not amenable to treatment and many have a poor prognosis. However, advances in the understanding of the functional problems associated with "active" congenital heart disease before birth are teaching us lessons in the evaluation of the fetus with a normal heart. For example, fetal constriction of the ductus arteriosus has long been suspected to cause persistent pulmonary hypertension of the newborn syndrome (PPHNS). By applying skills learned in the evaluation of congenital heart disease, it is now possible to evaluate the state of the ductus using Doppler fetal echocardiography (Fig. 15–10). Such skills may lead to reassessment of use of prostaglandin inhibitors in the treatment of preterm labor.[5]

Doppler techniques supplement imaging by providing a functional correlate to other findings in complicated pregnancies. Measurement of umbilical cord Doppler pattern is now being widely applied for the rough assessment of the placental resistance. A high systolic-to-diastolic ratio suggests a high placental resistance and is associated with growth retardation from placental insufficiency (Fig. 15–11).[14] A congenital malformation may lead to abnormalities of the velocity of flow on color Doppler, which are clues to the diagnosis (see Chapter 14).

Cost and Ethical Considerations

Regarding the cost of treatment of congenital heart defects, one often hears that from a societal point of view, it would be cost-effective to perform abortions in all cases that would otherwise need cardiac surgery under 1 year of age after birth. Some assumptions and a few calculations are in order to test this idea, for it violates the ethical and moral beliefs of many patients and seems diametrically opposed to the concept that physicians are to treat their patients and "do no harm."

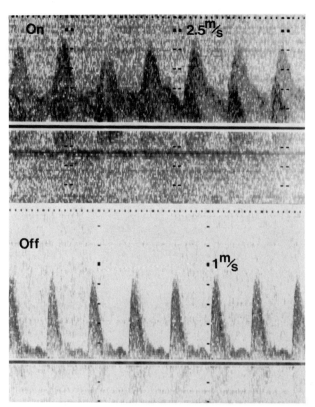

Figure 15–10. Fetal Doppler of a fetus at 27 weeks' gestation with constriction of the ductus arteriosus due to the use of indomethacin for the treatment of preterm labor. The increased systolic and diastolic velocities (upper panel) *on* indomethacin resolved completely, with reversion to the normal pattern (lower panel) after 36 hours *off* indomethacin. m/s = meters per second.

What If . . . ?

If we assume a country with 10 million people, nationalized health care, and mandatory abortion for certain defects (a situation currently existing in some countries today) and a birth rate of 18.5 per thousand population, or 185,000 births, then 1350 children (0.7 per cent) will be born per year with congenital heart disease, and approximately 385 (0.2 per cent) will require cardiac surgery in the first year. The cost of diagnosis and treatment includes cardiac centers numbering about one per 2 million population.[5] We will also assume that each will require a cardiac surgeon ($150,000), cardiologist ($50,000), house officer ($35,000), and operating room ($100,000) used only for surgery for infants under 1 year of age (a situation not unlike that existing in many U.S. low volume centers today). The cost of diagnosis, surgery, and postoperative care would be approximately $1.7 million. Alternatively, using cost figures for the first postnatal year obtained in the 1970s in this country from the New England Regional Infant Cardiac Program, each infant would cost an average of $6000[3] to treat. Therefore, the total cost for all 385 infants would be $2.3 million. We will assume that either the infant dies or survives without sequelae requiring more than routine follow-up visits.

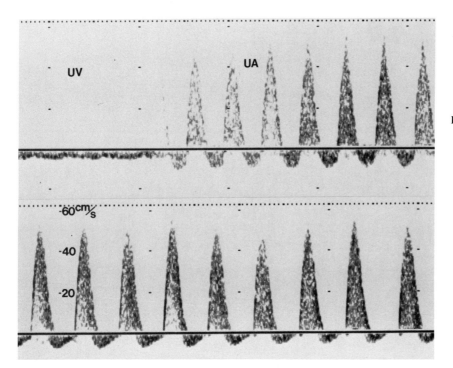

Figure 15–11. Umbilical cord Doppler in a severely growth retarded fetus, the infant of a mother with severe, cyanotic congenital heart disease. The umbilical vein Doppler (UV) shows continuous flow toward the baby (downward); moving the sampling site to the umbilical artery shows a biphasic pattern with systolic flow toward the placenta (upward) and reverse flow in diastole. This pattern suggests a marked increase in the placental resistance compared with the fetal systemic resistance.

Therefore, the latter figure would approximate the total national health cost of caring for these infants with severe congenital heart disease requiring treatment under 1 year of age.

Detection of all fetuses with life-threatening heart disease will require mandatory screening of all 185,000 pregnancies in our imaginary country. Let us assume that these pregnant women are ideally matched to the five major medical centers, and each center will screen 35,000 pregnancies and will require a specially trained staff, including three physicians ($50,000 each) to interpret 50 studies each per day and 10 technicians to perform them at $30,000 each (assumes 30 minutes per study = 15 studies per day per technician and 250 working days). Therefore, the cost of detection will be $450,000 times 5, or $2.25 million. The termination procedures would cost an average of $2000 (including autopsy) or $770,000. Therefore, the cost of prenatal detection and elimination of congenital heart disease requiring surgery in the first year of life would be about $3 million. There are no clear cost savings in such a hypothetical analysis, which ignores both the earning potentials of rehabilitated infants who are successfully treated and the costs of those survivors who are left with residual handicaps.

Since the first application of surgical treatment for congenital heart defects 50 years ago, over one-half million persons have been successfully treated by a combination of medical and surgical methods. Perhaps no group of patients with a congenital ailment are so well palliated or restored to normal lifestyles. Therefore, perhaps the most difficult decision in the scenario presented above (since only those fetuses with severe defects requiring surgery in the first year of life would be aborted) is "Who has *severe* congenital heart disease?" This question puts the physi-

cian in the untenable position of deciding which fetal patient, without an immediate threat to life, will be permitted to survive to term for postnatal treatment. Instead, the aim of in utero diagnosis should be the improvement of care for the babies and families affected by congenital heart disease.

References

1. Allan LD (1983): Early detection of congenital heart disease in prenatal life. Clin Obstet Gynaecol 10:507–14.
2. Allan LD, Crawford DC, Andersen RH, Tynan MJ (1984): Echocardiographic and anatomical correlations in fetal congenital heart disease. Br Heart J 52:542–548.
3. Fyler DC (1980): Report of the New England Regional Infant Cardiac Program. Pediatrics 65(Suppl):377–461.
4. Huhta JC (1986): Uses and abuses of fetal echocardiography: A pediatric cardiologist's view. J Am Coll Cardiol 8:451–8.
5. Huhta JC, Moise KJ, Fisher DJ, Sharif DS, Wasserstrum N, Martin C (1987): Detection and quantitation of constriction of the fetal ductus arteriosus by Doppler echocardiography. Circulation 75:406–412.
6. Kleinman CS, Hobbins JC, Jaffe CC, Lynch DC, Tainer NS (1980): Echocardiographic studies of the human fetus: Prenatal diagnosis of congenital heart disease and cardiac dysrhythmias. Pediatrics 65:1059.
7. Kleinman CS, Donnerstein RL (1985): Ultrasonic assessment of cardiac function in the intact human fetus. J Am Coll Cardiol 5 (Suppl 1):845–945.
8. Maulik D, Nanda NC (1985): Biological effects of ultrasound. In Nanda, DC (ed): Doppler Echocardiography. New York, Igaku-Shoin Medical Publishers, pp 453–475.
9. Sahn DJ (1985): Resolution and display requirements for ultrasound Doppler/evaluation of the heart in children, infants and the unborn human fetus. J Am Coll Cardiol 5(Suppl):125–195.
10. Sahn DJ, Shenker L, Reed KL, Valdes-Cruz LM, Sobonya R, Anderson C (1982): Prenatal ultrasound diagnosis of hypoplastic left heart syndrome in utero associated with hydrops fetalis. Am Heart J 104:1368–1372.
11. Silverman NH (1984): Fetal echocardiography: A technique and its

applications. In Friedman WF, Higgins CB (eds.): Pediatric Cardiac Imaging. Philadelphia, WB Saunders, pp 202–218.

12. Silverman NH, Kleinman CS, Rudolph AM, et al (1985): Fetal atrioventricular valve insufficiency associated with nonimmune hydrops: A two-dimensional echocardiographic and pulsed Doppler ultrasound study. Circulation 72:825–832.

13. Strasburger JF, Huhta JC, Carpenter RJ, Garson A Jr, McNamara DG (1986): Doppler echocardiography in the diagnosis and management of persistent fetal arrhythmias. J Am Coll Cardiol 7:1386–1391.

14. Trudinger BJ, Giles WB, Cook CM (1985): Fetal umbilical artery flow velocity waveforms and placental resistance: Clinical significance. Br J Obstet Gynaecol 92:23–30.

15. Turley K, Vlahakes GJ, Harrison MR, et al (1982): Intrauterine cardiothoracic surgery: The fetal lamb model. Ann Thorac Surg 34:422–426.

16. Wladimiroff JW, Stewart PA, Tonge HM (1984): The role of diagnostic ultrasound in the study of fetal cardiac abnormalities. Ultrasound Med Biol 10:457–463.

16 FETAL ARRHYTHMIAS

Lindsey D. Allan

A fetal arrhythmia can be defined as a fetal heart rate of less than 100 beats per minute (bpm) or greater than 200 beats per minute, or an irregular rhythm. The fetal heart rate is normally regular at about 140 bpm, but variation of fetal heart rate within the 100 to 200 bpm range is normal and physiological.

HISTORICAL PERSPECTIVE

As recently as 1979, Shenker wrote "A tentative diagnosis of the type of arrhythmia can be made during pregnancy utilizing abdominal lead electrocardiograms. A more precise diagnosis can be made once the scalp lead electrocardiogram is available during labour."[18] The abdominal fetal ECG was difficult to obtain in every patient, as the signal required filtering and amplification by 100 times. The abdominal fetal ECG could not demonstrate P waves, such that the elucidation of arrhythmias was not always clear. Despite these difficulties, Plant and Steven in 1944[16] reported the first case of complete heart block documented in intrauterine life; in 1968 Blumenthal et al[3] reported the first case of atrial flutter; and the first antenatal diagnosis of a ventricular tachycardia was made in 1959 by Muller-Schmid.[15] The observation that tachyarrhythmias could be associated with intrauterine cardiac failure or hydrops fetalis was first made in 1969 by Silber and Durnin.[19] There have been many reports of the benign nature of atrial or ventricular premature systoles, from a phonocardiographic study in 1930[5] to electrocardiographic studies in 1962[7] and 1977.[11]

The application of M-mode echocardiography to fetal arrhythmias has reduced uncertainty in the prenatal diagnosis of rhythm disturbances. Positioning the M-line to record atrial and ventricular contractions simultaneously permits accurate analysis of atrial activity in the same way as a postnatal ECG. The first report of M-mode analysis of fetal arrhythmias was by Kleinman et al in 1980[9] followed by a more detailed publication in 1982 by Allan et al.[1] Many authors have added similar experience and findings to this subject.[10,20] A more recent paper by Strasburger et al[22] reports on the use of Doppler echocardiography to record the relationship between atrial and ventricular contractions.

FETAL BRADYCARDIAS

A fetal heart rate of less than 100 bpm can be due to a sinus bradycardia or complete heart block or can be caused by blocked atrial ectopic beats.

Sinus Bradycardia

Sinus bradycardia is defined as a cardiac rhythm of less than 100 bpm, in which, when observed with M-mode echocardiography, the atria and ventricles are beating at the same rate, with a normal time interval of less than 100 msec between their contractions.

Short episodes of sinus bradycardia, lasting only a minute or two, are extremely common, particularly in the early fetus around 20 weeks' gestation. When observed by ultrasonography, the fetal heart appears to stop, then slowly starts up again. Such episodes are said to be related to cord compression and usually are followed by fetal movement. Episodic sinus bradycardia is absolutely physiologic and of no pathologic significance.

Occasionally, more prolonged sinus bradycardia is seen in the context of nonimmune hydrops fetalis. Prolonged sinus bradycardia probably reflects severe hypoxia and is a preterminal event. Congenital abnormalities are commonly present in this situation, and other poor prognostic signs, such as abnormal flow in the umbilical artery, are often detectable. All cases my department has seen of this kind were less than 24 weeks' gestation. The only intervention we have considered appropriate has been elective termination of pregnancy. In patients who considered this unacceptable, spontaneous intrauterine death occurred in each case.

Blocked Atrial Ectopics

Blocked atrial ectopic rhythms must be distinguished from complete heart block, as they have quite a different prognosis. Differentiation can be achieved by examining the relationship between atrial and ventricular contraction; M-mode tracings show that premature atrial escape beats are occurring close to the sinus beat. The atrial ectopics may be irregular but are often coupled to the sinus beat and occur too close to it to produce ventricular contraction. Thus, a ventricular bradycardia results. This sort of rhythm disturbance tends to disappear spontaneously as the pregnancy advances and is not associated with morbidity or mortality. The fetus appears otherwise well, and there is no associated structural heart disease. In our experience, this arrhythmia has not proved to be the precursor of a tachyarrhythmia.

Complete Heart Block

In complete heart block the echocardiogram shows complete dissociation between atrial and ventricular contractions. The ventricular rate can be between 50 and 100 bpm, but is usually about 60 bpm. The atrial rate will be regular at 140 bpm and will have no fixed time relationship to the ventricular contractions. An M-mode echocardiogram showing these features is seen in Figure 16–1. A varying ventricular rhythm with fetal movement may be a good prognostic sign. Complete heart block can complicate the management of labor, as the cardiotocograph is unreliable as an indicator of fetal well-being in this situation. Complete heart block either can be isolated or can occur in association with structural heart disease. In our series, 60 per cent of the cases of in utero complete heart block had cardiac malformations.[4]

Isolated Complete Heart Block

Of eight patients examined in this group, two had clinical evidence of connective tissue disease.[13] The remaining six patients all had serologic evidence of connective tissue disease, particularly anti-Ro antibody.[17] None of the affected fetuses developed evidence of intrauterine cardiac failure; therefore, none had any form of prenatal therapy. However, the development of intrauterine cardiac failure has been recorded in isolated complete heart block.[2] When hydrops fetalis occurred in a case presenting at 28 weeks' gestation to the Houston group, direct transventricular cardiac pacing was successfully achieved.[23] Although the fetus succumbed several hours later, this approach is obviously feasible if considered appropriate in the individual case. There was one death in our series of eight cases, but this death was thought to be due to obstetric causes rather than related to the fetal heart block. Thus, in general, isolated fetal complete heart block is associated with a good prognosis, and the need for intervention is rare. Complete heart block can recur in a subsequent pregnancy, although recurrences are not invariable. At our institution one of three patients who have had further pregnancies after isolated complete heart block has had a recurrence.

Complete Heart Block with Structural Heart Disease

Twelve fetuses have now been studied in this category. All have had complex intracardiac abnormalities, with ten also having left atrial isomerism. An atrioventricular septal defect has been present in nine of the cases, with additional anomalies of the great arteries in seven cases, double outlet right ventricle (three cases), transposition (one case), or valvular stenosis or atresia (three cases). Seven of the twelve cases have presented with intrauterine cardiac failure. In four of these seven, the pregnancy was terminated; in two, there was spontaneous intrauterine death. Only three of the twelve patients remain alive, and they are awaiting major cardiac surgery.

Thus, in complete heart block with congenital heart disease in the fetus, hydrops fetalis commonly develops. The prognosis is poor owing to the complexity of the associated heart disease, often occurring with left atrial isomerism. When the diagnosis of complete heart block

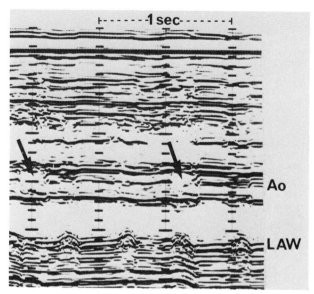

Figure 16–1. An M-mode tracing from a fetus with complete heart block. At the arrows the aortic valve opens (coincident with ventricular contraction) at a rate of approximately 60 beats per minute. Note atrial contractions at a rate of approximately 160 beats per minute immediately posterior to the aorta. Ao = aorta; LAW = left atrial posterior wall.

with structural heart disease is made in early gestation, termination of pregnancy is reasonable. In the hydropic fetus, such a course of action often preempts inevitable intrauterine death. If hydrops develops in late pregnancy, especially in association with operable congenital heart disease, early delivery may be of value, as it proved in one of our survivors. We feel that attempts at direct fetal pacing in the context of complex congenital heart disease are not appropriate.

FETAL TACHYCARDIAS

Sinus tachycardias of gradual origin to rates of 180 to 200 bpm are common, particularly in late pregnancy in association with fetal movement. However, a tachycardia that starts suddenly and reaches a rate of over 200 bpm, even if only intermittent, merits investigation. Fetal tachycardias can be divided into four different management groups: intermittent nonhydropic, sustained nonhydropic, intermittent hydropic, and sustained hydropic tachycardias. Before deciding on management, the rhythm disturbance must be recorded on M-mode echocardiography. A supraventricular tachycardia will show equal atrial and ventricular rates of over 200 bpm, with a fixed relationship between the contractions of each chamber. Atrial flutter will show an atrial rate of 400 to 500 bpm, with a ventricular response usually every second atrial beat, giving a ventricular rate of around 200 to 240 bpm. Atrial flutter is illustrated in Figure 16–2. A ventricular tachycardia will show the atrial and ventricular rates to be dissociated from each other, with the atrial rate slower than the ventricular rate. However, if there is retrograde conduction of every ventricular contraction, atrial and ventricular tachycardias

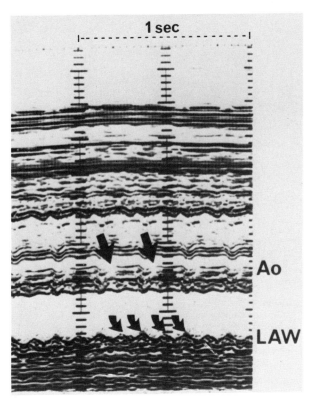

Figure 16–2. An M-mode tracing from a fetus with atrial flutter and 2:1 block. At the large arrows the aortic valve opens at a rate of approximately 240 beats per minute; at the small arrows atrial contractions at a rate of approximately 480 beats per minute are demonstrated. Ao = aorta; LAW = left atrial posterior wall.

could be confused. It is important to try to distinguish supraventricular tachycardias from ventricular tachycardias, as therapy for the one would not be appropriate for the other. Although ventricular arrhythmias are uncommon in fetal life, and we have not yet encountered one, they are recorded in the literature.[15] Therapy should not be started empirically before the arrhythmia has been recorded on M-mode echocardiography. Usually, fetal tachycardias present in the last 10 weeks of pregnancy, but a recent case presented at 22 weeks' gestation. Eleven of our 21 cases have presented in intrauterine cardiac failure. In 15 of these cases, the rhythm disturbance was atrial flutter. In none of our cases has there been structural heart disease in association with the fetal tachycardia. In one case, the fetus had evidence of multisystem viral infection at delivery. As viral infections can trigger fetal tachycardia, a viral screen of maternal serum should be carried out, and amniocentesis should be considered for viral studies when fetal tachycardia is detected.

Atrial Tachycardias

The Nonhydropic Fetus with Intermittent Tachycardia

Once the rhythm disturbance has been defined, management will depend on the gestational age and the frequency of the arrhythmia during 24 hours. The best method

for long-term monitoring is phonocardiography.[24] An overnight phonocardiographic recording can provide an estimate of the percentage of time that the rhythm disturbance will occur in an 8-hour period.

A case can be made for treating all patients with intermittent atrial tachycardias. One cannot predict whether an intermittent tachycardia will become sustained; if it does, it is unknown how long it will take for cardiac failure to develop. Once cardiac failure has developed, the fetus becomes more difficult to treat because of poorer placental transfer of maternal drugs. Also, the prognosis is less favorable once hydrops fetalis develops. However, despite these facts, we prefer not to treat if the arrhythmia is occurring less than 50 per cent of the time. If the rhythm disturbance occurs more than 50 per cent of the time and the patient is less than 36 weeks' gestation, the arrhythmia should be treated as a sustained nonhydropic tachycardia. If the fetus is not being treated, overnight monitoring and ultrasonographic evaluation for signs of hydrops fetalis should take place once a week, and fetal growth should be estimated fortnightly. Other indicators of fetal well-being, such as umbilical artery flow, should also be monitored.[25] As long as the fetus remains well, as estimated by these parameters, therapy can be withheld. If there is deterioration in the fetus of less than 36 weeks' gestation, pharmacologic therapy should be instituted. In a fetus greater than 36 weeks' gestation, we feel that delivery is the optimum course if deterioration occurs.

The Nonhydropic Fetus with a Sustained Tachycardia

Although the natural history of this condition is not yet clear in every case, our group feels that if the tachycardia is sustained, it should be treated. It is known that the outlook is unfavorable if hydrops fetalis ensues, but the time interval between a sustained tachycardia and the development of hydrops seems to differ among fetuses. We have observed a tachycardia of 240 bpm for up to 3 weeks before gaining therapeutic control, and yet hydrops did not develop. However, we believe a sustained tachycardia should be treated.

When an atrial tachycardia has been documented on M-mode echocardiography, the drug of choice is digoxin at the relatively high maternal dose of 0.5 to 0.75 mg per day. Dosage should be adjusted according to maternal tolerance of the drug. When hydrops is absent, fetal digoxin levels are probably equivalent to maternal serum levels, since equal digoxin levels have been found in simultaneously obtained maternal and cord blood samples. Thus, the fetus should respond within days of achieving an adequate maternal serum digoxin level. If there is no response, and conversion to sinus rhythm is the commonest response rather than slowing, we start verapamil at 40 to 120 mg three times per day orally in combination with digoxin. If therapeutic levels of both drugs have been documented for over a week with no response, other drugs such as procainamide or quinidine might be considered.[6,21] We have not yet used any of these alternatives. If control of the arrhythmia has not been achieved by 36 weeks' gestation, delivery might be considered the best alternative option.

The Hydropic Fetus with Intermittent Tachycardia

When presented with a case of hydrops fetalis in sinus rhythm, it is important to distinguish the cases of intermittent tachycardia from cases of hydrops due to noncardiac causes. If the heart is enlarged, there is some right ventricular dilation, and the pericardial and pleural components of the hydrops are moderate rather than severe, an intermittent arrhythmia should be considered as the possible cause. To identify this possibility, the patient should have overnight monitoring of the fetal heart rate by phonocardiography. Pharmacologic treatment should not be started until the type of rhythm disturbance has been recorded echocardiographically. Once the rhythm is documented as an atrial tachycardia, the patient should be treated in the same way as one with a sustained hydropic tachycardia.

The Hydropic Fetus with Sustained Tachycardia

When a sustained atrial tachycardia has resulted in hydrops fetalis, the fetus is at high risk of demise and should be treated as an emergency. When hydrops fetalis is present, we treat atrial tachycardias with intravenous verapamil. The dose is 10 to 20 mg given to the mother over half an hour. If the rhythm slows during the injection, this response is considered positive, the injection is stopped, and the mother is started on oral verapamil. Placental transfer is very variable and maternal clearance of this drug is faster in the pregnant than normal patient. Doses of up to 120 mg three times per day may be necessary. If control is not achieved on this regimen, digoxin can be added. However, in the hydropic fetus, placental digoxin transfer is poor, with fetal serum levels at simultaneous estimation being about 50 to 60 per cent of maternal levels. In recent cases, we have found fetal blood sampling by cordocentesis to provide useful management information, since the degree of hypoxia and acidosis can be measured as well as the fetal drug levels. Maternal drug dosages can be adjusted according to the fetal serum blood levels. The degree of fetal compromise may indicate a change in management, such as delivery, if the fetus is sufficiently mature, or direct fetal therapy, if the fetus is immature. In our experience, arrhythmia control has been most frequently achieved with combined digoxin and verapamil therapy, although this approach can take up to 3 weeks. Treatment must be carefully monitored by weekly maternal blood sampling, overnight heart rate recordings, and ultrasonographic evaluation of the degree of hydrops fetalis. In addition, fetal growth and umbilical artery blood flow should be regularly monitored. When combined therapy with digoxin and verapamil fails, other drugs should be considered, such as procainamide and quinidine or other forms of therapy. However, all antiarrhythmic drugs have a negative inotropic effect and are therefore hazardous in the fetus already in severe cardiac

failure. Further, conversion of fetal tachycardias by maternal drug therapy can be slow, and the hydropic fetus can be severely hypoxic. Thus, when hydrops fetalis is present, a case can be made for more immediate forms of treatment that avoid antiarrhythmic drugs. An intriguing suggestion was made by Martin et al.[14] They successfully converted two cases of supraventricular tachycardia by transabdominal cord massage. They felt this method acted by vagal stimulation. Certainly, direct cord compression using the ultrasonographic transducer on the maternal abdomen can produce bradycardia in the normal fetus, although we have been unsuccessful so far in converting a tachyarrhythmia by this means. However, umbilical cord compression seems to be an atraumatic method to try as a first option. The other options are delivery, direct current cardioversion, direct fetal drug therapy, or direct fetal pacing.

Delivery. If gestation is over 36 weeks, delivery is a reasonable option, as the arrhythmia and the hypoxia will be more quickly and easily controlled postnatally. However, early delivery is not without hazard in a hydropic fetus—one of our cases died after delivery at 36 weeks. Two cases delivered spontaneously at 31 and 33 weeks' gestation, the first being hydropic, the second nonhydropic. Although both infants survived, they suffered severe complications of prematurity. Elective delivery prior to 36 weeks' gestation should be avoided if possible.

Direct Current Fetal Cardioversion. Cardioversion with direct current is an attractive proposition, particularly for the conversion of atrial flutter, which is notoriously difficult to convert by drug therapy. However, the mother would require a general anesthetic, and there are theoretical risks of premature labor or placental abruption. To our knowledge, direct current cardioversion is as yet untried in the fetus. If effective, cardioversion with direct current would produce an immediate result, and hazardous drugs could be avoided. Perhaps direct current fetal cardioversion is a method that should be evaluated.

Direct Fetal Therapy. Using ultrasonographic control, it is possible to position a needle in the umbilical vein as it emerges from the placenta, and to take fetal blood samples. This route can also be used for fetal transfusion[5] or fetal injection of drugs. Direct fetal umbilical vein puncture permits immediate achievement of therapeutic drug levels in the fetus. A slow injection of digoxin or verapamil could be tried. We have not as yet been successful with direct umbilical vein drug injections, but it is a method that should be considered.

Direct Fetal Pacing. It is potentially possible to pass a pacing wire into the fetal heart by transventricular puncture.[23] A more attractive approach might be transvenous passage of a pacing catheter via fetal umbilical vein puncture. The umbilical vein leads to the inferior vena cava via the sinus venosus. The pacing wire could be passed from the inferior vena cava to the atria. This method might permit immediate cardioversion and avoid potentially hazardous drugs in the hydropic fetus. Potential disadvantages of transvenous fetal pacing include wire dislodgment, maintaining of the wire in situ for any length of time, and infection. However, perhaps transvenous fetal pacing should be an early option in the treatment of fetal tachycardias rather than being reserved for drug therapy failures as it has been until now. We have not yet attempted this form of treatment. In 60 per cent of our cases the rhythm disturbance has converted after maternal drug therapy. In the remainder, spontaneous (usually premature) labor has ensued prior to gaining rhythm control pharmacologically.

Ventricular Tachycardias

Ventricular tachycardias are uncommon in fetal life, but they must be differentiated from atrial tachycardias. Ventricular tachycardias are distinguished by slower atrial than ventricular rates on M-mode echocardiography. Appropriate therapy would be maternal administration of class I antiarrhythmic drugs. Our first choice would be diazopyramide given cautiously intravenously while watching for slowing of the ventricular rate. Any increase in the fetal heart rate after diazopyramide would suggest that the diagnosis of ventricular tachycardia is wrong and that in fact supraventricular tachycardia is present. An alternative drug might be lignocaine. If maternal therapy with these drugs fails, the more invasive methods described above could be considered.

Irregular Rhythms

Atrial and ventricular escape beats are common (particularly in the last 10 weeks of pregnancy) and produce irregular rhythms. Such escape beats can be very frequent or even coupled. Some authors have suggested that such irregular rhythms are strongly associated with structural heart disease, that such irregular rhythms are precursors of tachyarrhythmias,[10] or that such irregular rhythms are associated with a high incidence of perinatal morbidity.[12] However, our experience in the study of over 100 such patients has been that premature contractions are benign. It is important to exclude congenital heart disease when irregular rhythms are present, but if the heart is structurally normal, reassurance cen be provided to the mother.

SUMMARY

In conclusion, treatment of fetal tachycardias depends on the type and frequency of the arrhythmia, gestational age, and well-being of the fetus. A determined attempt should be made to control tachyarrhythmias prenatally, as in general these fetuses are otherwise normal. However, it is as yet unclear as to which mode or route of therapy will give the best long-term results.

References

1. Allan LD, Anderson RH, Sullivan ID et al (1983): Evaluation of fetal arrhythmias by echocardiography. Br Heart J 50:240–245.

2. Alterburger KM, Jedzliniak H, Roper WC, Hernandez J (1977): Congenital complete heart block associated with hydrops fetalis. J Pediatr 91:618–620.

3. Blumenthal S, Jacobs JC, Steer CM, Williamson SW (1968): Congenital atrial flutter. Report of a case documented by intrauterine electrocardiogram. Pediatrics 41:659–661.

4. Crawford DC, Chapman MG, Allan LD (1985): The assessment of persistent bradycardia in prenatal life. Br J Obstet Gynaecol 92:941–944.

5. Daffos F, Forestier F, Pavlovsky MC (1984): Fetal blood sampling during the third trimester of pregnancy. Br J Obstet Gynaecol 91:118–121.

6. Dumesic DA, Silverman NH, Tobias S et al (1982): Transplacental cardioversion of fetal supraventricular tachycardia with procainamide. N Engl J Med 307:1128–1133.

7. Hon EH, Huang HS (1962): The electronic evaluation of fetal heart rate. VII. Premature and missed beats. Obstet Gynecol 20:81–90.

8. Hyman AS (1930): Irregularities of the fetal heart. Am J Obstet Gynecol 20:332–347.

9. Kleinman CS, Hobbins JC, Jaffe CC, Lynch DC, Talner NS (1980): Echocardiographic studies of the human fetus: prenatal diagnosis of congenital heart disease and cardiac dysrhythmias. Pediatrics 65:1059–1066.

10. Kleinman CS, Donnerstein RL, Jaffe CC et al (1983): Fetal echocardiography: A tool for the evaluation of in utero cardiac arrhythmias and monitoring of in utero therapy: Analysis of 71 patients. Am J Cardiol 51:237–243.

11. Komaromy B, Gaal J, Lampe L (1977): Fetal arrhythmia during pregnancy and labour. Br J Obstet Gynaecol 84:492–496.

12. Lingman G, Lindstrom NR, Marsal K et al (1986): Fetal cardiac arrhythmia. Clinical outcome in 113 cases. Acta Obstet Gynecol Scand 65:263–267.

13. McCue CM, Mantakas ME, Tingelstad JB et al (1977): Congenital heart block in newborns of mothers with connective tissue disease. Circulation 56:82–90.

14. Martin CB, Nijhuis JG, Weijer AA (1984): Correction of fetal supraventricular tachycardia by compression of the umbilical cord: Report of a case. Am J Obstet Gynecol 150:324–326.

15. Muller-Schmid P (1959): Die paroxysmale tachykardie in utero. Geburtshilfe Frauenheilkd 19:401.

16. Plant RK, Steven RA (1945): Complete A-V block in a fetus. Am Heart J 30:615–618.

17. Scott JS, Maddison PH, Taylor PV et al (1983): Connective tissue disease, antibodies to ribonucleoprotein and congenital heart block. N Engl J Med 309:209–212.

18. Shenker L (1980): Fetal cardiac arrhythmias. Obstet Gynecol Survey 34:561–572.

19. Silber DL, Durnin RE (1969): Intrauterine atrial tachycardia (associated with massive edema in a newborn). Am J Dis Child 117:722–726.

20. Silverman NH, Enderlein MA, Stanger P, Teitel DF, Heymann MA, Golbus M (1985): Recognition of fetal arrhythmias by echocardiography. J Clin Ultrasound 13:255–263.

21. Spinnato JA, Shaver DC, Flinn GS et al (1984): Fetal supraventricular tachycardia: in utero therapy with digoxin and quinidine. Obstet Gynecol 64:730–735.

22. Strasburger JF, Huhta JC, Carpenter RJ, Garson A, McNamara DG (1986): Doppler echocardiography in the diagnosis and management of persistent fetal arrhythmias. J Am Coll Cardiol 7:1386–1391.

23. Strasburger JF, Carpenter R, Garson A , Smith RT, Deter R (1986): Fetal transthoracic pacing for advanced hydrops fetalis secondary to complete atrioventricular block. J Am Coll Cardiol 8:1434–1436.

24. Talbert DG, Davies WL, Johnson F et al (1986): Wide bandwidth fetal phonography using a sensor matched to the compliance of the mother's abdominal wall. Transactions Biomed Eng 33:175–181.

25. Trudinger BJ, Giles WB, Cook CM (1985): Flow velocity waveforms in the maternal uteroplacental and fetal umbilical placental circulations. Am J Obstet Gynecol 152:155–163.

17 FETAL DISTRESS

John W. Seeds

Deliberate interruption of pregnancy or labor because of evidence of fetal deterioration is a fairly recent practice. Before the widespread availability of blood banks and antibiotics, operative interruption of pregnancy or labor carried substantial maternal risks, and therefore obstetrical management was rarely based on fetal considerations.

HISTORICAL PERSPECTIVE

In a careful and scholarly review of the history of fetal distress, Fenton and Steer found that although published accounts of auscultated fetal heart sounds first appeared in 1650, fetal heart rate changes associated with fetal distress were not described until 1843 by Bodson.[15]

Encouraged by the reports of Hon[28] and others in the late 1950s and early 1960s, the techniques and the practice of continuous fetal heart rate monitoring before and during labor gained popularity. During these same years, the physiology of fetal respiratory gas exchange became more clearly understood and other interventions short of surgery, such as maternal oxygen supplementation, were introduced.

Severe unrelieved fetal hypoxia can result in fetal death or permanent neurologic damage. In a careful review of 765 stillbirths, Morrison and Olsen found direct evidence that hypoxia accounted for 43 per cent of the deaths.[55] Survival with disabilities can also result. Severe perinatal hypoxic-ischemic brain damage is considered by some observers to be responsible for 26 to 40 per cent of cases of acquired epilepsy.[4,46] The correlation, however, between fetal hypoxia and demonstrable physical or neurobehavioral damage is not precise. In the majority of cases of perinatal asphyxia with subsequent resuscitation, long-term follow-up of the infants shows normal intellect and absence of major neurologic handicap.[57] Furthermore, at least 50 per cent of cases of cerebral palsy have no documented history of depression at birth.[60] Nevertheless, it remains highly likely that early diagnosis and therapeutic relief of fetal asphyxia are critically important in reducing perinatal mortality and asphyxic morbidity. Low et al reported evidence suggesting that early diagnosis can be important in minimizing long-term damage.[44] A fetal hypoxic experience of less than 1 hour was not associated with long-term neurobehavioral deficit, but hypoxia lasting over 1 hour was associated with major motor or cognitive damage in 50 per cent of the infants studied.[44,46]

In order to understand fetal asphyxia, it is important to understand the normal fetal condition fully. The circumstances that allow the human fetus to thrive with an arterial partial pressure of oxygen that would threaten the welfare of any adult are unique. Since oxygen is the necessary recipient of electrons produced by aerobic metabolism, insufficient supplies of oxygen result in a metabolic shift to anaerobic systems that result in the production of lactic acid and eventually cause systemic acidosis and death if the oxygen deficiency is persistent or severe. Yet, the normal human fetus grows and develops in an environment of low oxygen tension without the development of acidosis. Oxygen is an element with small stores and a high rate of utilization in the human fetus.[35] Normal fetal respiratory physiology must be understood before any appreciation of the impact of the pathologic conditions influencing fetal oxygenation can be developed.

In this chapter, I will begin with a review of human placental structure and function and normal fetal respiratory physiology. Specific maternal and fetal conditions that might adversely influence fetal oxygenation will then be explored. Discussions of the fetal responses to chronic or acute oxygen deprivation and the clinical evidence of such deprivation as well as management options will integrate the basic physiology and pathophysiology into a clinically relevant summary of the condition known as fetal distress. Finally, a brief review of new techniques being developed for the monitoring of fetal oxygen sufficiency will give the reader a view of future directions.

NORMAL FETAL RESPIRATORY FUNCTION

Human Placental Structure and Function

Placenta

The human placenta is described as villose hemochorial.[61] Maternal blood enters the intervillous space from spiral arterioles at the base of each fetal cotyledon. The maternal arterial blood enters this space under arterial pressure, rises toward the chorionic plate, mixes with residual blood within the intervillous space, and bathes the fetal villi (Fig. 17–1).

The fetal villi are branching vascular structures that occupy the intervillous space with a core of fetal arterioles and veins. Respiratory gas exchange occurs as maternal blood circulates within the intervillous space, and fetal

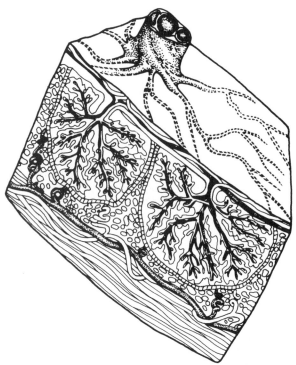

Figure 17–1. Shown is an artist's rendering of a placental cross-section. Two spiral arterioles are depicted entering the intervillous spaces of two fetal cotyledons.

blood is circulated through the branching network of vessels within the villi. Gas diffusion must transit at least three layers of tissue, including the trophoblastic outer layer of the villous tree, an intermediate stromal layer, and finally fetal vascular endothelium[61] (Fig. 17–2).

The trophoblastic layer undergoes continuous attenuation throughout gestation until it is quite thin late in pregnancy. The stromal element varies widely not only as a function of gestational age but also as a function of pathologic conditions including amnionitis or hydrops fetalis.

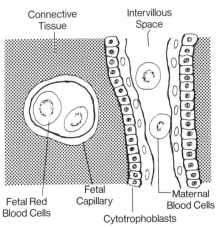

Figure 17–2. Shown is a schematic of the three tissue layers across which gases must diffuse from the intervillous space to the fetal red blood cells, and vice versa.

The size of the human placenta relative to the fetus drops as gestation progresses, finally being about 15 to 20 per cent of the weight of the fetus at term.[61] At any given time, approximately 40 per cent of the total fetal blood volume is found in the placenta. Fetal blood reaches the placenta via two umbilical arteries, which are branches of the fetal internal iliac arteries.[61] It has been estimated that 80 per cent of this fetal flow follows paths that allow for respiratory gas exchange, while about 20 per cent is shunted to paths that do not allow for exchange.[61] The uteroplacental unit receives approximately 10 per cent of the maternal cardiac output under normal circumstances, or about 700 ml per minute at term, via the uterine arteries and to a lesser extent, ovarian collateral arterial sources.[61] About 70 to 90 per cent of this flow enters the intervillous space with the remainder serving the myometrium.[61] Fetal venous drainage of the placenta is via the single umbilical vein to the ductus venosus and the right atrium, where the relatively oxygenated blood from the placenta mixes with venous blood from the superior and inferior vena cavae. A large fraction of the oxygenated blood crosses to the left atrium through the foramen ovale, and the rest enters the right ventricle. The mixed blood from the right ventricle then enters the systemic circulation through the ductus arteriosus, as the pulmonary circulation in the fetus is very small.

Maternal venous effluent leaves the intervillous space at the base of the cotyledon through venous channels that run parallel to the base and empty into tributaries of either the uterine or the ovarian veins.

Diffusion

Oxygen and carbon dioxide are exchanged between fetal and maternal blood by simple diffusion. The rate of diffusion is the result of several factors that result in a rate equilibrium described by Fick's diffusion equation.

$$\text{Rate of Diffusion} = \frac{K \cdot \text{area} \cdot \text{concentration gradient}}{\text{membrane thickness}}$$

*K = diffusion constant

It may be seen from this equation that the rate of transfer is proportional to the concentration gradient.[61] In the case of gas diffusion, the effective measure of concentration that influences the rate of exchange is the partial pressure of the gas in solution in blood. The rate of transfer is also proportional to a diffusion constant unique to a particular gas that describes the solubility of that gas in the substance of the effective diffusion barrier or membrane, in this case the three tissue layers previously described. Furthermore, the total rate of gas exchange is proportional to the total area of effective diffusion membrane. Finally, the rate of gas exchange is inversely proportional to the thickness of the diffusion membrane or the necessary distance of diffusion.

Many adaptive fetal physiologic mechanisms that permit survival in the intrauterine environment as well as many maternal and fetal disorders can influence fetal oxygenation either favorably or unfavorably by altering diffusion. Maternal hypoxemia would obviously decrease the effective concentration gradient at the placental exchange surface and adversely influence oxygen delivery to the fetus. A decrease in maternal or fetal placental flow, the result of either maternal hypotension or microvascular disease, would result in a drop in the effective concentration gradient between the two circulations and therefore a decrease in the effective transfer of gases. Hydrops fetalis from a variety of causes (see Chapters 18 and 19), including erythroblastosis, leads to villous stromal edema, thereby increasing diffusion membrane thickness and adversely affecting gas exchange. Furthermore, Naeye et al[56] found villous edema in 72 of 83 placentas with clinical and pathological chorioamnionitis. The degree of edema correlated well with fetal blood pH and Apgar scores. Subacute β-streptococcal infection has also been implicated in fetal asphyxia, at least partly through the mechanism of villous edema.[62] Finally, both partial placental abruption and infarction result in loss of effective membrane area, thereby potentially limiting exchange to an inadequate level.

Concurrent Versus Countercurrent Flow

When two circulations are in close enough approximation to allow for equilibrium of diffusible substances, such as respiratory gases, the direction of flow on each side of the diffusion barrier has profound influence on the nature of the final equilibrium.[51] In the case of countercurrent flow, the direction of flow is in opposite directions on either side of the dividing barrier and therefore arterial input from one source begins to equilibrate with venous effluent from the other. The final equilibrium, then, will depend on the respective rates of flow and the time of exposure but will finally be between the arterial input of the first and the venous effluent of the other (Fig. 17–3).

If the exchange circulation of the human placenta were of the countercurrent type, then the partial pressure of oxygen of the umbilical vein would be in rough equilibrium with the uterine arterial blood. Such is not the case.

The respiratory gas equilibrium between the maternal and fetal blood within the placenta follows the characteristics of a concurrent exchange model,[51,61] in which

blood of the two circulations flows in the same direction on either side of the dividing membrane. The oxygen and carbon dioxide partial pressures of the fetal blood in the umbilical vein achieve equilibrium with maternal uterine venous blood rather than maternal arterial blood. Such a relationship imposes an absolute limit to the maximum possible umbilical venous partial pressure of oxygen regardless of how much oxygen is given to the mother. The average partial pressure of oxygen (PO_2) in the umbilical vein in the normal patient is 30 to 35 mmHg, and the average normal partial pressure of carbon dioxide (PCO_2) is 35 to 40 mmHg.[51] Raising maternal PO_2 in the normal patient results in only a limited effect on fetal PO_2.[35] For instance, it has been shown that for each 21-mmHg rise over 100 in arterial PO_2 of the mother, only a 0.4 mmHg increase is seen in the fetus.[51] Thus increasing maternal arterial PO_2 to 600 mmHg in the normal mother by administering 100 per cent oxygen would be expected to increase fetal umbilical venous PO_2 only 11.5 mmHg and fetal arterial PO_2 substantially less. Despite this modest influence in the normal patient, however, in the case of maternal hypoxia, oxygen supplementation has a far more profound effect.[65]

Although the normally low fetal PO_2 and relative insulation from changes in maternal oxygenation might seem counterproductive, it is possible that a low fetal PO_2 is important in maintaining patency of the fetal ductus arteriosus as an effective right-to-left cardiovascular shunt during fetal life.[35] Changes in maternal PCO_2 related to maternal ventilation are more rapidly and effectively transmitted to the fetus and can have a significant effect on clinical management.

Fetal Adaptions to Low Oxygen Tension

The thriving existence of the human fetus at low oxygen tensions is the result of a variety of specific adaptions unique to the fetus (Table 17–1). At term, fetal tissues contain about 42 ml of O_2 and consume 21 ml per minute.[61] The per kilogram oxygen consumption of the undisturbed fetus is almost double the consumption of the adult.[53] Despite these considerations, fetal death does not automatically follow after 2 minutes of umbilical cord compression. Redistribution of fetal cardiac output, decreased oxygen consumption, and anaerobic metabolism allow the average fetus to survive undamaged for up to 10 minutes after its oxygen supply is terminated.[61]

The success of fetal development in a hypoxic environment hinges on oxygen content and net oxygen delivery per unit time, not the partial pressures of oxygen. Although

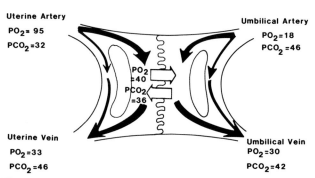

Figure 17–3. Shown is a schematic of the concurrent maternal and fetal blood flows. Normal gas tensions on the arterial and venous sides of the two circulations are depicted.

Table 17–1. FETAL ADAPTIONS TO LOW OXYGEN TENSION

Fetal Hemoglobin
  Binds more O_2 at lower tensions
  Higher concentration than adult hemoglobin

High Fetal Oxygen Extraction
  35 per cent normally versus 28 per cent in adult
  65 per cent maximum under stress

the partial pressures of oxygen represent the driving force in diffusion, oxygen content and net oxygen delivery are the critical limiting factors to aerobic metabolism.

Several fetal adaptions permit greater tissue oxygen delivery at a given oxygen partial pressure. These adaptions include fetal hemoglobin oxygen binding and concentration, fetal oxygen extraction, and local influences of respiratory acidosis near the diffusion membrane.

Fetal Hemoglobin

At a given oxygen tension, fetal hemoglobin demonstrates a higher binding affinity for oxygen than does adult hemoglobin (Fig. 17–4).

As a result, fetal hemoglobin binds and carries more oxygen at lower partial pressures and delivers more oxygen to fetal tissues at the same PO_2 than does adult hemoglobin.[61] The PO_2 at which fetal hemoglobin is 50 per cent saturated is 19 mmHg, compared with 25 mmHg for 50 per cent saturation in the adult.[53] At venous oxygen tensions similar to those of the uterine or umbilical vein, fetal blood is 80 to 90 per cent saturated, whereas adult blood is only 60 per cent saturated. Furthermore, at fetal tissue PO_2 levels of 16 to 18 mmHg, fetal hemoglobin delivers significant amounts of oxygen, whereas adult hemoglobin does not because it is largely unsaturated.[61] The steepest slope of the fetal dissociation curve is between 15 and 30 mmHg rather than 20 to 35 mmHg as in the adult. Finally, the concentrations of fetal hemoglobin are significantly greater than adult hemoglobin concentrations. While the average adult hemoglobin concentration might be 12 g%, fetal hemoglobin concentration is often 16 g%.[20,53] As a result, maximum oxygen capacity of adult blood is 15 ml of oxygen per 100 ml, compared with 19 to 20 ml of oxygen per 100 ml for fetal blood.

Oxygen Extraction

Fetal tissues can also extract a greater fraction of the available oxygen from fetal blood. While the adult typically extracts 25 to 28 per cent of the available oxygen,[16] fetal tissues normally extract 35 per cent, and under stress they can increase oxygen extraction to 65 per cent. In fact, some investigators have found in sheep that the fetus is capable of maintaining normal brain oxygen consumption until sagittal sinus PO_2 drops below 9 mmHg. Assuming a maximum extraction of 65 per cent and a constant flow, umbilical venous oxygen content would have to fall below 4.9 ml per 100 ml blood (vol %) to force a reduction in brain O_2 consumption.[3] Such a level of oxygen content would require reduction in oxygen tension to 12 mmHg.[50]

Bohr/Haldane Effect

Local biochemical factors can also encourage the exchange of oxygen and carbon dioxide between mother and fetus. As CO_2 rapidly crosses the placenta from fetus to mother it creates a local respiratory acidosis. In the face of decreasing pH, maternal hemoglobin shows reduced affinity for oxygen (Bohr effect), and oxygen release is encouraged, locally supporting diffusion of more O_2 across the diffusion membrane to the fetus.

Furthermore, as O_2 is released, maternal hemoglobin becomes an available blood buffer that removes H^+ from the local environment. Because of the Henderson-Hasselbalch equilibrium, the hemoglobin buffering capacity encourages the production of bicarbonate from H_2O and CO_2, thereby reducing local PCO_2 and encouraging CO_2 diffusion from fetus to mother. Additionally, there is an inverse relationship between oxygen and CO_2 hemoglobin binding (Haldane effect). Oxygenation of fetal blood therefore causes release of CO_2 and encourages fetal to maternal CO_2 diffusion. The reverse process occurs on the maternal side.

On the fetal side, the loss of CO_2 creates a local respiratory alkalosis that increases hemoglobin oxygen affinity and promotes O_2 diffusion to the fetus, while the uptake of oxygen removes the hemoglobin molecule from the buffer system and promotes the release of CO_2 from hemoglobin, promoting diffusion of carbon dioxide from fetus to mother.

ABNORMAL FETAL RESPIRATORY FUNCTION

Causes (Table 17–2)

Maternal Causes

Many investigators have shown that maternal intervillous flow is the single most powerful factor in the provision of sufficient oxygen to the fetus. Within the probable physiologic range of both factors, reduction of intervillous flow will have a far more profound effect on fetal oxygen delivery than reduction of maternal arterial PO_2.[61] If all else is held constant, maternal arterial PO_2 must fall to under 35 mmHg before fetal aerobic metabolism is hindered. On the other hand, if a 30 per cent reduction of uterine blood flow is sustained, fetal anaerobic metabolism and accumulation of titratable acid will result.

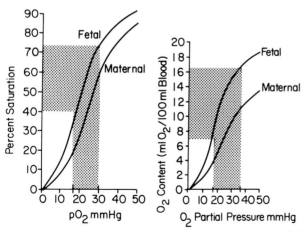

Figure 17–4. Shown are the maternal and fetal oxygen tension (left panel) and oxygen content (right panel) dissociation curves.

Clinically, both acute and chronic syndromes of fetal oxygen deprivation occur. Intrauterine growth retardation is a result of chronic intrauterine oxygen deficiency. In most pregnancies complicated by intrauterine growth retardation, uterine perfusion is usually adequate to support normal growth and development until a critical point in gestation unique for that particular fetomaternal unit. When gradually progressive uterine microvascular deterioration is present, the first manifestation of inadequate uteroplacental perfusion may be impaired fetal growth; clear evidence of fetal hypoxic distress may be a late event. In the case of sudden premature separation of a significant portion of the placenta, fetal growth may have been normal until the acute event of fetal hypoxemia. Some complications of pregnancy, such as chronic maternal hypertension, increase the probability of both gradual and sudden onset fetal compromise because such complications result in both a higher probability of chronic deprivation and a higher probability of abruption.[41]

Chronic hypertension, pregnancy-induced hypertension, chronic renal disease, and autoimmune diseases such as lupus erythematosus can all reduce uteroplacental perfusion through microvascular occlusion or constriction.[45] Both congenital and acquired maternal heart diseases also limit uteroplacental perfusion by limiting maternal cardiac output. Both restrictive and regurgitant valvular lesions limit the increase in maternal cardiac output necessary in pregnancy to sustain adequate uterine perfusion. Fetal growth retardation may be the earliest sign in such cases that perfusion is no longer adequate.

Uterine anomalies may contribute to uteroplacental insufficiency by limiting the development of collateral vascular competence. Normally, the uterus forms in the embryo by midline fusion of the bilateral müllerian systems. The sequence of fusion is from the cervix proximally. Failure of midline fusion will result in a bicornuate uterus, a uterus *Didelphis unicollis* (two uteri, one cervix), or, in the extreme, a uterus *Didelphis bicollis* (two uteri, two cervices). In cases of midline fusion defects, the main blood supply to a pregnancy will draw on the maternal pelvic vessels of only one side, rather than both, as in the case of the normally developed uterus with its extensive collateral connections. Intrauterine growth retardation and fetal distress in labor occur more often under such circumstances, presumably because total uteroplacental blood flow is limited. However, it is the common clinical experience that subsequent pregnancies of mothers with uterine anomalies fare better, perhaps because the uterine vessels involved are able to further hypertrophy with each gestation.

Maternal fever from almost any cause will result in fetal hyperthermia. The mother is the obligatory heat sink for the fetus. Fetal temperature averages about $1.5°$ higher than the mother. Since oxygen consumption increases as much as 10 per cent for every degree rise of temperature, the fetus doing well under normal circumstances but with marginal placental reserve might suffer relative hypoxemia during high maternal fever. Furthermore, maternal fever may cause redistribution of maternal cardiac output to peripheral vascular beds at the expense of uterine flow, and the consequent reduction in uteroplacental oxygen delivery

Table 17–2. CAUSES OF FETAL ASPHYXIA

Maternal Causes
  Chronic hypertension
  Pregnancy-induced hypertension
  Chronic renal disease
  Maternal heart disease
  Uterine anomalies
  Maternal fever
  Placental abruption

Fetal Causes
  Cardiovascular anomalies
  Hydrops fetalis
  Polyhydramnios
  Fetal infecton

Iatrogenic Causes
  Beta receptor blockade
  Uncorrected supine hypotension
  Oxytocin overstimulation
  Regional anesthetic-induced hypotension

can compound the problem of augmented fetal oxygen consumption.

Pregnancy induced hypertension, including preeclampsia, is a relatively common complication of pregnancy, with both acute and chronic implications for fetal well-being. When pregnancy-induced hypertension occurs, whether alone or superimposed on chronic maternal hypertension, arteriolar vasospasm reduces flow to the placental bed, among other areas. Many investigators have documented up to 50 per cent reductions in intervillous perfusion during preeclampsia. Furthermore, this reduction in intervillous flow has been shown to predate clinical hypertension by up to 10 weeks in some cases. Therefore intrauterine growth can be significantly affected before maternal hypertension develops. There is a strong correlation between decreasing fetal weight and increasing probability of intrapartum fetal acidosis as evidenced by umbilical cord blood gas values.[45] As birthweight drops below the third percentile for gestational age, the likelihood of cord acidosis rises to 50 per cent. Acute reductions in uterine blood flow related to exacerbation of the mother's condition cause additive effects that can result in fetal death in utero.[40,41]

Finally, although placental separation may occur with no warning and in the absence of other clinical complications, placental abruption is seen at a higher than expected rate in patients with both chronic hypertension and preeclampsia. Abruption compromises fetal oxygenation both by removing cotyledonary units from the maternal circulation (and therefore reducing the effective membrane diffusion area) and by causing an increase in uterine muscular tone. Subplacental blood is a myometrial irritant, and uterine hypertonia is commonly seen as a result. As intrauterine pressure rises first toward intervillous venous pressure and then approaches maternal arterial pressure, first venous drainage and later arterial inflow to the intervillous space are compromised.

Fetal Causes

Fetal causes for fetal distress are relatively few. Fetal cardiovascular anomalies that result in venous hypertension and hydrops fetalis also result in placental edema and therefore increase the probability of fetal hypoxia (see Chapters 18 and 19). Malformations of the fetal chest and abdomen that compromise fetal cardiac output may so reduce fetal perfusion of the placenta that hypoxemia and acidosis result. Congenital hydrothorax, congenital adenomatous malformation of the lungs, and thoracic lymphatic cysts are all capable of displacing the mediastinal structures and of compromising central venous return and thereby cardiac output. In addition, the consequent increase in intrathoracic pressure associated with some malformations can result in fetal venous hypertension, hydrops fetalis, and hypoxemia.

Polyhydramnios is associated with a broad family of fetal malformations and can increase to the point at which intrauterine pressure compromises intervillous perfusion;[1] fetal distress can result.

Finally, congenital infection with a variety of pathogens including syphilis, rubella, cytomegalovirus, and β-hemolytic-streptococcus, can lead to a stromal villositis, edema, and reduced placental respiratory efficiency. In addition, in some cases fetal infection increases fetal oxygen consumption beyond the compromised reserve of the infected placenta.[43]

Iatrogenic Causes

Therapeutic misadventures can lead to both chronic and acute uteroplacental insufficiency, and can result in either intrauterine growth retardation, acute fetal distress, or both.

The use of β-adrenergic blocking agents such as propranolol or related compounds may in certain cases be justified in the treatment of maternal chronic hypertension or dangerous maternal arrhythmias, but such therapy can also result in chronic elevation of uterine muscular tonus and a subtle but significant chronic reduction in intervillous perfusion.[37] Intrauterine growth retardation is seen more frequently in patients treated with such beta blockers, but absolute causation is difficult to prove, since in most cases the disease under treatment itself is associated with compromise of fetal growth.

Supine positional reduction in uteroplacental flow, maternal hypotension complicating regional anesthesia, and overstimulation of uterine contractility with oxytocin (Syntocinon) are all also known iatrogenic causes of fetal distress.

Simple supine positioning in the third trimester of pregnancy can result in up to a 29 per cent reduction in maternal cardiac output and a proportional reduction in uteroplacental flow. This reduction in maternal cardiac output is caused by uterine compression of the inferior vena cava and a consequent reduction in central venous return. The clinical team, therefore, must be constantly aware of maternal position, especially when fetal distress is suspected. The first therapeutic intervention in the case of fetal distress should consist of maternal positioning either on the left or right side to relieve maternal caval compression, which will in turn maximize central venous return and maternal cardiac output.

Acute fetal distress can also result from sudden maternal hypotension secondary to intrapartum anesthesia. Although most profound and most predictable with spinal anesthesia, maternal hypotension is also occasionally observed after lumbar epidural anesthesia. The sympathetic blockade that results from regional anesthesia leads to a direct reduction in systemic vascular resistance and a drop in arterial blood pressure. A proportional reduction in uteroplacental flow is to be expected as a result of this drop in perfusion pressure. Spinal anesthesia is used most often for cesarean delivery, but at one time it was commonly used for vaginal deliveries. The rare idiosyncratic reaction, or the equally rare inadvertent overdose, can produce not only profound hypotension but also apnea. Such events are not only emergencies for the fetus but also the mother. Treatment consists of first maternal respiratory and second maternal cardiovascular support. Delivery is accomplished as soon as the mother is stabilized. Crystalloid volume expansion is often all that is necessary to reverse the maternal hypotension from sympathetic blockade. If volume therapy does not reverse the drop in maternal arterial blood pressure, ephedrine hydrochloride is recommended. Ephedrine is chosen because the resulting generalized maternal vasoconstriction affects the uterine vasculature minimally and does not reduce uterine blood flow.

FETAL RESPONSE TO HYPOXEMIA

The clinical detection of fetal hypoxemia or fetal distress is based on a variety of observations, including abnormal changes in fetal heart rate or the absence of normally expected baseline fetal heart rate changes, impaired fetal growth, inadequate amniotic fluid volume (suggesting reduced fetal urine output), inappropriate levels of anaerobic metabolites in amniotic fluid or cord blood, decreased fetal movement, and finally, birth asphyxia with depressed Apgar scores and umbilical cord blood acidosis.

Fetal Heart Rate

Fetal heart rate is the result of a variety of interactive influences, including intrinsic sinoatrial nodal rhythm, intracardiac conduction, sympathetic and parasympathetic autonomic interaction at the atrioventricular node, and circulating catecholamine concentrations.[49] There is very little intrinsic variability in the heart rate of the very young fetus, as neither the sympathetic nor the parasympathetic influences exert significant effects before 20 weeks' gestation despite anatomic functional integrity.[49] The sympathetic system becomes progressively more active from 20 weeks' gestation onward.[49] Parasympathetic vagal influence is detectable by 15 weeks. Progressive slowing of the baseline rate and increased long-term variability become more apparent as parasympathetic influence grows into the third trimester[49] (see Chapter 13).

Long-term baseline variability in the form of accelerations and brief shallow decelerations indicates a normal healthy fetal central nervous system exerting normal control of heart rate. Accelerations that accompany fetal movement are normal. Immediate beat-to-beat variability is normal. Increases in heart rate can result from increased sympathetic tone or from decreased parasympathetic tone or both, and bradycardia can result from the reverse. Atropine causes not only an increase in baseline fetal heart rate but also a loss of short term variability, suggesting that variability may be more dependent on parasympathetic activity.[49]

Fetal hypoxemia may evolve gradually owing to a slowly progressive maternal microvascular compromise, or it may occur as the result of a sudden event such as placental abruption, uterine hypertonia, or umbilical cord compression secondary to cord prolapse. Any of these events can lead to pathologic alterations in fetal heart rate. The heart beat pattern observed may be related to the type of insult.

In the normoxemic fetus, the first observed response of the cardiovascular system to hypoxemia is a bradycardia mediated through aortic arch chemoreceptors when PO_2 drops below 20 mmHg.[44] In chronically hypoxic fetuses, several events contribute to the bradycardia: chemoreceptor stimulation, baroreceptor response to fetal hypertension, and direct myocardial depression from anoxia.[30] The reflex responses may be blocked with atropine. The direct myocardial depression is slow to recover and is not interrupted by atropine. Human fetal Doppler studies have confirmed changes in fetal blood velocity waveforms in the descending aorta during hypoxia, indicating increased peripheral vascular resistance.[33] If the insult is transient, as in the transient but repetitive influence of uterine labor contractions, the clinical pattern is that of a late deceleration.[49] Such a drop in heart rate begins after the contraction begins and persists after the uterus is relaxed. During late decelerations, which are normal unless greatly exaggerated, the fetal heart rate decreases slowly and returns to baseline slowly.

Such late declerations are to be contrasted with the rapid drop and rapid return of the variable deceleration associated with cord compression. (Variable decelerations are mediated solely through the hypertension-baroreceptor mechanism.)

The fetal hypertension seen with hypoxemia is the result of peripheral vasoconstriction.[34] However, fetal vasoconstriction in response to hypoxemia is not universal. The brain, adrenal, and coronary circulations are not affected.[51,53] Since overall fetal cardiac output changes little in response to hypoxemia, flow to those three vascular beds increases substantially at the expense of many others.[10,53] Such redistribution could possibly be detrimental if placental perfusion drops; indeed, Doppler studies in cases of fetal hypoxia or intrauterine growth retardation have shown decreased or even reversed umbilical vein blood flow.[32] There is also evidence that acute or chronic fetal asphyxia can serve as a stimulus to erythropoiesis and increase hematocrit. Increased numbers of immature red cell forms have been observed in the cord blood of asphyxiated newborns.[64]

In intrauterine growth retardation, analysis of the Doppler frequency shift profiles of reflected ultrasound pulses from blood in fetal umbilical vessels shows a dampening of the usual systolic-diastolic velocity relationship consistent with increased total peripheral resistance.[74]

Clinical correlates of the fetal redistribution of cardiac output in response to hypoxemia include reduced fetal urine excretion (because of decreased renal cortical perfusion), decreased amniotic fluid volume (because of decreased urine production), and asymmetric impairment of fetal somatic growth. The growth of the fetal brain is sustained while trunk growth is sacrificed. Catecholamine excretion is augmented, and metabolites have been identified in excess in amniotic fluid as well as cord blood samples of chronically stressed fetuses.[5,13,24,49,54] Hypoxanthine, an intracellular metabolite of adenyl monophosphate, is found in increased amounts in the plasma as well as in amniotic and other fluids after fetal asphyxia.[24-26,38,67,77] Saugstad and Gluck have reported there to be a good correlation between neonatal plasma hypoxanthine and pH and base deficit.[67] Beta endorphins have also been found to be increased in the plasma of asphyxiated infants.[20] Preliminary studies in rabbits seem to indicate that naloxone pretreatment in at least that animal model may be protective of the asphyxiated fetus.[8]

Metabolism in normal fetal tissue may be maintained despite substantial decrements in fetal capillary oxygen content by increasing oxygen extraction, but if the oxygen insufficiency is progressive, anaerobic metabolism will develop and metabolic acidosis will result.

Clinical Characteristics

Chronic Subacute Distress

The development of progressive, chronic, subacute distress is most often manifest as deprivational growth retardation.[70,71] As the fetus grows and nutritional and oxidative needs increase, maternal uteroplacental flow that was once adequate becomes inadequate. Usually, growth of the abdomen and trunk is impaired early, with normal brain and cranial growth sustained until late. Classically, transient or periodic fetal heart rate changes are not seen at this point.[70] Fetal blood sampling might not demonstrate acidosis or even substantial base deficit.

Eventually, however, a point of inadequacy is reached, at which even the slightest further deterioration in uteroplacental gas exchange results in bradycardia. Spontaneous central nervous system function is depressed, and baseline fetal heart rate variability, including the accelerations normally seen with fetal movement, is lost. Fetal adrenal stimulation from such progressive chronic stress leads initially to fetal heart rate accelerations after the additional new stresses and finally to a rise in baseline fetal heart rate.[49] Fetal heart rate variability in the early stages of hypoxia and after recovery appears to be mediated by the adrenal gland.[39,73] It is furthermore possible that such fetal heart rate responses actually represent adaptions to the stress stimulus. Beta receptor blockade in sheep results in reduced fetal tolerance for hypoxemic perturbations, suggesting the possible adaptive advantage of these influences.[36] Delprado and Baird found significantly different adrenal cellular pathology in stillborn infants depending on the duration of the clinical stress leading to death.[12] Longer periods of premortem fetal distress were associated with greater evidence of adrenal depletion.[12] Mild uterine contractions that would not represent a clinical stress to the uncompromised infant produce sufficient further reduction in uteroplacental flow in the compromised fetus, such that late decelerations are seen. As acidosis progresses, a fixed fetal tachycardia is often noted.[49]

CLINICAL DETECTION AND MANAGEMENT OF FETAL DISTRESS

As a result of chronic uteroplacental insufficiency, fetal distress may occur slowly and progressively long before the onset of labor, or it may develop acutely during labor. Appropriate clinical management of both conditions depends on sensitive and accurate diagnosis (Table 17–3).

Chronic Subacute Distress

Chronic subacute distress is often associated with chronic hypertension or maternal microvascular disease.

Diagnosis

The clinical diagnosis of chronic subacute fetal distress is based on a combination of clinical, biometric, and biophysical observations.

In any pregnancy, particularly in one with a known complication that suggests a higher than normal risk of fetal compromise, a significant discrepancy between uterine fundal size and gestational age might indicate fetal growth retardation. Ultrasonic evaluation should help clarify the clinical suspicion. If the clinical gestational age is accurate, fetal dimensions can either document normal fetal growth or confirm impaired development. If the gestational age is not accurately known, an observation interval of no less than 2 weeks may be necessary.[71] The most sensitive fetal dimension in the diagnosis of impaired fetal growth is the abdominal circumference. Estimation of

Table 17–3. PRENATAL SURVEILLANCE OF FETAL WELL-BEING

Clinical
    Uterine fundal growth
Electronic
    Nonstress fetal heart rate monitoring
    Contraction stress test
Ultrasonic
    Fetal growth
    Amniotic fluid volume
    Biophysical profile
    Doppler velocimetry

fetal weight using any of several methods has also been shown to be useful in the prenatal diagnosis of impaired growth.[59]

The frequency of daily fetal movement has been shown to be a sensitive indicator of fetal condition. If fetal movement is noted by the mother for a specified interval daily, and recorded, further evaluation is indicated if fewer than four movements are noted in a 1-hour interval.[31]

Other methods of fetal surveillance involve the use of electronic fetal heart rate monitoring. The earliest methods used continuous fetal heart rate recording during maternal physical stress or exercise. Fetal heart rate decelerations during maternal exertion indicated lack of uteroplacental respiratory reserve and the need for delivery. More commonly, the stress applied to detect marginal placental insufficiency is uterine contractions.[42] Contractions occurring spontaneously, or because of dilute oxytocin or nipple stimulation, produce the stress,[11,19,38,42] and fetal condition is inferred from heart rate responses. Late decelerations in response to uterine contractions indicate subacute distress.[2,23,42,58]

Nonstressed fetal heart rate testing evolved empirically from the observation that in most cases no late decelerations were seen when baseline accelerations were present with fetal movements. Such accelerations indicate functional competence of the autonomic nervous system.

The nonstress test (NST) assesses the functional competence of the fetal central nervous system at the time of testing. Such an assessment cannot predict the level of respiratory reserve of the placenta. If uterine activity increases or maternal uteroplacental perfusion deteriorates at some later time, the NST loses its predictive value. On the other hand, the contraction stress test, in measuring the fetal response to a given stress, is more reflective of fetal reserve and would retain some predictive value even if uterine activity increases or maternal condition deteriorates. The contraction stress test, therefore, is viewed by many as the more sensitive of the two.[19] Lin et al reviewed NST and stress test data from 85 growth retarded infants and concluded that the most accurate prediction of fetal compromise resulted from the combination of a nonreactive NST and a positive contraction stress test.[42]

Another commonly used clinical method for monitoring fetal condition is the sonographic biophysical profile (BPP).[3,48] Using real time ultrasound, the fetus is examined for fetal breathing movements as well as trunk and limb movements, and the volume of amniotic fluid is evaluated. These observations are combined with the results of the NST to provide a score of 0 to 10. Scores are evaluated as follow: 8 to 10 is normal, 4 to 6 is questionable (and the test should be repeated in 24 hours), and 0 to 2 indicates the need for immediate delivery.[47] Manning et al evaluated the BPP against the NST in 1184 high risk patients and concluded that a poor BPP better predicted fetal distress than a nonreactive NST. Manning et al also found that the predictive value of a normal BPP was comparable to that of the reactive NST.[47,48] When normal, both tests accurately predicted that the fetus was in good condition. When abnormal, the BPP was a more accurate predictor of subsequent fetal distress.

Clinical management of fetal compromise depends on the severity of the distress, the confidence of the diagnosis, and the maturity of the fetus. If fetal maturity is assured, delivery should be considered if distress is suggested.[71] If the fetus is not mature, or not likely to be, delivery may yet be indicated, but only if there is compelling evidence of immediate threat to either the mother or the fetus. In the case of the premature infant interventions short of delivery include maternal bedrest, augmented nutrition, and possibly maternal steroid therapy (the latter in an effort to accelerate fetal lung maturity and to improve outcome if delivery were mandated).

Acute Fetal Distress

Acute fetal distress is defined by such compromised uteroplacental respiratory function that metabolic acidosis and damage or death will occur unless intervention is undertaken. The diagnosis of fetal distress is based on a variety of observations, both direct and indirect, and management options range from the simple provision of additional oxygen to immediate cesarean delivery.

Diagnosis

As discussed previously, the fetal cardiovascular system responds to hypoxemia with hypertension, reflex autonomic bradycardia, and then direct myocardial depression. The fetal heart rate patterns associated with uteroplacental insufficiency include late decelerations, loss of beat-to-beat variability, and baseline tachycardia, as described in detail elsewhere.[49,76] The late type of periodic deceleration suggests that the fetus is responding to a hypoxic stress.[49] Maintenance of beat-to-beat variability indicates that although the fetus is stressed, metabolic acidosis and consequent depression of brain stem function have not yet occurred.[17,21,34,49,76] Some reports suggest that the fetus entering labor with no previous chronic deficiencies tolerates intermittent stress well, with prompt recovery of baseline heart rate after each contraction. The chronically stressed infant, whose baseline rate has adapted to chronic hypoxemia, demonstrates deeper and longer lasting decelerations when faced with further cuts in oxygen delivery during labor contractions.[17,38,49]

The positive predictive value of these abnormal fetal heart rate changes increases with time and is higher when all the heart rate changes are noted.[38,49] The combination of baseline tachycardia, late decelerations, and loss of beat-to-beat variability is associated with up to a 50 per cent incidence of fetal metabolic acidosis.[21] With sustained beat-to-beat variability and only late decelerations, one can safely conclude that although stress is present, fetal distress is not at hand, and a normally progressive labor might be observed further with only conservative interventions. Lack of baseline variability without periodic decelerations can by itself indicate fetal distress. Cibils noted that in the postterm fetus, fetal heart rate patterns prior to death may show only a fixed tachycardia with decreased beat-to-beat variability and no decelerations.[9]

Management

When electronic fetal heart rate monitoring suggests fetal compromise during labor, certain conservative measures may be employed with little risk and possible benefit while continued observation is underway. If a fetal heart rate pattern suggestive of fetal distress is seen during oxytocin augmentation or induction of labor, the oxytocin infusion should be stopped until the fetal condition is thoroughly evaluated. Uterine hyperstimulation is a common basis for fetal distress and can be easily corrected. Under such clinical circumstances, internal uterine pressure monitoring is indicated to evaluate accurately the level of uterine stimulation. Maternal position should be optimized to avoid pressure of the gravid uterus on the inferior vena cava. Left lateral positioning may be the only measure necessary to eliminate late decelerations, while in the case of significant variable decelerations, many different maternal positions might be explored to relieve pressure on the umbilical cord and to correct the fetal heart rate pattern. Sterile normal saline may be infused via the intrauterine pressure catheter to relieve cord compression secondary to oligohydramnios. Maternal oxygen supplementation should be started by mask. Although in the normal case hyperoxia in maternal arterial blood results in only a modest increase in fetal arterial oxygen tension, even a 10-mmHg rise in the PO_2 of fetal blood results in significant augmentation of fetal oxygen delivery. Several investigators have shown that nasal prongs are inadequate in the laboring woman; because of nasal congestion, most laboring patients breathe through the mouth.[77] In any given individual, maternal supplemental oxygen may correct the fetal distress and allow labor to continue.

Maternal volume resuscitation for maternal hypotension associated with regional obstetric anesthesia can be an immediate aid to the distressed fetus. Volume replacement may improve uteroplacental perfusion in severe maternal dehydration as well, but excessive glucose infusions should be avoided. Blomstrand and associates have reported a significant reduction in the tolerance of the fetal brain to asphyxia during hyperglycemia in sheep.[6] Intervillous flow is the single most influential element in fetal oxygenation. Modest decreases in maternal arterial blood pressure can cause substantial drops in fetal oxygenation.

Further Diagnostic Evaluation

If none of these conservative measures results in resolution of the abnormal fetal heart rate record, fetal scalp pH assessment may be helpful in further defining the condition of the fetus. Normally, the fetus enters labor with a scalp pH of 7.33 and experiences a slight drop to 7.25 by delivery.[19] A fetal scalp pH between 7.20 and 7.25 is possibly suggestive of impending compromise, and the test should be repeated. If a pH between 7.20 and 7.25 is confirmed and vaginal delivery is expected within a short time, labor may be safely continued. If vaginal delivery is not expected within a short time, cesarean delivery is considered prudent. A fetal scalp pH below 7.20 indicates fetal compromise, and delivery should be performed. However, fetal scalp pH is not perfect at predicting fetal condition, as up to 10 per cent of infants with a pH below 7.10 are vigorous at birth. Some investigators have shown that fetal scalp blood lactate levels correlate well with acidosis and low Apgar scores, but lactate levels are not better predictors than scalp blood pH or electronic fetal heart rate monitoring.[72]

The assessment of fetal scalp blood pH may prevent some cesarean deliveries that would be done on the basis of electronic fetal heart rate monitoring alone. The discovery of a normal fetal scalp blood pH might allow the continuation of labor when heart rate data alone suggest fetal distress. On the other hand, Perkins reviewed outcomes of 7100 births without the use of fetal scalp blood pH and reported no increase in either cesarean births or perinatal mortality. Perkins concluded that sensitive analysis of electronic fetal heart rate data alone can form the basis for successful perinatal management.[63]

It is possible for the maternal respiratory condition to influence fetal scalp pH.[52] Since CO_2 crosses the placenta rapidly, maternal respiratory alkalosis from hyperventilation is rapidly transmitted to the fetus and can mask a fetal metabolic acidosis.[52,68] Many authors, therefore, recommend comparison of fetal scalp pH to maternal mixed venous pH to confirm the diagnosis of fetal distress. Maternal-fetal pH differences less than 0.15 are normal; differences over 0.20 indicate fetal acidosis regardless of absolute pH.[68] Maternal-fetal pH differences between 0.15 and 0.20 are borderline, and the test should be repeated within 1 hour.

Delivery

The final assessment of fetal condition and the prognosis for delivery are unique to each case. The multigravida making rapid progress toward vaginal delivery at 7 cm of dilation might be observed with late decelerations and a fetal scalp pH of 7.22, whereas the fetus of a primagravida at 4 cm with late decelerations and a pH of 7.25 might be more safely managed with cesarean delivery. Scalp pH assessment can be instrumental in delaying cesarean delivery safely and in facilitating vaginal delivery in the face of fetal heart rate patterns that by themselves would be considered ominous.

At the time of delivery, double clamping of a length of umbilical cord for arterial and venous blood gas and pH measurement can be important to both pediatric management and evaluation of obstetric management. Blood gas and pH values of the blood in such an isolated segment of cord remain stable for up to 1 hour and can therefore be obtained after the delivery.

NEW DIRECTIONS

Estimates of inaccuracy of fetal heart rate monitoring alone in indicating fetal distress range to 50 per cent. Even fetal scalp pH is imperfect at predicting fetal condition. These imperfections may relate to the fact that fetal scalp capillary blood may be isolated from the mainstream of fetal circulation by stasis, edema, or extrinsic pressure from maternal tissue. Furthermore, scalp blood sampling is not always easily performed.

Techniques have been reported for the use of continuous fetal scalp pH monitoring and continuous fetal scalp PO_2 monitoring using special glass electrodes.[18,43,75] Although continuous monitoring might offer some theoretical advantages over intermittent sampling, such devices are not likely to become widely available because of the requirements for miniaturization of the fiberoptic light delivery and light detection apparatus. It is unlikely that such infrared light absorbance will be able to measure fetal brain oxygen in an absolute fashion but rather will provide relative information about oxygenation, from which patterns may be recognized that indicate fetal well-being or fetal distress. Development of such technical adaption and clinical evaluation will likely require considerable time.

References

1. Alexander ES, Spitz HB, Clark RA (1982): Sonography of polyhydramnios. AJR 138:343–346.
2. Baskett TF, Sandy EA (1979): The oxytocin challenge test: An ominous pattern associated with severe fetal growth retardation. Obstet Gynecol 54:365–366.
3. Baskett TF, Gray JH, Prewett SJ, Young LM, Allen AC (1984): Antepartum fetal assessment using a fetal biophysical profile score. Am J Obstet Gynecol 148:630–633.
4. Bergamasco B, Benna P, Ferrero P, Gavinelli R (1984): Neonatal hypoxia and epiletic risk: A clinical prospective study. Epilepsia 25:131–136.
5. Bissenden JG, Scott PH, Milner S, Doughty S, Ratnapala L (1979): The biochemistry of amniotic fluid with poor fetal growth. Br J Obstet Gynecol 86:540–547.
6. Blomstrand S, Hrbek A, Karlsson K, Kjellmer I, Lindecrantz K, Olsson T (1984): Does glucose administration affect the cerebral response to fetal asphyxia? Acta Obstet Gynecol Scand 63:345–353.
7. Brazy JE, Lewis DV, Mitnick MH, Jobsis vander Vliet FF (1986): Noninvasive monitoring of cerebral oxygenation in preterm infants: Preliminary observations. Pediatrics 75:217–225.
8. Naloxone reverses neonatal depression caused by fetal asphyxia [abstr]. (1982): Science 216:1252–1253.
9. Cibils LA (1977): Clinical significance of fetal heart rate patterns during labor. Am J Obstet Gynecol 129:833–844.
10. Cohn HE, Sacks EJ, Heymann MA, Rudolph AM (1974): Cardiovascular responses to hypoxemia and acidemia in fetal lambs. Am J Obstet Gynecol 120:817–824.
11. Crane J, Anderson B, Marshall R, Harvey P (1981): Subsequent physical and mental development in infants with positive contraction stress tests. J Repro Med 26:113–118.
12. Delprado WJ, Baird PJ (1984): The fetal adrenal gland: Lipid distribution with associated intrauterine hypoxia. Pathology 16:25–29.
13. Divers WA, Wilkes MM, Babaknia A, Hill LM, Quilligan EJ, Yen SSC (1981): Amniotic fluid catecholamines and metabolites in intrauterine growth retardation. Am J Obstet Gynecol 141:608–610.
14. Eaton JW, Skelton TD, Berger E (1974): Survival at extreme altitude: Protective effect of increased hemoglobin-oxygen affinity. Science 183:743–744.
15. Fenton AN, Steer CH (1962): Fetal distress. Am J Obstet Gynecol 83:354–362.
16. Finch CA, Lenfant C (1972): Oxygen transport in man. N Engl J Med 286:407–415.
17. Fleischer A, Schulman H, Jagani N, Mitchell J, Randolph G (1982): The development of fetal acidosis in the presence of an abnormal heart rate tracing. Am J Obstet Gynecol 144:55–60.

18. Flynn AM, Kelly J (1980): The continuous measurement of tissue pH in the human fetus during labour using a new application technique. Br J Obstet Gynaecol 87:666.

19. Freeman RK (1975): The use of the oxytocin challenge test for antepartum clinical evaluation of uteroplacental respiratory function. Am J Obstet Gynecol 121:481–489.

20. Fumia FD, Edelstone DI, Holzman IR (1984): Blood flow and oxygen delivery to fetal organs as functions of fetal hematocrit. Am J Obstet Gynecol 150:274–282.

21. Gilstrap LC III, Hauth JC, Toussaint S (1984): Second stage fetal heart rate abnormalities and neonatal acidosis. Obstet Gynecol 62:209–213.

22. Gosseye S, Golaire MC, Larroche JC (1982): Cerebral, renal and splenic lesions due to fetal anoxia and their relationship to malformations. Develop Med Child Neurol 24:510–518.

23. Grundy H, Freeman RK, Lederman S, Dorchester W (1984): Nonreactive contraction stress test: clinical significance. Obstet Gynecol 64:337–342.

24. Harkness RA, McFadyen IR (1983): Concentrations of hypoxanthine, xanthine, uridine and urate in amniotic fluid at caesarean section and the association of raised levels with prenatal risk factors and fetal distress. Br J Obstet Gynaecol 90:815–820.

25. Harkness RA, Coade SB (1983): Ratio of the concentration of hypoxanthine to creatinine in urine from newborn infants: A possible indicator for the metabolic damage due to hypoxia. Br J Obstet Gynaecol 90:447–452.

26. Harkness RA, Lund RJ (1983): Cerebrospinal fluid concentrations of hypoxanthine, uxanthine, uridine and inosine: high concentrations of the ATP metabolite, hypoxanthine, after hypoxia. J Clin Pathol 36:1–8.

27. Harkness RA, Whitelaw AGL, Simmonds RJ (1982): Intrapartum hypoxia: The association between neurological assessment of damage and abnormal excretion of ATP metabolites. J Clin Pathol 35:999–1007.

28. Hon EH (1962): Electronic evaluation of the fetal heart rate. Am J Obstet Gynecol 83:333–353.

29. Issel EP, Lun A, Pohle R, Gross J (1982): Hypoxanthine levels in amniotic fluid: An indicator of fetal hypoxia? J Perinat Med 10:221–225.

30. Itskovitz J, Goetzman BW, Rudolph AM (1982): The mechanism of late deceleration of the heart rate and its relationship to oxygenation in normoxic and chronically hypoxemic fetal lambs. Am J Obstet Gynecol 142:66–73.

31. Jarvis GJ, MacDonald HN (1979): Fetal movements in small-for-dates babies. Br J Obstet Gynaecol 86:724.

32. Jouppila P, Kirkinen P (1984): Umbilical vein blood flow as an indicator of fetal hypoxia. Br J Obstet Gynaecol 9:107–110.

33. Jouppila P, Kirkinen P (1984): Increased vascular resistance in the descending aorta of the human fetus in hypoxia. Br J Obstet Gynaecol 91:853–856.

34. Karinicmo V, Ammala P (1981): Short-term variability of fetal heart rate during pregnancies with normal and insufficient placental function. Am J Obstet Gynecol 139:33–37.

35. Kirschbaum TH, Lucas WE, DeHaven JC, Assali NS (1967): The dynamics of placental oxygen transfer. Am J Obstet Gynecol 98:429–443.

36. Kjellmer I, Dagbjartsson A, Hrbek A, Karlsson K, Rosen G (1984): Maternal beta-adreneceptor blockade reduces fetal tolerance to asphyxia. Acta Obstet Gynecol Scand (Suppl) 118:75–80.

37. Klink F, Grosspietzch R, Klitzing LV, Oberheuser F (1981): Uterine contraction intervals and transcutaneous levels of fetal oxygen pressure. Obstet Gynecol 57:437–440.

38. Krebs HB et al (1979): II. Multifactorial analysis of intrapartum fetal heart rate tracings. Am J Obstet Gynecol 133:773–780.

39. Lilja H, Karlsson K, Kjellmer I, Lindecrantz K, Olsson T, Rosen KG (1984): Heart rate variability and electro-cardiogram changes in the fetal lamb during hypoxia and beta-adrenoceptor stimulation. J Perinat Med 12:115–125.

40. Lin CC, Moawad AH, Rosenow PJ, River P (1980): Acid-base characteristics of fetuses with intrauterine growth retardation during labor and delivery. Am J Obstet Gynecol 137:553–559.

41. Lin CC, Lindheimer MD, River P, Moawad AH (1982): Fetal outcome in hypertensive disorders of pregnancy. Am J Obstet Gynecol 142:255–260.

42. Lin CC, Devoe LD, River P, Moawad A (1981): Oxytocin challenge test and intrauterine growth retardation. Am J Obstet Gynecol 140:282–288.

43. Lorijn RHW, Longo LD (1980): Clinical and physiologic implications of increased fetal oxygen consumption. Am J Obstet Gynecol 136:451–457.

44. Low JA, Galbraith RS, Muir DW, Killen HL, Pater EA, Karchmar EJ (1984): Factors associated with motor and cognitive deficits in children after intrapartum fetal hypoxia. Am J Obstet Gynecol 148:533–539.

45. Low JA, Karchmar J, Broekhover L, Leonard T, McGrath MJ, Pancham SR, Piercy WN (1981): The probability of fetal metabolic acidosis during labor in a population at risk as determined by clinical factors. Am J Obstet Gynecol 141:941–951.

46. Low JA, Galbraith RS, Muir DW, Killen HL, Pater EA, Karchmar EJ (1983): Intrapartum fetal hypoxia: A study of long-term morbidity. Am J Obstet Gynecol 145:129–134.

47. Manning FA, Lange IR, Morrison I, Harman CR (1984): Fetal biophysical profile score and the nonstress test: A comparative trial. Obstet Gynecol 64:326–331.

48. Manning FA, Baskett TF, Morrison I, Lange I (1981): Fetal biophysical profile scoring: A prospective study in 1,184 high-risk patients. Am J Obstet Gynecol 140:289–294.

49. Martin CB (1978): Regulation of the fetal heart rate and genesis of FHR patterns. Semin Perinatol 2:131–145.

50. Meschia G (1978): Evolution of thinking in fetal respiratory physiology. Am J Obstet Gynecol 132:806.

51. Meschia G (1979): Supply of oxygen to the fetus. J Reprod Med 23:160–165.

52. Miller FC, Petrie RH, Paul JJ (1974): Relationship of maternal acid-base balance to fetal oxygenation and pH. Am J Obstet Gynecol 120:489–495.

53. Milliez JM, James LS (1979): Fetal physiology. In Aladjem S, Brown A, Sureau C (eds): Clinical Perinatology. 2nd ed. St Louis, CV Mosby, pp 62–67.

54. Moniz CF, Nicolaides KH, Bamforth FJ, Rodeck CH (1985): Normal reference ranges for biochemical substances relating to renal, hepatic, and bone function in fetal and maternal plasma throughout pregnancy. J Clin Pathol 38:468–472.

55. Morrison I, Olsen J (1985): Weight-specific stillbirths and associated causes of death: An analysis of 765 stillbirths. Am J Obstet Gynecol 152:975–980.

56. Naeye RL, Maisels MJ, Lorenz RP, Botti JJ (1983): The clinical significance of placental villous edema. Pediatrics 71:588–594.

57. Niswander KR (1985): Quality of obstetric care and occurrence of fetal asphyxia and cerebral palsy. Is there a relationship? Postgrad Med 78:57–64.

58. Odendaal HJ (1979): The fetal and labor outcome of 102 positive contraction stress tests. Obstet Gynecol 54:591–596.

59. Ott WJ, Doyle S (1984): Ultrasonic diagnosis of altered fetal growth by use of a normal ultrasonic fetal weight curve. Obstet Gynecol 63:201–204.

60. Paneth N, Stark RI (1983): Cerebral palsy and mental retardation in relation to indicators of perinatal asphyxia. Am J Obstet Gynecol 147:960–966.

61. Parer JT (1979): Utero-placental circulation and respiratory gas exchange. In Shnider SM, Levinson G (eds): Anesthesia for Obstetrics 1979. Baltimore, Williams & Wilkins, pp 12–22.

62. Peevy KJ, Chalhub EG (1983): Occult group B streptococcal infection: An important cause of intrauterine asphyxia. Am J Obstet Gynecol 146:989–991.

63. Perkins RP (1984): Perinatal observations in a high-risk population managed without intrapartum fetal pH studies. Am J Obstet Gynecol 149:327–336.

64. Richards B, D'Souza SW, Black P, MacFarlane T, Jennison RF (1981): Haematological values in cord blood in relation to fetal hypoxia. Br J Obstet Gynaecol 88:129–132.

65. Rivard G, Motoyana EK, Acheson FM, Cook CD, Reynolds EOR (1967): The relation between maternal and fetal oxygen tensions in sheep. Am J Obstet Gynecol 97:925–930.

66. Sankaran K, Hindmarsh KW, Watson WG (1983): Hypoxic-ischemic encephalopathy and plasma β-endorphin. Dev Pharmacol Ther 7:377–383.

67. Saugstad OD, Gluck L (1982): Plasma hypoxanthine levels in

newborn infants: A specific indicator of hypoxia. J Perinatal Med 10:266–272.

68. Seeds AE (1978): Maternal-fetal acid-base relationships and fetal scalp-blood analysis. Clinical Obstet & Gynec 21:579–591.

69. Seeds JW, Cefalo RC (1984): The relationship of intra-cranial infrared light absorbance to fetal oxygenation. I: Methodology. Am J Obstet Gynecol 149:679–684.

70. Seeds JW (1984): Impaired fetal growth: Definition and clinical diagnosis. Obstet Gynecol 64:303–310.

71. Seeds JW (1984): Impaired fetal growth: Ultrasonic evaluation and clinical management. Obstet Gynecol 64:577–584.

72. Smith NC, McColl J (1983): Fetal scalp blood lactate as an indicator of intrapartum hypoxia. Br J Obstet Gynaecol 90:821–831.

73. Thaler I, Timor-Tritsch IE, Blumenfeld Z (1986): Effect of acute hypoxia on human fetal heart rate. Acta Obstet Gynecol Scand 64:47–50.

74. Trudinger BJ, Giles WB, Cook CM (1985): Flow velocity waveforms in the maternal uteroplacental and fetal umbilical placental circulations. Am J Obstet Gynecol 152:155–163.

75. Young BK, Noumoff J, Klein SA, Katz M (1979): Continuous fetal tissue pH measurement in labor. Obstet Gynecol 52:533–538.

76. Westgren M, Hormquist P, Ingemarsson I, Svenningsen N (1984): Intrapartum fetal acidosis in preterm infants: Fetal monitoring and long-term morbidity. Obstet Gynecol 63:355–359.

77. Willcourt RJ, King JC, Quennan JT (1983): Maternal oxygenation administration and the fetal transcutaneous PO_2. Am J Obstet Gynecol 146:714–715.

18 PATHOPHYSIOLOGY OF HYDROPS FETALIS

Alastair A. Hutchison

With general foetal dropsy, . . . the pathogenesis is very obscure, and
even the etiology is imperfectly known.

Ballantyne, 1902.

HISTORICAL PERSPECTIVE

The existence of hydrops fetalis has been known for centuries, but the modern era in the investigation of this condition began with the work of of Ballantyne in 1892 and 1902. Ballantyne described hydrops fetalis as a condition with edema, anemia, hepato-splenomegaly, and an enlarged placenta and noted its associations with bilirubin staining of the amniotic fluid and with multiple fetal deformities.[13,14]

In the first part of this century the major advances in understanding the etiology of hydrops fetalis were in the elucidation of the nature of immune hydrops fetalis. In 1938 Darrow proposed that the initiating event in hydrops fetalis was the production of a maternal antibody against a component of fetal blood.[51] In the following year Levine and Stetson suggested that the maternal antibody was directed against a fetal antigen inherited from the father and absent in the mother.[142] The description of the Rh antigen by Landsteiner and Weiner in 1940[136] led Levine and colleagues, in 1941,[141] to demonstrate that the Rh antigen was absent in more than 90 per cent of the mothers of affected neonates. The immune hemolysis theory of prior immunization and subsequent passage of antibodies from the mother to the fetus was proved in 1945 when the Coombs test confirmed the antibody's presence.[10,45] With the introduction of anti-D therapy by Finn et al in 1961[68] and Gorman et al in 1962,[87] prevention of hydrops fetalis due to Rh isoimmunization became a reality.

Hydrops fetalis due to causes other than fetomaternal blood group incompatibility was first categorized as nonimmune hydrops fetalis by Potter in 1943.[187]

The composition of fetal ascitic fluid was first reported by Dorland in 1919,[58] but it was not until the 1940s with the advent of radioisotopes that studies of transplacental fluxes were possible. In the 1950s Hutchison et al[111,112] and Friedman et al[72] carried out human and monkey studies using deuterium and tritium tracers to follow water fluxes in the pregnant mother and fetus and in amniotic fluid. They documented important differences in water fluxes both with advancing gestation and in pathologic states. However, much remains to be learned about the control of water transfer and the genesis of fetal edema.

In 1932, Diamond et al[56] proposed three etiologic mechanisms for the edema in Rh isoimmunization: chronic congestive heart failure secondary to chronic anemia, increased capillary permeability secondary to chronic hypoxia (a consequence of the anemia), and decreased colloid osmotic pressure secondary to hypoproteinemia. Although Jarvet[119] had noted in 1942 the association of hydrops fetalis with fetal hypoproteinemia, congestive heart failure due to chronic anemia was viewed as the key etiologic factor in edema secondary to Rh isoimmunization.[179-181] The importance of cardiac failure seemed to be corroborated by the finding that the incidence of nonimmune hydrops fetalis was reported to be 100 times increased when the fetal heart was malformed.[27]

The possibility that hypoproteinemia may be a more significant factor than anemia in hydrops fetalis was first suggested by Potter in 1961.[188] In 1968 McFadyen et al[151] could not produce edema in fetal sheep by inducing severe chronic anemia, but in 1970 Horger and Hutchinson[109] were able to produce fetal edema by giving a protein inhibitor to anemic fetal sheep. Driscoll suggested in 1966[59] that intense erythropoiesis in the hepatic sinusoids could result in ascites and impede umbilical venous flow, causing placental villous edema.

The primary etiologic role of congestive cardiac failure in hydrops fetalis was challenged further in the 1970s by Baum and Harris,[25] Phibbs et al,[180,181] and Barnes et al.[18] They cited the occurrence of hydrops without anemia as well as the occurrence of severe anemia without hydrops and emphasized the importance of low colloid osmotic pressure as the primary etiologic factor. Hypoproteinemia was postulated to result from liver dysfunction secondary to extramedullary erythropoiesis.[18]

On the other hand, supraventricular tachycardia was shown to cause fetal edema in utero,[126] and the fetal edema did resolve with in utero therapy for supraventricular tachycardia.[226] In a fetal sheep study, Stevens et al[220] in 1982 demonstrated that induction of supraventricular tachycardia without hypoproteinemia could produce fetal edema. Employing real time fetal ultrasonography, Fleischer et al[69] in 1981 and Kleinman et al[131,132] in 1982 and 1983 have increased the focus upon detection of in utero supraventricular tachycardia as a cause of nonimmune hydrops fetalis.

Thus, several factors are involved in the production of fetal edema. This chapter will review the mechanisms implicated in the production of fetal edema and will emphasize the important consequences of the edema, such as in utero hypoxia and acidosis, preterm delivery, and respiratory distress due to hyaline membrane disease and pulmonary hypoplasia.

INCIDENCE

In the United States the number of Rh-sensitized women of reproductive age has fallen from approximately 120,000 in 1968 to about 22,000 in 1986.[44] Fewer cases of hydrops fetalis due to Rh isoimmunization are seen today. During the 1960s and 1970s the incidence of nonimmune hydrops fetalis in level III neonatal units was approximately 1 in 3500.[110,153] Nonimmune hydrops fetalis has received more attention as the incidence of Rh isoimmunization has declined in the past decade. During the years 1970 to 1974, 26 per cent of hydropic perinatal deaths were due to nonimmune hydrops fetalis, whereas during 1975 to 1979 the number had risen to 57 per cent. A similar increase has been true for hydropic stillbirths (22 per cent Rh isoimmunized; 50 per cent nonimmune) and hydropic neonatal deaths (35 versus 68 per cent). The percentage of the total perinatal deaths due to nonimmune hydrops fetalis increased from 0.4 per cent in 1970 to 1974 to 0.7 per cent in 1975 to 1979.[8]

DEFINITION OF EDEMA

Edema results from an abnormal pattern of distribution of body water. Edematous patients have an excess of interstitial tissue water.

DETERMINANTS OF WATER DISTRIBUTION

In vivo water transfer is primarily determined by hydrostatic, osmotic, and electrochemical forces. Diffusional flow, defined as random movement of water molecules across a membrane to establish equal concentrations on both sides, also occurs. Flow of water across a porous membrane in response to osmotic or hydrostatic gradients is defined as nondiffusional or bulk flow.[236]

The control of the distribution of intracellular water is related to osmotic forces and the energy-dependent sodium transporter. The function of the transporter is influenced by many factors, including the activity of adenosine triphosphatase, adenosine triphosphate, sodium and potassium, glucose, acidosis, and hypoxia. The control of the distribution of extracellular water is determined by the integrity of capillary endothelium, Starling forces, the affinity of the interstitial gel for water, and the lymphatic drainage.[18]

The Starling equation states that

$$Qv,c = Kf,c\,[(Pc - Pti,f) - \sigma d(\pi p - \pi ti)]$$

where Qv,c = net volume flow across the capillary

Kf,c = capillary filtration coefficient

Pc = capillary pressure

Pti,f = interstitial tissue fluid pressure

σd = osmotic reflection coefficient of solute

πp = colloid osmotic pressure of the plasma

πti = colloid osmotic pressure of the tissues

In the adult, the osmotic pressure determining water flow is principally that due to colloid solutes (solutes of diameters 2×10^{-7} to 2×10^{-5} cm) that stay mainly in the vascular space. The reflection coefficient of the membrane for the solute gives a measure of the degree of permeability of the membrane for that solute, with a value of 0 indicating free permeability of the solute and a value of 1 indicating impermeability. If the membrane is completely impermeable to the solute ($\sigma = 1$), then the osmotic pressure difference due to that solute will equal that calculated by freezing point depression. The osmotic permeability to water will be generated by the osmotic gradient due to the solute. Osmotic pressure due to noncolloid solutes (diameter of 2×10^{-10} to 2×10^{-8} cm) is less important, since the membrane is permeable to such solutes. However, in the sheep fetus, noncolloids are responsible for the major part of the osmotic pressure difference between fetal and maternal blood.[17] The effect of the different membrane reflection coefficients for different solutes is such that transmembrane forces alter from those calculated on the basis of the osmotic pressures of the different solutes on either side of the membrane. In a system not in equilibrium, net flux across the membrane can alter so that the flow might even be opposite to that calculated.[236] The influence of the different amniochorial reflection coefficients for solutes may be important in determining maternofetal water flow.[236]

Movement of water is also determined by the movement of ions to balance the effect of nondiffusible charged particles—the Donnan effect. In sheep, the fetal plasma is electronegative with respect to maternal plasma early in pregnancy.[17] This electrical potential decreases later in gestation—one study reported its falling to zero.[17] In the human at term the transplacental electrical potential is minimal, about 2mV, with the fetus electropositive. The origin and site of the transplacental electrical potential are debated, but there is no relationship to ionic distribution.[17]

Water exchange at the placental membrane is influenced by hydrostatic and osmotic pressures. In addition, the red blood cell gives up water when oxygenation occurs. The nature of the placental barrier also affects water flux. With maturity, the thickness of the membrane decreases, as the cytotrophoblastic layer disappears, and its surface area increases. The porosity of the amniochorial membranes varies with hypoxia, ischemia, acidosis, and the effects of cortisol, prolactin, and antidiuretic hormone.[175,236,242]

Table 18–1. GESTATIONAL CHANGES IN WATER CONTRIBUTION TO TOTAL BODY MASS DURING FETAL LIFE

Gestational Age	Per cent
12 weeks	90
28 weeks	85
40 weeks	75
Adult	65

Modified from Friis-Hansen B (1971): Body composition during growth. Pediatrics 47:264–274.

Table 18–2. TRANSPLACENTAL WATER EXCHANGE (ml/hr)

	20 weeks	40 weeks
Mother to fetus	302	3,657
Fetus to mother	259	3,682

Modified from Hutchinson DL et al (1959:) The role of the fetus in the water exchange of the amniotic fluid of norml and hydramniotic patients. J Clin Invest 38:971–980.

MATERNOFETAL WATER EXCHANGE

Water transfer from fetus to mother is favored by hydrostatic pressure and colloid osmotic pressure gradients,[17] yet at term umbilical venous blood contains more water than umbilical arterial blood,[96] indicating water transfer to the fetus. It is not known if this transfer of water from the maternal to fetal circulation is influenced by the fetomaternal electrochemical gradient.[17] Diffusional flow occurs, but bulk flow is important since the flow is greater than would occur with diffusion alone.[236] Maternofetal water transfer in the sheep has been shown to be up to 500 times greater than that required for growth.[17] Fetal body water decreases as a percentage of fetal weight with advancing gestation[74] (Table 18–1). In human studies, the transfer rate of water from mother to fetus increases with advancing gestational age[111] (Table 18–2). Although differences in hydrostatic and osmotic pressures do not explain the water exchange,[17] the reported osmotic pressure differences vary and are decreased by hypocapnia and increased by acute hypoxia.[17,203] Under steady state conditions in sheep and goats the total osmotic pressure of fetal plasma equals or is slightly less than maternal osmotic pressure.[158] Very small differences are cited between human maternal vein and fetal umbilical vein total osmotic pressures.[23] As discussed above and as also discussed by Seeds,[203] the prediction of water fluxes on the basis of the measurement of total osmotic pressure by freezing point depression does not always determine the water fluxes that actually occur when different solutes are placed on either side of a semipermeable membrane. Thus small osmotic forces may exist that favor water transport to the fetus. Since the uterine arteriovenous volume of water transfer per milliliter of placental perfusion is only 0.66 µl, current techniques of measurement may not pick up the small differences in the forces required to achieve this transfer.[17]

DETERMINANTS OF FETAL EDEMA

Six factors are important in the production of fetal edema:

1. Alterations in hydrostatic pressure most likely result from heart failure or venous obstruction.

2. Alterations in colloid osmotic pressure most likely result from hypoproteinemia secondary to liver damage. Liver damage may result in portal hypertension and cause venous obstruction.

3. Alterations in membrane permeability may result from inflammatory, metabolic, genetic, or neoplastic causes.

4. Alterations in interstitial gel and its affinity for water may predispose to edema.[18] Little work has been done in this area, but abnormalities of mucopolysaccharide metabolism could decrease the buffering capacity of the interstitium for water.

5. Alterations in lymphatic drainage may result from congenital abnormalities of the lymphatic system or external obstructive lesions.

6. Alterations in water homeostasis of feto-placental-amniotic fluid compartments may occur.

ETIOLOGY OF HYDROPS FETALIS

General Considerations

1. Although a strong relationship exists between the severity of hydrops fetalis and the severity of colloid osmotic pressure reduction, edema at birth occurs rarely in neonates with congenital nephrotic syndrome and is not reported in those with analbuminemia. In these fetuses α-fetoprotein (fetal albumin) may compensate for the low concentrations of serum albumin. Alternatively, low colloid osmotic pressure may result from decreases in other small molecular weight proteins or from changes in the physicochemical behavior of albumin molecules.[18]

2. The fetus normally has a low colloid osmotic pressure compared with the adult. The extracellular fluid is larger than the intracellular fluid, and the urine is hypotonic, suggesting a state of water excess.[236]

3. At low protein concentrations, changes in the protein concentrations produce very little change in colloid osmotic pressure.[18] However, with the colloid osmotic pressure at a critical level, minor changes in hydrostatic pressure are very likely to produce large increases in the extracellular fluid volume.

4. Although changes in hydrostatic pressure can result from heart failure, it has been pointed out that edema at birth is seldom associated with the most severe forms of cardiac anomalies.[188]

5. Thus, it is unlikely that one cause is the sine qua non in the pathogenesis of hydrops fetalis (Fig. 18–1). The potential major role of several factors carries with it two implications: First, determination of etiology is important for therapeutic planning; second, therapeutic interventions

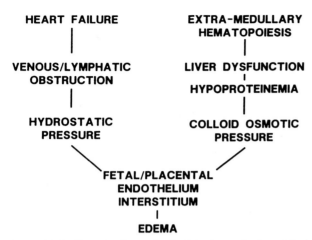

Figure 18–1. The main factors involved in the production of fetal edema. Several interactions are possible, and it is likely that edema results from a combination of factors rather than a single factor.

may correct one situation, e.g., anemia, but by expanding blood volume they may further compromise another, e.g., cardiac function.[180]

Maternal Factors and Water Homeostasis in Hydrops Fetalis

Of the maternal conditions associated with fetal edema, preterm birth (90 per cent) and polyhydramnios (75 per cent) are the commonest, with maternal anemia (39 per cent) and preeclamptic toxemia (34 per cent) also noted (Table 18–3).[110] Maternal hypoproteinemia can be present.[90,110] It is conceivable that the latter three conditions could result in alterations in the maternal hydrostatic pres-

Table 18–3. EVALUATION OF HYDROPS FETALIS

Maternal Associations with Hydrops Fetalis
Polyhydramnios
Anemia (Hb < 11g%)
Preeclamptic toxemia

Usual Investigations for Hydrops Fetalis
Blood group and type
Rh antibodies
Atypical antibodies
Full blood count
Kleihauer-Betke screen
Urinalysis
Real time ultrasonography of the fetus, placenta, and uterus
Fetal echocardiography and systematic assessment for congenital
    abnormalities (see reference 69)

Additional Diagnostic Tests
Urine culture
Serologic evaluation for viral, toxoplasma, syphilitic infection
Serum protein concentration
Hemoglobin electrophoresis
Red blood cell enzymes
Serum α-fetoprotein
Fasting serum glucose concentration
Amniocentesis for prenatal diagnoses

sure and colloid osmotic pressure favoring water transport to the fetus. Polyhydramnios is associated with esophageal atresia, lack of fetal swallowing, and continued urine output. However, this relationship has been questioned.[1] Experimental ligation of the esophagus in fetal sheep and monkeys does not result in chronic polyhydramnios.[242] Liley suggested that in Rh isoimmunization, hepatomegaly with venous obstruction resulted in both fetal ascites and polyhydramnios.[144] In later human pregnancy the principal direction of water exchange is from mother to fetus, fetus to amniotic fluid and amniotic fluid to mother.[111] In the human pregnancy complicated by polyhydramnios, it has been shown that water exchange between the mother and fetus decreases, although the result is a net fetal gain.[111] Despite the decreased maternofetal flux, water in the amniotic cavity in polyhydramnios arises primarily from the fetus. The rate of amniotic fluid water removal remains the same in polyhydramnios, but a greater percentage of the removal is by direct transfer to the mother.[111] Thus, the fetus appears to have an important role in the control of amniotic fluid volume; since no increase in fetal urine output has been documented in cases of polyhydramnios,[237] the umbilical cord may have a major role in the pathogenesis of polyhydramnios.[111,215] It should also be noted that hormonal influences may regulate both chorionic and amniotic membrane permeabilities.[175,236,242] Gordon reported an increase in the urinary excretion of human chorionic gonadotropin during development of hydrops fetalis in Rh isoimmunization.[86] It had been suggested that the persistence of the villous cytotrophoblastic layer in hydrops fetalis might result in an excess of chorionic gonadotropin and in turn might lead to the occurrence of theca lutein cysts of the ovaries both in the mother and female fetus.[59,70] Clearly, more work is needed in this area.

Etiology of Immune Hydrops Fetalis

Anti-D antibodies are the major cause of immune hemolysis, the severity of which is reflected by the degree of reticulocytosis and anemia.[10] The severity of the hemolytic process is related to the titer of maternal antibody (primarily IgG_1), the rate of transfer of antibody across the placenta ($IgG_1 > IgG_3$), the amount of antigen on fetal tissues, the capacity of the fetus's reticuloendothelial system to destroy antibody-coated cells, the ability of the infant to excrete bilirubin, and the erythropoietic response of the fetus.[199] Bilirubin staining of the amniotic liquor is used to assess the severity of immune hydrops fetalis in utero, although it is not always a sign of a hemolytic process, as it occurs in some cases of nonimmune hydrops fetalis.[154,245]

Currently the incidence of Rh isoimmunization as a cause of immune hydrops fetalis is falling, and other antibodies are assuming increasing importance. They include antibodies against the following blood antigens: Kell, c, E, Cw, Jka, S, M, k, and Fya.[73] Rare reports exist of hemolytic disease due to anti-D antibodies in the newborn of a Rh-positive Du-variant mother.[135a] An important implication of the immune etiology is recurrence of the condition in subsequent susceptible siblings.

Hemolytic anemia and its sequelae explain the findings in Rh isoimmunization. Extramedullary erythropoiesis is seen primarily in the liver and spleen. Metabolic dysfunction of the liver occurs and results in portal hypertension with ascites and umbilical venous obstruction.[18] The studies of Baum,[25] Phibbs[179–181] and Barnes et al[18] would argue that decreased colloid osmotic pressure, perhaps secondary to hypoproteinemia, is the key factor in the production of fetal edema. Low colloid osmotic pressure and hypoproteinemia are more closely related to the severity of fetal edema than is the fetal hemoglobin concentration, which can be normal in some cases.[18,25,168,180] If hemolysis is severe and cannot be compensated by increased red cell production, anemia occurs. The anemia and its accompanying tissue hypoxia are thought to result in high output cardiac failure. It should be noted that intrauterine transfusion with improvement of the oxygen-carrying capacity has not reversed hydrops fetalis,[179] and thus it is argued that the role of anemia in producing hydrops does not seem to be primarily through the production of tissue hypoxia and cardiac failure. The main impact of anemia may be through the accompanying extramedullary hematopoiesis. The resultant liver dysfunction and hypoproteinemia, combined with increases in local and generalized capillary hydrostatic pressure (due to cardiac failure or venous obstruction), result in a pattern of edema that is mainly centripetal, with ascites as a cardinal feature. Equally important as the major etiologic factors of fetal edema are the associated pathologies and conditions, which complicate transition from fetal to neonatal life (see Neonatal Cardiorespiratory Adaptation and Hydrops Fetalis).

The major findings of immune hydrops fetalis at autopsy include ascites, generalized edema, pleural effusions (sometimes with pulmonary hypoplasia and postnatally hyaline membranes), hepatosplenomegaly with evidence of marked extramedullary hematopoiesis, cardiomegaly with generalized dilation and hypertrophy, pancreatic islet cell hyperplasia, vacuolation and swelling of adrenal fetal zone cells, placental enlargement with villous edema, and some proliferation and persistence of the cytotrophoblastic layer. Extramedullary hematopoiesis is also evident in lungs, kidneys, heart, adrenals, and placenta. Reticulocytosis and thrombocytopenia are seen in peripheral blood, the latter probably being secondary to disseminated intravascular coagulation. Examination of the bone marrow reveals a relative hypoplasia of granulocytic precursors. Postnatally, kernicterus results in bilirubin staining primarily of basal nuclei but also may involve hippocampal, thalamic, pontine, cerebellar, and medullary nuclei. Fetuses with immune hydrops fetalis also have smaller body lengths than expected for their gestational ages.

Etiology of Nonimmune Hydrops Fetalis

Multiple factors are associated with the occurrence of nonimmune hydrops fetalis. The incidence of congenital abnormalities is high; chromosomal and genetic associations are also known,[127] and thus the potential for recurrence exists. Recurrence in idiopathic cases is rarely reported.[48,49,65,67,84,153,201,204,212] Typing of HLA antigens may be useful in such idiopathic cases.[107] In an autopsy study of 61 cases of nonimmune hydrops fetalis, a congenital abnormality was found in 65 per cent of those older than 28 weeks' gestation. Of these abnormalities, 40 per cent were assessed as lethal. The etiology of the remaining 35 per cent was described as "idiopathic."[110] A study of 44 cases calculated that the incidence of congenital abnormalities was 40 and 18 times higher than that expected for major and minor abnormalities, respectively.[27] The incidence of nonimmune hydrops fetalis was increased one hundred times when the fetal heart was malformed, although such malformations rarely occurred in isolation.[27]

Of the "idiopathic" cases it is thought that a large percentage may be accounted for by in utero cardiac arrhythmias.[4,57,131] Although supraventricular tachycardia has been frequently reported in otherwise normal neonates, prior to 1981 supraventricular tachycardia was infrequently associated with hydrops fetalis.[28,47,65,101,125,126,128,148,170,193,198,200,207,210,224,232,244] and was usually seen in association with underlying Wolff-Parkinson-White syndrome.[101,125,128,170,224,232] As opposed to atrial flutter and fibrillation,[29,103,131,173,190,198,200,207,234,243] hydrops fetalis secondary to supraventricular tachycardia is not usually seen in association with underlying structural cardiac abnormalities.[190,239] The advent of real time ultrasonography for fetal examination in utero has focused attention upon fetal supraventricular arrhythmias as a cause of hydrops fetalis.[69,129–133] Reports of hydrops fetalis secondary to supraventricular tachycardia and of in utero therapy have appeared more frequently since 1981.[3,4,31,52,57,61,69,89,90,100,110,114,115,129–132,192,208,233,241,243] The arrhythmia responsible for hydrops fetalis is not present all of the time, which makes the diagnosis difficult and perhaps explains the transient nature of some cases.[149,184,192] Maternal tocolytic therapy has been linked to the occurrence of supraventricular tachycardia and hydrops fetalis.[28] A review of neonatal ventricular arrhythmias indicated that in contrast to supraventricular arrhythmias none of the nine cases reported in utero had edema.[221] Hydrops fetalis complicating heart block has also been reported.[5,46,65,97,106,131,132,150,202]

Can cases of high output cardiac failure in the absence of other cardiac or extracardiac anomalies explain hydrops fetalis? Radford et al,[191] replying to a suggestion of Harkavy,[98] noted hypoproteinemia in two of three cases in which fetuses had developed hydrops fetalis as a result of paroxysmal supraventricular tachycardia. They supported the hypothesis that "pure" high output cardiac failure could be the sole cause of hydrops fetalis. Using a pacemaker to induce tachycardia in fetal sheep, Stevens et al[220] showed that cardiac failure without hypoproteinemia can result in fetal hydrops. Changes in blood gases during the pacing were minimal, and the hematocrit was unchanged. Stevens et al postulated that left atrial pacing was more detrimental than right atrial pacing, perhaps because of closure of the foramen ovale—a known association with nonimmune hydrops fetalis.[14,167,178] Thus, whether the supraventricular tachycardia originates in the left or right atrium might explain the variability in the clinical presentation of in utero paroxysmal atrial tachycardia.[220] In a similar study, Gest et al found a decrease in plasma protein in association with cardiac failure induced in utero with atrial pacing.[79] Since the ascitic fluid protein concentration was less than that of plasma, increased venous pressures were thought to be responsible. Thus, in cases of "pure" high output cardiac failure, hypoproteinemia may contribute to fetal edema.

High output cardiac failure is implicated in the etiology of nonimmune hydrops fetalis not only as a result of anemia but also from polycythemia and in situations in which large arteriovenous shunts exist, such as in a large sacrococcygeal tumor (in which microangiopathic anemia can coexist).[16,133,233,237] However, nonimmune hydrops fetalis has many causes other than cardiac failure.[163] Several of the associated conditions, especially infections, can result in hypoproteinemia from liver damage alone. Notable among these is syphilis, described by Ballantyne as a cause of hydrops fetalis.[14] In assessing the fetus with nonimmune hydrops fetalis, the diagnostic tests listed in Table 18–3 should be carried out. The association with diabetes mellitus has been stressed, and maternal glucose tolerance testing recommended.[114] However, some pediatricians and obstetricians would argue against the association of nonimmune hydrops fetalis and maternal diabetes mellitus.[152] It seems unlikely that in the absence of a cardiac or other malformation or umbilical vein thrombosis,[75] a fetal condition primarily characterized by carbohydrate excess such as diabetes mellitus should also have water excess. A list of known associations with nonimmune hydrops fetalis, arranged in potential etiologic categories,[81] is shown in Table 18–4. As in Rh isoimmunization, it is important to stress the associated pathologies and conditions, which complicate transition from fetal to neonatal life (see below).

Causes of low output cardiac failure are listed in Table 18–4. One major subgroup of this category is obstructed venous return, both above and below the diaphragm. The role of ascites in impeding umbilical venous return has been stressed. Any resulting placental and umbilical cord edema will limit that organ's capacity to correct the fetal fluid overload. This disturbance of water homeostasis may be important in the genesis of polyhydramnios. The accumulation of pleural fluid will also impede venous return and may lead to cardiac compression. Similarly, the accumulation of fluid in overdistended lungs may explain the occurrence of hydrops fetalis that accompanies experimental tracheal ligation or atresia.[183,187] A rare form of low output cardiac failure is that associated with arterial calcification,[122] which may be linked to inborn metabolic disease.[223]

Autopsy findings in nonimmune hydrops fetalis can include hepatomegaly, splenomegaly, cardiomegaly, and pulmonary hypoplasia, each occurring in about one fifth of cases.[110] The importance of quantifying pulmonary hypoplasia with radial alveolar counts has been stressed.[64] In hydrops fetalis secondary to α-thalassemia, pancreatic

Table 18–4. POTENTIAL ETIOLOGIC FACTORS ASSOCIATED WITH HYDROPS FETALIS

Alteration/Factor	References
Increased Hydrostatic Pressure	
High Output Cardiac Failure	
Severe Anemia	
Rh isoimmunization	10, 18, 44, 51, 56, 68, 73, 87, 136, 141, 179, 181
α-Thalassemia	33, 37, 40, 90, 91, 95, 106, 110, 144, 174, 206, 227, 233, 238
Other anemias	34, 43, 65, 83, 121, 127, 155, 157, 160, 164, 171, 176, 240
Arrhythmias	
Supraventricular tachycardia	3, 4, 28, 31, 47, 52, 57, 61, 62, 65, 69, 79, 89, 90, 100, 101, 106, 107, 110, 114, 124–126, 129–132, 146, 148, 170, 190–193,198, 207, 210, 220, 224, 226, 232, 233, 239, 241, 243, 244
Atrial flutter/fibrillation	29, 103, 131, 173, 190, 198, 200, 207, 234, 243
Fetofetal/maternal hemorrhages	
Fetofetal	27, 36, 59, 65, 89, 90, 106, 110, 114, 115, 131, 153, 154, 167, 187, 219, 230, 247
Fetomaternal	53, 59, 65, 110, 153, 177, 229
Maternofetal	35
Arteriovenous Shunts	
Tumors with large vascular supply	
Neuroblastoma	7, 32, 66, 120, 161, 164, 177, 216, 222, 233, 235
Placental chorangioma	24, 26, 69, 89, 121, 155, 209, 225, 228, 233
Sacrococcygeal teratoma	16, 78, 133, 177, 219, 233, 237
Hemangioendothelioma/hemangiomas	20, 50, 89, 155, 209
Wilms tumor	
Lymphangiomas	26, 107, 110, 230
Other Causes	
Pulmonary sequestration	65, 131, 135
Kasabach-Merritt syndrome	209
Parasitic fetus	99, 131, 166, 214

Table 18–4. POTENTIAL ETIOLOGIC FACTORS ASSOCIATED WITH HYDROPS FETALIS *(Continued)*

Alteration/Factor	References
Low Output Cardiac Failure	
Arrhythmias	
Bradyarrhythmias	5, 46, 65, 97, 106, 131, 132, 150, 202, 219
Structural Cardiac Abnormalities	
Valvular defects	27, 89, 106, 107, 114, 116, 131, 152, 161, 163, 217, 219
Hypoplastic ventricle	106, 110, 139, 197, 230, 248
Other structural abnormalities	14, 106, 114, 131, 154, 161, 163, 219, 248
Premature closure of foramen ovale	14, 167, 178
Premature closure of ductus arteriosus	9, 26, 162 (maternal indomethacin)
Other Causes	
Myocarditis/infarction	21, 27, 81, 114, 124, 131, 248
Endocardial fibroelastosis	27, 114, 131, 152, 161, 163
Tumors	15, 89, 110, 131, 173, 186, 218, 239
Increased Peripheral Resistance	
Arterial calcification	89, 110, 113, 114, 117, 122, 223
Obstructed Venous/Lymphatic Return	
Cystic adenomatoid and other cystic malformations of lungs	25, 26, 55, 59, 63, 65, 69, 110, 131, 135, 153, 161, 233
Diaphragmatic hernia	14, 27, 106, 110, 131, 152, 177, 187
Cystic hygroma	41, 65, 69, 92, 107, 110, 124
Lymphangiectasia	59, 69, 110, 134
Gastrointestinal abnormalities	27, 65, 76, 107, 110, 219
Meconium peritonitis, retroperitoneal fibrosis	14, 60, 65, 106, 110, 157
Neuroblastoma	(see above)
Genitourinary obstruction	14, 65, 67, 71, 106, 110, 147, 149, 219
Venous thrombosis	59, 75, 123, 196
Liver dysfunction (see below)	
Decreased Colloid Osmotic Pressure/ Hypoproteinemia	
Hepatic Dysfunction	
Extramedullary Hematopoiesis	
Rh isoimmunization	
α-Thalassemia	(see above)
Other	
Bone marrow dysfunction	
Gaucher disease	83, 223
?Dwarfing disorders	65, 69, 106, 107, 110, 127, 153, 154, 161
Liver Damage	
Hepatitis/cirrhosis	6, 14, 30, 110, 114, 152, 219, 231
Cytomegalovirus	65, 106, 110, 137, 154, 165, 189
Syphilis/other	14, 21, 26, 38, 59, 65, 102, 131, 187, 219, 231, 249
Inborn error of metabolism	2, 12, 65, 82, 83, 115a, 169, 223, 233
Renal Dysfunction	
Dysplastic/cystic kidneys	14, 65, 110, 187
Altered Capillary Endothelium	
Intrinsic Causes	
Genetic	
Turner syndrome	90, 106, 195 (see cystic hygroma)
Down syndrome	54, 76, 106, 110, 153, 161, 177
Trisomy 18, triploidy, other	27, 110, 131, 153
Metabolic	
Inborn error of metabolism	(see above)
Acquired Causes	
Hypoxia/ischemia	
Infection	
Neoplasia	

hyperplasia is seen. Placental examination is an important part of the fetal autopsy in hydrops fetalis, as evidence of the etiologic condition (e.g., an infection or a storage disease) may be found in that organ. Microscopically, the placenta appears immature, owing to persistence of the villous cytotrophoblastic layer.

NEONATAL CARDIORESPIRATORY ADAPTATION AND HYDROPS FETALIS

Three studies of neonatal cardiorespiratory adaptation in neonates with hydrops fetalis secondary to Rh iso-immunization were performed by Phibbs et al;[179–181] these studies are also relevant to nonimmune hydrops fetalis.

The conclusions of the first study were that survival varied with gestational age, severity of hydrops, and degree of asphyxia (Table 18–5). The degree of asphyxia was related to the mode of delivery and the time needed to achieve a pH higher than 7.30 and an arterial oxygen tension higher than 50 mmHg.[179] Survival was not correlated with the degree of anemia, although severe anemia was noted more frequently in those most severely affected. The authors also cited Hobel's observation that the anemic fetus can show no evidence of asphyxia early in labor[105] and focused upon the importance of perinatal events in the outcome of immune hydrops fetalis. They emphasized the problems of preterm delivery; perinatal asphyxia with early hypoxia and acidosis; respiratory distress due to hyaline membrane disease, pulmonary hypertension, and hemorrhage; disseminated intravascular coagulation; and hypoglycemia. To this list can be added pulmonary hypoplasia[67,69,106,110,182,212] and infection, the latter perhaps related to the lower concentrations of IgG in hydropic fetuses.[36,42] It is of note that hypoglycemia is also common in neonates with nonimmune hydrops fetalis, although pancreatic hyperplasia is not seen. The point was made that cardiac pathology, thought to be specific to Rh isoimmunization, was not specific to congestive heart failure from anemia and could be the consequence of perinatal stresses. The major practical thrust of this paper was to recommend intense monitoring and an aggressive approach to perinatal management, including prenatal steroid therapy, cesarean section, and immediate pediatric attention. The success of early resuscitation influenced survival (Table 18–6). A similar aggressive ap-

proach was applied effectively by Etches et al, who stressed that tapping ascitic fluid and, on occasion, pleural fluid could improve cardiac and respiratory function, respectively.[65]

The second study of Phibbs et al focused on blood and plasma volumes and the role of hypoalbuminemia in the etiology of fetal edema.[180] Blood volume was measured using ^{51}Cr-tagged red blood cells; the results were corrected to body weight postdiuresis. Plasma volume was measured using T^{1824} dye; precautions were taken to correct for loss from the circulation. Sampling times were appropriate.[180] In cases in which only plasma volume or red cell volume was measured, a total body-to-venous hematocrit ratio was used for the calculation of total blood volume.[180] Loss of albumin-tagged label in sick neonates was very evident, although the rates of loss for hydropic and nonhydropic and asphyxiated and nonasphyxiated neonates were not significantly different.

The investigations of Phibbs et al[179–181] were carried out after birth when major changes in arterial blood pressure, vasoactive catecholamines, peripheral resistance, and antidiuretic hormone secretion are occurring.[11,18,108] When hypoxia and even minor changes in hydrostatic pressure in the hypoproteinemic fetus accompany the cardiorespiratory changes at birth, a depletion of intravascular volume and an increase in extravascular fluid volume will occur. Acute hypoxia is known to result in an increase in serum osmolality as fluid leaves the vascular space.[22] In fact, Barr et al[19] demonstrated that the use of albumin infusions in sick preterm neonates can worsen their respiratory status, presumably by increasing pulmonary edema.[180] In addition, after cesarean section, as opposed to vaginal delivery, neonatal blood volume may be lower and total body water (primarily intracellular) may be increased.[39,246] The group of hydropic neonates studied by Phibbs et al was heterogeneous with regard to the mode of delivery and to the presence or absence of labor prior to cesarean section.[179] Thus, the application of findings from investigations of body water distribution in the sick neonate to the understanding of the nature of fetal edema is only a guide. However, the second study of Phibbs et al[180] is extremely important for understanding the pathophysiology of hydrops fetalis as it affects the neonate in the immediate perinatal period.

In that study the severity of hydrops fetalis varied inversely with the serum albumin concentration and the cord

Table 18–5. SEVERITY OF HYDROPS FETALIS, GESTATIONAL AGE, BIRTH ASPHYXIA, AND SURVIVAL

Hydropic State	Gestational Age (weeks)	Lived	Died	Severe Asphyxia
None	36 + 1	30 (97%)	1 (3%)	2
Mild	34 ± 2	7 (58%)	5 (42%)	3
Severe	33 ± 2	4 (22%)	14 (78%)	11

Modified from Phibbs et al (1972): Cardiorespiratory status of erythroblastotic infants. I. Relationship of gestational age, severity of hemolytic disease, and birth asphyxia to idiopathic respiratory distress syndrome and survival. Pediatrics 49:5–14.

Table 18–6. HYDROPS FETALIS, NEONATAL RESUSCITATION, IDIOPATHIC RESPIRATORY DISTRESS SYNDROME (IRDS), AND SURVIVAL

Recovery	Lived	Died	IRDS
(1) + (2)	24 (86%)	4 (14%)	5 (18%)
(1) or (2)	5 (45%)	6 (55%)	7 (64%)
Neither (1) nor (2)	3 (25%)	6 (75%)	9 (100%)

1. pH $\geq$ 7.30
2. PaO$_2$ $\geq$ 50 } by 30 minutes with later stability or improvement.

Modified from Phibbs et al (1972): Cardiorespiratory status of erythroblastotic infants. I. Relationship of gestational age, severity of hemolytic disease, and birth asphyxia to idiopathic respiratory distress syndrome and survival. Pediatrics 49:5–14.

venous hematocrit, the relationship with the former being stronger.[180] When the albumin concentration was less than 2.0 g/dl, ascites, with or without pleural effusions, was seen. The hypoalbuminemia was not related to birth asphyxia. Plasma volume increased as the venous cord blood hematocrit fell below 23 per cent. The plasma volume was related neither to the hydropic state nor to the hypoalbuminemia; that is, the hypoalbuminemia was due to a true decrease in albumin concentration and not to hemodilution. The decrease in red cell volume and the rise in plasma volume with increasing severity of the hydropic state produced a total blood volume in hydropic neonates that was similar to normal in moderate to severely affected cases and that was in the low normal range in mildly affected cases. Similar findings were reported in a case of nonimmune hydrops fetalis without hypoproteinemia, in which Cowan et al found a slight increase in plasma volume, with the major increase being in extracellular fluid.[47] Phibbs et al therefore concluded that routine phlebotomy should not be performed at birth and that the low colloid osmotic pressure from hypoalbuminemia was the major cause of the fluid volume changes in hydrops fetalis.[180] Individual case reports[119,168,231] and the work of Baum and Harris[25] and Barnes et al[18] support these conclusions, although the latter workers were unable to detect significant degrees of hypoalbuminemia as an explanation of the low colloid osmotic pressure.

The third study by Phibbs et al[181] concluded that asphyxia is associated with arterial hypertension and generalized vasoconstriction, which can result in a raised central venous pressure and thus worsen the tendency for ascites to develop. Upon recovery from asphyxia, vasodilation occurs, and both aortic blood pressure and central venous pressure fall despite a normal blood volume. Severe acidosis was an early feature that responded to therapy but recurred to some degree when peripheral perfusion improved and tissue acid was "washed" into the central circulation. The implications were that careful monitoring of arterial blood pressure and central venous pressure are required. For measurements of central venous pressure, particular emphasis was given to the following: (1) The venous catheter tip should not be in the portal system. (2) The ascitic fluid should be tapped. (3) If the catheter tip is in the right atrium assisted ventilation should be discontinued for 10 to 20 seconds for each measurement of the central venous pressure. (4) Bagging is required on recommencement of the assisted ventilation.

Phibbs et al stated that the colloid osmotic differences between infused blood and the hydropic neonates' extracellular fluid favor redistribution of water to the intravascular space.[181] If volume expansion is carried out in hydropic neonates (e.g., for shock), volume overload may occur. Phibbs et al noted volume overload during or following full exchange transfusions in hydropic neonates but not following albumin infusions. It should be noted that albumin infusions are seldom used currently because of their associations with worsening respiratory distress, rapid increase in blood volume, and intracranial hemorrhage.[19,85,138] The major neonatal problems to be anticipated in hydrops fetalis are outlined in Table 18–7.

Table 18–7. NEONATAL PROBLEMS RELATED TO HYDROPS FETALIS

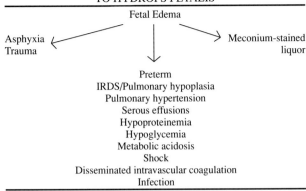

Fetal Edema

Asphyxia
Trauma

Meconium-stained liquor

Preterm
IRDS/Pulmonary hypoplasia
Pulmonary hypertension
Serous effusions
Hypoproteinemia
Hypoglycemia
Metabolic acidosis
Shock
Disseminated intravascular coagulation
Infection

CONCLUSIONS

Changes in hydrostatic and colloid osmotic pressures in fetal and placental circulations have been presented as the major etiologic factors in hydrops fetalis. From both clinical and experimental evidence it appears that each can have a primary role and that interactions are equally important. The role of other factors, such as anemia and increased capillary permeability secondary to hypoxia, appear to be less significant. However, since the fundamental mechanisms involved in the control of fetomaternal water fluxes remain unknown, definitive conclusions are premature. In nonimmune hydrops fetalis, the associations with congenital anomalies, especially cardiac, and other disease conditions are multiple. Therefore, the approach to therapy requires accurate diagnosis. The use of real time ultrasonography has identified a greater number of cardiac arrhythmias in fetuses with nonimmune hydrops fetalis. In turn these findings emphasize the need to be aware of maternal factors associated with hydrops fetalis as indicators for ultrasonography and potential therapy (see Table 18–3). The treatment of a tachyarrhythmia or even presumed cardiac failure and fetal edema with resolution of the hydrops[214,241] brings hope to approximately one third to one half of the fetuses previously described as having "idiopathic" nonimmune hydrops fetalis.[110] Fetal treatment, although not totally benign, is clearly preferable to delivery of a hydropic fetus. Such therapy has been applied to supraventricular arrhythmias without edema (and thus perhaps prior to the development of edema).[31,128] The presence of fetal and placental edema lowers the capacity of the fetoplacental unit to cope with labor and birth.[110] Postnatal transitions are complicated. Maternal postpartum hemorrhage and retained placenta occur commonly. For the optimum fetal outcome, especially in the absence of fetal abnormalities, prenatal steroids, perinatal monitoring, cesarean section, and aggressive pediatric management should be considered. Understanding the usual cardiorespiratory problems of the hydropic fetus in the postnatal period allows prenatal planning of postnatal ventilatory and cardiovascular support, which must be monitored carefully.

Ballantyne concluded "Let us here leave this subject; it is clear that it is obscure; this alone is clear."[14] The history of both immune and nonimmune hydrops fetalis demonstrates how understanding the pathophysiology of a condition can alter outcome for the better.

References

1. Abramovich DR, Garden A, Jandial L, Page KR (1979): Fetal swallowing and voiding in relation to hydramnios. Obstet Gynecol 54:15–20.
2. Abu-Dalu KI, Tamary H, Livni N, Rivkind AI, Yatziv S (1982): GM1 gangliosidosis presenting as neonatal ascites. J Pediatr 100:940–943.
3. Allan LD, Anderson RH, Sullivan ID, Campbell S, Holt DW, Tynan M (1983): Evaluation of fetal arrhythmias by echocardiography. Br Heart J 50:240–245.
4. Allan LD, Crawford DC, Sheridan R, Chapman MG (1986): Aetiology of non-immune hydrops: The value of echocardiography. Br J Obstet Gynaecol 93:223–225.
5. Altenburger KM, Jedziniak M, Roper WL, Hernandez J (1977): Congenital complete heart block associated with hydrops fetalis. J Pediatr 91:618–620.
6. Anand A, Gray ES, Brown T, Clewley JP, Cohen BJ (1987): Human parvovirus infection in pregnancy and hydrops fetalis. N Engl J Med 316:183–186.
7. Anders D, Kindermann G, Pfeifer U (1973): Metastasizing fetal neuroblastoma with involvement of the placenta simulating fetal erythroblastosis. J Pediatr 82:50–53.
8. Anderson HM, Drew JH, Beischer NA, Hutchison AA, Fortune DW (1983): Nonimmune hydrops fetalis: Changing contribution to perinatal mortality. Br J Obstet Gynaecol 90:636–639.
9. Arcilla RA, Thilenius OG, Ranniger K (1969): Congestive heart failure from suspected ductal closure in utero. J Pediatr 75:74–78.
10. Ascari WQ (1977): Serology of erythroblastosis fetalis. In Queenan JT (ed): Modern Management of the Rh Problem. 2nd ed New York, Harper & Row, pp 5–17.
11. Ashworth AM, Neligan GA (1959): Changes in the systolic blood pressure of normal babies during the first twenty-four hours of life. Lancet 1:804–807.
12. Aylsworth AS, Thomas GH, Hood JL, Malouf N (1980): A severe infantile sialidosis: Clinical, biochemical and microscopic features. J Pediatr 96:662–668.
13. Ballantyne JW (1892): In Diseases of the Fetus. Oliver, Edinburgh, pp 102–182.
14. Ballantyne JW (1902): In Manual of Antenatal Pathology and Hygiene. The Fetus 1902. Edinburgh, William Green and Sons, pp 288–354.
15. Banfield F, Dick M, Behrendt DM, Rosenthal A, Pescheria A, Scott W (1980): Intrapericardial teratoma: A new and treatable cause of hydrops fetalis. Am J Dis Child 134:1174–1175.
16. Barentsen S, Wladimiroff JW, Wallenburg HCS (1975): Sacrococcygeaal teratoom en hydramnion. Ned Tijdschr Geneesk 119:510–512.
17. Barnes RJ (1976): Water and mineral exchange between maternal and fetal fluids. In Beard RW, Nathanielsz PW (eds): Fetal Physiology and Medicine. Philadelphia, WB Saunders, pp 194–214.
18. Barnes SE, Bryan EM, Harris DA, Baum JD (1977): Oedema in the newborn. Molec Aspects Med 1:187–282.
19. Barr PA, Bailey PE, Sumners J (1977): Relation between arterial blood pressure and blood volume and effect of infused albumin in sick preterm infants. Pediatrics 60:282–289.
20. Barry FE, McCoy CP, Callahan WP (1951): Hemangioma of the umbilical cord. Am J Obstet Gynecol 62:675–680.
21. Bates HR (1970): Coxsackie virus B3 calcific pancarditis and hydrops fetalis. Am J Obstet Gynecol 106:629–630.
22. Battaglia FC, Meschia G, Hellegers AE, Barron DH (1959): The effects of acute hypoxia on the osmotic pressure of the plasma. Quart J Exp Pathol 43:197–208.
23. Battaglia FC, Prystowsky H, Smisson C, Hellegers AE, Bruns P (1960): The effect of the administration of fluids intravenously to mothers upon the concentrations of water and electrolytes in plasma of human fetuses. Pediatrics 25:2–10.
24. Battaglia FC, Woolever CA (1968): Fetal and neonatal complications associated with recurrent chorangiomas. Pediatrics 41:62–66.
25. Baum JD, Harris D (1972): Colloid osmotic pressure in erythroblastosis fetalis. Br Med J 1:601–603.
26. Becker MJ (1975): Hydrops fetalis [abstr]. Arch Dis Child 50:665.
27. Beischer NA, Fortune DW, Macafee J (1971): Nonimmunologic hydrops fetalis and congenital abnormalities. Obstet Gynecol 38:86–95.
28. Beitzke A, Winter R, Zach M, Grabbauer HM (1979): Kongenitales verhofflatero mit hydrops fetalis durch mutterliche tokolytikamedikaion. Klin Pediatr 191:410–417.
29. Belhassen B, Pauzer D, Blieden L, Sherez J, Zinger A, David M, Mutilbauer B, Laniado S (1982): Intrauterine and postnatal atrial fibrillation in the Wolff-Parkinson-White syndrome. Circulation 66:1124–1128.
30. Bellin LB, Bailit IW (1952): Congenital cirrhosis of the liver associated with infectious hepatitis of pregnancy. J Pediatr 40:60–63.
31. Bergmans MGM, Jonker GJ, Kock HCLV (1985): Fetal supraventricular tachycardia: Review of the literature. Obstet Gynec Surv 40:61–68.
32. Birner WF (1961): Neuroblastoma as a cause of antenatal death. Am J Obstet Gynecol 82:1388–1391.
33. Boer HR, Anido G (1979): Hydrops fetalis caused by Bart's hemoglobin. South Med J 72:1623–1624.
34. Bose C (1978): Hydrops fetalis and in utero intracranial hemorrhage. J Pediatr 93:1023–1024.
35. Bowman JM, Lewis M, deSa DJ (1984): Hydrops fetalis caused by massive maternofetal transplacental hemorrhage. J Pediatr 104:769–772.
36. Bryan EM (1977): IgG deficiency in association with placental oedema. Early Hum Dev 1:133–143.
37. Bryan EM, Chaimongkol B, Harris DA (1981): Alpha-thalassaemic hydrops fetalis. Arch Dis Child 56:476–478.
38. Bulova SI, Schwartz E, Harrer WV (1972): Hydrops fetalis and congenital syphilis. Pediatrics 49:285–287.
39. Cassady G (1971): Effect of cesarean section on neonatal body water spaces. N Engl J Med 285:887–891.
40. Chan V, Chan TK, Liang ST, Ghosh A, Kan YW, Todd D (1985): Hydrops fetalis due to an unusual form of HbH disease. Blood 66:224–228.
41. Chervenak FA, Issacson G, Blakemore KJ, Breg WR, Hobbins JC, Berkowitz RL, Tortora M, Mayden K, Mahoney MJ (1983): Fetal cystic hygroma. Cause and natural history. N Engl J Med 309:822–825.
42. Chiang W-T, Wei P-Y (1972): Immunoglobulins in hydrops fetalis. Am J Obstet Gynecol 114:816–818.
43. Clark DA (1981): Hydrops fetalis attributable to intra-uterine DIC Clin Pediatr 20:61–62.
44. Clewell WH (1986): Rh hemolytic disease: Forgotten but not gone. Perinatol-Nenatol 10:9–13/50.
45. Coombs RRA, Mourant AE, Race RR (1945): A new test for the detection of weak and "incomplete" Rh agglutinins. Br J Exp Pathol 26:255–266.
46. Cooke RWI, Mettau JW, Van Cappelle AW, De Villeneuve VH (1980): Familial congenital heart block and hydrops fetalis. Arch Dis Child 55:479–480.
47. Cowan RH, Waldo AL, Harris HB, Cassady G, Brans YW (1975): Neonatal paroxysmal supraventricular tachycardia with hydrops. Pediatrics 55:428–430.
48. Cowchock FS, Wapner RJ, Kurtz A, Chatzkel J, Barnhart S Jr, Lesnick C (1982): Brief clinical report: Not all cystic hygromas occur in the Ullrich-Turner syndrome. Am J Med Genet 12:327–331.
49. Cumming DC (1979): Recurrent nonimmune hydrops fetalis. Obstet Gynecol 54:124–126.
50. Daniel SJ, Cassady G (1968): Non-immunologic hydrops fetalis associated with a large hemangioendothelioma. Pediatrics 42:828–833.
51. Darrow RR (1938): Icterus gravis (erythroblastosis): neonatorum: Examination of etiologic considerations. Arch Pathol 25:378–417.

52. Davis CL (1982): Diagnosis and management of nonimmune hydrops fetalis J Reprod Med 27:594–600.

53. Debelle GD, Gillam GL, Tauro GP (1977): A case of hydrops fetalis due to feto-maternal hemorrhage. Aust Paediatr J 13:131–133.

54. de Crespigny LC, Robinson HP, McBain JC (1980): Fetal abdominal paracentesis in the management of gross fetal ascites. Aust NZ J Obstet Gynaecol 20:228–230.

55. Dempster AG (1969): Adenomatoid hamartoma of the lung in a neonate. J Clin Pathol 22:401–406.

56. Diamond LK, Blackfan KD, Baty JM (1932): Erythroblastosis fetalis and its associations with universal edema of fetus, icterus gravis neonatorum, and anemia of the newborn. J Pediatr 1:269–309.

57. Donnerstein RL, Allen HD (1986): Cardiac therapeutic implications from fetal echocardiography. Am J Dis Child 140:198.

58. Dorland WAN (1919): Watery accumulations in the fetal abdomen obstructing labor. Am J Obstet Gynecol 79:474–502.

59. Driscoll SG (1966): Hydrops fetalis. N Engl J Med 275:1432–1434.

60. Duffy JL (1966): Fetal retroperitoneal fibrosis associated with hydramnios: Case report with comments upon the factors controlling amniotic fluid volume. JAMA 198:993–996.

61. Dumesic DA, Silverman NH, Tobias S, Golbus MS (1982): Transplacental cardioversion of fetal supraventricular tachycardia with procainamide. N Engl J Med 307:1128–1131.

62. Dyggve H (1960): Hydrops fetalis without blood group incompatibility but associated with hydramnios. Acta Paediatr Scand 49:437–448.

63. Ehrlich JC, Goodfriend MJ, Shinohara Y, Seki M (1964): Fetal ascites and portal dysplasia of the liver (polycystic disease without cysts):. Pediatrics 33:216–226.

64. Emery JL, Mithal A (1960): The number of alveoli in the terminal respiratory unit of man during late intrauterine life and childhood. Arch Dis Child 35:544–547.

65. Etches PC, Lemons JA (1979): Nonimmune hydrops fetalis: Report of 22 cases including three siblings. Pediatrics 64:326–332.

66. Falkinburg LW, Kay MN (1953): A case of sympathogonioma (neuroblastoma): of the right adrenal simulating erythroblastosis fetalis. J Pediatr 42:462–465.

67. Feige A, Fiedler K, Rempen A, Osterhage HR (1984): Pranataldiagnose eines Prune-Belly-Syndroms, aufgetreten bei Geschwistern in zwei aufeinanderfolgenden Schwangerschaften. Z Gerburtshilfe Perinatol 188:239–243.

68. Finn R, Clarke CA, Donohoe WTA, McConnell RB, Sheppard PM, Lehane D, Kulke W (1961): Experimental studies on the prevention of Rh hemolytic disease. Br Med J 1:1486–1490.

69. Fleischer AC, Killam AP, Boehm FH, Hutchison AA, Jones TB, Shaff MI, Barrett JM, Lindsey AM, James AE Jr (1981): Hydrops fetalis: Sonographic evaluation and clinical implications. Radiology 141:163–168.

70. Fleming P, McLeary RD (1981): Nonimmunologic fetal hydrops with theca lutein cysts. Radiology 141:169–170.

71. France NE, Back EH (1954): Neonatal ascites associated with urethral obstruction. Arch Dis Child 29:565–568.

72. Friedman EA, Gray MJ, Hutchinson DL, Plentl AA (1959): The role of the monkey fetus in the exchange of the water and sodium of amniotic fluid. J Clin Invest 38:961–970.

73. Frigoletto FD Jr, Umansky I (1979): Erythroblastosis fetalis: Identification, management, and prevention. Clin Perinatol 6:321–330.

74. Friis-Hansen B (1971): Body composition during growth. Pediatrics 47:264–274.

75. Fritz MA, Christopher CR (1981): Umbilical vein thrombosis and maternal diabetes mellitus. J Reprod Med 26:320–324.

76. Fujimoto A, Ebbin AJ, Wilson MG (1973): Down's syndrome and nonimmunological hydrops fetalis [letter]. Lancet 1:329.

77. Garrett WJ, Kossoff G, Lawrence R (1975): Gray scale echography in the diagnosis of hydrops due to fetal lung tumor. J Clin Ultrasound 3:45–50.

78. Gergely RZ, Eden R, Schifrin BS, Wade ME (1980): Antenatal diagnosis of congenital sacral teratoma. J Reprod Med 24:229–231.

79. Gest A, Hansen T, Hartley C, Giesler M (1984): Atrial tachycardia causes hydrops in fetal lambs [abstr]. Pediatr Res 18:325A.

80. Ghorashi B, Gottesfeld KR (1976): Recognition of the hydropic fetus by gray scale ultrasound. J Clin Ultrasound 4:193–197.

81. Giacoia GP (1980): Hydrops fetalis (fetal edema). Clin Pediatr 19:334–339.

82. Gillan JE, Lowden JA, Gaskin K, Cutz E (1984): Congenital ascites as a presenting sign of lysosmal storage disease. J Pediatr 104:225–231.

83. Ginsburg SJ, Groll M (1973): Hydrops fetalis due to infantile Gaucher's disease. J Pediatr 82:1046–1048.

84. Goldberg JD, Mitty H, Dische MR, Berkowitz RL (1986): Prenatal shunting of fetal ascites in nonimmune hydrops fetalis. Am J Perinatol 3:92–93.

85. Goldberg R, Chung D, Goldman S (1980): The association of rapid volume expansion and intraventricular hemorrhage in preterm infants. J Pediatr 96:1060–1063.

86. Gordon H (1971): The diagnosis of hydrops fetalis. Clin Obstet Gynecol 14:548–560.

87. Gorman JG, Freda VJ, Pollack W (1962): Intramuscular injection of a new experimental gamma-2 globulin preparation containing high levels of anti-Rh antibody as a means of preventing sensitization to Rh. Proc 9th Cong Int Soc Hematology 2:545–549.

88. Gottschalk W, Abramson D (1957): Placental edema and fetal hydrops: A case of congenital cystic and adenomatoid malformation of the lung. Obstet Gynecol 10:626–631.

89. Gough JD, Keeling JW, Castle B, Iliff PJ (1986): The obstetric management of non-immunological hydrops. Br J Obstet Gynaecol 93:226–234.

90. Graves GR, Baskett TF (1984): Nonimmune hydrops fetalis: antenatal diagnosis and management. Am J Obstet Gynecol 148:563–565.

91. Gray CR, Towel ME, Wright VJ (1972): Thalassemic hydrops fetalis in two Chinese-Canadian families. Can Med Assoc 107:1186–1190.

92. Greenberg F, Carpenter RJ, Ledbetter DH (1983): Cystic hygroma and hydrops fetalis in a fetus with trisomy 13. Clin Genet 24:389–391.

93. Griscon NT, Colodny AH, Rosenberg HK, Fliegel CR, Hardy BE (1977): Diagnostic aspects of neonatal ascites: Report of 27 cases. AJR 128:961–969.

94. Hadlock FP, Deter RL, Garcia-Pratt J, Athey P, Carpenter R, Hinkley CM, Park SK (1980): Fetal ascites not associated with Rh incompatibility: Recognition and management with sonography. AJR 134:1225–1230.

95. Halbrecht I, Shabtai F (1975): An unusual case of Hb-Bart's hydrops fetalis. Acta Genet Med Gemellol 24:97–103.

96. Harbert GM Jr, Brame RG, McGaughey HS, Thornton WN Jr (1968): Fetomaternal water exchange. Obstet Gynecol 32:232–240.

97. Hardy JD, Solomon S, Banwell GS, Beach R, Wright V, Howard FM (1979): Congenital complete heart block in the newborn associated with maternal systemic lupus erythematosus and other connective tissue disorders. Arch Dis Child 54:7–13.

98. Harkavy KL (1977): Aetiology of hydrops fetalis [letter]. Arch Dis Child 52:338.

99. Harkavy K, Scanlon JW (1978): Hydrops fetalis in a parabiotic, acardiac twin. Am J Dis Child 132:638–639.

100. Harrigan JT, Kangos JJ, Sikka A (1981): Successful treatment of fetal congestive heart failure secondary to tachycardia. N Engl J Med 304:1527–1529.

101. Hedvall G (1973): Congenital paroxysmal tachycardia—a report of three cases. Acta Paediatr Scand 62:550–552.

102. Henderson JL (1942): Erythroblastosis fetalis or congenital syphilis. J Obstet Gynaecol Br Emp 49:499–511.

103. Hirata K, Kato H, Yoshioka F, Matsunaga T (1985): Successful treatment of fetal atrial flutter and congestive heart failure. Arch Dis Child 60:158–160.

104. Hobbins JC, Grannum PAT, Berkowitz RL, Silverman R, Mahoney MJ (1979): Ultrasound in the diagnosis of congenital anomalies. Am J Obstet Gynecol 134:331–345.

105. Hobel CJ (1970): The influence of anemia on the acid-base state of the fetus and newborn. Am J Obstet Gynecol 106:303–308.

106. Holzgreve W, Curry CJR, Golbus MS, Callen PW, Filly RA, Smith JC (1984): Investigation of nonimmune hydrops fetalis. Am J Obstet Gynecol 150:805–812.

107. Holzgreve W, Holzgreve B, Curry CJR (1985): Nonimmune hydrops fetalis: Diagnosis and management. Semin Perinatol 9:52–67.

108. Hoppenstein JM, Miltenberger FW, Moran WH (1968): The increase in blood levels of vasopressin in infants during birth and surgical procedures. Surg Gynecol Obstet 127:966–974.

109. Horger EO, Hutchinson DL (1970): Drug-induced hydrops in the fetal lamb. Obstet Gynecol 35:364–370.

110. Hutchison AA, Drew JH, Yu VYH, Williams ML, Fortune DW, Beischer NA (1982): Nonimmunologic hydrops fetalis: A review of 61 cases. Obstet Gynecol 59:347–352.

111. Hutchinson DL, Gray MJ, Plentl AA, Alvarez H, Caldeyro-Barcia R, Kaplan B, Lind J (1959): The role of the fetus in the water exchange of the amniotic fluid of normal and hydramniotic patients. J Clin Invest 38:971–980.

112. Hutchinson DL, Hunter CB, Nelson ED, Plentl AA (1955): The exchange of water and electrolytes in the mechanism of amniotic fluid formation and the relationship to hydramnios. Surg Gynecol Obstet 100:391–396.

113. Iff W (1931): Uber angeborene verkalkungen besonders der arterien. Virchows Arch Path Anat 281:377–395.

114. Iliff PJ, Nicholls JM, Keeling JW, Gough JD (1983): Nonimmunologic hydrops fetalis: A review of 27 cases. Arch Dis Child 58:979–982.

115. Im SS, Rizos N, Joutsi P, Shime J, Benzie RJ (1984): Nonimmunologic hydrops fetalis. Am J Obstet Gynecol 148:566–569.

115a. Irani D, Kim H-S, El-Hibri H, et al (1983): Postmortem observations on β-glucuronidase deficiency presenting as hydrops fetalis. Ann Neurol 14:486–490.

116. Ito T, Engle MA, Holswade GR (1961): Congenital insufficiency of pulmonic valve: A rare cause of neonatal heart failure. Pediatrics 28:712–718.

117. Ivemark BI, Lagergren C, Ljungqvist A (1962): Generalized arterial calcification associated with hydramnios in two stillborn infants. Acta Paediatr Scand (Suppl): 135:103–110.

118. Jacobi M, Litvak A, Gruber S (1946): The influence of human serum albumin on edema in erythroblastosis fetalis. J Pediatr 29:177–182.

119. Jarvet CT (1942): Erythroblastosis neonatorum. Surg Gynecol Obstet 74:1–19.

120. Johnson AT, Halbert D (1974): Congenital neuroblastoma presenting as hydrops fetalis. N Carol Med J 35:289–291.

121. Jones CEM, Rivers RPA, Taghizadeh A (1972): Disseminated intravascular coagulation and fetal hydrops in a newborn in association with a chorangioma of the placenta. Pediatrics 50:901–907.

122. Jones DED, Pritchard KI, Gioannini CA, Moore DJ, Bradford WD (1972): Hydrops fetalis associated with idiopathic arterial calcification. Obstet Gynecol 39:435–440.

123. Kanbour AI, Klionsky BL (1978): Idiopathic hydrops fetalis [abstr]. Lab Invest 38:390.

124. Keeling JW, Gough DJ, Iliff PJ. (1983): The pathology of nonrhesus hydrops. Diagn Histopathol 6:89–111.

125. Kerenyi TD, Gleicher N, Meurer J, Brown E, Steinfeld L, Chitkara U, Raucher H (1980): Transplacental cardioversion of intrauterine supraventricular tachycardia with digitalis. Lancet 2:393–395.

126. Kesson CW (1958): Foetal paroxysmal auricular tachycardia. Br Heart J 20:552–556.

127. King CR (1982): Hydrops fetalis and genetic disease. Birth Defects Original Article Series 18:101–113.

128. Klein AM, Holzman IR, Austin EM (1979): Fetal tachycardia prior to the development of hydrops—Attempted pharmacologic cardioversion: Case report. Am J Obstet Gynecol 134:347–348.

129. Kleinman CS, Copel JA, Weinstein EM, Santulli TV, Hobbins JC (1985): In utero diagnosis and treatment of fetal supraventricular tachycardia. Semin Perinatol 9:113–129.

130. Kleinman CS, Copel JA, Weinstein EM, Santulli TV Jr, Hobbins JC (1985): Treatment of fetal supraventricular tachycardias. J Clin Ultrasound 13:265–273.

131. Kleinman CS, Donnerstein RL, DeVore GR, Jaffe CC, Lynch DC, Berkowitz RL, Talner NS, Hobbins JC (1982): Fetal echocardiography for evaluation of in utero congestive heart failure. N Eng J Med 306:568–575.

132. Kleinman CS, Donnerstein RL, Jaffe CC, DeVore GR, Weinstein EM, Lynch DC, Talner NS, Berkowitz RL, Hobbins JC (1983): Fetal echocardiography. Amer J Cardiol 51:237–243.

133. Kohler HG (1976): Sacrococcygeal teratoma and "non-immunological" hydrops fetalis. Br Med J 2:422–423.

134. Kubinyi J, Pilishegyi (1974): Hydrops fetalis universalis ohne isoimmunization. Geburtshilfe Frauenheilkel 34:1012–1017.

135. Kucera H, Pollack A, Rudelstrorfer B (1975): Unusual case of congenital cystic adenomatoid malformation of the lung with hydrops universalis. Z Gynaekol 97:1142–1146.

135a. Lacey PA, Caskey CR, Werner DJ, Moulds JJ (1983): Fatal hemolytic disease of a newborn due to anti-D in an Rh-positive D" variant mother. Transfusion 23:91–94.

136. Landsteiner K, Weiner AS (1940): Agglutinable factor in human blood recognized by immune sera for rhesus blood. Proc Soc Exp Biol 43:223.

137. Lange I, Rodeck CH, Morgan-Capner P, Simmons A (1982): Prenatal serological diagnosis of cytomegalovirus infection. Br Med J 284:2673–2674.

138. Lay SK, Bancalari E, Malkus H (1980): Acute effects of albumin infusion on blood volume and renal function in premature infants with respiratory distress syndrome. J Pediatr 97:619–623.

139. Leake RD, Strimling B, Emmanouilides GC (1973): Intrauterine cardiac failure with hydrops fetalis: Case report of a twin with the hypoplastic left heart syndrome and a review of the literature. Clin Pediatr 12:649–651.

140. Levin DL (1979): Primary pulmonary hypoplasia. J Pediatr 95:550–551.

141. Levine P, Newmark NJ, Burnham L, Engelwood NJ, Katzin EM, Newmark NJ, Vogel P (1941): The role of iso-immunization in the pathogenesis of erythroblastosis fetalis. Am J Obstet Gynecol 42:925–937.

142. Levine P, Stetson RE (1939): Unusual cases of intra-group agglutination. JAMA 113:126–127.

143. Lie-Injo LE, Randhawa ZI, Kane JP, Ganesan J, George R (1979): Heterogeneity of hemoglobin gamma chains in normal newborns and in cases of alpha and beta thalassemia. Am J Hematol 6:17–25.

144. Liley AW (1972): Disorders of amniotic fluid. In Assali NS (ed): Pathophysiology of Gestation. Vol 11. New York, Academic Press, pp 157–206.

145. Linderkamp O (1982): Placental transfusion: determinants and effects. Clin Perinatol 9:559–592.

146. Lingman G, Ohrlander S, Ohlin P (1980): Intrauterine digoxin treatment of fetal paroxysmal tachycardia: Case report. Br J Obstet Gynaecol 87:340–342.

147. Lord JM (1953): Foetal ascites. Arch Dis Child 28:398–403.

148. Lorch V, Nelson RA, Meyers A, Carroll D, Mierau E (1979): Hydrops fetalis. J Kans Med Soc 80:503–520.

149. Lubinsky M, Rapoport P (1983): Transient fetal hydrops and "prune belly" in one identical female twin. N Engl J Med 308:256–257.

150. McCue CM, Mantakas ME, Tingelstad JB, Ruddy S (1977): Congenital heart block in newborns of mothers with connective tissue disease. Circulation 56:82–90.

151. McFadyen IR, Boonyaprokob U, Hutchinson DL (1968): Experimental production of anemia in fetal lambs. Am J Obstet Gynecol 100:686–695.

152. Macafee CAJ, Fortune DW, Beischer NA (1970): Non-immunological hydrops fetalis. J Obstet Gynaecol Br Comm 77:226–237.

153. Machin GA (1981): Differential diagnosis of hydrops fetalis. Am J Med Genet 9:341–350.

154. Maidman JE, Yeager C, Anderson V, Makabali G, O'Grady JP, Arce J, Tishler DM (1980): Prenatal diagnosis and management of nonimmunologic hydrops fetalis. Obstet Gynecol 56:571–576.

155. Mandelbaum B, Ross M, Riddle CB (1969): Hemangioma of the placenta associated with fetal anemia and edema. Obstet Gynecol 34:355–358.

156. Mayock DE, Hickok DE, Guthrie RD (1982): Cystic meconium peritonitis associated with hydrops fetalis. Am J Obstet Gynecol 142:704–705.

157. Mentzer WC, Collier E (1975): Hydrops fetalis associated with erythrocyte G-6-PD deficiency and maternal ingestion of fava beans and ascorbic acid. J Pediatr 85:565–567.

158. Meschia G, Battaglia FC, Barron DH (1957): A comparison of the freezing points of fetal and maternal plasmas of sheep and goat. Quart J Exper Physiol 42:163–170.
159. Merentstein GB (1969): Congenital cystic adenomatoid malformation of the lung. Am J Dis Child 118:772–776.
160. Miller DF, Petris SJ (1963): Fatal erythroblastosis fetalis secondary to ABO incompatibility. Obstet Gynecol 22:773–777.
161. Moerman F, Fryne J-P, Goddeeris P, Lauwerns JM (1982): Nonimmunologic hydrops fetalis. Arch Pathol Lab Med 106:635–640.
162. Mogilner BM, Ashkenazy M, Borenstein R, Lancet M (1982): Hydrops fetalis caused by maternal indomethacin treatment. Acta Obstet Gynecol Scand 61:183–185.
163. Moller JH, Lynch RP, Edwards JE (1966): Fetal cardiac failure resulting from congenital anomalies of the heart. J Pediatr 68:699–703.
164. Moss TJ, Kaplan L (1978): Association of hydrops fetalis with congenital neuroblastoma. Am J Obstet Gynecol 132:905–906.
165. Mostoufi-zadeh M, Driscoll SG, Biano SA, Kundsin RB (1984): Placental evidence of cytomegalovirus infection of the fetus and neonate. Arch Pathol Lab Med 108:403–406.
166. Naeye RL (1963): Human intrauterine parabiotic syndrome and its complications. N Engl J Med 268:804–809.
167. Naeye RL, Blanc WA (1964): Prenatal narrowing or closure of the foramen ovale. Circulation 30:736–742.
168. Nathan E (1968): Severe hydrops foetalis treated with peritoneal dialysis and positive-pressure ventilation. Lancet 1:1393–1396.
169. Nelson A, Peterson LA, Frampton B, Sly WS (1982): Mucopolysaccharidosis VII (B-glucuronidase deficiency) presenting as nonimmune hydrops fetalis. J Pediatr 101:574–576.
170. Newburger JW, Keane JF (1979): Intrauterine supraventricular tachycardia. J Pediatr 95:780–786.
171. Oie BK, Hertel J, Seip M, Friis-Hansen B (1984): Hydrops fetalis in 3 infants of a mother with acquired pure red cell aplasia: Transitory red cell aplasia in 1 infant. Scand J Hematol 33:466–470.
172. Ostor AG, Fortune DW (1978): Tuberous sclerosis initially seen as hydrops fetalis. Arch Pathol Lab Med 102:34–39.
173. Pearl W (1977): Cardiac malformations presenting as congenital atrial flutter. South Med J 70:622–624.
174. Pearson HA, Shanklin DR, Brodine CR (1965): Alpha-thalassemia as a cause of nonimmunologic hydrops fetalis. Am J Dis Child 109:168–172.
175. Perks AM, Vizsolyi E, Holt WF, Cassin S (1978): Hormonal influences on the movement and composition of amniotic fluid. In Gaillard PJ, Boer HH (eds). Comparative Endocrinology. Amsterdam, Elsevier/North Holland Biomedical Press, pp 231–234.
176. Perkins RP (1971): Hydrops fetalis and stillbirth in a male glucose-6-phosphate dehydrogenase–deficient fetus due to maternal ingestion of sulfisoxazole. Am J Obstet Gynecol 111:379–381.
177. Perlin BM, Pomerance JJ, Schrifrin BS (1981): Nonimmunologic hydrops fetalis. Obstet Gynecol 57:584–588.
178. Pesonen E, Haavisto H, Ammala P, Teramo K (1983): Intrauterine hydrops caused by premature closure of the foramen ovale. Arch Dis Child 58:1015–1016.
179. Phibbs RH, Johnson P, Kitterman JA, Gregory GA, Tooley WH (1972): Cardiorespiratory status of erythroblastotic infants. I. Relationship of gestational age, severity of hemolytic disease, and birth asphyxia to idiopathic respiratory distress syndrome and survival. Pediatrics 49:5–14.
180. Phibbs PH, Johnson P, Tooley WH (1974): Cardiorespiratory status of erythroblastotic newborn infants. II. Blood volume, hematocrit, and serum albumin concentration in relation to hydrops fetalis. Pediatrics 53:13–23.
181. Phibbs RH, Johnson P, Kitterman JA, Gregory GA, Tooley WH, Schlueter M (1976): Cardiorespiratory status of erythroblastotic newborn infants. III. Intravascular pressures during the first hours of life. Pediatrics 58:484–493.
182. Phillips RR, Batcup G, Vinall PS (1985): Non-immunologic hydrops fetalis [letter]. Arch Dis Child 60:84.
183. Pinon F, Sender A (1972): Anasarque foeto-placentaire. Pathologica 64:229–238.
184. Platt LD, Collea JV, Joseph DM (1978): Transitory fetal ascites: An ultrasound diagnosis. Am J Obstet Gynecol 132:906–908.
185. Platt LD, DeVore GR (1982): In utero diagnosis of hydrops fetalis: Ultrasound methods. Clin Perinatol 9:627–636.
186. Platt LD, Geierman CA, Turkel SB, Young G, Keegan KA (1981): Atrial hemangioma and hydrops fetalis. Am J Obstet Gynecol 141:107–109.
187. Potter EL (1943): Universal edema of the fetus unassociated with erythroblastosis. Am J Obstet Gynecol 46:130–134.
188. Potter EL (1961): In Pathology of the Fetus and Infant. 2nd ed. Chicago, Year Book Medical Publishers, pp 611–612.
189. Quagliarello JR, Passalaqua AM, Greco MA, Zinberg S, Young BK (1978): Ballantyne's triple edema syndrome: Prenatal diagnosis with ultrasound and maternal renal biopsy findings. Am J Obstet Gynecol 132:580–581.
190. Radford DJ, Izukawa T, Rowe RD (1976): Congenital paroxysmal atrial tachycardia. Arch Dis Child 51:613–617.
191. Radford DJ, Izukawa T, Rowe RD (1977): Aetiology of hydrops fetalis [letter]. Arch Dis Child 52:338.
192. Ramzin MS, Napflin S (1982): Transient intrauterine supraventricular tachycardia associated with transient hydrops fetalis. Case report. Br J Obstet Gynaecol 89:965–966.
193. Rees L, Vlies PR, Adams J (1980): Hydrops fetalis, an unusual case, presentation and method of diagnosis. Br J Obstet Gynaecol 87:1169–1170.
194. Riley P, Wittenberg DF, Riseborough J (1983): Non-immunological hydrops fetalis. A case report. S Afr Med J 63:334–336.
195. Robinow M, Spisso K, Buschi AJ, Brenbridge AN (1980): Turner syndrome: sonography showing fetal hydrops simulating hydramnios. AJR 135:846–848.
196. Rudolph N, Levin EJ (1977): Hydrops fetalis with vena caval thrombosis in utero. NY State J Med 77:421–423.
197. Sahn DJ, Shenker L, Reed KL (1982): Prenatal ultrasound diagnosis of hypoplastic left heart syndrome in utero associated with hydrops fetalis. Am Heart J 104:1368–1372.
198. Saint-Martin J, Lugassy G (1975): Tachycardies supraventriculaires du nouveau-ne. A propos de deux observations avec anasarque foeto-placentaire. Pediatrie 30:419–428.
199. Schanfield MS (1981): Antibody-mediated perinatal diseases. Clin Lab Med 1:239–263.
200. Schreiner RL, Hurwitz RA, Rosenfeld CR, Miller W (1978): Atrial tachy-arrhythmias associated with massive edema in the newborn. J Perinat Med 6:274–279.
201. Schwartz SM, Visekul C, Laxova R, McPherson EW, Gilbert EF (1981): Idiopathic hydrops fetalis report of 4 patients including two affected sibs. Am J Med Genet 8:59–66.
202. Schlotter CM, Kunz S (1978): Fetal parasystolia; uncommon cause of fetal arrhythmia with polyhydramnios and hydrops fetalis. Z Gerburtshilfe Perinatol 182:371–375.
203. Seeds AE Jr (1965): Water metabolism in the fetus. Am J Obstet Gynecol 92:727–743.
204. Seeds JW, Herbert WNP, Bowes WA, Cefalo RC (1984): Recurrent idiopathic fetal hydrops : Results of prenatal therapy. Obstet Gynecol 64:30S–33S.
205. Seward JF, Zusman J (1978): Hydrops fetalis associated with small bowel volvulus. Lancet 2:52–53.
206. Sharma RS, Yu V, Walters WAW (1979): Haemoglobin Bart's hydrops fetalis syndrome in an infant of Greek origin and prenatal diagnosis of alpha-thalassemia. Med J Aust 2:433–434.
207. Shenker L (1979): Fetal cardiac arrhythmias. Obstet Gynecol Surg 34:561–572.
208. Shirley IM, Richards BA, Ward RHT (1981): Ultrasound diagnosis of hydrops fetalis due to fetal tachycardia. Br J Radiol 54:561–572.
209. Shturman-Ellstein R, Greco MA, Myrie C, Goldman EK (1978): Hydrops fetalis, hydramnios and hepatic vascular malformation associated with cutaneous hemangioma and chorangioma. Acta Paediatr Scand 67:239–243.
210. Silber DL, Durbin RE (1969): Intrauterine atrial tachycardia. Am J Dis Child 117:722–726.
211. Silver HK, Huffman PJ, Nakashima II (1958): Fetal ascites. Am J Dis Child 96:268–271.
212. Silverstein AJ, Kanbour AI (1981): Repetitive idiopathic fetal hydrops. Obstet Gynecol 57:18S–21S.
213. Sim CC, Panny S, Combs J, Gutberlett R (1984): Hydrops fetalis associated with Gaucher disease. Pathol Res Pract 179:101–104.

214. Simpson PC, Trudinger BJ, Walker A, Baird PJ (1983): The intrauterine treatment of cardiac failure in a twin pregnancy with an acardiac, acephalic monster. Am J Obstet Gynecol 147:842–844.

215. Sloper KS, Brown RS, Baum JD (1979): The water content of the human umbilical cord. Early Hum Dev 3:205–210.

216. Smith DR, Chan HSL, de Sa DJ (1981): Placental involvement in congenital neuroblastoma. J Clin Pathol 34:785–789.

217. Smith RD, DuShane JW, Edwards JE (1959): Congenital insufficiency of the pulmonic valve including a case of fetal cardiac failure. Circulation 20:554–560.

218. Soltan MH, Keohane C (1981): Hydrops fetalis due to congenital cardiac rhabdomyoma. Case report. Br J Obstet Gynaecol 88: 771–773.

219. Spahr RC, Botti JJ, MacDonald HM, Holzman IR (1980): Nonimmunologic hydrops fetalis. Review of 19 cases. Int J Gynaecol Obstet 18:303–307.

220. Stevens DC, Hilliard JK, Schreiner RL, Hurwitz RA, Murrell R, Mirkin LD, Bonderman PW, Nolen PA (1982): Supraventricular tachycardia with edema, ascites and hydrops in fetal sheep. Am J Obstet Gynecol 142:316–322.

221. Stevens DC, Schreiner RL, Hurwitz RA, Gresham EL (1979): Fetal and neonatal ventricular arrhythmia. Pediatrics 63:771–777.

222. Strauss L, Driscoll SG (1964): Congenital neuroblastoma involving the placenta: Reports of two cases. Pediatrics 34:23–31.

223. Sun CC, Panny S, Combs J, Gutberlett R (1984): Hydrops fetalis associated with Gaucher's disease. Pathol Res Pract 179:101–104.

224. Sung RJ, Ferrer P, Garcia OL, Castellanos A, Gelband H (1977): A-V reciprocal rhythm and chronic reciprocating tachycardia in a newborn infant with concealed Wolff-Parkinson-White syndrome. Br Heart J 39:810–814.

225. Sweet L, Reid WD, Roberton NRC (1973): Hydrops fetalis in association with chorangioma of the placenta. J Pediatr 82:91–94.

226. Teuscher A, Bossi E, Inhof P, Erb E, Stocker FP, Weber JW (1978): Effect of propranolol on fetal tachycardia in diabetic pregnancy. Am J Cardiol 42:304–307.

227. Thumasathit B, Nondasuta A, Silpisornkosol S, Lousuebsakul B, Unchalipongse P, Mangkornkanok M (1968): Hydrops fetalis associated with Bart's hemoglobin in northern Thailand. J Pediatr 73:132–138.

228. Tonkin IL, Setzer ES, Ermocilla R (1980): Placental choriogangioma: A rare cause of congestive heart failure and hydrops fetalis in the newborn. AJR 134:181–183.

229. Tuberville PF, Killam AP, Davis PC Jr, Heath RE Jr, Fearnon RG, Pearson JW (1974): Nonimmunologic hydrops fetalis. Obstet Gynecol 43:567–570.

230. Turkel SB (1982): Conditions associated with nonimmune hydrops fetalis. Clin Perinatol 9:613–625.

231. Turski DM, Shahidi N, Viseskul C, Gilbert E (1978): Nonimmunologic hydrops fetalis. Am J Obstet Gynecol 131:586–587.

232. Valerius NH, Jacobsen JR (1978): Intrauterine supraventricular tachycardia. Acta Obstet Gynecol Scand 57:407–410.

233. Van Aerde J, Moerman P, Devlieger H, Dewolf F, Vandenberghe K, Jaeken J, Spitz B, Van Assche A, Eggermont E, Renaer M (1982): Congenital tumors and nonimmune hydrops fetalis [abstr]. J Perinat Med (Suppl) 2:78.

234. Van der Horst RL (1970): Congenital atrial flutter and cardiac failure presenting as hydrops foetalis at birth. South Afr J 44:1037–1039.

235. Van der Slikke JW, Balk AG (1980): Hydramnios with hydrops fetalis and disseminated fetal neuroblastoma. Obstet Gynecol 55:250–253.

236. Wallenburg HCS (1978): Water and electrolyte homeostasis of the amniotic fluid. In Developmental Aspects of Fluid and Electrolyte Homeostasis 1978. Mead Johnson Symposium on Perinatal and Developmental Medicine, No. 10, pp 9–17.

237. Wallenberg HCS, Wladimiroff JW (1978): Polyhydramnios and oligohydramnios. In Developmental Aspects of Fluid and Electrolyte Homeostasis 1978. Mead Johnson Symposium of Perinatal and Developmental Medicine, No. 10, pp 48–54.

238. Weatherall DJ, Clegg JB, Wong HB (1970): The haemoglobin constitution of infants with the haemoglobin Bart's hydrops fetalis syndrome. Br J Haematol 18:357–367.

239. Wedermeyer AL, Breitfeld V (1975): Cardiac neoplasm, tachyarrhythmia, and anasarca in an infant. Am J Dis Child 129:738–741.

240. Whitelaw AGL, Rogers PA, Hopkinson DA, Gordon H, Emerson PM, Darley JH, Reid C, Crawford M d'A (1979): Congenital anemia resulting from glucose phosphate isomerase deficiency: Genetics, clinical picture, and prenatal diagnosis. J Med Genet 16:189–196.

241. Wiggins JW, Bowes W, Clewell W, Manco-Johnson M, Manchester D, Johnson R, Appareti K, Wolfe RR (1986): Echocardiographic diagnosis and intravenous digoxin management of fetal tachyarrhythmias and congestive heart failure. Am J Dis Child 140: 202–204.

242. Wintour EM (1986): Amniotic fluid—our first environment. News Physiol Sci 1:95–97.

243. Wladimiroff JW, Stewart PA (1985): Treatment of fetal cardiac arrhythmias. Br J Hosp Med 34:134–140.

244. Wolff F, Breuker KH, Schlensker KH, Bolte A (1980): Prenatal diagnosis and therapy of fetal heart rate anomalies: With a contribution on the placental transfer of verapamil. J Perinat Med 8:203–208.

245. Wynn RJ, Schreiner RL (1979): Spurious elevation of amniotic fluid bilirubin in acute hydramnios with fetal obstruction. Am J Obstet Gynecol 134:105–106.

246. Yao AC, Wist A, Lind J (1967): The blood volume of the newborn infant delivered by cesarean section. Acta Paediatr Scand 56:585–592.

247. Young LW, Wexler HA (1978): Radiological case of the month: twin-twin transfusion syndrome. Am J Dis Child 132:201–02.

248. Zakanddin SS, Riemenschneider TA, Ikeda RM, Wennberg RP (1977): Hydrops fetalis in a preterm infant with Uhl's anomaly, pulmonary atresia and myocardial fibrosis and calcification [abstr]. Clin Res 25:192A.

249. Zuelzer WW (1944): Infantile toxoplasmosis. Arch Pathol 38: 1–19.

19 MANAGEMENT OF HYDROPS FETALIS

Nancy C. Chescheir
John W. Seeds

Hydrops fetalis is a pathologic condition of the fetus that includes generalized edema along with serous effusions of the pleural cavity and peritoneal and/or pericardial cavities. Historically, hydrops fetalis has most often been associated with fetomaternal blood group incompatibilities, such as Rh, Kell and Duffy isoimmunization, producing severe erythroblastosis fetalis. Nonimmune hydrops fetalis describes the occurrence of hydrops without hematologic evidence of fetomaternal blood group incompatibility.

HISTORICAL PERSPECTIVE

Fetal hydrops was first described by Ballantyne[4] in 1892, who reported a collection of 65 cases from the literature similar in appearance but with no uniformity in either maternal or fetal complications or conditions. Ballantyne concluded that "we are dealing with, not a pathologic entity, but with a group of symptoms common to several different morbid conditions." In 1943, Potter[27] first described nonimmune hydrops fetalis as a subset of this general syndrome. Of 17 hydropic infants without erythroblastosis in her study, four had anatomic and apparently unrelated abnormalities: One infant had a patent atrioventricular ostium; another had multiple anomalies, including facial clefting, diaphragmatic hernia, and clitoral hypertrophy; a third had tracheal atresia and polycystic kidneys; and the fourth had hypospadias.

Prophylactic administration of anti-D globulin to Rh-negative women in the perinatal period to prevent childbirth-associated Rh isoimmunization has become widespread. As a result, hydrops fetalis secondary to isoimmune erythroblastosis has decreased dramatically compared with nonimmunologic causes. In 1970, Macafee et al[19] reported that 17 per cent of hydrops fetalis was attributable to nonimmunologic causes. More recently,[3,21] up to 75 per cent of cases are reportedly the result of nonimmunologic causes. The overall reported incidence of nonimmune hydrops fetalis is estimated to be 1 in 2500 to 1 in 3500 neonates.[18,21]

Nonimmune hydrops fetalis (NIHF) has been associated clinically with an extremely poor fetal and neonatal prognosis, with perinatal mortality rates ranging from 50 to 98 per cent. As the number of different maternal, fetal, and placental conditions associated with NIHF grows, however, the development of a methodical and thorough approach to the management of these complex, high risk pregnancies may lead to improved outcomes.

In this chapter, we will explore prenatal diagnostic evaluation of hydrops fetalis, including sonographic appearance, etiology, perinatal management, and, briefly, neonatal care.

DIAGNOSIS

Prenatal detection of the general condition of hydrops fetalis is reliably accomplished with ultrasonographic visualization of the fetus. The diagnosis of a specific etiology for the hydrops fetalis may be more difficult. In a collected series of 289 patients, the correct prenatal diagnosis of hydrops fetalis was made in 243 (84 per cent).[35]

The initial ultrasonographic examination may be performed for a variety of clinical indications. In their review of 61 cases, Hutchinson et al[15] noted that anemia was present in 45 per cent of mothers, that pregnancy-induced hypertension or preeclampsia was present in 29 per cent, and/or polyhydramnios was present in 75 per cent. They propose that if any one of these symptoms is used as an indication to perform diagnostic ultrasonography, then 80 per cent of affected infants could be identified. In their series, approximately 20 per cent of the fetuses had a lethal abnormality, and another 25 per cent had a nonlethal congenital abnormality. Other reports have confirmed the high rate of hydramnios in cases of hydrops fetalis. Spahr et al[33] noted hydramnios in 57 to 76 per cent of cases.

Although there is not perfect agreement among investigators, the minimum criteria to establish the diagnosis of hydrops fetalis include generalized skin thickening (> 5 mm) and or two or more of the following: placental enlargement greater than 6 cm, ascites, pleural fluid, or pericardial fluid. Table 19–1 presents the ultrasonographic data from two groups of investigators and compares the frequency of a variety of ultrasonographic findings in their respective series of patients.

Table 19–1. ULTRASONOGRAPHIC CRITERIA FOR HYDROPS FETALIS

Ultrasound Finding	Mahoney[21] (N = 27 Patients) (Per Cent)	Fleischer[9] (N = 21 Patients) (Per Cent)
Scalp edema	59	–
Body wall edema	52	–
Anasarca	–	52
Polyhydramnios	48	52
Oligohydramnios	4	14
Ascites	85	76
Pleural fluid	33	–
Pericardial fluid	22	–
Placental thickening	55	67

Once the sonographic diagnosis of hydrops fetalis is made in a fetus, a methodical search for the etiology of the hydrops must be made. Rh isoimmunization or other hemolytic diseases such as Kell or Duffy immunization should be excluded by performing an antibody screening on the mother. If blood group incompatibilities are excluded, further evaluation should progress using the least invasive tests first. Table 19–2 lists some recommended initial studies and their rationale.

If these studies do not identify a cause for NIHF, it may be necessary to consider more invasive procedures. Amniocentesis may be performed to provide fetal fibroblasts for cell culture for identification of the aneuploid fetus. Pulmonary maturity studies may be performed on amniotic fluid to determine whether fetal lung maturity is present, an important variable in obstetric management.

It is possible to sample the fetal blood directly through either fetoscopy or umbilical vein aspiration with ultrasound guidance. Fetal blood sampling permits fetal hematologic and biochemical studies and also provides for rapid karyotyping (2 to 4 days as opposed to the 2 to 3 weeks necessary to obtain the karyotype from amniotic fluid fibroblasts). It is also possible to sample the serous fluid collections with fetal paracentesis or pleurocentesis for biochemical and microbiologic evaluation. Cell culture and karyotyping have been successfully performed on a variety of fetal fluids, including serous effusions of the chest and abdomen.

Nicolaides et al[23] reported on 30 patients in whom less invasive procedures had failed to uncover the etiology of the NIHF, prompting fetoscopic direct blood sampling at 16 to 32 weeks' gestation. In these 30 patients, a diagnosis was obtained in 43 per cent: 10 fetuses had chromosomal abnormalities, one fetus had an erythroblastic process (possibly erythroleukemia), one fetus had α-thalassemia, and one fetus had an in utero cytomegalovirus infection. In the 18 patients in whom it was sought, hypoproteinemia was identified.

In summary, antenatal attempts to diagnose the etiology of NIHF should proceed in a systematic fashion. The least invasive tests, such as maternal blood tests, ultrasonography, and fetal echocardiography, should be done first. If these fail to produce a diagnosis, amniocentesis may be considered for amniotic fluid karyotype. The most invasive procedures currently applicable are fetoscopy, fetal umbilical vein aspiration, and sampling of serous effusions. These should be used only for those fetuses in whom other investigations fail to produce a diagnosis.

ETIOLOGY

A constantly growing list of maternal, fetal, and placental abnormalities has been associated with NIHF. Many authors have attempted to define common pathophysiologic mechanisms to explain how hydrops can be the common end-stage manifestation of so many diverse conditions.

The most prominent theories postulate that the fetus has one of three possible pathophysiologic problems:

1. Profound fetal anemia. The mechanisms by which anemia is thought to lead to hydrops fetalis are threefold. First, severe anemia may lead to fetal tachycardia with resultant high output cardiac failure. Second, severe anemia may cause decreased colloid oncotic pressure with transudation of intravascular fluid to the extravascular spaces on an osmotic basis. Third, the fetal tissues may become hypoxic secondary to the decreased oxygen-carrying capacity; one of the pathologic responses to tissue hypoxia is capillary leakage, with transudation of fluid out of the intravascular spaces on this basis.

2. Congestive heart failure. Congestive heart failure is probably the cause of hydrops fetalis in those fetuses with in utero arrhythmias, such as supraventricular tachycardia, or heart block. Most structural congenital heart defects do not cause in utero congestive heart failure because the fetal circulation largely bypasses the left side of the heart. However, some structural defects will cause fetal heart failure. These include insufficiency of the atrioventricular valves, premature closure of the foramen ovale or ductus arteriosus, and intracardiac tumors, such as rhabdomyomas.

3. Decreased colloid oncotic pressure. In those fetuses with liver parenchymal distortion or hepatic dysfunction or in those fetuses who are losing a significant portion of

Table 19–2. SUGGESTED PRENATAL EVALUATION OF NIHF

1. Complete blood count. Maternal anemia is often found in association with NIHF (45 per cent). α-Thalassemia is a cause of NIHF, and women who are heterozygous for α-thalassemia will commonly have microcytic, hypochromic anemias.
2. Kleihauer-Betke screen. The Kleihauer-Betke is a test performed on maternal blood to detect the presence of fetal cells within the maternal circulation and therefore is useful in establishing the diagnosis of a significant fetomaternal hemorrhage. Massive fetomaternal hemorrhage with resultant profound fetal anemia can cause NIHF.
3. Hemoglobin electrophoresis. In women at high risk for hemoglobinopathies such as α-thalassemia, this test should be performed even in the absence of significant maternal anemia.
4. TORCH titres. Toxoplasmosis, rubella, cytomegalovirus, and herpes in utero infections can result in NIHF.
5. VDRL. Fetal syphilis, through either associated placental dysfunction or fetal myocardial dysfunction, is associated with NIHF.
6. Parental glucose-6-phosphate dehydrogenase (G-6-PD) and erythrocyte pyruvate kinase studies. Fetal red cell enzyme deficiencies in their homozygous form can cause NIHF. If both parents carry the gene for a deficiency of this kind, the fetus may be affected; such inherited fetal enzyme deficiencies may be the etiology for the hydrops fetalis.
7. Glucose tolerance evaluation. Maternal diabetes is associated with an increased incidence of congenital abnormalities, some of which are associated with NIHF. Infants of diabetic mothers are also at risk for dysfunction of structurally normal myocardiums.
8. Detailed real time ultrasonography. A careful fetal survey to document the degree of hydrops for later comparison during subsequent serial scans is very important. In infants of a gestational age compatible with extrauterine survival in whom the hydrops is worsening, delivery may be indicated. A careful search for fetal or placental anatomic abnormalities that may be responsible for NIHF is also very important.
9. Fetal echocardiography. Structural cardiac anomalies or fetal rhythm disturbances may be diagnosed by fetal real time echocardiography, M-mode echocardiography, or Doppler studies.

their plasma proteins to their serous fluid collections, reduced colloid osmotic pressure is probably an important contributing factor. As previously noted, Nicolaides et al[23] found significant hypoproteinemia in all of the fetuses in whom they searched.

Some observers, however, note the absence of hydrops fetalis in some infants with these same conditions. It is clear that in many cases of hydrops fetalis, these pathophysiologic conditions may exist alone or in association with one another, or they may in fact not be present. Thus, a diversity of conditions are associated with hydrops fetalis.

Table 19–3 lists conditions that have been associated with NIHF, along with the diagnostic tests that may prove most useful. Some of these conditions have appeared as isolated case reports only.

Despite the exhaustive diagnostic evaluation described above, in as many as 45 per cent of fetuses the etiology of hydrops fetalis will remain unknown[33] even after the birth of the infant. In a collection of 479 affected fetuses, described in 15 papers with more than five patients in each report,[6,7,9,13–16,19–24,30] 28.4 per cent of patients had idiopathic nonimmune hydrops fetalis.

Accurate diagnosis, if possible, facilitates perinatal care in several ways. First, some of the causes of hydrops fetalis are amenable to in utero treatment, which may improve outcome. Fetal arrhythmias are an example of a treatable cause of NIHF (see below). Second, if the diagnosis is made prior to 24 weeks' gestation and the associated abnormality is not compatible with extrauterine life, then termination of the pregnancy may be considered. Third, early delivery may benefit certain fetal conditions associated with NIHF, such as cases of twin-to-twin transfusion or fetomaternal hemorrhage. Fourth, if the diagnosis of a condition incompatible with extrauterine life is made after 24 weeks' gestation, then obstetric management could center on maternal welfare alone. Lastly, it is helpful to the neonatologist caring for these usually critically ill infants to have as much information as possible prenatally to permit rapid and efficient postnatal resuscitation.

Several of the etiologies listed in Table 19–3 deserve special mention, either because of relative frequency or because of availability of special treatments or diagnostic options.

Fetal Cardiac Anomalies or Dysfunctions

In the same series of 479 fetuses referred to above, the next largest groups of patients other than those with idiopathic hydrops fetalis were those fetuses with structural abnormalities of the heart or rhythm disturbances, composing 12.5 per cent and 4.0 per cent, respectively, of the 479 fetuses. This high frequency of cardiac abnormalities in association with NIHF mandates careful scrutiny of the fetal heart.

Three ultrasonographic modalities are presently available for this purpose: real time ultrasonography, M-mode echocardiography, and Doppler flow studies. These may be used to evaluate normal cardiac structure and function.

Table 19–3. CONDITIONS THAT HAVE BEEN ASSOCIATED WITH NIHF

Disorder	Diagnostic Studies
Cardiac Disorders	
Structural Defects	Real time ultrasonography
Premature closure of the	and M-mode
foramen ovale	echocardiography
Anomalies of the tricuspid or	
pulmonary valves	
Severe ASD	
Severe VSD	
Hypoplastic left heart	
Ebstein anomaly	
Aortic valve stenosis	
Subaortic stenosis	
Dilated heart	
Atrioventricular septal defect	
Single ventricle	
Tetralogy of Fallot	
Subendocardial fibroelastosis	
Intracardiac tumors	
Transposition of the great vessels	
Rhythm Disturbances	
Complete heart block	
Fetal bradycardia	
Supraventricular tachycardias	
Atrial flutter with rapid ventricular response	
Infections	
Myocarditis secondary to coxsackievirus	
Other	
Arteriovenous shunting with high output failure (hemangiomas of the cord or skin, arteriovenous malformations of the liver or brain)	
Hematologic Disorders	Maternal blood and ultrasound studies
Anemia	
α-Thalassemia	Hemoglobin electrophoresis
Fetomaternal transfusion	Kleihauer-Betke screen
Maternofetal transfusion	
Twin-to-twin transfusion	Ultrasonography
G-6-PD deficiency	Maternal enzyme analysis
Erythrocyte pyruvate kinase deficiency	Maternal enzyme analysis
In utero closed space hemorrhage	Ultrasonography
Other	
Vena caval, portal vein, or femoral thrombosis	Doppler flow studies of fetal vessels
Pulmonary Disorders	Ultrasonography or autopsy
Diaphragmatic hernias	
Congenital cystic adenomatoid malformation	
Pulmonary sequestration	
Pulmonary hypoplasia	
Pulmonary lymphangiectasia	
Mediastinal teratoma	
Hamartoma of the lung	
Thoracogastroschisis	
Congenital chylothorax	
Chromosomal Disorders	Fetal karyotype
Turner syndrome	
Trisomy 21	
Trisomy 18	
Triploidy	
Trisomy 13	

Table continued on following page

Table 19–3. CONDITIONS THAT HAVE BEEN
ASSOCIATED WITH NIHF *(Continued)*

Disorder	Diagnostic Studies
Congenital Disorders	Ultrasonography and neonatal assessment
Tuberous sclerosis	
Storage diseases (Gaucher)	
Achondroplasia	
Arthrogryposis multiplex congenita	
Osteogenesis imperfecta	
Neu-Laxova syndrome	
Saldino-Noonan syndrome	
Pena-Shokeir type 1 syndrome	
Renal Diseases	Maternal blood and ultrasound studies
Congenital nephrosis	α-Fetoprotein testing
Renal vein thrombosis	Ultrasonography
Renal dysplasia	Ultrasonography
Infection	Serology studies and/or cultures of mother, amniotic fluid, or fluid aspirated from fetal serous cavities
Chagas disease	
TORCH infections	
Leptospirosis	
Syphilis	
Congenital hepatitis	
Gastrointestinal (GI) and Hepatic Disorders	Ultrasonography and neonatal assessment
Meconium peritonitis	
GI obstruction	
Tracheoesophageal fistula	
Small bowel volvulus	
Prenatal bowel perforation	
Duplication of gut	
Twin Gestation	Ultrasonography
Twin-to-twin transfusion	
Parabiotic twin syndrome	
Placental and Cord Abnormalities	Ultrasonography, surgical pathology
Chorioangioma of placenta or cord	
Chorionic vein thrombosis	
Placental and umbilical vein thrombosis	
Umbilical cord torsion	
True cord knots	
Angiomyxoma of cord	
Aneurysm of cord	
Miscellaneous	Ultrasonography and neonatal assessment
Congenital neuroblastoma	
Polysplenia syndrome	
Torsion of ovarian cyst	
Sacral teratoma	
Fetal trauma	
Amniotic band syndrome	
Maternal diabetes	
Wilms tumor	
Fetal retroperitoneal fibrosis	
Idiopathic	

Beginning at 16 weeks' gestation and continuing until term, the anatomy of the normal fetal heart can be visualized using real time ultrasonography,[1] which is performed first to establish the normalcy of the anatomic structure and relationships. It is almost always possible to obtain four-chambered short-axis views of the fetal heart; in most fetuses, visualization of the pulmonary and aortic outflow tracts is also possible. Once these structures are identified with appropriate equipment (Figs. 19–1 to 19–5), the M-line (motion line) can be directed as desired through the cardiac valves or chambers. The efficacy of fetal cardiac ultrasonography depends in part on fetal position and activity as well as the experience and equipment of the ultrasonographer. Accurate measurements of the dimensions of the aortic root, left atrium, right and left ventricular dimensions, and septal size and motion are possible. In cases of suspected rhythm abnormalities, M-mode visualization of both atrial and ventricular contraction permits accurate assessment of rhythm disturbances, such as identification of supraventricular tachycardias, atrial flutter, complete heart block, and others.

Doppler flow studies have been used by various investigators to determine blood flow rates through the foramen ovale and through both aortic and pulmonary valves.[31]

Structural abnormalities of the fetal heart associated with NIHF that have been diagnosed in utero include a wide variety of problems. Sahn and colleagues[28] demonstrated a hypoplastic left heart with an echogenic mass, using real time ultrasonography, M-mode, and Doppler flow studies. At autopsy, this mass was shown to be an organized thrombus within a hypoplastic left ventricle.

Silverman and associates[31] performed M-mode echocardiography and pulsed Doppler ultrasonography on 466 patients referred to their prenatal diagnosis unit for evaluation of suspected congenital heart defects. Twenty-three of these patients had atrioventricular valve abnormalities, 16 of which were hydropic. Eleven of these 16 suffered in utero death, four had pregnancy terminations, and one survived the neonatal period. Those seven infants with atrioventricular valve insufficiency without hydrops fetalis survived.

Other structural cardiac abnormalities that have been diagnosed antenatally include congenital cardiac rhabdomyoma,[32] premature closure of the foramen ovale,[26] and hypoplastic left heart.[36] Hypoplastic left heart does not usually cause fetal heart failure, but in this instance it was associated with an extensive rete Chiari that occluded the tricuspid valve.

Fetal cardiac tachyarrhythmias including atrial flutter or atrial tachycardia are also amenable to evaluation using M-mode echocardiography. Tachyarrhythmias are potentially treatable causes of NIHF, which can completely resolve if a normal rhythm is re-established.

During prenatal auscultation of the fetal cardiac sounds, attention should be paid to the rate and rhythm. If a persistent abnormality in either is heard on two or more occasions, the patient should have ultrasonographic evaluation of fetal cardiac function.

Fetal congestive heart failure, with resultant hydrops fetalis, can occur from either tachy- or bradyarrhythmias.

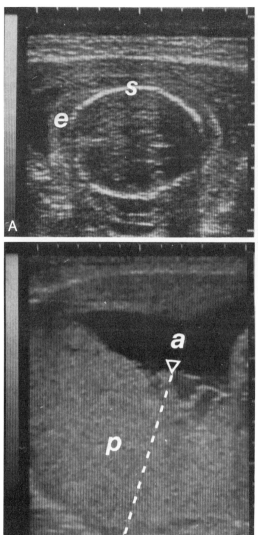

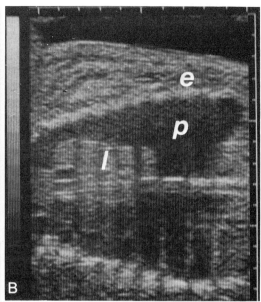

Figure 19–1. Typical examples of ultrasonographic findings of hydrops fetalis. *A,* Scalp edema of 1.2 cm thickness is seen as a "halo" around the skull. *B,* Longitudinal view of the fetal thorax and upper abdomen. It demonstrates bilateral pleural effusions, with the lung buds compressed to the mediastinum. The lungs usually are seen to fill the fetal chest on ultrasonographic examination. There is marked skin edema as well. *C,* The thickness of the placenta measures 8 cm; however, placental thickness should never exceed 5.5 cm. a = amniotic fluid; e = edema; l = lung; p = placenta in *C* and pleural effusion in *B*; s = skull.

Figure 19–2. *A,* Longitudinal view of the fetal thorax and upper abdomen. The cephalic end of the fetus is toward the right. This fetus has bilateral pleural effusions as well as ascites. The liver is clearly outlined by the effusions and ascites. The bowel is seen floating in the ascites. Skin edema is also present. *B,* This view represents a transverse scan of the fetal abdomen at the level of the fetal liver. Severe fetal ascites fills the abdomen and surrounds the liver. The vertical shadows are artifacts from the fetal spine. a = ascites; b = bowel; e = pleural effusions; li = liver.

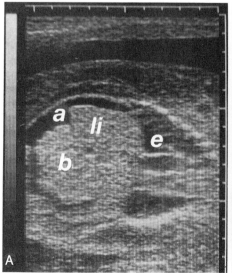

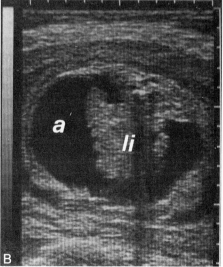

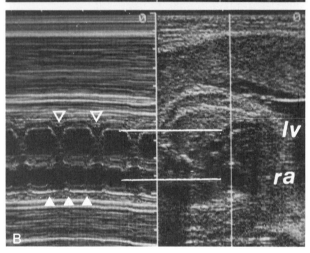

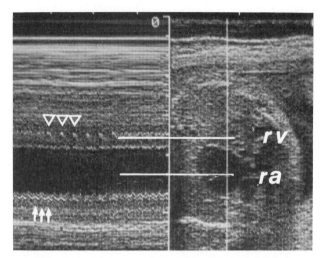

Figure 19–4. This echocardiogram demonstrates the findings in a fetus with atrial flutter. Note the enlarged right atrium, which is consistent with in utero heart failure. The atrial systole rate (closed arrows) is 480 per minute, while the right ventricular rate (open arrows) is approximately half that. ra = right atrium; rv = right ventricle.

Figure 19–3. *A*, Fetal echocardiogram of a normal fetus. On the right side the M-line is seen to be traversing the left ventricle, interventricular septum, and right ventricle. On the left side the M-mode echocardiogram shows normal motion of the left and right ventricles as well as normal motion of the septum. The small echodense spot (arrow) beneath the septum echo represents the motion of a papillary muscle. *B*, Fetal echocardiogram of a fetus with complete heart block. The M-line is traversing the left ventricle and right atrium. The atrial systoles are represented by the solid arrows and occur at a rate of 160 per minute (sweep speed is 3 seconds). The ventricular systoles are represented by the open arrows and occur at a rate of 80 per minute. No structural cardiac anomalies were noted. lv = left ventricle; ra = right atrium; rv = right ventricle; s = interventricular septum.

Complete heart block in the fetus can occur as a result of several pathologic processes. As many as 25 per cent of infants with congenital heart block have a structural abnormality of the heart, commonly endocardial fibroelastosis or transposition. There is a 30 to 60 per cent prevalence of connective tissue disorders in the mothers of infants with heart block.[18] Diagnosis of fetal complete heart block in the presence of hydrops fetalis indicates a very poor prognosis.

On the other hand, there are numerous case reports of successful in utero cardioversion of supraventricular tachycardia and atrial flutter by administering various agents

to the mother.[2,10] Some of the different medications used include digoxin, propranolol, procainamide, quinidine, and verapamil.

When administering these drugs to the mother in an attempt to convert the fetal tachycardia to a normal rhythm, there are several factors that must be considered. Guntheroth et al compare the use of several of these drugs in this setting.[11] They emphasize that fetal electrocardiograms do not include either P or T waves and therefore fetal atrial activity is not demonstrable by transabdominal electrocardiogram. They conclude that if the tachyarrhythmia is paroxysmal, as demonstrated by real-time and/or M-mode studies, it is safe to deduce a reciprocating atrioventricular mechanism. In the fetus, the upper limits of heart rate beyond which the clinician should assume an abnormal mechanism is 220 beats per minute. Table 19–4 summarizes their review of the use of antiarrhythmia therapy for fetal cardioversion.

In the fetus remote from term with NIHF secondary to supraventricular tachycardia, chemical cardioversion should be attempted. Digoxin is usually the first therapeutic option. A loading dose of digoxin, 0.75 to 1.25 mg in divided oral doses, or intravenous loading, is recommended. Often, larger loading doses are necessary in the pregnant woman to achieve therapeutic levels, owing to the increased clearance of the drug. If after a reasonable period of therapeutic blood levels in the mother, the fetus fails to respond, it may then be appropriate to try one of the other drugs. Based on the information summarized in Table 19–4, it would seem that quinidine is a reasonable second choice. Treatment of fetal arrhythmias is more fully considered in Chapter 16.

Thus, both structural fetal cardiac abnormalities and rhythm disturbances can cause NIHF. Accurate cardiac evaluation of fetuses with NIHF can provide information

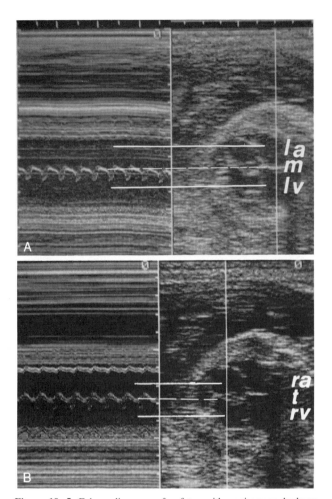

Figure 19–5. Echocardiograms of a fetus with nonimmune hydrops fetalis secondary to subendocardial fibroelastosis. *A*, The M-line traverses the left atrium, mitral valve, and the left ventricle. Note the minimal motion of the chamber sidewalls and the brief motion of the mitral valve into the left atrium, which is sustained through each cardiac cycle. Normally, the mitral valve is within the left ventricle during the majority of the cardiac cycle. *B*, The M-line traverses the right atrium, tricuspid valve, and right ventricle. Again, note the minimal motion of the chamber walls. la = left atrium; lv = left ventricle; m = mitral valve; ra = right atrium; rv = right ventricle; t = tricuspid valve.

important for subsequent fetal, maternal, and neonatal management.

Blood Dyscrasias

Of the hematologic disorders listed in Table 19–3, the one that most commonly causes nonimmune hydrops fetalis is α-thalassemia. In populations in which there is a large proportion of patients of Southeast Asian or Mediterranean origin, α-thalassemia can be a common cause of fetal and neonatal loss. The homozygous state for α-thalassemia is uniformly fatal, usually in the fetal period, but occasionally in the immediate neonatal period. The mothers of these fetuses are likewise at risk for perinatal morbidity and mortality. Maternal risk is in-

Table 19–4. SUMMARY OF FINDINGS OF THE USE OF ANTIARRHYTHMIC AGENTS FOR FETAL CARDIOVERSION*

Drug	Number of Cases	Cord Levels (Per Cent of Maternal)	Success
Digoxin	16	80	11
Propranolol	8	26	0 1 in combination with digoxin
Verapamil	NA	17 to 25	"not effective"
Procainamide	2	NA	temporary 1 time
Quinidine	3	24 to 94	3

*Reproduced with permission from Guntheroth et al (1985): Hydrops from reciprocating atrioventricular tachycardia in a 27 week fetus requiring quinidine for conversion. Obstet Gynecol 66:295–335.

creased because of the common occurrence of severe preterm maternal preeclampsia (which occurred in 100 per cent of patients in one report[12]) and complications from retained placentas.

Eleven per cent of the Southeast Asian population screened in this country carries α-thalassemia, and up to 39 per cent of these patients have some inherited hemoglobin disorder.[5,34] The initial screening procedure should be an evaluation of the maternal red blood cell indices and hemoglobin or hematocrit. If the mother has a microcytic anemia, then the father should be evaluated for the same problem. If both parents have such an anemia, not secondary to iron-deficiency, then hemoglobin electrophoresis should be performed on both parents. If they are heterozygous for α-thalassemia, the physician can offer prenatal diagnosis for their fetus using restriction endonuclease gene mapping of fetal cells from amniocentesis or, where available, chorionic villus biopsy. If the mother presents late in her pregnancy with a fetus having hydrops fetalis, confirmation of the fetal hemoglobinopathy can be performed by amniocentesis or fetal blood sampling. Since the homozygous state is uniformly fatal, this documentation allows the patient and her doctors to expedite delivery to avoid maternal morbidity secondary to preeclampsia, operative morbidity from an unnecessary cesarean birth, or hemorrhage from a retained placenta.

Miscellaneous

Congenital idiopathic hydrothorax in the fetus may cause nonimmune hydrops fetalis by increasing the intrathoracic pressure with obstructed venous return. In a patient whose fetus is preterm, diversion catheters have been placed into the fetal chest to allow drainage of the effusion into the amniotic fluid, thus decompressing the chest and permitting improved cardiac return.[29] In severe cases of congenital hydrothorax prior to 26 weeks' gestation, the fetus may have already suffered from a degree of pulmonary hypoplasia; however, the diagnosis of

Table 19–5. SUGGESTED EVALUATION OF THE
NEONATE WITH UNEXPLAINED NIHF

1. CBC with differential and platelet count
2. Blood type and Coombs test
3. Serolgy
4. IgM, TORCH studies
5. Liver function tests
6. Renal function tests
7. ECG, echocardiography
8. Karyotyping
9. Cultures (bacterial and viral)
10. Radiographs
11. Diagnostic thoracentesis and paracentesis
12. Placental histology and anatomy
13. Serum protein analysis
14. Hemoglobin electrophoresis

pulmonary hypoplasia can be made reliably only postnatally and should not be assumed antenatally.

DELIVERY

The perinatal issues involved in planning the place, time, and route of delivery in the pregnancy complicated by NIHF are complex. Attempting to maximize the well-being of one of the two patients involved, mother or fetus, may jeopardize the well-being of the other.

Frequent fetal assessments of well-being should occur. Serial ultrasonographic scans to follow the progression or remission of the hydrops and to continue searching for an etiology if none has yet been found are important. Weekly or biweekly nonstress testing of the fetus (an antenatal test that monitors the fetal heart rate responses to fetal movements) should be instituted around 30 weeks' gestation. Asking the mother to perform daily counts of perceived fetal movements is also helpful. Any decrease in fetal movements on a day-to-day basis should be an indication for further assessment. The mother should be on a program of bed rest either at home or in the hospital to maximize uteroplacental blood flow.

The timing of the delivery depends on evidence of maternal or fetal compromise. A progression in the severity of the hydrops or poor results on antenatal fetal well-being assessments are an indication to proceed with delivery. Maternal physiologic embarrassment or the onset of preeclampsia may also necessitate early delivery. If the mother and hydropic fetus are stable, delivery is delayed as long as possible. The goal of this approach is to achieve maximum safe retention in utero of the fetus to gain pulmonary maturity, stabilization of the germinal matrix in the brain, and maturity of other organ systems.

When either the patient goes into spontaneous labor or the obstetric team and patient decide to intervene to deliver the fetus, the mother should be at a hospital with a neonatal intensive care unit. Hydropic infants are commonly depressed at birth, may have associated congenital anomalies requiring immediate medical or surgical care, and may have problems with chest expansion because of serous fluid collections.

A uterus massively distended by polyhydramnios and a severely hydropic fetus can compromise maternal respiratory and renal function. Conservative clinical care often involves hospitalization and bed rest, and polyhydramnios may require either delivery or therapeutic amniocentesis for decompression of the uterus. When polyhydramnios is present, the uterus demonstrates poor contractility, and labor may be ineffective without drainage of some of the fluid. If amniotic fluid drainage is necessary for normal progression of labor, transabdominal drainage rather than amniotomy should be performed, so that the decompression of the uterus can proceed in a controlled fashion and so that the risks of placental abruption are minimized.

There may be a limited role for prenatal aspiration of fetal pleural or ascitic fluid to facilitate lung expansion at the time of delivery. If such fetal fluid aspiration is planned, it should be done as soon as possible prior to the delivery, as these fetal effusions commonly rapidly reform.

There is a debate regarding route of delivery when NIHF is present. Some would argue that in an illness with up to 98 per cent neonatal mortality cesarean section constitutes a heroic measure with little hope for benefit. On the other hand, the large edematous placenta has little reserve in NIHF and may not provide adequate fetal support during labor, perhaps leading toward a self-fulfilling prophecy of high perinatal mortality. These edematous fetuses, likewise, are at risk for shoulder dystocia and soft-tissue trauma. Postpartum hemorrhage from the large placenta is an additional hazard of vaginal delivery.

NEONATAL MANAGEMENT

The hydropic neonate admitted to the intensive care nursery is commonly extremely ill. The primary concern is usually ventilation. The fetus may experience respiratory distress from prematurity, external compression of fetal lungs from ascites, pleural effusions, pulmonary edema, or secondary pulmonary hypoplasia. Thoracentesis and paracentesis early in neonatal life may be life saving, but they should be undertaken cautiously as they can cause rapid fluid shifts from the intravascular to the extravascular compartment.[6]

The fluid status of the neonate with NIHF is also tenuous. Congestive heart failure, anemia, and intravascular fluid depletion may be present, and exchange transfusion, pressor support, and diuretics may be required.

Routine care of the neonate with NIHF is also important. Because of the severe edema, the neonate's skin may break down. To acheive adequate nutrition levels to obtain a positive nitrogen balance in infants who are hypoproteinemic may require total parenteral nutrition. Intensive ventilatory support is required, and chest tubes are often needed to drain the pleural effusions or air leaks.

Once the neonate with NIHF is delivered, further studies to find the cause should be conducted if the etiology of the NIHF has not been established prenatally. Recommended studies are included in Table 19–5.

PARENTAL COUNSELING

Many of the conditions associated with NIHF have a genetic basis, although the majority are multifactorial or sporadic. The parents of an affected infant should be counseled regarding the chance of recurrence in a future pregnancy as well as the possibilities for prenatal diagnosis. As chromosomal analysis and restriction endonuclease technology improve, the likelihood of early accurate prenatal diagnosis of conditions causing NIHF will increase.

Although in some instances NIHF is genetic, most cases are idiopathic or multifactorial, and the risk of a recurrence in a subsequent pregnancy is very small. However, there are reported cases[30] of recurrences in siblings of idiopathic NIHF, so careful surveillance of subsequent pregnancies is recommended.

References

1. Allan LD, Joseph M, Boyd E, Campbell S, Tynan M (1982): M-Mode echocardiography in the developing human fetus. Br Heart J 47:573–583.
2. Ambramowicz J, Jaffe R, Altaras M, Ben-Aderet N (1985): Fetal supraventricular tachycardia: Prenatal diagnosis and pharmacological reversal of associated hydrops fetalis. Gynecol Obstet Invest 20:109–112.
3. Anderson HM, Hutchison A, Fortune D (1983): Non-immune hydrops fetalis: Changing contribution to perinatal mortality. Br J Obstet Gynecol 90:636–639.
4. Ballantyne JW (1892): The Diseases and Deformities of the Fetus. Edinburgh, Olive and Boyd.
5. Craft J, Coleman D, Coulter H, Horwitz R, Barry M (1983): Hematologic abnormalities in Southeast Asian refugees. JAMA 249:3204–3206.
6. Davis CL (1982): Diagnosis and management of nonimmune hydrops fetalis. J Reprod Med 27:594–600.
7. Etches PC, Lemons JA (1979): Nonimmune hydrops fetalis: Report of 22 cases including three siblings. Pediatrics 64:326–332.
8. Evron S, Yagel S, Samueloff A, Margaliot E, Burstein P, Sadovsky E (1985): Nonimmunologic hydrops fetalis: A review of eleven cases. J Perinatal Med 13:147–151.
9. Fleischer AC, Killam A, Boehm F, Hutchison A, Jones T, Shaff M, Barrett J, Lindsey A, James A (1981): Hydrops fetalis: Sonographic evaluation and clinical implications. Radiology 141:163–168.
10. Graves GR, Baskett TF (1984): Nonimmune hydrops fetalis: Antenatal diagnosis and management. Am J Obstet Gynecol 148:563–565.
11. Guntheroth WG, Cyr D, Mack L, Benedetti T, Lenke R, Petty C (1985): Hydrops from reciprocating atrioventricular tachycardia in a 27 week fetus requiring quinidine for conversion. Obstet Gynecol 66:29S–33S.
12. Guy G, Coady D, Jansen V, Snyder J, Zinberg S (1985): Alpha-thalassemia hydrops fetalis: Clinical and ultrasonographic considerations. Am J Obstet Gynecol 153:500–504.
13. Hirsch M, Friedman S, Schoenfeld A, Ovadia J (1985): Nonimmune hydrops fetalis—a rational attitude of management. Eur J Obstet Gynecol Reprod Biol 19:191–196.
14. Holzgreve W, Holzgreve B, Curry C (1985): Nonimmune hydrops fetalis: Diagnosis and management. Semin Perinatol 9:52–67.
15. Hutchison AA, Drew J, Yu V, Williams M, Fortune D, Beischer N (1981): Non-immunologic hydrops fetalis: A review of 61 cases. Obstet Gynecol 59:347–352.
16. Iliff PJ, Nicholls JM, Keeling JW, Gough JD (1983): Non-immunologic hydrops fetalis: A review of 27 cases. Arch Dis Child 58:979–982.
17. Im SS, Rizos N, Joutsi P, Shime J, Benzie R (1984): Nonimmunologic hydrops fetalis. Am J Obstet Gynecol 148:566–569.
18. Lanham JG, Walport MJ, Hughes GV (1983): Congenital heart block and familial connective tissue disease. J Rheum 10:823–825.
19. Macafee CAJ, Fortune DW, Beischer NA (1972): Non-immunologic hydrops fetalis. J Obstet Gynecol Br Comm 77:226–237.
20. Machin GA (1981): Differential diagnosis of hydrops fetalis. Am J Med Genet 9:341–350.
21. Mahoney B, Filly R, Callen P, Chinn D, Golbus M (1984): Severe nonimmune hydrops fetalis: Sonographic evaluation. Radiology 151:757–761.
22. Maidman JE, Yeager C, Anderson V, Makabali G, O'Grady J, Arce J, Tishler D (1980): Prenatal diagnosis and management of non-immunologic hydrops fetalis. Obstet Gynecol 56:571–576.
23. Nicolaides K, Rodeck C, Lange I, Watson J, Gosden C, Miller D, Mibashan R, Moniz C, Morgan-Capner P, Campbell S (1985): Fetoscopy in the assessment of unexplained fetal hydrops. Br J Obstet Gynecol 92:671–679.
24. Pai S, Austin T (1985): Non-immune hydrops fetalis: A review of cases. S Carolina Med Assn 81:116–120.
25. Perlin BM, Pomerance JJ, Schifrin BS (1981): Non-immunologic hydrops fetalis. Obstet Gynecol 57:584–588.
26. Pesonen E, Haavisto H, Ammala P, Teramo K (1983): Intrauterine hydrops caused by premature closure of the foramen ovale. Arch Dis Child 58:1015–1016.
27. Potter E (1943): Universal edema of the fetus unassociated with erythroblastosis. Am J Obstet Gynecol 46:130–134.
28. Sahn D, Shenker L, Reed K, Valdes-Cruz L, Sobonya R, Anderson C (1982): Prenatal ultrasound diagnosis of hypoplastic left heart syndrome in utero associated with hydrops fetalis. Am Heart J 104:1368–1372.
29. Seeds JW, Bowes WA (1986): Results of treatment of severe fetal hydrothorax with bilateral pleuroamnionic catheters. Obstet Gynecol 68:577–579.
30. Sevitz H, Klein R, Sonnendecker E, Lubbe F, Merrell DA, Rothberg R (1982): Non-immunological hydrops fetalis. Report of six cases and a review. S Afr Med J 62:815–819.
31. Silverman J, Kleinman C, Rudolph A, Copel J, Weinstein E, Enderlein M, Golbus M (1985): Fetal atrioventricular valve insufficiency associated with non-immune hydrops: A two dimensional echocardiographic and pulsed Doppler ultrasound study. Circulation 72:825–832.
32. Soltan M, Keohane C (1981): Hydrops fetalis due to congenital cardiac rhabdomyoma. Case report. Br J Obstet Gynecol 88:771–773.
33. Spahr R, Botti J, MacDonald H, Holzman I (1980): Non-immunologic hydrops fetalis: A review of 19 cases. Int J Gynaecol Obstet 18:303–307.
34. Stein J, Berg C, Jones J, Detter J (1984): A screening protocol for a prenatal population at risk for hemoglobin disorders: Results of its application to a group of Southeast Asians and blacks. Am J Obstet Gynecol 150:333–341.
35. Turkel SB (1982): Conditions associated with nonimmune hydrops fetalis. Clin Perinatol 9:613–625.
36. Weinberg PM, Peyser K, Hackney JR (1985): Fetal hydrops in a newborn with hypoplastic left heart syndrome: Tricuspid valve "stopper." J Am Coll Cardiol 6:1365–1369.

PART 3
Neonatal Cardiology

20 CLINICAL EXAMINATION

Gregory L. Johnson

HISTORICAL PERSPECTIVE

The fact that certain clinical findings in newborn infants can be attributed to the presence of a congenital abnormality of the heart has been known at least since the time of Aristotle. Alterations in heart and respiratory rate, the presence of cyanosis or pallor, and palpation of a hyperactive precordial impulse have long been known as indicators of an underlying cardiac disorder in an otherwise healthy newborn infant. In the nineteenth century, the development of the stethoscope and improved cardiac auscultation led to an increased interest in clinical diagnosis of infants with signs of congenital cardiac abnormalities. By the time Holt published his landmark textbook of pediatrics at the end of the century he was not only able to describe several distinct types of cardiac murmurs audible in the newborn but also to point out correctly the high incidence of pulmonary stenosis and deficiency of the ventricular septum in infants with cyanosis and a systolic murmur audible at the cardiac base.[22]

Despite some similar attempts at clinicopathologic correlations, the ability to distinguish clinically between specific anatomic defects received little further attention over the next 30 years. The failure of clinical diagnosis to advance during this time was almost certainly due to the inescapable fact that neither prognosis nor treatment could be altered by such knowledge. In the second quarter of the twentieth century, however, an abrupt change in attitude led to the development of specific clinical criteria for the diagnosis of congenital heart disease. The improvement of clinical diagnosis in congenital heart disease was based largely on the work of Dr. Helen Taussig, who while at the Harriett Lane Home in the 1930s and 1940s devised the diagnostic schema based on clinical findings that continues to form the cornerstone of cardiac evaluation in infants and children. Dr. Taussig's work produced the first textbook addressing the clinical diagnosis of congenital heart disease[33] and led to the performance of the first Blalock-Taussig anastomosis in 1945.

Development of the Blalock-Taussig anastomosis coupled with the previous demonstration by Gross in 1938 that surgical closure of a patent ductus arteriosus could be safely performed created for the first time a need for accurate premortem diagnosis of specific anatomic lesions. The development of angiocardiography, introduced by Castellanos in 1937,[6] permitted precise clinicopathologic correlation to be performed during life and further contributed to the development of specific clinical differential diagnosis.

With the more recent advent of increasingly sophisticated means of both invasive and noninvasive evaluation, clinical examination in the newborn with suspected heart disease has become at times almost a forgotten tool. In the newborn, clinical examination must be performed in the context of changing physical findings that reflect normal postnatal changes in organ system function and organism homeostasis. The accurate diagnosis of intrinsic cardiac disease against this background can appear overly difficult, particularly to the less experienced examiner. The newborn, however, offers a unique opportunity for observation of cardiovascular physiology as expressed in findings on physical examination. Understanding of basic neonatal cardiovascular physiology and a good physical examination can frequently lead to a specific anatomic diagnosis in cases of neonatal congenital heart disease. Even in those cases in which a precise anatomic diagnosis is not possible, or in which true structural heart disease may be absent, careful evaluation of the infant's physical findings will nearly always result in an accurate assessment of both the overall severity of the condition and the expected future clinical course.

PERINATAL PHYSIOLOGY

A complete and detailed physical examination in an infant requires relatively little time. Interpretation of the examination is, however, based upon an understanding of the fact that neonatal physiology changes with time, albeit in a relatively predictable manner, and additionally that the physiology may be responding to multiple stimuli simultaneously. In order to be meaningful, data obtained from examination must take into account the presence and possible effects of all these stimuli. Even a complete and accurate physical examination will lead to false diagnoses if data are erroneously interpreted because the underlying physiology has been misinterpreted or because it has been ignored completely.

Autonomic Physiology

At delivery, the healthy infant appears to be in a hyper-sympathetic state. Assessment of physical findings at this time must be made in this setting. Tachycardia, rapid respiration, transient rales, grunting, flaring, and retractions are frequently noted in normal newborns during the first 20 to 30 minutes of life.[14] Hypertonia and alerting exploratory behavior are also seen.

Following this first period of reactivity, heart and respiratory rates decline, while diffuse motor activity reaches a peak and then diminishes. General responsiveness declines, and the infant sleeps. After sleep, the infant enters a second phase of reactivity marked by heightened responsiveness to both exogenous and endogenous stimuli. In some infants the secondary reactivity period results in waves of increased autonomic activity, causing wide swings in heart rate and irregular respiration with apneic pauses.[13] In most infants, this secondary period of reactivity is complete by 6 to 10 hours of age.

Circulatory Physiology

Simultaneously occurring with changes in autonomic physiology are those taking place in circulatory physiology, which are due to the change from a fetoumbilical circulation to a neonatal respiratory circulation. Systemic vascular resistance is suddenly increased with occlusion of the umbilical vessels and removal of the low resistance placental vascular bed. Pulmonary vascular resistance falls subsequent to the increase in PaO_2 and the decrease in PCO_2 associated with the onset of respiration. The rise in left atrial pressure resulting from increased pulmonary blood flow and pulmonary venous return coupled with the fall in inferior vena canal flow and pressure following occlusion of the umbilical vessels results in functional closure of the foramen ovale. Anatomic closure generally follows several weeks later[8] but may not occur at all in up to 15 to 20 per cent of normal individuals.[28] It is important to note that prior to the time of anatomic closure, continued functional closure is dependent on the maintenance of a higher pressure in the left atrium than in the right.

Similarly, the sudden postnatal changes in systemic and pulmonary vascular resistance can lead to transient left-to-right blood flow through the ductus arteriosus. Such shunting is common in the immediate neonatal period but generally ceases within 3 days after birth.[30] The ductus, however, remains anatomically open at 2 weeks of age in

65 per cent of normal infants and at 4 weeks in 44 per cent.[8] Clearly, ductal flow, either left to right or right to left, can occur under appropriate conditions during this period.

External Factors

The normal transitional physiology outlined in the preceding sections provides the substrate upon which cardiovascular examination of the newborn is based. Many factors external to the intrinsic cardiovascular physiology can, however, alter this substrate. An awareness of these factors and their effects is an essential part of any examination in a newborn. Acidosis, for example, whether a result of external (e.g., cold) or internal conditions, causes both systemic and pulmonary vasoconstriction as well as some diminution in ventricular performance. With correction of acidosis, physical findings associated with vasoconstriction may disappear, while other findings, which may have been masked by low cardiac output, may become prominent.

In infants with birth asphyxia, the normal drop in pulmonary vascular resistance may be delayed, and right-to-left shunting through the foramen ovale is commonly seen. Infants with anatomic reduction in the size of the pulmonary vascular bed, such as those with congenital lobar emphysema or diaphragmatic hernia, will also demonstrate persistent elevation of pulmonary vascular resistance. Similarly, pulmonary vascular resistance may remain near prenatal levels for several weeks in infants with Down syndrome. In those infants with Down syndrome–associated congenital heart disease, the onset of obstructive pulmonary vascular disease may preclude pulmonary vascular resistance from ever diminishing to levels approximating normal values.

SPECIAL CONSIDERATIONS IN PREMATURE INFANTS

In general, physical examination is more easily performed in the preterm infant as compared with the term infant, although interpretation of data obtained may be considerably complicated by the presence of other alterations in body homeostasis as well as by the effects of various life-support systems. As would be expected, the underlying normal physiology is different in infants of varying gestational age. Typically, the period of transitional circulation is prolonged in premature infants, with delayed closure of both the foramen ovale and the ductus arteriosus. In very premature infants (those less than about 32 weeks' gestation), pulmonary arteriolar smooth musculature is less well developed, and pulmonary vascular resistance falls much more rapidly after birth, leading to the potential for early and massive left-to-right shunting through a ductus or septal defect. In addition, blood volume for body weight is higher, and the left ventricular myocardium and its sympathetic innervation may be more poorly developed in premature infants, leading to a shifting of the Starling curve and to a greater tendency for ventricular dilation and cardiac failure.[27] Finally, premature infants are more sensitive to changes in the external environment, which might lead to vasoconstriction and acidosis.

GENERAL APPEARANCE AND BEHAVIOR

Physical examination must always begin with observation of the infant. Observation is of paramount importance in the newborn and is often best accomplished from a distance of several feet or more, so that the examiner is not tempted to pursue one or another observation until a full overall picture of the infant's appearance is obtained. If the infant is being monitored, resting respiratory and heart rates and, frequently, blood pressure can be assessed at this time. An assessment of the degree of "comfortableness" of the infant should also be made. An impression that an infant is not resting quietly can, when evaluated further, often be translated into the anxious facies and excessive diaphoresis of circulatory overload, the nasal flaring and intercostal retractions of pulmonary parenchymal disease, or the tachypnea without dyspnea that is the hallmark of pulmonary undercirculation. The infant's alertness and/or response to stimuli can also give a clue to the presence of circulatory compromise. Presence and distribution of cyanosis is often best appreciated from a distance. Finally, a systematic head to toe visual inspection for abnormal patterns to be further pursued on actual physical examination should be performed.

Extracardiac Malformations

Extracardiac defects are noted in up to 40 per cent of children born with congenital heart disease.[25] Such defects, particularly when presenting as a constellation forming a recognizable syndrome, can frequently be best appreciated on simple inspection of the infant.

Probably the most widely recognized of these syndromes is trisomy 21 (Down syndrome), in which between one third and one half of infants have congenital heart disease, usually atrioventricular septal defect or ventricular septal defect. Due to the persistence of high pulmonary vascular resistance in these infants, physical findings of congenital heart disease may be absent, and diagnosis depends on a high index of suspicion. The most common features noted on general physical examination include muscular hypotonia, hyperflexible joints, and a characteristic facies consisting of upward slanting palpebral fissures, epicanthal folds, a flat facial profile, small ears with overfolding of the helix, small nose with a flat bridge, and a tendency to keep the mouth open and tongue protruded. Other findings include a rounded skull with flat occiput and a short neck. Simian hand creases and a hypoplastic fifth middle phalanx are commonly noted on closer examination.

In trisomy 18, more than 90 per cent of infants have congenital heart disease, usually ventricular septal defect. Pulmonary hypertension frequently coexists.[34] A prominent occiput, low-set ears, short palpebral fissures, micrognathia, overlapping of index and fifth fingers, and rocker-bottom feet are characteristic. Similarly, congenital heart disease is noted in nearly all infants with trisomy 13, which is marked by polydactyly and central facial anomalies. Ventricular septal defect is again the most common cardiac malformation, although patent ductus arteriosus, atrial septal defect, and dextroposition also occur commonly.[34]

Several other extracardiac syndromes are associated with specific congenital heart defects and can be readily recognized by inspection during the newborn period. These include the Turner, Williams-Barrett, Noonan, and Holt-Oram syndromes; congenital rubella syndrome; fetal alcohol syndrome; and the mucopolysaccharidoses. These entities will be more fully discussed in Chapter 50.

COLOR AND OXYGENATION

Differences in skin color and perfusion can readily be noted on casual inspection of the newborn infant. Interpretation of skin color as an indicator of state of oxygenation can, however, be complicated by a number of conditions unrelated to oxygen saturation. Nursery lighting, wall paint, skin pigmentation, and even clothing are well-known examples. In addition, vasoconstriction associated with cold or acidosis can give the appearance of cyanosis even though PaO_2 may be well within the normal range.

Most normal newborns have peripheral cyanosis involving the hands and feet that may, on occasion, be marked, particularly when external cold is present. Such discoloration usually disappears by 48 hours and is rarely seen following 72 hours. Localized bruising, which appears as areas of bluish discoloration, may occur following forceps delivery or face presentation. Finally, transient skin mottling due to vasomotor instability is common in the newborn period and may recur for weeks to months.

Cyanosis

Although, contrary to widely held belief, peripheral cyanosis can affect the lips, true central cyanosis with hypoxemia can most easily be distinguished by examination of the tongue and oral mucosa, which are not involved in peripheral cyanosis.[17] Central cyanosis occurring shortly after birth is often a reflection of hypoventilation, either from the depressant effects of maternal analgesia or from unrecognized pneumothorax or choanal atresia. Following the first few minutes of life, central cyanosis often indicates congenital heart disease. Alternatively, right-to-left shunting through a patent foramen ovale or patent ductus arteriosus in the absence of other cardiac defects can lead to marked central cyanosis in those infants with persistent pulmonary hypertension, with or without associated pulmonary parenchymal disease. Even in the absence of pulmonary vascular hypertension, central cyanosis secondary to right-to-left shunting through these persistent fetal pathways can be noted intermittently, particularly with vigorous crying, through the first several days of life.

Cyanosis associated with congenital heart disease in the newborn may be caused by obstruction to pulmonary blood flow (e.g., pulmonary or tricuspid valve atresia), transposition of the great arteries, right-to-left shunting (e.g., truncus arteriosus), or pulmonary edema. Often, high concentrations of oxygen are administered in order to determine whether cyanosis improves. Infants with obstructed pulmonary blood flow, transposition of the great arteries, and most right-to-left shunts will experience only mild improvement in arterial oxygen concentration, whereas the improvement seen in infants with pulmonary edema or primary pulmonary parenchymal disease may be quite striking. Unfortunately, many infants with persistent patent ductus arteriosus associated with severe cyanotic congenital heart disease may experience a significant increase in arterial oxygen concentration following an administration of high ambient oxygen concentrations, while infants with some forms of pulmonary disease, particularly those associated with persistent pulmonary vascular hypertension, may experience little or no increase in arterial oxygen concentration under these conditions. Evaluation of breathing patterns and arterial carbon dioxide concentration may often be helpful in these cases.

In the evaluation of cyanosis in the newborn, it is important to recognize that the high proportion of fetal hemoglobin in the fetus and newborn results in a shift in the oxygen dissociation curve to the left, so that full saturation can be achieved at a lower PaO_2 level than in the older infant or child. Accordingly, in some newborn infants 95 per cent saturation may be reached with PaO_2 in the 45 to 50 mmHg range. Both oxygen saturation and PaO_2 values are necessary data if erroneous evaluation of suspected hypoxemia is to be avoided at this age. Normal PaO_2 rises to 70 to 80 mmHg by the second 24 hours of life.

Occasionally, differential cyanosis may be observed, and the distribution of cyanosis usually permits accurate delineation of the anatomy of the corresponding congenital defect. In infants with severe coarctation or interruption of the aortic arch, the lower extremities and, depending on the precise anatomy, the left arm may appear cyanotic because perfusion is from the pulmonary circulation through the ductus arteriosus, while perfusion of the right arm and upper body is from the ascending aorta, permitting these structures to remain pink. Occasionally, right-to-left ductal flow secondary to elevated pulmonary vascular resistance may mimic this situation, although associated right-to-left shunting through the foramen ovale generally results in a lower oxygen saturation in the distribution of the ascending aorta and hence minimizes the differential. In the presence of intracardiac left-to-right shunting, as with a coexisting ventricular septal defect, pulmonary artery oxygen saturation may be increased and differential cyanosis due to aortic arch obstruction masked. Rarely, the combination of aortic arch obstruction and transposition of the great arteries will result in reversal of the more common distribution of differential cyanosis, such that the right arm and upper body will be cyanotic, while the lower extremities will be pink.

Plethora

On initial inspection, plethora, generally associated with polycythemic states, may be mistaken for cyanosis. In many of these infants, a closer look will reveal ruddiness rather than true cyanosis, so that the distinction can be made. In the remainder, a normal PaO_2 and elevated hemoglobin and hematocrit usually serve to clarify the situation,[16] although occasional infants with very high hematocrit and subsequent hyperviscosity may have mild arterial oxygen desaturation secondary to diminished peripheral perfusion, low cardiac output, and metabolic acidosis.

Pallor

The appearance of the infant with poor peripheral perfusion and systemic vasoconstriction is easily distinguishable from that of the infant with cyanosis or plethora. Term infants usually present with a generalized pale gray color and mottling of the distal extremities. The mottling is due to poor capillary perfusion. The gray color probably represents a "white-on-blue" resulting from diminished vascular perfusion of the skin superimposed on the mild desaturation present when cardiac output is low and tissue extraction results in a wide arteriovenous oxygen difference. The extremities are cool to the touch and the infant often appears somnolent, probably reflecting diminished cerebral perfusion. The most common cause is probably hypoplastic left-heart syndrome, although intrauterine myocarditis, hypoxic myocardial damage, or intrauterine arrhythmia can have a similar presentation.

A special circumstance exists in the premature infant with a large left-to-right shunt through a patent ductus arteriosus. In these infants cardiac output is normal or, often, increased, so that the arteriovenous oxygen difference is normal or narrow, and cyanosis, in the absence of overt pulmonary edema, is not seen. The run-off through the ductus into the pulmonary artery, however, results in a "washed-out" appearance, with peripheral vasoconstriction and a marked pallor to the skin. These changes are often accompanied by a mild but persistent metabolic acidosis as peripheral tissue oxygen extraction is diminished. Further investigation to confirm the presence of a left-to-right ductal shunt is warranted, however, as other conditions, notably sepsis or intracranial hemorrhage, can produce a similar appearance.

RESPIRATORY ACTIVITY

Observation of the pattern of respiration is an integral part of the examination of any newborn but can be particularly valuable in providing clues to the etiology of hypoxemia in cyanotic infants. In most newborn infants, the work of breathing is done principally with the diaphragm so that respiratory movement and excursion are most easily judged from the lateral view of the upper abdomen and chest.

In the first hour of life the average respiratory rate is about 60 breaths per minute. Transient variations from 20 to 100 breaths per minute occur normally. Between 2 and 6 hours of age the average rate decreases to 50 breaths per minute (range 20 to 80) and then to 30 to 40 breaths per minute (range 20 to 60) after 6 hours.[13] Throughout the first 12 to 24 hours of life breathing is more often irregular than regular, and recurrent, brief (less than 3 seconds) pauses are common.

As noted, normal transient variations in respiratory rate encompass a wide range of values. Most infants with heart disease will not have respiratory rates outside these ranges. They will, however, often maintain a rate that is consistently near the upper end of the normal range. Additionally, the normal irregularity of the breathing pattern may be lost. Infants with diminished pulmonary blood flow or with transposition of the great arteries will most often demonstrate a rapid shallow respiratory pattern, with rates persistently between 50 and 60 breaths per minute in term infants and between 60 and 80 breaths per minute in preterm infants. The rate will often increase, rather than decrease, with increasing age. Respiration will, however, still be primarily performed utilizing the diaphragm, so that rapid shallow movements of the abdominal wall may be the most striking feature on observation. In contrast, in infants with pulmonary edema, primary pulmonary parenchymal disease or airway obstruction tachypnea will be accompanied by a pattern of irregular respiratory effort with deeper breathing (hyperpnea) and intercostal and subcostal retractions.

HEART RATE

Range of Normal Rates

Wide variability in heart rate is also normal in the neonate.[12] The resting rate averages 120 to 130 beats per minute (bpm) over the first week of life in the term neonate, increasing to about 150 bpm during the second to fourth weeks. During the first week, resting rates below 100 bpm or above 160 bpm are present in less than 5 per cent of normal term infants. Transient fluctuations in rate to as high as 220 bpm or as low as 59 bpm (measured over 9 beats) have, however, been reported to occur normally in healthy term newborns during the first 3 days of life.[31] The transient nature of this variability is underscored by the fact that when measured over 3 beats, the lowest heart rate noted in the same group of infants was 53 bpm. It is also of note that the mean variability in newborn heart rate over a 24-hour period has been reported to be as high as 100 beats per minute.[24] Accordingly, it would be expected that with newer monitors digitally displaying instananeous changes in R-R interval, rates that are both higher and lower than those tradi-

tionally viewed as normal would be transiently noted in healthy newborns.

The mean heart rate observed in premature infants is slightly higher than that noted in term infants, even when both groups are of similar weight and body surface area. Additionally, the heart rate is somewhat less variable in preterm as compared with term infants. In the first 48 hours of life, median resting heart rate noted in 1388 normal premature infants evaluated as part of the national collaborative study on patent ductus arteriosus was 151 bpm in infants weighing less than 750 g. The median rate gradually declined with increasing body weight to 140 bpm in infants weighing between 1500 and 1750 g. Resting rates above 180 bpm or below 110 bpm lay two standard deviations outside the mean, regardless of weight or gestational age, and may therefore be considered abnormal in the preterm infant.

Sinus Bradycardia

In my institution, sinus bradycardia is defined as a heart rate less than 90 bpm in term infants and less than 110 bpm in preterm infants. As might be expected from the normal variability, short-lived episodes that meet these definitions are common, particularly in term infants. The episodes are nearly always benign and are perhaps due to the predominant parasympathetic innervation of the sinus node in the newborn. These short periods of sinus bradycardia have been most frequently noted in association with nasopharyngeal suctioning[9] but are also often associated with eating, defecating, or hiccuping. Prolonged periods of bradycardia are associated with generalized abnormalities, including asphyxia and intracranial hemorrhage, and carry a grave prognosis. Bradycardia is generally not an indication of primary cardiac disease.

Sinus Tachycardia

Sinus tachycardia has been associated with a variety of stimuli and is generally considered to be due to increased adrenergic activity. Persistent tachycardia may be an indication of congestive heart failure or may be associated with infection, dehydration, anemia, or hyperthyroidism.[7]

Isolated premature beats are noted occasionally in otherwise normal newborns but appear to be more common in term than in preterm infants.[35] Premature beats may be of atrial, junctional, or ventricular origin and by themselves are nearly always benign.

BLOOD PRESSURE

Method

Neonatal blood pressure has long been evaluated utilizing the flush method described by Goldring and Wohltmann.[18] In this technique the hand or foot is gently squeezed to express blood and the blood pressure cuff then rapidly inflated, resulting in a blanched appearance of the extremity distal to the cuff. As the cuff is released, the extremity will suddenly flush as mean arterial pressure is realized.

More recently, in many centers Doppler techniques have replaced more traditional blood pressure measurement tools. The Doppler ultrasound principle allows detection of blood flow by the ultrasonic frequency shift produced by moving blood particles. A cuff and sphygmomanometer are employed in the usual manner, and blood flow is detected by an ultrasonic probe placed over the artery distal to the cuff. As with more standard methods of measurement, cuff size is all-important. The cuff bladder should encircle the extremity and be the widest that can be applied to the upper arm (or leg).[32] For the term neonate, this generally means that a 4- or 5-cm cuff should be used.

When comparing blood pressure values, it must be kept in mind that while indwelling arterial catheters provide both systolic and diastolic pressures, Doppler readings, as well as those readings obtained by simple palpation of the pulse, give only systolic pressure, and the flush method provides an estimate of mean arterial pressure only.

Normal Values

When measured by direct arterial catheterization, systolic blood pressure in normal full-term neonates averages 70 to 75 mmHg (range 55 to 90), and diastolic pressure in these infants averages 40 to 45 mmHg (range 30 to 55).[36] Systolic pressures obtained by Doppler techniques are similar, averaging 66 mmHg in one study of term infants.[37] In premature infants, values are more or less directly proportional to size and gestational age, with mean values in infants weighing 1000 g being 50 mmHg systolic and 30 mmHg diastolic.[36]

Blood pressure in infants can be greatly affected by body temperature, activity, and posture. For example, both systolic and diastolic pressures average 10 to 12 mmHg higher in newborns who are awake and sucking compared with those who are sleeping quietly.[23] Readings may be falsely elevated if the extremity in which the reading is taken is lower than the heart. In the immediate neonatal period, the method of delivery, degree of placental transfusion, and amount of birth asphyxia can alter blood pressure readings significantly. Pressure is also slightly lower in the first 3 to 4 hours of life than subsequently, presumably because of fluid shifts into and out of the vascular space.

Pressures obtained in the leg are generally slightly higher than those in the arm but can be equal or slightly lower. A systolic pressure in the upper extremities that is more than 20 mmHg higher than that in the lower extremities is highly suggestive of aortic coarctation. It should be noted, however, that in the presence of a patent ductus arteriosus or a ductus diverticulum that permits free passage of blood around the coarcted area, the pressure difference in coarctation may be masked. In cases of interrupted aortic arch, aortic coarctation involving the left subclavian artery or coarctation with aberrant right subclavian artery, there may be a differential pressure between the arms as well as between upper and lower extremities. If aortic arch anomalies are suspected, careful, and preferably simultaneous, measurement in both arms and at least one leg is indicated.

Neonatal Hypertension

As a general rule, neonatal hypertension (see Chapter 39) has been arbitrarily defined as systolic pressure higher than 90 mmHg and diastolic pressure higher than 60 mmHg in resting full-term neonates and systolic pressure higher than 80 mmHg and diastolic pressure higher than 50 mmHg in quietly resting preterm infants.[2] Virtually all reported hypertension in neonates has been secondary, with renal artery thrombosis, generally secondary to high umbilical artery catheter placement, being by far the most common etiologic factor.[1] Renal parenchymal anomalies, renal artery stenosis, and coarctation of the aorta are less common anatomic causes.

Among miscellaneous causes of neonatal hypertension are increased intracranial pressure, fluid and electrolyte overload, drug administration such as corticosteroids or ocular phenylephrine, and hypertension following genitourinary surgery or closure of abdominal wall defects.[2,3] Hypotension in the neonate is generally a reflection of shock, with or without congestive heart failure.

Pulse Pressure

Pulse pressure is defined as the difference between systolic and diastolic blood pressure and averages 25 to 30 mmHg in term neonates and 15 to 25 mmHg in premature infants. Narrow pulse pressures are seen in infants with myocardial failure, peripheral vasoconstriction, or generalized vascular collapse. Wide pulse pressure can be normal or can be associated with arteriovenous malformation (see Chapter 35), truncus arteriosus (see Chapter 46), aorticopulmonary window (see Chapter 35), or patent ductus arteriosus (see Chapter 30). In the term neonate with well-developed pulmonary arteriolar musculature, run-off into the systemic venous bed rather than into the pulmonary arterial bed is more likely to cause a wide pulse pressure. Arteriovenous malformations should be carefully sought. In preterm infants, in contrast, a widened pulse pressure is often among the first signs of a left-to-right shunt through the patent ductus arteriosus.

PERIPHERAL PULSES

Findings on examination of the peripheral pulses in neonates generally reflect those found on measurement of systemic blood pressure. The infant should be warm and resting quietly. Pulses in the brachial and femoral arteries should always be palpated simultaneously on each side in turn. Pulses thus palpated should be synchronous and of equal intensity. Discrepancies should alert the examiner to the possibility of abnormalities of the aortic arch. In infants with an indwelling umbilical artery catheter, lower extremity pulses may feel weaker than those in the upper extremities; blood pressure measurements are necessary for evaluation.

Weak pulses generally reflect low systemic output, as in myocardial failure, shock, or left-heart obstructive lesions such as hypoplastic left-heart syndrome or critical aortic stenosis. Strong, jerky pulses are often indicative of aortic run-off into the systemic venous or pulmonary arterial bed. The collapsing quality of the pulse in such conditions can often be appreciated by the experienced examiner in the absence of a widened pulse pressure.

VENOUS PULSE

Evaluation of the jugular venous pulse in neonates is hard to perform, primarily because of the difficulty associated with achievement of the proper degree of extension of the neck to permit visualization of the veins without disturbing the infant. The jugular venous pulse can, however, occasionally be visualized in the sleeping infant, and individual a and v waves may be recognized.[29] A prominent presystolic a wave, when visualized, may indicate obstruction to right atrial emptying. Similarly, a pulsating liver can occasionally be palpated (or, on occasion, visualized) in a cyanotic infant, suggesting the presence of right atrial or right ventricular obstructive lesions.

EDEMA

Mild transient peripheral edema is noted at birth in many normal neonates and appears to be of minimal clinical significance. Lymphedema and the edema associated with the Noonan and Turner syndromes also can be present at birth. The massive edema of hydrops fetalis can frequently be related to intrauterine myocarditis or arrhythmia.

Edema occurring postnatally is dependent and, therefore, most prominent in the presacral area, although edema of the eyelids, lower legs, and feet can be seen. Cardiac disease is a rare cause of peripheral edema in neonates. When cardiac disease does cause edema in the newborn, it is generally in the context of associated abnormalities of renal blood flow as occur in coarctation, interrupted aortic arch, or the hypoplastic left-heart syndrome.

ABDOMINAL EXAMINATION

In normal infants, the hepatic edge may be palpated as much as 3 cm below the right costal margin. In addition, the liver may occasionally be displaced even further inferiorly by hyperexpansion of the lungs. If hepatic enlargement is suspected, therefore, the upper edge of the liver should be percussed.

While hepatic enlargement is an important sign of congestive heart failure, particularly left ventricular failure, it must be realized that other causes of hepatomegaly, particularly hemolytic disease, also occur in the newborn period. Even in the presence of cardiac disease capable of producing congestive heart failure, hepatic enlargement is a late development. Of 331 premature infants with clinically significant patent ductus arteriosus in whom hepatomegaly was sought, only 15 (5 per cent) had a liver edge palpable 3 cm or more below the costal margin.[15] While the spleen tip is easily palpable in most newborn infants, splenomegaly as a consequence of cardiac disease is extremely rare.

A clearly left-sided liver is, of course, indicative of situs inversus abdominalis. A centrally placed liver, or a right-sided liver that clearly extends across the midline is suggestive of malposition (Ivemark syndrome), and the possibility of asplenia or polysplenia with accompanying complex congenital heart disease should be thoroughly pursued.

PRECORDIAL EXAMINATION

Asymmetrical Thorax

The precordial bulge noted in older infants and children with cardiomegaly is rarely observed in the neonatal period. When present, precordial prominence in the neonate is associated with lesions in which hemodynamic alterations existed prenatally despite the presence of an adequate placental circulation. These include arteriovenous malformations (see Chapter 35), Ebstein anomaly of the tricuspid valve with severe tricuspid regurgitation (see Chapter 44), tetralogy of Fallot with absent pulmonary valve (see Chapter 45), and intrauterine arrhythmia (see Chapter 16) or myocarditis.

More frequently, asymmetry of the thorax associated with noncardiac disease may produce a precordial bulge. Atelectasis, emphysema, pneumothorax, and diaphragmatic hernia all can result in an asymmetrical thoracic contour in the newborn.

Precordial Impulse

A visible precordial impulse along the lower left sternal border is frequently present in normal newborns during the secondary period of reactivity. In the absence of cardiopulmonary disease this sign has generally disappeared by 4 to 6 hours of life. The persistence of a visible impulse beyond 12 hours of age is generally associated with volume overload lesions such as in the various types of aortopulmonary shunts but is also a prominent feature in transposition of the great arteries.

In premature infants in whom there is less development of anterior thoracic musculature, a slight precordial impulse is not infrequently visible in the absence of significant circulatory overload. In those infants who subsequently develop a left-to-right shunt through a patent ductus arteriosus, the precordial activity visibly increases and can frequently be noted from some distance away.

On palpation, the cardiac impulse in newborns is nearly always best felt in the parasternal area. Even in those infants with large aortopulmonary or arteriovenous shunts, in whom findings of left ventricular overload would be expected, the anticipated "apical" lift is absent, and physical findings are those of increased parasternal activity.

A palpably increased precordial impulse is notably absent in most cases of pulmonary atresia, tetralogy of Fallot, or tricuspid atresia. Absence of an increased precordial impulse serves as an important negative finding in distinguishing these cyanotic lesions from transposition of the great arteries, in which an easily palpable parasternal lift is nearly invariably present.

Displacement of the cardiac impulse to the right side of the chest should alert the examiner to the possible presence of dextrocardia. Palpation of the abdominal viscera in this situation will often provide confirmatory evidence for either situs inversus totalis or malposition syndrome. In the presence of a right-sided cardiac impulse and normal abdominal viscera, cardiac dextroposition, as in pneumothorax or congenital lobar emphysema, must also be considered. It is important to note that not infrequently the cardiac impulse may seem to be best palpated in the usual left parasternal position, even in those infants with proven dextrocardia.

Thrills

Thrills are rarely palpable in the newborn. When present, they generally indicate gross insufficiency of an atrioventricular valve. Thrills can also be occasionally noted in newborns with severe pulmonary stenosis or with tetralogy of Fallot and absent pulmonary valve.

AUSCULTATION

Method

If the remainder of the examination has been performed with appropriate care, the main role of auscultation will be to confirm initial impressions or to make the final distinction between a small number of possible diagnoses. Accordingly, auscultation should be performed with specific questions in mind, and specific information should be sought.

Cardiac auscultation must be performed as carefully as possible in as quiet an environment as possible. Except in true emergencies, the infant should be examined when he is sleeping. Outside noises should be kept to a minimum. If the infant is being mechanically ventilated, temporarily disconnecting the endotracheal tube from the ventilator is imperative for adequate cardiac auscultation. In the very sickest premature infants, assessing the location of possible abnormal findings as well as overall rate and rhythm can be done prior to disconnecting the ventilator in order to keep the actual time off mechanical ventilation to an absolute minimum. With a good feel for rate and rhythm,

a surprising amount of information can be gathered in the space of 6 to 10 heart beats. Slowing of the rate indicates deterioration, and the ventilator should be reconnected at that time. If necessary, auscultation can be repeated after several minutes of assisted ventilation.

Choice of stethoscope is largely a matter of personal preference, but the examiner should be familiar with the characteristics of the specific instrument being used. For this reason, each examiner should use his or her personal stethoscope. To obtain the best results, tubing should be as short as possible. Many stethoscopes have a "newborn head," which consists of a small diaphragm and bell that replace the normal head. Although these heads are occasionally useful in the evaluation of very small premature infants in whom a good seal cannot be obtained because of lack of subcutaneous tissue, the attenuation in sound associated with the smaller surface makes them poor tools for the evaluation of larger premature and term infants.

Most sounds and murmurs audible in the newborn are relatively high pitched. Accordingly, the diaphragm is generally used for initial auscultation. Even with use of a large diaphragm, location and radiation of murmurs can be easily delineated in most newborn infants. The bell can then be used for further evaluation of lower frequency sounds initially heard with the diaphragm or when listening for sounds known to have low frequency, such as mid-diastolic atrioventricular valve flow murmurs. Heart sounds, clicks, and abnormal sounds and murmurs should be evaluated separately and in turn.

Evaluation of information gained from auscultation requires synthesis of auscultory data with physiologic changes that are occurring in the newborn. A full understanding of the transitional circulation as well as knowledge of external factors that may affect the cardiovascular physiology in the newborn is necessary for accurate integration of auscultory findings.

Heart Sounds

The first heart sound is produced by closure of the mitral and tricuspid valves. While mitral valve closure generally precedes tricuspid valve closure, the difference is slight and, particularly in light of the rapid heart rates of most newborns, the sound is usually single. Rarely, delayed closure of the tricuspid valve in Ebstein anomaly can produce audible splitting of the first heart sound at the lower left sternal border. Physiologic splitting can occasionally be heard in infants with very low heart rates such as those with congenital complete heart block.

Normally, the first heart sound is accentuated at birth[10] and is further accentuated in conditions in which there is increased flow across an atrioventricular valve. These include patent ductus arteriosus, mitral insufficiency, and ventricular septal defect (increased mitral flow) as well as total anomalous pulmonary venous drainage and arteriovenous malformation (increased tricuspid flow). The first heart sound is also accentuated, particularly at the lower left sternal border, in infants with tetralogy of Fallot with or without pulmonary valve atresia. In congestive heart failure or prolonged atrioventricular conduction, the first heart sound may be diminished in intensity.

The second heart sound arises from closure of the aortic and pulmonary valves and, consequently, is usually best heard at the upper left sternal border. While on first impression the second heart sound may seem to be single in most neonates, with practice and patience, splitting can nearly always be heard. Often, the splitting is appreciated only as a slurring or prolongation of the second heart sound as compared with the discrete sound of a single valve closure. Time invested in learning to appreciate the difference is well spent, as splitting of the second heart sound is usually absent in a number of significant cardiac defects, including aortic atresia, pulmonary atresia, truncus arteriosus, and transposition of the great arteries.

Wide splitting of the second heart sound is rarely heard in term newborns but can occur in pulmonary stenosis, Ebstein anomaly, total anomalous pulmonary venous drainage, and tetralogy of Fallot. The wide splitting of the second heart sound noted in older children with atrial left-to-right shunting is rarely heard in term newborns because of the relatively decreased compliance of the right ventricle and consequent reduction in atrial shunting. Left-to-right atrial shunts can, however, occasionally produce wide splitting of the second heart sound in premature infants.

A loud second heart sound is indicative of high resistance in either the systemic or pulmonary vascular system. In practice, a loud second heart sound is generally a sign of persistent pulmonary hypertension of the newborn syndrome, and narrow splitting of the sound can be appreciated.

Third heart sounds in the newborn are nearly always a reflection of increased atrioventricular valve flow and are commonly heard in premature infants with patent ductus arteriosus. Third heart sounds are also heard, but rarely, in infants with overt congestive heart failure.

Fourth heart sounds are rarely heard in the newborn and, when present, usually indicate the presence of significant primary myocardial disease and diminished left ventricular compliance.

Clicks

Early systolic ejection clicks, audible at the lower left sternal border, are often detected in the first several hours of life and appear to be benign.[4] After this brief initial period, ejection clicks are always abnormal.

Pathologic ejection clicks in the newborn occur as a result either of dilation of a great vessel or deformity of a semilunar valve. The conditions associated with dilation of a great vessel are generally more serious. Clicks that are probably related to dilation of the ascending aorta are frequently heard in infants with truncus arteriosus as well as in those with tetralogy of Fallot, although in the absence of pulmonary valve atresia, the click heard in tetralogy of Fallot may be obscured by the murmur. Clicks associated with dilation of the pulmonary artery can be

heard in infants with hypoplastic left-heart syndrome or with pulmonary stenosis and poststenotic dilation. Ejection clicks arising from the semilunar valves can occasionally be heard in the absence of dilation of the great vessel in infants with valvular aortic stenosis, coarctation of the aorta, or valvular pulmonary stenosis.

Distinguishing clicks that arise from the aortic valve or ascending aorta from those that arise from the pulmonary valve or artery is extremely difficult in most newborns. Occasionally, particularly with milder degrees of obstruction, the timing of the click in relation to the first heart sound can be noted to vary with respiration, indicating a right heart origin of the click. Also, ejection clicks heard at the apex generally are of left heart origin. Most clicks heard in newborns, however, are best heard at the cardiac base and left sternal border, and a distinction cannot be made on the basis of localization. Additionally, the rapid respiratory rate noted in newborns makes evaluation of lesser degrees of respiratory variation impossible.

Nonejection clicks are occasionally audible in the newborn at the lower left sternal border or apex. They are nearly always transient findings and seem more common in infants with a history of a brief acute insult, such as birth asphyxia or transient fluid overload. While my colleagues and I and others have documented mitral valve prolapse echocardiographically in some of these infants, no clear-cut etiology for these sounds has yet been proved.

Physiologic Murmurs

Heart murmurs have been noted in 60 per cent of infants who were examined an average of nine times during the first 48 hours of life.[4] A similar report noted murmurs in 33 per cent of normal infants examined on the first day of life and in 70 per cent after 1 week.[21] The vast majority of these murmurs are physiologic. Such murmurs can be separated into several main types.

A murmur secondary to transient left-to-right flow through the ductus arteriosus can often be noted during the period that pulmonary vascular resistance is falling but ductal closure has not yet been accomplished. Such murmurs are occasionally continuous but more often are crescendo systolic. When present, the ductal murmur is best heard at the cardiac base and over the left scapula. It is estimated that such murmurs occur in up to 15 per cent of normal infants and occur most often at about 5 to 6 hours of age.[4]

Occasionally, soft ejection systolic murmurs are heard at the cardiac base, with wide radiation to both lung fields. The quality and distribution of the murmur resemble those of the murmur of very mild bilateral peripheral pulmonary arterial stenosis. It is known that at birth the diameter of the left and right pulmonary arteries is much less than that of the main pulmonary trunk, and small pressure differences have been recorded between the main trunk and the right and left branches.[11] In addition, the angle of origin of the branch pulmonary arteries is more acute in newborns than in older infants and children, and it is possible that more turbulent blood flow in this area can be produced by this sharper angle. Accordingly, it has been postulated that the murmur noted over the cardiac base and lung fields of some infants is related to turbulent flow at the site of origin of the left and right pulmonary arteries. Regardless of etiology, this murmur nearly always disappears by 6 to 8 months of age.

An ejection systolic murmur that peaks early in systole and ends well before the second heart sound is probably the most common physiologic heart murmur heard in newborn infants. The murmur is best heard along the mid and upper left sternal border and is generally only grade 1 or 2 on a 1 to 6 scale. It can occasionally be heard over the left back but does not have the wide distribution of the murmur that has been attributed to turbulent flow at the origin of the branch pulmonary arteries. Similarly, this particular murmur lacks the crescendo or continuous quality of the murmur attributed to left-to-right ductal flow, and most resembles the benign systolic flow murmur heard in older children. Its existence in infants has been attributed to the marked increase in flow across the pulmonary valve associated with rapidly falling pulmonary vascular resistance. Up to 56 per cent of normal term infants have been reported to develop this murmur within the first 2 days of life, and the murmur appears to be somewhat more common in infants with lower hemoglobin concentration.[4] The murmur generally disappears by the end of the second week of life.

Vibratory systolic murmurs resembling a Still murmur are also heard in some newborns. Such murmurs are generally heard between the mid left sternal border and the apex, are usually grade 1 or 2 but may be louder, and are thought to arise from the chordae tendineae cordis within the left ventricular cavity. My colleagues and I have followed several infants in whom these murmurs have persisted up to 1 to 2 years of life with no evidence of associated heart disease. Because of the potential for confusion between this murmur and that associated with mild degrees of ventricular outlet obstruction, follow-up examination is strongly encouraged.

Pathologic Murmurs

Murmurs associated with pathologic conditions derive their characteristics not only from the anatomic abnormality but also from the normal changes associated with the transitional circulation and from alterations in circulatory dynamics that might be produced by noncardiac pathology.

Pathologic murmurs audible in the first hours of life are generally related to some form of obstruction to ventricular outflow. Such murmurs are invariably crescendo-decrescendo, or ejection, in quality, begin following the first heart sound, and are usually grade 2 or 3. Both aortic and pulmonary valve stenosis can present with loud systolic ejection murmurs in the first day of life, and it is often quite difficult to distinguish between the two on auscultation. A similar murmur is heard in many infants of diabetic mothers and is related to turbulent flow across the subaortic region produced by the thickened interventricular

septum and hypercontractile left ventricular outflow tract of many of these infants.[19,20] The right ventricular infundibular stenosis of tetralogy of Fallot results in turbulent flow across the right ventricular outflow tract, and a systolic ejection murmur is nearly always audible in the first day of life in infants with this abnormality.

Infants with structural abnormalities resulting in an increased volume of flow across a normal semilunar valve, as in atrial septal defect or unobstructed total anomalous pulmonary venous drainage, will present during the newborn period only if pulmonary vascular resistance and right ventricular compliance are abnormally low. Infants with these defects usually do not develop murmurs typical of their defect until at least several weeks of age.

Even in the presence of significant anatomic obstruction, a murmur will not be heard if flow across the area of obstruction is sufficiently reduced. In cases of severe valvular stenosis with minute openings, the volume of flow may not be great enough to create the degree of turbulence necessary for an audible murmur. In severe aortic stenosis particularly, the relatively underdeveloped left ventricular myocardium may fail to generate the output required to create turbulent flow even in the presence of slightly less severe obstruction. Clearly, cold, acidosis, or hypoxia will also diminish myocardial contractility. Murmurs of outlet obstruction may be absent in these situations and become audible only when the abnormality of homeostasis has been corrected.

Systolic murmurs that include, or obscure, the first heart sound are termed pansystolic. They generally have a less crescendo-decrescendo quality than systolic ejection murmurs. In the newborn, such murmurs generally are associated with atrioventricular valve insufficiency or with the presence of a left-to-right shunt through a ventricular septal defect. Since left-to-right shunting through a ventricular septal defect is dependent on the presence of falling pulmonary vascular resistance, pansystolic murmurs audible at or shortly after birth usually indicate tricuspid or mitral valve insufficiency.

The murmur of tricuspid insufficiency is heard fairly often in infants who have suffered birth asphyxia (see Chapter 40). Tricuspid valve insufficiency in this situation is usually attributed to transient ischemia of the right ventricular papillary muscles.[5] The murmur is best heard just to the left of the xiphosternal junction, usually radiates only minimally, and has a sound that is somewhat blowing in quality. The murmur of neonatal mitral valve insufficiency has a similar quality but is somewhat higher pitched and is located at the cardiac apex. Radiation to the axilla and the back is sometimes heard. Mitral valve insufficiency murmurs are much less often heard than murmurs of tricuspid valve insufficiency and may indicate intrauterine stress, as with arrhythmia or myocarditis, as opposed to perinatal stress. A murmur of mitral valve insufficiency can also occasionally be present before overt left ventricular failure occurs in infants with critical left ventricular outlet obstruction.

The occurrence of the murmur of ventricular septal defect is usually delayed until late in the first day or into the second or third day of life. The murmur may initially appear unremarkable, resembling a benign flow murmur, but as pulmonary vascular resistance continues to fall, the murmur rapidly evolves and becomes typical. In infants with ventricular septal defect, the first heart sound is totally obscured and the murmur is harsh, high pitched, and generally grade 3. It is most audible at the mid or lower left sternal border and can be well localized in some infants and widely distributed in others.

Short, harsh early systolic murmurs that begin with the first heart sound and are well-localized to the lower left sternal border have been noted as a transient finding during the first 1 to 2 days of life in up to 5 per cent of normal newborns.[4] It is hypothesized that these murmurs arise from trivial muscular ventricular septal defects that undergo early spontaneous closure.

Diastolic Murmurs

Diastolic murmurs are rarely heard in the newborn. The early diastolic blow of semilunar valve insufficiency may occasionally be present at birth in infants with truncus arteriosus (see Chapter 46). A similar murmur can be heard in those rare infants with tetralogy of Fallot and absent pulmonary valve (see Chapter 45) or in those with a ruptured sinus of Valsalva aneurysm.

Continuous Murmurs

Continuous murmurs represent aortopulmonary or arteriovenous communication and are heard in 20 to 25 per cent of premature infants with patent ductus arteriosus. Owing to the higher pulmonary vascular resistance in the term newborn, presence of a patent ductus arteriosus in these infants is generally accompanied only by a systolic murmur. Continuous murmurs can be heard, regardless of gestational age, in infants with arteriovenous fistulas.

Arteriovenous fistulas are most commonly located within the lung (either singly or multiply), within the liver, intracranially, or between the subclavian artery and vein. In addition to creating a continuous murmur, the massive shunts that can be associated with these malformations may result in neonatal congestive heart failure. Accordingly, auscultation of the head, liver, and lungs for the presence of a murmur should be a part of the examination of every infant with suspected circulatory overload. In addition, such auscultation should be carried out in any infant with a precordial murmur. Occasionally, a precordial systolic murmur will be found to be a portion of the radiation of a louder continuous murmur audible over the liver or head.

Absence of Murmur

The potential for the existence of serious congenital heart disease in the absence of a murmur cannot be overemphasized. Studies have shown that as many as 20 per cent of infants who died from proven heart abnormalities during the first month of life did not have heart murmurs during life.[26] Particularly in infants with ductus-dependent pulmonary blood flow, such as those with tricuspid or pulmonary valve atresia, absence of a murmur is an ominous sign. It is not uncommon for a murmur to be noted early in these infants, then for rapid clinical deterioration to occur coincident with the disappearance of the murmur, presumably indicating closure of the ductus arteriosus. It is also of note that most patients with transposition of the great arteries do not have an audible murmur during the newborn period.

Absence of a murmur in acyanotic heart disease can also be an ominous prognostic sign. As noted above, absence of an audible murmur in cases of semilunar valve stenosis may indicate severe obstruction and consequent reduction in flow or may be secondary to external influences, such as acidosis, which might reduce cardiac output. In shunt lesions, absence of a murmur generally indicates the presence of hypertensive pulmonary vascular disease. Ventricular septal or atrioventricular septal defects without murmurs are particularly common in infants with Down syndrome. The potential for a severe defect to exist in the absence of a murmur is so great in this latter group of infants that my institution routinely advises that all infants with Down syndrome have an electrocardiogram performed during the newborn period regardless of whether signs suggesting heart disease are present. The characteristic superior electrical axis associated with atrioventricular septal defect is often the only clue present during the newborn period, suggesting the existence of a major cardiac defect in these infants.

CONGESTIVE HEART FAILURE

In the newborn, congestive heart failure presents as a clinical syndrome involving multiple organ systems. While the common unifying concept is that of failure of the myocardial pump, the clinical manifestations of the pump's inability to dispose adequately of venous return and/or to supply the body with the cardiac output it demands can be quite variable. Additionally, myocardial reserve in the newborn is minimal and very rapid progression of congestive heart failure is not uncommon. The clinician must be alert to early indications of myocardial failure so that appropriate therapy can be instituted in a timely fashion.

Cardiac failure presenting at birth is rare and is generally a manifestation of hydrops fetalis associated with intrauterine hemolysis, arrhythmia, or myocarditis. Congestive heart failure in the first day of life is also uncommon but is occasionally seen in infants with structural heart disease. In this group, hypoplastic left-heart syndrome, obstructed total anomalous pulmonary venous drainage, and severe tricuspid or pulmonary valve regurgitation are the most common etiologies. Myocardial hypoxia related to birth asphyxia can also produce early signs of congestive heart failure, as can other extracardiac disturbances that result in diminished metabolic substrate being delivered to the myocardium. Hypoglycemia and anemia are the main entities in this latter category.

Beyond the first 24 hours of life, congestive heart failure may be seen in infants with severe left ventricular outlet obstruction, most commonly critical aortic stenosis (see Chapter 36), interrupted aortic arch (see Chapter 38), or severe aortic coarctation (see Chapter 37). Congestive heart failure secondary to left-to-right shunts can be seen in the first week of life in those cases in which the shunt feeds into a low resistance vascular bed, such as in patent ductus arteriosus in the premature infant (see Chapter 30) or in arteriovenous malformation (see Chapter 35). Systemic-to-pulmonary shunting through a patent ductus arteriosus or ventricular septal defect in a term infant generally does not cause signs of congestive heart failure until the second to fourth weeks of life, owing to the persistence of the relatively high pulmonary vascular resistance in these infants.

Recognition of congestive heart failure depends on first appreciating that findings that might not be abnormal in themselves can form a constellation indicative of the clinical syndrome of congestive heart failure. Clinical findings also generally follow a temporal sequence. Tachycardia and tachypnea are both invariably present in infants with congestive heart failure, but neither the heart rate nor the respiratory rate exceeds values generally accepted as upper limits of normal. Rather, the typical finding is that of persistence of values near the upper end of the normal range, with loss of normal variability. A gallop rhythm may or may not be present, but when present, it generally indicates more advanced dysfunction. Pallor, with peripheral vasoconstriction, is almost invariably present and is often the most striking early finding, particularly in premature infants. Pulses are poorly felt, and the pulse pressure is narrow, even in infants in whom failure is a result of systemic run-off into a low resistance circulation. Oliguria and weight gain are also very common, although somewhat later findings, but peripheral edema is rarely seen. Hepatomegaly, when it occurs, is a late finding, and splenomegaly is almost never noted. Cyanosis and rales indicate overt pulmonary edema and are markers of far-advanced myocardial failure.

It is important to recall that findings of congestive heart failure may mask findings that might permit accurate elucidation of the underlying lesion responsible for the development of myocardial dysfunction. Accordingly, appropriate treatment of congestive heart failure may cause marked changes in clinical findings. Interpretation of findings observed in the presence of congestive heart failure should be performed only with great caution. Frequently, definitive diagnosis of the underlying lesion that has precipitated myocardial failure must either await resolution of congestive heart failure or be carried out using other methods.

References

1. Adelman RD (1978): Neonatal hypertension. Pediatr Clin North Am 25:99–110.

2. Adelman RD (1984): Neonatal hypertension. Annales Nestle 42:32–42.

3. Adelman RD, Sherman MP (1980): Hypertension in the neonate following closure of abdominal wall defects. J Pediatr 97:642–644.

4. Braudo M, Rowe RD (1961): Auscultation of the heart—early neonatal period. Am J Dis Child 101:575–586.

5. Bucciarelli RL, Nelson RM, Egan EA, Eitzman DV, Gessner IH (1977): Transient tricuspid insufficiency of the newborn: A form of myocardial dysfunction in stressed newborns. Pediatrics 59:330–337.

6. Castellanos A, Pereiras R, Garcia A (1937): La angio-cardiografia radio-opaca. Arch Soc Estud Clin Habana 31:9–10.

7. Chameides L, Diana DJ, Dougherty J (1978): Neonatal cardiac rhythm abnormalities. Perinatal Care 2:4–13.

8. Christie A (1930): Normal closing time of the foramen ovale and the ductus arteriosus: An anatomic and statistical study. Am J Dis Child 40:323–326.

9. Cordero L, Hon EH (1971): Neonatal bradycardia following nasopharyngeal stimulation. J Pediatr 78:441–447.

10. Craige E, Harned HS (1963): Phonocardiographic and electrocardiographic studies in normal newborn infants. Am Heart J 65:180–189.

11. Danilowicz D, Rudolph AM, Hoffman JIE (1965): Vascular resistance in the large pulmonary arteries in infancy (abstr). Circulation 32:II–74.

12. Davignon A, Rautaharju P, Boiselle E, Soumis F, Megelas M, Choquette A (1980): Normal ECG standards for infants and children. Pediatr Cardiol 1:123–131.

13. Desmond MM, Franklin RR, Vallbora C, Hill RM, Plumb R, Arnold H, Watts J (1963): The clinical behavior of the newly born. J Pediatr 62:307–325.

14. Desmond MM, Rudolph AJ, Phitaksphraiwan P (1966): The transitional care nursery. Pediatr Clin North Am 13:651–668.

15. Ellison RC, Peckham GJ, Lang P, Talner NS, Lerer TJ, Lin L, Dooley KJ, Nadas AN (1983): Evaluation of the preterm infant for patent ductus arteriosus. Pediatrics 71:364–372.

16. Gatti RA, Muster AJ, Cole RB, Paul MH (1966): Neonatal polycythemia with transient cyanosis and cardiorespiratory abnormalities. J Pediatr 69:1063–1072.

17. Goldman HI, Maralit A, Sun S, Lanzkowski P (1973): Neonatal cyanosis and arterial oxygen saturations. J Pediatr 82:319–324.

18. Goldring D, Wohltmann HJ (1952): "Flush" method for blood pressure determinations in newborn infants. J Pediatr 40:285–289.

19. Gutgesell HP, Mullins CE, Gillette PC, Speer M, Rudolph AJ, McNamara DG (1976): Transient hypertrophic subaortic stenosis in infants of diabetic mothers. J Pediatr 85:120–125.

20. Gutgesell HP, Speer ME, Rosenberg HS (1980): Characterization of the cardiomyopathy in infants of diabetic mothers. Circulation 61:441–450.

21. Halladie-Smith KA (1960): Some auscultory and phonocardiographic findings observed in early infancy. Br Med J 1:756–759.

22. Holt LE (1897): The Diseases of Infancy and Childhood. New York, D. Appleton and Company, pp 566–568.

23. Lee Y-H, Rosner B, Gould JB, Lowe EW, Kass EH (1976): Familial aggregation of blood pressures of newborn infants and their mothers. Pediatrics 58:722–729.

24. Montague TJ, Taylor PG, Stockton R, Roy DL, Smith ER (1982): The spectrum of cardiac rate and rhythm in normal newborns. Pediatr Cardiol 2:33–38.

25. Noonan JA (1978): Association of congenital heart disease with syndromes or other defects. Pediatr Clin North Am 25:797–816.

26. Ober WB, Moore TE (1955): Congenital cardiac malformations in the neonatal period: An autopsy study. N Engl J Med 253:271–75.

27. Romero TE, Friedman WF (1979): Limited left ventricular response to volume overload in the neonatal period: A comparative study with the adult animal. Pediatr Res 13:910–915.

28. Rowe RD, Freedom RM, Mehrizi A, Bloom KR (1981): The Neonate with Congenital Heart Disease. 2nd ed. Philadelphia, WB Saunders, p 33.

29. Ibid, p 55.

30. Rudolph AM, Drorbaugh JE, Auld PAM, Rudolph AJ, Nadas AS,

Smith CA, Hubbell JP (1961): Studies on the circulation in the neonatal period. Pediatrics 27:551–566.

31. Southall DP, Richards J, Mitchell P, Brown DJ, Johnston PGB, Shinebourne EA (1980): Study of cardiac rhythm in healthy newborn infants. Br Heart J 43:14–20.

32. Steinfeld L, Dimich I, Reder R, Cohen M, Alexander H (1978): Sphygmomanometry in the pediatric patient. J Pediatr 92:934–938.

33. Taussig HB (1947): Congenital Malformations of the Heart. New York, Commonwealth Fund.

34. Taylor AI (1968): Autosomal trisomy syndrome. A detailed study of 27 cases of Edwards syndrome and 27 cases of Patau's syndrome. J Med Genet 5:227–252.

35. Valimaki I, Tarco PA (1971): Heart rate patterns and apnea in newborn infants. Am J Obstet Gynecol 110:343–349.

36. Versmold HT, Kitterman JA, Phibbs RH, Gregory GA, Tooley WH (1981): Aortic blood pressure during the first 12 hours of life in infants with birth weight of 610 to 4220 grams. Pediatrics 67:607–613.

37. Zachman RD, Bauer CR, Boehm J, Korones SB, Rigatto H, Gustafson NF (1986): Neonatal blood pressure at birth by the Doppler method. Am Heart J 111:189–190.

21 ELECTROCARDIOGRAPHY

D. Woodrow Benson, Jr.
C. Elise Duffy

HISTORICAL PERSPECTIVE

The basic concepts utilized in recording and interpreting the electrocardiogram (ECG) were formulated near the turn of this century. Waller is credited with making the observation that electrical activity of the heart could be recorded from the body surface, and in 1887 he obtained the first ECG in a human being.[17] Interpretation of these early recordings was hampered by the poor frequency response of the available recording device, the capillary electrometer. Einthoven, considered the father of electrocardiography, directed his early efforts toward understanding the physical laws governing the movements of the mercury column in the capillary electrometer and providing correction factors for reconstructing the recorded waveforms. The recordings that Einthoven reconstructed provided an accurate depiction of the ECG and showed five waves, which Einthoven termed P, Q, R, S, and T. In 1901, Einthoven published a description of the string galvanometer, a device ideally suited for recording the rapidly changing and weak currents of cardiac electrical activity present on the body surface. This instrument proved useful for the study of the ECG, and subsequent reports described the utility and techniques for ECG recording from a variety of extracardiac sites, including the report by Cremer in 1906 of ECG recording from the esophagus.[3]

Most of the early reports of the use of the ECG appeared in the German literature. The first report of ECG recording in infants and children was published by Nicolai and Funaro in 1908[50] and evaluated lead I recordings in 45 subjects. In 1913, Hecht published a "comprehensive" study utilizing all three standard bipolar leads (I, II, III) using records from hundreds of premature infants, term infants, and children with normal and abnormal hearts.[27]

Chest lead ECGs have been recorded in infants and children since 1934, 2 years after the introduction of their use in clinical electrocardiography.[76] By the late 1930s, the distinctive ECG changes that occur in normal infants and children had been described. These include right axis deviation and the presence of prominent R waves in leads from the right precordium in infants, which resolve during childhood, and the frequent occurrence of inverted T waves in leads recorded from the right and midportion of the precordium in children, which change with adulthood.[76] Subsequently, many studies reported surface ECG findings in infants and children with known or suspected cardiac disease, but for decades there was relatively little application of the esophageal ECG.[3,74]

GENERAL PRINCIPLES

The ultimate goal of clinical electrocardiography is to detect normal and abnormal electrical events within the myocardium using waveforms recorded from the body surface during depolarization and repolarization of the atria and ventricles. Atrial depolarization normally commences in the right atrium and terminates in the left atrium. The first half of the P wave is associated with depolarization of the right atrium and the second half with depolarization of the left atrium. When atrial depolarization is "nonsinus," as may happen during certain tachycardias, the shape of the P wave will be altered. Usually, atrial repolarization (Ta wave) is inapparent, since it occurs simultaneously with the QRS waveform. As opposed to atrial depolarization, which tends to be sequential (right, then left), right and left ventricular depolarization proceeds virtually simultaneously. The major determinants of the QRS waveform at a given site on the body surface are the sequence of ventricular depolarization and the geometric relationship between the myocardium (cardiac generator) and the torso (volume conductor). On the other hand, under ordinary circumstances, the principal determinant of the ST-T wave is the sequence of ventricular depolarization.

Thus, in electrocardiography the body surface potentials are used to make deductions about the electrical activity of the heart. From a clinical standpoint, the deduced electrical activity is used to make inferences about cardiac pathology. The deductions, or ECG interpretations, have been based primarily on the empirical association of specific changes in certain leads with findings at cardiac catheterization, surgery, and autopsy. Cardiac potentials recorded from the body surface may be displayed as a group of scalar tracings (standard ECG tracings), as a vectorcardiogram, or as a series of instantaneous maps of the surface potentials (body surface maps). The initial idea, based on the concepts of Waller and Einthoven, was that the cardiac potentials recorded from the body surface could be accounted for by considering electrical events in the heart to be equivalent to those generated by a dipole source. Electrocardiography is based on the idea that cardiac electrical activity can be represented by an equivalent dipole, as is vector electrocardiography. The dipolar model has had a major influence on electrocardiographic research. However, numerous studies have shown the inadequacies of the equivalent dipole model, which cannot account for all the electrical information available on the body surface.[2,69] Much of electrocardiographic research has been directed at development of lead systems to minimize the extent of the "lost" information.

From the standpoint of interpreting selective intracardiac electrical events, a disadvantage in evaluating an individual scalar tracing as obtained in a standard ECG is that the voltage variation is the result of a change in time rather than in variation in the electrical sources at a single intracardiac location. Thus, for example, it is not possible to examine a single scalar tracing and make inferences about selective right or left ventricular effects. This disadvantage may be overcome by examining potential variation in space, rather than time, since the relationship between the spatially distributed electrical sources within the heart and the potential distributions produced on the epicardial or body surfaces for any instant in time can be considered independently of the relationship that exists at any other time. Such voltage variation in space is the basis of body surface maps. Thus, rather than selection of one lead system, this approach permits evaluation of all electrical information at the body surface.

RECORDING TECHNIQUE

Surface ECG

Standard ECG recording in active neonates and infants is a technical challenge. However, artifact-free recordings are essential for accurate interpretation. The quality of the recordings may be enhanced by using two technicians. The relatively rapid resting heart rates of neonates and infants make high fidelity recorders essential. The technical aspects of ECG recording have been outlined by Thomas,[71] and the performance specifications for direct-writing electrocardiographs have been outlined in the report of the American Heart Association's Committee on Electrocardiography.[53]

The standard electrocardiographic record consists of 12 leads recorded from nine body surface positions. These include the three bipolar limb leads (I, II, III) originally designated by Einthoven as well as the three unipolar

Table 21–1. LOCATION OF PRECORDIAL LEADS

V Lead	Location
1	Fourth intercostal space, right sternal border
2	Fourth intercostal space, left sternal border
3	Midway between V_2 and V_4
4	Fifth intercostal space, midclavicular line
5	Same level as V_4, anterior axillary line
6	Same level as V_4 and V_5, midaxillary line
7	Same level as V_4, V_5, and V_6, posterior axillary line
3R	Same as V_3 on right chest
4R	Same as V_4 on right chest

limb leads (R, L, F) and the six unipolar left chest leads (V_1 to V_6) as specified by Wilson. The standard configuration is sometimes modified by recording additional chest leads on the left (V_7) and/or right (V_3R, V_4R) chest (Table 21–1 and Fig. 21–1). Simultaneous recording of three or more surface leads is essential for facilitating rhythm analysis and for measuring intervals and assessing morphology of the P, QRS, and ST-T wave complexes.

Transesophageal ECG

There has been considerable documentation of the utility of transesophageal ECG recording. Electrode placement is a practical consideration in utilization of the technique. In neonates and infants, placement of catheter electrodes is similar to esophageal intubation for nasogastric tube placement. From the patient's standpoint, the procedure can be considerably improved and discomfort minimized with use of a soft, flexible catheter, which may be passed either through the nares or, since these young patients are edentulous, through the mouth (Fig. 21–2). Our experience has been that there is less electrode movement during the recording if the catheter

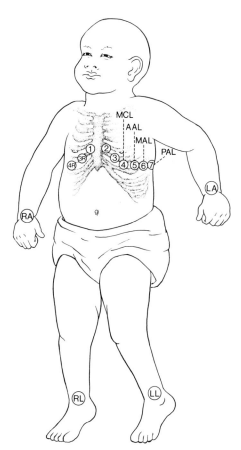

Figure 21–1. Torso depicting location of electrodes for recording standard ECG. AAL = anterior axillary line; LA = left arm; LL = left leg; MAL = midaxillary line; MCL = midclavicular line; PAL = posterior axillary line; RA = right arm; RL = right leg.

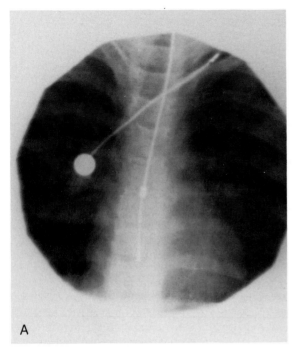 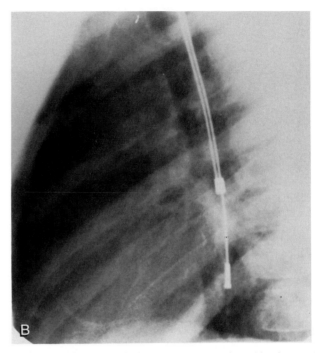

Figure 21–2. Anteroposterior (*A*) and lateral (*B*) chest radiographs showing a silicone rubber-coated bipolar electrode catheter in position for recording an esophageal ECG.

is positioned through the nares. The electrode insertion depth for recording the largest esophagoatrial deflection can be estimated from infant height.[4]

The principal technical difficulty in obtaining artifact-free transesophageal ECG is elimination of respiratory artifact, which may be accomplished by appropriate filtering

of the recording. Consequently, faithful reproduction of the electrocardiographic waveform may be accomplished by using an instrument with a band width of 10 to 100 Hz. It is the low frequency filter that is most important for eliminating the respiratory artifact (Fig. 21–3).

NORMAL ELECTROCARDIOGRAM OF TERM INFANT

The hallmark of the ECG changes in the normal newborn and infant are the age-related transitions of QRS morphology, QRS duration, and the pattern of the ST-T wave.[5,12,38,54] The focus has been on changes that occur in the first few days of life[5,12,26,38,70,73] as well as those occurring during the first and second years.[5,12,38,54] Because of these age-related changes, abnormalities of QRS morphology and duration as well as changes in the ST-T wave may be difficult to recognize.

In the normal infant, the gradual decrease in heart rate, increase in P wave duration, increase in PR interval, and increase in QRS duration have been well described. QRS voltages are low in the newborn but gradually increase during the first several months of life. The mean QRS axis in the frontal plane moves from a rightward direction to the left. Slight elevations of the ST segment followed by decrease before the T wave are very common. True ST segment elevation is considered to be present if greater than 2 mm in the chest leads and 1 mm in the limb leads.

The "right ventricular dominance" of the infant as compared with the older child or adult is widely known, and the effects on the QRS and T wave complexes have been well described. The changes in depolarization of the

Figure 21–3. Effect of filtering on esophageal ECG. The high cutoff filter is fixed at 1000 HZ. The low cutoff filter varies, as shown on the lower right of each panel. Filtering at 10 Hz provides adequate elimination of respiratory artifact in most patients. II = lead II; ESO = esophageal ECG.

ventricles during the first year of life occur as an orderly progression. In the newborn, the principal QRS potentials are determined by currents from the right ventricle, while at 9 months of age currents from the left ventricle play a major role. While the well-known normal transitional change in the right ventricular peak systolic pressure from systemic levels to much lower levels occurs in hours to days, the ECG transition lags considerably. Benson and Spach[5] observed the first identifiable currents from the left ventricle around 1 month of age, and left ventricular current gradually becomes dominant during the first year.

Age-related patterns of repolarization are more difficult to interpret. However, in the first day of life the major feature (positive T wave in lead V_1) most likely results from early appearance of repolarization in the left ventricle and the late termination of depolarization in the right ventricle. Thereby, an overall left ventricle to right ventricle repolarization sequence would result, and this would account for the well-known upright T wave in lead V_1 in the normal term infant. After 1 month, qualitative ECG features of repolarization are similar to those of normal adults. The age-related changes in repolarization are most likely due to changes in the sequence of repolarization secondary to changes in the sequence of ventricular depolarization.[5]

NORMAL ELECTROCARDIOGRAM OF PREMATURE INFANT

When compared with the ECG of term infants, the initial ECG of the premature infant is notable for a shorter QRS duration. The PR interval and QT interval are also shorter, but these observations may reflect a faster heart rate. The electrocardiogram of the premature infant shows less right ventricular predominance at birth than the electrocardiogram of the full-term infant.[67,72] At 1 year the heart rate of the premature infant exceeds that of the term infant. Further, precordial voltages are reduced in the 1-year-old infant who was premature.[72] The reduced precordial voltages may be observed in the absence of bronchopulmonary dysplasia. Whether these differences are related to intrinsic myocardial differences of the premature versus term infant or to altered cardiac-torso geometry has not been determined.

VENTRICULAR HYPERTROPHY

Criteria for an ECG determination of ventricular hypertrophy rely primarily on whether QRS voltages in specific leads exceed some normal value. The criteria have been empirically derived, based on studies of normal infants or on comparison of ECG measurements with findings at cardiac catheterization, surgery, or autopsy. Interpretation of criteria for hypertrophy depends on the assumption that cardiac-torso geometry is normal or near normal and that the ventricular depolarization sequence is normal (i.e., no bundle branch block). These assumptions limit the sensitivity and specificity of ECG diagnosis of hypertrophy,

since the closer the heart is to a particular lead, the greater the observed voltage, regardless of the underlying cardiac pathology.[39] The proximity effect is particularly important in infants (i.e., relatively thin chest) and may cause an unequal emphasis on the magnitude of the voltage in some leads but not in others. The right chest lead voltage may be particularly distorted by proximity, and thus cloud even further the issue of right ventricular hypertrophy in the neonate and infant.

From a clinical standpoint, not all criteria for ventricular hypertrophy carry equal weight in evaluating underlying pathology; use of a point scoring system has been advocated by some investigators.[19,56] Following the recommendation of Liebman,[39] we advocate not using ventricular hypertrophy criteria based on intrinsicoid deflection.

In general, tests for left ventricular hypertrophy derive from two considerations: amplitude tests and strain tests. The amplitude tests evaluate voltage increase, while strain tests monitor the shift of the ST-T wave axis in a direction opposite to the QRS. Amplitude tests utilize R and S waves in leads V_1, V_2, V_5, and V_6, the ratio of R and S waves in lead V_1, and Q wave amplitude in lead V_6. There has not been general agreement on the amplitude of Q, R, S waves in defining what might be considered abnormal. The strain tests evaluate T wave negativity in the lateral precordial leads and the angle (greater than 100 degrees) between the frontal plane QRS and T axis.

Criteria for right ventricular hypertrophy tend to be more specific than those for left ventricular hypertrophy, and they include an amplitude test for the S wave in left precordial leads (V_5, V_6), an amplitude test for the R wave in the right precordial leads (V_1, V_2), an RSR′ pattern with R taller than R′ in lead V_1, and a positive T wave in lead V_1. Right axis deviation also indicates right ventricular hypertrophy. Finally, evaluation of the R:S ratio in lead V_6 may be useful for detecting right ventricular hypertrophy, especially when lung disease is present.

In the neonate and infant, hypertrophy of both ventricles may be present. Electrocardiographically, biventricular hypertrophy may be inferred when criteria for both left and right ventricular hypertrophy are met. An alternative criterion uses prominent midprecordial voltage to diagnose biventricular hypertrophy (so-called Katz-Wachtel criteria).[33]

ATRIAL ENLARGEMENT

Determination of atrial enlargement can be difficult and is usually based on increased P wave voltage or P wave duration. For example, increased voltage in leads II, V_1, and V_2 indicates right atrial enlargement; these voltage increases would be expected in the early portion of the P wave. On the other hand, increased voltage in the terminal portion of the P wave may manifest primarily as prolonged P wave duration, usually in lead II or V_1. In the neonate and infant, both right and left atrial enlargement may be present simultaneously; biatrial enlargement may be diagnosed if criteria for both left and right atrial enlargement are present.

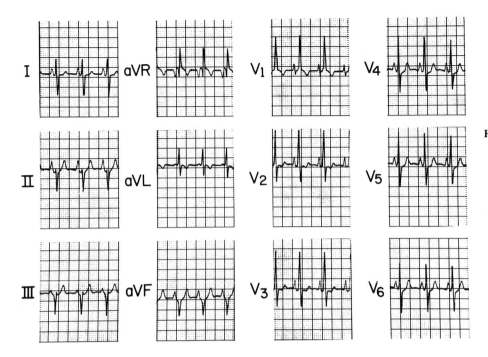

Figure 21–4. Electrocardiogram demonstration of features of ventricular preexcitation. Specifically, note the short PR interval, delta wave, and prolonged QRS duration. The delta wave may be positive (V5), negative (AVF), or isoelectric (II). The atrial enlargement in this case is most likely the result of prolonged tachycardia (not shown).

DISTURBANCES OF RHYTHM AND CONDUCTION

Much of the classic framework of rhythm and conduction disturbance analysis is based on the standard ECG. In spite of many other advances in the evaluation of disturbances of rhythm and conduction, the ECG is still of fundamental diagnostic importance. In the neonate and infant suspected of having rhythm and conduction abnormalities, careful attention should be addressed to the measurement of the basic age- and heart rate-dependent intervals during sinus rhythm.[12] The utility of this approach is obvious in the case of an infant with a history suggesting undocumented tachycardia in whom the ECG during sinus rhythm demonstrates the classic features of ventricular preexcitation, as seen in the Wolff-Parkinson-White syndrome (Fig. 21–4).

A limitation of ECG diagnosis of disorders of rhythm and conduction is that the ECG documentation may not be sufficient to permit a precise electrophysiologic diagnosis. For example, the combination of tachycardia with a regular rate, no evidence of atrioventricular (AV) dissociation, and a normal QRS is commonly known as paroxysmal atrial tachycardia (PAT). However, it is now known that this rhythm disturbance may be the result of several different electrophysiologic mechanisms, which cannot be specifically inferred from the ECG. Use of the esophageal ECG to evaluate the temporal relationship between atrial and ventricular depolarization and the standard ECG to evaluate the pattern of ventricular depolarization is critical for establishing a differential diagnosis of rhythm disturbances, and it is in this context that the ECG is most useful.

During conduction disturbances, the ECG should be examined for the pattern of conduction abnormality. To determine whether first, second, or third degree heart block is present, particular attention should be given to whether the PR interval and P-QRS relationship are appropriate for age and heart rate. The QRS duration should be examined to determine whether it is prolonged, and if so, then an effort should be made to determine whether a specific pattern (e.g., right or left bundle branch block) is present. Finally, examination of the ST-T wave may reveal important abnormalities. These might be due to changes in ventricular depolarization or they may be the result of a primary abnormality in repolarization. For example, the prolonged QT interval syndrome is thought to represent a primary repolarization abnormality, since the QRS complex is thought to be normal.[13]

ABERRANCY

Altered QRS configuration associated with depolarization initiated via the normal conduction system is a well-recognized electrocardiographic entity, which is termed "aberrancy."[60] Aberrancy is thought to occur relatively infrequently in the neonate and infant, but recognition of it is important in assessing disorders of conduction and rhythm. The initial step in recognizing aberrancy is to observe that QRS duration is prolonged. This may be difficult, since prolonged QRS duration in neonates and infants is relatively short compared with that in older children and adults.

Right bundle branch block (RBBB) results from delay in right ventricular depolarization. Consequently, ventricular depolarization is sequential (left then right) rather than nearly simultaneous, as is characteristic for normal ventricular depolarization. In neonates and infants, the electrocardiographic patterns for RBBB characteristically

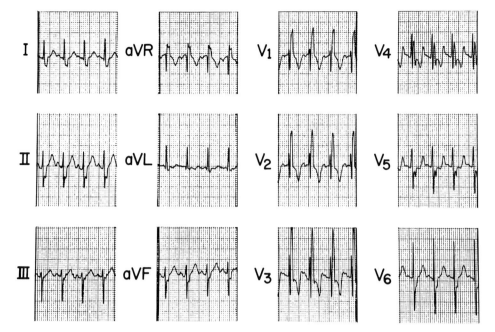

Figure 21–5. Right bundle branch block following cardiac surgery in an infant. The QRS duration is unusually prolonged for an infant. Note the dominant R wave in lead V_1 and S wave in lead V_6. The left axis deviation was present prior to surgery.

include a QRS of prolonged duration (exceeding 80 msec, 0.08 sec), a dominant R wave in lead V_1, and a dominant S wave in lead V_6 (Fig. 21–5). In infants, RBBB may be transiently or permanently observed during tachycardia,[21] particularly in association with Ebstein anomaly of the tricuspid valve (Fig. 21–6)[23,61] or following cardiac surgery.[29]

RBBB is probably most frequently observed in the neonate and infant following cardiac surgery for congenital heart disease, especially following right ventriculotomy. Horowitz et al[29] demonstrated that RBBB following cardiac surgery was the result of conduction block at three specific sites, which they termed as "proximal RBBB," "distal RBBB," and "terminal RBBB." The site of proximal RBBB was between the bundle of His and the RBB immediately distal to the ventricular septal defect. Distal RBBB resulted from conduction block distal to the moderator band. Terminal RBBB resulted from block in the terminal ramifications of the RBB.

The term "incomplete RBBB" is often used to describe ECGs in which QRS morphology resembles RBBB but in which the QRS duration is normal. As the name suggests, the implication is that an abnormality exists in the right-sided peripheral Purkinje conduction system. However, as pointed out by Moore et al,[46] this term is probably a misnomer, since the ECG pattern may be due to variation in right ventricular free-wall thickness rather than an abnormality of the specialized conduction system.

Left bundle branch block (LBBB) results from delay in left ventricular depolarization. In neonates and infants this conduction defect is most often observed as rate-dependent block at the onset of paroxysmal atrial tachycardia[21] (Fig. 21–7), but it may be seen following cardiac surgery. In infants, ECG evidence of LBBB is characterized by prolonged QRS duration, a dominant S wave in lead V_1, and a dominant R wave in lead V_6. LBBB may be associated with normal or left axis deviation.

While the concept of fascicular block (hemiblock)[57] has been important in ECG interpretation of conduction abnormalities of the left bundle branch, the anatomic description of fascicular block is overly simplified.[16,35] In the ECGs of neonates and infants, it is well known that frontal plane QRS axis deviation, the principal ECG feature of fascicular block, is often not due to conduction system impairment or block. For example, Kulangara et al[34] found that left axis deviation in tricuspid atresia patients was due to early right ventricular activation with relative delay, primarily in the base, of left ventricular depolarization. On the other hand, left axis deviation in atrioventricular septal defect is due to early depolarization of the diaphragmatic surface of the left ventricle, a finding consistent with the known posterior and inferior

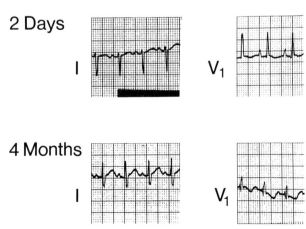

Figure 21–6. ECG features of Ebstein anomaly of the tricuspid valve. In the top tracing (at age 2 days), right atrial enlargement and right ventricular hypertrophy are present. By 4 months of age (bottom tracing), the QRS duration is prolonged and right bundle branch block is present.

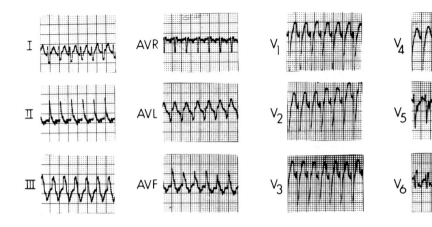

Figure 21–7. Rate-related left bundle branch block during infant tachycardia. The QRS duration is prolonged (100 msec). Note the dominant S wave in lead V_1 and dominant R wave in V_6.

displacement of the specialized conduction system in atrioventricular septal defects.[7,10]

The diagnosis of intraventricular conduction delay is made when the QRS duration is prolonged for age but a definite pattern of bundle branch block or other specific conduction abnormality is not present. Associated ST-T wave changes may be observed. The presence of intraventricular conduction delay is not associated with any specific underlying cardiac abnormality, and it does not appear to be otherwise associated with any particular rhythm disturbance.

PREEXCITATION

Preexcitation, a term first proposed by Ohnell[51] and subsequently modified by Durrer et al,[15] is said to be present "if in relation to atrial events, the whole or some part of the ventricular muscle is activated earlier by the impulse originating from the atrium than would be expected if the impulse reached the ventricles by way of the normal specific conduction system only."[22] In this chapter the discussion is limited to ventricular preexcitation.

The contribution of the European Study Group[1] has proved valuable in establishing precise terminology for structures permitting ventricular preexcitation. This classification utilizes the term "connection" for accessory conduction pathways inserting into ordinary, working myocardium, and the term "tract" to describe accessory conduction tissue that inserts into the specialized cardiac conduction system.

The two principal features of the ECG in preexcitation syndromes may occur alone or in combination: shortening for age of the PR interval and/or prolongation for age of the QRS duration. Different combinations of these features prevail for the different anomalous conducting pathways, as depicted in Figure 21–8. Since ventricular depolarization is altered by ventricular preexcitation, associated changes in the ST-T wave changes are predictable. In fact, the associated ST-T wave changes have been shown to be useful in predicting the location of accessory AV connections.[6]

Ventricular preexcitation in the Wolff-Parkinson-White syndrome is the result of fusion of ventricular depolarization via the normal conduction system and the accessory AV connection. Accessory AV connections are the most common preexcitation syndromes reported in neonates and infants, and consequently, have been the most studied. The electrophysiologic and morphologic bases of accessory AV connections have been well-described; the PR interval shortening is the result of early ventricular activation, inscribed by the delta wave via the accessory connection.

ECTOPIC VENTRICULAR DEPOLARIZATION

The prolonged QRS duration that results from ectopic ventricular depolarization is the result of protracted ventricular muscle depolarization. Ectopic ventricular depolarization is infrequently encountered in the neonate and infant but does occur during ventricular extrasystoles, ventricular tachycardia, and ventricular pacing. It is possible to estimate crudely the site at which ectopic ventricular depolarization began by noting the electrocardiographic similarity of the QRS morphology to that of RBBB (early depolarization of the left ventricle) or to that of LBBB (early depolarization of the right ventricle). From an electrophysiologic standpoint, there is little similarity between intraventricular conduction disorder (bundle branch block) and initiation of ventricular activation from an ectopic site on the contralateral ventricle, but the electrocardiographic similarity is well recognized.

PROLONGED QT INTERVAL

The significance of a prolonged QT interval on the ECG of an asymptomatic neonate or infant is unknown but has been subject to a variety of interpretations. Factors known to affect the QT interval include heart rate, metabolic derangement, and drug administration. Thus, at times, a prolonged QT interval may indicate a therapeutic effect of antiarrhythmic drug administration (e.g., procainamide). On the other hand, QT interval prolongation may indicate a metabolic disturbance such as hypocalcemia. However, in other neonates and infants, an idiopathic prolongation of the QT interval may be associated

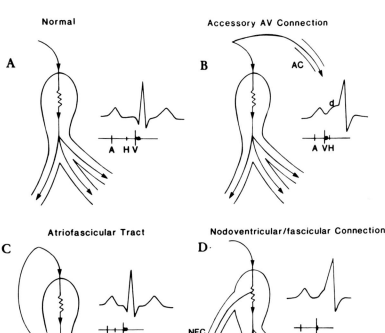

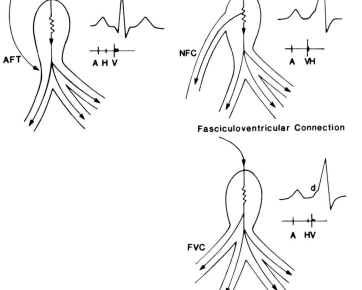

Figure 21–8. *A* to *D*, Diagrammatic depiction of types of preexcitation with associated ECG and His bundle electrocardiogram changes. (Reproduced with permission from Gornick CC, Benson DW Jr [1986]: Electrocardiographic aspects of the preexcitation syndrome. In Benditt DG, Benson DW Jr (eds): Cardiac Preexcitation Syndromes: Origins, Evaluation and Treatment. Boston, Martinus-Nijhoff Publishing, pp 43–73.)

with an ominous prognosis and the risk of syncope or sudden death due to ventricular tachycardia (torsade de pointes).[30,31,47,48,55,63,68,75] In previously reported cases, symptoms rarely occurred until the infant was a toddler (18 months or more). However, symptoms in a fetus[47] and in neonates have been described,[63] with second degree heart block commonly associated[52,63] (Fig. 21–9). A link of sudden infant death syndrome and prolonged QT interval has been suggested[41,63] but not well documented.[25]

Burchell[8] has reviewed the historical developments involved in the measurement of the QT interval and the QT interval corrected for heart rate, the so-called corrected QT interval. In the fetus, neonate, and infant, the problem is more complex, since the work of Davignon et al[12] has clearly demonstrated the relationship of both age and heart rate to the QT interval in young patients. A simple explanation for this association might be the well-known dependence of cardiac action potential duration on both age and heart rate.[62] A major technical problem with meas-

uring the QT interval is that in young patients with relatively rapid resting heart rates, it is difficult to determine the end of the T wave, since it may overlap with the succeeding P wave.

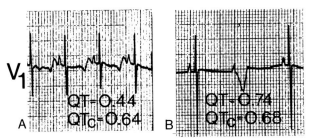

Figure 21–9. Prolonged QT interval in a neonate. ECG lead V$_1$ is shown in both *A* and *B*. *A*, 1:1 atrioventricular conduction. *B*, 2:1 atrioventricular conduction. The corrected QT interval (QTc) is extraordinarily long and nearly the same in *A* and *B*.

ELECTROCARDIOGRAPHIC FEATURES OF SPECIFIC SYNDROMES

Bronchopulmonary Dysplasia

Bronchopulmonary dysplasia is a relatively common disorder of infants born prematurely. It usually follows severe hyaline membrane disease, but the primary cause is unknown. The principal ECG abnormalities include right atrial enlargement and right ventricular hypertrophy. ECG abnormalities reflecting the development of atrial enlargement and ventricular hypertrophy may be obscured by the development of an increase in the anteroposterior diameter of the chest.

Respiratory Distress Syndrome

Hyaline membrane disease is the most common cause of severe, acute respiratory distress in the perinatal period. Electrocardiographic features are nonspecific or absent. In fact, the principal value of the ECG may be in establishing a specific diagnosis of heart disease, since the diagnosis of hyaline membrane disease may be one of exclusion.

Birth Asphyxia

In the neonatal period, asphyxia is usually defined by low Apgar scores, but asphyxia may occur in a silent fashion. A wide spectrum of symptoms can result from the cardiovascular sequelae of asphyxia, including severe cardiogenic shock.[37] ECG findings are quite variable and may be absent.

Persistent Pulmonary Hypertension of the Newborn Syndrome

In infants with persistent pulmonary hypertension of the newborn syndrome, the fetal pattern of right-to-left shunting persists; consequently, idiopathic cases are sometimes known as persistent fetal circulation. The association of persistent pulmonary hypertension of the newborn syndrome with a variety of entities,[18,28] including congenital heart disease,[36] has been well documented. In idiopathic cases, electrocardiographic changes may be absent but, when present, are nonspecific and include right ventricular hypertrophy and right atrial enlargement. As the diagnosis of idiopathic persistent pulmonary hypertension of the newborn syndrome is one of exclusion, the value of the ECG is related to establishing a diagnosis of other specific heart disease.[18,49] In fact, Linday et al[40] found the ECG to be 100 per cent sensitive and 90 per cent specific for detecting cardiovascular abnormalities in patients with underlying congenital heart disease causing persistent pulmonary hypertension of the newborn syndrome. Murphy et al[49] found the ECG to be less sensitive but highly specific for identifying infants in whom persistent pulmonary hypertension of the newborn syndrome was secondary to congenital heart disease.

Systemic Diseases

Cardiac involvement is common in a variety of systemic diseases, including neuromuscular, collagen vascular, and storage diseases.[44] Electrocardiographic abnormalities are often nonspecific or absent in young infants with these disorders, but a few conditions are associated with characteristic ECG abnormalities. Although nonspecific ECG abnormalities have been reported in glycogen storage diseases types III, IV and V, in type IIA (Pompe disease), characteristic ECG abnormalities are commonly found;[9] these include a short PR interval and high QRS voltages, which may be interpreted as left or biventricular hypertrophy. The short PR interval is the result of shortened AV nodal conduction time.[20]

Congenital Heart Disease

ECG abnormalities are present in a variety of congenital cardiac defects. Our purpose here is to review abnormalities associated with distinctive ECG features that may permit a specific diagnosis to be made.

Dextrocardia

One of the fundamental assumptions in the interpretation of the standard ECG is that the cardiac-torso relationship is the same from person to person. Dextrocardia provides an extreme situation demonstrating the importance of this relationship (Fig. 21–10). Altered cardiac-torso geometry is clinically important in a number of other situations, including chronic lung disease as well as cases of dextroversion. Obviously, an alteration in the cardiac-torso relationship severely limits interpretation of the ECG, since all the usual criteria for hypertrophy depend on a specific relationship between electrode and cardiac position.

In general, it is probably sufficient to recognize the limitation of the ECG when the cardiac-torso relationship is altered rather than trying to correct for it. In interpretation of the ECG, one of the initial questions to ask is whether the cardiac-torso relationship is normal.

Ebstein Anomaly of the Tricuspid Valve

The electrocardiographic features of Ebstein anomaly are valuable in establishing the diagnosis.[58] The principal QRS abnormalities are either low voltage with right bundle branch block or evidence of ventricular preexcitation (Figs. 21–6 and 21–11). In patients with Ebstein anomaly, ventricular preexcitation results from either accessory atrioventricular connections in a right lateral to posteroseptal connection or a nodoventricular connection.[61] Occasionally, the ECG may be normal.[23,59] The PR interval is often prolonged, usually because of an increased duration of the P wave. The P waves often show

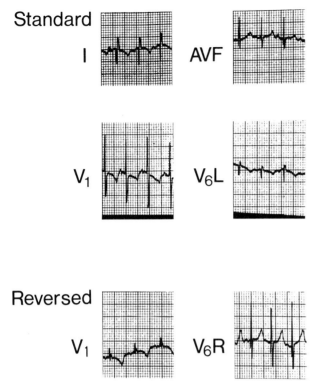

Figure 21–10. ECG features of dextrocardia. An altered P wave axis is present in standard leads I and AVF. Note the diminished voltage in the standard lead V₆ (V₆L) compared with that recorded in a right-sided V₆.

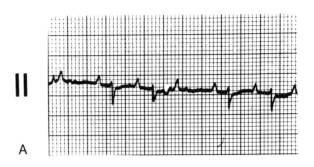

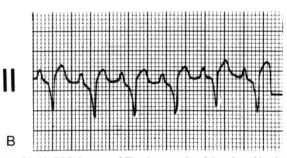

Figure 21–11. ECG features of Ebstein anomaly of the tricuspid valve. *A*, Second degree heart block with normal duration QRS is present. *B*, In tracing taken a few hours later, 1:1 conduction with ventricular preexcitation is present.

right atrial enlargement. Both the large P wave and the prolonged PR interval correlate with the size of the right atrium.[23]

Hypoplastic Right-Heart Syndromes

There is considerable anatomic variation in hypoplastic right-heart syndromes. The principal lesions are tricuspid and pulmonary valve atresia. Absent or markedly diminished right ventricular forces (reduced R wave in lead V₁) with normal left ventricular forces are a characteristic ECG finding. The additional ECG features of tricuspid atresia are superior and leftward frontal plane QRS axis and right atrial enlargement[11,14] (Fig. 21–12). In pulmonary atresia with intact septum, right atrial enlargement is usually present, but the QRS axis is normal or rightward.

Atrioventricular Septal Defects

The presence of a mean QRS axis in the frontal plane of −30 to −90 degrees is a characteristic ECG feature of atrioventricular septal defects (Fig. 21–13). Anatomic and electrophysiologic studies have shown this ECG pattern to be associated with posterior and inferior displacement of the atrioventricular conduction system.[7,10] Additional features typically include prolonged PR interval, right atrial enlargement, and hypertrophy of the right and/or left ventricles, depending on the extent of septal defects and associated cardiac anomalies.

Anomalous Left Coronary Artery

In this anomaly, there are characteristic Q waves and T wave inversions in leads I, aVL, and the left precordial leads (Fig. 21–14). The prominent Q waves and T wave inversions can represent severe hypertrophy and strain or infarction. Similar ECG patterns may be seen in other conditions resulting in ventricular dilation (e.g., cardiomyopathy). On the other hand, ST elevation is a reliable sign of infarction (or pericarditis) and in infants with ventricular dilation, ST elevation may be virtually pathognomonic of anomalous left coronary artery. In cases with infarction, the infarct is located anteriorly and anterolaterally along the distribution of the left coronary artery.

SUDDEN INFANT DEATH SYNDROME

ECG abnormalities have been considered in the evaluation of sudden infant death syndrome (SIDS).[66] In recent years, there has been a perception that the pathologic basis for apnea and bradycardia[43] was similar to that of victims of SIDS. For example, in eight infants with near-miss SIDS, Guilleminault et al[24] found shoulder muscle hypotonia, mixed apneas in clusters, and significant cardiac arrhythmias, predominantly bradycardia. An analogy was made to adult obstructive sleep apnea, and it was concluded that the major rhythm disturbance, sinus arrest,

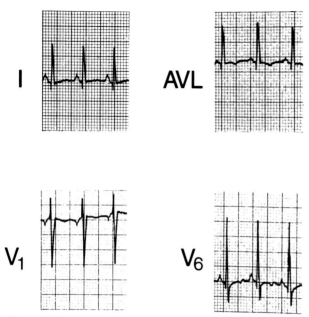

Figure 21–12. ECG features of tricuspid atresia. The most noticeable features include diminished R wave in lead V_1, right atrial enlargement, and left axis deviation for a neonate.

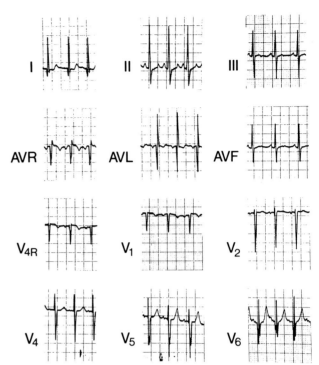

Figure 21–14. ECG features of anomalous origin of left coronary artery. Prominent Q waves and biphasic T waves are present in leads I and AVL. There is also a prominent Q wave in lead V_6. In anomalous origin of left coronary artery, these changes are usually interpreted as evidence of myocardial infarction, but they may represent hypertrophy with strain. ST elevation, a highly specific electrocardiographic feature of anomalous origin of the left coronary artery, is absent.

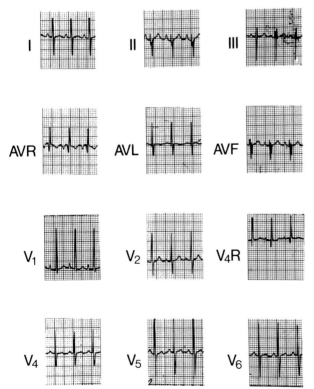

Figure 21–13. ECG features of atrioventricular septal defect. In this example, the left axis deviation and right and left ventricular hypertrophy are evident.

was the result of increased vagal tone during hypoxia. The precise causes of apnea and bradycardia, SIDS, and near-miss SIDS are not known, but other investigators have noted autonomic nervous system dysfunction in some patients considered to be at risk for SIDS.[32,45]

Maron et al[41] found QT interval prolongation (QT interval exceeding ninety-seventh percentile) in 26 per cent of parents of SIDS victims. In families in which QT interval prolongation was found in a parent, QT interval prolongation was found in 39 per cent of siblings of SIDS victims. However, other investigators have failed to note this association.[64] Montague et al[45] noted that ventricular repolarization was abbreviated, rather than prolonged, in at risk infants and therefore suggested that this might represent an increase in sympathetic tone.

In a prospective study of SIDS, Southall et al[65] examined records of 24-hour tape recordings of ECG and breathing movements of 16 term infants (evaluated at 2 to 40 [mean = 12] days) who were subsequent SIDS victims at 27 to 457 (mean = 137) days of age; results were compared with those obtained in a large control group. In the 16 SIDS victims, heart and respiratory rates during regular breathing as well as quantities of periodic breathing and apneic breathing compared well with the normal range; in fact, there was no significant difference between SIDS victims and control infants. While this study does not eliminate the possibility that primary disorders of cardiac rhythm or respiratory function are mechanisms for SIDS, it does highlight the difficulty in prospectively identifying at risk patients.[64]

In conclusion, the cause of SIDS is not known, but based on available clinical and epidemiologic observations, SIDS is not due to unrecognized occult heart disease[42] or the specific ECG abnormalities seen in the prolonged QT interval syndrome or preexcitation syndromes.

References

1. Anderson RG, Becker AL, Brechenmacher C, Dawes MJ, Rossi L (1975): Ventricular preexcitation: A proposed nomenclature for its substrates. Eur J Cardiol 3:27–35.
2. Barr RC, Spach MS (1983): Construction and interpretation of body surface maps. Prog Cardiovasc Dis 26:33–42.
3. Benson DW Jr (1987): Transesophageal electrocardiography and cardiac pacing: State of the art. Circulation 75:III-86–III-90.
4. Benson DW Jr, Sanford M, Dunnigan A, Benditt DG (1984): Transesophageal atrial pacing threshold: Role of interelectrode spacing, pulse width and catheter insertion depth. Am J Cardiol 53:63–67.
5. Benson DW Jr, Spach MS (1982): Evolution of QRS and ST-T wave body surface potential distributions during the first year of life. Circulation 65:1247–1258.
6. Benson DW Jr, Sterba R, Gallagher JJ, Walston A II, Spach MS (1982): Localization of the site of ventricular preexcitation with body surface maps in patients with Wolff-Parkinson-White syndrome. Circulation 65:1259–1268.
7. Boineau JP, Moore EN, Patterson DF (1973): Relationship between the ECG, ventricular activation and the ventricular conduction system in ostium primum ASD. Circulation 48:556–564.
8. Burchell HB (1983): The QT interval historically treated. Pediatr Cardiol 4:139–148.
9. Caddell JL, Whittemore R (1962): Observations on generalized glycogenosis with emphasis on electrocardiographic changes. Pediatrics 29:743–763.
10. Campbell RM, Dick M II, Hees P, Behrendt DM (1983): Epicardial and endocardial activation in patients with endocardial cushion defect. Am J Cardiol 51:277–281.
11. Davachi F, Lucas RV Jr, Moller JH (1970): The electrocardiogram and vectorcardiogram in tricuspid atresia: Correlation with pathologic anatomy. Am J Cardiol 25:18–27.
12. Davignon A, Rautaharju R, Boiselle F, Soumis F, Megelas M, Aroquette A (1980): Normal ECG standards for infants and children. Pediatr Cardiol 1:123–131.
13. DeAmbroggi L, Bertoni T, Locati E, Stramba-Badiale M, Schwartz PJ (1986): Mapping of body surface potentials in patients with the idiopathic long QT syndrome. Circulation 74:1334–1345.
14. Dick M, Fyler DC, Nadas AS (1975): Tricuspid atresia: Clinical course in 101 patients. Am J Cardiol 36:327–337.
15. Durrer D, Schuilenberg RM, Wellens HJJ (1970): Preexcitation revisited. Am J Cardiol 25:690–701.
16. Esmond WA, Mailton A, Cowley RA, Attar S, Blair E (1963): Peripheral ramification of the cardiac conduction system. Circulation 27:732–738.
17. Fournier M (1976): Willem Einthoven—The electrophysiology of the heart. Medicamundi 21:65–70.
18. Fox WW, Duara S (1983): Persistent pulmonary hypertension in the neonate: Diagnosis and management. J Pediatr 105:505–514.
19. Francis DB, Miller BL, Benson DW Jr (1981): A new computer program for the analysis of pediatric scalar electrocardiograms. Computers Biomed Res 14:63–77.
20. Gillette PC, Nihill MR, Singer D (1974): Electrophysiological mechanism of the short PR interval in Pompe disease. Am J Dis Child 128:622–626.
21. Goldstein MA, Dunnigan A, Benson DW Jr (1968): Transient bundle branch block during paroxysmal atrial tachycardia onset in infants. (Abstr) Circulation 74:II–119.
22. Gornick CC, Benson DW Jr (1986): Electrocardiographic aspects of the preexcitation syndromes. In Benditt DG, Benson DW Jr (eds): Cardiac Preexcitation Syndromes: Origins, Evaluation and Treatment. Boston, Martinus-Nijhoff Publishing, pp 43–73.
23. Guilani ER, Fuster V, Brandenburg RO, Mair DD (1979): The clinical features and natural history of Ebstein's anomaly of the tricuspid valve. Mayo Clin Proc 54:163–173.
24. Guilleminault C, Ariagno R, Coons S, Winkle R, Koroblum R, Baldwin R, Sougnet M (1985): Near-miss sudden infant death syndrome in eight infants with sleep-apnea related cardiac arrhythmias. Pediatrics 76:236–242.
25. Guntheroth WG (1977): Sudden infant death syndrome (crib death). Am Heart J 93:784–793.
26. Hait G, Gasul BM (1963): The evolution and significance of T-wave changes in the normal newborn during the first seven days of life. Am J Cardiol 12:494–504.
27. Hecht AF (1913): Der mechanismus der harzaktion im kindesalter, seine physiologie und pathologie. Ergebr d inn Med u Kinderh 11:324 (cited in reference 5).
28. Henry GW (1984): Noninvasive assessment of cardiac function and pulmonary hypertension in persistent pulmonary hypertension of the newborn. Clin Perinatol 11:627–640.
29. Horowitz LN, Alexander JA, Edwards LH (1980): Postoperative right bundle branch block: Identification of three levels of block. Circulation 62:319–328.
30. Jervell A, Lange-Neilson F (1957): Congenital deaf-mutism, functional heart disease, with prolongation of the Q-T interval and sudden death. Am Heart J 54:59–68.
31. Jervell A, Thingstad R, Endsjo TO (1966): The surdo-cardiac syndrome. Am Heart J 72:582–593.
32. Kahn A, Riazi J, Blum D (1983): Oculocardiac reflex in near-miss for sudden infant death syndrome. Pediatrics 71:49–52.
33. Katz LN, Wachtel H (1937): The diphasic QRS type of electrocardiogram in congenital heart disease. Am Heart J 13:202–206.
34. Kulangara RJ, Boineau JP, Moore HV, Rao S (1981): Ventricular activation and genesis of QRS in tricuspid atresia. (abstr) Circulation 64:IV–225.
35. Kulbertus HE, Demoulin JC (1976): Pathological basis of concept of left hemiblock. In Wellens HJJ, Lie KI, Janse MJ (eds): The Conduction System of the Heart. Philadelphia, Lea and Febiger, pp 3–28.
36. Long WA (1984): Structural cardiovascular abnormalities presenting as persistent pulmonary hypertension of the newborn. Clin Perinatol 11:601–626.
37. Lees MH, Sunderland CO (1983): Heart disease in the newborn. In Adams FH, Emmanouilides BC (eds): Moss' Heart Disease in Infants, Children and Adolescents. 3rd ed. Baltimore, Williams & Wilkins, pp 658–669.
38. Liebman J (1982): The normal electrocardiogram. In Liebman J, Plonsey R, Gillette PC (eds): Pediatric Electrocardiography. Baltimore, Williams & Wilkins, pp 82–133.
39. Liebman J (1982): Ventricular hypertrophy. In Liebman J, Plonsey R, Gillette PC (eds): Pediatric Electrocardiography. Baltimore, Williams & Wilkins, pp 144–171.
40. Linday LA, Ehlers KH, O'Laughlin JE, La Gamma E, Engle MA (1983): Noninvasive diagnosis of persistent fetal circulation versus congenital cardiovascular defects. Am J Cardiol 52:847–851.
41. Maron BJ, Clark EC, Goldstein RE, Epstein SE (1976): Potential role of QT interval prolongation in sudden infant death syndrome. Circulation 54:423–430.
42. Maron BJ, Fisher RS (1977): Sudden infant death syndrome (SIDS): Cardiac pathologic observations in infants with SIDS. Am Heart J 93:762–766.
43. McBride JT (1984): Infantile apnea. Pediatr Rev 5:275–283.
44. Moller JH, Pierpont ME (1983): Cardiac manifestations of systemic diseases. In Adams FH, Emmanouilides GC (eds): Moss' Heart Disease in Infants, Children and Adolescents. 3rd ed. Baltimore, Williams & Wilkins, pp 626–645.
45. Montagne TJ, Finley JP, Mukdabai K, Black SA, Rigby SM, Spencer CA, Horacek MB (1984): Cardiac rhythm, rate and repolarization properties in infants at risk for sudden infant death syndrome: Comparison with age- and sex-matched control infants. Am J Cardiol 54:301–307.
46. Moore EN, Boineau JP, Patterson DP (1971): Incomplete right bundle branch block. An electrocardiographic enigma and possible misnomer. Circulation 44:678–687.

47. Morville P, Mauran P, Motte J, Digeon B, Coffin R (1985): Torsades de pointe foetales et syndrome du QT long. Arch Mal Coeur 78:781–784.

48. Moss AJ, Schwartz PJ, Crampton RS, Locati E, Carleen E (1985): The long QT syndrome: A prospective international study. Circulation 71:17–21.

49. Murphy DJ Jr, Meyer RA, Kaplan S (1985): Noninvasive evaluation of newborns with suspected congenital heart disease. Am J Dis Child 139:589–594.

50. Nicolai, Funaro (1908): Das electrokardiogram des sauglings. Zentralb f Physiologie 22:58 (cited in reference 76).

51. Ohnell RF (1944): Preexcitation, a cardiac abnormality. Acta Med Scand (Suppl) 152:1–167.

52. Pellegrino A, Ho SY, Anderson RH, Hegerty A, Goodman MJ, Michaelson M (1986): Prolonged QT interval and the cardiac conduction tissues. Am J Cardiol 58:1112–1113.

53. Piperberger HV, Arzbaecher RC, Benson AS, Briller SA, Brody DA, Flowers NC, Geselowitz DB, Lepeschkin E, Oliver GC, Schmitt OH, Spach M (1975): Recommendations for standardization of leads and of specifications for instruments in electrocardiography and vectorcardiography. Report of the Committee on Electrocardiography, American Heart Association. Circulation 52:11–31.

54. Rautaharju PM, Davignon A, Soumis F, Boiselle E, Choquette A (1979): Evaluation of QRS-T relationship from birth to adolescence in Frank-lead orthogonal electrocardiograms of 1491 normal children. Circulation 60:196–204.

55. Romano C, Gemme G, Pongiglione R (1963): Aritmie cardiache rare dell ete pediatria. Clin Pediatr (Bologna) 45:656–683.

56. Romhilt DW, Bove KE, Norris RJ, Conyers E, Conradi S, Rowlands DT, Scott RC (1969): A critical appraisal of the electrocardiographic criteria for the diagnosis of left ventricular hypertrophy. Circulation 40:185–195.

57. Rosenbaum MB (1970): The hemiblocks: Diagnostic criteria and clinical significance. Mod Concepts Cardiovasc Dis 39:141–146.

58. Schiebler GL, Adams P Jr, Anderson RC, Amplatz K, Lester RO (1959): Clinical study of twenty-three cases of Ebstein's anomaly of the tricuspid valve. Circulation 19:165–187.

59. Sealy WC, Gallagher JJ, Pritchett ELC, Wallace AG (1978): Surgical treatment of tachyarrhythmias in patients with both an Ebstein anomaly and a Kent bundle. J Thorac Cardiovasc Surg 75:847–853.

60. Singer DH, Ten Eick RE (1971): Aberrancy: Electrophysiologic aspects. Am J Cardiol 28:381–401.

61. Smith WM, Gallagher JJ, Kerr CR, Sealy WC, Kasell JH, Benson DW Jr, Reiter MJ, Sterba R, Grant AO (1982): The electrophysiologic basis and management of symptomatic recurrent tachycardia in patients with Ebstein's anomaly of the tricuspid valve. Am J Cardiol 49:1223–1234.

62. Smith WM, Gallagher JJ (1979): Q-T prolongation syndromes. Practical Cardiol 5:118–130.

63. Southall DP, Arrowsmith WA, Oakley JR, McEnery G, Anderson RH, Shinebourne EA (1979): Prolonged QT interval and cardiac arrhythmias in two neonates: Sudden infant death syndrome in one case. Arch Dis Child 54:776–779.

64. Southall DP and participants in a multicentered prospective study into the sudden infant death syndrome (1983): Identification of infants destined to die unexpectedly during infancy: Evaluation of predictive importance of prolonged apnea and disorders of cardiac rhythm or conduction. Br Med J 286:1092–1096.

65. Southall DP, Richards JM, Stebbens V, Wilson AJ, Taylor V, Alexander JR (1986): Cardiorespiratory function in 16 full-term infants with sudden infant death syndrome. Pediatrics 78:787–796.

66. Southall DP, Richards JM, Rhoden KJ, Alexander JR, Shinebourne EA, Arrowsmith WA, Cree JE, Fleming PJ, Goncalves A, Orme RL (1982): Prolonged apnea and cardiac arrhythmias in infants discharged from neonatal intensive care units: Failure to predict an increased risk for sudden infant death syndrome. Pediatrics 70:844–851.

67. Sreenivasan V, Fisher BJ, Liebman J, Downs TD (1973): Longitudinal study of the standard electrocardiogram in the healthy premature infant during the first year of life. Am J Cardiol 31:57–63.

68. Surawicz B, Knoebel SB (1984): Long QT: Good, bad or indifferent? J Am Coll Cardiol 4:398–413.

69. Taccardi B, De Ambroggi L, Viganotti C (1976): Body surface mapping of heart potentials. In Nelson CV, Geselowitz DB (eds): The Theoretical Basis of Electrocardiology. Oxford, Clarendon Press, pp 436–466.

70. Tazawa H, Yoshimoto C (1969): Electrocardiographic potential distribution in newborn infants from 12 hours to 8 days after birth. Am Heart J 78:312–305.

71. Thomas CW (1982): Electrocardiographic measurement system response. In Liebman J, Plonsey R, Gillette PC (eds): Pediatric Electrocardiography. Baltimore, Williams & Wilkins, pp 40–59.

72. Walsh EP, Long P, Ellison RC, Zierler S, Harned HS, Miettinen OS (1986): Electrocardiogram of the premature infant at 1 year of age. Pediatrics 77:353–356.

73. Walsh SZ (1963): The electrocardiogram during the first week of life. Br Heart J 25:784–794.

74. Walsh SZ (1967): The esophageal electrocardiogram during the first week of life. Acta Pediatrica Scand (Suppl) 173:1–33.

75. Ward OC (1964): New familial cardiac syndrome in children. J Irish Med Assoc 54:103–106.

76. Ziegler RF (1951): Electrocardiographic studies in normal infants and children. Springfield, Charles C Thomas, pp 3–9.

22 CHEST RADIOGRAPHY

Hrudaya Nath
Benigno Soto

Approximately one third of the patients with congenital heart disease present in the newborn period.[26,34,47] The major problem in recognizing these infants is distinguishing the symptoms caused by heart disease from those caused by the more frequent primary lung disease. The symptoms of tachypnea, tachycardia, edema, and cyanosis are common to both heart and lung disease at this age. Auscultation and electrocardiography may sometimes be of limited use in the newborn period, but radiographs of the chest are a very useful tool in distinguishing between heart and lung disease. However, recent widespread use of echocardiography has partially eclipsed the role of chest films in diagnosing heart disease in the newborn. In this chapter we will briefly discuss the technique of radiographic examination of the chest, the normal appearance of the newborn chest, the role of chest radiographs in distinguishing between primary lung and heart disease, and the pertinent radiographic features of common cardiac diseases in the newborn period.

HISTORICAL PERSPECTIVE

Less than 1 year following the discovery of the x-ray, Dr. Francis H. Williams of Boston described the use of roentgenology in cardiac diagnosis. In a paper entitled "Notes on X-rays in Medicine" read before the Association of American Physicians on April 30, 1896, he reported visualization of an enlarged heart in a man through the fluoroscope.[8] By the end of 1898 Dr. Williams had used fluoroscopy to study virtually all the cardiac diseases known at that time and described the radiographic features of most of them. In 1898 Qinn published a case of persistent ductus arteriosus in which the clinical diagnosis was confirmed by the fluoroscopic evidence of enlargement of the pulmonary artery.[25] Soon the hazards of fluoroscopy were discovered, and its use waned. By 1905 Kohler introduced teleroentgenography, which soon became the standard method of radiologic diagnosis and was ranked behind history, physical examination, and electrocardiography by Paul Dudley White.[25] A combination of fluoroscopy and roentgenography was used by many cardiologists in diagnosing congenital heart disease until 1950. Helen Taussig[64] relied heavily on fluoroscopy in the evaluation of her patients. Rib notching in coarctation of the aorta was described by Roesler[49] in 1928. Rigler[48] described the role of the esophagram in the diagnosis of heart disease in 1929.

RADIOGRAPHIC TECHNIQUE

An optimal chest radiograph is essential for proper interpretation. This assertion is particularly true in a newborn infant because of the infant's small size. The radiograph should provide adequate detail of the lung parenchyma, vasculature, and mediastinum. The film should be exposed at about 110 to 120 kVp to suppress the bone contrast. This exposure will aid in better visualizing the mediastinal structures. A medium speed screen and film combination, such as Kodak Lanex Regular Screen combined with Ortho-G film, provides a good compromise between patient dose and image sharpness. Wolf et al[74] described a technique employing high kilovoltage, special compositive (tin, copper, and aluminum) filtration, and geometric magnification to visualize the tracheal air column in patients suspected of having a right aortic arch (see Fig. 22–16A). The composite filter is not essential, and similar results can be obtained without sacrificing the detail of the lung parenchyma by employing a simple 0.35-mm thick copper or brass filter. Ablow et al[1] described the use of a magnification technique for radiographing newborn infants with dedicated x-ray equipment situated next to the newborn intensive care unit. This technique will certainly produce an optimal image, as the area of interest is exposed to a larger area of the film; this technique, when combined with the air gap, eliminates most of the scatter radiation, resulting in a larger, sharper image. The disadvantages are the need for dedicated equipment and moving the baby out of the incubator to the x-ray unit. The radiation dose also is increased by a factor of four, resulting in average entrance skin exposure of about 15 mR per film. Radiation to the infant should be minimized as much as possible, since these patients usually require numerous radiographic examinations during their life. Adequate collimation should be used to exclude areas other than lower neck, thorax, and upper abdomen. Gonads should be shielded with a shadow shield or lead glove. Most of the time, a single frontal projection is adequate; esophagography is not necessary as a routine but may be an essential investigation when a vascular abnormality is suspected. In such cases, performing a barium swallow examination under fluoroscopy and obtaining spot films are superior and safer.

THE NORMAL CHEST FILM

In the newborn there is little difference in the appearance of optimally exposed chest films obtained in supine

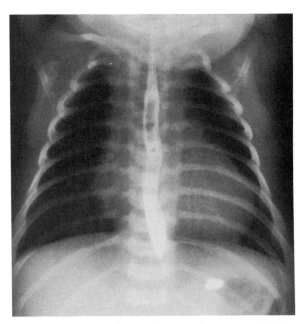

Figure 22–1. Normal PA view of chest in supine posture with barium swallow. Pulmonary vascularity is normal. Hilar pulmonary arteries are well seen. Notice the slightly upturned cardiac apex. The tracheal air column is to the left of the midline, the esophagus is to the left of the trachea, and the descending aorta is to the left of the vertebral column. Compare with Figure 22–16.

or erect postures. Hence, there is little advantage in attempting to obtain an upright chest film in a sick infant. Aeration of the lungs is complete in the first few breaths after delivery.[22,38] The adequacy of inspiration is better judged by the uniformity of aeration rather than by the rib

count. The diaphragm maintains a convex outline. Lung markings are usually well visualized into the middle one third of the lungs. Hilar pulmonary arteries are often recognized (Fig. 22–1). Normal pleural fissures are seen in 60 per cent of newborn infants.[5] The width of the fissures is variable, and it is not uncommon normally to see small fissural effusions during the first 48 hours of life. However, these regress as the infant gets older. Increasing size of the effusion is more significant than the presence of small amounts of fluid on one film.[39]

The trachea, carina, and main bronchi, including lobar divisions, are routinely identifiable on well-exposed posteroanterior (PA) views. The position of the trachea at the thoracic inlet is variable and easily influenced by the position of the neck. Buckling of the trachea at the thoracic inlet is common and normal. Similarly, on the lateral projection, a slight anterior impression upon the trachea as it enters the thorax is not necessarily pathological.[59] Although the position of the trachea superiorly is variable, at the level of the carina it is constant and is determined most frequently by the aortic arch. In a well-positioned infant, the supracarinal trachea is clearly to the right of the midline (see Fig. 22–22B). As the aortic knob or the descending thoracic aorta is infrequently seen in the newborn position of the trachea is an important landmark for determining the location of the aortic arch[74] (see Figs. 22–1 and 22–15). Likewise, the carina and the central bronchi are also visualized in most instances. The length of the main bronchi can usually be determined as an aid in evaluating the atrial situs.[55] In our experience in this age group, the relationship of the pulmonary arteries to their respective bronchi is not always well defined, and bronchial morphology is better evaluated by the asymmetry

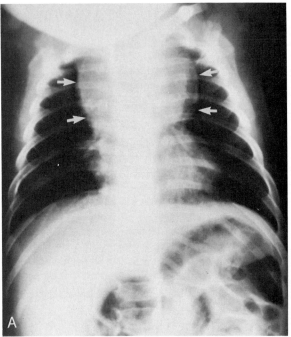
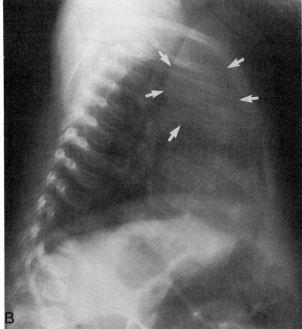

Figure 22–2. A normal 1-week-old child. *A,* AP view. *B,* Lateral view. Notice the unusually prominent right and left lobes of the thymus (arrows) mimicking TAPVC to left superior vena cava. In the lateral view the thymus is anterior, and there is no tubular pretracheal density. The left lobe is larger than the right. Compare with Figure 22–5B and *C.*

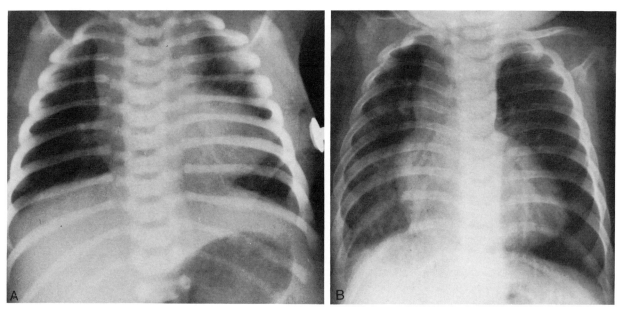

Figure 22–3. Complete transposition with intact ventricular septum. (*A*) One day of age. The heart size is normal. Notice the prominently upturned cardiac apex. Pulmonary vascularity is at the upper limits of normal. Thymus is not atrophic. Pulmonary artery segment is concave. *B*, Two months. The heart is larger, and shunt vascularity is more obvious.

in length of bronchi; i.e., the right main stem bronchus is shorter than the left (see Fig. 22–22*B*).

The thymus should be visible in most normal chest films of newborns and is usually identified by its wavy or lobulated margins[44,63] (Figs. 22–2 and 22–3*A*). The normal thymus usually obscures the structures at the base of the heart, such as the ascending aorta, pulmonary trunk, and the more cephalic great vessels, including the superior vena cava and aortic arch. The thymus is inapparent when it is atrophic in conditions of perinatal stress, such as asphyxia, heart disease (see Fig. 22–24*A*), and sepsis, as well as when it is absent, as in DiGeorge syndrome. Thymic enlargement can simulate cardiac enlargement (Fig. 22–4).

Normally, heart size is slightly larger in newborns period than in older children and adults. The CT ratio is estimated to be 0.56 in the perinatal period.[9,10] There is no appreciable difference in the heart size between systole and diastole.[20] Shape of the cardiac silhouette is very variable in the newborn, as it is greatly influenced by patient position and x-ray beam angle.[62] It is very common for the newborn chest to be filmed in a slightly lordotic projection, which can make the cardiac apex appear upturned, thereby mimicking right ventricular hypertrophy, as in tetralogy of Fallot. Hence, radiographic detection of an abnormal cardiac shape should prompt further cardiac evaluation, not diagnosis of congenital heart disease.

PHYSIOLOGIC BASIS FOR RADIOGRAPHIC ABNORMALITIES IN THE NEWBORN PERIOD

Difficulties in plain film identification of congenital heart disease and plain film characterization of the type

of malformation present in newborns are well known. Severe malformations such as complete transposition of great arteries can be present with a normal-appearing chest radiograph, while conditions like erythroblastosis fetalis or perinatal asphyxia can produce cardiac enlargement and abnormal pulmonary vascularity without any structural heart disease. These discrepancies exist because of the differences in the fetal and neonatal circulations and the transitional period that occurs between the two. The pathway of blood in the fetus is determined by the presence of high resistance in the pulmonary vascular bed, low resistance in the systemic vascular bed (as the

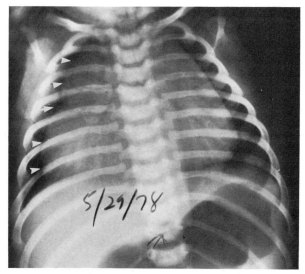

Figure 22–4. Huge thymus. The right lobe of the thymus is larger. Notice the wavy outline (arrowheads) and the characteristic notch in its midportion (arrow).

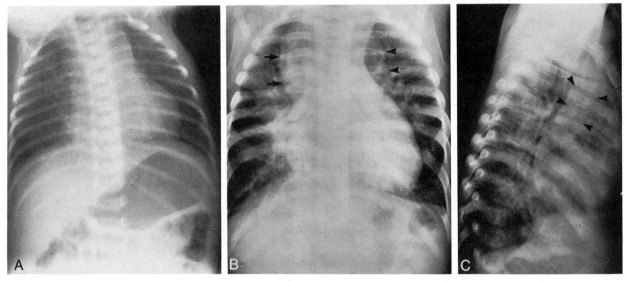

Table 22–1. CONDITIONS THAT CAN LEAD TO HEART FAILURE IN THE FETUS

Volume Overload
Extracardiac AV malformation (aneurysm of vein of Galen, hepatoblastoma)
Left ventriculoaortic tunnel
Erythroblastosis fetalis
Twin to twin transfusion
Premature closure of foramen ovale
Premature closure of ductus arteriosus
Severe atrioventricular valve regurgitation

Pressure Overload
Aortic valvular stenosis

Miscellaneous
Rhythm disturbances (congenital heart block, supraventricular tachycardia)
Postmaturity
Severe thoracic cage abnormalities

result of the placenta), and patency of the foramen ovale and ductus arteriosus. The presence of flow obstructions such as stenosis of a semilunar valve or atresia of an atrioventricular valve is easily bypassed by the fetal pathways. Similarly, the presence of most lesions that result in left-to-right shunts postnatally after pulmonary vascular resistance falls and systemic vascular resistance rises has no obvious prenatal effects; examples include ventricular and atrial septal defects. Hence, the fetal heart is not aware, in hemodynamic terms, of many developmental malformations. Table 22–1 lists the very few cardiovascular defects that may cause cardiac failure during fetal life. For a substantial period after birth, the foramen ovale is only physiologically closed and can allow right-to-left shunting if right atrial pressure exceeds left atrial pressure; as a result, lung vascularity can diminish. Further, if the left atrium is dilated and the foramen ovale is

stretched, postnatal elevations in left atrial pressure can result in left-to-right atrial shunts; as a result, lung vascularity can increase. Similarly, the ductus arteriosus, though normally functionally closed within hours of birth, can either remain open or reopen during postnatal hypoxia and permit either right-to-left or left-to-right shunts, depending on the pulmonary and systemic vascular resistances; as a result, lung vascularity can either decrease or increase. For example, in neonates with critical aortic stenosis or mitral atresia, a stretched foramen ovale can allow a left-to-right shunt at the atrial level, thus producing shunt vascularity instead of the expected pulmonary venous hypertension or pulmonary edema (Fig. 22–20). Another factor that complicates early chest film diagnosis is the usual absence of cardiac chamber enlargement or vascular dilation in the immediate newborn period, for these structures were not affected in the intrauterine period. A typical example is total anomalous pulmonary venous connection (TAPVC) to the left vertical vein. In the older child this lesion is recognizable from posteroanterior and lateral views of the chest by the typical "figure eight" or "snowman" appearance (Fig. 22–5B and C). However, since these anomalous pathways did not receive any excess blood flow during fetal life, they are not dilated in the neonate (Fig. 22–5A).

DISTINGUISHING HEART DISEASE FROM OTHER CAUSES OF RESPIRATORY DISTRESS

As mentioned earlier, noncardiac pathology frequently causes respiratory distress and produces cyanosis in the newborn. Radiographs of the chest are valuable in demonstrating the noncardiac pathology that can account for

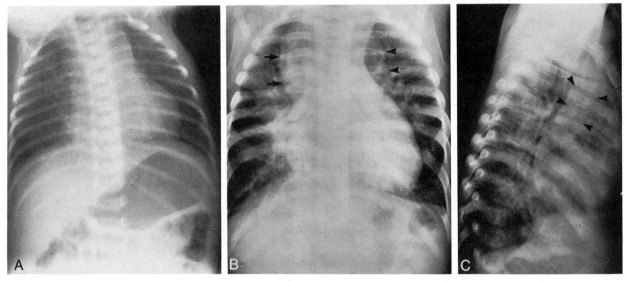

Figure 22–5. Total anomalous pulmonary venous connection to the left superior vena cava. *A,* Four-day-old infant. Heart size is normal. The left or right superior vena cava is not enlarged. Pulmonary vascularity is unremarkable. *B,* A different patient at age 1 year. Now, the shunt vascularity is obvious. The left superior vena cava (arrowheads) and the right superior vena cava (arrows) are dilated. The right superior vena cava is larger than the left. *C,* The same child as in *B.* Lateral view of the chest. Notice a tubular vascular shadow in front of the trachea (arrowheads), which represents the dilated cavae.

Table 22–2. RADIOGRAPHIC ABNORMALITIES
CAUSED BY BOTH CARDIAC AND EXTRACARDIAC PATHOLOGY

Radiographic Abnormality	Cardiovascular Causes	Extracardiac Causes
Pulmonary edema	Left-heart obstructive lesions, such as aortic stenosis Pulmonary venous obstruction, such as TAPVC to portal vein Excessive pulmonary blood flow, such as tricuspid atresia with transposition Nonstructural heart disease, such as myocarditis, asphyxia in the newborn	TTNB Pneumonia HMD Iatrogenic fluid overload Neurogenic pulmonary edema Lymphangiectasia
Focal hyperaeration or emphysema	Vascular rings Pulmonary artery sling Absent pulmonary valve	Congenital lobar emphysema Diaphragmatic hernia with air in intestine Pneumothorax
Focal or unilateral opaque lung	Vascular rings Pulmonary artery sling Agenesis of pulmonary artery Interruption of pulmonary artery	Diaphragmatic hernia without air in intestine Pulmonary agenesis Sequestration Cystic adenomatoid malformation Pleural fluid Tumors
Cardiomegaly	Congenital heart disease causing volume overload, such as Ebstein malformation Pericardial effusion Nonstructural heart disease, such as myocardial ischemia	Large thymus Mediastinal cysts

*HMD = Hyaline membrane disease; TAPVC = total anomalous pulmonary venous connection; TTNB = transient tachypnea of the newborn.

respiratory distress and/or cyanosis. A detailed discussion of all of the causes of respiratory distress in the newborn period is beyond the scope of this book, and the interested reader is referred to the many excellent reviews on this subject.[3,30,54,60]

A number of conditions like meconium aspiration or tracheoesophageal fistula are clinically obvious, and chest films confirm the clinical diagnosis. However, several cardiac and noncardiac diseases can produce identical radiographic appearances. Table 22–2 summarizes four important radiographic abnormalities that can occur in either cardiac or extracardiac lesions.

Pulmonary Edema

Pulmonary edema is diagnosed when chest films demonstrate either diffuse ill-defined air space opacities suggestive of alveolar edema or linear streaky opacities, or peribronchial and/or perivascular haziness associated with Kerley B lines suggestive of interstitial edema. Such abnormalities imply the presence of fluid in the interstitium and/or air spaces, which can result from several extracardiac causes. Transient tachypnea of the newborn (TTNB) is a condition in which there is delayed clearance of nor-

mal intrapulmonary fluid.[58] The presence of this fluid impairs normal respiratory physiology, leading to tachypnea. Radiographic abnormalities range from slight hyperaeration and interstitial fluid (Fig. 22–6) to pleural effusions and air space opacities.[33,70] Heart size is usually normal but may be enlarged. These opacities typically disappear in 24 to 48 hours.

A variety of congenital and perinatal pneumonias can cause diffuse pulmonary opacities mimicking pulmonary edema. While β-hemolytic streptococcal infection is often considered the common offender,[2] any pneumonia causing sepsis can produce similar abnormalities. Pleural effusion may be present. Again, the heart is not enlarged, and clinical signs of sepsis will be evident.

Hyaline membrane disease (HMD) or infant respiratory distress syndrome can closely mimic pulmonary edema. Clinical diagnosis is often easy. During the early stages of HMD when clinical diagnosis may be difficult, lung volumes are small (Fig. 22–7) because the lung compliance is decreased. On the contrary, in cardiogenic pulmonary edema, the lungs are hyperinflated, which is attributed to air hunger. HMD can be complicated by patent ductus arteriosus (PDA), resulting in cardiogenic pulmonary edema and cardiac chamber enlargement (Fig. 22–7). Wesenberg et al[71] described three radiographic patterns in PDA

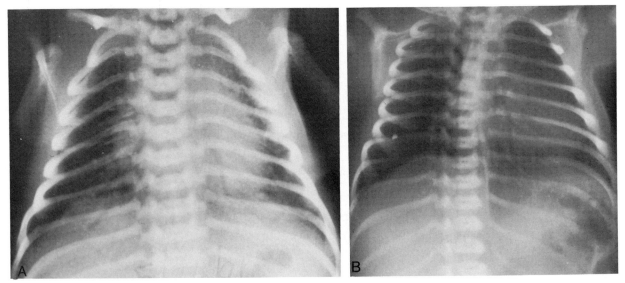

Figure 22–6. Transient tachypnea of newborn. *A*, First day of life. Heart is mildly enlarged. There is pulmonary edema. *B*, Same infant, 2 days later. Heart size has returned to normal, and pulmonary edema has resolved.

complicating HMD: (1) a pattern of congestive heart failure in which massive cardiac enlargement, increased pulmonary vascularity, and pleural effusions are present; (2) a pattern of purely left-sided heart failure manifest by increased vascularity and streaky perihilar and interstitial opacities; and, (3) uncommonly hyperaeration associated with cystic spaces in the lungs, which they describe as

pseudo–Wilson-Mikity syndrome. However, these features may not be evident, and Burney et al[12] found no correlation between radiographic findings and the presence of PDA in a group of 50 premature infants. Our experience has been similar as well, and a high index of clinical suspicion and the results of Doppler echocardiography are more sensitive indicators than radiographs of the chest.

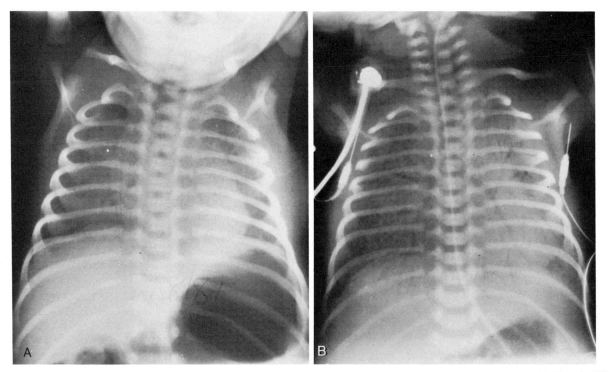

Figure 22–7. Hyaline membrane disease complicated by patent ductus arteriosus. *A*, Fourth day of life. Lung volumes are small. There is diffuse, bilateral pulmonary haziness. *B*, Same infant seventh day of life. Pulmonary edema has significantly worsened. It is difficult to appreciate the shunt vascularity.

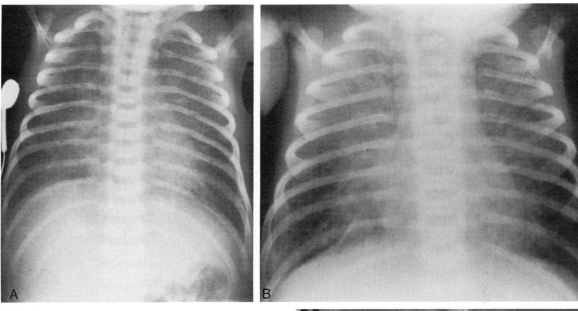

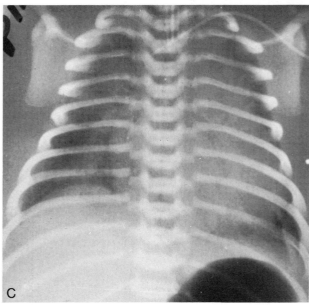

Figure 22–8. *A,* Total anomalous pulmonary venous connection to the portal vein. Heart size is normal. Lungs are hyper-aerated. There is diffuse, bilateral pulmonary edema. *B,* Primary pulmonary lymphangiectasia. There are streaky, ill-defined, interstitial opacities in both lungs, with a small right pleural effusion. Notice the similarity of radiographic appearance to that in Figure 22–8*A*. *C,* Viral myocarditis in a 2-week-old infant. The heart is enlarged, and there is bilateral pulmonary edema.

Pulmonary lymphangiectasia has been classified into three groups.[24] One group consists of a primary, isolated abnormality of the lungs. A more common second group includes those patients in whom pulmonary venous obstruction is present, such as TAPVC to the portal vein or pulmonary venous atresia. In the third group, generalized lymphangiectasia is present. This last group usually presents later in life with protein-losing enteropathy. The first two groups manifest in the newborn period with severe respiratory distress, cyanosis and bilateral, diffuse streaky nodular and reticular interstitial opacities, hyperaeration, and normal heart size (Fig. 22–8). There is usually no difficulty in distinguishing this condition from HMD, but it is often not possible to distinguish the primary form from that secondary to heart disease based on radiographic appearances (Fig. 22–8).

Focal Hyperaeration or Emphysema

Cardiovascular causes of hyperaeration are uncommon. They include vascular rings, pulmonary artery sling, or absent pulmonic valve (Fig. 22–9). Both the cardiovascular and the extracardiac etiologies can involve a single lobe or the whole lung. Congenital lobar emphysema is the most important noncardiac cause. The pathogenesis is often underdevelopment of bronchial cartilage resulting in collapse of the bronchial wall leading to redundancy and crinkling of the mucosa that produces ball-valve obstruction.[13] Lobar emphysema may also result from bronchial stenosis, intraluminal mucous plugs, or obstructing mediastinal tumors, cysts, or vessels. The left upper lobe, right upper lobe, and right middle lobe are most commonly involved. Lower lobe involvement is very rare.

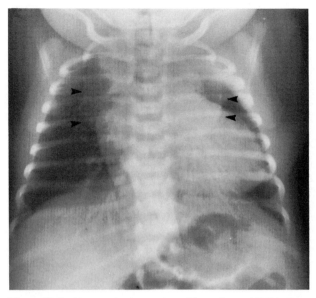

Figure 22–9. Absent pulmonary valve with tetralogy of Fallot. Heart is slightly enlarged. Cardiac apex is upturned. There is pulmonary hyperaeration. The superior mediastinum is dilated owing to massive dilation of both pulmonary arteries (arrowheads).

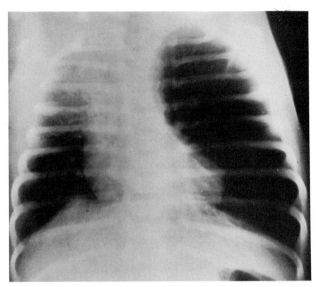

Figure 22–10. Congenital lobar emphysema of the left upper lobe. There is mediastinal shift to the right. The left lung is hyperlucent, with crowding of the lung markings in the medial portion of the left lower lobe. Compare with Figure 22–11.

Radiographically, there is hyperlucency of the involved lobe, and the remaining ipsilateral lung is compressed and often herniates across the midline (Fig. 22–10). Diagnosis is usually easy. Gas-filled, distended intestine in a diaphragmatic hernia should not cause confusion, as mucosal markings can frequently be seen, and lower lobe involvement in congenital lobar emphysema is unusual.

Vascular rings causing obstructive emphysema more frequently involve the right lung. In the absent pulmonary valve syndrome, the dilated proximal pulmonary arteries can compress both bronchi (Fig. 22–9), but unilateral obstructive emphysema may result.[7] Vascular rings usually have additional radiographic abnormalities. Right aortic arch or double arch is common. However, their recognition from plain chest films may be difficult because of mediastinal shift caused by the emphysematous lung. In patients with pulmonary artery sling, the aberrant left pulmonary artery courses posterior to the trachea to reach the left lung and produces a soft tissue density between the trachea and esophagus, which may be recognized on lateral chest films[14,73] (Fig. 22–11). An esophagram is essential when a vascular ring or pulmonary artery sling is suspected and allows diagnosis of most of these anomalies. An aberrant subclavian artery produces a posterior impression on the esophagus (Fig. 22–16). In pulmonary artery sling, the characteristic abnormality is an anterior impression on the esophagus[73] (Fig. 22–11). However, it must be realized that when severe obstructive emphysema is present, this condition may produce a lateral impression on the esophagus or no impression at all.[56]

Focal or Unilateral Opaque Lung

While vascular rings may cause atelectasis of a lung or lobes, noncardiovascular causes are more frequent. Pleu-

ral fluid is a common offender but is usually obvious on the chest films. Diaphragmatic hernia and lobar emphysema in the early stages can appear uniformly opaque.[21] Cystic adenomatoid malformation is also variably opaque. All these conditions cause mediastinal shift to the contralateral side.

Pulmonary hypoplasia or agenesis can be unilateral or bilateral. The majority of cases of bilateral pulmonary hypoplasia are the result of lung compression from extra- or intrathoracic causes. In this context we are more interested in unilateral pulmonary hypoplasia, which can be frequently associated with other cardiovascular anomalies. The unilateral process may involve a lobe or an entire lung (Fig. 22–12). While either lung may be involved, agenesis of the right lung is associated with greater mediastinal shift to the right, with consequent impingement on bronchovascular structures and resultant cardiorespiratory embarrassment.[41] When pulmonary hypoplasia is associated with absence of the pulmonary artery, it appears to be more frequently contralateral to the aortic arch, that is, absence of the left pulmonary artery with right aortic arch and vice versa.[32] Radiographically, the involved lung is opaque, with mediastinal shift to the affected side. Hypoplasia of the right lung may be associated with anomalous pulmonary venous connection and/or systemic arterial supply, which may also be detected on chest films (Fig. 22–13).

Sequestration and bronchopulmonary foregut malformations are related congenital anomalies.[61] These often do not cause symptoms until later in infancy or childhood, but severe cases can cause respiratory distress and congestive heart failure in the newborn period.[43,65,72] Pulmonary sequestration results from isolation of a portion of the lung from the developing lung bud and usually involves the lower lobes. There is systemic arterial supply to the involved lung, and venous return may be to the pulmonary

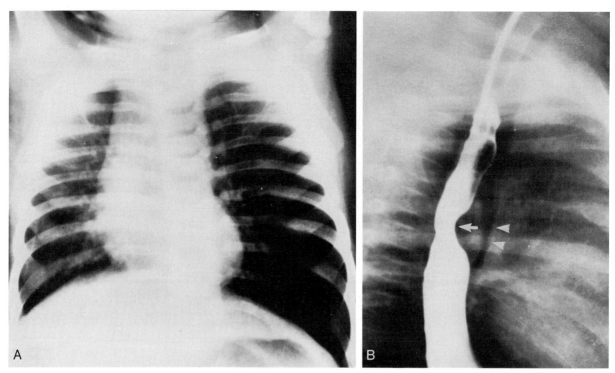

Figure 22–11. Pulmonary artery sling. *A*, PA view of the chest. The left lung is hyperinflated, with mediastinal shift to the right. *B*, Lateral view of the esophagram. There is characteristic indentation of the anterior wall of the esophagus (arrow) caused by the anomalous origin of the left pulmonary artery, which courses between the trachea and the esophagus to reach the left lung. Also notice the soft tissue density separating the esophagus (tip of arrowheads) from the right bronchus (base of arrowheads).

or systemic veins. If the area of involvement is large, it may cause volume overload and congestive heart failure. Radiographically, a triangular- or oval-shaped basal lung mass is present. Bronchoesophageal fistula may be present,[36] and the involved lung may be hypoplastic.

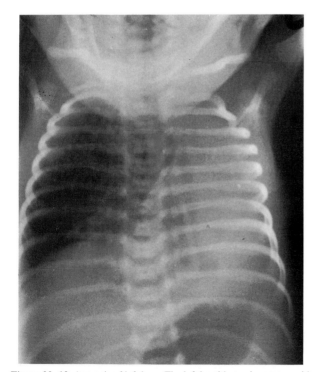

Figure 22–12. Agenesis of left lung. The left hemithorax is opaque, with mediastinal shift to the left. Left ribs are crowded.

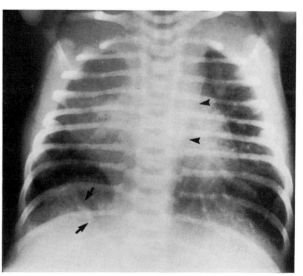

Figure 22–13. Systemic arterial supply to the lung. AP view of the chest. The heart is enlarged. Density in right upper lung field is thymus. Lungs exhibit prominent vascularity. Descending aorta is prominent (arrowheads). A tubular opacity is seen in the right base (arrows), which represents a systemic artery supplying the right lung.

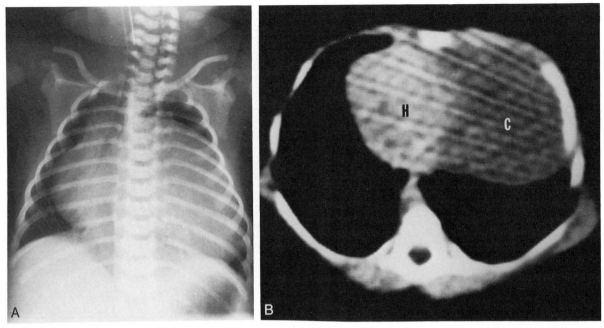

Figure 22–14. Bronchogenic cyst in a newborn. *A,* Supine AP view of the chest. The cardiac silhouette is massively enlarged. Lung vascularity is normal. Compare with Figures 22–17 and 22–18. *B,* Same patient. Computed tomogram of the chest. There is a large paracardial cystic structure (*C*) to the left of the heart, displacing the cardiac structures (*H*). Notice that there is no pericardial effusion, which would make the diagnosis of pericardial teratoma less likely.

Cardiomegaly

Rarely, cardiac enlargement may be simulated by an unusual thymus (see Fig. 22–4) or a mediastinal cyst (Fig. 22–14). The thymus can be distinguished by its wavy outline and anterior mediastinal location as seen on the lateral chest radiograph. Mediastinal masses can be difficult to diagnose based on chest radiographs but can be easily differentiated with echocardiography and confirmed by computed tomography (Fig. 22–14*B*).

CONGENITAL HEART DISEASE

The precise diagnosis of a specific congenital heart defect from chest radiographs is difficult in the neonate. However, chest films provide sufficient information, which when interpreted with knowledge of the frequency of various cardiac defects in the newborn period and a few clinical findings, can provide a useful differential diagnosis. The following description provides the basis for such an approach. Detailed descriptions of the radiographic features of individual malformations are not given. Interested readers are encouraged to refer to the appropriate cited literature.

It has been repeatedly shown that a limited number of cardiac defects are encountered in symptomatic neonates.[26,34,35] The more common forms of congenital heart disease, such as atrial and ventricular septal defects, and also many complex defects, such as single ventricle, truncus arteriosus, and unobstructed TAPVC, do not usually cause symptoms during the neonatal period because the normal postnatal elevation in pulmonary vascular resistance limits left-to-right shunt until 6 to 8 weeks of age. Table 22–3 lists the common cardiac defects presenting during the first week and month of life. In analyzing the chest film of an infant with suspected heart disease, the following areas should be evaluated.

Bony Thorax

Abnormalities of the bony thorax, including the ribs, spine, and clavicles, can occur in a variety of syndromes[46] that are known to be associated with congenital heart disease. Alternatively, severe thoracic deformities like asphyxiating thoracic dystrophy[31] can cause clinical symptomatology mimicking heart disease. Many of the syndromes associated with skeletal abnormalities like Holt-Oram syndrome and trisomy-18 have simple cardiac defects such as ventricular and atrial septal defects, which do not commonly manifest in the newborn period. A few exceptions include trisomy 21 (Down syndrome), Turner syndrome and Noonan syndrome.[15,45,68] In Down syndrome as well as trisomy 18 there are 11 pairs of ribs. Multiple ossification centers in the sternum are noted in trisomy 21.[27] In Turner syndrome, a characteristic soft tissue web is seen at the cervicothoracic region, and the rib cage is deformed.[45] Similar soft tissue and skeletal abnormalities exist in Noonan syndrome, and hence the term pseudo-Turner syndrome has been used to describe this entity. However, unlike in Turner syndrome no chromosomal anomalies are seen in Noonan syndrome (Chapters 48 and 50).

Table 22–3. SYMPTOMATIC CARDIAC DEFECTS
IN THE NEWBORN PERIOD*

Cyanotic Lesions†	Heart Failure Lesions†
First Week of Life	
Complete transposition	Hypoplastic left-heart syndrome
Pulmonary atresia or severe	Patent ductus arteriosus
pulmonary stenosis with intact	Obstructed TAPVC
ventricular septum	Interruption of aortic arch
Pulmonary atresia or severe	Large arteriovenous
pulmonary stenosis with	malformations
ventricular septal defect	Intrauterine asphyxia
Ebstein's malformation	Pericardial effusion
Tricuspid atresia	
Persistent pulmonary	
hypertension of the newborn	
syndrome secondary to	
structural cardiovascular	
lesions	
First to Fourth Week of Life	
Unobstructed TAPVC	Ventricular septal defect
Truncus arteriosus	AV canal
Single ventricle	Aortic valve stenosis
	Cor triatriatum
	Vascular rings
	Coarctation

*Depending on the severity and associated anomalies, all of the lesions may
present earlier or later.
†The dominant symptom.
TAPVC = total anomalous pulmonary venous connection.

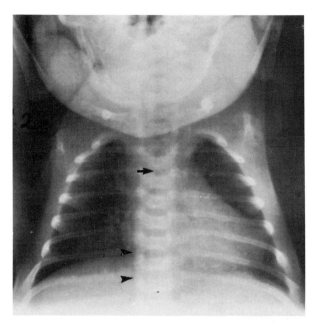

Figure 22–15. Tetralogy of Fallot. There is mild cardiac enlargement. Cardiac apex is elevated. Pulmonary vascularity is diminished (compare with Fig. 22–1). Trachea is displaced to the left (arrow) by the right aortic arch. The descending thoracic aorta is on the right (arrowheads).

Mediastinum

Examination of the mediastinum should focus on the trachea and its bifurcation, including the main bronchi; the great vessels encompassing the aortic arch, pulmonary trunk, and superior vena cava as well as the azygos vein; and, of course, the thymus. If the thymus is prominent, analysis of many of the above structures may be difficult. The thymus is often atrophied or absent in severely distressed infants, such as those with complete transposition of the great vessels or pulmonary atresia (Fig. 22–24A). The thymus is absent in DiGeorge syndrome, which may be associated with interruption of the aortic arch.

Recognizing the presence of a right aortic arch is valuable, as its presence is frequently associated with either pulmonary outflow tract obstruction (in which case the pulmonary vascularity is diminished) or truncus arteriosus (in which case shunt vascularity is present if pulmonary vascular resistance has fallen). In the newborn period, a right arch is most easily recognized by the displacement of the tracheal air column (Figs. 22–15 and 22–16).[74] If the esophagus is opacified with barium in the presence of a right arch, the esophagus overlies the left third of the vertebral column, as it is displaced to the left by the aortic arch (see Figs. 22–1 and 22–16).[16] The barium esophagram can also demonstrate the presence of any aberrant vessels (Fig. 22–16), which may be recognized on the frontal projection as an oblique impression and in the lateral projection by a posterior indentation. The impression formed by the aberrant left subclavian artery is larger than that caused by the right.[52] Usually, when a right arch is seen with an aberrant left subclavian artery, no cardiac defects are present. It has been shown that when an aberrant subclavian artery is associated with pulmonary outflow tract obstruction, such as tetralogy of Fallot, the impression formed by the aberrant subclavian artery is usually shallow.[66]

The distal trachea may be narrowed when tracheal stenosis is present associated with pulmonary artery sling[6] or an obstructing vascular ring.[74] Atrial situs can be diagnosed by analyzing the length of the main bronchi.[55] Normally, the right main stem bronchus is shorter than the left (see Fig. 22–22B). As the longer left bronchus continues as the upper lobe bronchus, the contour resembles a U, while the right main stem bronchus courses inferiorly, almost straight, as the bronchus intermedius. When thoracic situs inversus is present, the right-to-left relationship is inverted; in thoracic isomerism, both main bronchi resemble either the normal right- or left-sided bronchus. Because right isomerism is more frequently associated with severe congenital heart disease (commonly pulmonary atresia and/or TAPVC) than left isomerism, bilateral short bronchi are far more commonly seen than bilateral long bronchi in neonates with congenital heart disease.

In the normal newborn, the main pulmonary artery is usually not visible. However, total absence of the main pulmonary trunk can be striking in pulmonary atresia (see Figs. 22–15 and 22–24). Similarly, abnormal position of the pulmonary trunk can be obvious in transposition of the great arteries after the thymus has shrunk (see Fig. 22–3). Many of the conditions with increased pulmonary blood flow in the newborn period, particularly in the first

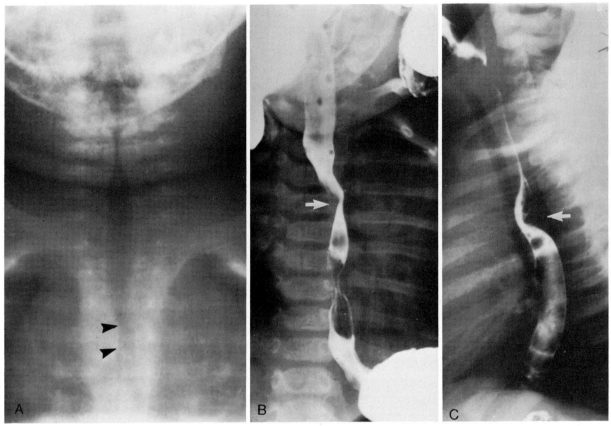

Figure 22–16. Right aortic arch with aberrant left subclavian artery. *A*, A magnification film of the airway. There is a focal deviation of the trachea, above the carina, to the left (arrowheads). *B*, Same patient, esophagram (AP view). There is an oblique impression on the esophagus (arrow) at the level of the carina (compare with Fig. 22–1). *C*, Lateral view after the barium swallow. There is a deep posterior indentation on the esophagus caused by the aberrant left subclavian artery (arrow).

week of life, are cyanotic lesions, and the pulmonary trunk may not be apparent even though it is dilated; an example is seen in Figure 22–20, which shows a case of hypoplastic left-heart syndrome in which the branch pulmonary arteries are large but the main pulmonary artery (though dilated) is not seen. The main pulmonary artery can appear unusually large in cases of absent pulmonary valve (see Fig. 22–9) and aneurysm of the ductus arteriosus.

Systemic venous abnormalities are rare in infancy. The superior vena cava is prominent with an aneurysm of the vein of Galen. Occasionally, inferior vena caval shadow is prominent with lesions associated with severe tricuspid regurgitation such as Ebstein malformation. The systemic veins are occasionally dilated in patients with unobstructed TAPVC. The "snowman" configuration is rarely encountered in a neonate with TAPVC to the left superior vena cava. Weaver et al[69] described a tubular opacity anterior to the trachea in these patients before a "snowman" configuration is seen on the PA view (see Fig. 22–5C). In our experience, this sign also is uncommon in neonates. A mediastinal contour resembling the "snowman" configuration in a newborn is most likely caused by a large thymus (see Fig. 22–2). The azygos vein may be dilated with TAPVC to this structure.[23] The more com-

mon anomaly of interruption of inferior vena cava with azygos continuation is rarely encountered in the newborn period.

Heart Size, Shape, and Position

The heart is considered to be enlarged if the cardio-thoracic ratio exceeds 0.58. Cardiac enlargement is a reliable sign of heart disease, whether structural, functional, or pericardial. If structural heart disease is responsible for cardiac enlargement, lesions without pulmonary outflow obstruction, such as hypoplastic left-heart syndrome, PDA, or tricuspid regurgitation (with or without pulmonary outflow tract obstruction) are usually found. Neonates with tricuspid regurgitation can have massive cardiomegaly (Figs. 22–17 and 22–18), largely because tricuspid regurgitation is worsened by the normally elevated pulmonary vascular resistance of the neonatal period. As the pulmonary vascular resistance falls, the tricuspid regurgitation and the heart size also decrease (Fig. 22–17). Heart size is typically normal with complete transposition, obstructed TAPVC, and severe tetralogy of Fallot, but exceptions to these generalizations are common. Mild cardiac enlargement is found in 20 per cent of newborns with tetralogy of Fallot or pulmonary atresia with ventricular septal defect.

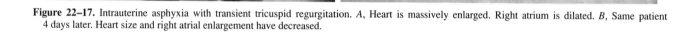

Figure 22–17. Intrauterine asphyxia with transient tricuspid regurgitation. *A,* Heart is massively enlarged. Right atrium is dilated. *B,* Same patient 4 days later. Heart size and right atrial enlargement have decreased.

The cardiac shape is usually not of much benefit in diagnosing the specific form of heart disease. Although it is reported that the "egg on a side" configuration is commonly found in transposition of the great arteries[42] and that an upturned cardiac apex is commonly found in tetralogy of Fallot, it has been our experience that any cardiac shape can occur with any heart disease. Minor projectional errors can cause abnormal cardiac configuration even in normal newborns.[62]

Normally, the cardiac apex and stomach are on the left side and the liver on the right. Cardiac malposition with normal abdominal and atrial situs may occur secondary to abnormalities in the thoracic cage, lungs, or diaphragm. In such instances, associated cardiac defects are uncommon. Cardiac malpositions may also occur without thoracic, pulmonary, or diaphragmatic abnormalities; such cardiac malpositions may occur with or without abnormalities of atrial situs, such as situs inversus (as judged by bronchial morphology; see the preceding). In situs inversus totalis (bronchial situs inversus, along with right-sided cardiac apex, aortic arch, and stomach) heart disease need not be present.[42] However, if there is discordance between atrial (bronchial) and abdominal situs, complex congenital heart disease is almost always present (Fig. 22–19); interested readers are referred to several excellent reviews for further discussion.[18,19,53,57]

Pulmonary Vascular Pattern

In all age groups, the assessment of pulmonary vascularity is the key to the functional diagnosis of heart disease, and the newborn is no exception. However, characterizing the abnormal pulmonary vascularity is more difficult in the neonate than in the older child or adult. Hence, in practical terms, neonatal pulmonary vascular patterns can be

identified as being one of four types: (1) normal, (2) prominent vascularity, (3) pulmonary venous obstruction, and (4) decreased pulmonary blood flow.

Normal

A surprising number of severe cardiac defects can be associated with normal vascularity in the first week of life. This observation is particularly true of complete transposition of the great vessels (see Fig. 22–3A).[42] Nonstructural heart disease[50] (asphyxia, arrhythmias) and pericardial effusion can cause cardiac enlargement, but pulmonary vascularity can be normal (Fig. 22–7).

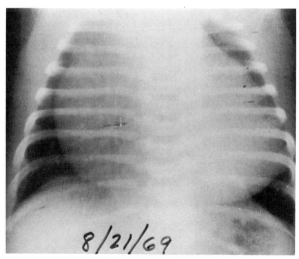

Figure 22–18. Ebstein anomaly. AP view of the chest in a 4-day-old infant. Notice the massive cardiac enlargement, particularly that of the right atrium.

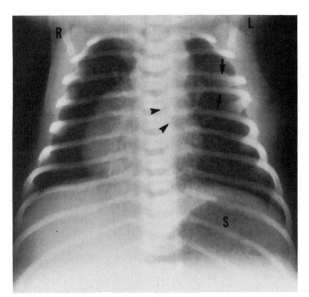

Figure 22–19. Cardiac malposition. A cyanotic 7-day-old infant. The heart size is normal, and the cardiac apex is on the right. There is deformity of the left ribs (arrows) due to a recent Blalock-Taussig shunt. There is atrial situs solitus (notice the long left main stem bronchus) (arrowheads). The stomach (S) is on the left. Pulmonary vascularity appears normal owing to the palliative shunt. The child had complete transposition and pulmonary atresia.

Prominent Vascularity

In adults, increased pulmonary vascularity is subdivided into shunt vascularity, pulmonary venous hypertension, and systemic pulmonary collaterals. These patterns can often be distinguished from one another in older children and adults. However, in neonates, it is often

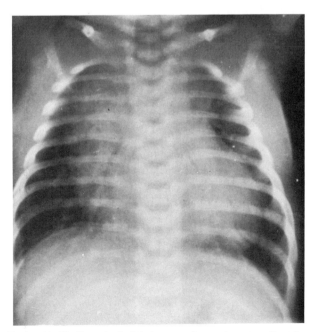

Figure 22–20. Hypoplastic left heart syndrome due to aortic valve atresia. Heart is enlarged. There is prominent vascularity with pulmonary edema. Notice the left-sided descending aorta.

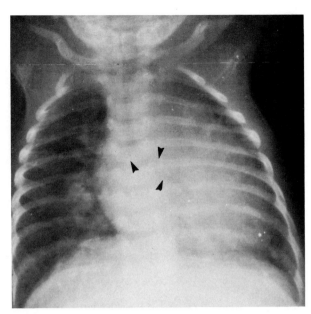

Figure 22–21. Ventricular septal defect. A 2-week-old baby. The heart is enlarged, and prominent vascularity is obvious. The arrowheads point out the carina, and the normally longer left-sided bronchus.

impossible to distinguish one type from another because quite frequently interstitial edema and increased pulmonary blood flow coexist, as seen in infants with PDA and congestive heart failure. In conditions grouped under the category prominent vascularity, pulmonary markings are simply increased in size and number; often the markings may be indistinct (Fig. 22–20). The pulmonary trunk may be prominent. Heart size is usually increased, and pleural effusions may be noted.

ACYANOTIC LESIONS

Several types of acyanotic congenital heart disease can cause pulmonary vascularity to be prominent in newborn infants. The most frequent acyanotic left-to-right shunts encountered during infancy are PDA, ventricular septal defect (Fig. 22–21), and atrioventricular septal defects (Fig. 22–22). The age at which infants present with these lesions depends on the rate of decrease in pulmonary vascular resistance.[51] If the pulmonary vascular resistance drops rapidly (as occurs in the premature infant), PDA, ventricular septal defect, and atrioventricular septal defects may be encountered in the neonatal period. These three conditions cannot be differentiated on chest films in neonates. Left atrial enlargement, which should help differentiate atrioventricular septal defect from other left-to-right shunts with intact atrial septum, is difficult to detect in neonates.

Left-sided obstructive lesions cause prominent vascularity as a result of pulmonary venous hypertension; typical neonatal causes include coarctation of the aorta, hypoplastic left-heart syndrome, and cor triatriatum. These conditions also produce varying degrees of cardiac enlargement, shunt vascularity, and pulmonary edema

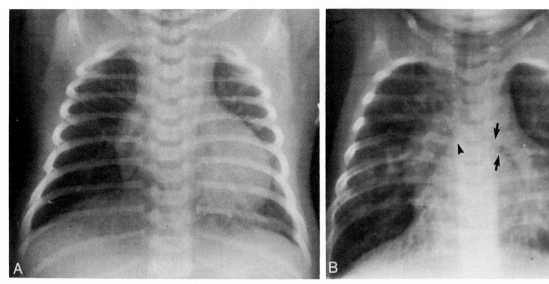

Figure 22–22. Atrioventricular septal defect. *A,* A 2-week-old infant. Heart is mildly enlarged. Lungs exhibit prominent vascularity but no pulmonary edema. *B,* One-month-old patient. Prominent vascularity (due to shunt) is more obvious. There is also pulmonary edema. Both main bronchi are well seen. Notice that the right main bronchus (arrowhead) is shorter than the left (arrows).

(see Figs. 22–20 and 22–23). The magnitude of pulmonary congestion in such lesions depends on the size of interatrial communication because the ventricular septum is usually intact. The age of presentation varies somewhat; hypoplastic left-heart syndrome tends to manifest earlier than coarctation of aorta or aortic stenosis.[34] Apart from these temporal events, radiographic features are almost identical in all neonatal left-sided obstructive lesions.

CYANOTIC LESIONS

Complete transposition of the great vessels is the most important cyanotic lesion in neonates with prominent vascularity. However, our experience parallels that of Moes,[42] who found normal vascularity in over one half of patients with transposition. The lung vascularity is greater in patients with transposition and ventricular septal defect (about 50 per cent of patients) and in older infants (see Fig. 22–3*B*). Pulmonary stenosis is present and limits pulmonary blood flow in about 20 per cent of patients with transposition.

Another important cyanotic lesion in neonates with prominent vascularity is truncus arteriosus. However, patients with truncus arteriosus tend to present later in infancy and with less cyanosis than patients with complete transposition of the great vessels. About 30 to 50 per cent of patients with truncus arteriosus have a right aortic arch, a helpful radiographic finding in distinguishing truncus arteriosus from complete transposition. A right aortic arch was found in only 2 to 3 per cent of patients with transposition at the Hospital for Sick Children.[42] Heart size and the magnitude of pulmonary blood flow tend to be greater in truncus arteriosus, but the cardiac shape is often not helpful.[67]

Less commonly, many other congenital anomalies that permit mixing at the atrial or ventricular level but are un-

accompanied by pulmonary stenosis present in the neonatal period. Examples include double-outlet right ventricle (particularly with subpulmonic ventricular septal defect), single ventricle, and unobstructed TAPVC. None of these disorders exhibits specific radiographic findings useful in differential diagnosis.

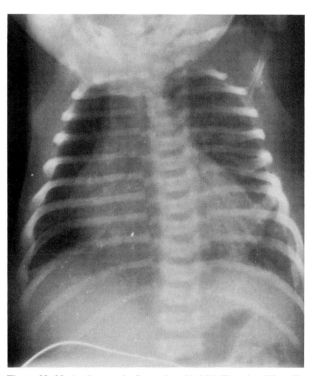

Figure 22–23. Aortic stenosis. Seven-day-old child. There is mild cardiomegaly. Pulmonary vascular markings are prominent with pulmonary edema.

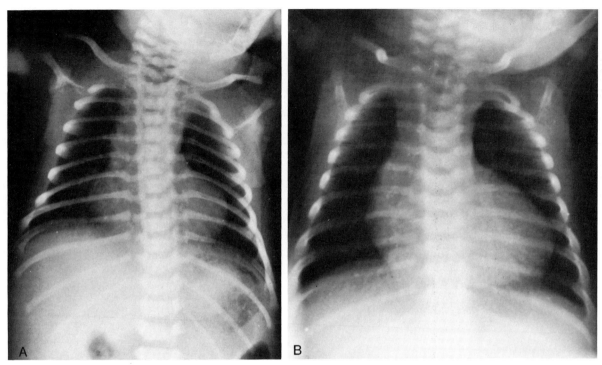

Figure 22–24. *A,* Pulmonary atresia with ventricular septal defect. Heart size is normal. The pulmonary vascularity is diminished and the pulmonary artery segment is concave. *B,* Pulmonary atresia with intact ventricular septum and moderate tricuspid regurgitation. Compared with *A* the heart is larger. Right heart border is prominent. Lung vascularity is not particularly diminished.

Pulmonary Venous Obstruction

Pulmonary venous obstruction has many causes in the newborn period, but most cardiac types of pulmonary venous obstruction present similarly because the site of obstruction is nearly always at or proximal to the mitral valve. The single most common lesion presenting as pulmonary venous obstruction in the neonate is total anomalous pulmonary venous connection (TAPVC) to the portal vein. Babies with TAPVC to the portal vein present early in life with severe respiratory distress and heart failure. Chest films, which are remarkably similar no matter what the location of the pulmonary venous obstruction, exhibit normal heart size, small central pulmonary arteries, severe pulmonary edema manifest by hazy-appearing lungs, streaky opacities radiating from the hili, and occasionally Kerley B lines, which are interlobular septa thickened by distended lymphatics and edema fluid.[28,29,37] The heart may occasionally be enlarged. Eisen and Elliott[17] described an anterior impression upon the lower esophagus just above the diaphragm in TAPVC with connection below the diaphragm; the impression is caused by the common pulmonary venous channel as it traverses the diaphragm through the esophageal hiatus to reach the portal vein. Other cardiac causes of neonatal pulmonary venous obstruction include obstructed TAPVC to other structures (such as the inferior vena cava or left superior vena cava), atresia of the common pulmonary vein, and congenital abnormalities of the mitral valve (including mitral atresia, severe congenital mitral stenosis, and supravalvular mitral ring).[40] In neonates presenting with radiographic signs of pulmonary venous obstruction, it is very important to distinguish cardiac from extracardiac causes (see Fig. 22–8 and preceding discussion).

Decreased Pulmonary Blood Flow

Most commonly, infants presenting with decreased pulmonary blood flow have either pulmonary atresia or severe pulmonary stenosis with or without other accompanying lesions. Infants with pulmonary outflow obstruction are normal at birth, but become profoundly hypoxemic as the ductus arteriosus begins to close. Two examples of pulmonary atresia, one with and the other without ventricular septal defect, are shown in Figure 22–24.

When the ventricular septum is intact, the clinical and radiographic features are dependent upon the size of interatrial communication and competence of the tricuspid valve.[26] Pulmonary vascularity is typically diminished with a flat or concave pulmonary trunk (Fig. 22–24B). If the tricuspid valve is competent, the right ventricle is hypoplastic, and the heart size is typically normal. However, if the tricuspid valve is incompetent, the heart is moderately enlarged and the right atrium is very prominent in the frontal and lateral projections. Similar appearances can be seen in infants with Ebstein anomaly who have similar physiology when they present at this age (Fig. 22–18).

In contrast, infants with pulmonary atresia and ventricular septal defect usually exhibit normal heart size or only mild cardiac enlargement. An upturned cardiac apex is often seen (Fig. 22–24*A*), but this finding is not constant. A right aortic arch is seen in about 30 per cent of patients.

Another important condition in which pulmonary blood flow may be diminished is persistent pulmonary hypertension of the newborn syndrome (PPHNS), earlier known as persistent fetal circulation (PFC). In the newborn, pulmonary hypertension may result from many factors, including congenital heart disease and primary pulmonary disease, or it may arise without any apparent cause. The term idiopathic persistent pulmonary hypertension of the newborn syndrome (idiopathic PPHNS) is used in this book for the last group, that is, persistent, severe pulmonary hypertension resulting in ductal right-to-left shunting without underlying structural heart disease, lung disease, or other predisposing causes.[11] Chest films in idiopathic PPHNS typically demonstrate a normal to mildly enlarged heart size and hyperaerated lungs with small central and peripheral pulmonary arteries (Fig. 22–25).[4] However, cardiac causes of PPHNS cannot be excluded by plain film radiography. The diagnosis, pathology, and treatment of PPHNS are considered in Chapters 51, 52, and 55, respectively.

CONCLUSION

Despite remarkable advances in other diagnostic modalities, chest radiography remains valuable in the clinical evaluation of newborns with cyanosis or respiratory distress. While in several instances the chest film may appear normal or may show nonspecific findings in infants who have underlying cardiac disease, in the majority of cases with underlying cardiovascular disorders, a functional, if not an accurate, anatomic diagnosis can be suggested when the radiographic findings are evaluated in light of a few clinical signs. Most importantly in the neonate with cyanosis or respiratory distress, chest radiography can identify obvious noncardiac causes (such as diaphragmatic hernia or pneumothorax) and can provide a reliable differential diagnosis when radiographic abnormalities with both cardiovascular and noncardiovascular causes are identified.

References

1. Ablow RC, Greenspan RH, Gluck L (1969): The advantages of direct magnification techniques in the newborn chest. Radiology 92:745–750.
2. Ablow RC, Gross I, Effmann EL, Uauy R, Driscoll S (1977): The radiographic features of early onset group B streptococcal neonatal sepsis. Radiology 124:771–777.
3. Avery ME (1968): The Lung and Its Disorders in the Newborn Infant. Philadelphia, WB Saunders, pp 143–150.
4. Bauer CR, Tsipuras D, Fletcher BD (1974): Syndrome of persistent pulmonary vascular obstruction of the newborn: Roentgen findings. AJR 120:285–290.
5. Bean WJ, Jordan RB, Gentry H, Nice CM (1969): Fissure lines in the pediatric roentgenogram. AJR 106:109–112.
6. Berdon WE, Baker DH, Wung JT, Chrispin A, Kozlowski K, de Silva M, Bales P, Alford B (1984): Complete cartilage–ring tracheal stenosis associated with anomalous left pulmonary artery: The ring–sling complex. Radiology 152:57–64.
7. Borg SA, Young LW, Roghair GD (1975): Congenital avalvular pulmonary artery and infantile lobar emphysema: A diagnostic correlation. AJR 130:1149–1151.
8. Brecher E, Brecher R (1969): The Rays. Baltimore, Williams & Wilkins, pp 70–77.
9. Burnard ED, James LS (1961): Radiographic heart size in apparently healthy newborn infants: Clinical and biochemical correlations. Pediatrics 27:726–739.
10. Burnard ED, James LS (1961): The cardiac silhouette in newborn infants: A cinematographic study of the normal range. Pediatrics 27:713–725.
11. Burnell RH, Joseph MC, Lees MH (1972): Progressive pulmonary hypertension in newborn infants: A report of two cases with no identifiable respiratory or cardiac disease. Am J Dis Child 123:167–170.
12. Burney B, Smith WL, Franken EA, Smith JA, Klatte EC (1978): Chest film diagnosis of patent ductus arteriosus in infants with hyaline membrane disease. AJR 130:1149–1151.
13. Campbell PE (1969): Congenital lobar emphysema. Aust Paediatr J 5:226–233.
14. Capitanio MA, Ramos R, Kirkpatrick JA (1971): Pulmonary sling: Roentgen observations. AJR 112:28–34.
15. Cassidy SB, McGee BJ, Eyes JV, Nance WE, Engel E (1975): Trisomy 18 syndrome. Pediatrics 56:826–831.
16. Deutsch V (1970): Right aortic arch diagnosis in the radiogram of the neonate. Clin Radiol 21:306–307.
17. Eisen S, Elliott LP (1968): A plain film sign of total anomalous pulmonary venous connection below the diaphragm. AJR 102:372–378.
18. Elliott LP (1978): An angiographic and plain film approach to complex congenital heart disease: Classification and simplified nomenclature. Current Prob Cardiol 3:1–64.
19. Elliott LP, Jue KL, Amplatz KA (1966): A roentgen classification of cardiac malpositions. Invest Radiol 1:17–28.
20. Emmanouilides GC, Moss AJ, Duffie ER, Adams FH (1964): Pulmonary arterial pressure changes in human newborn infants from birth to 3 days of age. J Pediatr 65:327–332.
21. Fagan CJ, Swischuk LE (1972): The opaque lung in lobar emphysema. AJR 114:300–304.
22. Fawcitt J, Lind J, Wegelius C (1960): The first breath. Acta Paediatr (Suppl 123) 49:5–17.

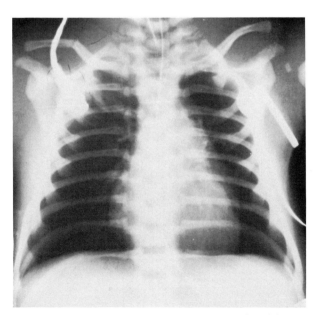

Figure 22–25. Idiopathic persistent pulmonary hypertension of the newborn syndrome. Lungs are hyperinflated. Heart size is normal. Pulmonary vascular markings are small, and their margins are sharply defined.

23. Fellows KE, Sigmann J, Stern AM, Bookstein JJ (1970): Coronary sinus enlargement in infants. Radiology 94:347–349.

24. Felman AH, Rhatigan RN, Pierson KK (1972): Pulmonary lymphangiectasia: Observations in 17 patients and proposed classification. AJR 116:548–558.

25. Fulton H (1956): Sixty years of cardiovascular roentgenology. AJR 76:657–663.

26. Gardner TH (1971): Cardiac emergencies in the newborn period. Radiol Clin North Am 9:385–394.

27. Hall B (1966): Mongolism in newborn infants. Clin Pediatr 5:4–12.

28. Harris GBC, Neuhauser EBD, Giedion A (1960): Total anomalous pulmonary venous return below the diaphragm. AJR 84:436–440.

29. Haworth SG, Reid L, Simon G (1977): Radiological features of the heart and lungs in total anomalous pulmonary venous return in early infancy. Clin Radiol 28:561–569.

30. Kachaner J (1973): Iatrogenic diseases related to the treatment of respiratory distress in the neonatal period. Radiological diagnosis: Part 1. Pleuro–pulmonary lesions. Ann Radiol 16:57–87.

31. Keats TC, Riddervald HO, Michaelis LL (1970): Thanatophoric dwarfism. AJR 108:473–480.

32. Kieffer SA, Amplatz K, Anderson RC, Lillehei CW (1965): Proximal interruption of a pulmonary artery. AJR 95:592–597.

33. Kuhn JP, Fletcher BD, LeLemos RA (1969): Roentgen findings in transient tachypnea of the newborn. Radiology 92:751–757.

34. Lambert EC, Canent RV, Hohn AR (1966): Congenital cardiac anomalies in newborn: Review of conditions causing death or severe distress in first month of life. Pediatrics 37:343–351.

35. Lambert EC, Tingelstad JB, Hohn AR (1966): Diagnosis and management of congenital heart disease in the first week of life. Pediatr Clin North Am 13:943–982.

36. Leithiser RE, Capitanio MA, Macpherson RI, Wood BP (1986): "Communicating" bronchopulmonary foregut malformations. AJR 146:227–231.

37. Levin B, White H (1961): Total anomalous pulmonary venous drainage into the portal system. AJR 76:894–901.

38. Lind J, Tahti E, Hirvensalom M (1960): Roentgenologic studies of the size of the lungs of the newborn baby before and after aeration. Ann Pediatr Fenn 12:20.

39. Long WA, Lawson EE, Harned HS Jr, Kraybill EN (1984): Pleural effusion in the first days of life: A prospective study. Am J Perinatol 1:190–194.

40. Lucas R, Anderson R, Amplatz K, Adams P, Edwards J (1963): Congenital causes of pulmonary venous obstruction. Pediatr Clin North Am 10:781–836.

41. McCormick TL, Kuhns LR (1979): Tracheal compression by a normal aorta associated with right lung agenesis. Radiology 130:659–660.

42. Moes CAF (1975): Analysis of the chest in the neonate with congenital heart disease. Radiol Clin North Am 13:251–275.

43. Mortensson W, Lundstrom NR (1971): Broncho–pulmonary vascular malformation syndrome causing left heart failure during infancy. Acta Radiologica 11:449–457.

44. Mulvey RB (1963): The thymic "wave" sign. Radiology 81:834–837.

45. Nora JJ, Sinha AK (1968): Direct familial transmission of the Turner phenotype. Am J Dis Child 116:343–350.

46. Poznanski AK, Stern AM, Gall JC (1971): Skeletal anomalies in genetically determined congenital heart disease. Radiol Clin North Am 9:435–456.

47. Richards MR, Merrit KK, Samuels MH, Langman AG (1955): Congenital malformations of the cardiovascular system in a series of 6053 infants. Pediatrics 15:12–29.

48. Rigler LG (1929): The visualized esophagus in the diagnosis of diseases of the heart and aorta. AJR 21:563–572.

49. Roesler H (1937): Clinical Roentgenology of the Cardiovascular System; Anatomy, Physiology, Pathology, Experiments and Clinical Applications. Springfield, Charles C Thomas Publishers.

50. Rowe RD, Izukawa T, Mulholland HC, Bloom KR, Cook DH, Swyer PR (1978): Nonstructural heart disease in the newborn. Arch Dis Child 53:726–730.

51. Rudolph AM (1970): The changes in the circulation after birth. Circulation 41:343–357.

52. Salonomowitz E, Edwards JE, Hunter DW, Castaneda–Zuniga WR, Lund G, Gragg AH, Amplatz K (1984): The three types of aortic diverticula. AJR 142:673–679.

53. Shaher RM, Moes CAF, Khoury GH (1967): The significance of the atrial situs in the diagnosis of positional anomalies of the heart. II. An angiocardiographic study of 29 patients. Am Heart J 73:41–48.

54. Singleton EB (1967): Respiratory distress syndrome. In Kaufman HJ (ed): Progress in Pediatric Radiology 1967. Chicago, Year Book Medical Publishers, pp 108–134.

55. Soto B, Pacifico AD, Souza AS, Bargeron LM, Ermocilla R, Tonkin IL (1978): Identification of thoracic isomerism from the plain chest radiograph. AJR 131:995–1002.

56. Sprague PL, Kennedy JC (1976): Anomalous left pulmonary artery with an unusual barium swallow. Pediatr Radiol 4:188–189.

57. Stanger P, Rudolph AM, Edwards JE (1977): Cardiac malpositions. Circulation 56:159–172.

58. Swischuk LE (1970): Transient respiratory distress of the newborn (TRDN). AJR 108:557–563.

59. Swischuk LE (1971): Anterior tracheal indentation in infancy and early childhood: Normal or abnormal? AJR 112:12–17.

60. Swischuk LE (1978): Acute respiratory distress in the infant. Radiol Clin North Am 16:77–90.

61. Swischuk LE (1980): Radiology of the Newborn and Young Infant. 2nd ed. Baltimore, Williams & Wilkins, p 143.

62. Ibid, p 214.

63. Tausend ME, Stern WZ (1965): Thymic patterns in the newborn. AJR 95:125–130.

64. Taussig H (1947): Congenital Malformations of the Heart. New York, The Commonwealth Fund.

65. Telander RL, Lennox C, Sieber W (1976): Sequestration of the lung in children. Mayo Clin Proc 51:578–583.

66. Velasquez G, Nath PH, Castaneda–Zuniga WR, Amplatz K, Formanek A (1980): Aberrant left subclavian artery in tetralogy of Fallot. Am J Cardiol 45:811–818.

67. Victorica BE, Elliott LP (1968): The roentgenologic findings and approach to persistent truncus arteriosus in infancy. AJR 104:440–451.

68. Warkany J, Passaarge B, Smith LB (1966): Congenital malformations in autosomal trisomy syndromes. Am J Dis Child 112:502–517.

69. Weaver MD, Chen JTT, Anderson PAW, Lester RG (1976): Total anomalous pulmonary venous connection to the left vertical vein. Radiology 118:679–683.

70. Wesenberg RL, Graven SN, McCabe EB (1971): Radiological findings in wet-lung disease. Radiology 98:69–74.

71. Wesenberg RL, Wax RE, Zachman RD (1972): Varying roentgenographic patterns of patent ductus arteriosus in the newborn. AJR 114:340–349.

72. White JJ, Donahoo JS, Ostrow PT, Murphy J, Haller JA (1974): Cardiovascular and respiratory manifestations of pulmonary sequestration in childhood. Ann Thoracic Surg 18:286–294.

73. Williams RG, Jaffe RB, Condon VR, Nixon GW (1979): Unusual features of pulmonary sling. AJR 133:1065–1069.

74. Wolf EL, Berdon WE, Baker DH (1978): Improved plain film diagnosis of right aortic arch anomalies with high kilovoltage–selective filtration-magnification technique. Pediatr Radiol 7:141–146.

23 CARDIAC ENZYMES

Richard L. Bucciarelli

Serum creatine kinase and lactate dehydrogenase isoenzyme activity have become important tests in the diagnosis of acute myocardial infarction in adults, but the elevation of these isoenzymes is by no means specific to myocardial injury. In fact, many insults result in isoenzyme patterns identical to those seen in patients with isolated acute myocardial infarction. In order to use these enzymes as biochemical markers of myocardial infarction, the clinician must be aware of all conditions causing alterations in enzyme patterns and must exercise caution when interpreting specific isoenzyme patterns in certain situations.

The significance of isoenzyme pattern alterations in asphyxiated neonates has had a similar history as that in adults. Initial studies attempting to establish normal standards for neonatal isoenzyme activity revealed wide ranges of activity in apparently normal, nonstressed full-term infants. Further investigation linked this variability to subtle peripartal hypoxia as well as to rhabdomyolysis during parturition.

With the discovery that myocardial ischemia and infarction are relatively common events in stressed neonates, studies were performed to identify the pattern of isoenzyme changes in these infants and to evaluate whether the observed patterns could aid in diagnosing neonatal myocardial necrosis. Data gathered to date indicate that in neonates, just as in adults, variations in isoenzyme activity can be used to confirm the diagnosis of myocardial injury, provided the pediatrician is aware of the other conditions that may also result in elevation and alteration in the pattern of cardiac isoenzyme activity.

BIOCHEMISTRY OF CREATINE KINASE AND ISOENZYMES OF CREATINE KINASE

Biochemical Properties

Creatine kinase is a dimeric molecule consisting of two subunits with a combined molecular weight of approximately 86,000 daltons. The subunits are identified as either B or M, based on their net ionic charge at pH 8.0.[55] Thus, three creatine kinase isoenzymes may be present in plasma: BB, MB, and MM. These subunits are loosely associated and may be subject to dissociation and random recombination both in vivo and in vitro.[72]

Since the B subunit carries a net negative charge at pH 8.0, the movement of the homologous BB isoenzyme is

most rapid in an electrophoretic field, migrating with albumin; movement of the MB fraction is intermediate, migrating with the α_2–globulins. MM is neutral, migrating only slightly from the cathode with the γ–globulins (Fig. 23–1).

Appreciable activity of creatine kinase is found in skeletal muscle (3200 IU/g), myocardium (1600 IU/g), brain (200 IU/g), and gastrointestinal tract (150 IU/g); other tissues, including the lung, liver, kidney, uterus, placenta, prostate, and tongue, possess less activity.[41,55] The predominant isoenzyme in skeletal muscle is MM, but significant activity of MB has also been reported. The predominant isoenzyme of creatine kinase activity present in the heart is of the MB type, but considerable quantities of MM are also present.[13] BB isoenzyme activity appears to be most highly concentrated in the brain but is also found in the gastrointestinal tract, adrenal gland, lung, and kidney[55] (Table 23–1).

Recently, several investigators have reported the existence of a fourth band of creatine kinase activity that migrates toward the cathode. This band has been termed the mitochondrial band, since it appears to be released from the mitochondria of myocardial cells.[30,31,60,63,65]

Biochemical Activity

Creatine kinase participates in a reversible reaction transferring phosphate from creatine phosphate to adenosine diphosphate (ADP), forming creatine plus high energy adenosine triphosphate (ATP). ATP in the presence of glucose and hexokinase produces glucose-6-phosphate and regenerates ADP; glucose-6-phosphate is then available for glycolysis (Fig. 23–2).

Assay of Total Creatine Kinase Activity

Rosalki's method[56] of serum creatine phosphokinase assay utilizes the glucose-6-phosphate generated in the presence of creatine kinase as a substrate to be converted into 6-phosphogluconate. The reaction requires nicotinamide-adenine dinucleotide (NAD) and glucose-6-phosphate dehydrogenase (G6PDH) as coenzymes. The NAD is reduced to NADH, which can be assayed spectrophotometrically. The intensity of the fluorescence produced is directly proportional to the concentration of the glucose-6-phosphate and, hence, is proportional to the concentration of the creatine kinase that catalyzed the original reaction (Fig. 23–2).

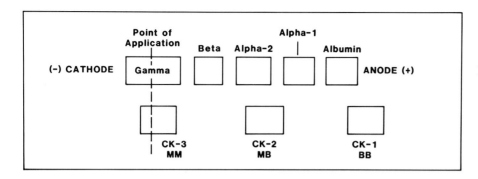

Figure 23–1. Comparison of the electrophoretic mobilities of the major human serum proteins and serum creatine kinase isoenzymes.

Table 23–1. CREATINE KINASE ISOENZYME PROFILE
AND CLINICAL RELEVANCE

CK Isoenzyme Fraction	Normal Range (Per Cent of Total)	Tissue Distribution	Elevated
CK-1 (BB)	< 5 %	Central nervous system, biliary tree, adrenal gland, lung, kidney	Cerebral infarct, biliary atresia, subarachnoid hemorrhage, renal infarct
CK-2 (MB)	2 to 10 %	Myocardium, skeletal muscle, liver, tongue	Myocardial injury, extensive ischemic rhabdomyolysis
CK-3 (MM)	90 %	Skeletal muscle, myocardium, central nervous system, prostate, placenta, uterus	Ischemic rhabdomyolysis, central nervous system injury, cardiac injury

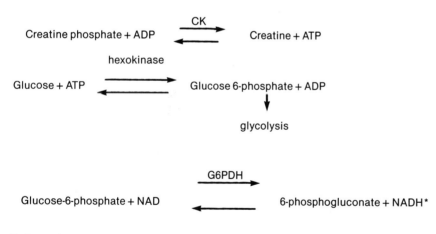

Figure 23–2. Biochemical pathway utilizing creatine kinase to generate ATP for the conversion of glucose to glucose-6-phosphate. The Rosalki assay[56] for creatine kinase activity converts glucose-6-phosphate to 6-phosphogluconate in the presence of glucose-6-phosphate dehydrogenase (G6PDH) and generates fluorescent NADH.

*Indicates flourescence

Assay of Creatine Kinase Isoenzyme Activity

Techniques to separate creatine kinase isoenzymes and to identify the MB fraction include the use of radioimmunoassay, glass bead separation, immunoinhibition, and gel electrophoresis.[1,25,28,74] Each has been used clinically and has advantages and disadvantages. Perhaps the most widely available system uses gel electrophoresis with a scanning fluorometric densitometer to quantify isoenzyme activity. In this system, serum undergoes electrophoresis in either an agarose or an acetate medium. The resulting bands, corresponding to the three isoenzymes, are scanned with a fluorometric densitometer. Bands are compared with each other and are reported as a percentage of total activity. When the total creatine kinase enzyme activity is known, the fraction of each band can be multiplied by the total enzyme activity to semiquantify isoenzyme activity[16,72] (Fig. 23–3).

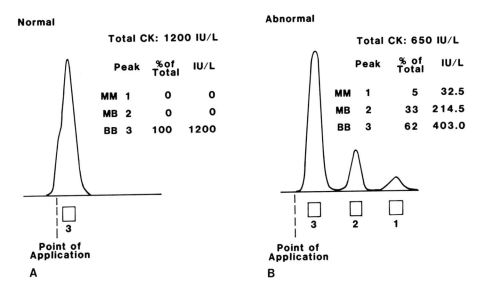

Figure 23–3. *A,* Fluorometric scan of creatine kinase (CK) showing the normal pattern of 100 per cent CK-MM (CK-3) activity. The semiquantitative calculation of the activity of each fraction appears to the right of the scan. *B,* Fluorometric scan of creatine kinase (CK) after a generalized hypoxic insult. CK-MB (CK-2) and CK-BB (CK-1) are also present. The semiquantitative calculation of isoenzyme activity appears to the right of the scan.

Release After Injury

The half-life of the circulating creatine kinase isoenzymes is 10 to 12 hours for MM and 6 to 8 hours for MB. BB has an extremely short half-life and is rarely detected in adult plasma.[55]

Within 4 to 6 hours after myocardial infarction, total creatine kinase, MB, and MM activities are increased. The MB activity peaks at 24 to 48 hours and returns to normal after approximately 72 hours. The MM activity rises within a similar time frame but often remains high for 4 to 5 days after the episode.[22] Sufficient data are not available to permit comment about the pattern of response of the mitochondrial band after myocardial injury.

BIOCHEMISTRY OF LACTATE DEHYDROGENASE AND ISOENZYMES OF LACTATE DEHYDROGENASE

Biochemical Properties

Lactate dehydrogenase is a tetramer composed of the five possible combinations of two distinct monomers, H

chains and M chains. The combined molecular weight is approximately 140,000 daltons.[16] Each isoenzyme possesses a unique electrophoretic mobility based on the number of H chains present. The H monomer carries a negative charge at pH 8.6, and as a result, the isoenzymes containing the most H components move fastest from the cathode (Fig. 23–4). Lactate dehydrogenase 1 (LDH-1) is a tetramer of four H chains and migrates with the α_1–globulins and albumin. LDH-2 migrates next fastest, moving with the α_2– and α_1–globulins. Normally, these two isoenzymes account for 17 to 27 per cent and 28 to 38 per cent, respectively, of serum lactate dehydrogenase activity, with LDH-2 having a higher concentration than LDH-1. They are concentrated in the myocardium, erythrocytes, and renal cortex. LDH-3 moves with intermediate speed from the cathode, migrating with the β–globulins. LDH-3 is composed of two H and two M chains and is found in a variety of tissues. It is responsible for 19 to 27 per cent of total serum lactate dehydrogenase activity. LDH-4 and LDH-5 are the slowest moving, migrating with the γ–globulins. They are found in serum in equal quantities and make up 5 to 16 per cent of total lactate dehydrogenase activity. These isoenzymes are concentrated in liver tissue and skeletal muscle[16] (Table 23–2).

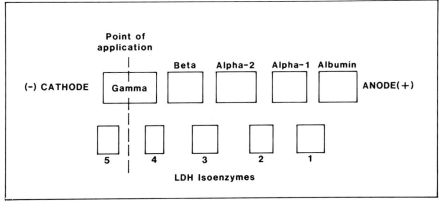

Figure 23–4. Comparison of the electrophoretic mobilities of the major human serum proteins and serum lactate dehydrogenase isoenzymes.

Table 23–2. LACTATE DEHYDROGENASE ISOENZYME PROFILE
AND CLINICAL RELEVANCE

LDH Isoenzyme Fraction	Normal Range (Per Cent of Total)	Tissue Distribution	Elevated
LDH-1 (HHHH)	17 to 27 %	Myocardium, erythrocytes, central nervous system	Myocardial infarction, hemolysis, cerebral infarct, renal cortical necrosis
LDH-2 (HHHM)	28 to 38 %	Erythrocytes, gastrointestinal tract, lung	Pulmonary infarct
LDH-3 (HHMM)	19 to 27 %	Lung, liver	Pulmonary infarct, hepatopathy
LDH-4 (HMMM)	5 to 16 %	Liver, kidney	Hepatopathy, renal tubal necrosis
LDH-5 (MMMM)	5 to 16 %	Liver, skeletal muscle, kidney	Ischemic rhabdomyolysis, liver infarct

Biochemical Activity

Lactate dehydrogenase is required to convert lactate to pyruvate. It uses NAD as a coenzyme. In the reaction, NAD is reduced to NADH (Fig. 23–5).

Assay of Total Lactate Dehydrogenase Activity

Elevitch[16] adapted Rosalki's methods for the determination of creatine kinase and used them to assay for

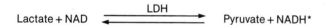

$$\text{Lactate} + \text{NAD} \underset{\longleftarrow}{\overset{\text{LDH}}{\longrightarrow}} \text{Pyruvate} + \text{NADH*}$$

*Indicates flourescence

Figure 23–5. Biochemical reaction involving lactate dehydrogenase (LDH) in the conversion of lactate to pyruvate. This reaction is also the basis for the Elevitch assay[16] for LDH activity.

lactate dehydrogenase activity. His method also employed NADH fluorescence as an indication of enzyme activity.

Lactate Dehydrogenase Isoenzyme Determination

Like creatine kinase, lactate dehydrogenase can be separated into its isoenzymes by a variety of methods. The most widely accepted method is the scanning fluorometric technique utilizing an agarose gel system. As in creatine kinase, the isoenzymes are expressed as a percentage of total lactate dehydrogenase activity. When the total activity is known, isoenzyme activity can be semiquantified[16,29] (Fig. 23–6).

Release After Injury

After myocardial injury, serum lactate dehydrogenase activity rises markedly. In addition, the ratio of LDH-1 to

Figure 23–6. A, Fluorometric scan of lactate dehydrogenase (LDH) showing the normal pattern of isoenzyme activity. The semiquantitative calculation of isoenzyme activity appears to the left of the scan. Note that LDH-2 activity exceeds the activity of LDH-1. B, Fluorometric scan of lactate dehydrogenase (LDH) after an acute myocardial infarction. The semiquantitative calculation of isoenzyme activity appears to the left of the scan. Note that while total activity is increased, the major change is that the LDH-1 activity now exceeds that of the LDH-2 fraction.

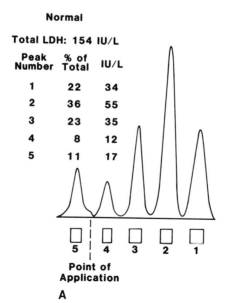

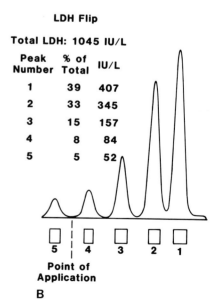

LDH-2, normally less than 1, exceeds 1 after 12 to 24 hours, resulting in the so-called "flipped LDH pattern." After peak activity is reached, usually within 48 hours, the concentrations of all the isoenzymes decline, reaching normal within 1 to 2 weeks. The LDH-1 to LDH-2 ratio of greater than 1 persists until approximately 1 week after the injury, when the normal profile of LDH-2 being greater than LDH-1 returns.[16]

MYOCARDIAL INFARCTION AND CARDIAC ENZYME ACTIVITY IN THE ADULT

Changes in serum enzyme activity after myocardial injury result from the movement of the various enzymes from damaged myocardial cells into the systemic circulation. The first phase of this process is postulated to be the escape of enzymes from the cell into the interstitium. This release of enzyme is regulated by both the amount of cell damage and the intracellular binding of the enzymes to various cellular proteins. Once in the interstitium, the enzymes are denatured and metabolized, so that most never reach the general circulation. Those enzymes that escape damage gain entry into the circulation via the lymphatics and the coronary circulation of the heart. Once in the circulation, each class of enzymes has a unique coefficient of distribution and mechanism of clearance. The majority of the isoenzymes are cleared by the reticuloendothelial system in conjunction with the kidneys and biliary tree.[21]

In 1955, Karmen and associates[33] described the presence of elevated glutamic-oxaloacetic transaminase activity in human serum after acute myocardial infarction. Later in the 1960s and early 1970s, several investigators published data demonstrating the value of assays for serum total creatine kinase and lactate dehydrogenase as a means of confirming the diagnosis of myocardial infarction. With further experience, however, many investigators reported other circumstances and disease states that caused increases in the serum activity of these enzymes. Thus, serum creatine kinase and lactate dehydrogenase activity appeared to be sensitive indicators of myocardial injury but not specific enough to be used clinically.[26,37,40,43,45,47,64]

The measurement of serum creatine kinase activity became more accurate when Rosalki[56] developed a standardized method for quantification. However, the usefulness of these measurements was not appreciated until 1974 when Roberts and associates[50] described the kinetic fluorometric method for separating and quantifying serum creatine kinase isoenzyme activity. This technique provided a rapid, reliable, reproducible, and clinically available method for analyzing these serum isoenzymes. Later, the same method was applied to the separation and quantification of the isoenzymes of lactate dehydrogenase.[39,46] With the kinetic fluorometric method, the measurement of enzyme activity of creatine kinase and lactate dehydrogenase and their isoenzymes became extremely useful for diagnosing acute myocardial infarction and estimating infarct size.[22–24,35,49,50–54,69] By 1975, the efficacy of these serum enzyme and isoenzyme measurements led Galen[21] to the conclusion that the routine use of α–hydroxybutyrate dehydrogenase and serum glutamic oxaloacetic transaminase could be abandoned if creatine kinase and lactate dehydrogenase isoenzyme assays were available.

MYOCARDIAL INFARCTION AND CARDIAC ENZYME ACTIVITY IN THE NEONATE

Although the presence of myocardial infarct in infants and children with and without congenital heart disease was described in the 1960s, it was not until the mid to late 1970s that the true significance of myocardial necrosis in the neonate was appreciated.[14,17,19,27] In 1972, Rowe and Hoffman[57] described three infants presenting with congestive heart failure who had suffered severe perinatal asphyxia. Evidence of left ventricular dysfunction in combination with electrocardiographic changes consistent with myocardial ischemia led the investigators to conclude that these infants suffered a transient form of myocardial ischemia related to their birth stress.

In 1977, Bucciarelli and colleagues[6] identified 14 term infants who had transient tricuspid insufficiency secondary to perinatal asphyxia. Two infants who died had extensive necrosis of the papillary muscles of the tricuspid valve. The authors postulated that transient tricuspid insufficiency of the newborn is secondary to myocardial ischemia and necrosis. In 1978, Nelson and associates[44] showed that the serum creatine kinase MB fraction was markedly elevated in infants with transient tricuspid insufficiency and was highest in infants with confirmation of papillary muscle infarcts at postmortem examination. These findings prompted their suggestion that the creatine kinase MB fraction could help identify infants with underlying transient atrioventricular valve insufficiency secondary to asphyxial myocardial ischemia as the cause of cardiopulmonary symptoms.[44] Later, Bucciarelli and LaPine[8] reported changes in the fractions of lactate dehydrogenase in infants with asphyxial myocardial dysfunction similar to those seen after acute myocardial infarction in adults. In Bucciarelli and LaPine's study, the diagnosis of myocardial dysfunction syndrome with atrioventricular valve insufficiency was more accurate when both creatine kinase and lactate dehydrogenase isoenzyme patterns were consistent with recent myocardial necrosis.

Several other groups have confirmed the presence of myocardial infarcts and ischemia in stressed term and preterm infants with normal coronary arteries.[34,71] Donnelly and coworkers[15] as well as Setzer and associates[61] retrospectively studied large populations of infants who died during the first week of life from a variety of diseases. Both groups found that myocardial necrosis was very common in this age group. The papillary muscles of both ventricles were most vulnerable to infarction, while additional lesions were scattered throughout the free wall of both the right and left ventricles and the interventricular septum. In most patients, the lesions were multiple and bilateral.

CLINICAL RELEVANCE OF CARDIAC ENZYMES IN THE NEONATE

Because many diseases and conditions cause the release of creatine kinase and lactate dehydrogenase, the value of the serum activities of these enzymes as adjuvants for diagnosing acute myocardial injury in the neonate is limited if other conditions known to release these enzymes are also present (Tables 23–1 and 23–2).

In order to apply cardiac enzymology to the neonate, one must determine whether the distribution of the isoenzymes and the factors regulating their clearance from serum are similar to those in adults.

Researchers investigating the prenatal and early postnatal diagnosis of the various muscular dystrophies discovered that fetal and neonatal skeletal muscle contains greater quantities of creatine kinase MB than are found in the muscles of adults.[68] Ziter[73] showed that in skeletal muscle of the developing rat, the predominant isoenzyme of creatine kinase found early in gestation is creatine kinase BB, with creatine kinase MB appearing next and dominating at birth. Similarly, Foxall and Emery[18] analyzed human fetal skeletal muscle and found that at 8 weeks' gestation 82 per cent of the creatine kinase activity could be identified as creatine kinase MB. By term, this value had fallen to 22 to 30 per cent.[18]

The ontogeny of the enzyme activity of the developing myocardium shows similar changes. Ziter's analysis[73] of developing rat myocardium showed that creatine kinase BB is the dominant isoenzyme early in gestation. By term, the dominant isoenzyme is creatine kinase MM, although significant amounts of creatine kinase MB are present. Likewise, Cao et al[9] found large amounts of creatine kinase BB activity in the human fetal myocardium, which decreased to undetectable levels by 4 years of age. Although the human myocardium contains large amounts of creatine kinase MB throughout late gestation and early childhood, the dominant isoenzyme is creatine kinase MM. Takahashi and coworkers[67] confirmed these evolutions in isoenzyme activity in both human skeletal and cardiac muscle.

These findings explain why any stress that causes ischemic rhabdomyolysis results in the elevation of *both* creatine kinase MM and creatine kinase MB in the serum. The consequent increase in serum creatine kinase MB may be misinterpreted as being cardiac in origin, even though it was released from skeletal muscle.[59] Likewise, isolated myocardial injury will result in an increase in *both* the creatine kinase MB and creatine kinase MM fractions. Creatine kinase BB, on the other hand, appears to be concentrated in brain tissue and is the *only* creatine kinase isoenzyme to rise after isolated brain injury in preterm and term neonates, children, and adults.[2,10,38,63]

Like creatine kinase activity, lactate dehydrogenase activity is affected by a variety of stresses in the neonate.

Total lactate dehydrogenase activity and the activity of certain of the isoenzymes increase after ischemic muscle injury, liver trauma, and hemolysis—conditions common to the neonate. Data suggest that the flipped pattern (LDH-1 > LDH-2) remains characteristic of neonates with myocardial damage, but it may also be present in extreme hemolysis.[8]

An important difference between the neonate and the adult in serum activity of isoenzymes after injury is the rate of enzyme clearance. In the neonate, the microsomal fraction of the liver fails to clear enzymes as efficiently as it does in the older infant or adult. Also, glomerular filtration rate of the neonatal kidney is approximately one half that of the adult rate. Thus, it is not surprising that many biologic products and drugs have longer half-lives in the neonatal period than during later life. Furthermore, many endogenous and exogenous compounds may compete with the isoenzymes in the various degradation pathways, leading to maintenance of serum activity due to decreased rate of excretion of these proteins from the serum. These factors may explain why Shields and Feldman[62] found evidence of creatine kinase BB, the isoenzyme with the shortest half-life, in the peripheral circulation up to 3.5 days after intraventricular hemorrhage in the neonate.

ASSAY OF CREATINE KINASE AND LACTATE DEHYDROGENASE ACTIVITY IN NONSTRESSED NEONATES

Since a variety of frequently occurring circumstances can lead to elevation of creatine kinase and lactate dehydrogenase activity, one must contrast enzyme levels between nonstressed and stressed infants to determine the normal neonatal range of activity and the patterns of release of these enzymes.

Creatine Kinase Activity in Nonstressed Neonates

Rudolph and Gross[58] reported that total creatine kinase activity varied greatly in neonates, with its being highest in infants born to primiparous mothers after long, difficult deliveries. However, some infants with apparently benign intrapartum courses had unexplained rises in enzyme activity. The lowest levels were observed in infants born by cesarean section without labor. These findings were supported by the work of Bodensteiner and Zellweger[4] and Blum and Brauman,[3] who reported similar results when analyzing cord and venous blood samples in the first 24 hours of life. Thus, it seems that the labor and delivery process results in rhabdomyolysis and the release of creatine kinase. These studies analyzed blood samples obtained at birth or within the first 24 hours after delivery for total creatine kinase activity; neither the isoenzymes of creatine kinase nor those of lactate dehydrogenase were evaluated.

Table 23–3. DISTRIBUTION OF MEAN (AND SD) CREATINE KINASE ISOENZYME ACTIVITIES
AT DIFFERENT TIMES AFTER BIRTH

Time After Birth (Hours)		CK Total	CK-MM	CK-MB	CK-BB	CK-MM	CK-MB	CK-BB
Range	Mean		Activity (IU/liter)				Per Cent of Total Activity	
Cord blood	0	185 (73)	173 (71)	3 (3)	9 (9)	92.9 (5.1)	1.4 (1.4)	5.5 (5.3)
5 to 8	6.3	536 (236)	468 (218)	25 (18)	43 (22)	86.3 (5.6)	4.6 (3.0)	9.1 (5.0)
24 to 33	28.7	494 (254)	450 (24)	18 (14)	25 (12)	90.6 (3.5)	3.4 (1.6)	5.9 (3.3)
71 to 100	77.3	288 (163)	252 (152)	11 (9)	25 (15)	86.3 (6.5)	3.4 (1.9)	10.3 (6.6)

Notes: Reprinted with permission from Jedeikin R et al (1982): Creatine kinase isoenzyme activity in serum from cord blood of healthy full-term infants during the first three postnatal days. Clin Chem 28:317–322.

Cao and coworkers[11] performed serial analyses of creatine kinase and found levels exceeding the adult standards in cord blood and in infants up to 10 days old. The serial data indicated that total creatine kinase activity tended to peak at 24 to 48 hours after delivery, returning to cord values by 72 hours. The magnitude of peak activity correlated with the type of delivery. The levels did not fall to adult standards until 10 days post partum. In this study, creatine kinase MB was not detected in any of the infants' sera. The entire rise in creatine kinase activity was due to increases in the creatine kinase MM isoenzyme. Kristensen and associates,[36] while establishing norms of a variety of enzymes in newborns and peripartous women, also found elevated cord creatine kinase activity entirely of the MM type. Freer and associates[20] found cord creatine kinase to range from 28 to 475 IU/liter, with only 1 of 38 samples positive for creatine kinase MB activity.

More recently, Jedeikin and associates[32] published longitudinal data on the serial changes in creatine kinase and its isoenzymes in the sera of 45 healthy full-term infants at 5 to 8 hours, 24 to 33 hours, and 72 to 100 hours after delivery (Table 23–3). Creatine kinase MB was detected in the sera of these infants but reached a mean maximum activity of only 25 IU/liter. The 97.5 percentile at 24 to 48 hours was less than 63 IU/liter (Table 23–4). In this series, the creatine kinase MB activity accounted for 1.4 to 7.6 per cent of total creatine kinase activity. Again, total creatine kinase activity and the activity of the isoenzymes correlated with the type of delivery, with their being higher in vaginally delivered infants at all time intervals except at birth in the cord samples. These values are in agreement with norms for neonates published by Mertes[41] in 1981. In a study of 150 normal term infants within 24 hours of birth, Bucciarelli and LaPine[7] observed that the mean total creatine kinase activity was 248 ± 140 IU/liter (± SD), while the creatine kinase MB mean was 17 ± 3 IU/liter (± SD), accounting for 2 to 20 per cent of total creatine kinase activity.

Lactate Dehydrogenase in Nonstressed Neonates

Much less has been written about the activity of lactate dehydrogenase in normal term infants. Blum and Brauman[3] reported total lactate dehydrogenase levels of 472 ± 30 IU/liter (± SEM) at 4 days after delivery. Total lactate dehydrogenase levels remained high by adult standards at 395 ± 84 IU/liter (± SEM) at 10 days after delivery.[3] Similarly they reported total lactate dehydrogenase levels to be 200 to 850 IU/liter with an LDH-2 dominant pattern.[8] Mertes[42] reported levels in excess of 500 U/liter at birth and 208 to 473 IU/liter up to 18 months following delivery. Freer and colleagues[20] found cord lactate dehydrogenase activity ranging from 337 to 871 IU/liter. In their study of 24 infants, the LDH-1 fraction (heart) was lower than adult levels, while LDH-5 (muscle) exceeded adult levels (Table 23–5).

ASSAY OF CREATINE KINASE AND LACTATE DEHYDROGENASE ACTIVITY IN STRESSED NEONATES

Creatine Kinase in Stressed Neonates

Nelson and associates[44] first reported increases in serum creatine kinase and its isoenzymes in the sera of acutely stressed neonates with clinical evidence of myocardial dysfunction and transient atrioventricular valve insufficiency. Since that report, several groups have questioned the application of serum creatine kinase MB determinations in the neonate, as this isoenzyme is found in the sera of newborn infants without clinical evidence of myocardial damage.[32,48,70] Sutton and coworkers[66] studied 10 ill neonates with congenital heart disease or persistent

Table 23–4. REFERENCE INTERVALS FOR CREATINE KINASE ISOENZYME ACTIVITIES

Time After Birth (Hours)	Total CK	CK-MM	CK-MB	CK-BB
Range		Activity (IU/liter)		
Cord blood	70 to 380	60 to 363	0 to 11	> 5 to 35
5 to 8	214 to 1175	166 to 1096	< 5 to 76	12 to 126
24 to 33	158 to 1230	130 to 1200	< 5 to 63	10 to 52
72 to 100	87 to 725	68 to 676	< 5 to 30	8 to 63

Notes: 2.5th to 97.5th percentiles of log gaussian distribution. Reprinted with permission from Jedeikin R et al (1982): Creatine kinase isoenzyme activity in serum cord blood of healthy full-term infants during the first three postnatal days. Clin Chem 28:317–322.

Table 23–5. TOTAL LACTATE DEHYDROGENASE (LDH)
AND ISOENZYME ACTIVITY IN THE NEONATE

	Activity (IU/liter)		
	Range	*Mean*	*Tolerance Interval*
Total LDH	327 to 874	444	337 to 871

	Activity (IU/liter)		LDH/total LDH × 100	
Isoenzyme	*Mean*	*Range*	*Mean*	*Range*
LDH-1	61	16 to 130	11	4 to 19
LDH-2	151	102 to 288	30	17 to 40
LDH-3	131	84 to 245	26	15 to 35
LDH-4	67	23 to 122	13	6 to 21
LDH-5	83	14 to 200	17	4 to 30

Notes: Data modified with permission from Freer DE et al (1979): Reference values for selected enzyme activities and protein concentrations in serum and plasma derived from cord-blood specimens. Clin Chem 25:565–569.

pulmonary hypertension of the newborn syndrome and found detectable serum levels of creatine kinase MB in five of them. The peak creatine kinase MB activity was 40 IU/liter, occurring in an infant with atrial septal defect and tricuspid insufficiency. In all other cases, creatine kinase MB activity was less that 25 IU/liter. In contrast, Warburton and coworkers[70] showed that creatine kinase MB activity remained low in term infants with sustained metabolic acidosis, despite increases in creatine kinase MM and creatine kinase BB on serial determinations. Similarly, Cuestas' data[12] from sick high-risk preterm and term infants indicated that the creatine kinase MB fraction does not exceed 20 IU/liter ± 23 (± SD) in the first 15 days after delivery.

In the original report of Nelson et al,[44] the infants with clinical evidence of myocardial dysfunction syndrome with atrioventricular valve insufficiency presented with a mean creatine kinase MB value of 113 IU/liter and a range of 29 to 587 IU/liter. Thirty-two additional infants with myocardial dysfunction syndrome (as previously defined) demonstrated creatine kinase MB fractions from 15 to 183 IU/liter at 0 to 24 hours, peaking at 57 to 1054 IU/liter at 24 to 36 hours.[7] Similarly, Primhak and coworkers[48] studied 20 asphyxiated and 43 normal term newborns and found that the mean creatine kinase MB fractions were high in all asphyxiated infants, with the highest elevations in those with the most severe asphyxia. Although several control infants had creatine kinase MB activity detectable in their sera, the activity was significantly lower than that of those who were asphyxiated. Of particular interest was the extensive myocardial necrosis found in all five of the infants who died. In each case, significant activity of creatine kinase MB was present, with four infants having values above the established mean and three exceeding the upper limit of normal for age.[48] Thus, it appears that although creatine kinase MB can be detected in normal and stressed neonates, the levels seen in normal neonates and stressed neonates without myocardial dysfunction are usually considerably below those found in infants with clinical signs of acute myocardial dysfunction and atrioventricular valve insufficiency or autopsy-proven myocardial necrosis.

Although most of the reported data involve creatine kinase MB release after acute hypoxic stress, Boucek and colleagues[5] indicated that creatine kinase MB fractions can be chronically elevated in infants and children with congenital heart defects that produce congestive heart failure. They concluded that pressure-volume overload or chronic, severe hypoxemia can lead to myocardial cell injury and release of enzymes.

Lactate Dehydrogenase in Stressed Neonates

In the only report of lactate dehydrogenase activity in stressed neonates, the mean level of total activity was 1697 IU/liter in infants with clinical myocardial dysfunction, while those experiencing asphyxia without myocardial dysfunction demonstrated a mean level of 845 IU/liter.[8]

SUMMARY

Sufficient data are available to indicate that neonates with myocardial infarcts respond like adults with elevations in creatine kinase. This response includes an increase in total creatine kinase activity as well as in both the creatine kinase MM and creatine kinase MB fractions. Similarly, total lactate dehydrogenase activity rises with the formation of a "flipped pattern" (LDH-1 > LDH-2), further supporting the diagnosis of myocardial injury. Like adults, neonates may have low levels of creatine kinase MB activity after a variety of stresses that result in enzyme release from muscle (creatine kinase MM and creatine kinase MB) and from myocardium (creatine kinase MB and creatine kinase MM). Because a number of these stresses occur during and after the birth process, many neonates demonstrate increased levels of all cardiac enzymes in their sera. Consequently, it is important to recognize that the range of isoenzyme activity seen in neonates is broader than that seen in normal adults. However, it appears that a creatine kinase MB fraction in excess of the established norms for a given postnatal age and/or a LDH-1 to LDH-2 ratio of higher than 1 identifies most infants who have sustained significant myocardial damage and differentiates them from other infants who may have had similar stress but whose myocardium was spared.

References

1. Bayer PM, Boehm M, Hajdusich P, Hotschek H, Koehn H, Unger W, Wider G (1982): Immunoinhibition and automated column chromatography compared for assay of creatine kinase isoenzyme MB in serum. Clin Chem 28:166–169.
2. Becker M, Menzel K (1978): Brain-typical creatine kinase in the serum of newborn infants with perinatal brain damage. Acta Pediatr Scand 67:177–180.
3. Blum D, Brauman J (1975): Serum enzymes in the neonatal period. Biol Neonate 26:53–57.
4. Bodensteiner JB, Zellweger H (1971): Creatine phosphokinase in normal neonates and young infants. J Lab Clin Med 77:853–858.
5. Boucek RJ, Kasselberg AG, Boerth RC, Parrish MD, Graham TP (1982): Myocardial injury in infants with congenital heart disease: Evaluation by creatine kinase MB isoenzyme analysis. Am J Cardiol 50:129–135.
6. Bucciarelli RL, Nelson RM, Egan EA II, Eitzman DV, Gessner IH (1977): Transient tricuspid insufficiency of the newborn: A form of myocardial dysfunction in stressed newborns. Pediatrics 59:330–337.
7. Bucciarelli RL, LaPine T (1988): Serial creatine kinase activity in cord blood and blood of stressed and nonstressed neonates (in preparation).
8. Bucciarelli RL, LaPine T (1982): Serum lactic dehydrogenase isoenzyme patterns in infants with myocardial dysfunction syndrome (abstr). Clin Res 30:111a.
9. Cao A, De Virgiliis S, Falorni A (1969): The ontogeny of creatine kinase isoenzymes. Biol Neonate 13:375–380.
10. Cao A, De Virgiliis S, Lippi C, Trabalza N (1969): Creatine kinase isoenzymes in serum of children with neurological disorders. Clin Chim Acta 23:475–478.
11. Cao A, Trabalza N, De Virgiliis S, Furbetta M, Coppa G (1971): Serum creatine kinase activity and serum creatine kinase isoenzymes in newborn infants. Biol Neonate 17:126–134.
12. Cuestas RA (1980): Creatine kinase isoenzymes in high-risk infants. Pediatr Res 14:935–938.
13. Dawson DM, Fine IH (1967): Creatine kinase in human tissues. Arch Neurol 16:175–180.
14. DeSa DJ (1977): Myocardial changes in immature infants requiring prolonged ventilation. Arch Dis Child 52:138–147.
15. Donnelly WH, Bucciarelli RL, Nelson RM (1980): Ischemic papillary muscle necrosis in stressed newborn infants. J Pediatr 96:295–300.
16. Elevitch FR (1973): Fluorometric techniques in clinical chemistry. 1st ed. Boston, Little Brown & Co, pp 163–169.
17. Esterly JR, Oppenheimer EH (1966): Some aspects of cardiac pathology in infancy and childhood. I. Neonatal myocardial necrosis. Bull Johns Hopkins Hosp 119:191–199.
18. Foxall CD, Emery AEH (1975): Changes in creatine kinase and its isoenzymes in human fetal muscle during development. J Neurol Sci 24:483–492.
19. Franciosi RA, Blanc WA (1968): Myocardial infarcts in infants and children. I. A necropsy study in congenital heart disease. J Pediatr 73:309–319.
20. Freer DE, Statland BE, Johnson M, Felton H (1979): Reference values for selected enzyme activities and protein concentrations in serum and plasma derived from cord-blood specimens. Clin Chem 25:565–569.
21. Galen RS (1975): The enzyme diagnosis of myocardial infarction. Hum Pathol 6:141–155.
22. Galen RS, Reiffel JA, Gambino R (1975): Diagnosis of acute myocardial infarction. JAMA 232:145–147.
23. Galen RS (1977): Myocardial infarction: A clinician's guide to the isoenzymes. Resident Staff Physician 26:67–74.
24. Gerhardt W, Waldenstrom J, Horder M, Hofvendahl S, Billstrom R, Ljungdahl R, Berning H, Bagger P (1982): Creatine kinase and creatine kinase B–subunit activity in serum in cases of suspected myocardial infarction. Clin Chem 28:277–283.
25. Gerson B, LaBrie J (1979): Relative reliability of visual scanning and densitometer scanning in detection of CK–MB by agarose electrophoresis. Lab Med 10:670–673.
26. Griffiths PD (1966): ATP: Creatine phosphotransferase in the diagnosis of acute chest pain. Br Heart J 28:199–203.
27. Guller B, Bozic C (1972): Right-to-left shunting through a patent ductus arteriosus in a newborn with myocardial infarction. Cardiology 57:348–357.
28. Henry PD, Roberts R, Sobel BE (1975): Rapid separation of plasma creatine kinase isoenzymes by batch absorption on glass beads. Clin Chem 21:844–849.
29. Jacobs DS, Clark GM, Beers AL, Palmer G (1979): Automation of interpretive clinical laboratory reports: Isoenzymes of serum lactate dehydrogenase. Lab Med 10:636–639.
30. Jacobs H, Heldt HW, Klingenberg M (1964): High activity of creatine kinase in mitochondria from muscle and brain and evidence for a separate mitochondrial isoenzyme of creatine kinase. Biochem Biophys Res Commun 16:516–521.
31. James GP, Harrison RL (1979): Creatine kinase isoenzymes of mitochondrial origin in human serum. Clin Chem 25:943–947.
32. Jedeikin R, Makela SK, Shennan AT, Rowe RD (1982): Creatine kinase isoenzymes in serum from cord blood and the blood of healthy full-term infants during the first three postnatal days. Clin Chem 28:317–322.
33. Karmen A, Worblewski F, LaDue JS (1955): Transaminase activity in human blood. J Clin Invest 34:126–131.
34. Kilbride H, Way GL, Merenstein GB, Winfield JM (1980): Myocardial infarction in the neonate with normal heart and coronary arteries. Am J Dis Child 134:759–762.
35. Konttinen A, Somer H (1973): Specificity of serum creatine kinase isoenzymes in diagnosis of acute myocardial infarction. Br Med J 1:386–389.
36. Kristensen SR, Horder M, Pedersen GT (1979): Reference values for six enzymes in plasma from newborns and women at delivery. Scand J Clin Lab Invest 39:777–784.
37. Medias JE, Chahine RA, Gorlin R, Blacklow DJ (1974): A comparison of transmural and nontransmural acute myocardial infarction. Circulation 49:498–507.
38. Madsen A (1972): Creatine phosphokinase isoenzymes in human tissue with special reference to brain extract. Clin Chim Acta 36:17–25.
39. McKinzie D, Clark PI, Henderson AR (1976): How accurate are lactate dehydrogenase isoenzyme estimations by the thin-layer agarose fluorescent technique? Clin Chem 22:1995–1998.
40. Meltzer HY, Mrozak S, Boyer M (1970): Effect of intramuscular injections on serum creatine phosphokinase activity. Am J Med Sci 259:42–48.
41. Mertes S (1981): Pediatric Clinical Chemistry. 2nd ed. Washington, D.C., American Association for Clinical Chemistry, pp 167–170.
42. Mertes S (1981): Pediatric Clinical Chemistry. 2nd ed. Washington, D.C., American Association for Clinical Chemistry, pp 300–306.
43. Munsat TL, Baloh R, Pearson CM, Fowler W (1973): Serum enzyme alterations in neuromuscular disorders. JAMA 226:1536–1543.
44. Nelson RM, Bucciarelli RL, Eitzman DV, Egan EA II, Gessner IH (1978): Serum creatine phosphokinase MB fraction in newborns with transient tricuspid insufficiency. N Engl J Med 298:146–149.
45. Nevins MA, Saran M, Bright M, Lyon LJ (1973): Pitfalls in interpreting serum creatine phosphokinase activity. JAMA 224:1382–1387.
46. Papadopoulos NM, Kintzios JA (1966): Quantitative electrophoretic determination of lactate dehydrogenase isoenzymes. Am J Clin Pathol 47:96–99.
47. Pearce J (1965): Serum creatine kinase and exercise. Br Med J 2:167.
48. Primhak RA, Jedeikin R, Ellis G, Makela SK, Gillan JE, Swyer PR, Rowe RD (1985): Myocardial ischaemia in asphyxia neonatorum: Electrocardiographic, enzymatic and histologic correlation. Acta Paediatr Scand 74:595–600.

49. Pyle RB, Blomberg DJ, Burke MD, Lindsay WG, Nicoloff DM (1976): CPK–MB isoenzyme: Use in diagnosis of acute myocardial infarction in the early postoperative period. J Thorac Cardiovasc Surg 71:884–890.

50. Roberts R, Henry PD, Witteeveen SAGJ, Sobel BE (1974): Quantification of serum creatine phosphokinase isoenzyme activity. Am J Cardiol 33:650–654.

51. Roberts R, Gowda KS, Ludbrook PA, Sobel BE (1975): Specificity of elevated serum MB creatine phosphokinase activity in the diagnosis of acute myocardial infarction. Am J Cardiol 36:433 437.

52. Roberts R, Henry PD, Sobel BE (1975): An improved basis for enzymatic estimation of infarct size. Circulation 52: 743–754.

53. Roberts R, Sobel BE (1976): Elevated plasma MB creatine phosphokinase activity. Arch Intern Med 136:421–424.

54. Roberts R, Sobel BE, Ludbrook PA (1974): Determination of the origin of elevated plasma CPK after cardiac catheterization. Cathet Cardiovasc Diagn 2:329–336.

55. Roberts R, Sobel BE (1978): Creatine kinase isoenzymes in the assessment of heart disease. Am Heart J 95:521–527.

56. Rosalki SB (1967): An improved procedure for serum creatine phosphokinase determination. J Lab Clin Med 69:696–705.

57. Rowe RD, Hoffman T (1972): Transient myocardial ischemia of the newborn infant: A form of severe cardiorespiratory distress in full-term infants. J Pediatr 81:243–250.

58. Rudolph N, Gross RT (1966): Creatine phosphokinase activity in serum of newborn infants as an indicator of fetal trauma during birth. Pediatrics 38:1039–1046.

59. Russell SM, Bleiweiss S, Brownlow K, Elevitch FR (1976): Ischemic rhabdomyolysis and creatine phosphokinase isoenzymes. JAMA 235:632–633.

60. Sanders JL, Joung JI, Rochman H (1976): The further heterogeneity of creatine kinase presence of isoenzymes of cathodic mobility in rat tissues. Biochim Biophys Acta 438:407–411.

61. Setzer E, Ermocilla R, Tonkin I, John E, Sansa M, Cassady G (1980): Papillary muscle necrosis in a neonatal autopsy population: Incidence and associated clinical manifestations. J Pediatr 96:289–294.

62. Shields WD, Feldman RC (1982): Serum CK–BB isoenzyme in pre-term infants with periventricular hemorrhage. J Pediatr 100:464–468.

63. Sobel BE, Shell WE, Klein MS (1972): An isoenzyme of creatine phosphokinase associated with rabbit heart mitochondria. J Mol Cell Cardiol 4:367–380.

64. Sobel BE, Shell WE (1972): Serum enzyme determinations in the diagnosis and assessment of myocardial infarction. Circulation 45:471–482.

65. Somer H, Uotila A, Konttinen A, Saris N (1974): Creatine kinase activity and its isoenzyme pattern in heart mitochondria. Clin Chim Acta 53:369–372.

66. Sutton TM, O'Brien JF, Kleinberg F, House RF, Feldt RH (1981): Serum levels of creatine phosphokinase and its isoenzymes in normal and stressed neonates. Mayo Clin Proc 56:150–154.

67. Takahashi K, Ushikubo S, Oimomi M, Shinko T (1972): Creatine phosphokinase isoenzymes of human heart muscle and skeletal muscle. Clin Chim Acta 38:285–290.

68. Van Der Veen KJ, Willebrands AF (1966): Isoenzymes of creatine phosphokinase in tissue extracts and in normal and pathological sera. Clin Chim Acta 13:312–316.

69. Wagner GS, Roe CR, Limbird LE, Rosat RA, Wallace AG (1973): The importance of identification of the myocardial-specific isoenzyme of creatine phosphokinase (MB form) in the diagnosis of acute myocardial infarction. Circulation 52:263–269.

70. Warburton D, Singer DB, Oh W (1981): Effects of acidosis on the activity of creatine phosphokinase and its isoenzymes in the serum of newborn infants. Pediatrics 68:195–197.

71. Way GL, Pierce JR, Wolfe RR, McGrath R, Wiggins J, Merenstein GB (1979): ST depression suggesting subendocardial ischemia in neonates with respiratory distress syndrome and patent ductus arteriosus. J Pediatr 95:609–611.

72. Wolf PL, Kearns T, Neuhoff J, Lauridson J (1974): Identification of CPK isoenzyme MB in myocardial infarction. Lab Med 5:48–50.

73. Ziter FA (1974): Creatine kinase in developing skeletal and cardiac muscle of the rat. Exp Neurol 43:539–546.

74. Zweig MH, Van Steirteghem AC, Schecter AN (1978): Radioimmunoassay of creatine kinase isoenzymes in human serum: Isoenzyme BB. Clin Chem 24:422–428.

24 BLOOD GASES

Enid R. Kafer

During the past 2 decades, major progress has been made in neonatal cardiology and in the management of neonatal cardiac surgical patients. This progress is the result not only of improved understanding of neonatal physiology and the physiology of prematurity but also of improved ability to adapt and develop technology suitable for diagnosis, management, and monitoring of gas exchange and oxygen transport in neonates and premature infants. Nevertheless, major advances in invasive and noninvasive diagnostic and monitoring techniques that measure blood gases and pH or oxygen saturation and that are continuous, rapid in response, and accurate are required to optimize cardiac diagnosis and management, particularly during anesthesia, cardiac surgery, and critical care.

The physiologic factors that in neonates necessitate continuous measurement technology are (1) complexity of congenital cardiac malformations; (2) hemodynamic characteristics that allow changes in the direction and magnitude of shunt with changes in pressure and flow and that result in rapid changes in oxygenation; and (3) the relatively high metabolic rate that increases rapidly in response to increased physical or psychologic stress. The recent development of the transcutaneous oxygen ($PtcO_2$) and carbon dioxide ($PtcCO_2$) technology improved neonatal critical care.[64] Unfortunately, this technology is not ideal because of the instability of the polarographic $PtcO_2$ technology, multifactorial perturbations of the relationship between the arterial and the transcutaneous measurements, and relatively long response time. In addition, it has little if any role in cardiac diagnosis or anesthetic management. However, recent advances in pulse oximetry (which measures arterial oxygen saturation coincident with the arterial pulsation) and the development of vascular probes (fluorescent probes and reflective oximetry) suitable for neonates and premature infants are anticipated to contribute to both critical care monitoring and diagnosis. The parallel developments of more reliable respired gas oxygen (polarographic and paramagnetic) and carbon dioxide analyzers (mass spectrometry and infrared) have also improved ventilatory management during critical care and anesthesia. Although invasive technology has been used with difficulty in neonates and premature infants because of patient size and vascular access limitations, advances such as reflective oximetry that have an established role in adult cardiology[87] and critical care are technologically adaptable to infants for critical care and anesthesia.

The clinical blood gas laboratory, whether within the cardiac laboratory or critical care area or centrally located, has enabled accurate measurements of blood gases and oxygen content and saturation within the vascular system. However, such measurements from a single vessel at a single time have limited value in neonates because patency of the foramen ovale and ductus arteriosus permit dramatic swings in blood flow and arterial blood gases during changes in pulmonary and systemic vascular resistance. In neonates the demonstration of the effects of both anatomic congenital cardiac abnormalities and changes in pulmonary and extrapulmonary shunt on oxygenation requires both continuous and multisite measurements. Therefore, instruments designed to adequately monitor the rapid changes that occur in neonatal blood gas exchange will move measurement from the central clinical chemistry laboratory to the cardiac catheter laboratory, critical care area, and operating room. Currently, invasive biosensors designed to measure pH and blood gases as well as other biologic products (e.g., glucose, electrolytes) are undergoing preclinical evaluation.[100,124] Advances in the design of transducers and in signal processing and transmission using integrated circuits and fiberoptics are making possible the development of improved monitoring technology.[133]

The goals of this chapter are to provide a historical perspective on the development of in vivo and in vitro blood gas and associated technology; to describe the current methods of blood gas, pH, and oxyhemoglobin measurement; and to summarize methods and problems of invasive arterial monitoring and obtaining and interpreting blood gas values. The focus is on measurements relevant not only to the cardiac diagnostic laboratory but also on those made during critical care and cardiac surgery.

HISTORICAL PERSPECTIVE

Clinical Diagnosis and Cardiac Surgery

The early methods of diagnosis of cyanotic congenital heart disease were based on the clinical observation of cyanosis, which is usually associated with polycythemia and clubbing of the fingers. An early description of cyanosis is attributed to the Smith papyrus, which Breasted translated as "his lips are ruddy." Luckardt, a collaborator of Breasted, added, "I am inclined to the view that the

I gratefully acknowledge the secretarial contribution of Diena Burton and the artistic excellence of Ann Jennings of Medical Illustration. I also thank Herbert Harned, Jr., MD, for his constructive criticism of the manuscript.

Table 24–1. PARALLEL DEVELOPMENT OF BLOOD GAS TECHNOLOGY, PHYSIOLOGIC CALCULATIONS
AND CONCEPTS, INVASIVE TECHNOLOGY, AND SURGERY FOR CONGENITAL HEART DISEASE

Date	Blood Gas Measurement	Physiologic Measurements And Concepts	Invasive Technology	Pediatric Cardiac Surgery
1870–1900	Spectrophotometric and manometric measurement of O_2Hb, CO_2, and O_2 contents	Fick principle: A. Fick, 1870; dilution technique: Stewart, 1893, 1897	Isolated organ perfusion: Bunge, 1876, and Schroder, 1882	
1900–1929	Blood O_2 content: Van Slyke and Neill, 1924	Dilution technique for cardiac output: Stewart, 1921, Hamilton et al, 1928	Right-sided heart catheterization in humans: Forssman, 1929	Attempted closed pulmonary valvotomy: Doyen, 1923
1930		$a\bar{v}O_2D$ in humans: Jimenez Diaz and Sanchez Cuenco, 1930; cardiac output by Fick principle in patients: Klein, 1930	Pulmonary angiography; cardiopulmonary bypass in cats: Gibbon, 1937	Successful repair of patent ductus arteriosus: Gross and Hubbard, 1938
1940	Measurement of oxygen content in the right atrium, right ventricle, and pulmonary artery in congenital heart disease: Dexter et al, 1947	Measurement of cardiac output, shunt and gas exchange in patients; concepts of alveolar ventilation and maldistribution of ventilation perfusion: Richards, 1945; Rahn, 1949; Cournand, Riley 1949	Right-sided heart catheterization: Cournand, 1941; disc oxygenation: Bjork, 1948	Palliative shunt: Blalock and Taussig, 1945; Potts shunt, 1946
1950	Evolution of blood gas electrodes: pH, PCO_2 by Astrup, 1954; PO_2 by Clark, 1956; PCO_2 by Gertz and Loeschcke, 1958, Stow, 1957, and Severinghaus and Bradley, 1958	Thermodilution in anesthetized animals: Fegler, 1954; evolution of gas exchange concepts: Farhi, Rahn, 1955	Modern bubble oxygenator: Clark, 1950; application of thermodilution to postcardiac surgery pediatric patients, Boyd et al, 1959	Hypothermia for repair of atrial septal defect: Lewis, 1953; cardiopulmonary bypass in humans: Gibbon, 1954
1960	Development of $PtcO_2$: Huch, Huch, and Lübbers, 1969		Development of intra-arterial polarographic electrodes, invasive reflectance oximetry: Polanyi and Hehir, 1962; Hugenholtz et al, 1965	
1970	Advances in noninvasive transmittance oximetry: Hewlett-Packard	Continuous distributions of ventilation perfusion ratios: Wagner, West, 1974	Flow-directed thermodilution pulmonary artery catheters: Ganz, Swan, and associates 1970	Advances in cardiopulmonary bypass techniques: membrane oxygenations, filters, priming solution
1980	Pulse oximetry: Yoshiya et al, 1980; Yelderman and New, 1983	Clinical evaluation of oxygen transport using $S\bar{v}O_2$	Refinement of invasive reflective oximetry: Sperinde and Senelly, 1985	

References: 4, 14, 16, 25, 29, 30, 34–36, 42, 44, 52, 53, 58, 61, 64, 66, 68, 70, 71, 75, 87, 90, 97, 102, 103, 106, 107, 118, 132, 139, 152–154.

colour meant is the one medical men have in mind when they say a person is cyanotic. It is a mixture of a red and a blue." Human figures with blue skin are portrayed in many ancient Egyptian frescoes.[106]

The advent of surgical correction and palliation of congenital heart disease and the associated technology of cardiopulmonary bypass surgery necessitated both anatomic and functional diagnoses (Table 24–1).[14,19,58] In 1929, Forssmann successfully catheterized the right side of his own heart.[44] The technique of right-sided heart catheterization together with the measurement of blood oxygen contents was soon applied to the measurement of arteriovenous oxygen contents and the cardiac output in patients.[68,71] However, subsequent criticism of the safety of right-sided heart catheterization resulted in discontinuance of these procedures until Cournand and his associates advanced right-sided heart catheterization in the 1940s.[30] Cournand's studies with Baldwin and Himmelstein resulted in the publication of *Cardiac Catheterization in Congenital Heart Disease* in 1949.[29]

During the following decade, cardiac surgical procedures advanced with the development of palliative procedures to increase pulmonary blood flow by creation of a shunt[14,103] or creation of an atrial septal defect (ASD)[13] and reduction of pulmonary flow by banding.[85] Further development depended on the ability to stop the heart (hypothermia) and on cardiopulmonary bypass technology.[53,70,107] Subsequent refinements in cardiopulmonary bypass techniques and technology and in the associated anesthetic and critical care management of neonates and children have resulted in the surgical correction of an increasing number of congenital heart lesions. In addition, it is now possible to correct these lesions at an earlier age before irreversible changes in pulmonary vasculature or impairment of mental or physical development. These events have made the accurate functional and anatomic diagnosis of paramount importance, together with the ability to optimize anesthetic and critical care. The development of the technology to provide functional diagnoses as well as to optimize critical care was essential to these advances, as it will be to future progress.

History of Blood Gas and Oxyhemoglobin Measurement

The early history of the measurement of oxygen and carbon dioxide in the blood in the late 19th century parallels the development of chemical and spectrophotometric methods of studying hemoglobin (Hoppe-Seyler, 1825–1895), and manometric measurement of oxygen and carbon dioxide in the blood (Bohr, 1855–1911; Krogh, 1874–1949; and Hasselbalch, 1874–1962). Hoppe-Seyler obtained crystalline hemoglobin, attributed oxygen carrying capacity to hemoglobin, and demonstrated the absorption spectra for oxygenated and reduced hemoglobin.[97] Holmgren, in 1863, reported that the content and partial pressure of oxygen were higher in arterial than venous blood and that as the oxygenation of blood increased the partial pressure of carbon dioxide in the gas with which it was equilibrated also increased.[97] The latter was rediscovered by Christiansen, Douglas, and Haldane in 1914.[24] Bert, during the course of studies on the effects of hypoxia using barometric chambers, demonstrated the oxyhemoglobin dissociation curve by plotting partial pressures or equivalent percentages of oxygen against the oxygen content of blood.[12] Studies on the oxyhemoglobin dissociation curve were extended by Bohr, who observed the S-shaped curve, and by Krogh and Hasselbalch, who also reported that carbon dioxide reduced the oxygen binding to hemoglobin (Bohr effect).[15,97] Henderson, based on the data of Christiansen and coworkers, calculated the hydrogen ion dissociation constants for reduced and oxygenated hemoglobin and reported that the change in the dissociation constant for reduced hemoglobin was responsible for the "isohydric" uptake of carbon dioxide in the venous blood.[83]

As a result of systematic intense efforts by Henderson at Yale and by van Slyke at the Rockefeller Institute, knowledge of the steady-state reactions of oxygen and carbon dioxide were comprehensive by the 1920s.[98,99] The publications of these researchers demonstrate the application of laboratory methods to clinical medicine. Similar quantitative methods of gas and blood analysis were used by August and Marie Krogh and their associates in their studies on the role of diffusion in carbon dioxide and oxygen exchange in the lung, on nitrous oxide measurement of the cardiac output, and on exercise and comparative physiology. Barcroft (1872–1947), whose research spanned both organ and whole-body metabolism, together with pulmonary gas exchange and oxygen transport, used similar methods.[7] He also obtained arterial blood from his own radial artery for gas analysis in order to resolve the oxygen lung secretion controversy (1912). Barcroft subsequently turned his energies to a study of the respiration and circulation of fetal lambs and the mechanisms of the first breath.

Oxygen Content Measurement and Oximetry in Cardiac Diagnosis

The van Slyke manometric method of measuring the oxygen and carbon dioxide content of arterial and mixed venous blood was used extensively in measurement of the cardiac output (Fick principle),[30] in calculation of shunt, and also in measurement of step changes in oxyhemoglobin saturation (O_2Hb) in the right side of the heart.[139] The van Slyke technique is an absolute method of measuring the oxygen content in arterial or mixed venous blood. The amount of oxygen is measured by the height of a column of mercury (manometer) and results from the release of oxygen. The technique requires considerable technical skill and time. Dexter subsequently reported the vascular pressures and oxygen content in the right atrium, ventricle, and pulmonary artery in children with congenital heart disease.[34–36] The Fick principle was also used for measuring the cardiac output postoperatively following surgery for congenital heart disease.[16]

Cardiac Output and Shunt

The Fick principle states that the uptake or release of a substance by an organ is the product of the blood flow to that organ and the arteriovenous difference. The Fick principle as generally applied to oxygen uptake by the body or lungs, $\dot{V}O_2$, can be written mathematically as follows:

$$\dot{V}O_2 = \dot{Q}_t (CaO_2 - C\bar{v}O_2)$$

where CaO_2 = arterial oxygen content,

$C\bar{v}O_2$ = mixed venous oxygen content obtained from the pulmonary artery, and

$\dot{Q}p$ = pulmonary blood flow

$\dot{Q}_t$ = total blood flow or cardiac output.

In the absence of shunt, $\dot{Q}_t = \dot{Q}_p$, and cardiac output and pulmonary blood flow are equal. The $\dot{V}O_2$ was usually obtained by a 3-minute collection period of expired gas during stable, resting conditions. The above general equation was, therefore, expressed as follows:

$$\dot{Q}_t = \frac{\dot{V}O_2}{CaO_2 - C\bar{v}O_2}$$

The accumulative errors in measurement even under ideal resting and steady-state conditions were at least 10 per cent. Therefore, when the indicator dilution technique became available for patient studies it was widely accepted[2,134,150] and it remains in use as the principle of the thermodilution technique. However, inaccuracy of thermodilution measurement of cardiac output is increased in low cardiac output states, valvular regurgitation (non-exponential decay of indicator), or early recirculation. Nevertheless, although the indicator dilution technique was readily accepted in the measurement of the cardiac output, in vitro measurement of arterial and mixed venous blood oxygen content directly by manometry (van Slyke),[29,30,139] by oximetry (spectrophotometric), or by in-line measurement of arterial oxyhemoglobin (SaO_2)[59,149] continued to be used in cardiac catheterization to estimate the amount of shunt ($\dot{Q}_{sh}/\dot{Q}_t$) and to detect the level of the shunts.

Detection of the Level of Left-to-Right Shunt

Left-to-right shunts were demonstrated by obtaining sequential samples as a catheter was withdrawn from the pulmonary artery to the venae cavae. The criteria for a step increase in oxyhemoglobin saturation depended on the chamber in which the sample was obtained (mixing increases from the venae cavae to the pulmonary artery).[3] However, oximetry is only able to detect shunts greater than 25 per cent of the cardiac output. Therefore, when angiography became available it was combined with oximetry to improve the identification of the level of the shunts. The accuracy of identifying smaller left-to-right shunts was improved by inhaling an inert gas and detecting its early arrival in the right-sided heart circulation.[47,67] Although the use of in vitro oximetry made the measurement of shunt and detection of step changes in saturation in the right side of the heart more rapid, it did not contribute to the critical care of the neonate with heart disease. Wood and his group at the Mayo Clinic, however, used early in vivo models of ear oximetry to examine exercise tolerance in children with cyanotic congenital heart disease.[149]

Nevertheless, it should be noted that on examination of the oxyhemoglobin dissociation curve for normal adult hemoglobin (at pH 7.40 and 37°C) (see Fig. 24–7) it is evident that in the region of venous partial pressures of oxygen (30 to 60 mmHg) the oxyhemoglobin dissociation curve approaches linearity with a slope that ranges from 0.7 to 0.8 ($\Delta S\bar{v}O_2/\Delta P\bar{v}O_2$). Therefore, in this region, measurement of the O_2Hb for the purposes of detecting the level of a small left-to-right shunt is only minimally less sensitive than that of measuring the partial pressure of oxygen (PO_2). However, outside this region changes in O_2Hb do not linearly reflect the magnitude of shunt. In contrast, measurement of partial pressure of oxygen in arterial blood (PaO_2) and calculation of the alveolar-arterial difference (AaO_2P) are sensitive measures of shunt and ventilation–blood flow maldistribution. The sensitivity of using the venous O_2Hb in the premature or full-term neonate will depend on the position of the O_2Hb curve and the venous PO_2.

Evolution of Polarography and Blood Gas Electrodes

The modern era of blood gas and related measurement technology spans the past 30 years (see Table 24–1). The results of the evolution of these technologies were both a greater availability of blood gas measurements for critical care and anesthetic management (with improved reliability and accuracy and less demand for technical expertise) and a greater suitability for neonates as a result of the development of micromethods and more rapid measurement. The Danish poliomyelitis epidemic of 1952 provided the motivation for simpler and faster methods of pH and CO_2 measurement.[5] Similarly, progress in artificial organ perfusion, also in the 1950s, led to the modification of polarographic technology in order to measure oxygen in biologic fluids.[25] These changes were paralleled by the development of more rapid methods of gas analysis,[46] which enhanced the study of physiology and pathophysiology, including the measurement of transient events. Discussion of the modern evolution of the technology of blood gas and gas exchange measurements and their clinical and diagnostic laboratory application covers three main areas: (1) in vitro and in vivo measurement of arterial and transcutaneous blood gases and pH using conventional polarography and pH electrode technology, (2) rapid respired gas analysis together with its application to transcutaneous and arterial blood gas measurement, and (3) reflective and transmittance oximetry.

Polarographic Method of Measuring Oxygen Tension

The polarographic method of measuring oxygen at a metal surface was first demonstrated in Nernst's laboratory by Salomon (1897), Danneel (1897–1898), and others,[80] and 25 years later Heyrovský enunciated the principle.[62] Another 20 years were to elapse before Davies and Brink (1942)[31] were to make the platinum polarographic cathode a reliable instrument, and it was not until 1956 when Clark advocated the use of a membrane that the polarographic oxygen electrode could be used for measuring biologic fluids.[25] The Clark electrode involved the placement of a membrane permeable to O_2 over a platinum wire exposed by polishing and sealed in glass. The principle of polarography involves the application of a constant voltage to the polarographic cell and the generation of an electric current by the electrochemical reduction of oxygen. The current is directly proportional to the availability of oxygen. Subsequent refinements in design and performance of the polarographic electrode have resulted in smaller electrodes and use of less permeable membranes, which reduced the oxygen consumption of the electrode; in more accurate temperature control at 37°C; and in improved reliability.

Measurement of PCO_2 and pH

The pH and PCO_2 electrode underwent a series of refinements during the same time period. The bulb-type pH glass electrode that was originally used for blood gas analysis was replaced by the microcapillary glass electrode. The pH ultramicrocapillary electrode is composed of "pH sensitive" glass. The hydrogen ions in the unknown solution on the sample side of the glass electrode displace metal ions from the glass lattice work. This displacement establishes an electromagnetic force across the glass membrane of the electrode that is measured as a potential difference on the measuring electrode side of the glass.[1,123]

The PCO_2 is measured by three methods: (1) calculation from the pH of the blood and the plasma CO_2; (2) the interpolation method of Astrup and Siggaard-Andersen;[125,127] and (3) directly using a membrane-covered pH electrode. In the evolution to rapid, accurate, small sample volume and readily available technology to measure the arterial PCO_2 ($PaCO_2$) for patient care, the interpolation method played a critical role.[4,5,125,127] The interpolation method involved measurement of the arterial pH (pHa) and measurement of the pH of that blood that had been equilibrated with two known partial pressures of PCO_2 or at one known PCO_2 where the hemoglobin was known. The resulting pH–log PCO_2 line was then plotted onto a Siggaard-Andersen plot.[125] The "actual" $PaCO_2$ was obtained from the pH–log PCO_2 line ($PaCO_2$ at the pHa) and the base excess or deficit was obtained from the intersection of the pH–log PCO_2 line with the base excess/deficit curve. The success of this technology depended on an accurate micro-pH electrode as well as on a suitable microtonometer. In spite of the apparent complexity of the technology and procedures, the interpolation method made a major contribution to the development of clinical blood gas measurement and was rapidly available to anesthesiologists in many cardiac surgical facilities during the 1960s. In spite of theoretical objections, the base excess/deficit estimation of the buffer-base status of the body became a convenient guide for acid-base correction during anesthesia and surgery, particularly cardiac surgery.[113] The principle of the modern CO_2 electrode was demonstrated in 1957 by Gertz and Loeschcke[52,53] and by Stow[135] and subsequently described by Severinghaus and Bradley in 1958.[118] The CO_2 electrode consists of a pH electrode covered by a membrane permeable to CO_2 that holds a thin film of electrolyte solution containing sodium bicarbonate.

Clinical Applications

During the late 1950s and early 1960s, the technology and the clinical application of these in vitro blood gas measurements rapidly advanced. The application of the measurements was focused on respiratory physiologic and clinical studies, particularly on gas exchange (see Table 24–1) and, to a lesser extent, on respiratory control as well as on acute care during and following cardiac surgery.[50,144] As a result, during the 1960s an enormous volume of data on gas exchange in pulmonary, cardiac, and systemic disease was reported. The majority of these studies, because of the use of arterial cannulation, were in adults. However, a number of papers reported preoperative and postoperative gas exchange and blood gas measurement following cardiac surgery,[144] and a few included postoperative data on children.[50] Therefore, although these technologies were available to cardiac diagnostic laboratories, to measure shunts cardiologists continued to use the van Slyke manometric method to measure contents directly or to calculate the contents from the saturation obtained oximetrically, together with the hemoglobin concentration.[149]

The current generation of in vitro blood gas instruments that measure pH and blood gases at 37°C have performance characteristics of a short response time and accuracy within the full pathophysiologic range and can accept a sample size as small as 85 µl or 40 µl split sample (Corning Medical Systems, Medfield, MA). Unfortunately, these in vitro systems do not provide continuous measurement of the arterial blood gases, and the growing distance between the critical care unit, the operating room, the cardiac diagnostic laboratory, and the central blood gas laboratory does not facilitate rapid correction of clinical problems or rapid diagnosis. During the past 2 decades considerable effort has been devoted to the development of in vivo technology to measure the oxygen tension or oxyhemoglobin saturation. However, the practical problems include the relative large size of the cannulas, thrombi formation, electrode "drift," and difficulties in in vivo recalibration.[23] Nevertheless, a number of studies have reported the use of continuous intra-arterial monitoring in neonates.[136] The technology has now widened to include reflective oximetry (Oximetrix, Inc, Mountain View, CA) and fluorescence photometry. The latter is now undergoing development and evaluation prior to clinical application[81] (Cardiovascular Devices, Inc, Irvine, CA).

Transcutaneous Oxygen and Carbon Dioxide Measurement

In 1951, Baumberger and Goodfriend measured the PO_2 in heated phosphate buffer sealed in a test tube in which a finger was immersed.[11] They demonstrated that oxygen could pass through the skin in both directions depending on the gradient between the surface and the blood and that the PO_2 in the solution surrounding the finger was similar to that of the arterial blood. These studies were confirmed by Rooth and associates using a heated, bare platinum electrode.[109] Huch and associates, in 1969, using a special-surface polarographic electrode, demonstrated that the PaO_2 could be measured at selected sites in newborns after drug-induced hyperemia.[63]

Following the development of heated transcutaneous polarographic oxygen electrodes ($PtcO_2$) and the rapid application of these noninvasive devices to "trend" PaO_2, during the next decade transcutaneous oxygen measurement became a normal standard of practice in neonatal and premature critical care units.[117] Peevy and Hall reported that during the 4 years of application of $PtcO_2$ (1979–1982), $PtcO_2$ monitoring significantly contributed to a reduction in health care cost attributed to reduced blood gas analyses in neonates.[95] The transcutaneous oxygen electrode was soon complemented by the development of the transcutaneous CO_2 electrode ($PtcCO_2$). The $PtcCO_2$ electrodes were of two principles of design: the Stow-Severinghaus CO_2 electrode[119] and the infrared CO_2 absorption system.[39] Subsequently, the polarographic and Stow-Severinghaus CO_2 electrodes were combined.[116]

Although the $PtcO_2$ measurement was noninvasive, was continuous, and could be used to measure regional differences in $PtcO_2$, the technique had a number of practical problems, including electrode drift, complexity of the relationship between PaO_2 and the $PtcO_2$ and the prolonged response time. However, the advocates of the $PtcO_2$ technology claim that analysis of the factors that contribute to the difference between the PaO_2 and the $PtcO_2$, as well as the heat energy required to maintain a stable electrode temperature, provide additional information on the patient's hemodynamic status and tissue oxygenation.[8] In spite of these claims, the role of the $PtcO_2$ as a diagnostic tool in the cardiac laboratory and for monitoring during diagnostic studies or anesthesia for cardiac surgery is extremely limited.

Respired Gas Analysis

Development of continuous and short response time–respired gas analysis has had a less direct impact on neonatal care, including ventilatory management, than has the development of blood gas technology. Nevertheless, during anesthetic management, respired gas analysis (CO_2 and O_2) is rapidly becoming an essential standard of monitoring. A number of technical advances were essential and these included (1) the development of respired gas analysis devices whose performance characteristics included reliability and accuracy, small sample volume, specificity (i.e., noninterference by anesthetic gases), and short response time; (2) reduction in unit price and/or economic multiplexed systems; and (3) modification of the sampling system to reduce dilution of the expirate by the "fresh gas flow." The most important technical development in respired gas analysis was the design of the respiratory mass spectrometer by Fowler in the 1950s[46] and the subsequent technical advances that enabled the respiratory-anesthesia mass spectrometer to become a "user friendly" instrument. During the past 5 years, a number of manufacturers have offered multiplexed systems for the operating room and critical care areas. More recently, a number of advances in conventional gas analysis technology (i.e., infrared carbon dioxide and paramagnetic oxygen analysis) now offer acceptable individual gas

analysis systems (Datex/Instrumentarium OY, Helsinki; marketed by Puritan-Bennett Corporation, Wilmington, MA).

Oximetry

The principle of the oximetric measurement of oxygen saturation depends on the large difference in absorption between oxyhemoglobin and reduced hemoglobin in the red region of the spectrum (650 nm), whereas in the infrared spectrum (800 nm) the absorption is similar (isobestic point). The techniques of measurement are transmittance (cuvette or ear oximetry) and reflectance (cuvette or in vivo catheter).

Transmittance Oximetry

Transmittance oximetry that was to be applied to the noninvasive measurement of arterial oxygen saturation was developed separately by Mathes and Kramer in 1935.[59,149] The measurement site was intact blood vessels in the ear through which light could be transmitted and the arterial blood flow increased to minimize interference from venous blood. Deviations from the Lambert-Beer law between whole blood in vessels and hemolyzed or hemoglobin solution necessitated calibration for the red cell concentration. A series of commercial instruments were developed, and the technique was used extensively in studies at high altitudes, in aviation medicine, and in physiologic studies in children with congenital heart disease.[21,59,149] However, when the arterial oxygen saturation measured by the standard van Slyke method was compared with ear oximetry, the deviation of ear oximetry was 2 to 4 per cent.[59] Although the blood flow of the ear could be increased to minimize the error from venous blood, other variables including skin pigmentation, ear thickness, blood flow, and hemoglobin concentration contributed to the inaccuracy.

Attempts were made to improve the accuracy of noninvasive transmission spectroscopy by measurement of SaO_2 at multiple wavelengths,[74] but it was not until the technology was developed to measure absorption at multiple wavelengths and to process the data electronically that the accuracy became acceptable. In the 1960s Hewlett-Packard developed an ear oximeter that measured absorption at eight different wavelengths (650–1050 nm), and that was designed to eliminate the effects of skin pigmentation, ear thickness, incident light, and ear motion artifacts (HP 47201A, Hewlett-Packard, 2/75).[61] Over the range of 70 to 90 per cent saturation, when the SaO_2 obtained by ear oximetry was compared with measured SaO_2 (IL Co-Oximeter), the Hewlett-Packard 47201A was within acceptable accuracy for black subjects and for white and Asian subjects. The accuracies were 100 to 90 ± 1.7 per cent, 90 to 80 ± 2.0 per cent, 80 to 70 ± 2.3 per cent and 70 to 60 ± 2.6 per cent. Because the in vivo response time depends on light transmission, the response is immediate, and the instrument can be adjusted to average the SaO_2 over one or several cardiac pulsations (i.e., from 1.5 to 4.7 seconds).

Clinical studies confirmed the instrument's accuracy,[112,129] although in the presence of COHb or SaO_2 less than 65 per cent, the Hewlett-Packard 47201A overreads or underreads, respectively, the SaO_2.[38] The instrument became the standard for adult studies in sleep, exercise, and respiratory control. However, even for adults the ear probe was bulky. No suitable technology was developed for infants or children.

Recent advances in microprocessor and electronic technology have resulted in the development of an oximeter that measures the SaO_2 by transmittance absorption at the red and infrared wavelengths coincident with the pulse (pulse oximetry).[153] Probes are available for all patient sizes including neonates and may also be used for different regions of the body (Nellcor, Inc, Hayward, CA).

Reflectance Oximetry

The development of technology to measure in vivo oxyhemoglobin saturation by reflectance oximetry was an extension of the demonstration that in vitro reflectance oximetry was accurate[18] and of the manufacture of a satisfactory instrument for clinical evaluation.[102,143] More recently, as a result of advances in fiberoptics and microelectronics, intravascular reflectance oximetry now provides the ability to continuously monitor the mixed venous oxygen saturation ($S\bar{v}O_2$) together with pulmonary artery pressures and thermodilution measurement of cardiac output (Oximetrix Opticath, Oximetrix, Inc, Mountain View, CA). This technology has rapidly become an essential tool in the management of critically ill patients, including during cardiac anesthesia. The $S\bar{v}O_2$ is used as an index of the adequacy of cardiac output for oxygen transport in relation to the oxygen consumption.[6,82,142] It is interesting to note that fiberoptic reflectance oximetry was initially developed to provide continuous intra-arterial (umbilical artery) monitoring in neonates with pulmonary disease[137,146,147] (size 4 F catheter with a single lumen for pressure monitoring). As the technology advanced and the accuracy improved, invasive reflectance oximetry was applied in critical care, in anesthetic management of high-risk patients including cardiac patients, and in both the diagnosis and management of congenital heart disease.[40,49,66,94,102,142]

CURRENT MEASUREMENT METHODS

Arterial Oxygen Tension

In Vitro Measurement of the PaO2

PRINCIPLE

The polarographic cell is the basis of measurement of the PaO_2 in blood gas analyzers. Polarography produces an electrochemical reaction in which oxygen molecules are reduced and the resulting current is proportional to the availability of oxygen. The polarographic cell consists of a cathode (noble metal such as gold, silver, or platinum of

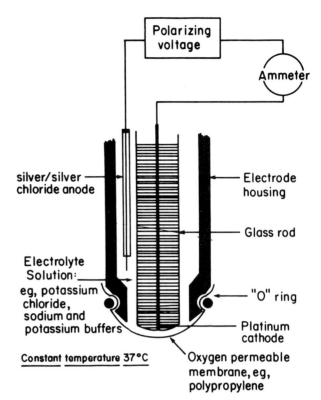

Figure 24–1. Schematic of an oxygen polarographic electrode system. The schematic demonstrates the platinum wire (cathode) imbedded in a glass rod, silver/silver chloride anode, electrolyte solution, polymer membrane with retaining "O" ring and housing. The polarographic oxygen electrode system is maintained at a constant temperature of 37°C.

20-μm diameter), an anode, an electrolyte solution, a membrane, and an external circuit for applying a constant voltage (−600 to −800 mV range) (Fig. 24–1). Each substance that is reduced by polarography has a characteristic sigmoid-shaped current-voltage curve (polarogram), and for oxygen the current-voltage curve is flat in the region of −500 to −800 mV (Fig. 24–2). Therefore, in this region of the plateau (e.g., −650 mV), polarization with a constant voltage results in a direct linear relationship between the oxygen available to the cathode and the current. Oxygen diffuses from the blood sample through the membrane and is dissolved in the electrolyte solution, through which it diffuses to the cathode. In practice, the polarizing voltage is fixed so that the cathode is operating within the diffusion-limited zone and, therefore, the current is directly and linearly related to the PO_2 in the sample or calibration gas.[1] In the majority of the commercial systems, the anode is a silver/silver chloride electrode. The electrolyte solution consists of potassium chloride, sodium, and potassium buffers with potassium hydroxide. The pH of the electrolyte solution is usually in the region of pH 7. The membrane that separates the sample from the electrolyte solution is permeable to oxygen but impermeable to water, electrolytes, and proteins. A number of different membrane polymers have been used, including polyethylene, polypropylene, Mylar, and Teflon (20 μm

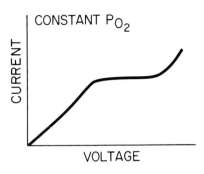

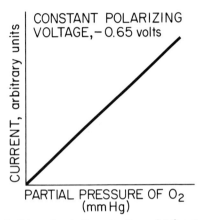

Figure 24–2. Schematic. *A,* Current-voltage plot for constant partial pressure of oxygen (polarogram) showing the "plateau" between –400 and –800 mV polarization. *B,* The linear relationship between partial pressure of oxygen and current where the constant polarization voltage is within the plateau region (e.g., –650 mV).

thick). Polypropylene is used in most modern blood gas analyzers. Modern blood gas systems control the temperature to within 0.1°C of 37°C.

TECHNICAL PROBLEMS

The technical problems include instrumentation, calibration, effects of other gases, and sampling problems. The modern blood gas instrument is the product of 2 decades of design development that optimizes stability, sensitivity, response time, and acceptance of small samples.[123] In order to optimize performance the operator should adhere strictly to the manufacturer's recommendations for maintenance, membrane replacement, cathode cleaning, and quality assurance. Errors in calibration include allowing air to mix with oxygen calibration gas, residual debris in the cuvette, unstable temperature control, and the theoretical difference between liquid and gas calibration.[1] The two most important gases that are reduced by a polarographic cell are nitrous oxide and halothane.[120] At the polarizing voltage used by most manufacturers, the effects of nitrous oxide and halothane are small but nevertheless may result in an erroneously high PO_2 measurement.[104] In the clinical environment, sampling problems are the most important and include failure to obtain an anaerobic sample, failure to clear a sample line or catheter in order to obtain a current sample, pulling against a negative pressure, excess heparin, and

prolonged transport time.[123] The use of liquid heparin in syringes, which is common in the clinical environment and aggravated by small blood samples that are used for neonates, results in a dilutional error. The direction of the dilutional error for oxygen depends on the actual PO_2 in the gas with which the heparin has been equilibrated. Although a number of different types of dry heparin have been evaluated for use in prepared syringes or capillary tubes, some of this heparin dissolves poorly or has a limited shelf life. The current recommended standards are the use of lithium lyophilized heparin in syringes (1, 3, 5 ml) and a similar preparation of heparin in capillary tubes that are used for neonates (Radiometer America, Inc, Westlake, OH; Corning Medical Instruments, Medfield, MA; Marquest Medical Products, Inc, Englewood, CO).

In Vivo Measurement of PaO₂

Devices designed for intravascular, specifically arterial, measurement of the PO_2 as well as tissue measurement of PO_2 are available for clinical or experimental application. The goal has been to provide continuous on-line measurement of the PaO_2, particularly in critically ill patients in whom hemodynamic or gas exchange deterioration may result in a rapid decrease in the PaO_2. These clinical problems include neonatal and adult respiratory distress syndromes. The problem of rapid deterioration of oxygenation is critical in neonates in whom hyperoxia results in retrolental fibroplasia and hypoxia causes brain damage.[60,93,108,136] Three types of intravascular devices that measure PaO_2 are available or undergoing preclinical evaluation: (1) in vivo polarographic electrode, (2) in vivo mass spectrometer probe, and (3) optical fluorescence probe.

IN VIVO POLAROGRAPHIC OXYGEN ELECTRODE

The polarographic oxygen electrode is the most common intravascular system used for measuring PO_2.[60,93,136] The tip of the catheter with the cathode is covered by an oxygen-permeable polymer, and the anode is placed either behind the cathode or with a reference electrode (anode) on the skin.[93,138] In addition to calibration prior to insertion, the electrodes are also calibrated in vivo by withdrawing a blood sample through the lumen proximal to the cathode and then analyzing it with an in vitro blood gas instrument. The major problems include instability, variable response time, thrombi formation, technical difficulty in production, and relatively large size of the catheter and electrode. Manufacture with an antithrombogenic polymer[138] or bonding or coating the polymer with heparin theoretically reduces the incidence of thrombi formation. Although electrodes small enough to pass through an 18-gauge cannula with sufficient space to sample blood (22 gauge) or measure pressure have been developed, an 18-gauge cannula is a larger size than is the normal standard of practice for radial artery sampling in children or adults. Intravascular polarographic oxygen probes are available (Neocath 100, Biomedical Sensors, Inc, Kansas

City, MO). These bi-lumen catheters are 5 F (1.7 mm OD), 50 cm long, and 4 F (1.35 mm OD), 35 cm long. The latter are designed for the umbilical artery of the neonate.

IN VIVO MEASUREMENT OF BLOOD GASES BY MASS SPECTROMETRY

Since Woldring and associates, in 1966, described the use of the mass spectrometer to measure the PaO_2 and $PaCO_2$ in the aorta of the cat, a number of researchers have reported the validation, the technical aspects of the diffusion membrane (Teflon or Silastic coated with heparin), and the design of catheters for the application of this technique.[17,43,148] The majority of these studies have been in experimental animals, and the clinical application has therefore been limited. More recently, attention has been directed to the use of mass spectrometry technology in the transcutaneous measurement of PO_2 and CO_2.[92,151]

IN VIVO MEASUREMENT OF OXYGEN USING AN OPTICAL FLUORESCENCE PROBE

Oxygen quenches fluorescence by colliding with the fluorescent molecule (e.g., pyrene-3-butyric acid) when it is in an activated state. The quenching is proportional to the amount of oxygen present and may be measured electronically using an optical probe.[78,81,84,101,140] Optical fluorescence technology has primarily been used to measure PO_2 in tissues such as the brain.[78,84,101] However, recent advances in fiberoptic technology have enabled the development of an experimental oxygen fluorescence probe for intravascular use.[51] Concurrently, a commercial in-line multimodality measurement system using optical fluorescence technology that measures the pH, PO_2 and PCO_2 in the cardiopulmonary bypass circuit is now available (CDI System 200 Extracorporeal Blood Gas Monitoring System, Cardiovascular Devices, Inc, Irvine, CA). In addition, a module for intra-arterial measurement in adults is also available (CDI Intravascular Blood Gas Monitoring System). It is anticipated that the manufacturer will extend the development of this technology to clinical intravascular probes suitable for placement in the umbilical artery of neonates (personal communication, 1987).

Arterial Carbon Dioxide Tension and Blood pH Measurement

As described in the history of measurement of the $PaCO_2$, three methods are available for measuring the $PaCO_2$: (1) calculation from the pHa and the CO_2 content, (2) the interpolation method, and (3) direct measurement using a membrane-covered pH electrode (Stow-Severinghaus electrode). The last method is now used almost exclusively in commercial blood gas instruments (e.g., Corning Medical Instruments, Medfield, MA; Radiometer America, Inc, Westlake, OH).

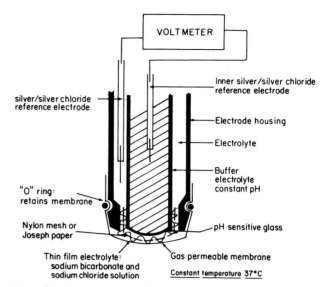

Figure 24–3. Schematic of a CO_2 electrode demonstrating the circuit, voltmeter, pH sensitive glass electrode, electrolyte with nylon mesh or Joseph paper, membrane with retaining "O" ring, reference electrodes, and housing. The CO_2 electrode system is maintained at a constant temperature of 37°C.

Carbon Dioxide Electrode

PRINCIPLE

The carbon dioxide electrode consists of a pH electrode (pH-sensitive glass with an inner silver/silver chloride reference electrode) housed behind a membrane permeable to carbon dioxide and enclosing a bicarbonate electrolyte solution in continuity with a reference electrode. The circuit is completed by a voltmeter (Fig. 24–3). The carbon dioxide diffuses across the membrane into the electrolyte solution adjacent to the pH electrode and by reaction with water changes the pH gradient across the electrode. By designing the instrument with only a very thin layer of electrolyte solution between the membrane and the pH electrode, only a small fraction of carbon dioxide molecules have to diffuse into the area to effect a change in pH. The bulk of the electrolyte does not participate in the equilibration process and, therefore, serves as a reservoir and an electrical conductor.

DESIGN

The pH glass electrode contains a silver/silver chloride reference electrode, and its glass surface is adjacent to the membrane (see Fig. 24–3). The Teflon membrane that separates the glass electrode from the sample solution holds a thin film of electrolyte (0.1 molar sodium bicarbonate and 0.1 molar sodium chloride) within a nylon or Joseph paper mesh. The electrode system is housed within a constant temperature system at 37°C. In order to optimize the equilibration process with the electrolyte beneath the membrane, a calibration solution should always be kept in the sample chamber between readings. It should be noted that because all the reactions are reversible and no component is consumed as in a polarographic oxygen

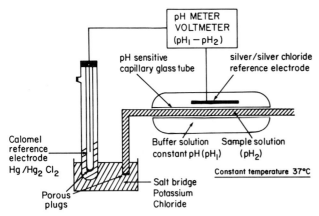

Figure 24–4. Schematic of a micro pH capillary tube electrode showing the circuit, blood sample solution (pH_2), pH sensitive capillary tube, constant pH buffer solution (pH_1), silver/silver chloride reference electrode, potassium chloride salt bridge with ceramic plugs, calomel reference electrode (Hg/Hg_2Cl_2), and pH meter (voltmeter). (Adapted with permission of Adams AP, Hahn CEW: Principles and Practice of Blood Gas Analysis. London, Churchill Livingstone, 1982, and Franklin Scientific Projects, London, 1979.)

electrode, both gases and liquid solutions will have the same PCO_2. That is, there is no so-called liquid-gas difference as described for the PO_2 electrode.

TECHNICAL PROBLEMS

The potential technical problems are similar to the polarographic electrode and are concerned with maintenance, calibration, and sampling. The PCO_2 electrode measurement is not interfered with by anesthetics such as nitrous oxide or halothane.

Blood pH Measurement

The principle of the glass pH electrode is based on the Nernst equation for the development of an electromotive force across a membrane. The "membrane" is the glass electrode, which responds quantitatively and specifically only to hydrogen ions. The electrode is not influenced by dissolved gases, such as oxygen or carbon dioxide, or by oxidizing or reducing agents. The potential difference that develops between the "inner" and "outer" (sample side) surfaces of the glass microcapillary electrode is directly related to the corresponding hydrogen ion gradient. The characteristics of the glass are important, and they include a relatively high degree of purity as well as a thin wall (0.003 inch). The circuit is completed by a silver/silver chloride reference electrode in contact with the inner surface of the pH electrode, a potassium chloride solution between the sample and the calomel reference electrode, and a pH meter (voltmeter) between the silver/silver chloride and calomel reference electrodes (Fig. 24–4).[123] As in the use of other blood gas electrodes, the temperature is maintained at 37°C. The sources of error are attributed to design, maintenance and calibration errors, and sampling problems. The design of the pH measuring device (which includes the junctions between the sample and the potassium chloride, and between the potassium chloride and

the calomel electrode) and the specifications of the potassium chloride solution result in a reduction of artifacts and minimize maintenance problems.[123] Proper maintenance and recognition of slow or erratic responses and testing for cracks in the electrode are important. Sampling problems are equally important for pH measurement as they are for the blood gas measurements.

In Vivo Arterial PCO_2 and pH Measurement Systems

In vivo arterial PCO_2 systems (membrane-covered pH electrode or mass spectrometer systems) and pH systems have been developed. However, the use of these systems has primarily been in experimental animals.[26,27,76,89] As described previously, multimodality probes that measure pH, PCO_2 and PO_2 are now under development for intravascular monitoring (Cardiovascular Devices, Inc, Irvine, CA).

Calculated Acid-Base Parameters

Several calculated acid-base parameters are derived from the arterial blood pH, blood gases, and hemoglobin concentration. The modern blood gas analyzers that use microprocessors "automatically" print out and transmit the blood gas and derived data via hospital information systems to the critical care areas and operating rooms. Although controversy exists as to the theory, interpretation, and practical application of these derived variables, they are frequently used as a guide to management, particularly during anesthesia and critical care. The following calculations of the plasma bicarbonate, standard bicarbonate, and base excess/deficit are based on the Henderson-Hasselbalch equations and other equations that characterize the buffer systems of the blood and the body fluids. These equations incorporate "constants" and coefficients of equilibrium that vary between individual patients and may vary over time within a patient. Additional problems include corrections for temperature deviations, which are particularly important in the management of accidental or induced hypothermia.[1,123]

The standard bicarbonate level is the bicarbonate level referenced to a $PaCO_2$ of 40 mmHg at a temperature of 37°C with fully oxygenated hemoglobin. The normal value is between 22 and 26 millimole·liter^{-1}. The base deficit or excess is the titratable acid or base to a pH of 7.40 at a PCO_2 of 40 mmHg and temperature of 37°C (normal value ± 2.5 millimole·liter^{-1}). The actual bicarbonate level is the bicarbonate ion concentration in the blood or plasma, and the exact value depends on the method of measurement. When derived from the $PaCO_2$ and pHa, the value of plasma bicarbonate in arterial blood ranges from 22 to 26 millimole·liter^{-1}. The total carbon dioxide content in blood includes bicarbonate ion (plasma and red cell), dissolved carbon dioxide, carbonate ion, carbamate ion, and carbamino groups on proteins. In plasma, the amounts of the last three are negligible. Therefore, in modern blood gas analyzers, the total plasma carbon dioxide content refers to the bicarbonate ion and the

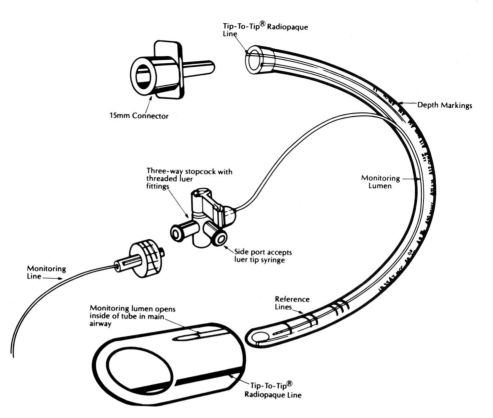

Figure 24–5. Drawing of an uncuffed Mallinckrodt Critical Care (MCC) pediatric endotracheal tube showing the monitoring lumen for respired CO_2 measurement. (Reproduced with permission of Mallinckrodt, Mallinckrodt Critical Care Division, Glens Falls, New York.)

dissolved carbon dioxide. Normal total plasma carbon dioxide content is 25.2 millimole·liter^{-1} (24 + [0.0306 × 40]).

Respired Gas Analysis

As a result of improved technology, clinical advantages of continuous respired gas analysis, and risk-limiting standards of monitoring, the continuous monitoring of both respired carbon dioxide and oxygen is today normal practice during general anesthesia and controlled mechanical ventilation. The recent advances in respired gas analysis include a reduced sampling rate with maintenance of 90 per cent response time for both carbon dioxide and oxygen of 200 to 300 msec. In addition, several manufacturers have developed pediatric size endotracheal tubes that have a sample port at the tracheal end, thus minimizing the problem of inadequate end-tidal sampling (Mallinckrodt, Inc, Glens Falls, NY; Sheridan Catheter Corporation, Argyle, NY). Therefore, respired gas analysis can now be used to optimize ventilatory management in the operating room and during critical care in neonates (Fig. 24–5). The respired carbon dioxide measurement provides four categories of information: (1) the end-tidal carbon dioxide value, which usually is 5 to 12 mmHg lower than the $PaCO_2$ and is a reasonable guide over time to the direction of the $PaCO_2$; (2) the slope and shape of the alveolar plateau, which are indicative of pulmonary function or severe airway obstruction; (3) short-term trends in end-tidal carbon dioxide (video display or recorder), such as decreases parallel to decreases in cardiac output (delivery

of carbon dioxide to the lungs); and (4) long-term trends in end-tidal carbon dioxide, such as decreases parallel to increases in alveolar ventilation (relative to carbon dioxide production), or increases parallel to decreases in alveolar ventilation (relative to the carbon dioxide production) (e.g., a decrease in minute ventilation or increase in ventilation–blood flow maldistribution, V_D/V_T). In addition, an inspired carbon dioxide measurement greater than zero indicates malfunction of the breathing circuit or insufficient fresh gas flow. Therefore, in ventilatory management monitoring, display of respired carbon dioxide with "trending" is now recognized as an extremely informative clinical tool.

Oxyhemoglobin Dissociation Curve and Blood Oxygen Content

The arterial or other blood hemoglobin oxygen saturation is obtained by in vitro measurement, or by calculation from the blood gases and from the oxyhemoglobin dissociation curve (ODC), or by measurement in vivo by either transmittance or reflectance absorption spectroscopy. The measurement of hemoglobin concentration (THb), oxyhemoglobin (O_2Hb) saturation and dyshemoglobins, if present, by transmission absorption spectroscopy depends on the principles of the Lambert-Beer law and on differences and similarities in the absorptions (extinction coefficients) of hemoglobin, oxyhemoglobin, and the dyshemoglobins at different wavelengths in the red and infrared wavelengths. Variations of this principle are used in vitro (e.g., IL Co-Oximeter, Instrumentation Laboratory, Inc,

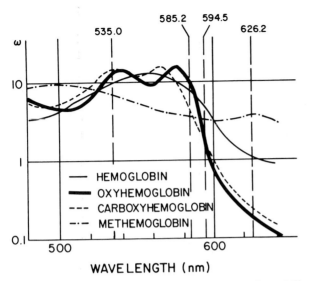

Figure 24–6. Extinction coefficients (ε) for hemoglobin, oxyhemoglobin, carboxyhemoglobin, and methemoglobin in the range of wavelengths of 480 to 640 nm showing the wavelengths at which absorption is measured in the IL-282 Co-Oximeter. (Redrawn with permission of Instrumentation Laboratory, Lexington, Massachusetts. Copyright 1977, Instrumentation Laboratory.)

Lexington, MA) (Fig. 24–6)[20,33,149] and in vivo (e.g., Nellcor Pulse Oximeter, Nellcor Inc, Hayward, CA). The absorption spectra depend on both the ligand status of heme moiety and the structure of the globin molecule. Therefore corrections are also made for different animal species and human globins.[28,33,65,110,155]

Oximeter Measurement of Oxyhemoglobin Saturation

The current standard in vitro method of measurement depends on the characteristic absorption patterns for oxyhemoglobin (O_2Hb), reduced hemoglobin (RHb), and the dyshemoglobins, carboxyhemoglobin (COHb) and methemoglobin (MetHb) (IL282 Co-Oximeter, Instrumentation Laboratory, Inc, Lexington, MA) (see Fig. 24–6).[20,33,123] It is assumed that any other hemoglobin species are present in negligible quantity. The concentrations of O_2Hb, RHb, COHb, and MetHb are calculated from four independent measurements with four independent equations. The specific absorption spectral lines were selected to minimize error from wavelength shift (535.0, 585.2, 594.5 and 626.6 nm) (see Fig. 24–6). These wavelengths are fixed by the properties of the sources and, therefore, so also are the extinction coefficients (ε) (IL282 Co-Oximeter Operations Manual, 1977).[20] The total hemoglobin is the sum of all the hemoglobin species, and each species is expressed as a percentage of the total hemoglobin. The oxygen content is obtained by adding the product of the hemoglobin concentration oxygen saturation and the hemoglobin oxygen binding capacity (1.34 ml·g⁻¹) to the dissolved oxygen. The hemoglobin oxygen binding capacity, however, may vary from 1.30 to 1.45 ml·g⁻¹ both within and between different animal species. The IL282 Co-Oximeter also offers the software to calculate the

THb, Rhb, O_2Hb, and dyshemoglobins if they are present for other animal species.[33] Sources of error from the spectrophotometric measurement of O_2Hb and the dyshemoglobins include errors in calibration, use of incorrect algorithms for animal species, and spectral interfering substances. By eliminating wavelengths shorter than 500 nm and longer than 630 nm, interference from bilirubin and Cardiogreen, respectively, are eliminated.[20] However, hyperlipidemia may interfere with the measurements.[123] High concentrations of methemoglobin interfere with the measurement of O_2Hb, particularly if O_2Hb is less than 60 per cent.[126] High levels of COHb also interfere with the measurement of O_2Hb. In addition, because of the similarity in absorption spectra between COHb and fetal hemoglobin (HbF), high concentrations of HbF may demonstrate falsely high concentrations of COHb and therefore low O_2Hb (Instrumentation Laboratory, Inc, Lexington, MA, personal communication).[28,65,110,155] Cornelissen and associates report a method for correcting the values of COHb and O_2Hb in the presence of HbF, and this correction algorithm is incorporated into the software of the new IL-482 Co-Oximeter (Instrumentation Laboratory, Inc, Lexington, MA, personal communication).

Oxyhemoglobin Dissociation Curve and Oxygen Affinity

The position of the ODC and therefore the affinity for oxygen is dependent on the structure of the globin molecule (e.g., HbF in comparison with HbA), the ligand status of the heme moiety, the pH, the PCO_2, the concentration of organic phosphates (e.g., 2,3-diphosphoglycerate [2,3-DPG]) within the erythrocyte, and also the temperature. The position of the curve, with corrections for pH, PCO_2, and temperature may be expressed mathematically or graphically.[114,115] The affinity of hemoglobin for oxygen is also expressed as the P_{50}, which is the partial pressure at which 50 per cent of the hemoglobin is saturated with oxygen.[9,10] For normal adult humans the P_{50} is 26 mmHg (37°C, pH 7.40, PCO_2 40 mmHg, and normal hemoglobin concentration), and in neonates the P_{50} increases with age from 19.9 in the premature infant to 27.2 at 6 years of age (Table 24–2 and Fig. 24–7).[111,141] The increase in P_{50} parallels the decrease in HbF and the increase in 2,3-DPG in the erythrocyte. Therefore, in order to calculate the O_2Hb from the PO_2, in addition to the pH, PCO_2, and body temperature, the P_{50} or the position of the ODC should also be known. An increase in P_{50} decreases the affinity of hemoglobin for oxygen, whereas a decrease in P_{50} increases the affinity. Therefore, as a result of all these variables, particularly in neonates, where the P_{50} varies with the HbF and the erythrocyte 2,3-DPG concentration, calculation of the oxygen hemoglobin saturation may be inaccurate.

Pharmacologic Influences on the Oxyhemoglobin Dissociation Curve

Shifts in the ODC and changes in P_{50} have been attributed to a number of drugs used in anesthesia or cardiac

Table 24–2. HEMOGLOBIN CONCENTRATION, BLOOD O_2 CAPACITY, AND P_{50} OF NEONATAL, INFANT, AND ADULT BLOOD

Age	Hemoglobin Concentration (g·dl⁻¹)	Blood Oxygen Capacity (ml·dl⁻¹)	HbF (%)	P_{50} (mmHg)
Premature	16.26	21.80 ± 2.30	74.8 ± 3.8	19.91 ± 1.44
Full term	17.65	23.65 ± 2.51	59.1 ± 7.9	21.50 ± 1.57
5–10 days	16.89	22.63 ± 2.51	53.7 ± 6.6	22.87 ± 1.40
11–20 days	15.87	21.26 ± 2.58	50.3 ± 4.5	23.60 ± 1.33
21–30 days	13.54	18.14 ± 2.94	42.8 ± 6.2	24.60 ± 1.45
60–120 days	11.00	14.74 ± 1.83	19.4 ± 6.2	26.74 ± 2.64
6 months	11.12	14.90 ± 0.88	4.1 ± 2.1	27.47 ± 2.43
6 years	13.10	17.55 ± 1.37	1.2 ± 0.8	27.15 ± 1.59
Adult	14.28	19.13 ± 1.65	0	25.87 ± 1.28

Notes: Mean ± SD; n = 6 to 12 infants. Adapted with permission from Versmold H et al (1973): Blood oxygen affinity in infancy: The interaction of fetal and adult hemoglobin oxygen capacity and red cell hydrogen ion and 2,3-diphosphoglycerate concentration. Respir Physiol 18:14–25.

management. Diethyl ether, enflurane, nitrous oxide, and cyclopropane were reported to shift the curve to the right in vivo,[130] and an increase in P_{50} of 0.5 to 7 mmHg was also shown for halothane.[54] However, halothane is polarographically reduced, and this accounts for the shift in the P_{50}.[145] Conflicting evidence continues to be reported on the effect of nitrous oxide in vitro on the P_{50}.[45,121] Again, polarographic reduction of nitrous oxide could cause a small shift to the right. Lidocaine in vitro has no effect on the ODC.[22] Propranolol, both in vivo and in vitro, has been reported to increase the P_{50}.[96]

Blood Oxygen Content

The relationship between the oxyhemoglobin saturation (S%), oxygen tension (PO_2) and oxygen content (CaO_2, $CćO_2$ or $C\bar{v}O_2$) is written as follows:

$$\text{Oxygen content} = \frac{S\%}{100} \times Hb \times 1.34 + \alpha PO_2$$

where Hb is the hemoglobin concentration, 1.34 is the hemoglobin oxygen binding capacity, and α is the solubility coefficient of oxygen in the blood. The oxygen content variables are those conventionally used in the equations for shunt and cardiac output using the Fick equation. Therefore, until the availability of dye and thermodilution techniques, measurement of oxygen content was of fundamental importance in calculation of the cardiac output and shunt. However, although cardiac output is now usually measured by thermodilution and the site(s) and magnitude of shunts are identified by angiography, by radionuclide techniques, or by echocardiography, measurement of the mixed venous oxygen saturation

($S\bar{v}O_2$) and indices of oxygen transport are a valuable guide to management in critical care.[87]

Until recently, the arterial and mixed venous oxygen contents were measured by the van Slyke manometric technique.[139] Because this technique requires considerable skill and time it became impracticable. In order to obviate the error in calculation of the blood oxygen content and as a result of the availability of the polarographic oxygen

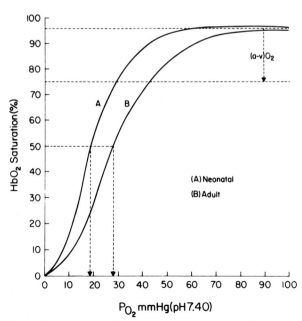

Figure 24–7. Oxyhemoglobin dissociation curves and P_{50} for adult hemoglobin (HbA) and fetal hemoglobin (HbF). (Reproduced with permission of Sacks LM, Delivoria-Papadopoulos M [1984]: Hemoglobin-oxygen interactions. Semin Perinatol 8:168–183.)

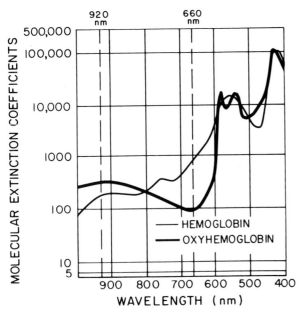

Figure 24–8. Absorption coefficients for oxyhemoglobin and reduced hemoglobin and the wavelength measurements within the infrared and red spectrum in a pulse oximeter.

electrode, a number of methods of directly measuring the oxygen content of blood were developed. These methods involve the release of oxygen from hemoglobin (saponin ferricyanide) and the polarographic measurement of oxygen. A number of techniques and devices have been developed in order to improve the efficiency and accuracy of these methods.[1,72,123]

Noninvasive Continuous Transmission Oximetry

Pulse Oximetry

Pulse oximetry, a noninvasive, optical method of measuring the arterial oxygen saturation was first described by Yoshiya and associates in 1980.[122,154] There are now a large range of pulse oximeters commercially available that use similar principles of operation (Fig. 24–8). They do, however, differ concerning the details of operation; processing, display, and transmission of physiologic variables; default and selectable alarm values; probes, including the availability of neonatal and infant probes; and reported accuracy of measurement of the SaO_2. Several oximeters are compact, lightweight, as well as battery operated and thus suitable for transport monitoring within the hospital and air or surface transport monitoring.

THEORY OF OPERATION

Although the pulse oximeters are similar in principle, they differ in the details of operation. The following description will be based on the Nellcor N-100 (Figs. 24–8 to 24–11). The pulse oximeter combines the technique of transmittance spectroscopy at two wavelengths (660 nm and 940 nm),[152] with measurement of absorption coincident with the arterial pulsation, thus eliminating the confounding variables of venous blood, skin pigmentation, and skin thickness. The probe (or transducer) consists of two light-emitting diodes (LEDs), one in the visible red (660 nm) spectrum and one in the infrared (940 nm) spectrum, and a photodiode (photodetector). The three components are mounted in the finger receptacle (reusable) or one of a series of disposable probes (see Fig. 24–10) that supports them and maintains contact with the finger. The LEDs alternate through a high frequency on/off state, and therefore the microprocessor analyzes the photodiode detection of the light from only one diode at a time. The microprocessor executes an algorithm to determine the pulse amplitude at each wavelength, and the oxyhemoglobin saturation is calculated from the ratio of the two wave amplitudes. The conventional display represents the average saturation and heart rate from the last five to seven beats (the frequency of response of the Nellcor N-100 may also be altered to three selectable values). The Nellcor N-100 displays the pulse height in an LED bar, the SaO_2 and the heart rate digitally, as well as an audible tone whose pitch is related to the saturation (see Fig. 24–9). The display in the OhMEDA Pulse Oximeter (OhMEDA, Boulder, CO) is a backlit liquid crystal dis-

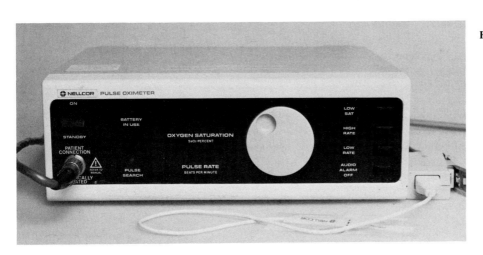

Figure 24–9. Photograph of a Nellcor Pulse Oximeter demonstrating the front panel controls: on/standby switch, vertical bar pulse (digital), oxygen saturation (SaO_2) (per cent), readout for pulse rate (beats per minute), control (dial) for audio and visual alarm units for low SaO_2, high and low heart rates, and adjustable audio alarm off control (30 to 120 seconds, preset 60 seconds). The Nellcor Pulse Oximeter provides an audible beat signal whose sound quality correlates with the saturation. The adapter, which connects the reusable adult probe or disposable probes to the monitor, is also shown. (Instrument courtesy of Nellcor, Inc. Hayward, California.)

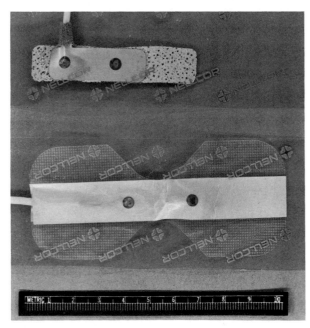

Figure 24–10. Photograph of the Nellcor Pulse Oximeter disposable finger or foot probes, which are suitable for neonates and infants (Courtesy of Nellcor, Inc, Hayward, California).

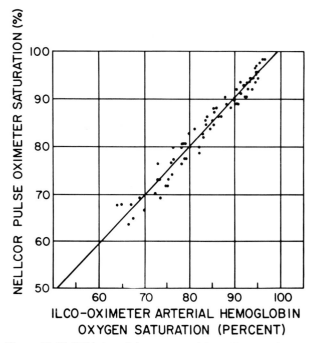

Figure 24–11. Validation of the accuracy of the Nellcor N-100 pulse oximeter in comparison with arterial oxygen saturation meaured by the IL-282 Co-Oximeter. (Redrawn from Yelderman M, New W [1983]: Evaluation of pulse oximetry. Anesthesiology 59:349–352.)

play (LCD) of the arterial waveform. The pulse oximeter probes do not require heating or special skin preparation. The accuracy of the Nellcor N-100 SaO_2 measurement is 70 to 100 ± 2 per cent, 50 to 70 ± 3 per cent, and below 50 per cent unspecified (see Fig. 24–11).[153] The instrument does not require calibration; however, Nellcor now provides an optical test device. Significant levels of dyshemoglobins (COHb and MetHb) may interfere with the accuracy of measurement of the SaO_2. In the presence of COHb, the pulse oximeter measures the SaO_2 as a per cent of the "functional" hemoglobin.[152] The validity of measurement of SaO_2 in neonates and infants with pulse oximetry was examined in two studies.[32,41] In both studies the pulse SaO_2 was compared with in vitro measurement obtained from the IL-282 Co-Oximeter and regression lines were demonstrated close to the line of identity. However, neither study discussed the possible underestimation of O_2Hb by the IL-282 Co-Oximeter in the presence of high concentrations of fetal hemoglobin or any attempt to correct the values.[28,65,110,155] Failure to measure the SaO_2 was infrequent, and it was noted that the pulse oximeter detected desaturation before reflex changes in heart rate occurred (bradycardia).[41] A recent improvement (Nellcor N-200) incorporates a QRS detector designed to verify the pulse and eliminate artifacts, particularly those arising from patient movement.

CLINICAL APPLICATION

Following its introduction, the pulse oximeter has rapidly become an essential standard of monitoring during anesthesia and a desirable standard in the recovery room environment. The rapid response of the instrument enables immediate recognition of early desaturation and is, therefore, a major advance in monitoring for hypoxemia.

The ease and rapidity of setting up and absence of calibration or drift are major technical advances over the transcutaneous oxygen tension sensors. However, low perfusion from shock or cold environment may result in failure to obtain an adequate pulse for analysis. Several pediatric studies have documented the value of the pulse oximeter in specific clinical situations: (1) during surgery for congenital heart disease;[37,48] (2) in the pediatric intensive care unit,[41] including monitoring of premature infants;[32] (3) in hypoxemia during sleep or feeding in children;[131] and (4) in home monitoring for sudden infant death syndrome.[69] Frieson recommended the use of the pulse oximeter during surgery in neonates for congenital heart defects in order to optimize banding of the pulmonary artery[37] or placement of a Blalock-Taussig shunt. The pulse oximeter enabled immediate recognition of desaturation and correction of surgical manipulation without having to wait for laboratory results or deterioration of clinical signs.[48] Similarly, during cardiac catheterization when procedures, arrhythmias, sedation, local anesthesia, and contrast medium may result in a decrease in cardiac output or an increase in right-to-left shunt, continuous monitoring for desaturation is essential to safety.[86] In addition, placement of multiple probes, such as on nose or finger (aortic arch distribution) and toes (lower aorta distribution), in the neonate provides continuous information on the magnitude of right-to-left ductal shunting in response to changes in hemodynamics or inspired oxygen concentration.

The disadvantages of the pulse oximeter, as in all measurements of arterial oxygen saturation, are that above 99 ± 1 per cent saturation, there is no change in SaO_2 and therefore, any change in PaO_2 or alveolar-arterial oxygen

Table 24–3. NORMAL ARTERIAL BLOOD GASES
IN FULL TERM NEONATES BREATHING AIR

Age	PaO$_2$ (mmHg)	PaCO$_2$ (mmHg)	pHa	Standard Bicarbonate Concentration (mequiv·liter^{-1})	Hematocrit (%)
Birth, 5–10 minutes	49.6	46.1	7.207	16.7	53.0
	± 9.9	± 7.0	± 0.051	± 1.6	± 5.0
1 hour	63.3	36.1	7.332	19.2	54.1
	± 11.3	± 4.2	± 0.031	± 1.2	± 4.9
5 hours	73.7	35.2	7.339	19.4	52.4
	± 12.0	± 3.6	± 0.028	±1.2	± 5.9
24 hours	72.7	33.4	7.369	20.2	54.8
	± 9.5	± 3.1	± 0.032	± 1.3	± 7.2
5 days	72.1	34.8	7.371	20.6	50.1
	± 10.5	± 3.5	± 0.031	± 1.7	± 6.9
7 days	73.1	35.9	7.371	21.8	51.0
	± 9.7	± 3.1	± 0.026	± 1.3	± 7.8

Notes: Mean ± SD; n = 30 to 42 neonates. Adapted with permission from Koch G, Wendel H (1968): Adjustment of arterial blood gases and acid-base balance in the normal newborn infant during the first week of life. Biol Neonate 12:136–161.

difference (AaO$_2$P) cannot be detected. This problem is further aggravated when the ODC is shifted to the left with a decrease in P$_{50}$ as in fetal hemoglobin (see Fig. 24–7 and Table 24–3). Therefore, as when any measurement or monitoring device is used, both the advantages and the limitations must be fully recognized. Thus, the pulse oximeter must be regarded as primarily a safety monitor during anesthesia,[90] critical care, and diagnostic studies. Pulse oximetry may supplement but is unlikely to replace invasive measurement of the PaO$_2$ and calculation of the AaO$_2$P. When arterial access is limited during critical care, particularly following cardiac surgery, the pulse oximeter is essential to management, especially during "weaning" from supplemental oxygen and mechanical ventilation.

Reflectance Oximetry

The principles of reflectance oximetry are similar to those of transmittance oximetry and involve measurement of absorption at a number of wavelengths with the light signals separated in time. During the development of the current technology (Oximetrix Inc, Mountain View, CA) a number of problems were overcome, including (1) non-linearity of O$_2$Hb to the ratio of reflected light intensities and the effect of physiologic factors (pH, hematocrit, and flow); (2) calibration problems as a result of optical limitations in design and construction and which were resolved by the arrangement of the transmitting and receiving fibers; and (3) stiffness and fragility of the catheter, which was minimized by the introduction of plastic optical fibers. The current Oximetrix reflectance catheters measure absorption at three wavelengths in the range of 600 to 800 nm, use a single monofilament optical fiber for each of the transmitting and receiving fibers, and have close control of the optical spacing. An optical standard is issued to calibrate each catheter before use (Figs. 24–12 to 24–15). The catheter may also be calibrated in vivo by comparison with a simultaneous blood sample taken and measured in a laboratory by a suitable method. However, this in vivo calibration has all the inherent inaccuracies of errors in sampling, measurement errors, and calculation of oxyhemoglobin saturation as described previously.

The reflectance oximeter that has been incorporated into a 7.5 F triple-lumen flow-directed pulmonary artery catheter (110 cm) has rapidly become an essential moni-

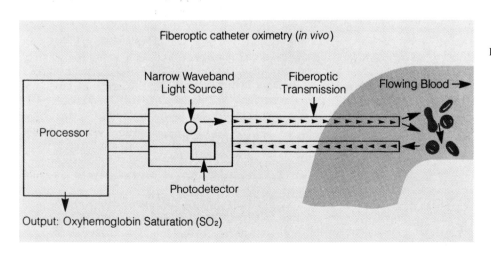

Figure 24–12. Schematic of the design for reflectance spectrometry used in invasive reflective oximetrix catheters. (Reproduced with permission of Sperinde JM, Senelly KM [1985]: The Oximetrix and Opticath oximetry system: Theory and development. In Fahey JM (ed): Continuous Measurement of Blood Oxygen Saturation in the High Risk Patient. Theory and Practice in Monitoring Mixed Venous Oxygen Saturation. Vol 2. San Diego, Beach International, Inc, pp 59–80, and Oximetrix, Inc [a subsidiary of Abbott Laboratories], Mountain View, California.)

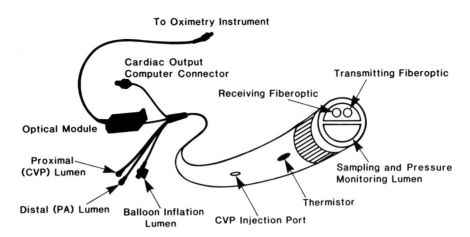

Figure 24–13. Schematic of the Oximetrix flow-directed pulmonary artery catheter (7.5 French, 110 cm), demonstrating the dual fiberoptic transmission system together with the pressure monitoring lumen and thermodilution cable. (Reproduced with permission of Sperinde JM, Senelly KM [1985]: The Oximetrix and Opticath oximetry system: Theory and development. In Fahey JM (ed): Continuous Measurement of Blood Oxygen Saturation in the High Risk Patient. Theory and Practice in Monitoring Mixed Venous Oxygen Saturation. Vol 2. San Diego, Beach International, Inc, pp 59–80, and Oximetrix, Inc [a subsidiary of Abbott Laboratories], Mountain View, California.)

toring tool in the management of critically ill patients as well as during anesthesia for cardiac surgery and postoperative management.[6,87,142] The advantages include (1) a multifunction catheter incorporating pressure and thermodilution capability as well as S$\bar{v}$O$_2$; (2) continuous measurement of both pressure and S$\bar{v}$O$_2$, providing an indication of transient as well as steady-state events; and (3) the sensitivity of the adult oxyhemoglobin dissociation curve within the range of the mixed venous blood (S$\bar{v}$O$_2$, 60 to 80 per cent) in indicating adequacy of the cardiac output. Two size 4 F fiberoptic umbilical artery catheters (25 and 40 cm long) with a lumen for pressure monitoring and blood sampling are also available.[137,146,147] Rah and associates reported the successful use of the 4 F Opticath (40 cm), which was inserted into the pulmonary artery for continuous S$\bar{v}$O$_2$ monitoring in pediatric patients (3

months to 12 years of age) following cardiac surgery.[105] The catheter was inserted into the pulmonary artery via the right ventricular outflow tract and brought out through the anterior chest wall. As in adult management, continuous measurement of the S$\bar{v}$O$_2$ provided a method to optimize management and an early warning system for impaired oxygen delivery.

The Oximetrix system, which measures the absorption at three wavelengths, does not measure the concentration of dyshemoglobins such as COHb and MetHb; therefore, the O$_2$Hb is expressed as a percentage of the total "functional" hemoglobin. In addition, high concentrations of COHb interfere with the measurement of O$_2$Hb, but the effect is relatively small. A COHb of 14 per cent would result in only a 1 per cent increase in O$_2$Hb.[132] Similarly,

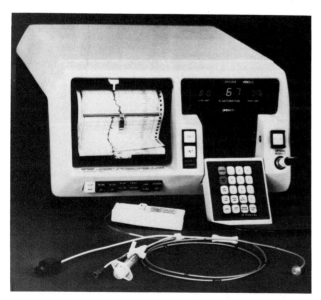

Figure 24–14. Schematic of the Oximetrix monitor, demonstrating the calibration and control pad, digital readout for SO$_2$ (S$\bar{v}$O$_2$ for pulmonary artery catheter or SaO$_2$ for sites in the arterial system), strip chart recorder and catheter with pressure monitoring/sample lumen, and the dual fiberoptic cables. (Reproduced with permission from Oximetrix, Inc [a subsidiary of Abbott Laboratories], Mountain View, California.)

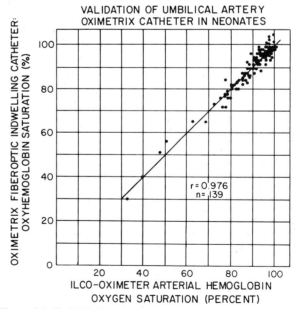

Figure 24–15. Validation of the accuracy of the in vivo reflective oximeter, Opticath (Oximetrix, Inc, Mountain View, California), by comparison with the IL-282 Co-Oximeter in measurement of intraarterial (umbilical artery) SaO$_2$. The Il-282 values were corrected for "COHb." (Redrawn with permission of Wilkinson AR et al [1978]: Continuous measurement of oxygen saturation in sick newborn infants. J Pediatr 93:1016–1019.)

Table 24–4. ARTERIAL BLOOD GASES IN NORMAL PRETERM INFANTS BREATHING AIR

Age	PaO$_2$ (mmHg)	PaCO$_2$ (mmHg)	pHa
Birth			7.32
3–5 hours	59.5 ± 7.7	47.0 ± 8.5	7.329 ± 0.038
13–24 hours	67.0 ± 15.2	27.2 ± 8.4	7.464 ± 0.064
5–10 days	80.3 ± 12.0	36.4 ± 4.2	7.378 ± 0.043

Notes: Mean ± SD. Adapted from Gregory GA (1983): Anesthesia for premature infants. In Gregory GA (ed): Pediatric Anesthesia. New York, Churchill-Livingstone, pp 579–606; and Orzalesi MM, Mendicini M, Bucci G, Scalamandre A, Savignoni PG (1967): Arterial oxygen studies in premature newborns with and without mild respiratory disorders. Arch Dis Child 42:174–180.

the effect of HbF on the measurement of the HbO$_2$, although present, is small (Oximetrix, Inc, personal communication). Comparative studies on continuous oxygen monitoring in neonates demonstrated that the SaO$_2$ obtained from an Oximetrix catheter placed in the umbilical artery was close to the line of identity of measurement obtained from the IL-282 Co-Oximeter (see Fig. 24–15).[136,146]

Arterial Blood Gases and Acid-Base Values in the Neonate

In both premature infants and neonates there is a rise in PaO$_2$ and pH and a fall in PaCO$_2$ during the initial hours after birth (see Table 24–3 and 24–4). In the full-term infant the PaO$_2$ plateaus after 5 hours, but in the premature infant the PaO$_2$ continues to increase over several days.[57,73,91] As the neonate establishes and maintains an adequate level of gas exchange, coincident changes occur in the pH, standard bicarbonate value, and PaCO$_2$. The AaO$_2$P is approximately three times greater in the neonate than in the adult (average, 25 mmHg).[88] Because the washout of nitrogen in the neonate was rapid and the AaO$_2$P breathing oxygen was high, Nelson and associates concluded that the major contributor to the increased AaO$_2$P was intracardiac or intrapulmonary right-to-left shunt.[88] The decrease in hematocrit and hemoglobin concentration occurs more slowly. By 30 days, the hemoglobin concentration approaches the adult concentration, and during childhood it is usually lower than the normal adult value. An increase in P$_{50}$, which is dependent on the replacement of fetal hemoglobin by adult hemoglobin, and an increase in the erythrocyte 2,3-DPG concentration occur over a 6-month period (see Table 24–2).

Placement and Maintenance of Arterial Monitoring Catheters in Neonates

ARTERIAL CANNULATION IN THE NEONATE

Arterial access enables measurement of arterial blood gases and pH as well as continuous monitoring of the arterial pressure and pulse wave contour. In neonates, it is usually possible to place a 3.5 F (< 1500 g) or 5 F (> 1500 g) catheter in the umbilical artery,[56] although, after several days of life, surgical dissection may be necessary. The selection of other sites for arterial cannulation is dependent on the adequacy of the collateral circulation and other factors. The most common sites for placement are the radial artery, the dorsalis pedis artery, and the posterior tibial arteries. Because thrombi may occlude the sites of collateral vessels above the elbow, the brachial artery is not ideal for prolonged cannulation in neonates. Although in adults the axillary artery has been used and the complications are infrequent, there are no data on the use of the axillary artery in neonates. Cannulation of the femoral artery is not recommended in neonates because of the proximity of the hip joint and the risk of septic arthritis, and prolonged cannulation is associated with thrombotic or embolic complications to the leg. The temporal artery has been used in the neonate; however, the risk of embolization of the internal carotid artery should be noted. Simmons and associates report a correlation between the use of the temporal artery and clinical and computed tomographic evidence of neurologic abnormalities.[128]

ANTICOAGULATION

A relationship between the use of heparin to maintain patency of vascular catheters in neonates and intracerebral hemorrhage has been reported by Lesko and associates,[77] who reviewed the incidence of intracerebral hemorrhage in infants with birthweight under 2000 g in three neonatal intensive care units. They observed an association between the use of heparin to maintain patency of the umbilical artery catheters and intraventricular or germinal matrix (periventricular) hemorrhage or hemorrhage at both sites. Although the maximal safe or optimal amount of heparin recommended is not documented, extrapolation from adult dosage to maintain patency in a heparin-lock device should not exceed 5 to 10 units of heparin or a concentration of greater than 1 unit per ml.[56,79]

TECHNIQUE OF PERIPHERAL ARTERY CANNULATION IN THE NEWBORN

The technique of placement of radial artery cannula in the neonate is similar to that in the adult. The wrist should be *gently* extended by placing a small roll under the wrist with the forearm and palm fixed. Marked extension flattens the artery, makes cannulation difficult, and may abolish the radial pulse. The radial artery can usually be cannulated with a 24- or 22-gauge, nontapered vascular cannula in infants weighing more than 700 g. In addition to palpation, the radial artery may be identified with a Doppler study or by transillumination with a *cold* fiber-optic light through the wrist. After successful cannulation, the cannula is connected to a Luer-lok "T-connector" (Medex, Inc, Hilliard, OH), which has been flushed with saline (1 unit of heparin per milliliter) and is connected to the monitoring tubing, controlled constant infusion system, and transducer. Because several volumes of the connector and vascular tubing must be removed to obtain a representative arterial blood gas sample, and reinfusion of this blood/crystalloid solution may occlude small vessels in the arm, sampling via a stopcock at the T-connector junction with the monitoring tubing or from the latex bung via a 25-gauge needle has been recommended to reduce the volume of blood withdrawn.[56] As in adults, it is desirable to verify the presence of collateral circulation to the hand via the ulnar artery prior to radial artery cannulation. However, in neonates the conventional Allen test is difficult to interpret. Several alternatives have been recommended, which include both clinical or Doppler examination after occlusion of the radial artery, and finger plethysmography.[79]

COMPLICATIONS

The complications of arterial cannulation are both immediate and delayed. The immediate complications include hemorrhage, hematoma, clot and air emboli, distal occlusion, and excess fluid administration. This last complication may be minimized by using an accurate constant infusion pump with suitable alarms for air and occlusion and flushing with a known volume (0.1 to 0.2 ml). A significant percentage of peripheral arteries will be occluded by prolonged cannulation; however, adequate circulation is usually provided by collateral vessels. Permanent occlusion is more frequent following a cutdown on a vessel. The most frequent delayed complication of cannulation of the radial artery is occlusion of a small distal end-branch, which may result in an area of necrosis and sloughing. An area of ischemia or pale mottled skin of the forearm is an indication for prompt removal of the catheter.[79] *No drugs should be administered via any peripheral artery.* Therefore, the T-connector should be clearly identified as arterial in order to avoid confusion with a peripheral intravenous line to which a T-connector in a neonate may be also connected.

OTHER INTRAVASCULAR MONITOR LINES

During the past decade a number of pediatric cardiac surgical groups have gained considerable experience with transthoracic intracardiac monitoring for postcardiac surgical management.[55] Their experience indicates that with careful selection, placement, and maintenance both right and left atrial catheters offer helpful information for hemodynamic management. The incidence of complications was low (bleeding and retention complications), and when these problems were recognized early and treated effectively the morbidity was low. The value of these hemodynamic monitors will be enhanced by using reflectance oximetry to give continuous intravascular O_2Hb measurement.

STANDARDS OF PATIENT MONITORING: RISK AND COST

As the technology to diagnose and to monitor critically ill patients improves and offers more appropriate information, so also do the monitors that become recognized as

"normal" standards of care. During the past decade the safety of the technology to manage critically ill patients during anesthesia and surgery as well as during critical care and diagnostic procedures has improved. As evidenced by advances in pulse and invasive reflectance oximetry, as well as in respired gas analysis, current technology provides continuous, rapid response and accurate information on gas exchange, oxygenation, and the adequacy of the cardiac output. In addition, both pulse oximetry and respired gas analysis are noninvasive. Therefore, these technologies are now recognized as both valuable and essential instruments for managing the critically ill patient. When applied with an understanding of the physiology and pathophysiology, these devices should prevent life-threatening hypoxemia or cerebral damage. As in transcutaneous oxygen monitoring, their cost to patient care may be less than that of traditional technologies.

ABBREVIATIONS

AaO_2P	=	alveolar-arterial oxygen pressure gradient, mmHg
$a\bar{v}O_2D$	=	arterial-mixed venous oxygen content difference, ml·dl^{-1}
AVO_2	=	oxygen availability or delivery, ml·min^{-1} or ml·min^{-1}·kg^{-1} = $\dot{Q}_t \times CaO_2 \times 10$
CaO_2	=	arterial oxygen content, ml·dl^{-1}
$C\acute{c}O_2$	=	end-pulmonary capillary oxygen content, ml·dl^{-1}
$C\bar{v}O_2$	=	mixed venous oxygen content, ml·dl^{-1}
CO	=	cardiac output, ml·min^{-1} or ml·min^{-1}·kg^{-1}
O_2ER	=	oxygen extraction, ratio, or percentage, $\dot{V}O_2/CO \times CaO_2$
P_{50}	=	partial pressure of oxygen at which hemoglobin is 50% saturated with oxygen, pH 7.40 and 37°C
PAO_2	=	alveolar oxygen tension, mmHg
PaO_2	=	arterial oxygen tension, mmHg
$PaCO_2$	=	arterial carbon dioxide tension, mmHg
PCO_2	=	partial pressure of carbon dioxide
pHa	=	arterial pH
PO_2	=	partial pressure of oxygen
$PtcO_2$	=	transcutaneous oxygen tension, mmHg
$PtcCO_2$	=	transcutaneous carbon dioxide tension, mmHg
$P\bar{v}O_2$	=	mixed venous oxygen tension, mmHg
$\dot{Q}_p$	=	pulmonary blood flow, l or ml·min^{-1}
$\dot{Q}_{sh}$	=	shunt flow, l or ml·min^{-1}

$\dot{Q}_t$ = total organ flow or cardiac output, l or ml·min^{-1}

$\dot{Q}_{sh}/\dot{Q}_t$ = shunt fraction, %

SaO_2 = arterial oxygen hemoglobin saturation, %

$S\bar{v}O_2$ = mixed venous oxyhemoglobin saturation, %

V_D = dead space, ml BTPS

V_T = tidal volume, ml BTPS

V_D/V_T = dead space/tidal volume ratio

$\dot{V}O_2$ = oxygen consumption, ml·min^{-1} or ml·min^{-1}·kg^{-1}, STPD

$\dot{V}CO_2$ = carbon dioxide production, ml·min^{-1}·kg^{-1}, STPD

HbA = adult hemoglobin

HbF = fetal hemoglobin

ODC = oxyhemoglobin dissociation curve

O_2Hb = oxyhemoglobin, % (SO_2 %)

COHb % = carboxyhemoglobin, %

MetHb % = methemoglobin, %

RHb % = reduced hemoglobin, %

THb = total hemoglobin concentration, g·dl^{-1}

ASD = atrial septal defect

VSD = ventricular septal defect

PDA = patent ductus arteriosus

MANUFACTURERS

Biomedical Sensors, Inc
10737 Ambassador Drive
Kansas City, MO 64153
Telephone: (800) 826-7112

OhMEDA
4765 Walnut Street
Boulder, CO 80300
Telephone: (800) 652-2469

Cardiovascular Devices, Inc
2801 Burranca Road
Irvine, CA 92714
Telephone: (714) 786-8001

Corning Medical Instruments
Corning Glass Works
Medfield, MA 02052
Telephone: (617) 359-7711

Datex/Instrumentarium OY
P.O. Box 357
SF-00101
Helsinki 10
Finland

Hewlett-Packard Company
Medical Products Group
3000 Minuteman Road
Andover, MA 01810
Telephone: (617) 687-1501

Instrumentation Laboratory, Inc
113 Hartwell Avenue
Lexington, MA 02173
Telephone: (617) 861-0710

Mallinckrodt, Inc—Critical Care Division
73 Quaker Road
Glens Falls, NY 12801
Telephone: (518) 793-6671

Marquest Medical Products, Inc
11039 East Lansing Circle
Englewood, CO 80112
Telephone: (800) 525-7044

Medex, Inc
3627 Lakehorn Road
Hilliard, OH 43026
Telephone: (614) 876-2413

Nellcor, Inc
25495 Whitesell Street
Hayward, CA 94545
Telephone: (415) 887-5858

Oximetrix, Inc
1212 Terra Bella Avenue
Mountain View, CA 94043
Telephone: (415) 961-4380

Puritan-Bennett Corporation
Boston Division
265 Ballardvale Street
Wilmington, MA 01887
Telephone: (617) 935-4954

Radiometer America, Inc
811 Sharon Drive
Westlake, OH 44145-9990
Telephone: (800) 321-9484

Sheridan Catheter Corporation
RT 40
Argyle, NY 12809
Telephone: (518) 638-6101

References

1. Adams AP, Hahn CEW (1982): Principles and Practice of Blood Gas Analysis. 2nd ed. London, Churchill.

2. Alfieri O, Subramanian S (1975): Cardiac output determination in infants and small children after open intracardiac operations. Ann Thorac Surg 19:322–326.

3. Antman EM, Marsh JD, Green LH, Grossman W (1980): Blood oxygen measurements in the assessment of intracardiac left to right shunts: A critical appraisal of methodology. Am J Cardiol 46:265–271.

4. Astrup P (1961): A new approach to acid-base metabolism. Clin Chem 7:1–15.

5. Astrup P, Gotzsche H, Neukirch F (1954): Laboratory investigation during treatment of patients with poliomyelitis and respiratory paralysis. Br Med J 1:780–786.

6. Baele PL, McMichan JC, Marsh HM, Sill JC, Southorn PA (1982): Continuous monitoring of mixed venous oxygen saturation in critically ill patients. Anesth Analg 61:513–517.

7. Barcroft J (1914): The Respiratory Function of the Blood. Cambridge, Cambridge University Press.

8. Barker SJ, Tremper KK (1985): Transcutaneous oxygen tension: A physiological variable for monitoring oxygenation. J Clin Monit 1:130–134.

9. Bartels H, Harms H (1959): Sauerstoffdissoziationskurven des Blutes von Saugertieren. Pflugers Arch Ges Physiol 268:334–365.

10. Bauer Ch, Ludwig M, Ludwig I, Bartels H (1969): Factors governing the oxygen affinity of human adult and foetal blood. Respir Physiol 7:271–277.

11. Baumberger JP, Goodfriend RB (1951): Determination of arterial oxygen tension in man by equilibration through intact skin (Abstr). Fed Proc 10:10–11.

12. Bert P (1878): Barometric Pressure Research in Experimental Physiology. Translated by Hitchcock MA, Hitchcock FA (1943). Columbus, College Book Company.

13. Blalock A, Hanlon CR (1950): The surgical treatment of complete transposition of the aorta and pulmonary artery. Surg Gynecol Obstet 90:1–15.

14. Blalock A, Taussig H (1945): The surgical treatment of malformations of the heart in which there is pulmonary stenosis or pulmonary atresia. JAMA 128:189–202.

15. Bohr C, Hasselbalch K, Krogh A (1904): Ueber einen in biologischer Beziehung wichtigen Einfluss, den die Kohlensäurespannung des Blutes auf dessen Sauerstoffbindung übt. Scand Arch Physiol 16:402–417.

16. Boyd AD, Tremblay RE, Spencer FC, Bahnson HT (1959): Estimation of cardiac output soon after intracardiac surgery with cardiopulmonary bypass. Ann Surg 150:613–626.

17. Brantigan JW, Dunn KL, Albo D (1976): A clinical catheter for continuous blood gas measurement by mass spectrometry. J Appl Physiol 40:443–446.

18. Brinkman R, Zylstra WG (1949): Determination and continuous registration of the percentage oxygen saturation in clinical conditions. Arch Chir Neerl 1:177–183.

19. Brock RC (1948): Pulmonary valvotomy for the relief of congenital pulmonary stenosis: Report of three cases. Br Med J 1:1121–1126.

20. Brown LJ (1980): A new instrument for simultaneous measurement of total hemoglobin, % oxyhemoglobin, % carboxyhemoglobin, % methemoglobin, and oxygen content in whole blood. IEEE Trans Biomed Eng BME-27:132–138.

21. Burchell HB, Wood EH (1949): Reproducibility of values for oxygen saturation in arterial blood and magnitude of venous-arterial shunts in pediatric patients with congenital cardiac malformations. J Appl Physiol 1:560–566.

22. Carden WD, Petty WC (1973): The lack of effect of lidocaine on oxyhemoglobin dissociation. Anesthesiology 38:177–180.

23. Charlton G, Read D, Read J (1963): Continuous intra-arterial PO_2 in normal man using flexible microelectrode. J Appl Physiol 18:1247–1251.

24. Christiansen J, Douglas CG, Haldane JS (1914): The absorption and dissociation of carbon dioxide by human blood. J Physiol (Lond) 48:244–271.

25. Clark LC Jr (1956): Monitor and control of blood and tissue oxygen tensions. Trans Am Soc Art Intern Org 2:41–48.

26. Coon RL, Lai NCJ, Kampine JP (1976): Evaluation of a dual-function pH and PCO_2 in vivo sensor. J Appl Physiol 40:625–629.

27. Coon RL, Zuperku EJ, Kampine JP (1978): Systemic arterial blood pH servocontrol of mechanical ventilation. Anesthesiology 49:201–204.

28. Cornelissen PJH, Woersel CLM van, Oel WC van, Jong PA de (1982): Correction factors for hemoglobin derivatives in fetal blood, as measured with the IL282 Co-Oximeter (letter). Clin Chem 29:1555–1556.

29. Cournand A, Baldwin JS, Himmelstein A (1949): Cardiac Catheterization in Congenital Heart Disease. New York, Commonwealth Fund.

30. Cournand A, Riley RL, Breed ES, Baldwin E deF, Richards DW Jr (1945): Measurement of cardiac output in man using the technique of catheterization of the right auricle or ventricle. J Clin Invest 24:106–116.

31. Davies PW, Brink F Jr (1942): Microelectrode for measuring local oxygen tensions in animal tissues. Rev Sci Instrum 13:524–533.

32. Deckardt R, Steward DJ (1984): Noninvasive arterial hemoglobin oxygen saturation versus transcutaneous oxygen tension monitoring in the preterm infant. Crit Care Med 12:935–939.

33. Dennis RC, Valeri CR (1980): Measuring percent oxygen saturation of hemoglobin, percent carboxyhemoglobin and methemoglobin, and concentrations of total hemoglobin and oxygen in blood of man, dog and baboon. Clin Chem 26:1304–1308.

34. Dexter L, Haynes FW, Burwell CS, Eppinger EC, Sagerson RP, Evans JM (1947): Studies of congenital heart disease: I. Venous catheterization as a diagnostic aid in patent ductus arteriosus, tetralogy of Fallot, ventricular septal defect and auricular septal defect. J Clin Invest 26:561–576.

35. Dexter L, Haynes FW, Burwell CS, Eppinger EC, Sagerson RP, Evans JM (1947): Studies of congenital heart disease: II. The pressure and oxygen content of blood in the right auricle or ventricle and pulmonary artery in control patients, with observations on the oxygen saturation and source of pulmonary "capillary" blood. J Clin Invest 26:554–560.

36. Dexter L, Haynes FW, Burwell CS, Eppinger EC, Sosman MC, Evans JM (1947): Studies of congenital heart disease: III. Venous catheterization as a diagnostic aid in patent ductus arteriosus, tetralogy of Fallot, ventricular septal defect, and auricular septal defect. J Clin Invest 26:561–576.

37. Doty DB (1983): Pulmonary artery banding. In Glenn WWL (ed): Thoracic and Cardiovascular Surgery. Norwalk, Appleton-Century-Crofts, pp 681–687.

38. Douglas NJ, Brash HM, Wraith PK, Calverley PMA, Legett RJE, McElderry L, Flenley DC (1979): Accuracy, sensitivity to carboxyhemoglobin and speed of response of the Hewlett-Packard 47201A ear oximeter (notes). Am Rev Respir Dis 119:311–313.

39. Eletr S (1980): Cutaneous gas measurements. In Gravenstein JS, Newbower RS, Ream AK, Smith NT (eds): Essential Noninvasive Monitoring in Anesthesia. New York, Grune & Stratton, pp 63–181.

40. Enson Y, Jameson AG, Cournand A (1964): Intracardiac oximetry in congenital heart disease. Circulation 29:499–507.

41. Fanconi S, Doherty P, Edmonds JF, Barker GA, Bohn DJ (1985): Pulse oximetry in pediatric intensive care: A comparison with measured saturations and transcutaneous oxygen tension. J Pediatr 107:362–366.

42. Fick A (1870): Ueber die Messung des Blutquantums in der Herzventrikeln: Sitzungberichte der Physikalisch—Medizinischen Gesellschaft in Wurzburg 16.

43. Foex P, Burt G, Maynard P, Ryder WA, Hahn CEW (1979): Continuous measurement of blood gases in vivo by mass spectrometry. Br J Anaesth 51:999–1005.

44. Forssmann W (1929): Die Sondierung des rechten Herzens. Klin Wochenschr 8:2085–2087.

45. Fournier L, Major D (1984): The effect of nitrous oxide on the oxyhaemoglobin dissociation curve. Can Anaesth Soc J 31:173–177.

46. Fowler KT (1969): The respiratory mass spectrometer. Phys Med Biol 14:185–199.

47. Fowles RE (1982): Interpretation of cardiac catheterization. In Ream AK, Fogdall RP (eds): Acute Cardiovascular Management Anesthesia and Intensive Care. Philadelphia, JB Lippincott, pp 69–138.

48. Friesen RH (1985): Pulse oximetry during pulmonary artery surgery. Anesth Analg 64:376.

49. Gamble WJ, Hugenholtz PG, Monroe RG, Polanyi M, Nadas AS (1965): The use of fiberoptics in clinical cardiac catheterization: I. Intracardiac oximetry. Circulation 31:328–343.

50. Geha AS, Sessler AD, Kirklin JW (1966): Alveolar-arterial oxygen gradients after open intracardiac surgery. J Thorac Cardiovasc Surg 51:609–615.

51. Gehrich JL, Lubbers DW, Opitz N, Hansmann DR, Miller WW, Tusa JK, Yafusa M (1986): Optical fluorescence and its application to an intravascular blood gas monitoring system. IEEE Trans Biomed Eng BME-33:117–132.

52. Gertz KH, Loeschcke HH (1958): Elektrode zur Bestimmung des CO_2-Drucks. Naturwissenschaften 45:160–161.

53. Gibbon JH (1954): Application of a mechanical heart and lung apparatus to cardiac surgery. Minn Med 37:171–180.

54. Gilles IDS, Bird BD, Norman J, Gordon-Smith EC, Whitwam JG (1970): The effect of anesthesia on the oxyhemoglobin dissociation curve (Abstr). Br J Anaesth 42:561.

55. Gold JP, Jonas RA, Lang P, Elixson EM, Mayer JE, Castaneda AR (1986): Transthoracic intracardiac monitoring lines in pediatric surgical patients: A ten-year experience. Ann Thorac Surg 42:185–191.

56. Gregory GA (1983): Monitoring during surgery. In Gregory GA (ed): Pediatric Anesthesia. New York, Churchill-Livingstone, pp 381–401.

57. Gregory GA (1983): Anesthesia for premature infants. In Gregory GA (ed): Pediatric Anesthesia. New York, Churchill-Livingstone, pp 579–606.

58. Gross RE, Hubbard JP (1938): Surgical ligation of a patent ductus arteriosus. Report of first successful case. JAMA 112:729–731.

59. Harned HS Jr, Lurie PR, Crothers CH, Whittemore R (1952): Use of the whole blood oximeter during cardiac catheterization. J Lab Clin Med 40:445–456.

60. Harris TR, Nugent M (1973): Continuous arterial oxygen tension monitoring in the newborn infant. J Pediatrics 82:929–939.

61. Hewlett-Packard Ear Oximeter 47201A (1975): Technical Information. Waltham, Hewlett-Packard Medical Products Group. 2/75. 5925–5942.

62. Heyrovsky J (1923–1924): The processes at mercury dropping cathode. Part II. The hydrogen potential. Trans Farady Soc 19:785–788.

63. Huch A, Huch R, Lübbers DW (1969): Quantitative polarographische Sauerstoffdruckmessung auf der Kopfhaut des Neugeborenen. Arch Gynaekol 207:443–451.

64. Huch R, Huch A, Lübbers DW (1981): Transcutaneous PO_2. New York, Thieme-Stratton.

65. Huch R, Huch A, Tuchschmid P, Zylstra WG, Zwart A (1983): Carboxyhemoglobin concentration in fetal cord blood (letter to editor). Pediatrics 71:461–462.

66. Hugenholtz PG, Gamble WJ, Monroe RG, Polanyi M (1965): The use of fiberoptics in clinical cardiac catheterization: II. In vivo dye-dilution curves. Circulation 31:344–355.

67. Hyman AL, Myers W, Hyatt K, deGaff AC Jr, Quiroz AC (1962): A comparative study of the detection of cardiovascular shunts by oxygen analysis and indicator detection methods. Ann Intern Med 56:535–544.

68. Jimenez Diaz C, Sanchez Cuenca B (1930): El sondaje del corazon derecho. Arch Latinoam Cardiol Hematol 11:105–108.

69. Josten KU (1985): Hausliche Uberwachung nach dem plotzlichen Sauglingstod: Der personliche Erfahrungsbericht eines Anasthesisten. Klin Padiatr 197:127–129.

70. Kirklin JW, Dushane JW, Patrick RT, Donald DE, Hetzel PS, Harshbarger HG, Wood EH (1955): Intracardiac surgery with the aid of a mechanical pump oxygenator system (Gibbon type): Report of eight cases. Mayo Clin Proc 30:201–206.

71. Klein O (1930): Zur Bestimmung des zirkulatorischen Minuten Volumen nach dem Fickschen Prinzip. Munchener Med Wochensch 77:1311–1312.

72. Klingenmaier CH, Behar MG, Smith TC (1969): Blood oxygen content measured by oxygen tension after release by carbon monoxide. J Appl Physiol 26:653–655.

73. Koch G, Wendel H (1968): Adjustment of arterial blood gases and acid-base balance in the normal newborn infant during the first week of life. Biol Neonate 12:136–161.

74. Kramer K, Elam JO, Saxton GA, Elam WM Jr (1951): Influence of oxygen saturation, erythrocyte concentration and optical depth upon the red and near-infrared light transmittance of whole blood. Am J Physiol 165:229–246.

75. Krogh A, Krogh M (1910): On the tensions of gases in the arterial blood. Scand Arch Physiol 23:179–192.

76. LeBlanc OH Jr, Brown JF Jr, Klebe JF, Niedrach LW, Slusarczuk GMJ, Stoddard WH Jr (1976): Polymer membrane sensors for continuous intravascular monitoring of blood pH. J Appl Physiol 40:644–647.

77. Lesko SM, Mitchell AA, Epstein MF, Louik C, Giacoia GP, Shapiro S (1986): Heparin use as a risk factor for intraventricular hemorrhage and low birth weight infants. N Engl J Med 314:1156–1160.

78. Longmuir JS, Knopp JA (1976): Measurement of tissue oxygen with a fluorescent probe. J Appl Physiol 41:598–602.

79. Loomis JC (1983): Pediatric intensive care. In Gregory GA (ed): Pediatric Anesthesia. New York, Churchill-Livingstone, vol 2, pp 915–1020.

80. Lübbers DW (1966): Methods of measuring oxygen tensions of blood and organ surfaces. In Payne JP, Hill DW (eds): A Symposium on Oxygen Measurements in Blood and Tissues and Their Significance. London, J & A Churchill, pp 103–128.

81. Lübbers DW, Opitz N (1976): Quantitative fluorescence photometry with biological fluids and gases. Adv Exp Med Biol 75:65–68.

82. McArthur KT, Clark LC Jr, Lyons C, Edwards S (1962): Continuous recording of blood oxygen saturation in open-heart operations. Surgery 51:121–126.

83. McLean FC, Murray HA Jr, Henderson LJ (1920): The variable acidity of hemoglobin and the distribution of chlorides in the blood. Proc Soc Exp Biol Med 17:180–182.

84. Mitnick MH, Jobsis FF (1976): Pyrenebutyric acid as an optical oxygen probe in the intact cerebral cortex. J Appl Physiol 41:593–597.

85. Muller WH Jr, Damman JF Jr (1952): Treatment of certain malformations of the heart by creation of stenosis to reduce pulmonary hypertension and excessive blood flow. Surg Gynecol 95:213–219.

86. Neagley SR, Vought MB, Wiedner WA, Zwillich CW (1986): Transient oxygen desaturation following radiographic contrast medium administration. Arch Intern Med 146:1094–1097.

87. Nelson LD (1987): Mixed venous oximetry. In Snyder JV, Pinsky MR (eds): Oxygen Transport in the Critically Ill. Chicago, Year Book Medical Publishers, pp 235–248.

88. Nelson NM, Prod'hom LS, Cherry RB, Lipsitz PJ, Smith CA (1963): Pulmonary function in the newborn infant: The alveolar-arterial oxygen gradient. J Appl Physiol 18:534–538.

89. Neumark J, Bardeen A, Sulzer E, Kampine JP. Miniature intravascular PCO_2 sensors in neurosurgery. J Neurosurg 43:172–176, 1975.

90. New W (1985): Pulse oximetry. J Clin Monit 1:126–129.

91. Orzalesi MM, Mendicini M, Bucci G, Scalamandre A, Savignoni PG (1967): Arterial oxygen studies in premature newborns with and without mild respiratory disorders. Arch Dis Child 42:174–180.

92. Parker D, Delphy D, Reynolds EOR (1978): Transcutaneous blood gas measurement by mass spectrometry. Acta Anaesthesiol Scand [Suppl] 68:131–136.

93. Parker D, Soutter LP (1975): In vivo monitoring of blood PO_2 in newborn infants. In Payne JP, Hill DW (ed): Oxygen Measurement in Biology and Medicine. London, Butterworths, pp 269–283.

94. Parr GVS, Blackstone EH, Kirklin JW (1975): Cardiac performance and mortality early after intracardiac surgery in infants and children. Circulation 51:867–874.

95. Peevy KJ, Hall MW (1985): Transcutaneous oxygen monitoring: Economic impact on neonatal care. Pediatrics 75:1065–1067.

96. Pendleton RG, Newman DJ, Sherman SS, Brann EG, Maya WE (1972): Effect of propranolol upon the hemoglobin oxygen dissociation curve. J Pharmacol Exp Ther 180:647–656.

97. Perkins JF Jr (1964): Historical Development of Respiratory Physiology. In Fenn WO, Rahn H (ed): Handbook of Physiology, Section 3, Respiration. Washington, American Physiological Society, vol 1, pp 1–62.

98. Peters JP, Van Slyke DD (1931): Hemoglobin and oxygen. Carbonic acid and acid-base balance. In Quantitative Clinical Chemistry, Volume I, Interpretations. Baltimore, Williams & Wilkins, pp 518–652, 868–1018. Reprinted 1963. Baltimore, Waverly Press.

99. Peters JP, Van Slyke DD (1932): Quantitative Clinical Chemistry, Volume II, Methods. Covent Garden, Bailliere, Tindall & Cox.

100. Pickup JC (1985): Biosensors: A clinical perspective. Lancet 2:817–820.

101. Podgorski GT, Longmuir IS, Knopp JA, Benson DM (1981): Use of an encapsulated fluorescent probe to measure intracellular PO_2. J Cell Physiol 107:329–334.

102. Polanyi ML, Hehir RM (1962): In vivo oximeter with fast dynamic response. Rev Sci Instrum 33:1050–1054.

103. Potts WJ, Smith S, Gibbon S (1946): Anastomosis of the aorta to a pulmonary artery: Certain types in congenital heart disease. JAMA 132:627–631.

104. Rafferty TD, Schachter EN, Mentelos RA, Yoker RE (1981): In vitro evaluation of a transcutaneous CO_2 and O_2 monitor: The effects of nitrous oxide, enflurane, and halothane. Med Instrum 15:316–318.

105. Rah KH, Dunwiddie WC, Lower RR (1984): A method for continuous postoperative measurement of mixed venous oxygen saturation in infants and children after open heart procedures. Anesth Analg 63:873–881.

106. Rashkind WJ (1980): A Backward Glance. In Graham G, Rossi E (eds): Heart Disease in Infants and Children. London, Edward Arnold, pp 3–12.

107. Ream AK (1982): Cardiopulmonary bypass period. In Ream AK, Fogdall RP (eds): Acute Cardiovascular Management. Philadelphia, JB Lippincott, pp 420–455.

108. Rolfe P (1976): Arterial oxygen measurement in the newborn with intravascular transducers. In Hill DW, Watson BW (eds): IEEE Medical Electronics Monographs. Stevenge, Peter Peregrenus, pp 18–22.

109. Rooth G, Sjostedt S, Caligara F (1957): Bloodless determination of arterial oxygen tension by polarography. Science Tools: LKW Instrum J 4:37–42.

110. Ryan CA, Barrington KJ, Vaughan D, Finer NJ (1986): Directly measured arterial oxygen saturation in the newborn infant. J Pediatr 109:526–529.

111. Sacks LM, Delivoria-Papadopoulos M (1984): Hemoglobin-oxygen interactions. Semin Perinatol 8:168–183.

112. Saunders NA, Powles ACP, Rebuck AS (1976): Ear oximetry: Accuracy and practicability in the assessment of arterial oxygenation. Am Rev Respir Dis 113:745–749.

113. Schwartz WB, Relman AS (1963): A critique of the parameters used in the evaluation of acid base disorders: "Whole-blood buffer base" and "standard bicarbonate" compared with blood pH and plasma bicarbonate concentration. N Engl J Med 268:1382–1387.

114. Severinghaus JW (1966): Blood gas calculator. J Appl Physiol 21:1108–1116.

115. Severinghaus JW (1979): Simple, accurate equations for human O_2 dissociation computations. J Appl Physiol Respir Environ Exer Physiol 46:599–620.

116. Severinghaus JW (1981): A combined transcutaneous PO_2–PCO_2 electrode with electrochemical HCO_3 stabilization. J Appl Physiol 51:1027–1032.

117. Severinghaus JW (1982): Transcutaneous blood gas analysis. Respir Care 27:152–159.

118. Severinghaus JW, Bradley AF (1958): Electrodes for blood PO_2 and PCO_2 determination. J Appl Physiol 13:515–520.

119. Severinghaus JW, Stafford M, Bradley AF (1978): $tcPCO_2$ electrode design, calibration, and temperature gradient problems. Acta Anesthesiol Scand Suppl 68:118–123.

120. Severinghaus JW, Weiskopf RB, Nishimura M, Bradley AF (1971): Oxygen electrode errors due to polarographic reduction halothane. J Appl Physiol 31:640–642.

121. Shah MV, Anderson LK, Bergman NA (1986): The influence of nitrous oxide on oxyhemoglobin dissociation and measurement of oxygen tension. Anaesthesia 41:586–588.

122. Shimada Y, Yoshiya I, Oka N, Hamaguri K (1984): Effect of multiple scattering and peripheral circulation on arterial oxygen saturation measured with a pulse-type oximeter. Med Biol Eng Comput 22:475–478.

123. Shrout JB (1985): Blood gases, pH, and buffer systems. In Bishop ML, Duben-von Laufen JL, Fody EP (eds): Clinical Chemistry: Principles, Procedures, Correlations. Philadelphia, JB Lippincott, pp 241–262.

124. Sibbald A (1985): Chemical biosensors and on-line patient monitoring. Med Instrum 19:164–167.

125. Siggaard-Andersen O (1963): The Acid-Base Status of the Blood. Copenhagen, Munksgaard.

126. Siggaard-Andersen O (1977): Experiences with a new direct reading oxygen saturation photometer using ultrasound for hemolyzing the blood. Scand J Clin Lab Invest 37 (suppl 146):45–50.

127. Siggaard-Andersen O, Engel K, Jorgensen K, Astrup P (1960): A micro method for determination of pH, carbon dioxide tension, base excess and standard bicarbonate in capillary blood. Scand J Clin Lab Invest 12:172–176.

128. Simmons MA, Levine RL, Lubchenco LO, Guggenheim MA (1978): Warning: Serious sequelae of temporal artery catheterization (clinical note). J Pediatr 92:284.

129. Slutsky AS, Strohl KP (1980): Quantification of oxygen saturation during episodic hypoxemia. Am Rev Respir Dis 121:893–895.

130. Smith TC, Colton ET III, Behar MG (1970): Does anesthesia alter hemoglobin dissociation? Anesthesiology 32:5–10.

131. Southall DP, Johnson P, Salmons S, Talbert DG, Morley CT, Miller J, Helms PJ (1985): Prolonged expiratory apnoea: A disorder resulting in episodes of severe arterial hypoxaemia in infants and young children. Lancet 2:571–577.

132. Sperinde JM, Senelly KM (1985): The Oximetrix Opticath Oximetry System: Theory and development. In Fahey PJ (ed): Continuous Measurement of Blood Oxygen Saturation in the High Risk Patient, Volume 2, Theory and Practice in Monitoring Mixed Venous Oxygen Saturation. San Diego, Beach International, pp 59–80.

133. Spiegel J van der (1985): The impact of integrated and intelligent sensor systems on medical equipment and methods. Med Instrum 19:153–157.

134. Stanger P, Heymann MA, Hoffman, JIE, Rudolph AM (1972): Use of the Swan-Ganz catheter in cardiac cathterization in infants and children. Am Heart J 83:749.

135. Stow RW, Baer RF, Randall BF (1957): Rapid measurement of the tension of carbon dioxide in blood. Arch Phys Med Rehabil 38:646–650.

136. Strauss AW, Escobedo M, Goldring D (1974): Continuous monitoring of arterial oxygen tension in newborn infants. J Pediatr 85:254–261.

137. Strauss J, Bancalari E, Feller R, Gannon J, Beran AV, Baker R (1979): Clinical aspects of continuous neonatal oxygen monitoring. Fed Proc 38:2478–2483.

138. Sugioka K (1975): Theoretical and clinical consideration in the use of a new in vivo oxygen electrode. In Payne JP, Hill DW (eds): Oxygen Measurements in Biology and Medicine. London, Butterworths, pp 111–120.

139. Van Slyke DD, Neill JM (1924): The determination of gases in blood and other solutions by vacuum extractions and manometer measurements. J Biol Chem 61:523–573.

140. Vaughan WM, Weber G (1970): Oxygen quenching of pyrenebutyric acid fluorescence in water: A dynamic probe of the microenvironment. Biochemistry 9:464–473.

141. Versmold H, Seifert G, Riegel KP (1973): Blood oxygen affinity in infancy: The interaction of fetal and adult hemoglobin oxygen capacity and red cell hydrogen ion and 2,3-diphosphoglycerate concentration. Respir Physiol 18:14–25.

142. Waller JL, Kaplan JA, Bauman DI, Carver JM (1982): Clinical evaluation of a new fiberoptic catheter oximeter during cardiac surgery. Anaesth Analg 61:676–679.

143. Ware PF, Polanyi ML, Hehir RM, Stapelton JF, Sanders JI, Kocot SL (1961): A new reflection oximeter. J Thorac Cardiovasc Surg 42:580–588.

144. Weintraub HD, Sullivan SF, Malm JR, Bowman FO, Papper EM (1965): Lung function and blood-gas exchange, before and after cardiac surgery. J Appl Physiol 20:483–487.

145. Weiskopf RB, Nishimura M, Severinghaus JW (1971): The absence of an effect of halothane on blood hemoglobin O_2 equilibrium in vitro. Anesthesiology 35:579–581.

146. Wilkinson AR, Phibbs RH, Gregory GA (1978): Continuous measurement of oxygen saturation in sick newborn infants. J Pediatr 93:1016–1019.

147. Wilkinson AR, Phibbs RH, Gregory GA (1979): Continuous in vivo oxygen saturation in newborn infants with pulmonary disease: A new fiberoptic catheter oximeter. Crit Care Med 7:232–236.

148. Woldring S, Owens G, Woolford DC (1966): Blood gases: Continuous in vivo recording of partial pressures by mass spectrography. Science 153:885–887.

149. Wood EH, Sutterer WF, Cronin L (1966): Oximetry. In Glasser O (ed): Medical Physics. Chicago, Year Book Medical Publishers, vol 3, pp 416–445.

150. Wyse SD, Pfitzner J, Rees A, Lincoln JCR, Branthwaite MA (1975): Measurement of cardiac output by thermal dilution in infants and children. Thorax 30:262–265.

151. Yamamoto K, Watanabe Y, Mikami T (1985): Characterization of steady-state and transient responses of transcutaneous PO_2 and PCO_2 by mass spectrometry. Med Biol Eng Comput 23:572–578.

152. Yelderman M, Corenmem J (1983): Real time oximetry. In Prakask O, Mey SH, Patterson RW (eds): Computing in Anesthesia and Intensive Care. Boston, Martinus Nijhoff.

153. Yelderman M, New W (1983): Evaluation of pulse oximetry. Anesthesiology 59:349–352.

154. Yoshiya I, Shimada Y, Tanaka K (1980): Spectrophotometric monitoring of arterial oxygen saturation in the fingertip. Med Biol Eng Comput 18:27–32.

155. Zwart A, Buursma A, Oeseburg B, Zijlstra WG (1981): Determination of hemoglobin derivatives with the IL-282 Co-Oximeter as compared with a manual spectrophotometric 5-wavelength method. Clin Chem 27:1903–1907.

25 ECHOCARDIOGRAPHY

Stephen P. Sanders

Since its introduction into clinical medicine in the 1960s, cardiac ultrasonography has become the preeminent imaging technique in pediatric cardiology. Unlike most new medical technologies, which are designed for and most useful in adult patients, cardiac ultrasonography is custom made for pediatric patients: First, the image resolution is superior in infants and children. The resolving power of sonic imaging techniques is, in part, a function of the frequency of the transmitted ultrasound. The higher the frequency the better the resolution but the poorer the penetration. The shorter distance from the body surface to the heart in infants and children permits use of higher frequency ultrasound, thus enhancing the image quality. Second, cardiac ultrasonography is especially good at defining cardiac anatomy. It is predominantly in infants and children that one encounters complex anatomic abnormalities. Third, Doppler echocardiography works better over the shorter distances encountered in pediatric patients. The signal-to-noise ratio deteriorates with increasing distance, so that much cleaner signals can be obtained in smaller patients.

HISTORICAL PERSPECTIVE

The history of echocardiography in pediatric cardiology reflects the technological development of medical ultrasound. Until the mid 1970s only A-mode or M-mode echocardiography was available.[26] As will be discussed later, M-mode echocardiography affords an unidimensional or "icepick" view of the heart. Despite the obvious limitations of this technology for viewing cardiac anatomy, M-mode echocardiography was used extensively for anatomic diagnosis. Even complex anomalies such as total anomalous pulmonary venous connection,[2,80,87,88] abnormalities of the atrioventricular canal,[5,11,24,54,66,79] tricuspid atresia,[106,111] transposition of the great arteries,[6,22,35,37] hypoplastic left-heart syndrome,[25] pulmonary atresia with intact septum,[61] and single ventricle,[104] were diagnosed using M-mode echocardiography. The works of Solinger et al,[126,127] which describe a deductive approach to the use of M-mode echocardiography for segmental analysis of cardiac anatomy, epitomize this era.

The use of M-mode echocardiography for anatomic diagnosis should be viewed simply as a function of the chronology of the development of cardiac ultrasonography. Today, with the general availability of two-dimensional echocardiography, M-mode echocardiography has no place in the diagnosis of structural heart defects. This does not mean that M-mode echocardiography has no place in pediatric cardiology. In fact, M-mode echocardiography is used extensively for evaluation of ventricular function and for timing of cardiac events, such as valve opening and closing.

Development of two-dimensional echocardiography in the mid and late 1970s ushered in a new era of cardiac imaging. For the first time wide, cross-sectional cuts of the beating heart could be imaged in real time. The motion of the heart valves could actually be observed in the intact subject. Early two-dimensional echocardiographic machines were crude, with poor resolution and primitive image display technology. As transducers and image processing improved, excellent quality real time pictures of the heart became available. One major advance was the introduction of digital image processing. Digital images can be enhanced by techniques not applicable to analog images, such as adjacent pixel averaging, interpolation, border enhancement, and variation of gray scale assignment.

Today, two-dimensional echocardiography is the method of choice for diagnosing most congenital heart defects. The aspects of cardiac morphology for which angiography remains superior to two-dimensional echocardiography are imaging of the muscular ventricular septum, branch pulmonary arteries, and aortopulmonary collaterals.

Although not a new technology, Doppler echocardiography did not become popular until the 1980s. While some investigators such as Hatle and Angelsen[41] used continuous wave Doppler echocardiography without concomitant imaging quite successfully, general use of Doppler echocardiography depended upon the development of duplex imaging Doppler systems. Such systems allow the operator to interrogate specific areas within the heart and great vessels using the two-dimensional echocardiographic image to guide placement of the Doppler sample volume.

Currently, Doppler echocardiography is used qualitatively to detect valvular regurgitation, atrial and ventricular septal defects, persistent ductus arteriosus, and coarctation. Perhaps more important, Doppler echocardiography can be used to quantify systemic and pulmonary blood flow, to determine the severity of stenotic lesions, and in some cases, to estimate right ventricular or pulmonary artery pressure. The physiologic information provided by Doppler echocardiography complements the anatomic data obtained from two-dimensional echocardiography. These two modalities used in concert provide a very complete evaluation of infants suspected of having a congenital heart defect.

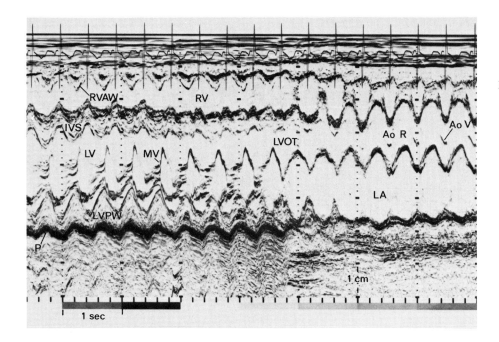

Figure 25–1. A standard M-mode echocardiographic sweep from the left ventricle to the aortic root. Distance from the transducer is shown along the vertical axis, and time is shown along the horizontal axis. Ao R = aortic root; Ao V = aortic valve; IVS = interventricular septum; LA = left atrium; LV = left ventricle; LVOT = left ventricular outflow tract; LVPW = left ventricular posterior wall; MV = mitral valve; P = pericardium; RV = right ventricle; RVAW = right ventricular anterior wall.

M-MODE ECHOCARDIOGRAPHY

Background

M-mode echocardiography displays motion of the heart along a single dimension as a function of time (Fig. 25–1), affording an "icepick" view of the heart. The transducer, a piezoelectric crystal that converts electrical

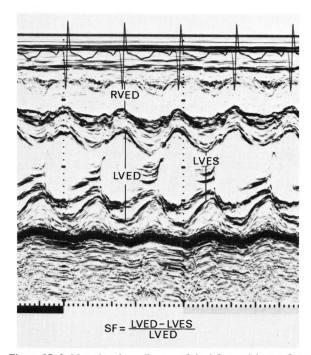

$$SF = \frac{LVED - LVES}{LVED}$$

Figure 25–2. M-mode echocardiogram of the left ventricle at a faster paper speed illustrating the method for measuring ventricular dimensions and calculating the left ventricular shortening fraction. LVED = left ventricular end-diastolic dimension; LVES = left ventricular end-systolic dimension; RVED = right ventricular end-diastolic dimension; SF = shortening fraction.

energy to sound energy and vice versa, transmits a short burst of ultrasound (~ 1 μsec in duration) into the subject. The transducer then acts as a receiver, "listening" for reflected sound energy until the next pulse is sent. Typically, the pulse rate is 1 kHz, or 1000 pulses per second. As each pulse of sound energy is transmitted, a clock is started in the ultrasound machine. As reflected sound energy returns to the transducer, the clock measures the time required for the sound waves to make the round trip back to the reflector. Then, based on the speed of propagation of sound in tissue (1560 m/sec), the distance between the transducer and the reflector is calculated, and a "dot" is drawn at the corresponding position on the display. The intensity of the "dot" is proportional to the amplitude of the reflected sound energy. This process is repeated many times to build up an image. The usual display plots distance from the transducer along the y axis and time on the x axis. This unidimensional view of the heart is excellent for measuring chamber dimension or wall thickness but is obviously quite limited for investigating cardiac anatomy.

Left Ventricular Performance

The most important use of M-mode echocardiography today is in assessment of left ventricular performance. M-mode echocardiography permits very accurate measurement of left ventricular dimension and wall thickness. The rapid sampling rate provides an essentially continuous record of the motion of the ventricular septum and left ventricular free wall, allowing determination of chamber dimension, wall thickness, and rate of change of these variables over the course of the cardiac cycle.

The most commonly used echocardiographic index of left ventricular performance is the shortening fraction, or the relative change in short axis dimension from diastole to systole. This index is easily measured (Fig. 25–2) and under certain conditions provides a reliable and reproducible estimate of ventricular performance. Since the ex-

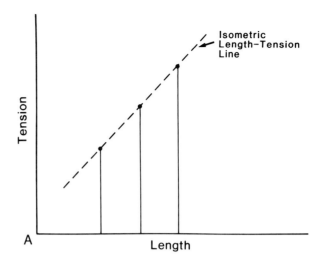

Figure 25–3. Schematic pressure-volume loops illustrating the effect of varying preload with constant afterload. Note that the stroke volume ($SV_2 > SV_1$) and ejection fraction ($EF_2 > EF_1$) increase with increasing preload as long as the end-systolic point remains constant. EDV = end-diastolic volume; EF = ejection fraction; ESV = end-systolic volume; SV = stroke volume.

In figure 25-3: $SV_1 = EDV_1 - ESV$; $SV_2 = EDV_2 - ESV$; $EF_1 = SV_1/EDV_1$; $EF_2 = SV_2/EDV_2$

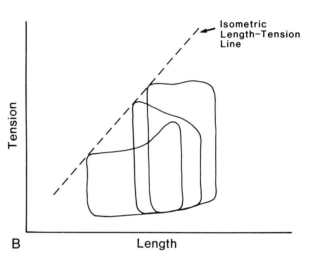

Figure 25–4. *A,* Length-tension relation for isolated papillary muscle contracting isometrically. For each starting length there is a maximum tension that can be generated. The line joining these points is the isometric length-tension line. *B,* Length-tension relation for shortening contractions. Note that the muscle contracts until the length–tension loop intersects the isometric length–tension line irrespective of the conditions at the onset of contraction or trajectory of the loop.

aminer is attempting to measure the pumping efficiency of the left ventricle, the short axis dimension must be related to left ventricular volume in some constant and predictable fashion for the shortening fraction to be useful. The usual shape of the left ventricle, the prolate ellipsoid, satisfies this condition, since the minor or short axis is predictably related to volume, and the shortening fraction is correlated with the ejection fraction. If, however, the shape of the left ventricle deviates significantly from an ellipsoid, then the short axis dimension no longer bears a predictable relation to volume, and the shortening fraction is not a reliable index of performance. Notice that the shape of the left ventricle must be ellipsoidal in both diastole and systole for the shortening fraction to be a valid index of performance. Factors that tend to alter the shape of the left ventricle include right ventricular volume loading, right ventricular systolic hypertension, and left ventricular regional wall motion abnormalities, as may be seen in ischemic heart disease. Of note, the septal flattening seen in normal newborns for the first few days of life invalidates the shortening fraction as an index of left ventricular performance in newborn infants.[95]

Given the proper conditions, then, the echocardiographic shortening fraction provides an excellent measure of left ventricular performance. Ventricular performance, however, has three major determinants: namely, loading conditions, contractility, and heart rate.[68,145] Consequently, one cannot determine from the shortening fraction alone if abnormal performance is due to depressed contractility or unusual loading conditions. The implications of these two alternatives are quite different.

Loading Conditions

Preload, or the length of the myofibers at the beginning of contraction, is largely determined by the end-diastolic volume and the compliance of the left ventricle. Although relatively easy to assess in an acute preparation, preload is very difficult to track chronically because the diastolic

pressure-volume relation may not be constant over time. Hypertrophy or dilation, which may occur in response to altered hemodynamics, affects the pressure-volume relation. Ventricular performance is highly dependent upon preload (Fig. 25–3).[68] According to the Frank-Starling mechanism, an increase in preload augments performance and vice versa. Acute infusion of a blood volume expander such as dextran into an intact animal results in an increase in performance, whereas reduction of circulating blood volume depresses performance, provided the sympathetic nervous system is not reflexly stimulated.

Afterload can be thought of as the force on the myofibers resisting shortening. Another, and potentially more useful, way to think of afterload is as the unique relation between myofiber tension and length that limits contraction.[38,132,144] If an isolated papillary muscle is stimulated to contract isometrically, there is a maximum tension that it can generate for each starting length (Fig. 25–4A). If the muscle is allowed to shorten, contraction proceeds

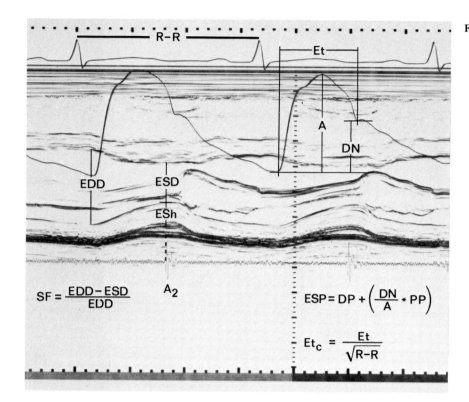

Figure 25–5. An M-mode echocardiogram of the left ventricle with simultaneously recorded electrocardiogram, carotid pulse tracing, and phonocardiogram used for calculating end-systolic wall stress and velocity of fiber shortening. The end-diastolic and end-systolic dimensions of the left ventricle and the end-systolic posterior wall thickness are derived from the echocardiogram using the largest cavity dimension and the aortic component of the second heart sound to mark end-diastole and end-systole, respectively. The end-systolic pressure is determined from the carotid pulse tracing by linear interpolation. The pulse tracing is calibrated using cuff blood pressure measurements. The ejection time is measured from the carotid pulse tracing and the R-R interval from the electrocardiogram. A = distance from the nadir to the apex of the pulse tracing; A_2 = aortic component of the second heart sound; DN = distance from the nadir of the pulse tracing to the dicrotic notch; DP = diastolic blood pressure; EDD = end-diastolic dimension; ESD = end-systolic dimension; ESh = end-systolic wall thickness; ESP = end-systolic pressure; Et = ejection time; Et_c = ejection time adjusted for heart rate; PP = pulse pressure; R-R = R-R interval.

until the length-tension loop intersects the maximum length-tension line, at which point contraction stops (Fig. 25–4B).[144] Thus, the end-systolic tension felt by each myofiber (end-systolic wall stress) is an extremely useful expression of afterload. In addition, this measure of afterload is independent of preload.[132] Notice that the end-systolic length-tension point is unaffected by the previous trajectory of the length-tension loop or by the conditions at the onset of contraction (Fig. 25–5).

Practically, the end-systolic meridional wall stress can be estimated as the following:[20,39]

$$ESS = \frac{0.34 \cdot ESD \cdot ESP}{ESh \cdot \left(1 + \frac{ESh}{ESD}\right)}$$

where: ESS is end-systolic wall stress (g/cm^2)

ESP is end-systolic pressure (mmHg)

ESD is end-systolic dimension (cm)

ESh is end-systolic wall thickness (cm)

The end-systolic dimension and wall thickness can be measured readily from an M-mode echocardiogram. The end-systolic pressure can be derived from a simultaneously recorded carotid or axillary pulse tracing calibrated with a cuff blood pressure measurement (Fig. 25–5). Using this technology, the end-systolic wall stress can be measured noninvasively, providing an excellent index of afterload. It must be pointed out, however, that Mirsky's formula for wall stress holds only if the left ventricle is ellipsoidal in shape.

Increasing afterload decreases performance as evaluated by the shortening fraction or velocity of fiber shortening, while lowering afterload does the opposite.[20] For example, infusion of methoxamine, a pure α-adrenergic agonist, raises blood pressure, increases end-systolic wall stress, and lowers shortening fraction and velocity of shortening. In fact, there is an inverse linear relationship between end-systolic wall stress and shortening fraction or velocity of shortening.

Contractility

Contractility may be defined as the intrinsic ability of muscle fibers to generate force. Practically, contractility may be assessed by relating performance to the loading conditions under which performance was measured. This concept is illustrated by examining the effect of altered contractile state on the end-systolic pressure-volume relation. If a ventricle is allowed to contract to various end-systolic pressure-volume points, these points define a straight line, provided the inotropic state remains constant (Fig. 25–6). The slope of this line (E_{max}) uniquely describes the contractile state of the ventricle.[38,132,133] Administration of an inotropic drug such as dobutamine increases the slope of the end-systolic pressure-volume line, indicating augmentation of the inotropic state. On the other hand, heart failure is associated with reduction of the slope of the end-systolic pressure-volume line, indicating reduced contractile state. In other words, the maximum tension or pressure that can be generated at a given fiber length is a function of the contractile state.

Heart Rate

Normal variation in heart rate appears to have a small but reproducible effect on performance, probably mediated through rate-related changes in contractility.[69] In the intact animal, an increase in heart rate is associated with a reduction in preload due to diminished left ventricular filling time, resulting in a reduction in ejection fraction, despite a small increase in contractility. Since the effects are small under usual physiologic conditions, heart rate will not be discussed further.

Indexes of Performance and Contractility

SHORTENING FRACTION

The echocardiographic shortening fraction (see Fig. 25-2) is derived from the end-diastolic and end-systolic short axis dimensions as the following:

$$SF = \frac{EDD - ESD}{EDD}$$

where: SF is shortening fraction

EDD is end-diastolic dimension

ESD is end-systolic dimension

Recall that the shortening fraction is valid only when the left ventricle is ellipsoidal in shape and there are no regional wall motion abnormalities. Normal values should be established for each laboratory. The normal range of values for our laboratory is 28 to 34 per cent.

The shortening fraction is a measure of performance, which is dependent on preload, afterload, contractility, and heart rate. Loading conditions and contractility cannot be independently assessed by the shortening fraction alone.

VELOCITY OF FIBER SHORTENING

The mean velocity of fiber shortening is an estimate of the average rate of change of the left ventricular circumference in diameters per second. This parameter (see Fig. 25-5) is calculated as the following:

$$VCF_c = \frac{EDD - ESD}{EDD \cdot ET_c}$$

where: ET_c is the ejection time divided by the square root of the R-R interval.

Use of the heart rate adjusted ejection time (ET_c) removes the small but definite effect of heart rate on velocity of fiber shortening. Since calculation of the velocity of fiber shortening is dependent on the short axis dimension of the left ventricle, this parameter is valid only when the left ventricle is ellipsoidal in shape. In our laboratory the normal range of values for rate-adjusted velocity of fiber shortening is > 0.9 diameters/sec. The heart rate-adjusted mean velocity of fiber shortening is dependent on afterload and contractility but is independent of preload.[68,83,92]

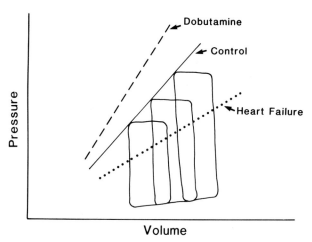

Figure 25-6. Pressure-volume loops for a ventricle contracting under various levels of afterload. The slope of the line connecting the end-systolic points of the loops is E_{max}. The dashed line indicates the effect of an inotropic drug (dobutamine) and the dotted line the effect of heart failure on E_{max}.

END-SYSTOLIC PRESSURE-DIMENSION RELATION

The slope of the end-systolic pressure-volume line (E_{max}), as discussed previously, is the current gold standard for assessment of contractility. This parameter, however, cannot be readily calculated noninvasively. As previously noted, if the left ventricle is ellipsoidal in shape, the short axis dimension is linearly related to volume over the physiologic range and can be substituted for volume. It should be noted, however, that use of the end-systolic pressure-volume relation is not subject to these geometrical constraints regarding left ventricular shape. Use of the end-systolic pressure-dimension relation has been validated in animal studies[65] and in humans.[14] Needed for this calculation are an M-mode echocardiogram, an electrocardiogram, a phonocardiogram showing the aortic component of the second heart sound, and a carotid (or in infants an axillary) indirect pulse tracing, all recorded simultaneously (see Fig. 25-5). Also, the blood pressure is measured by an arm cuff for calibration of the indirect pulse tracing. The endocardial borders of the left ventricle are digitized into a computer, and the instantaneous left ventricular dimension is calculated over the course of the cardiac cycle. The pulse tracing is also digitized and calibrated by assigning the systolic blood pressure to the peak and the diastolic blood pressure to the nadir of the pulse tracing. The instantaneous pressure over the course of ejection is then calculated by linear interpolation. The time delay of the pulse tracing is corrected by aligning the dicrotic notch with the aortic component of the second heart sound. The ejection portion of the pressure-dimension loop is then generated by the computer.

This procedure is repeated several times as the blood pressure is increased 40 to 50 per cent by infusing methoxamine. Pretreatment with atropine is necessary to prevent reflex bradycardia. The end-systolic points of the ejection pressure-dimension loops so generated are

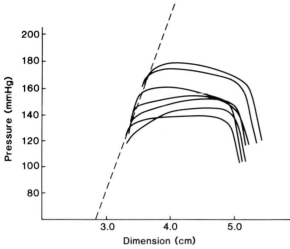

Figure 25–7. The ejection portion of several pressure–dimension loops generated by augmenting afterload with methoxamine. The point of maximum change of slope at the left side of each ejection loop is considered the end-systolic point. The best fit line through these points is the end-systolic pressure–dimension line, the slope of which (Pes-Des) is analogous to E_{max} as a load-independent index of contractility.

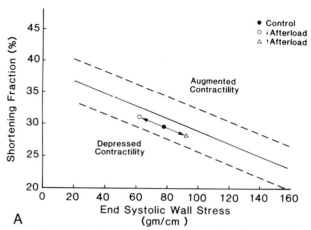

A

Figure 25–8. *A*, The shortening fraction–end-systolic wall stress relation. The normal range (mean ± 2 standard deviations) for our laboratory is shown. Changes in afterload move the relation parallel to the normal range, while changes in contractile state move the relation above or below the normal range.

connected by the best-fit line and the slope of the line (pes-des) determined (Fig. 25–7). The normal value for the slope of the end-systolic pressure-dimension line in our laboratory is > 90 mmHg/cm/M².

The slope of the end-systolic pressure-dimension line is difficult and time consuming to measure. Since this index is dependent upon the short axis dimension of the left ventricle, the same constraints on left ventricular shape and wall motion as stated for the shortening fraction prevail. However, the slope of the end-systolic pressure-dimension line is an index of contractility, which is independent of loading conditions.

END-SYSTOLIC WALL STRESS–
SHORTENING FRACTION RELATION

The relation between the end-systolic wall stress and the shortening fraction is an index of contractility that takes into account afterload.[13] The shortening fraction is calculated as described previously from the M-mode echocardiogram (see Fig. 25–5). The end-systolic wall stress is calculated as previously described using Mirsky's formula, deriving the end-systolic dimension and wall thickness from the M-mode echocardiogram and the end-systolic pressure from the indirect pulse tracing (see Fig. 25–5).

There is a linear relation between shortening fraction and the end-systolic wall stress, which is sensitive to the contractile state and which takes into account afterload (Fig. 25–8A). However, this index is also sensitive to preload (Fig. 25–8B).[20]

END-SYSTOLIC WALL STRESS–VELOCITY
OF FIBER SHORTENING RELATION

The relationship between end-systolic wall stress and velocity of shortening is also an index of contractility that

takes into account afterload (Fig. 25–9A).[20] This relationship is calculated much like the end-systolic wall stress–shortening fraction relation. The two additional items (ejection time and R-R interval) required are derived from the indirect pulse tracing (see Fig. 25–5).

The end-systolic wall stress–velocity of shortening relation has two advantages over the end-systolic wall stress–shortening fraction relation. First, the former is insensitive to preload because mean velocity of fiber shortening is insensitive to preload (see Fig. 25–9B). Second, adjustment of the velocity of fiber shortening for heart rate removes the small but potentially confounding effects of heart rate on performance.[20] Thus, the end-systolic wall stress–velocity of fiber shortening relation is an easily measured index of contractility that adjusts for afterload and heart rate and is insensitive to preload.

Pulmonary Artery Pressure

Attempts have been made to estimate pulmonary artery pressure using systolic time intervals derived from the pulmonary valve echogram. Pulmonary artery hypertension increases the afterload on the right ventricle. An increase in ventricular afterload lengthens the preejection period and shortens the ejection time.[142] Several investigators have reported a strong positive correlation (r = 0.6 to 0.85) between the ratio of the right ventricular preejection period to the right ventricular ejection time (RVPEP/RVET) and the pulmonary artery pressure.[48,85,97] Although the systolic time interval ratio, or some function of the ratio, is correlated with the pulmonary artery pressure (usually most closely with the diastolic pressure), all investigators report that the predictive value for an individual subject is less than what would be expected from the correlation coefficient, with a 16 to 20 per cent false prediction rate in one study.[85] This relatively poor predictive value appears to be due to rather broad scatter of the data points about the regression line, with one or two

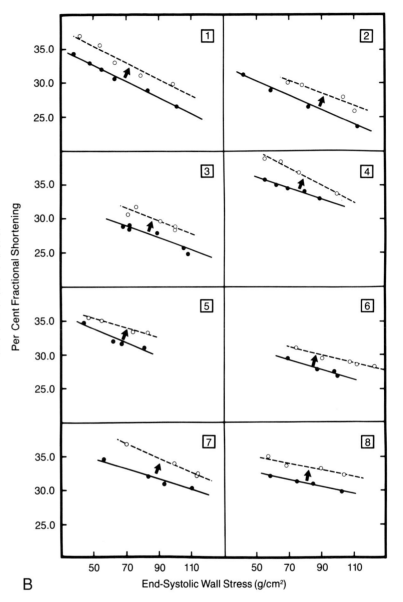

Figure 25–8 *Continued B,* The effect on the shortening fraction–end-systolic wall stress relation of augmenting preload by infusion of dextran. The closed circles are baseline measurements, and the open circles are measurements made after preload augmentation. Note that increased preload cannot be distinguished from enhanced contractility by this parameter alone. (Reprinted with permission from the American College of Cardiology. Colan SD et al [1984]: Left ventricular end-systolic wall stress—velocity of fiber shortening relation: A load-independent index of myocardial contractility. J Am Coll Cardiol 4:715–724.)

outlying points contributing heavily to the correlation coefficient. The ratio of the right ventricular to left ventricular systolic time interval ratios (RVPEP/RVET to LVPEP/LVET) offers no advantage over the RVPEP/RVET alone.[85]

A well-designed study by Silverman et al[115] in which right ventricular systolic time intervals, measured directly from the pulmonary artery pressure tracing obtained using a manometer-tipped catheter and from the pulmonary valve echogram, were compared with simultaneously measured pressure. While the invasively and noninvasively derived systolic time intervals were highly correlated (r = 0.91), neither was predictive of pulmonary artery pressure (r = 0.54). Although we have not rigorously tested right ventricular systolic time intervals for estimating pulmonary artery pressure, the variability of this index seems too large to use in place of direct pressure measurement.

TWO-DIMENSIONAL ECHOCARDIOGRAPHY

Two-dimensional echocardiographic images can be thought of as a collection of adjacent M-mode echocardiographic views of the heart obtained by rapidly rotating a single transducer through an arc of 30 to 90 degrees. The imaging device keeps track of the orientation of the transducer as it is being rotated and displays each M-mode line in the correct position. This process is, in fact, how mechanical scanners work. Phased-array scanners contain a number of fixed transducer elements (usually 32 or 64 elements) that can be activated individually, allowing the sound beam to be steered electronically to achieve the same effect. Various image processing techniques are then used to blend adjacent lines, producing a more coherent image.

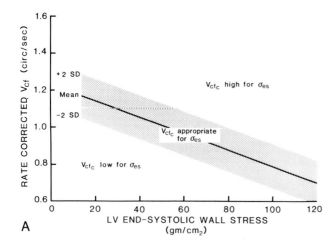

Figure 25–9. *A,* The velocity of fiber shortening–end-systolic wall stress relation. The shaded area is the normal range for our laboratory. Changes in afterload move the relation in a linear manner parallel to the normal range. Changes in contractility move the relation above or below the normal range. *B,* Unlike the shortening fraction–end-systolic wall stress relation, augmentation of preload has no effect on the velocity of fiber shortening–end-systolic wall stress relation. Closed circles are baseline measurements, while open circles are measurements made after preload augmentation. (Reprinted with permission from the American College of Cardiology. Colan SD et al [1984]: Left ventricular end-systolic wall stress—velocity of fiber shortening relation: A load-independent index of myocardial contractility. J Am Coll Cardiol 4:715–724.)

Structural Heart Defects

Two-dimensional echocardiography is currently the imaging technique of choice for diagnosing structural heart defects in infants. Nearly any defect can be diagnosed using two-dimensional echocardiography if a comprehensive and systematic examination is performed. The examination technique my colleagues and I have found most useful is based on multiple plane imaging of the heart and great vessels.[149] While the examination is generally started with standard subxiphoid, apical, parasternal, and suprasternal notch views, we improvise as needed to investigate the cardiac anatomy.

Subxiphoid long axis, short axis,[8–10,100] and oblique views[71,72] of the heart are usually obtained first because these views afford an overview of the cardiac anatomy, including the segmental combination. The importance of displaying the subxiphoid (and apical) views in an anatomically correct orientation[40] cannot be overemphasized.

Visceroatrial situs is first determined from a transverse view of the abdomen at the diaphragm, which shows the relative positions of the inferior vena cava, the descending aorta, and the spine (Fig. 25–10A).[51] Angling the transducer cranially tracks the inferior vena cava to the right atrium and allows imaging of both atria and the atrial septum (Fig. 25–10B).[10] Further cranial and anterior an-

gulation of the transducer successively shows the atrioventricular valves, the ventricles, and the outflow tracts and great arteries (Fig. 25–10C to E).[100]

Rotation of the transducer 90 degrees about its long axis provides a short axis, or parasagittal plane, view of the heart. Angling the transducer from the right heart border toward the apex sequentially displays the atria, the atrioventricular valves, the outflow tracts, and the ventricles in cross-section (Fig. 25–11A to E).[8,100] Rotation of the transducer 20 to 30 degrees counterclockwise or clockwise from the short axis view produces left and right oblique views, respectively.[71,72]

Once the general anatomic survey has been completed, other views[91,136] are used to fill in details. The parasternal long axis view is especially useful for imaging the left and right ventricular outflow tracts, while the parasternal short axis view allows for detailed investigation of the aortic and mitral valves. Parasternal short axis views from the first or second intercostal space display the branch pulmonary arteries. A parasagittal plane view from this transducer position is excellent for imaging a persistent ductus arteriosus (Fig. 25–12). Since the apical four-chamber view displays all four chambers of the heart and the atrioventricular valves simultaneously, the ventricular morphology and atrioventricular alignments can be determined readily using this view.[113] The pulmonary veins and left

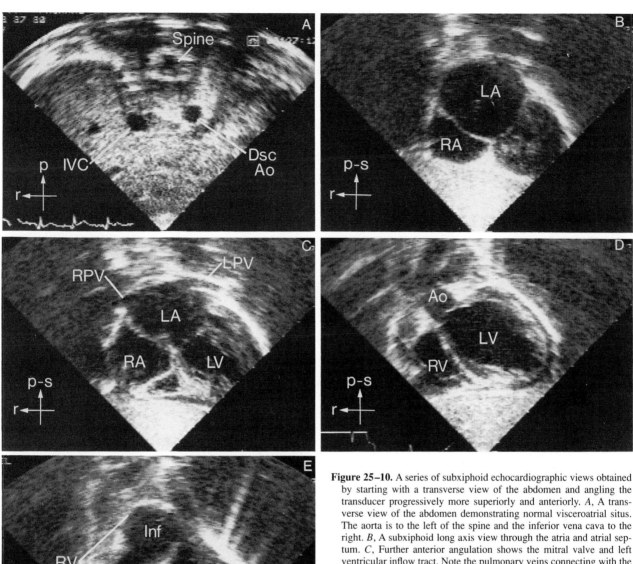

Figure 25–10. A series of subxiphoid echocardiographic views obtained by starting with a transverse view of the abdomen and angling the transducer progressively more superiorly and anteriorly. *A*, A transverse view of the abdomen demonstrating normal visceroatrial situs. The aorta is to the left of the spine and the inferior vena cava to the right. *B*, A subxiphoid long axis view through the atria and atrial septum. *C*, Further anterior angulation shows the mitral valve and left ventricular inflow tract. Note the pulmonary veins connecting with the left atrium. *D*, Next is the right ventricular inflow tract and the left ventricular outflow and aorta. *E*, Finally, a coronal plane view of the right ventricle showing the sinus and infundibular portions. Ao = aorta; Dsc Ao = descending aorta; Inf = infundibulum; IVC = inferior vena cava; LA = left atrium; LPV = left pulmonary vein; RPV = right pulmonary vein; LV = left ventricle; p = posterior; p-s = posterior-superior; r = right; RA = right atrium; RPA = right pulmonary artery; RV = right ventricle; s = superior; Si = right ventricular sinus.

atrium also are usually seen well in this view. The apical two-chamber, or long axis, view is the most sensitive for detecting a membrane in the left ventricular outflow tract.[23] Also, both apical views are useful for detecting muscular ventricular septal defects. Suprasternal notch views (Fig. 25–13) generally display the aortic arch and brachiocephalic vessels, the systemic veins of the upper mediastinum, the pulmonary veins, and the branch pulmonary arteries.[123] Right sternal border views, with the patient in a steep right decubitus position, are valuable for displaying the atrial septum, particularly the sinus venosus portion.[137]

As the various views are obtained, the examiner mentally constructs a three-dimensional image of the heart from the two-dimensional "slices." Accurate diagnosis of congenital heart defects requires not only high quality images of the heart and vessels in multiple planes but also a thorough understanding of and familiarity with pathologic cardiac anatomy. Given all these elements, two-dimensional echocardiography is an indispensable tool in the practice of pediatric cardiology.

The remainder of this section will discuss the diagnosis of a few specific defects that commonly present in the neonate, some of which may be confused with other neonatal

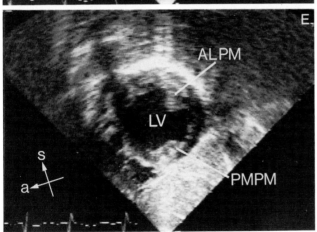

Figure 25–11. A series of subxiphoid short axis or parasagittal plane views of the heart, starting at the right atrium and angling to the apex of the heart. *A*, Right parasagittal plane view showing the junction of the inferior and superior vena cavae with the right atrium. *B*, Subxiphoid short axis view through the mid portion of the atrial septum showing the fossa ovalis (triangle). *C*, Further leftward angulation shows the left ventricular outflow tract. Mitral-to-aortic continuity can be seen (arrow). *D*, Next, the right ventricular outflow tract is seen. *E*, A short axis view at midventricular level showing the left ventricular papillary muscles. a = anterior; ALPM = anterolateral papillary muscle; Ao = aorta; IVC = inferior vena cava; LA = left atrium; LV = left ventricle; MPA = main pulmonary artery; PMPM = posteromedial papillary muscle; RA = right atrium; RPA = right pulmonary artery; RV = right ventricle; s = superior; SVC = superior vena cava.

problems. Excellent textbooks are available that detail the general use of two-dimensional echocardiography for diagnosing congenital heart defects.[114,149]

Cyanotic Heart Defects

TOTAL ANOMALOUS PULMONARY
VENOUS DRAINAGE

In this condition none of the pulmonary veins connect with the left atrium. Rather, some or all of the pulmonary veins form a confluence or collecting vessel that usually lies posterior to the left atrium. There may be one or more sites of connection between the pulmonary venous confluence or individual pulmonary veins and the systemic venous circuit.

The two-dimensional echocardiographic diagnosis of this anomaly depends on adequate imaging of the pulmonary veins and their connections. When the pulmonary veins connect normally, their junction with the left atrium can be seen using subxiphoid, apical, or suprasternal notch views (see Figs. 25–10*C* and 25–13*B*). In contrast, the diagnosis of anomalous venous connection is based on detection of a pulmonary venous confluence posterior to and distinct from the left atrium,[16,99,121,124] in addition to failure to detect normal pulmonary venous connection with the left atrium (Fig. 25–14A). The next task is to determine the site(s) of connection between the pulmonary venous confluence and the systemic veins. When the connection is subdiaphragmatic or cardiac (to the right atrium or coronary sinus), subxiphoid views are generally superior (Fig. 25–14B and C). Apical and parasternal views are alternatives for imaging cardiac connections. Supracardiac connections are usually seen best using suprasternal notch views (Fig. 25–14D). If the route of the connection is lengthy, as is often the case in supracardiac connection, it generally does not lie in a single plane, so that scanning or multiple plane imaging may be required to display the venous pathway adequately.

There are now a number of reports in the literature that document the reliability of two-dimensional echocardiography for diagnosing total anomalous pulmonary venous drainage and for determining the site(s) of connection with the systemic veins. In our laboratory over the last 3 years,[16] two-dimensional echocardiography has been 100 per cent accurate for diagnosing total anomalous pulmonary venous drainage in infants. Further, the site of connection with the systemic veins was determined correctly in 95 per cent of the cases.

d-TRANSPOSITION OF THE GREAT ARTERIES

Transposition refers to that condition in which the great arteries are aligned with the opposite ventricle from normal. The most common type is d-transposition, in which the atria and ventricles are normally positioned but the aorta is anterior and rightward ("d" for dextro) and aligned with the right ventricle while the pulmonary artery is posterior and leftward and aligned with the left ventricle. This condition seems to be related to abnormal development of the infundibulum.

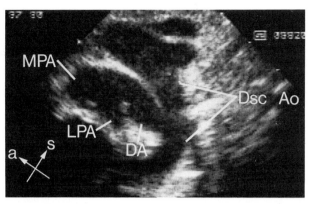

Figure 25–12. A high parasternal, parasagittal plane view for imaging the ductus arteriosus. a = anterior; DA = ductus arteriosus; Dsc Ao = descending aorta; LPA = left pulmonary artery; MPA = main pulmonary artery; s = superior.

The echocardiographic diagnosis of d-transposition of the great arteries is based on determining the ventriculoarterial alignments. The ventricles are identified on the basis of morphology.[28] The morphologically left ventricle is ovoid in shape, with fine trabeculations, free wall papillary muscles (usually two), a smooth septal surface, and a more basal septal insertion of its atrioventricular valve. In contrast, the morphologically right ventricle is more triangular in shape, with coarse trabeculations, septal attachments of the atrioventricular valve, a moderator band, and a more apical septal insertion of its atrioventricular valve. Next, the great arteries are identified by the branching pattern. The aorta is an arch-forming artery that gives rise to the brachiocephalic arteries (usually three), while the pulmonary artery bifurcates early into the right and left pulmonary arteries. The ventriculoarterial alignments are then determined by simultaneously imaging the ventricles and great arteries (Fig. 25–15).[9,72,100]

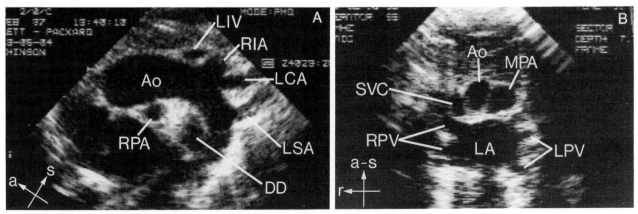

Figure 25–13. Suprasternal notch views. A, The aortic arch and bracheocephalic vessels. B, Pulmonary veins connecting with the left atrium. a = anterior; Ao = aorta; a-s = anterior-superior; DD = ductus diverticulum; LA = left atrium; LCA = left carotid artery; LIV = left innominate vein; LPV = left pulmonary vein; LSA = left subclavian artery; MPA = main pulmonary artery; RIA = right innominate artery; RPA = right pulmonary artery; RPV = right pulmonary vein; s = superior; r = right; SVC = superior vena cava.

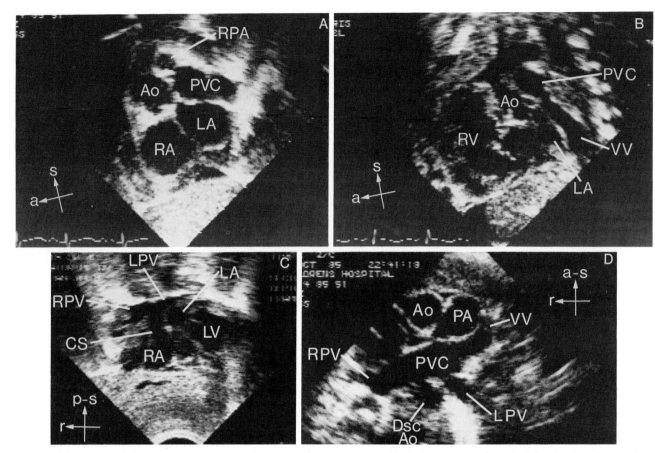

Figure 25–14. *A,* Subxiphoid short axis view showing the pulmonary venous confluence behind, and separate from, the left atrium in total anomalous pulmonary venous connection. *B,* Subxiphoid short axis view of the venous confluence and the descending vertical vein in subdiaphragmatic total anomalous pulmonary venous connection. *C,* Subxiphoid long axis view of anomalous pulmonary venous connection to the coronary sinus. *D,* Suprasternal notch view showing the pulmonary venous confluence and part of the ascending vertical vein in supracardiac total anomalous pulmonary venous connection. a = anterior; Ao = aorta; CS = coronary sinus; Dsc Ao = descending aorta; LA = left atrium; LPV = left pulmonary vein; LV = left ventricle; p = posterior; PA = pulmonary artery; p-s = posterior-superior; PVC = pulmonary venous confluence; RA = right atrium; RPA = right pulmonary artery; RPV = right pulmonary vein; RV = right ventricle; s = superior; r = right; VV = vertical vein.

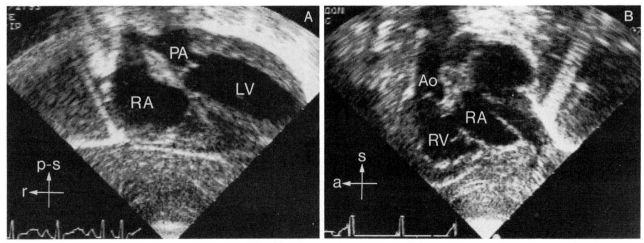

Figure 25–15. Subxiphoid views in an infant with d-transposition of the great arteries. *A,* Long axis view showing the bifurcating pulmonary artery aligned with the left ventricle. *B,* Alignment of the aorta with the right ventricle is seen in this short axis view. a = anterior; Ao = aorta; LV = left ventricle; PA = pulmonary artery; p-s = posterior-superior; RA = right atrium; RV = right ventricle; s = superior; r = right.

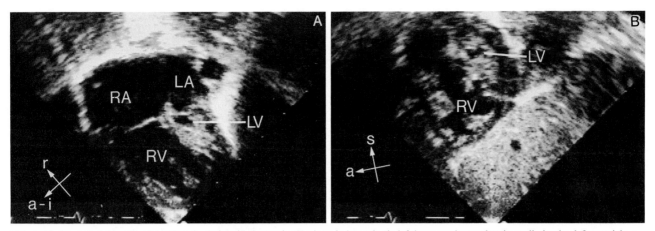

Figure 25–16. Apical four-chamber (*A*) and subxiphoid short axis (*B*) views in hypoplastic left heart syndrome showing a diminutive left ventricle. a = anterior; a-i = anterior-inferior; LA = left atrium; LV = left ventricle; r = right; RA = right atrium; RV = right ventricle; s = superior.

Associated features that must be investigated include the status of the ventricular septum,[8] the presence and nature of left ventricular outflow tract obstruction,[17] and, in the era of the arterial switch operation, the anatomy of the coronary arteries.[89]

Left Heart Obstructive Lesions

HYPOPLASTIC LEFT-HEART SYNDROME

This anomaly is characterized by extreme hypoplasia of all left heart structures. The mitral valve is diminutive or atretic. The left ventricular cavity is usually tiny, although the walls may be thick. In some cases the left ventricle is too small to be imaged by two-dimensional echocardiography. The aortic valve is usually atretic with variable hypoplasia of the aortic root and ascending aorta. In the typical case the diagnosis is straightforward, based on the appearance of the left ventricle, aortic valve, and aortic root.[4,60] Occasionally, the left heart hypoplasia is only moderate in severity, what we have termed the "not-so-hypoplastic left-heart syndrome." In such cases the over-riding question is "How small is too small?" There are no definitive answers, owing to the variability of factors such as left ventricular outflow tract obstruction, left ventricular performance, and arch obstruction. Nonetheless, we have found that as a general rule, a left ventricle with a volume less than 15 to 20 ml/M^2 or an aortic root smaller than 5 mm in diameter is very unlikely to support adequate cardiac output.

The diagnosis is usually obvious from the initial subxiphoid or apical scans, which show the mitral hypoplasia or atresia and the tiny left ventricle (Fig. 25–16). The ascending aorta is usually seen best from a parasternal, parasagittal view. The aortic arch and ductus arteriosus are optimally seen from suprasternal or high left or right parasternal views. The branch pulmonary arteries, which may be hypoplastic, can be imaged using a high left sternal border or suprasternal notch transverse view.

Two-dimensional echocardiography has been considered a reliable technique for making this diagnosis for several years.[60] Even now in the era of surgical palliation of infants with hypoplastic left-heart syndrome, two-dimensional echocardiography continues to provide all the information necessary to undertake palliative surgery.[4] In those infants in whom the left ventricular size is borderline, however, angiographic volume measurements may provide information useful in making difficult management decisions.

COARCTATION OF THE AORTA

Coarctation in the neonate typically presents at 7 to 10 days with absent lower extremity pulses and congestive heart failure or a shock-like syndrome. The diagnosis can readily be confirmed with two-dimensional and Doppler echocardiography,[50,119] and other lesions in the differential diagnosis, such as aortic arch interruption, hypoplastic left-heart syndrome, or critical aortic stenosis, can be excluded.

Right sternal border, suprasternal notch, or left sternal border views are best for defining the coarctation echocardiographically (Fig. 25–17). Typically, a "shelf" is seen

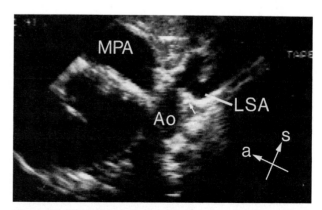

Figure 25–17. A high, left sternal border view showing a discrete coarctation just distal to the left subclavian artery. Note the shelf (arrow) projecting into the lumen from the posterior aortic wall. a = anterior; Ao = aorta; LSA = left subclavian artery; MPA = main pulmonary artery; s = superior.

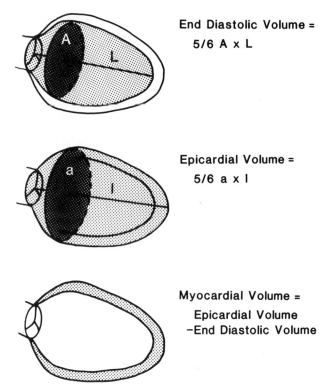

End Diastolic Volume =

5/6 A x L

Epicardial Volume =

5/6 a x l

Myocardial Volume =

Epicardial Volume

−End Diastolic Volume

Figure 25–18. Schematic of the method for calculating left ventricular volume and mass using the ⅚ area × length algorithm.

protruding from the posterior wall of the aorta opposite the remnant of the ductus arteriosus and just distal to the left subclavian artery. If the ductus arteriosus is widely patent, at least at the aortic end, the coarctation may be missed or its severity underestimated. The presence of a posterior shelf should alert the examiner to the possibility that arch obstruction will develop with closure of the ductus arteriosus. Serial examinations are useful in such situations. In addition, there may be variable hypoplasia of the transverse arch.

Persistent Ductus Arteriosus

Probably the most common cardiac abnormality in the neonate, especially the preterm neonate, is persistence of the ductus arteriosus. Since the excess pulmonary blood flow and pressure associated with persistence of the ductus arteriosus may adversely affect the course of the neonate with or without lung disease, it is important to make the diagnosis expeditiously. Combined use of two-dimensional and Doppler echocardiography is currently the method of choice for diagnosing persistent ductus arteriosus[49,120,141] as well as for monitoring medical therapy.[118]

The most useful view for diagnosing a persistent ductus is a high (first or second interspace) parasagittal, parasternal view (see Fig. 25–12).[120] This view is in the plane of the ductus arteriosus and displays its entire length. While the ductus may be seen from the suprasternal notch or the subxiphoid space, these views are not as reliable as

the parasagittal view. Misunderstanding of the anatomic location of the ductus often hinders imaging. The ductus actually lies superior and nearly parallel to the left pulmonary artery. It does not arise between the branch pulmonary arteries, as often depicted.

The newly closed ductus may appear patent by imaging, since the necrosing intima and media and associated thrombus do not reflect ultrasound efficiently. Therefore, we require further evidence for patency, such as the Doppler flow pattern or a contrast injection.

Ventricular Performance

Two-dimensional echocardiography can be used to measure ventricular volume, mass, stroke volume, and ejection fraction, to assess ventricular conformation, and to evaluate regional performance.

Left Ventricular Volume

Estimation of left ventricular volume is often used in evaluating volume overload lesions, in determining the adequacy of the size of the left ventricle, and in calculating the ejection fraction. While many algorithms[112] are available for the calculation of left ventricular volume, we have found the ⅚ area × length method to be both simple and reliable for infants and children (Fig. 25–18). This method requires one long axis and one short axis view of the left ventricle. Subxiphoid views are most satisfactory in infants. The subxiphoid long axis view provides a full-length view of the left ventricle without truncation. Apical views, on the other hand, may foreshorten the left ventricle, resulting in falsely low volumes. Use of an algorithm that includes a short axis view seems to improve reliability if the ventricular conformation is unusual, since the true cross-sectional topography of the ventricle is included in the calculation. The subxiphoid view provides a true short axis cut, which may be difficult to obtain using parasternal views in infants because of the horizontal orientation of the heart.

Volume calculations are performed using whichever method is preferred at end-diastole and end-systole. The definitions of end-diastole and end-systole vary, but largest and smallest cavity area, respectively, are simple and reproducible definitions. Stroke volume is then calculated as the end-diastolic volume minus end-systolic volume.

Ventricular volumes must be related in some way to the size of the patient for any meaningful interpretation. The most widely accepted method is to divide the raw volume (ml) by the body surface area, yielding an indexed volume (ml/M^2). The normal range of values in our laboratory for end-diastolic volume index in infants less than 2 years of age is $45 \pm 15 \ ml/M^2$.

Gordon et al[34] tested the reproducibility of echocardiographic measurements of left ventricular volume. While the intraobserver variability was low, there was significant interobserver and beat-to-beat variability. Further, serial volume measurements by the same observer on successive days varied by as much as 15 per cent for end-diastolic volume and 25 per cent for end-systolic volume, thought to be due mostly to biologic variation. The authors recommend that the end-diastolic volume measurement change by at least 15 per cent and the end-systolic volume measurement by at least 25 per cent before such changes are considered to reflect real changes in volume. Because intraobserver variability is low compared with interobserver variability, more consistent results can be obtained if one examiner makes serial measurements in an individual patient.

Right Ventricular Volume

Because of the shape of the right ventricle, measurement of volume is much less straightforward than for the left ventricle. Nonetheless, evaluation of right ventricular size and function is often of great importance in pediatric cardiology. Methods have been devised for measurement of right ventricular volume from the two-dimensional echocardiogram using one or two apical views.[47,110] Although an excellent correlation has been reported between the right ventricular volume measured by two-dimensional echocardiography and angiography, some correction procedure is necessary to obtain numerically comparable values.

We have used subxiphoid coronal and parasagittal plane views of the right ventricle for volume calculations in infants and small children. A biplane Simpson's rule algorithm, defining the pulmonary valve-to-diaphragmatic free wall dimension as the long axis of the ventricle, has proved most suitable. In our laboratory, the normal values for right ventricular end-diastolic volume in infants under 1 year of age using this technique are 30 ± 5 ml/M^2. This method probably underestimates the right ventricular volume slightly. We prefer it because the subxiphoid views are readily obtained and easily standardized using anatomic landmarks. Also, this technique makes no assumptions regarding the relative contributions of the sinus and infundibulum to the total right ventricular volume.

Left Ventricular Mass

Left ventricular myocardial volume can be measured from the two-dimensional echocardiogram in a manner similar to cavitary volume (see Fig. 25–18).[93] First, the combined cavitary and myocardial volume is calculated using the epicardial border. Then the cavitary volume is subtracted from the combined volume, leaving the myocardial volume. Mass can be calculated by multiplying the myocardial volume by the density of muscle (1.05 g/ml). Like volume, the myocardial mass must be related to body size, usually by dividing by body surface area to yield the mass index (g/M^2). The mass-to-volume ratio (normally ~ 1 for the left ventricle) is useful for determining whether the myocardial mass is appropriate for the size of the cavity. Values significantly greater than 1 indicate left ventricular hypertrophy, while values lower than 0.85 indicate inadequate muscle development, as is usually seen in congestive cardiomyopathy or an acutely imposed pressure or volume load. Normal values for left ventricular mass index in infants less than 2 years of age for our laboratory are 48 ± 8 g/M^2.

Ejection Fraction

The most commonly used index of global ventricular performance is the ejection fraction. The ejection fraction is calculated using the end-diastolic and end-systolic volumes derived from the two-dimensional echocardiogram (see Fig. 25–18) as the following:

$$EF = \frac{EDV - ESV}{EDV}$$

where: EF is ejection fraction

EDV is end-diastolic volume

ESV is end-systolic volume

The ejection fraction is an index of performance, which is highly dependent upon loading conditions (see Figs. 25–3 and 25–6) as well as contractile state. The range of normal values for ejection fraction varies with the ventricle being evaluated and the method for volume measurement used. Normal values should be established for each laboratory. The normal values for our laboratory in infants less than 2 years of age for left ventricular ejection fraction are 60 ± 6 per cent and for right ventricular efection fraction are 65 ± 7 per cent.

As for volume, there may be significant interobserver and beat-to-beat variability in the ejection fraction,[34] the latter probably due largely to biologic variation. A measured change in ejection fraction should be at least 10 per cent before the measurement is considered to reflect a real change in performance. As noted above for volume measurements, serial measurements of ejection fraction are more consistent if made by a single observer.

Regional Performance

Evaluation of regional ventricular performance assumes importance not only in pathologic conditions in which there is regional variation in the functional level of the ventricle but also in some normal states. For example, the elevated right ventricular pressure seen in the the early neonatal period is associated with distortion of left ventricular shape. Further, the pattern of wall motion seen in newborn infants is clearly different from that seen in older infants, children, and adults. Regional evaluation of function may also be of value in assessing performance of the right ventricle and may even provide clues to the etiology of ventricular dysfunction.

Regional wall motion analysis of the left ventricle was originally undertaken in adults with coronary artery disease to evaluate the location and extent of disease.[46,62,96,146] While this technology has not been applied widely in infants and children, the few studies performed indicate that regional analysis of function may provide insights into ventricular mechanics in infants and children with and without heart defects.

Rein et al[95] investigated the regional left ventricular performance of normal neonates over the first week of life. Striking regional variation in performance was noted

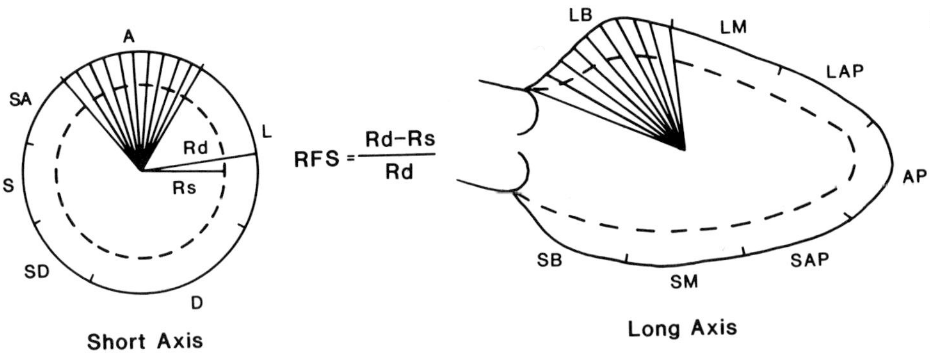

Figure 25–19. Schematic of a method for analysis of regional wall motion using a floating center of mass model. Sixty-four radii are drawn outward from the center of mass of the cavity to their intersection with the end-diastolic and end-systolic endocardial borders. The shortening fraction is then calculated for each radius. Short axis: A = anterior free wall; D = diaphragmatic free wall; L = lateral free wall; S = midseptum; SA = anterior septum; SD = diaphragmatic septum. Long axis: AP = apical; LAP = apical lateral free wall; LB = basal lateral free wall; LM = midlateral free wall; SAP = apical septum; SB = basal septum; SM = midseptum. (Reproduced by permission of Rein AJ et al [1987]: Regional and global left ventricular function in infants with anomalous origin of the left coronary artery from the pulmonary trunk: Preoperative and postoperative assessment. Circulation 75:115–123.)

before day 4 or 5, probably related to elevated right ventricular systolic pressure. A major implication of this finding is that a single-dimension measurement of performance, such as the M-mode echocardiographic shortening fraction, is not a valid index of global performance in most infants before day 4 or 5 of life because of the regional variation in function. While it is not necessary to perform formal regional wall motion analysis, it is advisable to assess regional performance qualitatively using two-dimensional echocardiography in all subjects before using M-mode echocardiography to measure global performance.

Trowitzsch et al[138] applied similiar analytical techniques to the right ventricle in patients with transposition of the great arteries following an atrial baffle repair. As expected, the pattern of motion of the right ventricle differed from that seen in age-matched controls. An unexpected finding, however, was that the few patients included in the study who had congestive heart failure also had regional wall motion abnormalities of the right ventricle. This finding suggests some local injury to the ventricle rather than a globally acting agent such as cyanosis or volume overload.

Analysis of regional wall motion requires a computer-based device designed for this purpose. The cardiac cycles to be analyzed, usually one long axis and one or two short axis views of the ventricle, are selected and recorded. Then, the end-diastolic and end-systolic frames are selected, using the largest and smallest enclosed cavity area, respectively, as markers. The endocardial and epicardial borders of these and the intervening frames are digitized by hand or by using an automatic edge detection algorithm. If an automatic edge detector is used, it is imperative that the operator be able to correct the digitized borders if necessary. Adjustment can be made for rotational motion of the heart by aligning anatomic landmarks such as the anterior and posterior insertion points of the right ventricular free wall, the left ventricular papillary muscles, the anterior and posterior borders of the aortic root, or the apex of the left ventricle.

Either a fixed reference or a floating center of mass model can be used for analysis, but we prefer the latter. Using the floating center point model, the center of mass

is calculated for each frame of the cycle and superimposed one upon the other. Then 16 to 64 radii are drawn outward from the center of mass to their intersection with the endocardial border for each frame (Fig. 25–19). The length of each radius is then plotted for each frame of the cardiac cycle (Fig. 25–20), and the shortening fraction of each radius is calculated using the end-diastolic and end-systolic lengths. Superimposition of the centers of mass adjusts for overall cardiac motion as well as any instability of the video image. On the negative side, this method tends to average the motion of opposing segments, which may obscure subtle wall motion abnormalities.

Alternatively, wall thickness can be determined over the course of the cardiac cycle in an analogous manner using the endocardial and epicardial borders.[84] Then, thickening fraction instead of shortening fraction can be determined along each radius. Use of the thickening fraction does not appear to have advantages over the shortening fraction and, in our laboratory, is less reproducible in children because of the relatively large error associated with measuring thin ventricular walls.

The fixed reference method, in contrast, uses an external reference point and records motion of the endocardium and epicardium relative to this point. Correction for rotational and translational motion of the heart is much more difficult with this technique. While this may be of little importance in adult subjects,[81] the overall cardiac motion seen in infants and children cannot be ignored. On the other hand, the fixed reference technique may be more sensitive for detection of subtle wall motion abnormalities. We have not found this method to be as reproducible as the floating center point method in children. Further, the range of normal for regional shortening fraction for the fixed reference method is much broader than for the floating center point method, making interpretation difficult.

Pulmonary Artery Pressure

Because of the importance of pulmonary artery pressure in pediatric cardiology and neonatology, various methods have been devised to estimate pulmonary pres-

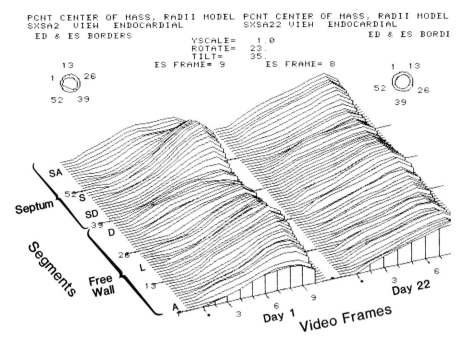

Figure 25–20. Typical display of the frame-by-frame shortening fraction for each of the 64 radii in a normal neonate on the first day of life and at 22 days of age. Note the exaggerated septal motion on day 1. The small insert showing the end-diastolic and end-systolic borders indicates how this appears as septal flattening on the two-dimensional echocardiogram. On day 22 the wall motion is more uniform, and both the end-diastolic and end-systolic borders are circular.

sure noninvasively. King et al[56] have shown that the right ventricular pressure can be estimated from the radius of curvature of the ventricular septum at end-systole. As right ventricular pressure increases, the radius of curvature of the septum increases, that is, the septum flattens. This flattening can be observed readily in either a subxiphoid or a parasternal short axis view of the left ventricle. While a more precise estimate of right ventricular pressure can be obtained by actually measuring the radius of curvature, simply observing the septum at end-systole provides a rough estimate. If the left ventricle maintains a circular contour throughout systole, the right ventricular pressure is less than one half of the left ventricular pressure. Flattening of the septum by end-systole indicates that the right ventricular pressure is at least one half of but

not greater than left ventricular pressure (Fig. 25–21A). Reversal of the septal curvature, with the convex portion toward the left ventricle, indicates that right ventricular pressure is greater than left ventricular pressure (Fig. 25–21B).

CONTRAST ECHOCARDIOGRAPHY

Background

In the late 1960s, Gramiak et al[36] noted that intravascular injection of most any solution resulted in a contrast effect detectable by echocardiography. The initial use of this technique was for identification of structures seen by

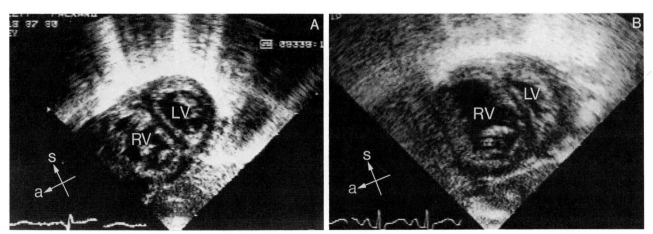

Figure 25–21. Subxiphoid short axis views of the left ventricle at end-systole in an infant with near systemic right ventricular pressure showing flattening of the ventricular septum (A) and suprasystemic right ventricular pressure where the septum becomes convex toward the left ventricle (B). a = anterior; LV = left ventricle; RV = right ventricle; s = superior.

M-mode echocardiography.[27,36] Subsequently, intracardiac injection of contrast material was employed during cardiac catheterization as an adjunct to angiography for diagnosis of congenital heart defects.[55,107] Later investigation demonstrated that injection of a solution of indocyanine green into a peripheral vein produced excellent intracardiac contrast effect.[105,140] Contrast echocardiography has been used in this manner, with both M-mode and two-dimensional echocardiography, for diagnosis of systemic[19,52,122,123] and pulmonary venous anomalies[124] and for detection of intracardiac[29,30,103,147] and great artery level[1] shunts.

Commonly used contrast agents include physiologic saline, 5 per cent dextrose, indocyanine green, blood, and mixtures of blood and saline. Experimental agents used in animal studies include hydrogen peroxide, supersaturated solutions of carbon dioxide or other gases, collagen or polysaccharide microspheres, and perflourocarbon compounds. These compounds are generally cleared by the lungs, so that only right heart chambers are opacified by a contrast injection into a systemic vein. A safe contrast agent that will opacify the left heart from a systemic venous injection is being sought. However, no such agent is currently available for general use.

The cause of the contrast effect is not completely understood, but it appears to be due to microbubbles of gas suspended in the liquid, which act as very efficient reflectors of ultrasound. The large mismatch in acoustic impedance between the liquid and gas results in reflection of almost all the incident sound energy. Other potential explanations for the contrast effect include a density gradient between the blood and the injectate or an induction of rouleaux formation.

Technique

Contrast echocardiography requires a stable intravenous line in an extremity that drains to the vein or heart chamber of interest. For example, if the objective is to determine the connection of a left superior vena cava, then the intravenous line must be in the left arm or left side of the head. Any type of intravenous device is suitable. If the intravenous line is only for the contrast injection, then a 23- or 21-gauge butterfly device is most convenient. A T connector or 3-way stopcock is attached to the tubing of the butterfly. Two 3 or 5 ml syringes (or a single 1 or 3 ml syringe in a newborn) are filled with contrast agent and attached to the T connector or to the stopcock, with care taken to eliminate air bubbles. Two smaller bore syringes are used instead of a single large bore syringe to increase the speed of injection so that the contrast is delivered as a bolus. The volume of contrast used varies with the size of the patient; 1 ml in a newborn, 3 to 6 ml in a child, and 10 ml in an adult. The vessel or chamber of interest is then imaged while an assistant injects both syringes as rapidly as possible. Imaging is continued until the contrast effect has passed or become attenuated. Recordings may be made using M-mode or two-dimensional echocardiography. Careful, even frame-by-frame, examination of the recorded contrast echocardiogram is often necessary for correct interpretation.

The contrast agent used depends upon the preference of the examiner. While any of the agents previously listed are suitable, we prefer a mixture of the patient's blood in sterile saline (0.5 ml of blood in 10 ml of saline) shaken vigorously. The mixture should be used within a few minutes to avoid loss of contrast effect. We prefer this agent because it is readily available and produces a dense contrast effect. In our hands, saline or dextrose solutions alone are not reliable and indocyanine green is not as readily available.

Structural Heart Defects

Systemic Venous Anomalies

An important use of contrast echocardiography is in defining the drainage of anomalous systemic veins, most commonly a persistent left superior vena cava.[19,52,122] Usually, the left vena cava drains to the right atrium via the coronary sinus, but it may terminate in the left atrium. In most cases two-dimensional imaging indicates the site of drainage of the left superior vena cava. Contrast echocardiography is useful for confirming the findings of two-dimensional echocardiography. Injection of contrast agent through a peripheral vein in the left arm or left side of the head opacifies the left superior vena cava. Passage of contrast directly from the left superior vena cava to the left atrium indicates that the cava connects with the left atrium (Fig. 25–22). On the other hand, if contrast passes instead into the coronary sinus and right atrium, then the more common drainage pattern for the left superior vena cava (to the coronary sinus) is present.

In the presence of a large innominate vein, contrast may not fill the left superior vena cava, particularly if the vena cava connects with the left atrium. Rather, there may be a left-to-right shunt through the innominate vein and vena cava so that flow is upward in the left superior vena cava. A coronary sinus septal defect may be difficult to distinguish from direct connection of the left superior vena cava to the left atrium. Contrast material may pass from the coronary sinus directly into the left atrium through the coronary sinus septal defect. In such cases the distinction must be made by imaging.[151]

Pulmonary Venous Anomalies

Contrast echocardiography may be useful for identifying the pulmonary venous confluence in total anomalous pulmonary venous drainage.[122,124] Since this is a common mixing lesion, that is, the systemic and pulmonary venous bloods are completely mixed at the atrial level, a systemic venous contrast injection will opacify all four heart chambers and both great arteries. However, the contrast agent does not cross the pulmonary capillary bed, so the pulmonary venous confluence remains unopacified. Therefore, the structure that remains unopacified after a dense systemic venous contrast injection is the pulmonary venous confluence.

Atrial Septal Defect

Contrast injections are useful for identifying transseptal shunts at the atrial level.[29,103,147] In particular, an atrial

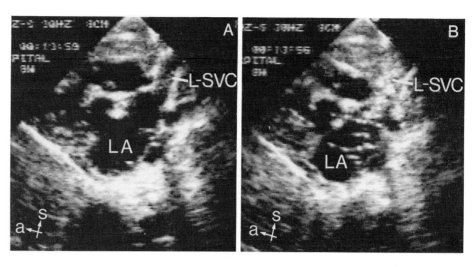

Figure 25–22. Left parasternal view in a patient with connection of a persistent left superior vena cava to the left atrium before (*A*) and after (*B*) contrast injection in the left arm. Note contrast filling the left superior vena cava and entering the left atrium. a = anterior; LA = left atrium; L-SVC = left superior vena cava; s = superior.

right-to-left shunt, often a question in infants suspected of having persistent pulmonary hypertension of the newborn syndrome, can be documented or excluded confidently using venous contrast injection[103] (Fig. 25–23). Most patients with a predominant left-to-right shunt exhibit a small right-to-left shunt by contrast echocardiography, permitting documentation of an interatrial connection. The "negative contrast effect" produced by the unopacified blood traversing the atrial defect from left to right is also an excellent marker for an interatrial connection.[147]

Persistent Ductus Arteriosus

Although a persistent ductus arteriosus can usually be diagnosed using two-dimensional and Doppler echocardiography, contrast echocardiography may be useful in questionable cases.[1] A catheter in the proximal descending thoracic aorta is required for this technique. The ductus arteriosus, main pulmonary artery, and descending aorta are imaged in a parasternal, parasagittal plane. Alternatively, suprasternal notch M-mode imaging of the transverse aorta and the right pulmonary artery may be used. A forceful injection of contrast agent is then made through the arterial catheter, so that the transverse aortic arch is opacified. If there is a left-to-right shunt through the ductus arteriosus, contrast will be seen in the main or right pulmonary artery. If the aorta is not opacified, then an adequate contrast effect was not achieved and the examination cannot be interpreted. An adequate contrast injection may fail to demonstrate a persistent ductus arteriosus in the presence of markedly elevated pulmonary vascular resistance.

A right-to-left shunt through the ductus arteriosus is more difficult to demonstrate because it is usually accompanied by a right-to-left shunt at the atrial level. Thus, the source of contrast in the aorta may be impossible to determine. A contrast injection in the pulmonary artery is the most reliable method, but this requires a catheter in the pulmonary artery.

DOPPLER ECHOCARDIOGRAPHY
Principles

As described in previous sections, sound energy transmitted into the body is reflected by tissue interfaces and

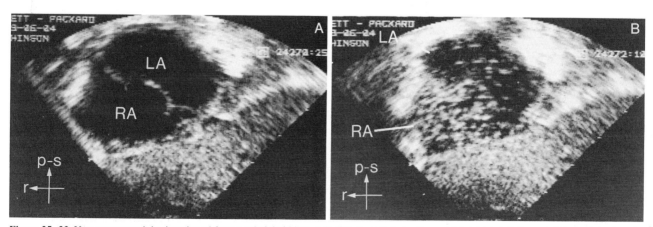

Figure 25–23. Venous contrast injection viewed from a subxiphoid long axis view in an infant with an atrial right-to-left shunt. *A*, Prior to injection, the foramen ovale can be seen in the mid portion of the atrial septum. *B*, After injection the RA is opacified and contrast is seen in the left atrium. LA = left atrium; p-s = posterior-superior; r = right; RA = right atrium; s = superior.

returns to the transducer. The spatial information contained in the temporal pattern of the returning sound energy allows construction of the echocardiographic image. In addition, the returning signal contains other information gained from the interaction of the sound energy with reflecting tissue interfaces. If the reflector is moving with respect to the transducer, then the frequency of the reflected sound energy is altered in proportion to the velocity of the reflector, as described by the Doppler equation. A detailed explanation of Doppler echocardiography can be found in a textbook on the topic.[33,41]

The Doppler equation describes the interaction of sound waves with a moving target:

$$f_d = \frac{2f_o \cdot V \cdot \cos(\Theta)}{c}$$

where: f_d is the Doppler frequency shift

f_o is the transmitted frequency

V is the velocity of the reflector

Θ is the Doppler angle

c is the speed of sound in tissue

As can be seen, the Doppler frequency shift is directly proportional to the velocity of the reflector as long as the other variables remain constant. Notice also that the Doppler frequency shift is directly proportional to the frequency of the transmitted ultrasound. The higher the transmitted frequency (e.g., 5 mHz versus 3 mHz), the larger the Doppler shift for any given reflector velocity. The importance of this concept will become apparent later when pulsed Doppler echocardiography is discussed. Finally, the angle between the ultrasound beam and the direction of motion of the reflector (Θ or the Doppler angle) also determines the Doppler shift. If the Doppler beam is parallel to the direction of motion of the reflector ($\Theta = 0$ degrees), then $\cos \Theta$ is 1, and this term has no effect on the Doppler shift. As Θ increases, the cosine function progressively decreases, resulting in a smaller Doppler shift for any reflector velocity. For practical purposes, angles less than 20 degrees ($\cos \Theta > 0.95$) produce a negligible effect on the Doppler shift.

The sign of the Doppler frequency shift produced by a moving reflector indicates the direction of motion of the reflector. If the reflector is moving toward the transducer, the frequency of the reflected sound waves is higher than the transmitted frequency (+ shift), while motion away from the transducer results in lower frequency reflected sound waves (− shift).

Generally, in clinical use the velocity of the reflector is the unknown variable in the equation. Rearranging the Doppler equation to solve for velocity yields the following:

$$V = f_d \cdot \frac{1}{\cos(\Theta)} \cdot \frac{c}{2f_o}$$

The right side of the equation is composed of three terms. The last term is a constant for each transducer frequen-

cy. The middle term approaches unity as Θ approaches 0 degrees. As noted above, for angles less than 20 degrees this term is sufficiently close to unity that it can be ignored. Thus, if the incident angle is small, the velocity of the reflector is the product of the Doppler frequency shift and a constant derived from the transmitted frequency and the speed of sound in tissue.

Doppler Instruments

CONTINUOUS WAVE DOPPLER ECHOCARDIOGRAPHY

This technique uses two transducers, one transmitter and one receiver. The transmitter continuously sends out sound energy and the receiver continuously "listens" for reflected sound energy. Any reflector in the path of the ultrasound beam contributes to the total Doppler shift recorded. There is no way to determine which reflector has contributed what portion of the total Doppler shift. In other words, continuous wave Doppler has no spatial resolution. On the other hand, since sampling occurs continuously, theoretically there is no limit to the velocity that can be measured with this device. In clinical practice, the processing equipment imposes a limit on the peak velocity, but the limit is well above the range of velocities encountered under physiologic conditions. Therefore, continuous wave Doppler is excellent for measuring high velocities often associated with a stenotic valve, a ventricular septal defect, or a patent ductus arteriosus. The lack of spatial resolution is overcome by using another technique, such as pulsed Doppler echocardiography (see below), to localize the high velocity jet. Continuous wave Doppler echocardiography is then used simply to measure the peak velocity in the jet.

PULSED DOPPLER ECHOCARDIOGRAPHY

This technique is analogous to M-mode echocardiography as previously described. A single transducer acts alternately as a transmitter and a receiver. A short pulse of sound energy (~ 1 μsec in duration) is transmitted, after which time the transducer is available to act as a receiver until the next pulse is sent. Spatial resolution is introduced by allowing the transducer to receive reflected signals only during a brief time interval corresponding to the distance from the transducer to the reflector of interest. This is called time gating. The time interval required for the sound waves to make the round trip between the transducer and the reflector is calculated based on the measured distance and the speed of sound in tissue. Once this is accomplished, the receiver function is activated at this interval after transmission of the ultrasound pulse. The sampling location can easily be changed by changing the interval between the pulse transmission and activation of the receiver function. The shorter the length of time that the receiver is active, the smaller the length of the sampling site or sample volume and vice versa. The diameter of the sample volume is determined by the width of the ultrasonic beam.

The rate at which ultrasonic pulses are sent by the transducer (the sampling rate) is determined by the distance between the transducer and the sample volume. The greater the distance, the lower the sampling rate because of the finite time interval required for sound energy to travel to the reflector and back. The sampling rate is extremely important because it determines the maximum Doppler shift that can be measured unambiguously. The sampling theorem states that the sampling rate must be at least twice the frequency of the wave phenomenon to be recorded. Therefore, the maximum Doppler shift that can be measured with pulsed Doppler echocardiography is one half the sampling rate. Attempting to measure a higher Doppler shift results in aliasing, or registration of falsely low frequencies of opposite sign. A familiar example of aliasing is the apparent change in direction and slowing of the blades of a fan as the motor accelerates.

Since the Doppler frequency shift is directly proportional to the reflector velocity, the sampling rate also limits the maximum velocity that can be measured. Several techniques have been employed to overcome this limitation. First, use of a lower transmitted frequency results in a lower Doppler frequency shift for any given reflector velocity[102] (see above). Thus, use of 1 mHz ultrasound instead of 5 mHz results in one fifth as large a Doppler shift for the same reflector velocity. Second, increasing the Doppler angle also decreases the Doppler shift for any reflector velocity.[129] This technique is less useful because one must measure the Doppler angle and correct for it. At large angles, even small measurement errors have large effects on the measured velocity. Also, increasing the Doppler angle lowers the signal-to-noise ratio. Third, the sampling rate may be increased arbitrarily (for example, doubled or tripled), increasing the maximum velocity that can be measured.[44] The tradeoff for the higher maximum velocity is some degree of range ambiguity. Since there are multiple ultrasonic pulses in the field, one cannot determine with certainty which one gave rise to the recorded reflection. This technique, known as extended range or multiple sample volume pulsed Doppler echocardiography, can be thought of as intermediate between continuous wave and pulsed Doppler echocardiography.

DOPPLER COLOR FLOW MAPPING

This technique is the newest application of Doppler technology.[12,86] In essence, in Doppler color flow mapping pulsed Doppler echocardiography is performed at many points along some or all scan lines of the two-dimensional image. A tremendous number of data points are generated for each frame. Spectral analysis of the Doppler signal from each point would be impossible because of the time required. Instead, a much faster but less precise method called autocorrelation is used, which can be thought of as comparing succeeding Doppler signals from each sampling site. Only the sound waves reflected by moving structures will differ in frequency between the two signals. The difference in phase between the two signals, then, indicates the direction and frequency of the Doppler shift. The temporal variance between succeeding Doppler signals from each sample volume is determined as an index of turbulence.

In Doppler color flow mapping, the velocity and directional information are superimposed in color on the two-dimensional image. On most instruments, reds arbitrarily indicate flow toward the transducer, and blues indicate flow away from the transducer (BART – Blue Away Red Toward). Higher velocities are displayed as lighter shades of red or blue. Color flow mapping employs pulsed Doppler echocardiography so that aliasing may occur as described above. In fact, since so many points are being sampled, the sampling rate for each point is lower than conventional pulsed Doppler echocardiography. Thus, aliasing occurs at even lower velocities in color flow mapping. When aliasing occurs, flow is registered in the opposite direction from what is actually occurring. Thus, in color flow mapping, aliasing results in color reversal. For example, aliasing of the left ventricular inflow signal seen from the apex would appear as an area of blue in the midportion of the ventricle (aliased signal) surrounded by red (nonaliased signal). Turbulence is displayed as green and usually appears speckled.

The attractive feature of Doppler color flow mapping is the ability to image flow over a broad two-dimensional slice of the heart and to display the flow image superimposed on the two-dimensional anatomic image. In theory, such capability should greatly facilitate detection and localization of shunt lesions and valvular regurgitation, allow for determination of the orientation of stenotic jets, and enhance our understanding of flow dynamics under normal and pathologic conditions. Nonetheless, it is still too early to know the role of Doppler color flow mapping in pediatric cardiology.

Clinical Uses

QUANTIFICATION OF BLOOD FLOW

Doppler echocardiography combined with two-dimensional echocardiography can be used to measure both systemic and pulmonary blood flow.[3,53,57,94,102,139,143] As noted previously, the velocity of blood flow can easily be measured with Doppler echocardiography. If the Doppler angle is maintained at less than 20 degrees, the Doppler frequency shift can be converted directly to velocity of blood flow. The two-dimensional image can be used to align the Doppler cursor with the vessel in which a flow measurement is to be made. If continuous wave Doppler without imaging is being used, the transducer position and orientation must be slowly and carefully adjusted to yield the highest velocity and strongest signal.[94] Usual transducer locations for measuring aortic flow are the apex (two-chamber view) or the suprasternal notch. For pulmonary flow, a parasternal short axis view is usually suitable.[102] If the velocity measurements are confined to the annulus or immediate supravalvular area for semilunar valves, the velocity profile across the vessel is blunt, so that the midline flow velocity closely approximates the average velocity across the vessel.[31] The diameter of the vessel in which flow is occurring can be measured from the two-dimensional echocardiogram. Stroke volume can then be calculated from the integral of the Doppler velocity curve and the cross-sectional area of the vessel[102] as the following:

$$SV = A_x \cdot \int_{O}^{E} \vec{V} \, dt$$

where: SV is stroke volume (ml)

A_x is vessel cross-sectional area (cm^2)

V is flow velocity (cm/sec)

O is onset of flow

E is end of flow

Then:

$$Q = SV \cdot HR$$

where: Q is cardiac output (ml/min)

HR is heart rate (beats/min)

It is also possible to calculate flow using the integral of the Doppler velocity curve for an atrioventricular valve and the cross-sectional area of the valve annulus as described above for semilunar valves.[3,139] However, we have found this method less reliable, possibly because of difficulties in measuring the cross-sectional area of a noncircular orifice such as an atrioventricular valve. The systemic-to-pulmonary flow ratio can be determined by measuring blood flow in the pulmonary artery and the aorta and by calculating the ratio.

Limitations of this technology include outflow tract obstruction, which produces flow disturbance and increased flow velocity. If the method for measuring semilunar valve velocity is used in the presence of a persistent ductus arteriosus, the systemic flow will be overestimated and the pulmonary flow underestimated. In theory, aortic flow should be a measure of pulmonary blood flow and pulmonary artery flow a measure of systemic blood flow. However, we have not tested this approach. In patients with a dilated aortic root, the annulus measurement must be used to calculate the cross-sectional area, since use of the root dimension would lead to overestimation of the cardiac output. Use of this method in the presence of semilunar regurgitation will also lead to overestimation of flow. Under these circumstances the atrioventricular valve method may be useful.

ESTIMATION OF PRESSURE DROP

Since most of the energy derived from the drop in pressure across a stenosis is dissipated in accelerating the blood through the stenosis, the change in velocity correlates closely with the pressure drop.[42] Therefore, it is possible to estimate the difference in pressure by measuring the change in velocity across the stenosis. Practically, the upstream velocity is generally quite low compared with the downstream velocity and can be ignored. Thus,

the pressure drop can be calculated using a modification of the Bernoulli equation as follows:

$$p_1 - p_2 = 4 \cdot v^2$$

where: $p_1 - p_2$ is the pressure drop in mmHg

v is the peak velocity in the jet in m/sec

This technique works nicely for discrete lesions such as semilunar stenosis and atrioventricular valve stenosis. There is a tendency for this method to overestimate the pressure drop across coarctation, possibly because the upstream velocity is relatively high and should be used in the calculation.[77]

It is important to keep in mind that the Doppler method measures the instantaneous pressure difference, which may be quite different from the peak-to-peak pressure difference often reported at cardiac catheterization. In fact, the peak-to-peak gradient never actually exists, since the peaks of the left ventricular and aortic pressure contours are not coincident.

Structural Heart Defects

Total Anomalous Pulmonary Venous Drainage

While the diagnosis of total anomalous pulmonary venous drainage (see Chapter 34) is made on the basis of imaging, Doppler echocardiography can provide additional useful information. Pulsed Doppler has been used in cardiac, infracardiac and supracardiac drainage to confirm the diagnosis on the basis of the flow pattern in the anomalous venous channels.[21,90,116,131] More recently, Smallhorn and Freedom[117] showed that the flow pattern in the individual veins and venous confluence is useful for detecting obstruction (Fig. 25–24). Flow upstream from an obstruction, whether in an individual pulmonary vein or the venous confluence, is nonphasic and varies only with respiration. At, and just distal to, the point of obstruction, flow becomes disturbed, and the velocity increases markedly.

Multiple sites of connection between the pulmonary and systemic veins may be difficult to detect by two-dimensional imaging alone. Perhaps pulsed Doppler or Doppler color flow mapping will be of value in detecting the secondary drainage sites.

Atrial Septal Defect

Both pulsed Doppler echocardiography[43,75] and Doppler color flow mapping[134] appear to be of value in diagnosing interatrial communications. Shunting in either direction can be detected (see Color Plate 6). Either method could be used instead of contrast echocardiography to detect a right-to-left shunt, although contrast echocardiography is probably more definitive. The best views are the subxiphoid, apical, and right sternal border views.

Ventricular Septal Defect

Flow through a ventricular septal defect can be detected readily by either pulsed Doppler echocardiography[67,130] or

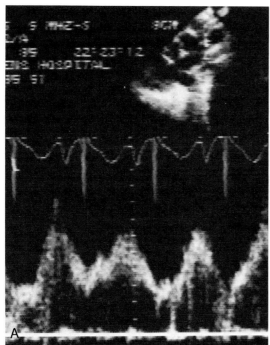

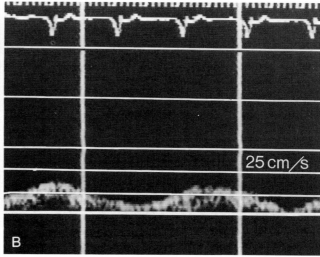

Figure 25–24. *A,* Typical phasic flow pattern in the vertical vein recorded from the suprasternal notch in a patient with unobstructed supracardiac total anomalous pulmonary venous drainage. *B,* Continuous flow pattern in the descending vertical vein in a patient with obstructed subdiaphragmatic total anomalous pulmonary venous drainage.

Doppler color flow mapping (see Color Plate 7).[109] Detection is enhanced if the pressures in the ventricles differ by at least 15 to 20 mmHg. If the pressure difference is less, the flow through the ventricular septal defect may be difficult to distinguish from a normal flow pattern. Doppler color flow mapping may avoid this problem.

Once the defect is detected, the interventricular pressure difference is estimated using the peak velocity in the jet as described above.[76] Continuous wave Doppler echocardiography may be necessary to measure the peak velocity if the defect is small. Although preliminary data suggest that Doppler color flow mapping is able to detect multiple defects, the final word is not yet in, especially if one of the defects is large.

Persistent Ductus Arteriosus

Combined use of two-dimensional imaging and Doppler echocardiography is extremely sensitive for detection of a persistent ductus arteriosus.[49,118,141] A high parasternal, parasagittal view is best for both imaging and Doppler. As illustrated by Doppler color flow mapping, the jet through the persistent ductus often hugs the superior wall of the main pulmonary artery (see Color Plate 8A). This feature may make detection by pulsed Doppler echocardiography difficult if this area is not carefully searched. Elevated pulmonary vascular resistance due to severe lung disease may result in a small shunt even in the presence of a large ductus and hinder detection by Doppler echocardiography. Under these circumstances, however, the physiologic significance of the ductus is unclear. Usually, flow is bidirectional in the ductus in infants with severe lung disease, facilitating detection.

The pressure drop across the persistent ductus may be estimated as described above, using the peak velocity in the jet[78] (see Color Plate 8B). In our hands, this method tends to underestimate the pressure drop, possibly because of the inability to align the ultrasonic beam parallel to flow through the ductus.

The timing of closure of the ductus arteriosus has been investigated in normal newborns using Doppler echocardiography.[32,70] On the first day of life the ductus was found to be patent in over 90 per cent of the subjects studied. The proportion of infants with detectable flow through the ductus progressively decreased over the first 3 or 4 days of life. By 72 to 96 hours the ductus appeared to be closed in virtually all subjects.

The pattern of flow in the ductus arteriosus may vary depending on the pulmonary artery pressure and associated defects.[18] Flow in an isolated persistent ductus arteriosus, in the absence of significant pulmonary artery hypertension, is continuously from aorta to pulmonary artery. This pattern is also seen in patients with ductus-dependent pulmonary blood flow (severe pulmonary stenosis or pulmonary atresia). In infants with persistent pulmonary artery hypertension, flow in the ductus is typically bidirectional. Flow from the pulmonary artery to the aorta always occurs in systole, with reversal of flow in late systole or early diastole. This pattern is also typical for infants with severe left heart obstructive lesions.

Several investigators have studied the effects of a persistent ductus arteriosus on flow in the carotid arteries and descending aorta in an attempt to explain the propensity for premature infants with a persistent ductus to develop intraventricular hemorrhage or necrotizing enterocolitis.[73,148] Retrograde diastolic flow was detected in both locations in nearly all infants with a large ductus, suggesting that blood flow to both the brain and the gastrointestinal tract may be reduced in the presence of a significant shunt

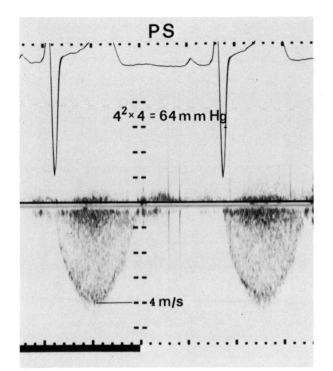

Figure 25–25. Continuous wave Doppler recording of the stenotic jet in an infant with severe valvar pulmonary stenosis (PS). The method for calculating the valve gradient is illustrated.

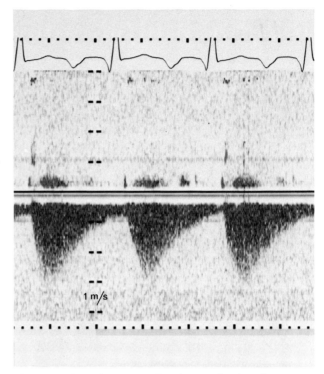

Figure 25–26. Continuous wave Doppler recording from the suprasternal notch in an infant with coarctation. Note the high velocity, continuous flow pattern.

through the ductus arteriosus. While no attempt was made to quantify flow, the abnormal pattern is highly suggestive of a steal phenomenon.

Atrioventricular Valve Regurgitation

Tricuspid regurgitation is relatively common in neonates,[70] especially in the presence of severe lung disease and/or birth asphyxia.[15,82] Usually tricuspid regurgitation is secondary and resolves as right ventricular hypertension or dysfunction abates. Apical four-chamber and parasternal views are excellent for detecting tricuspid regurgitation. Likewise, either pulsed Doppler echocardiography or Doppler color flow mapping (see Color Plate 9) is equally able to detect the regurgitant flow.[135] The size of the regurgitant jet may be determined more easily and quickly with Doppler color flow mapping. However, a close correlation between the size of the regurgitant jet by flow mapping and the severity of regurgitation has not been demonstrated.

The peak velocity in the regurgitant jet is useful for predicting right ventricular pressure.[152] The pressure drop across the valve in systole is calculated as described above, using the peak regurgitant velocity. Next, the atrial pressure is estimated or measured and added to the calculated pressure drop across the atrioventricular valve, yielding right ventricular systolic pressure.

Semilunar Valve Stenosis

Aortic (see Chapter 36) and pulmonary (see Chapter 45) stenosis are readily diagnosed by combined use of two-dimensional and Doppler echocardiography.[7,45,63,64,125,128,129,153] The Doppler findings include delayed up-

stroke of the Doppler velocity curve in the subvalvular area, abnormally high flow velocity in the valve and the immediate supravalvular area and flow disturbance more distal in the great artery as a result of dispersion of the jet. Associated findings often include atrioventricular valve regurgitation on the same side of the heart as the semilunar valve stenosis, hypoplasia and/or dysfunction of the associated ventricle, and dependence on the ductus arteriosus for systemic or pulmonary blood flow.

The pressure drop across the valve can be determined from the peak velocity in the valve jet, as described previously[42] (Fig. 25–25). However, the peak pressure drop may be misleading in assessing the severity of stenosis. A small gradient may be associated with severe stenosis in the presence of low ventricular output. In patients with critical aortic stenosis, for example, much or most of the systemic output may be supplied by the right ventricle through the ductus arteriosus. We have found Doppler color flow mapping to be of value in assessing how much of the systemic output is supplied by the left ventricle. Doppler flow imaging of the aortic arch from the right sternal border or suprasternal notch allows determination of the direction of flow in the ascending, transverse, and descending aorta (see Color Plates 10A and 10B). If flow is retrograde in the proximal descending and transverse arch, then most of the systemic output is from the right ventricle. Doppler flow mapping or pulsed Doppler echocardiography in the ductus arteriosus is also useful for determining the proportion of the cardiac cycle in which blood flows from the ductus into the aorta. Similar techniques may be applied in patients with critical pulmonary stenosis.

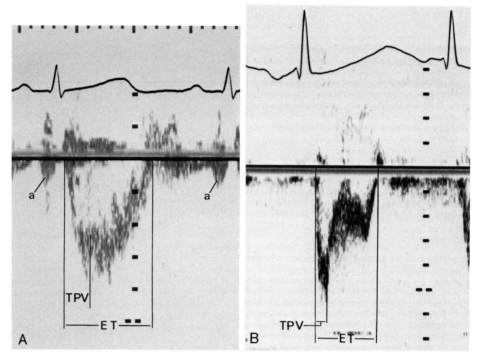

Figure 25–27. Doppler recording from the main pulmonary artery. *A,* Normal pulmonary artery pressure. Note the presence of atriosystolic flow and the rounded contour and slow upstroke of the systolic flow wave. *B,* Pulmonary artery hypertension. Note the more rapid upstroke and the notching of the deceleration limb. The time to peak velocity decreases with increasing pulmonary artery pressure. a = atriosystolic flow wave; ET = ejection time; TPV = time to peak velocity.

Coarctation of the Aorta

Coarctation (see Chapter 37) usually presents in the first 7 to 10 days of life in association with closure of the ductus arteriosus. The diagnosis is usually suspected on the basis of absent femoral pulses and congestive heart failure and can be confirmed readily using two-dimensional[119] and Doppler echocardiography.[98,101,108,150] Right sternal border or suprasternal notch imaging of the aortic arch shows the typical posterior "shelf" opposite the small residual ductus arteriosus or ligamentum arteriosum. Pulsed or continuous wave Doppler echocardiography from this transducer position demonstrates a large increase in flow velocity at and just distal to the narrow area (Fig. 25–26). The pressure drop across the coarctation can be estimated using the peak velocity in the jet, as described previously. Marx and Allen[77] have recently shown that this technique slightly overestimates the pressure drop. Including the upstream velocity in the calculation seems to improve the accuracy of the method.

In the absence of a persistent ductus arteriosus with a right-to-left shunt, the flow pattern in the descending aorta at the diaphragm is also useful for detection of coarctation.[101,108] In the typical case, the upstroke time of the Doppler velocity curve is long and there is continuous anterograde flow throughout the cardiac cycle. While this method is not useful for quantifying the severity of the coarctation, it is of value in those patients in whom the aortic arch cannot be adequately imaged.

Pulmonary Artery Pressure

Cardiologists and neonatologists are often interested to know the pulmonary artery pressure in an infant with either pulmonary disease or a heart defect. The standard method for measuring pulmonary artery pressure is by cardiac catheterization. Consequently, Doppler echocardiography, in addition to the various methods discussed in previous sections, has been investigated as a technique for estimating pulmonary artery pressure noninvasively.

The contour of the Doppler velocity curve recorded from the right ventricular outflow tract or main pulmonary artery is a fair qualitative index of pulmonary artery pressure[58,59] (Fig. 25–27). A small anterograde flow wave, corresponding temporally to atrial systole, is seen in most subjects with normal pulmonary artery pressure (systolic pressure < 30 mmHg) but not in those with pulmonary artery hypertension. A notch or dip in the deceleration limb of the Doppler velocity curve is seen in about one half of patients with pulmonary artery hypertension. However, this finding may be present in subjects with normal pulmonary pressure and idiopathic dilation of the pulmonary artery.

Quantitative indexes that have been proposed include the time to peak velocity, or acceleration time, and the time to peak velocity divided by the right ventricular ejection time.[58,59,74] As the pulmonary artery pressure increases, peak velocity occurs earlier, so that the time to peak velocity decreases. While investigators have reported fair to good correlation (r = −0.75 to −0.90) between pulmonary artery pressure and time to peak velocity, the scatter about the regression line is too large to use this index in place of directly measured pressure.

A more direct measurement of pulmonary artery pressure can be obtained in some patients with congenital heart defects and in those with tricuspid regurgitation. In patients with a ventricular septal defect, the peak velocity in the jet through the defect is used to determine the pressure difference between the ventricles.[76] The left ventricular systolic pressure can be determined by measuring the blood pressure. The right ventricular pressure and, in the absence of right ventricular outflow tract obstruction, the pulmonary arterial pressure are calculated by subtracting the interventricular pressure difference from the left ventricular systolic pressure. The right ventricular pressure can be estimated in patients with tricuspid regurgitation by adding the measured or estimated right atrial pressure to the systolic pressure drop across the tricuspid valve, determined by using the peak velocity in the regurgitant jet.[152] Finally, in patients with a persistent ductus arteriosus or other aortopulmonary communication, the pulmonary artery pressure can be determined by using the peak velocity through the aortopulmonary connection to estimate the pressure difference between the aorta and the pulmonary artery.[78] This pressure difference is then subtracted from the measured systemic arterial pressure to determine the pulmonary arterial pressure. Potential sources of error in these techniques include inability to align properly the ultrasound beam with the flow jet and inaccurate sphygmomanometric blood pressure measurements.

References

1. Allen HD, Sahn DJ, Goldberg SJ (1978): New serial contrast technique for assessment of left to right shunting patent ductus arteriosus in the neonate. Am J Cardiol 41:288–294.
2. Aziz KU, Paul MH, Bharati S, Lev M, Shannon K (1978): Echocardiographic features of total anomalous pulmonary venous drainage into the coronary sinus. Am J Cardiol 42:108–113.
3. Barron JV, Sahn DJ, Valdes-Cruz LM, Lima CO, Goldberg SJ, Grenadier E, Allen HD (1984): Clinical utility of two-dimensional echocardiographic techniques for estimating pulmonary to systemic flow ratios in children with left to right shunting atrial septal defect, ventricular septal defect or patent ductus arteriosus. J Am Coll Cardiol 3:169–178.
4. Bash SE, Huhta JC, Vick GW, Gutgesell HP, Ott DA (1986): Hypoplastic left heart syndrome: Is echocardiography accurate enough to guide surgical palliation? J Am Coll Cardiol 7:610–616.
5. Bass JL, Bessinger FB, Lawrence C (1978): Echocardiographic differentiation of partial and complete atrioventricular canal. Circulation 57:1144–1150.
6. Bass NM, Roche AHG, Brandt PWT, Neutze JM (1978): Echocardiography in assessment of infants with complete d-transposition of the great arteries. Br Heart J 40:1165–1173.
7. Berger M, Berdoff RL, Gallerstein PE, Goldberg E (1984): Evaluation of aortic stenosis by continuous wave Doppler ultrasound. J Am Coll Cardiol 3:150–156.
8. Bierman FZ, Fellows K, Williams RG (1980): Prospective identification of ventricular septal defects in infancy using two-dimensional echocardiography. Circulation 62:807–817.
9. Bierman FZ, Williams RG (1979): Prospective diagnosis of d-transposition of the great arteries in neonates by subxiphoid two-dimensional echocardiography. Circulation 60:1469–1502.
10. Bierman FZ, Williams RG (1979): Subxiphoid two-dimensional imaging of the interatrial septum in infants and neonates with congenital heart disease. Circulation 60:80–90.
11. Bloom KR, Freedom RM, Williams CM, Trusler GA, Rowe RD (1979): Echocardiographic recognition of atrioventricular valve stenosis associated with endocardial cushion defect: Pathologic and surgical correlates. Am J Cardiol 44:1326–1331.
12. Bommer WJ (1985): Basic principles of flow imaging. Echocardiography 2:501–509.
13. Borow KM, Green LH, Grossman W, Braunwald E (1982): Left ventricular end-systolic stress-shortening and stress-length relations in humans. Normal values and sensitivity to inotropic state. Am J Cardiol 50:1301–1308.
14. Borow KM, Propper R, Bierman FZ, Grady S, Inati A (1982): Left ventricular end-systolic pressure-dimension relation in patients with thalassemia major: A new noninvasive method of assessing contractile state. Circulation 66:980–985.
15. Bucciarelli R, Nelson RM, Egan EA II, Eitzman DV, Gessner IH (1977): Transient tricuspid insufficiency of the newborn: A form of myocardial dysfunction in stressed newborns. Pediatrics 59:330–337.
16. Chin AJ, Sanders SP, Sherman F, Lang P, Norwood WI, Castaneda AR (1987): Accuracy of subcostal 2-dimensional echocardiography in prospective diagnosis of total anomalous pulmonary venous connection. Am Heart J 113:1153–1159.
17. Chin AJ, Yeager SB, Sanders SP, Williams RG, Bierman FZ, Burger BM, Norwood WI, Castaneda AR (1985): Accuracy of prospective two-dimensional echocardiographic evaluation of left ventricular outflow tract in complete transposition of the great arteries. Am J Cardiol 55:759–764.
18. Cloez JL, Isaaz K, Pernot C (1986): Pulsed Doppler flow characteristics of ductus arteriosus in infants with associated congenital anomalies of the heart or great arteries. Am J Cardiol 57:845–851.
19. Cohen BE, Winer HE, Kronzon I (1979): Echocardiographic findings in patients with left superior vena cava and dilated coronary sinus. Am J Cardiol 44:158–161.
20. Colan SD, Borow KM, Neumann A (1984): Left ventricular end-systolic wall stress–velocity of fiber shortening relation: A load-independent index of myocardial contractilty. J Am Coll Cardiol 4:715–724.
21. Cooper MJ, Teitel DF, Silverman NH, Enderlein, MA (1984): Study of the infradiaphragmatic total anomalous pulmonary venous connection with cross-sectional and pulsed Doppler echocardiography. Circulation 70:412–416.
22. Dillon JC, Feigenbaum H, Konecke LL, Keutel J, Hurwitz RA, Davis RH, Chang S (1973): Echocardiographic manifestations of d-transposition of the great vessels. Am J Cardiol 32:74–78.
23. Disessa TG, Hagan AD, Isabel-Jones JB, Ti CC, Mercier JC, Friedman WF (1981): Two-dimensional echocardiographic evaluation of discrete subaortic stenosis from the apical long axis view. Am Heart J 101:774–782.
24. Driscoll DJ, Gutgesell HP, McNamara DG (1976): Echocardiographic features of congenital mitral stenosis. Am J Cardiol 42:259–266.
25. Farooki ZQ, Henry JG, Green EW (1976): Echocardiographic spectrum of the hypoplastic left heart syndrome. Am J Cardiol 38:337–343.
26. Feigenbaum H (1983): Echocardiography: An overview. J Am Coll Cardiol 1:216–224.
27. Feigenbaum H, Stone JM, Lee DA, Nasser WK, Chang S (1970): Identification of ultrasound echos from the left ventricle by use of intracardiac injection of indocyanine green. Circulation 41:615–621.
28. Foale R, Stefanini L, Rickards A, Somerville J (1982): Left and right ventricular morphology in complex congenital heart disease defined by two dimensional echocardiography. Am J Cardiol 49:93–99.
29. Fraker TD, Harris PJ, Behar VS, Kisslo JA (1979): Detection and exclusion of interatrial shunts by two-dimensional echocardiography and peripheral venous injection. Circulation 59:379–384.
30. Funabashi T, Yoshida H, Nakaya S, Maeda T, Taniguchi N (1981): Echocardiographic visualization of ventricular septal defect in infants and assessment of hemodynamic status using contrast technique. Comparison of M-mode and two-dimensional imaging. Circulation 64:1025–1031.
31. Gabe IT, Gault JH, Ross J, Mason DT, Mills CJ, Schillingford JP, Braunwald E (1969): Measurement of instantaneous blood flow velocity and pressure in conscious man with a catheter tip velocity probe. Circulation 40:603–614.
32. Gentile R, Stevenson G, Dooley T, Franklin D, Kawabori I, Pearlman A (1981): Pulsed Doppler echocardiographic determination of time of ductal closure in normal newborn infants. J Pediatr 98:443–448.
33. Goldberg SJ, Allen HD, Marx GR, Flinn CJ (1985): Doppler Echocardiography. Philadelphia, Lea & Febiger.
34. Gordon EP, Schnittger I, Fitzgerald PJ, Williams P, Popp RL (1983): Reproducibility of left ventricular volumes by two-dimensional echocardiography. J Am Coll Cardiol 2:506–513.

35. Gramiak R, Shah PM (1968): Echocardiography of the aortic root. Invest Radiol 3:356–366.

36. Gramiak R, Shah PM, Kramer DH (1969): Ultrasound cardiography: Contrast study in anatomy and function. Radiology 92:939–948.

37. Gramiak R, Chung KJ, Nanda N, Manning J (1973): Echocardiographic diagnosis of transposition of the great vessels. Radiology 106:187–189.

38. Grossman W, Braunwald E, Mann T, McLaurin LP, Green LH (1977): Contractile state of the left ventricle as evaluated from the end-systolic pressure-volume relation. Circulation 56:845–852.

39. Grossman W, Jones D, McLaurin LP (1975): Wall stress and patterns of hypertrophy in the human left ventricle. J Clin Invest 56:56–64.

40. Gutgesell HP (1985): Cardiac imaging with ultrasound: Rightside up or upside down? (editorial) Am J Cardiol 56:479–480.

41. Hatle L, Angelsen B (1985): Doppler Ultrasound in Cardiology. Physical Principles and Clinical Applications. 2nd ed. Philadelphia, Lea & Febiger.

42. Ibid, pp 22–26.

43. Ibid, pp 228–236.

44. Ibid, pp 98–101.

45. Hatle L, Angelsen BA, Tromsdal A (1980): Noninvasive assessment of aortic stenosis by Doppler ultrasound. Br Heart J 43:284–292.

46. Heger JJ, Weyman AE, Wann LS, Rogers EW, Dillon JC, Feigenbaum H (1980): Cross-sectional echocardiographic analysis of the extent of left ventricular asynergy in acute myocardial infarction. Circulation 61:1113–1118.

47. Hiraishi S, DiSessa TG, Jarmakani JM, Nakanishi T, Isabel-Jones JB, Friedman WF (1982): Two-dimensional echocardiographic assessment of right ventricular volume in children with congenital heart disease. Am J Cardiol 50:1368–1375.

48. Hirschfeld S, Meyer R, Schwartz DC, Korfhagen J, Kaplan S (1975): The echocardiographic assessment of pulmonary artery pressure and pulmonary vascular resistance. Circulation 52:642–650.

49. Huhta JC, Cohen M, Gutgesell HP (1984): Patency of the ductus arteriosus in normal neonates: Two-dimensional echocardiography versus Doppler assessment. J Am Coll Cardiol 4:561–564.

50. Huhta JC, Gutgesell HP, Latson LA, Huffines FD (1984): Two-dimensional echocardiographic assessment of the aorta in infants and children with congenital heart disease. Circulation 70:417–424.

51. Huhta JC, Smallhorn JF, Macartney FJ (1982): Two-dimensional echocardiographic diagnosis of situs. Br Heart J 48:97–108.

52. Huhta JC, Smallhorn JF, Macartney FJ, Anderson RH, De Leval M (1982): Cross-sectional echocardiographic diagnosis of systemic venous return. Br Heart J 48:388–403.

53. Huntsman LL, Stewart DK, Barnes SR, et al (1983): Noninvasive Doppler determination of cardiac output in man. Circulation 67:593–602.

54. Johnson GL, Twyman RE, Todd EP, Cottrill CM, Noonan JA (1981): Echocardiographic classification of complete atrioventricular canal defects. Am Heart J 101:612–618.

55. Kerber RE, Kioschos JM, Lauer RM (1974): Use of an ultrasonic contrast method in the diagnosis of valvular regurgitation and intracardiac shunts. Am J Cardiol 34:722–727.

56. King ME, Braun H, Goldblatt A, Liberthson R, Weyman AE (1983): Interventricular septal configuration as a predictor of right ventricular systolic hypertension in children: A cross-sectional echocardiographic study. Circulation 68:68–75.

57. Kitabatake A, Inoue M, Asao M, Ito H, Masuyama T, Tanouchi J, Morita T, Hori M, Yoshima H, Ohnishi K, Abe H (1984): Noninvasive evaluation of the ratio of pulmonary to systemic flow in atrial septal defect by duplex Doppler echocardiography. Circulation 69:73–79.

58. Kitabatake A, Inoue M, Asao M, Masuyama T, Tanouchi J, Morita T, Mishima M, Uematsu M, Shimazu T, Hori M, Abe H (1983): Noninvasive evaluation of pulmonary hypertension by a pulsed Doppler technique. Circulation 68:302–309.

59. Kosturakis D, Goldberg SJ, Allen HD, Loeber C (1984): Doppler echocardiographic prediction of pulmonary arterial hypertension in congenital heart disease. Am J Cardiol 53:1110–1115.

60. Lange LW, Sahn DJ, Allen HD, Ovitt TW, Goldberg SJ (1980): Cross-sectional echocardiography in hypoplastic left ventricle: Echocardiographic-angiographic-anatomic correlations. Ped Cardiol 1:287–299.

61. Lewis BS, Amitai N, Simcha A, Merin G, Gotsman MS (1979): Echocardiographic diagnosis of pulmonary atresia with intact ventricular septum. Am Heart J 97:92–95.

62. Lieberman AN, Weiss JL, Jugdutt BI, Becker LC, Bulkley BH, Garrison JG, Hutchins GM, Kallman CA, Weisfeldt ML (1981): Two-dimensional echocardiography and infarct size: Relationship of regional wall motion and thickening to the extent of myocardial infarction in the dog. Circulation 63:739–746.

63. Lima CO, Sahn DJ, Valdes-Cruz LM, Allen HD, Goldberg SJ, Grenadier E, Barron JV (1983): Prediction of the severity of left ventricular outflow tract obstruction by quantitative two-dimensional echocardiographic Doppler studies. Circulation 68:348–354.

64. Lima CO, Sahn DJ, Valdes-Cruz LM, Goldberg SJ, Barron JV, Allen HD, Grenadier E (1983): Noninvasive prediction of transvalvar pressure gradient in patients with pulmonary stenosis by quantitative two-dimensional echocardiographic Doppler studies. Circulation 67:866–871.

65. Little WC, Freeman GL, O'Rourk RA (1985): Simultaneous determination of left ventricular end-systolic pressure-volume and pressure-dimension relationships in closed-chest dogs. Circulation 71:1301–1308.

66. Lundstrm NR (1972): Ultrasound cardiographic studies of the mitral valve region in young infants with mitral atresia, mitral stenosis, hypoplasia of the left ventricle, and cor triatriatum. Circulation 45:324–334.

67. Magherini A, Azzolina G, Weichmann V, Fantini F (1980): Pulsed Doppler echocardiography for diagnosis of ventricular septal defects. Br Heart J 43:143–147.

68. Mahler F, Ross J, O'Rourke RA, Covell JW (1975): Effects of changes in preload, afterload, and inotropic state on ejection and isovolumic phase measures of contractility in the conscious dog. Am J Cardiol 35:626–634.

69. Mahler F, Yoran C, Ross J Jr (1974): Inotropic effect of tachycardia and poststimulation potentiation in the conscious dog. Am J Physiol 227:569–575.

70. Mahoney LT, Coryell KG, Lauer RM (1985): The newborn transitional circulation: A two-dimensional Doppler echocardiographic study. J Am Coll Cardiol 6:623–629.

71. Marino B, Ballerini L, Marcelletti C, Piva R, Pasquini L, Zacch C, Giannico S, De Simone G (1984): Right oblique subxiphoid view for two-dimensional echocardiographic visualization of the right ventricle in congenital heart disease. Am J Cardiol 54:1064–1068.

72. Marino B, De Simone G, Pasquini L, Giannico S, Marcelletti C, Ammirati A, Guccione P, Boldrini R, Ballerini L (1985): Complete transposition of the great arteries: Visualization of left and right outflow tract obstruction by oblique subcostal two-dimensional echocardiography. Am J Cardiol 55:1140–1145.

73. Martin CG, Snider AR, Katz SM, Peabody JL, Brady JP (1982): Abnormal cerebral blood flow patterns in preterm infants with a large patent ductus arteriosus. J Pediatr 101:587–593.

74. Martin-Duran R, Larman M, Trugeda A, Vazquez de Prada JA, Ruano J, Torres A, Figueroa A, Pajaron A, Nistal F (1986): Comparison of Doppler-determined elevated pulmonary arterial pressure with pressure measured at cardiac catheterization. Am J Cardiol 57:859–863.

75. Marx GR, Allen HD, Goldberg SJ (1985): Transatrial septal velocity measurement by Doppler echocardiography in atrial septal defect—correlation with QP:QS ratio. Am J Cardiol 55:1162–1167.

76. Marx GR, Allen HD, Goldberg SJ (1985): Doppler echocardiographic estimation of systolic pulmonary artery pressure in pediatric patients with interventricular communications. J Am Coll Cardiol 6:1132–1137.

77. Marx GR, Allen HD (1986): Accuracy and pitfalls of Doppler evaluation of the pressure gradient in aortic coarctation. J Am Coll Cardiol 7:1379–1385.

78. Marx GR, Allen HD, Goldberg SJ (1986): Doppler echocardiographic estimation of systolic pulmonary artery pressure in patients with aortico-pulmonary shunts. J Am Coll Cardiol 7:880–885.

79. Mehta S, Hirschfeld S, Riggs T, Liebman J (1979): Echocardiographic estimation of ventricular hypoplasia in complete atrioventricular canal. Circulation 59:888–893.

80. Moodie DS (1981): Spectrum of M-mode echocardiographic findings in total anomalous pulmonary venous return. Cleveland Clinic Quart 48:315–324.

81. Moynihan PF, Parisi AF, Feldman CL (1981): Quantitative detection of regional left ventricular contraction abnormalities by two-dimensional echocardiography. I. Analysis of methods. Circulation 63:752–760.

82. Nelson RM, Bucciarelli RL, Eitzman DV, Egan EA II, Gessner IH (1978): Serum creatine phosphokinase MB fraction in newborns with transient tricuspid insufficiency. N Engl J Med 298:146–149.

83. Nixon JV, Murray RG, Leonard PD, Mitchell JH, Blomqvist CG (1982): Effect of large variations in preload on left ventricular performance characteristics in normal subjects. Circulation 65:698–703.

84. O'Boyle JE, Parisi AF, Nieminen M, Kloner RA, Khuri S (1983): Quantitative detection of regional left ventricular contraction abnormalities by 2-dimensional echocardiography. Comparison of myocardial thickening and thinning and endocardial motion in a canine model. Am J Cardiol 51:1732–1738.

85. Oberhnsli I, Branden G, Girod M, Friedli B (1982): Estimation of pulmonary artery pressure by ultrasound. A study comparing simultaneously recorded pulmonary valve echogram and pulmonary arterial pressures. Ped Cardiol 2:123–130.

86. Omoto R, Kasai C (1986): Basic principles of Doppler colorflow imaging. Echocardiography 3:463–473.

87. Orsmond GS, Ruttenberg HD, Bessinger FB, Moller JH (1978): Echocardiographic features of total anomalous venous connection to the coronary sinus. Am J Cardiol 41:597–601.

88. Paquet M, Gutgesell H (1975): Echocardiographic features of total anomalous pulmonary venous connection. Circulation 51:599–605.

89. Pasquini L, Sanders SP, Parness I, Colan SD (1987): Echocardiographic diagnosis of coronary artery anatomy in transposition of the great arteries. Circulation 75:557–564.

90. Pickoff AS, Sequeira R, Ferrer PL, Tamer D, Bennett V, Fojaco R, Gelband H (1980): Pulsed Doppler echocardiographic findings in total anomalous pulmonary venous drainage to the coronary sinus. Cathet Cardiovasc Diagn 6:247–254.

91. Popp RL, Fowles R, Coltart J, Martin RP (1979): Cardiac anatomy viewed systematically with two dimensional echocardiography. Chest 75:579–585.

92. Quinones MA, Gaasch WH, Cole JS, Alexander JK (1975): Echocardiographic determination of left ventricular stress-velocity relations in man. With reference to the effects of loading and contractility. Circulation 51:689–700.

93. Reichek N, Helak J, Plappert T, St. John Sutton M, Weber KT (1983): Anatomic validation of left ventricular mass estimates from clinical two-dimensional echocardiography: Initial results. Circulation 67:348–352.

94. Rein AJJT, Hsieh KS, Elixson M, Colan SD, Lang P, Sanders SP, Castaneda AR (1986): Cardiac output estimates in the pediatric intensive care unit using a continuous-wave Doppler computer: Validation and limitations of the technique. Am Heart J 112:97–103.

95. Rein AJJT, Sanders SP, Colan SD, Parness IP, Epstein MF (1987): Left ventricular mechanics in the normal newborn. Circulation 76:1029–1036.

96. Rein AJJT, Sapoznikov D, Lewis N, Halon DA, Gotsman MS, Lewis BS (1982): Regional left ventricular ejection fraction from real-time two-dimensional echocardiography. Int J Cardiol 2:61–70.

97. Riggs T, Hirschfeld S, Borkat G, Knoke J, Liebman J (1978): Assessment of the pulmonary vascular bed by echocardiographic right ventricular systolic time intervals. Circulation 57:939–947.

98. Robinson PJ, Wyse RKH, Deanfield JE, Franklin R, Macartney FJ (1984): Continuous wave Doppler velocimetry as an adjunct to cross sectional echocardiography in the diagnosis of critical left heart obstruction in neonates. Br Heart J 52:552–556.

99. Sahn DJ, Allen HD, Lange LW, Goldberg SJ (1979): Cross-sectional echocardiographic diagnosis of the sites of total anomalous pulmonary venous drainage. Circulation 60:317–325.

100. Sanders SP, Bierman FZ, Williams RG (1982): Conotruncal malformations: Diagnosis in infancy using subxiphoid 2 dimensional echocardiography. Am J Cardiol 50:1361–1367.

101. Sanders SP, MacPherson D, Yeager SB, (1986): Temporal flow velocity profile in the descending aorta in coarctation. J Am Coll Cardiol 7:603–609.

102. Sanders SP, Yeager S, Williams RG (1983): Measurement of systemic and pulmonary blood flow and Qp/Qs ratio using Doppler and two-dimensional echocardiography. Am J Cardiol 51:952–956.

103. Serruys PW, van den Brand M, Hugenholtz PG, Roelandt J (1979): Intracardiac right-to-left shunts demonstrated by two-dimensional echocardiography after peripheral vein injection. Br Heart J 42:429–437.

104. Seward JB, Tajik AJ, Hagler DJ, Giuliani ER, Gau GT, Ritter DG (1977): Echocardiogram in common (single) ventricle: Angiographic-anatomic correlation. Am J Cardiol 39:217–225.

105. Seward JB, Tajik AJ, Hagler DJ, Ritter DG (1977): Peripheral venous contrast echocardiography. Am J Cardiol 39:202–212.

106. Seward JB, Tajik AJ, Hagler DJ, Ritter DG (1978): Echocardiographic spectrum of tricuspid atresia. Mayo Clin Proc 53:100–112.

107. Seward JB, Tajik AJ, Spangler JG, Ritter DG (1975): Echocardiographic contrast studies: Initial experience. Mayo Clin Proc 50:163–192.

108. Shaddy RE, Snider AR, Silverman NH, Lutin W (1986): Pulse Doppler findings in patients with coarctation of the aorta. Circulation 73:82–88.

109. Sherman FS, Sahn DJ, Valdes-Cruz LM, Chung KJ, Elias W, Swensson RE (1986): Two-dimensional Doppler color flow mapping for detecting atrial and ventricular septal defects. Echocardiography 3:527–531.

110. Silverman NH, Hudson S (1983): Evaluation of right ventricular volume and ejection fraction in children by two-dimensional echocardiography. Pediatr Cardiol 4:197–204.

111. Silverman NH, Payot M, Stanger P (1978): Simulated tricuspid valve echoes in tricuspid atresia. Am Heart J 95:761–765.

112. Silverman NH, Ports TA, Snider AR, Schiller NB, Carlsson E, Heilbron DC (1980): Determination of left ventricular volume in children; echocardiographic and angiographic comparisons. Circulation 62:548–557.

113. Silverman NH, Schiller NB (1978): Apex echocardiography. A two-dimensional technique for evaluating congenital heart disease. Circulation 57:503–511.

114. Silverman NH, Snider AR (1982): Two-dimensional Echocardiography in Congenital Heart Disease. Norwalk, Appleton-Century-Crofts.

115. Silverman NH, Snider AR, Rudolph AM (1980): Evaluation of pulmonary hypertension by M-mode echocardiography in children with ventricular septal defect. Circulation 61:1125–1132.

116. Skovrnek J, Tuma S, Urbancov D, Sam nek M (1980): Range-gated pulsed Doppler echocardiographic diagnosis of supracardiac total anomalous pulmonary venous drainage. Circulation 61:841–847.

117. Smallhorn JF, Freedom RM (1986): Pulsed Doppler echocardiography in the preoperative evaluation of total anomalous pulmonary venous connection. J Am Coll Cardiol 8:1413–1420.

118. Smallhorn JF, Gow R, Olley PM, Freedom RM, Swyer PR, Perlman M, Rowe RD (1984): Combined noninvasive assessment of the patent ductus arteriosus in the preterm infant before and after indomethacin treatment. Am J Cardiol 54:1300–1304.

119. Smallhorn JF, Huhta JC, Adams PA, Anderson RH, Wilkinson JL (1983): Cross-sectional echocardiographic assessment of coarctation in the sick neonate and infant. Br Heart J 50:349–361.

120. Smallhorn JF, Huhta JC, Anderson RH, Macartney FJ (1982): Suprasternal cross-sectional echocardiography in assessment of patent ductus arteriosus. Br Heart J 48:321–330.

121. Smallhorn JF, Sutherland GR, Tommasini G, Hunter S, Anderson RH, Macartney FJ (1981): Assessment of total anomalous pulmonary venous connection by two-dimensional echocardiography. Br Heart J 46:613–623.

122. Snider AR, Ports TA, Silverman NH (1979): Venous anomalies of the coronary sinus: Detection by M-mode, two-dimensional and contrast echocardiography. Circulation 60:721–727.

123. Snider AR, Silverman NH (1981): Suprasternal notch echocardi-

ography: A two-dimensional technique for evaluating congenital heart disease. Circulation 63:165–173.

124. Snider AR, Silverman NH, Turley K, Ebert PA (1982): Evaluation of infradiaphragmatic total anomalous pulmonary venous connection with two-dimensional echocardiography. Circulation 66:1129–1132.

125. Snider AR, Stevenson JG, French JW, Rocchini AP, Dick M II, Rosenthal A, Crowley DC, Beekman RH, Peters J (1986): Comparison of high pulse repetition frequency and continuous wave Doppler echocardiography for velocity measurement and gradient prediction in children with valvular and congenital heart disease. J Am Coll Cardiol 7:873–879.

126. Solinger R, Elbl F, Minhas K (1973): Echocardiography in the normal neonate. Circulation 47:108–118.

127. Solinger R, Elbl F, Minhas K (1974): Deductive echocardiographic analysis in infants with congenital heart disease. Circulation 50:1072–1096.

128. Stamm RB, Martin RP (1983): Quantification of pressure gradients across stenotic valves by Doppler ultrasound. J Am Coll Cardiol 2:707–718.

129. Stevenson JG, Kawabori I (1984): Noninvasive determination of pressure gradients in children: Two methods employing pulsed Doppler echocardiography. J Am Coll Cardiol 3:179–192.

130. Stevenson JG, Kawabori K, Dooley T, Guntheroth W (1978): Diagnosis of ventricular septal defect by pulsed Doppler echocardiography. Circulation 58:322–326.

131. Stevenson, JG, Kawabori I, Guntheroth WG (1979): Pulsed Doppler echocardiographic detection of total anomalous pulmonary venous return: Resolution of the left atrial line. Am J Cardiol 44:1155–1158.

132. Suga H, Kitabatake A, Sagawa K (1979): End-systolic pressure determines stroke volume from fixed end-diastolic volume in the isolated left ventricle under a constant contractile state. Circ Res 44:238–249.

133. Suga H, Sagawa K (1974): Instantaneous pressure-volume relationships and their ratio in excised, supported canine left ventricle. Circ Res 35:117–126.

134. Suzuki Y, Kambara H, Kadota K, Tamaki S, Yamazato A, Nohara R, Osakada G, Kawai C, Kubo S, Karaguchi T (1985): Detection of intracardiac shunt flow in atrial septal defect using a real-time two-dimensional color-coded Doppler flow imaging system and comparison with contrast echocardiography. Am J Cardiol 56:347–350.

135. Suzuki Y, Kambara H, Kadota K, Tamaki S, Yamazato A, Nohara R, Osakada G, Kawai C, Kubo S, Karaguchi T (1986): Detection and evaluation of tricuspid regurgitation using a real-time, two-dimensional, color-coded Doppler flow imaging system: Comparison with contrast two-dimensional echocardiography and right ventriculography. Am J Cardiol 57:811–815.

136. Tajik AJ, Seward JB, Hagler DJ, Mair DJ, Lie JT (1978): Two-dimensional real-time ultrasonic imaging of the heart and great vessels. Mayo Clin Proc 53:271–303.

137. Tei C, Tanaka H, Kashima T, Yoshimura H, Minagoe S, Kanehisa T (1979): Real-time cross-sectional echocardiographic evaluation of the interatrial septum by right atrium–interatrial septum–left atrium direction of ultrasound beam. Circulation 60:539–546.

138. Trowitzsch E, Colan SD, Sanders SP (1985): Global and regional right ventricular function in normal infants and infants with transposition of the great arteries after Senning operation. Circulation 72:1008–1014.

139. Valdes-Cruz LM, Horowitz S, Mesel E, Sahn DJ, Fisher DC, Larson D (1984): A pulsed Doppler echocardiographic method for calculating pulmonary and systemic blood flow in atrial level shunts: Validation studies in animals and initial human experience. Circulation 69:80–86.

140. Valdes-Cruz LM, Pieroni DR, Roland JMA, Varghese PJ (1976): Echocardiographic detection of intracardiac right-to-left shunts following peripheral vein injection. Circulation 54:558–562.

141. Vick GW, Huhta JC, Gutgesell HP (1985): Assessment of the ductus arteriosus in preterm infants utilizing suprasternal two-dimensional/doppler echocardiography J Am Coll Cardiol 5:973–977.

142. Wallace AG, Mitchell JH, Skinner NS, Sarnoff SJ (1963): Duration of the phases of the left ventricular systole. Circ Res 12:611–619.

143. Walthers FJ, Siassi B, Ramadan NA, Ananda AK, Wu PYK (1985): Pulsed Doppler determinations of cardiac output in neonates: Normal standards for clinical use. Pediatrics 76:829–833.

144. Weber KT, Janicki JS, Hefner LL (1976): Left ventricular force-length relations of isovolumic and ejecting contractions. Am J Physiol 231:337–343.

145. Weber KT, Janicki JS, Hunter WC, Shroff S, Pearlman ES, Fishman AP (1982): The contractile behavior of the heart and its functional coupling to the circulation. Prog Cardiovasc Dis 24:375–400.

146. Weiss JL, Bulkley BH, Hutchins GM, Mason SJ (1981): Two-dimensional echocardiographic recognition of myocardial injury in man: Comparison with post-mortem studies. Circulation 63:401–408.

147. Weyman AE, Wann LS, Caldwell RL, Hurwitz RA, Dillon JC, Feigenbaum H (1979): Negative contrast echocardiography: A new method for detecting left-to-right shunts. Circulation 59:498–505.

148. Wilcox WD, Carrigan TA, Dooley KJ, Giddens DP, Dykes FD, Lazzara A, Ray JL, Ahmann PA (1983): Range-gated pulsed Doppler ultrasound evaluation of carotid arterial blood flow in small preterm infants with patent ductus arteriosus. J Pediatr 102:294–298.

149. Williams RG, Bierman FZ, Sanders SP (1986): Echocardiographic Diagnosis of Cardiac Malformations. Boston, Little, Brown and Company, pp 4–33.

150. Wyse RKH, Robinson PJ, Deanfield JE, Pedoe DST, Macartney FJ (1984): Use of continuous wave Doppler ultrasound velocimetry to assess the severity of coarctation of the aorta by measurement of aortic flow velocities. Br Heart J 52:278–283.

151. Yeager S, Chin AJ, Sanders SP (1984): Subxiphoid two-dimensional echocardiographic diagnosis of coronary sinus septal defects. Am J Cardiol 54:686–687.

152. Yock PG, Popp RL (1984): Noninvasive estimation of right ventricular systolic pressure by Doppler ultrasound in patients with tricuspid regurgitation. Circulation 70:657–662.

153. Young BJ, Quinones MA, Waggoner AD, Miller RR (1980): Diagnosis and quantification of aortic stenosis with pulsed Doppler echocardiography. Am J Cardiol 45:987–994.

26 RADIONUCLIDE ANGIOCARDIOGRAPHY

Roger A. Hurwitz

Radionuclide angiocardiography is a relatively non-invasive technique used extensively in adults to study the central cardiovascular system. The procedure has also been applied to the study of children with cardiac abnormalities. Neonates and young infants have been less commonly studied with radionuclide techniques than older children, mainly because most cardiac diagnostic problems in very young children are structural rather than functional and because other noninvasive diagnostic modalities provide better anatomic definition. However, newer radionuclide technology has made it possible to obtain useful cardiac information in small, ill neonates.

HISTORICAL PERSPECTIVE

In 1927, Blumgart and colleagues used radium-C and a radiation detector to analyze the velocity of blood flow.[3] Prinzmetal and associates, using sodium iodide iodine-131 and a Geiger-Müller counter, first described patients with congenital heart disease in 1948.[22]

Since that period numerous diagnostic and therapeutic modalities have been developed to salvage, treat, and even cure cardiac malformations. In early palliative and corrective surgery the surgeon must have a precise knowledge of the anatomy and physiology of the cardiovascular system. To provide this knowledge, shorter-lived radiopharmaceuticals and portable gamma cameras with "zoom" magnification make possible low radiation imaging in even the most severely ill neonate. Dedicated computer assist and multicrystal and digital cameras offering high count acquisition allow precise quantitation of physiologic measurements.

Radionuclide angiocardiography can now be performed and evaluated in a few minutes at the patient's bedside. It provides information on anatomy, right-to-left and left-to-right shunting, ventricular performance, myocardial integrity, and pulmonary perfusion. Information obtained by radionuclide angiocardiography may supplement or replace information requiring more invasive and dangerous procedures. Radionuclide techniques can be useful before and after surgery to assess the natural history of cardiac lesions and the results of medical or surgical intervention in neonates with cardiac lesions.

TECHNIQUE

First pass radionuclide angiocardiography provides anatomic and quantitative data from the initial transit of radioactivity through the central circulation. A compact radionuclide bolus is injected rapidly into a vein, preferably through an indwelling venous catheter, and dynamic imaging (which takes advantage of the temporal characteristics of flow) is performed in an anterior or right anterior oblique projection. The first pass technique provides excellent visualization of venous and right-sided heart structures, identification and quantitation of intracardiac shunts, and estimates of ventricular function and cardiac output.

Equilibrium ventriculography is an ECG-gated blood pool scintigram that allows repetitive sampling of all or selected portions of the cardiac cycle. Sequential studies after a single radionuclide bolus are possible, but decay of the isotope injected limits the length of time that repeat studies may be performed. Technetium-99m, which permits at least 6 hours of repeat study, is routinely used.

Imaging in any projection is possible, but to separate structures a left anterior oblique projection with caudal tilt (often supplied by a slant-hole collimator) is commonly employed. Despite both loss of septal resolution and depth distortion, a converging or pinhole collimator may be preferred when the procedure is used in infants.[11] Although only a gross indication of anatomy is provided by equilibrium ventriculography, the technique provides precise quantitation of ventricular systolic and diastolic function, valvular regurgitation, and reasonable estimates of ventricular volumes.

Myocardial perfusion scintigraphy is presently performed with thallium-201, which has a physical half-life of 73 hours, resulting in a radiation dose to the newborn's kidneys of approximately 1.5 rad after injection of a standard imaging dose.[28] Maximal myocardial uptake generally occurs at 10 minutes during rest and earlier after exercise. Perfusion scintigraphy is useful for evaluation of relative size and shape of the ventricles, myocardial integrity, and functional reserve.

Determination of myocardial reserve usually involves examination of images acquired during exercise (stress) and rest (reperfusion). As a substitute for exercise in small children, crying and/or infusion of isoproterenol have been used.[9] Responsiveness of the compromised coronary arterial system has also been investigated during infusion of a vasodilatory agent (e.g., dipyridamole).[1]

Pulmonary blood flow is readily assessed. A visual estimate can be made from standard radionuclide studies, although precise quantitation is determined by counts of activity in each lung after injection of macroaggregated albumin. Determination of time activity curves over different anatomic areas may isolate partial or complete great vessel anomalies.[16] Liver-spleen imaging, which is done most precisely with denatured red blood cells, can be definitive in the diagnosis of asplenia or polysplenia associated with major cardiovascular malformations.[5]

LIMITATIONS IN RADIONUCLIDE EVALUATION OF THE NEONATE

Radionuclide angiocardiography has technical limitations similar to those of many other modalities in the study of the neonate. Most of these concern the size of the patient. The isotope must be injected through a secure, relatively large-bore intravenous line, with persistence of activity often limiting the evaluation to one or two injections. Radiation exposure, although small, is additive. A "critical mass" of isotope is required, necessitating at least 2 mCi of technetium-99m for each study; this dose results in 200 to 500 mrad total body radiation. The usual myocardial perfusion agent (thallium-201), with a longer half-life, causes increased radiation exposure to the neonate's kidneys. Standard stress-intervention testing in a neonate is not possible; crying or drug infusion must provide the necessary stress.

CLINICAL APPLICATIONS

Angiographic Anatomy

Anatomic delineation is often possible during first pass radionuclide imaging (Fig. 26–1). Great vessel anatomy is most easily determined. Inspection of vena cavae during initial transit of the bolus of activity demonstrates the location and patency of these veins. In my experience at Indiana University, persistence of a left superior vena cava was identified by radionuclide study in 3 per cent of patients with cardiac lesions requiring cardiopulmonary bypass. Moderate or severe venous obstruction has been identified (Fig. 26–2) in approximately 20 per cent of patients following intra-atrial baffle procedures for repair of transposition of the great vessels.[14] Diagnosis of partial and complete anomalous pulmonary venous connection can be made by inspection of time activity curves and anatomic images. Long and coworkers used the technique to define infradiaphragmatic pulmonary venous drainage by demonstrating nuclide recirculation in the right atrium 3 to 6 seconds after initial passage and visualization of the anomalous trunk as a "tail" below the diaphragm.[16] Radionuclide angiography may also be used to demonstrate obstruction or perforation of intravascular catheters.

Although precise anatomic diagnosis often requires cardiac catheterization and cineangiography, radionuclide studies may provide important information on intracardiac structures and great arteries. An important application in newborns is differentiation of cardiac from pulmonary causes of cyanosis. In patients with normal cardiac anatomy and elevated pulmonary resistance, right-to-left shunting through a foramen ovale or patent ductus arteriosus may be identified on the radionuclide angiogram. Although

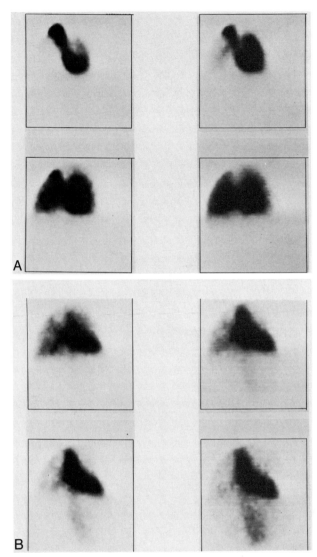

Figure 26–1. A and B, First pass radionuclide angiocardiograms showing normal circulation through right and left heart. Each image represents sequential data obtained at 1 second intervals collected in the right anterior oblique projection.

similar early appearance of aortic filling will be noted in cyanotic cardiac lesions, some of these defects show an anatomic pattern distinct enough for radionuclide angiocardiographic recognition. A hypoplastic right ventricle can be diagnosed by absence of activity in the tricuspid valve region, with early appearance of radionuclide in the left atrium and large left ventricle (Fig. 26–3). The absence of the right ventricle or the presence of a single large ventricle may also be seen by equilibrium ventriculography.

Pulmonary blood flow can be estimated by inspection of radionuclide angiocardiograms using technetium-99m or xenon-133. Relative flow is more precisely quantitated after injection of macroaggregated albumin, which deposits in the first capillary bed it enters. These studies are valuable in the diagnosis of congenital abnormalities of the lung and pulmonary emboli. Infants with transposition

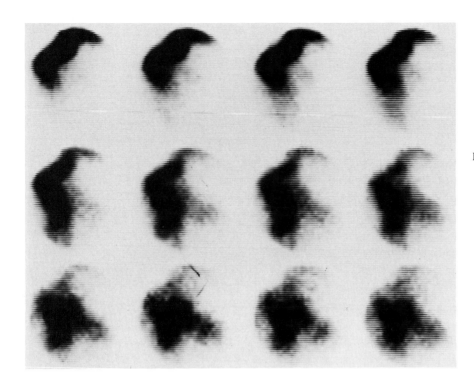

Figure 26–2. First pass radionuclide angiocardiogram in patient following Mustard repair for transposition of great arteries. Most activity courses below the diaphragm via the azygous vein, demonstrating severe obstruction to the superior limb of the intra-atrial baffle.

of the great arteries have been shown by radionuclide studies to have discrepant pulmonary vascularity, with increasing flow to the right lung as the infant ages.[19] The radionuclide technique is especially valuable in determining relative flow to each lung as supplied by collateral vessels (natural or surgical) in patients with severe or total pulmonary ventricular outflow obstruction. Such studies have been used to evaluate relative pulmonary flow after the initial surgical procedure for treatment of hypoplastic left-heart syndrome (Fig. 26–4).

Shunt Quantitation

If left-to-right shunting is present, the first pass angiogram shows persistent radioactivity in the lungs due to early re-circulation. The pulmonary time activity curve may be analyzed to quantitate the pulmonary-to-systemic flow ratio (Qp:Qs) by the gamma variate technique (Fig. 26–5). Estimate of the Qp:Qs ratio by the gamma variate method correlates well with the Qp:Qs ratio determined during cardiac catheterization.[17] Most studies have been used to quantitate intracardiac shunts as an aid in determining whether further invasive procedures are needed.

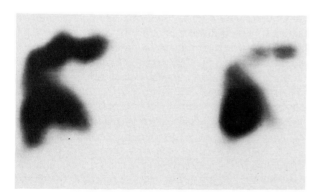

Figure 26–3. First pass radionuclide angiocardiogram in patient with hypoplastic right heart. In the image on the left, note absent tricuspid flow with left heart filling. In the systolic image on the right, a large right atrium and left ventricle are demonstrated.

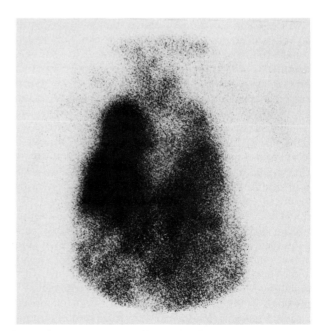

Figure 26–4. Pulmonary perfusion studied after injection of macro-aggregated albumin. Right lung has greater perfusion than left lung following creation of a right Blalock-Taussig shunt.

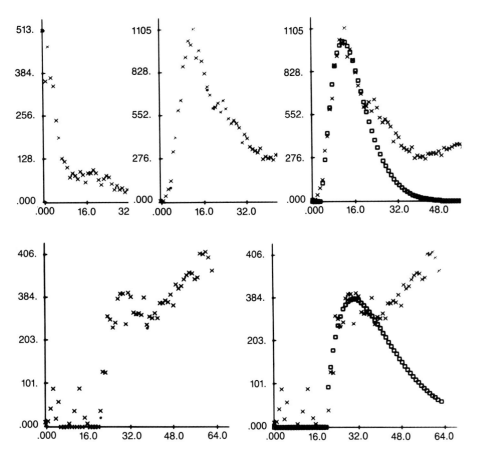

Figure 26–5. Radionuclide shunt study. Top left shows sharp, single spike determined from time activity curve over superior vena cava, documenting a compact injection bolus. Top middle is time activity curve over lung, demonstrating recirculation into lung. Top right is gamma variate curve derived from lung-time activity curve. Bottom left is time activity curve produced by subtracting gamma variate curve from original. Bottom right is second (recirculation) gamma variate curve. Note change in scale between first and second lung curves. Patient has moderate left-to-right shunt, with Qp:Qs of 1.9.

Anderson and associates have shown that age has no limitation on shunt quantitation; in 23 infants the correlation of radionuclide shunt studies with Fick shunt determinations was similar to the correlation found in 65 older children.[2]

The determination of the Qp:Qs ratio associated with the presence of a patent ductus arteriosus in full-term and premature neonates with respiratory distress can help estimate the contribution of ductal shunting to the infant's condition. Fifteen premature infants were studied by Treves and coworkers, and radionuclide estimates of the Qp:Qs ratio were helpful in the management of these neonates.[26] Determinations of the Qp:Qs ratio are useful in the selection of infants who might benefit from ductal closure, as well as in assessment of residual shunting after previous pharmacologic or surgical treatment of the ductus. Similarly, Qp:Qs determinations can also help differentiate a significant shunt from an atrial septal defect from the smaller shunt associated with a stretched patent foramen ovale.

Radionuclide shunt studies have certain limitations. Separate sites of shunt cannot be determined; the Qp:Qs ratio is the summation of all left-to-right shunting. Shunt studies cannot accurately assess other cardiac abnormalities, such as the severity of pulmonary stenosis or the magnitude of pulmonary hypertension. Further, shunt studies may overestimate pulmonary blood flow in the presence of severe tricuspid regurgitation, pulmonary regurgitation, or severe congestive heart failure and extremely low cardiac output.

Ventricular Function

Both right and left ventricular function may be assessed by radionuclide angiocardiography. Different techniques are often employed because each laboratory has its own preference for a specific first pass or blood-pool technique. Systolic function, as estimated by ventricular ejection fraction, is most commonly determined in infants and children; ventricular volumes and diastolic function (ventricular filling rate) are also being evaluated and used. Evaluation of left ventricular volume and ejection fraction in infants and children by equilibrium ventriculography (Fig. 26–6) has shown good correlation (r > 0.90) with measurements obtained during cardiac catheterization.[21] Because of overlap of the right atrium on the right ventricle in equilibrium studies, many laboratories prefer first pass angiography for determination of right ventricular function. The first pass technique uses flow dynamics to help define chambers; once the chambers are accurately defined, a more reliable estimate of ventricular function can be obtained. A shortcoming in radionuclide assessment of ventricular function has been the relatively low number of counts afforded by conventional gamma cameras; thus, use of multicrystal cameras and new single-crystal digital

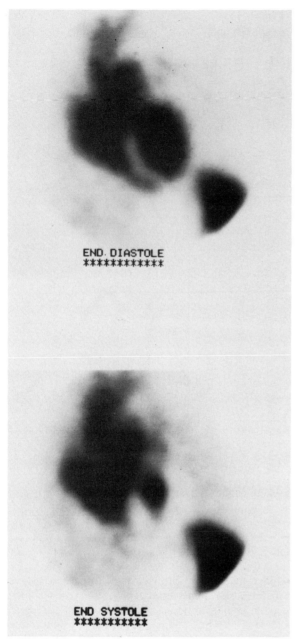

Figure 26–6. End-diastolic and end-systolic frames of equilibrium ventriculogram imaged in left anterior oblique projection. Left ventricle is large but contracts well.

systems achieves the greater counts necessary for more reliable quantitation of ventricular function.[7]

Normal values for radionuclide cardiac function are difficult to obtain in pediatrics. Nevertheless, normal values are vital for each laboratory performing such studies, so that recognition of abnormal values will be facilitated. By using first pass radionuclide angiocardiography, ventricular function was determined for 74 infants and children with normal cardiovascular systems who were undergoing skeletal scintigraphy.[15] Infants had a right ventricular ejection fraction of 0.54 ± 0.09 and a left ventricular ejection fraction of 0.68 ± 0.13.

Evaluation of ventricular function helps in the management of patients facing surgery. As surgical techniques improve, the frequency of neonatal cardiac surgery is increasing. New operations are being performed in attempts both to treat previously uncorrectable lesions (see Chapter 62) and to improve long-term outcome in correctable lesions (see Chapter 66). In addition, well-established operations are being performed in younger patients (see Chapter 64). Similar right ventricular ejection fractions have been found in patients with ventricular septal defects palliated by pulmonary artery banding and unoperated ventricular septal defects, suggesting that pulmonary artery banding has no deleterious effect on ventricular function. However, when definitive surgery is undertaken, postoperative right ventricular ejection fractions are better if the ventricular septal defect is repaired through the tricuspid valve rather than by using a right ventricular incision.

Similarly, reduced right ventricular ejection fractions have been demonstrated in patients following repair of tetralogy of Fallot in which a transannular outflow tract patch is necessary versus those patients who require only infundibular augmentation. However, many older children who have undergone surgical repair of tetralogy of Fallot and have normal right ventricular ejection fractions at rest decrease their right ventricular ejection fractions during dynamic exercise.[24]

Right ventricular ejection fractions in patients with transposition of the great arteries are often in the 0.50 to 0.60 range; these ejection fractions are similar to normal values for the normally connected right ventricle. Following intra-atrial baffle procedures for transposition, right ventricular ejection fractions seldom rise and often show a blunted response to exercise.[12,20] Thus, after physiologically corrective atrial rerouting operations that eliminate hypoxemia, the right ventricular ejection fraction does not increase to levels commonly present when the normal left ventricle is in the systemic circuit. Absence of normal ventricular ejection fraction for the systemic ventricle after venous repair is one factor in consideration of the anatomic correction (arterial switch) for treatment of transposition of the great arteries.

Evaluation of left ventricular ejection fraction may help in the management of infants with lesions whose course is greatly dependent on left ventricular function, such as those with the hypoplastic right-heart syndrome. There is reluctance to disregard criteria of age (more than 5 years) and normalcy of left ventricular function in the selection of patients for the Fontan procedure.[4] Yet there is worry that the left ventricle, chronically stressed by volume overload and hypoxemia, may deteriorate in patients with hypoplastic right-heart syndrome. Some patients have had successful surgery despite not meeting the ideal characteristics for the Fontan procedure,[8, 13] but it is preferable that left ventricular function and pulmonary arterial pressures are normal. Therefore, an abnormal left ventricular ejection fraction even in infancy, or a decrease in ejection fraction shown by serial radionuclide studies, may signal the need for early surgery. Although left ventricular function has not always been normal in the few infants studied with low or normal pulmonary blood flow, radionuclide

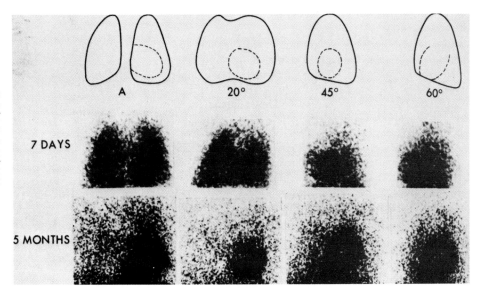

Figure 26–7. Thallium-201 perfusion study in 7-day-old infant, demonstrating poor cardiac uptake of isotope. At 5 months, the study has normalized. (Reprinted with permission of Finley JP et al [1979]: Transcient myocardial ischemia of the newborn infant demonstrated by thallium myocardial imaging. J Pediatr 94:263–270.)

data suggest that the presence of mild-to-moderate pulmonary hypertension from excessive pulmonary blood flow is frequently associated with abnormal left ventricular ejection fraction. Thus, performance of Fontan-type surgery in the hypoplastic right-heart syndrome must be considered relatively early in patients with large pulmonary blood flow.

Radionuclide scintigraphy has been used to assess functional myocardial integrity. Finley and colleagues injected thallium-201 into seven newborns (five term infants and two premature infants) with congestive heart failure and ECG changes suggestive of myocardial ischemia.[6] There was poor global perfusion in all; at repeat evaluation the clinical course and perfusion study had normalized (Fig. 26–7).

Myocardial perfusion imaging has been investigated as an aid in diagnosing other cardiac abnormalities in infants and children. When right ventricular uptake was quantitated to assess the degree of right ventricular hypertrophy, a reasonable prediction of right ventricular pressure was established.[23] Myocardial scintigraphy has also been employed in an effort to assess patients with the difficult diagnostic problems of anomalous or compromised coronary artery flow. Gutgesell and colleagues demonstrated focal abnormalities in seven patients with anomalous coronary arteries and myocardial ischemia; unfortunately there was also a focal defect in one and diffuse irregularity in three of nine patients with congestive cardiomyopathy without coronary anomalies.[10] Similar diffuse irregularities were reported in one infant and in 11 children imaged 1 week to 13 months after the onset of viral myocarditis.[25] These patients have been compared with those with mucocutaneous lymph node syndrome. The latter have shown no perfusion abnormalities when coronary angiography has been normal, but scintigraphy has demonstrated a large filling defect in a 4-month-old child following an infarct.[29] Recently developed radiopharmaceuticals, such as gallium-67 citrate and indium-111, also show promise in the identification of myocardium affected by an inflammatory process.[30]

CLINICAL UTILITY

Radionuclide angiography is "relatively" noninvasive, requiring an intravenous injection of a radiopharmaceutical, which results in a small accumulation of radioactivity. Current technology provides important cardiovascular data with minimal risk, but there are certain inherent drawbacks. Other imaging techniques, such as magnetic resonance imaging, can provide excellent anatomic detail; however, equipment is costly and each study requires the subject to be very quiet for a considerable time period, necessitating sedation in infants and small children. Two-dimensional echocardiography is an essentially noninvasive technique that provides excellent anatomic delineation. Complementary Doppler flow studies provide additional hemodynamic measurements, but the studies can be technically difficult to perform and interpret.

Radionuclide angiography is excellent for imaging of the venae cavae but is of limited value in defining intracardiac structures. However, when patients are injected with a radionuclide for noncardiac diagnostic problems or for ventricular function analysis, major structural abnormalities of the heart and great vessels can be readily identified. Even though specific cardiac anatomy can be best evaluated by two-dimensional echocardiography and Doppler flow studies or magnetic resonance imaging, quantitation of shunt and determination of relative pulmonary blood flow are quickly and precisely ascertained by nuclear techniques. Radionuclide angiocardiography is capable of accurately quantitating valvular regurgitation but is less valuable in estimating the severity of valvular stenosis. The severity of valvular stenosis is best made noninvasively with Doppler flow techniques. Assessment of relative pulmonary pressure is also available with the use of two-dimensional echocardiography and Doppler techniques.

Noninvasive estimates of systolic ventricular function, diastolic ventricular function, and wall motion are being made with radionuclide, magnetic resonance imaging, and echocardiography and Doppler methods. Estimating right ventricular function from first pass radionuclide angiocardiography and left ventricular function from radionuclide equilibrium ventriculography can be done with confidence. Wall motion can also be assessed with these studies. Although coronary perfusion and myocardial integrity can be evaluated by several radionuclide techniques, perfusion scintigraphy has been successfully used for many years and is probably the radionuclide method of choice.

FUTURE DIRECTIONS

Further improvements in diagnostic techniques for evaluation of the neonatal cardiovascular system will depend on methodologies that are simple, reproducible, and free from side effects. Such improvements are necessary to complement the major advances taking place in neonatal cardiac surgery and to define the contribution of the ductus to the respiratory distress syndrome in premature infants. Nuclear technology is continually improving. Newer digital cameras[7] and advanced collimators offer higher count acquisitions; the better resolution that results allows improved imaging in small patients with rapid heart rates. Computed tomography has improved radionuclide assessment of myocardial integrity by adding spatial information. Biochemical myocardial substructure may be defined with positron emission tomography, which is increasingly available.

Perhaps of greatest importance in increasing the use of radionuclide techniques for evaluation of neonates with cardiovascular problems will be the development of radiopharmaceuticals possessing very low radioactivity. Krypton-81m, a rare gas with a 13-second half-life, is excreted via the lung but can be used to evaluate right-sided heart function. Gold-195m, with a half-life of 30.5 seconds, and iridium-191m, with a half-life of 5 seconds, also have applicability to the study of right- and left-sided ventricular function.[18,27]

References

1. Albro PC, Gould KL, Westcott RJ, Hamilton GW, Ritchie JL, Williams DL (1978): Non-invasive assessment of coronary stenosis by myocardial imaging during pharmacologic coronary vasodilatation: III. Clinical trial. Am J Cardiol 42:751–760.
2. Anderson PAW, Bowyer KW, Jones RH (1984): Effects of age on radionuclide angiographic detection and quantitation of left-to-right shunts. Am J Cardiol 53:879–883.
3. Blumgart HL, Yens OC (1927): Studies of the velocity of blood flow: I. The method utilized. J Clin Invest 4:1–13.
4. Choussat A, Fontan F, Besse P, Vallot F, Chauve A, Bricaud H (1970): Selection criteria for Fontan's procedure. In Anderson RH, Shinebourne EA (eds): Pediatric Cardiology. Edinburgh, Churchill Livingstone, pp 559–566.
5. Ehrlich CP, Papanicolaou N, Treves S, Hurwitz RA, Richards P (1982): Splenic scintigraphy using Tc-99m labelled heat denatured red blood cells in pediatric patients. J Nucl Med 23:209–213.
6. Finley JP, Howman-Giles RB, Gilday DL, Bloom KR, Rowe RD (1979): Transient myocardial ischemia of the newborn infant demonstrated by thallium myocardial imaging. J Pediatr 94:263–270.
7. Gal R, Grenier RP, Carpenter J, Schmidt DH, Port SC (1986): High count rate first-pass radionuclide angiography using a digital gamma camera. J Nucl Med 27:198–206.
8. Gale AW, Danielson GK, McGoon DC, Wallace RB, Mair DD (1981): Fontan procedure for tricuspid atresia. Circulation 62:91–96.
9. Girod DA, Faris J, Hurwitz RA, Caldwell RL, Burt RW, Siddiqui A (1979): Thallium 201 assessment of myocardial perfusion in coronary anomalies in children (abstr). Am J Cardiol 43:402.
10. Gutgesell HP, Pinsky WW, Depuey EG (1980): Thallium-201 myocardial perfusion imaging in infants and children. Circulation 61:596–599.
11. Hannon DW, Gelfand MJ, Bailey UW, Hall JW, Kaplan S (1986): Pinhole radionuclide ventriculography in small infants. Am Heart J 111:316–321.
12. Hurwitz RA, Caldwell RL, Girod DA, Mahony L, Brown J, King H (1985): Ventricular function in transposition of the great arteries: Evaluation by radionuclide angiocardiography. Am Heart J 110:600–605.
13. Hurwitz RA, Caldwell RL, Girod DA, Wellman H (1986): Left ventricular function in tricuspid atresia: A radionuclide study. J Am Coll Cardiol 8:916–921.
14. Hurwitz RA, Papanicolaou N, Treves S, Keane JF, Castaneda A (1982): Radionuclide angiocardiography in evaluation of patients after surgical repair of transposition of the great arteries. Am J Cardiol 49:761–765.
15. Hurwitz RA, Treves S, Kuruc A (1983): Right ventricular and left ventricular ejection fraction in pediatric patients with normal hearts: First pass radionuclide angiocardiography. Am Heart J 107:726–732.
16. Long WA, Lawson EE, Perry JR, Harned HS Jr, Henry GW (1985): Radionuclide diagnosis of infradiaphragmatic total anomalous pulmonary venous drainage. Pediatr Cardiol 6:69–76.
17. Maltz DL, Treves S (1972): Quantitative radionuclide angiocardiography: Determination of Qp:Qs in children. Circulation 47:1049–1056.
18. Mena I, Narahara KA, DeJong R, Maublant J (1983): Gold-195m an ultra short lived generator produced radionuclide: Clinical application in sequential first pass ventriculography. J Nucl Med 24:139–144.
19. Muster AJ, Paul MH, Van Grondelle A, Conway JJ (1976): Asymmetric distribution of the pulmonary blood flow between the right and left lungs in d-transposition of the great arteries. Am J Cardiol 38:352–361.
20. Parrish MD, Graham TP Jr, Bender HW, Jones JP, Patton J, Partain CL (1983): Radionuclide angiographic evaluation of right and left ventricular function during exercise after repair of transposition of the great arteries. Circulation 67:178–183.
21. Parrish MD, Graham TP Jr, Born ML, Jones JP, Boucek RJ Jr, Partain CL (1982): Radionuclide ventriculography for assessment of absolute right and left ventricular volumes in children. Circulation 66:811–819.
22. Prinzmetal M, Corday E, Bergman HC, Schwarz L, Spritzler RJ (1948): Radiocardiography: A new method for studying the blood flow through the chambers of the heart in human beings. Science 108:340–341.
23. Rabinovitch M, Fischer KC, Treves S (1982): Quantitative thallium-201 myocardial imaging in assessment of right ventricular pressure in patients with congenital heart defects. Br Heart J 45:198–205.
24. Reduto LA, Berger JH, Johnstone DE, Hillenbrand W, Wackers FJ, Whittemore R, Cohen LS, Gottschalk A, Zaret BL (1980): Radionuclide assessment of right and left ventricular exercise reserve after total correction of tetralogy of Fallot. Am J Cardiol 45:1013–1018.
25. Saji T, Matsuo N, Hashisuchi R, Sato K, Umezawa T, Morishita K, Yamazaki J, Kawamura Y, Okuzumi K, Yabe Y (1985): Radionu-

clide imaging for assessment of myocarditis and postmyocarditic state in infants and children. Jpn Heart J 26:413–423.

26. Treves S, Collins-Nakai R, Ahnberg D, Lang P (1976): Quantitative radionuclide angiocardiography (RAC) in premature infants with patent ductus arteriosus (PDA) and respiratory distress syndrome (RDS)(abstr). J Nucl Med 17:554.

27. Treves S, Fyler D, Fujii A, Kuruc A (1982): Low radiation iridium-191m radionuclide angiography: Detection and quantitation of left-to-right shunts in infants. J Pediatr 101:210–215.

28. Treves ST, Hurwitz R, Kuruc A, Strauss HW (1985): Heart. In Treves ST (ed): Pediatric Nuclear Medicine. New York, Springer-Verlag, p 272.

29. Ueda K, Saito A, Nakano H, Yano M (1980): Thallium 201 scintigraphy in an infant with myocardial infarction following mucocutaneous lymph node syndrome. Pediatr Radiol 9:183–185.

30. Yasuda T, Palacios IF, Khaw BA, Dec W, Gold HK, Leinbach RC, Fallon JT, Barlai-Kouach M, Strauss HW, Haber EC (1985): Myoclonal indium-111 antimyosin antibody imaging versus right ventricular biopsy in diagnosing acute myocarditis (abstr). Circulation 72(suppl III):110.

27 CARDIAC CATHETERIZATION

Michael R. Nihill

The role of cardiac catheterization in the management of cardiovascular disease has changed considerably over the past 20 years, particularly in neonates with cardiovascular or pulmonary disorders. These changes have been brought about by the development of new invasive and noninvasive diagnostic and therapeutic techniques.

Until the late 1970s, when high quality two-dimensional echocardiography became widely used, the main reasons to catheterize a newborn infant were to determine the anatomy of the heart and great vessels and to rule out congenital heart disease as a cause of symptoms, particularly in neonates with severe respiratory distress. High resolution two-dimensional echocardiography and Doppler echocardiography can define cardiovascular anatomy with 95 per cent accuracy in the neonatal period.[44,77,93] Neonatal cardiac catheterization is now performed to obtain information other than cardiovascular anatomy. Accurate precatheterization assessment of the infant's clinical problems is essential in deciding whether neonatal catheterization is even indicated and what procedures should be performed.

Catheterization procedures should be goal oriented. After the precise nature of the patient's problem is clearly identified noninvasively, catheterization should be carefully planned to further elucidate the nature of the problem as well as to set the background for future therapeutic maneuvers.

HISTORICAL PERSPECTIVE

Since its inception, cardiac catheterization has been used as an investigative and diagnostic tool by diverse disciplines in medicine and physiology. J. R. Dieffenbach[24] has been credited with the first use of a cardiac catheter in a human in the treatment of a patient with cholera. Physiologist Claude Bernard[3] measured intracardiac temperature and Pavy[72] in 1836 coined the term "cardiac catheterism" to describe his experiences in passing a catheter into the right ventricle in humans and animals. A double lumen catheter was used by physiologists Chauveau and Marey in 1861[16,17] to measure simultaneous pressures in the right ventricle and right atrium.

Werner Forssmann[33] is acknowledged as the first to undertake a systematic study of the technique of cardiac catheterization and angiography using himself as the subject. His early experiments were published in 1929 and shortly afterwards in the early 1930s.[34] The first body of work on central and peripheral angiography in children was published by Castellanos and his colleagues in Havana.[11,12,13]

By the early 1940s, angiography of congenital cardiac defects was a well-established investigation.

The methodology and techniques of cardiac catheterization were standardized and extensively used by Cournand[20] and others[2,4,6,23] in New York in the early and late 1940s, and there soon followed several papers and monographs[15,19,25,46,90,103] on the use of cardiac catheterization to diagnose congenital heart defects in children and infants. Catheterization of neonates was sporadic, and little was published until the late 1950s[80,81] and 1960s when Adams,[1] Emmanouilides, and others[27,28,55,82] catheterized normal and sick infants to establish the foundations of our knowledge of fetal and neonatal cardiovascular physiology.

As surgical techniques for the repair and palliation of congenital heart defects were developed in the 1950s[65] and 1960s, there were rapid developments and refinements of catheterization techniques, especially in younger children, infants, and newborns.[5,14,82,83,84,99]

Changes and improvements in imaging, catheterization, and surgical techniques have mandated that a constantly evolving management approach be used in infants and children with cardiovascular and pulmonary disease.[48,93]

CLINICAL APPROACH

Precatheterization Assessment

In addition to a thorough history, a complete physical examination is essential to assess the infant's condition and stability. A physical examination will identify the overall clinical status of the patient, state of hydration, cyanosis, respiratory distress, and adequacy of the peripheral circulation. Physical examination together with complementary laboratory investigations will determine whether the infant needs endotracheal intubation prior to the catheterization and whether other therapy, such as inotropic support, diuretics, or prostaglandins, should be started prior to catheterization.

An electrocardiogram is useful in evaluating arrhythmias that may require therapy prior to the catheterization. The electrocardiogram can also reflect disturbances of electrolytes, pH, and blood sugar.[42]

Arterial blood gases indicate whether acidosis or hypoxemia is present. Any abnormalities in acid-base balance, oxygenation, or electrolytes should be corrected insofar as possible before the catheterization. Hemoglobin and hematocrit should be measured prior to the catheterization, and blood volume or hemoglobin should be corrected as necessary. Using measured arterial oxygen saturation, the

Table 27–1. INDICATIONS FOR CARDIAC CATHETERIZATION
IN THE NEWBORN INFANT

Define cardiovascular anatomy, including the morphology, position, relations, and
   connections of the following:
   1. Systemic and pulmonary veins
   2. Atria
   3. Atrioventricular valves
   4. Ventricles and outflow tracts
   5. Proximal pulmonary and systemic arteries
   6. Peripheral pulmonary and systemic arteries
Measure and calculate central and peripheral hemodynamics
   1. Measure blood pressure in the systemic and pulmonary arteries and veins
   2. Measure blood flow in the systemic and pulmonary circulations
   3. Calculate shunts
   4. Calculate vascular resistance in the pulmonary and systemic beds
   5. Calculate valve areas
Monitor changes in hemodynamics in response to drug, respirator, or surgical
   interventions
Monitor cardiac pump function, especially in response to inotropic drugs
Monitor cardiac muscle function
Conduct electrophysiologic studies and assess antiarrhythmic therapy
Biopsy the myocardium

hemoglobin should be adjusted to produce an oxygen-carrying capacity of at least 15 ml O_2 per 100 ml blood (content = Hb g/dl × 1.34 × O_2 sat). Blood should be typed and cross-matched and available before the start of the catheterization; a volume of at least 20 ml/kg of body weight should be available during the catheterization.

A current two-dimensional echocardiogram should be reviewed before the catheterization to evaluate the basic anatomy of the heart so that excessive use of contrast material is not required. Any anomalies of systemic venous return should also be noted in planning the venous access route.[51–53]

Echocardiography can define the basic anatomy of the heart and great arteries and help determine the need for further anatomic studies such as angiography. An echocardiogram is also useful in evaluating the contractility of the myocardium prior to the catheterization. The patency of the ductus arteriosus can be determined and can be monitored in response to prostaglandin administration.[47,97]

A written outline or plan of the catheterization procedures should be made so that none is omitted during the course of the catheterization. A wide variety of information may be obtained during cardiac catheterization (Table 27–1).

Not all of the procedures outlined in Table 27–1 are a required part of a cardiac catheterization; one must formulate a protocol and must design the catheterization to obtain needed information in the least traumatic and time-consuming manner possible. Cardiac catheterization is no longer a "fishing expedition" in critically ill neonates but a goal-oriented, carefully designed investigation performed in an optimally stabilized infant.

Prior to catheterization, a thorough two-dimensional echocardiographic study with Doppler (see Chapter 25) will help to plan the various angiographic studies. Two-dimensional echocardiography will be able to diagnose accurately most of the anatomic features under ideal conditions.[44] Echocardiography, however, is still an art, and the echocardiographer requires great experience in order

to demonstrate, and more importantly to recognize, intracardiac and extracardiac anatomy. Demonstration of intrathoracic anatomy may be especially difficult in those sick newborns with severe pulmonary disease, particularly those with emphysematous lungs in whom an adequate echo window is difficult to find. In infants with severe hyaline membrane disease, anomalous connection of the pulmonary veins may be especially difficult to rule out,[49] and catheterization may be required for this single piece of information (see Chapter 34).

Catheterization Data

Cardiovascular Anatomy

The anatomy of the various parts of the heart and great vessels is demonstrated at cardiac catheterization using angiography (see Chapter 28) and the course of the catheter through the heart and great vessels.[96]

Hemodynamics

BLOOD PRESSURES IN THE CENTRAL
AORTA AND PULMONARY ARTERY

The principles of data acquisition and waveform analysis during cardiac catheterization have been well established and standardized for a number of years.[102] Dynamic changes in the normal pulmonary and systemic circulations occur up to and immediately after birth,[27,50,68] and normal vascular pressures in the newborn infant depend on both gestational and postnatal age (see Chapters 7, 20, and 39). In this chapter I will confine myself to guidelines and modifications of the various techniques for acquisition of vascular pressure data during cardiac catheterization in premature and newborn infants.

In order to obtain accurate and reproducible blood pressure measurements with a fluid-filled measuring system, one should have a well-balanced and optimally damped transducer that is matched to the catheter size and length of the connection tubing.[30] Catheters with side and end holes are preferred with the widest, shortest path possible to the transducer. Great care should be taken when using small, balloon-directed Swan-Ganz catheters, which have only an end hole; the small lumen size and relatively long length of these multilumen catheters usually produce over-damped pressure tracings. Other factors that may influence the accuracy and reproducibility of the pressure recordings are (1) severe airway obstruction with marked inspiratory and expiratory swings in intrathoracic pressure and (2) high mean airway pressure produced by high respirator settings necessary for adequate oxygenation.

Pulmonary artery and wedge pressures may be obtained with balloon-directed catheters,[64,94] which can be floated out to the pulmonary artery at the bedside after percutaneous sheath insertion.[74] However, this procedure may be difficult in small premature babies, even with echocardiographic guidance;[73] the bulk of the balloon itself may hinder passage through the tricuspid valve or right ventricular outflow tract. The catheter may also pass into the left atrium and left ventricle during blind manipulation. Fluoroscopy may be necessary to manipulate the catheter into the pulmonary artery and into one or another pulmonary artery branches; blind insertion may result in the balloon catheter passing through the ductus arteriosus into the descending aorta. If cardiac output is not to be measured, higher fidelity pressures may be obtained with a regular wedge type Swan-Ganz catheter rather than the extralumen thermodilution catheter.

If the pulmonary artery catheter is to be used for long-term monitoring of pulmonary artery pressure during drug administration (such as tolazoline or prostacyclin), the catheter tip should be placed in the proximal part of a branch pulmonary artery. Leaving a catheter in the right ventricle will promote premature ventricular contractions and ventricular arrhythmias, particularly if it is positioned in the right ventricular outflow tract, and may cause right ventricular perforation. When measuring central aortic pressure after retrograde passage of a catheter, one should make sure that the catheter tip does not pass into the main pulmonary artery via the patent ductus arteriosus. Pulmonary artery placement can be detected most reliably by an injection of a small amount of contrast material rather than by looking at the pressure curve or the oxygen saturation.

BLOOD FLOW IN THE SYSTEMIC AND PULMONARY CIRCULATIONS

Blood flow may be measured by the Fick principle[32] or by indicator dilution techniques.[59] The direct Fick principle requires measurement of oxygen consumption; there are commercially available flow-through hoods that measure oxygen extracted by the infant.[66] However, these hoods cannot be used if the infant is intubated or is receiving added oxygen. Assumed oxygen consumption from tables[63] may be quite inaccurate in infants with respiratory distress or unstable metabolic and hemodynamic states.

The thermodilution method[31] may be used to measure systemic blood flow, providing there is no right-to-left or left-to-right shunt. With a large left-to-right shunt, a reasonably accurate measurement may be made of pulmonary blood flow if the cold indicator is injected into the right atrium and sampling is performed in the pulmonary artery distal to any shunting.[89] The accuracy of this measurement of pulmonary blood flow in neonates has not been demonstrated. However, if one wants to follow trends or changes in pulmonary blood flow, the thermodilution method is acceptable. The injectate port is usually 15 cm from the tip of a 5 French catheter and may lie in the sheath or iliac vein in small premature babies; unpredictable results will be obtained if the cold indicator is not injected as a central bolus. Likewise, if the proximal injectate port is in the right atrium and there is right-to-left shunting, the quantity of the cold injectate that reaches the distal thermistor may vary with changes in pulmonary resistance.

SHUNT CALCULATION

Other indicators, such as indocyanine green, are used in older children to measure blood flow by the indicator dilution technique.[10,98] This method is time consuming and requires withdrawing relatively large amounts of blood; it is not generally used in small premature or sick neonates.

If one is confident in the accuracy of systemic and pulmonary blood flow measurements,[87] the amount of left-to-right or right-to-left shunting can be calculated. The amount of shunting can be expressed as liters/minute/m^2 or as a percentage of the flow through the pulmonary or systemic circulation.

RESISTANCE

The calculation of systemic or pulmonary resistance requires the simultaneous measurement of both flow and pressure. As already discussed, the measurement of pulmonary or systemic blood flow in neonates may be fraught with inaccuracies.[87] In addition, great care should be taken to verify the position of the catheter tip when pressure is being measured. Flow-directed balloon catheters can drift into unexpected positions, become wedged, or drift back to the right ventricle (where a damped pressure may resemble a pulmonary arterial tracing).

VALVE AREAS

Accurate calculations of valve areas are difficult to make in neonates, since such calculations require accurate measurements of both blood flow and pressure. Infants who develop symptoms due to severe outflow obstruction from the heart usually have a low cardiac output. Pressure gradients alone give no real indication of the severity of the obstruction; a valve area should be calculated using both flow and pressure parameters, if possible.

Pump Function

Cardiac pump function can be assessed by measuring cardiac output and calculating various derived indices of pump function such as mean systolic ejection rate and stroke volume.[102] These measurements are useful in monitoring the action of inotropic drugs during an acute intervention. One must be sure of the reproducibility of cardiac output measurements.

Cardiac Muscle Function

Catheterization-derived indices of cardiac muscle function such as V_{max}, systolic pressure–volume ratios, and dp/dt may also be useful in monitoring the acute effects of a drug.[102] A more simple and practical estimate of muscle function can be obtained from the shortening fraction measured from an echocardiogram.

Electrophysiologic Studies and Therapy

Electrophysiologic studies in the premature and neonatal infant are rarely required to diagnose and to manage cardiac arrhythmias.[38,39] However, multiple catheter studies can be performed in neonates to localize the site of origin of ventricular tachycardia.[37] Small submacroscopic tumors may initiate recurrent ventricular tachycardia, and intracardiac mapping may be required prior to surgical exploration and excision.[36,41]

Diagnostic intracardiac mapping of supraventricular tachycardias has not proved useful in the neonatal period;[40] however, insertion of a pacing catheter into the atrium to overdrive and suppress recurrent uncontrollable supraventricular tachycardias can be therapeutic.

Myocardial Biopsy

Myocardial biopsy can be performed even in neonates. I have used the long sheath technique (6 French) and a malleable Cordes bioptome in small infants to biopsy a right ventricular tumor.[78] Some intracardiac tumors, such as rhabdomyomas, may initially appear to be quite obstructive but may regress in size in the first few months of life. However, other tumors, such as fibromas, will not shrink and may need surgical excision. Tumor biopsy may prove useful in identifying the type of tumor. Inflammatory myocarditis is extremely rare in the neonatal period (see Chapter 47); most congestive cardiomyopathies in neonates (see Chapter 40) are a result of previous hypoxia or severely decompensated congenital cardiac defects.[8]

Preparation for Catheterization

Transport to the Catheterization Laboratory

The basic principles of neonatal transport as they are used in extramural transport should be applied to intrahospital transport.

1. Hemodynamics. The baby's hemodynamics should be as stable as possible, and blood volume replacement should be completed before transport. Inotropic or other cardiovascular support drugs should be at a stable infusion rate, with no adjustments required during the time of transport.

2. Vascular access. All intravenous lines should be secured, and intravenous infusion pumps should be stabilized for safe transport. Infusions of prostaglandins should be via a dedicated intravenous line; flushing of this line should be avoided because of apnea and hypotension with bolus injections of prostaglandins.

3. Body temperature control. The infant should be transported in a stable thermal environment such as an incubator or warming stand, since rapid heat loss can occur in an uncovered infant during transport through cold hospital corridors. Insulated wrappers such as Thinsulate (manufactured by the 3M Company and referred to as "Neonatal Bunting") are excellent for neonatal transport and are also radiolucent; the infant can be kept wrapped in this bunting during the catheterization with no degradation of radiograph quality.

4. Ventilator support. An intubated or ventilated infant should be transported to the catheterization lab with handbagging done by one operator. The infant's respirator or another respirator should be set up in the catheterization lab prior to transport so that it is ready to receive the baby on arrival.

5. Monitoring. Electrocardiographic monitoring is the only form of monitoring necessary during transport. Arterial lines should be secured with three-way stopcocks and flush syringes during transport.

6. Premedication. Most neonates do not require sedatives or narcotics prior to cardiac catheterization. Infants are particularly susceptible to the central nervous system depressant effects of narcotics; in particular, morphine may destablize the hemodynamics of an infant with low cardiac output by producing vagotonic bradycardia and venous dilation. Any sedation should be administered under the direct supervision of the attending physician in the catheterization laboratory.

Arrival in the Catheterization Laboratory

The catheterization laboratory is warmed to an ambient temperature of 80 to 85° F prior to arrival. The infant should be placed on a warming device, such as a Mul·T·Pad (Gaymar Industries Inc., New York). The warming device and the bunting, together with an infrared heating lamp, should be sufficient to keep the infant warm until he is draped for the catheterization. The Mul·T·Pad is not as radiopaque as older rubber heating pads; if heat loss is persistent, the baby can be sandwiched between two Mul·T·Pads without significant loss of radiograph quality.

A respirator must be placed for easy access. Some modern biplane C-arm laboratories have insufficient access to the head of the table or insufficient room for a respirator to be placed at the head of the table. Catheterization laboratory personnel should be drilled in a resuscitation routine so that obstructing radiograph equipment can be rapidly moved for access to the infant's head for respirator management and/or cardiopulmonary resuscitation.

Restraints are placed on the infant's limbs if paralyzing agents have not been used, so that there will be no movement of limbs or body after draping. The quality of respiration is assessed with a stethoscope after the infant is placed on the catheterization table and the respirator is connected. Adjustments to endotracheal tube position with or without the use of fluoroscopy are performed before the infant is draped and while there is adequate access to the head. Arterial lines are connected to the catheterization lab transducers. Blood pressure and the electrocardiogram are evaluated for stability prior to starting any procedure.

Intravenous infusion sites should be inspected and be available for visual monitoring during catheterization to guard against extravasation of fluid and drugs, particularly those containing calcium.

Monitoring During Catheterization

The heart rate, electrocardiogram, blood pressure, temperature, respiratory rate, respirator settings, chest movement, and air entry and infusion sites are monitored during the catheterization. Very soon after the baby enters the catheterization laboratory, arterial blood gases are drawn to make sure that there has been no significant deviation from the previous values.[91]

A respiratory therapist or physician is assigned to monitor the respirator, endotracheal tube, chest movement, and air entry during the catheterization. The position of the endotracheal tube, diaphragm movement, and presence of pneumothorax can be checked by fluoroscopy. Central temperature is monitored via a rectal probe, with the monitor visible at all times. Excessive withdrawal of blood for blood gas measurements can be avoided by the use of a pulse oximeter placed over the toe, palm of the hand, or ear lobe for constant monitoring during catheterization. Blood sampling should be carefully monitored, and excessive loss should be replaced during the catheterization with fresh packed red cells. Two ECG leads are displayed, one for monitoring heart rate and one for diagnostic interpretation, to observe the P waves and ST segments.

Monitoring urine output is important, especially in those babies with prerenal azotemia. A bladder catheter can be inserted, or the diaper can be weighed prior to catheterization.

Blood pressure can be monitored via an umbilical artery catheter, radial artery line, or femoral artery line. Marked fluctuations of blood pressure can occur during drug infusions given during catheterization, such as administration of prostaglandins or injection of hyperosmolar contrast material.

Right Heart Catheterization

Catheter Insertion

The femoral route is the preferred approach for diagnostic catheterization in infants. Percutaneous insertion of a sheath into the femoral vein allows multiple catheter exchanges with minimal trauma to the vein.[22,43,68,71,95] Relatively large sheaths can be used even in small infants; for example, a 7 French sheath is used to insert a balloon septostomy catheter in infants as small as 1.5 kg.

The percutaneous approach to the femoral vessels is now a standard procedure. Special short bevel needles of 21 gauge should be used in small infants for easy insertion of guide wires. Longer bevel needles tend to lacerate

the vessels; blood return can be obtained with longer bevel needles even if the lumen of the needle is not completely within the blood vessel lumen. Guide wires of 0.018 inch diameter should be used for the initial insertion of a small 5 French sheath. If a larger sheath (7 French) is to be used, a larger diameter guide wire (0.025 inch) is used for greater stability of the dilator as it enters the vein at the pelvic brim.

The umbilical vein can usually be quickly cannulated and is often patent up to 1 week after birth.[86] To avoid prolonged probing of the umbilical vein and the portal veins, a small injection of contrast material after insertion of the catheter will demonstrate whether the ductus venosus is still patent. A 5 French sheath and dilator can be passed over a guide wire through the ductus venosus in a similar fashion to femoral vein cannulation. This technique avoids spasm of the ductus venosus if catheter changes are necessary. Intracardiac manipulation of the catheter from the umbilical vein is more difficult, as the catheter tends to lie more posteriorly in the right atrium, and it is often difficult to enter the tricuspid valve and right ventricle from this approach. It is relatively easy to enter the left atrium and left ventricle from the umbilical vein, and the umbilical vein approach is a useful one from which to perform balloon atrial septostomy fairly quickly.

The brachial or axillary approach can be used if the femoral veins are not accessible.[45] The axillary vein can be punctured percutaneously about 0.5 to 1.0 cm below the distal axillary crease. The vein usually lies medial to the axillary artery, but the position can be variable. There is a greater risk of damaging the brachial plexus or axillary artery with a percutaneous approach because of lack of supporting subcutaneous tissue. If the axillary approach is necessary, it may be more expedient and safer to perform a cutdown just distal to the distal axillary crease. The vein or artery can be cannulated with a needle and guide wire under direct vision to avoid performing a cutdown on these small vessels.

The anterior brachial vein can be entered percutaneously or by cutdown, but in small neonates and premature babies this vein is usually too small to accommodate even a 5 French catheter. Also, there is a greater risk of spasm of the brachial vein, and there is more difficulty in manipulating the catheter through the long course from the arm to the superior vena cava.

The right jugular vein can be entered percutaneously and a relatively large sheath can be placed into the superior vena cava. Catheter manipulation from the jugular vein can be more difficult for operators used to the femoral approach. A flow-guided balloon catheter is very useful from this approach.

Catheter Types

Standard 5 French woven Dacron catheters are optimal for catheterizing newborns and small premature babies. Softer, flow-guided balloon catheters are perhaps less traumatic but have much less torque control; in small babies the balloon size itself can be obstructive and limit catheter manipulation. Smaller catheters, such as a 4 French Dacron catheter or a 4 French balloon-guided catheter, have very small fluid lumina, causing pressure tracings usually to be overdamped. The catheters can clot very quickly. Recent improvements in small catheter design have extended the usefulness of 4 French catheters.[56,57]

Catheter manipulation should be performed very carefully by a skilled operator, especially when passing through the right ventricular outflow tract. In newborn and premature babies, the myocardium is very soft, without much tactile feedback through the catheter. The myocardium is easily perforated, especially the medial wall of the right atrial appendage, which is very thin with little muscle. Perforation of the ventricle is especially likely with a dilated right ventricular outflow tract. There is often a diverticulum-like pouch just proximal to the pulmonary annulus, which appears to be more cranial than the pulmonary artery itself. Forceable manipulation of the catheter in this position can result in perforation of the right ventricular outflow tract. Where the anatomy of the heart is uncertain, small hand injections of 0.5 to 1 ml of contrast material will outline the anatomy adequately for safe catheter manipulation and advancement.

Hemodynamic measurements are performed with an end and side hole catheter for more accurate pressure recordings as well as to reduce the likelihood of clotting. After blood sampling and hemodynamic measurements are made, a fresh, clean angiographic side hole catheter is inserted for performance of angiography.

Guide wires may be used to help manipulate or bend the catheter,[68,95] especially to gain access to the left ventricle from the left atrium. Prolonged use of guide wires, even teflon-coated guide wires, can result in thrombosis of the catheter lumen; guide wires should be used sparingly, with catheters carefully aspirated and flushed after guide wire use. Guide wires with preformed tight curves are difficult to pass through small catheters, and usually the curve is lost in the attempt. The use of a deflector wire and handle (Cook catheters) has been very helpful and avoids the passage of a tightly curved wire into a relatively straight catheter. The deflector wires are manufactured with a tight 5-mm or a larger 10-mm curve. They are particularly useful in entering the left ventricle from the left atrium. In small hearts, manipulation of a catheter by itself, even with a balloon, can be difficult and traumatic.

Echocardiography and Catheter Manipulation

Echocardiography has been used to help guide the catheter into the heart and into various chambers[73] and has also been used to assist in balloon atrial septostomy. Echocardiographic guidance may be a useful technique to help in the performance of an emergency balloon atrial septostomy in the neonatal intensive care ward or in catheterization laboratories not adequately equipped with high quality biplane fluoroscopy. Echo guidance of catheters, even with skilled operators, is more time consuming than fluoroscopic guidance of catheterization. The benefits of echo-guided catheterization have yet to be demonstrated. The small decrease in fluoroscopic radiation time is inconsequential compared with the extended time and lack

of precision in catheter manipulation when echocardiographic guidance is used.

Left Heart Catheterization

Arterial Cannulation

Blood pressure monitoring is usually performed through a 21-gauge polyethylene femoral artery catheter. A retrograde catheterization is performed at the end of the procedure to minimize the time the catheter is in the artery.

Arterial access can be facilitated by the use of a small Doppler probe over the groin to locate the site of the artery.[88] Continuous wave Doppler echocardiographic monitoring of the arterial pulse has been used as an early warning of arterial compromise.

The umbilical artery can usually be cannulated in an infant less than 5 days of age.[86] In small infants, when there is spasm of the artery, or if the artery has begun to close, a small 3.5 French umbilical artery catheter can be used initially. The umbilical artery can be further dilated with a 5 French feeding tube or catheter to allow for passage of a larger angiographic catheter, if necessary. I have used the umbilical artery to insert a 5 mm balloon catheter for dilation of a coarctation. If the umbilical artery or vein is not accessible from the umbilical stump, a cutdown can be made at the base of the umbilicus to locate the vein or artery.

Left Ventricular Catheterization

I prefer the transseptal puncture with a long sheath technique to enter the left atrium and left ventricle when the atrial septum is intact, even in small infants.[26,69] This technique is preferred to retrograde arterial catheterization for entry into the left ventricle, as it avoids traumatizing small arteries and allows for use of a larger, shorter catheter for left ventriculography and other maneuvers. Transseptal left atrial catheterization has been performed in infants as small as 1.5 kg.

Recent improvements in catheter design and material have resulted in smaller (3.2 and 4 French) catheters,[56,57] which deliver adequate amounts of contrast material at a fast enough rate for adequate visualization of the heart chambers and great vessels in infants with a rapid heart rate and high cardiac output. These catheters have less torque control than larger catheters, and newer formulations of catheter material have resulted in less kinking during manipulation. They are best used for retrograde aortic and left ventricular angiography, in which little catheter manipulation is required.

If it is anticipated that a retrograde catheter will be in place for longer than 20 to 30 minutes, I recommend systemic heparinization at 50 units/kg. Routine heparinization for all retrograde catheterizations has been recommended by some authors.[35]

Imaging

Biplane fluoroscopy and cineangiography are essential for optimal catheterization of infants and children with congenital cardiovascular defects. Magnification fluoroscopy in the 5 or 6 inch mode is necessary for small infants; a small focal spot of 0.3 to 0.6 mm is required for optimal resolution. A high quality videotape or disk recorder is necessary to review angiograms immediately to avoid unnecessary repeat angiography. Cineangiograms should be developed and viewed immediately after the catheterization, as the resolution of cineangiograms is higher than most currently available video recording systems. Small details not visualized on the video recorder may become apparent when the developed film is viewed.

Two-dimensional echocardiography with Doppler facility is a useful adjunct to imaging in the catheterization laboratory. Contrast echocardiograms can localize shunting in any direction and have virtually replaced indocyanine green dye curves for shunt detection in our laboratory.

Physiologic Recordings

A minimum of four channels of simultaneous records should be available to record two electrocardiograms, with at least two simultaneous pressures. The pressure measuring and recording system should be evaluated prior to catheterization to optimize pressure signal recording. Small caliber catheters will produce overdamped pressures in a fluid-filled system. Tubing length, caliber, and rigidity should be tested prior to the catheterization to minimize over- or underdamping. The recording device should produce an instantaneous record for review. If photographic paper is used, it must be available for immediate review after the catheterization.

Electrophysiologic studies in premature and newborn infants are rarely indicated; if they are required, specially filtered channels on the recorder are necessary. The catheterization room itself should be electrically silent, with careful shielding and placement of cables.

Overdrive pacing may be necessary to convert tachyarrhythmias to sinus rhythm. Special overdrive pacemakers with rates up to 600 beats per minute may be required to convert atrial flutter to sinus rhythm. A 4 French bipolar catheter is recommended, since larger catheters tend to be stiffer and more traumatic because of the wire core.

Hemostasis and Anticoagulants

Precatheterization clotting studies are performed on all newborns with suspected congenital heart disease. Most newborns require the administration of vitamin K. Some patients may have disorders of blood clotting or platelets due to infection or shock. Vitamin K is administered intramuscularly as long as possible before the catheterization; fresh frozen plasma and fresh platelets are ordered if clotting disorders are identified. One unit of fresh packed red cells, or at least 20 ml/kg, should also be available during all catheterizations of infants under 5 kg because of the relatively large blood loss when exchanging catheters or sheaths in infants compared with other children.

The use of hemostasis or bleed-back valves on percutaneous sheaths will minimize blood loss during catheter exchanges or when there is poor tolerance between the catheter and sheath size. When using a small catheter in a larger sheath, back flow of blood into the sheath around the catheter may result in thrombosis inside the sheath; this clot could be flushed into the circulation during catheter exchanges or flushing of the side arm of the hemostasis valve. I have used a constant slow infusion of heparinized saline through a bleed-back valve in patients who have required prolonged catheter manipulation.

If a femoral or saphenous cutdown is performed, the distal vessel is ligated or secured with a heavy suture if later repair is planned. A temporary hemostasis suture is placed around the proximal part of the common femoral vein while the catheter is in the heart. This proximal suture prevents back bleeding during the catheterization and also helps in repairing the vein after the catheterization.

Anticoagulants are not routinely used during a right-sided venous approach. Patients with marked polycythemia may have accelerated clotting if the hematocrit is over 60 per cent;[61,100] phlebotomy with plasma replacement will reduce this tendency.

Polycythemia and Anemia

Patients who are markedly polycythemic have a marked elevation of blood viscosity when the hematocrit is above 65 per cent. If the hemoglobin is above 20 g/dl, it is recommended that a centrifuged hematocrit be obtained using central venous blood to measure the true packed cell volume. An oxygen-carrying capacity of 14 to 19 ml of oxygen per 100 ml of blood is maintained (assuming 95 per cent saturation in a normal patient with 10 to 15 g of hemoglobin). If the hematocrit is 65 per cent or greater, erythropheresis before angiography is recommended to reduce the centrifuged hematocrit to 60 per cent.[79] The amount of blood withdrawn is replaced with fresh plasma or 5 per cent albumin in Ringer's lactate solution, which has the same osmolality as plasma. Patients with secondary polycythemia have an elevated blood volume owing to the increased red cell mass of the order of 90 to 110 ml/kg of body weight (average 100 ml/kg).

$$\text{Blood volume to withdraw} = \text{wt(kg)} \times 100 \times \frac{\text{Observed Hct} - \text{Desired Hct}}{\text{Observed Hct}}$$

A similar calculation can be used to increase the patient's oxygen-carrying capacity if there is a systemic hypoxemia and low oxygen-carrying capacity.

Reduction of the oxygen-carrying capacity and blood viscosity is performed cautiously in all patients with obstruction to pulmonary blood flow, such as tetralogy of Fallot, or those with high pulmonary resistance. A reduction in blood viscosity will result in a greater fall in systemic resistance than in pulmonary resistance, and this may induce more right-to-left shunting with systemic hypoxemia. On the other hand, patients with transposition physiology tend to improve their systemic saturation with reduction in the hematocrit to 60 per cent.[79]

Drugs

Intravenous drug infusions are maintained on arrival at the catheterization laboratory. Once monitoring catheters have been inserted, the infusion rate of these drugs may be changed and the effects recorded. Maintenance fluid in these infants and in premature babies is 10 per cent glucose with one quarter to one fifth normal saline. Regular checks of the blood glucose level are made during the catheterization, since the stress of the illness or the catheterization may cause hypoglycemia even with 10 per cent glucose administration. If required, bolus doses of glucose are given intravenously at a concentration of 25 per cent; more concentrated solutions may cause hypotension due to hyperosmolality.

Half the calculated dose of a drug is administered initially, and the effect upon the patient is observed to make sure that no idiosyncratic or untoward reactions occur. The rest of the calculated dose may then be administered in small aliquots with interval flushing until the desired effect is achieved.

Infants are more susceptible to the central nervous system depressant effects of narcotics and drugs such as ketamine. I have found that a total dose of 0.1 mg of morphine is adequate for sedation in infants under 6 months of age rather than the usually recommended dose of 0.1 mg/kg.

A bolus flush of ketamine of 0.5 to 1 mg/kg may result in apnea or extrapyramidal seizures in infants. This dose causes few problems or changes in hemodynamics when infused over 30 to 60 seconds.[29]

The dose of lidocaine used for local anesthesia infiltration is carefully monitored. No more than 5 mg/kg should be given subcutaneously, or seizures may result.

Antibiotics are not routinely given prior to catheterization, as bacterial endocarditis in an otherwise noninfected child is extremely rare after cardiac catheterization. If indicated, cardiac catheterization can be safely carried out in a child who has other signs of sepsis while the usual therapeutic antibiotics are being administered. If a cutdown is needed for venous access, topical antibiotics can be applied to the wound at closure.

My colleagues and I have found an increased incidence of wound and systemic infections in children who have prostaglandin E_1 (PGE_1) infusions for ductal-dependent congenital heart defects. We recommend the routine administration of broad spectrum antibiotics in all children receiving PGE_1 and also recommend that the use of this drug be limited to as short a time as possible, with as low a dose as possible.

Emergency medications should be drawn up in administration syringes and be made available during the catheterization. Table 27–2 lists emergency drugs and their doses that should be available during a cardiac catheterization.

Complications

The mortality and morbidity associated with cardiac catheterization in neonates are directly related to the underlying cardiopulmonary defect and the general condition of the patient rather than his or her age and size.[18] The moribund, acidotic, hypoxic neonate with poor perfusion who has not responded to precatheterization medications and management has a poor chance of survival with or without cardiac catheterization. Such infants are likely to have very complex or inoperable cardiopulmonary defects and usually die in spite of, rather than because of, the catheterization.

The type and incidence of complications and the causes of death from cardiac catheterization in neonates and premature babies have changed over the past 20 years as a result of advances in cardiac catheterization techniques, vascular access, catheter design and materials, quality and type of imaging, and type of contrast materials used for imaging. The indications for cardiac catheterization have also changed with the introduction of other imaging modalities such as two-dimensional echocardiography.

Mortality

There have been several well-designed prospective studies of the complications of cardiac catheterization, all of which have included a significant number of neonates.[7,18,85,92] These studies were from three different eras of catheterization and medical and surgical therapy of infants.

The mortality findings in these studies were remarkably similar in some respects: very few deaths were related directly to the procedure of catheterization itself. The major determinant of death was the underlying cardiopulmonary defect and the condition of the patient at the time of the catheterization.

In a national cooperative study on cardiac catheterization, data were collected for 24 months between 1963 and 1965,[7,85] and 325 neonates less than 30 days of age were included in the study. Twenty of these neonates (6.2 per cent) died, and complications occurred in 50 neonates. Thirteen of the deaths were associated with complications during the catheterization procedure; there was a 26 per cent mortality rate if complications occurred.

Those infants assessed prior to catheterization as having a low risk (20 per cent of the neonates) had a mortality rate of 6.7 per cent, while those assessed as having a moderate (30 per cent) or a high (49 per cent) risk had mortality rates of 9 and 23.3 per cent, respectively.

The causes of death associated with the catheterization procedure itself were cardiac perforation and tamponade (five patients, two moribund at the time of catheterization and one with aortic atresia), ventricular fibrillation or asystole (five patients, three moribund at the time of catheterization), and progressive deterioration and hypotension during the catheterization (four patients, one moribund and one with aortic atresia).

Stanger et al[92] studied the complications of cardiac catheterizations in neonates, infants, and children for a 36-month period from January 1970 to December 1972. There were 218 neonates in this group, and 20 died (9.2 per cent) within 24 hours of catheterization. Forty-seven neonates were severely ill prior to the catheterization, as defined by profound hypoxemia (PO_2 less than 25 mmHg),

Table 27–2. EMERGENCY DRUGS AND DOSAGES

Drug	Intravenous Dose	Comment
Albumin	1.0 g/kg	Volume replacement
Aminophylline	Bolus: 3.0 mg/kg	
	Infusion: 0.7 mg/kg/hour	Hypotension, tachycardia
Atropine	0.01–0.04 mg/kg	Tachycardia, spells in tetralogy
Bretylium tosylate	5.0 mg/kg, up to 20 mg/kg	
Calcium chloride	50–100 mg/kg	Vagal stimulation
Chloral hydrate	Rectal, PO: 25–80 mg/kg	
Chlorpromazine	IM: 1.0 mg/kg	
	IV: 0.25 mg/kg	Hypotension, hypothermia
Cryoprecipitate	1 unit (bag) = 250 ml FFP	
Dextrose 25 per cent	2.0 ml/kg	
Diazepam	0.10 mg/kg	Vasoconstriction in pulmonary hypertension
Digoxin	IV digitalizing dose: 20–30 mcg/kg	
Diphenhydramine	2.0–5.0 mg/kg	
Dobutamine	1–40 mcg/kg/min	
Dopamine	1–30 mcg/kg/min	Tachycardia, arrhythmias at higher doses
	Renal dose: 2–5 mcg/kg/min	
Epinephrine	Infusion: 0.10 mcg/kg/min	
Epinephrine 1:10000	Bolus: 0.10 ml/kg	
Fresh plasma	10–15 ml/kg	Hypotension, Ca^{2+} reverses
Furosemide	1–5 mg/kg/dose	
Hydralazine	0.20–1.2 mg/kg	Hypotension
Isoproterenol	0.10 mcg/kg/min	Tachycardia, hypotension
Ketamine	0.5–1.0 mg/kg	Apnea, seizures
Lidocaine	Bolus: 1–5 mg/kg	Seizures
	Infusion: 20–40 mcg/kg/min	
Mannitol	0.5–1.0 g/kg	
Meperidine HCl	1–2 mg/kg	Hypoventilation
Methoxamine	0.05–0.1 mg/kg	Vasoconstriction
Morphine	0.01–0.1 mg/kg	Hypoventilation, apnea
Nalorphine	0.1–0.2 mg/kg	
Naloxone HCl	0.01 mg/kg	
Neostigmine	0.025–0.05 mg/kg	
Nitroglycerin	0.1–1.0 mcg/kg/min	Hypotension
Nitroprusside	0.5–10 mcg/kg/min	Hypotension, cyanide
Pancuronium	0.1 mg/kg	
Pentothal	10–30 mg/kg	Apnea
Phenobarbital	1–5 mg/kg	Apnea
Phenylephrine	0.01–0.10 mg/kg	Vasoconstriction
Procaine	10–15 mg/kg over 40 minutes	Hypotension
Propranolol	0.01–0.025 mg/kg	Bradycardia, hypotension
Solu-Medrol (methylprednisolone)	30 mg/kg	
Succinylcholine	1.0 mg/kg	
Tolazoline	1–2 mg/kg	Hypotension, gastric hyperacidity
Verapamil	0.10 mg/kg	Bradycardia, hypotension

FFP = fresh frozen plasma.

acidemia (pH less than 7.1) with poor peripheral perfusion, or requirement for mechanical ventilation during catheterization. Two of these patients died during the catheterization (one with hypoplastic left-heart syndrome and one with pulmonary disease), and 15 others died within 24 hours of the catheterization, giving a mortality rate of 36.2 per cent among severely ill neonates. Only two of these patients had remedial cardiac defects. The authors felt that only one patient died as a direct result of the catheterization itself, and in another patient the relationship was not clear.

A similar study of 194 neonates catheterized at less than 1 week of age was conducted at Texas Children's Hospital between January 1971 and July 1976.[75] There were 10 deaths (5 per cent), of which three (1.6 per cent) were related to the catheterization procedure itself, resulting from perforation of the right ventricular outflow tract, right atrium, and umbilical artery. Three patients with pulmonary disease and pulmonary hypertension died within 24 hours of catheterization, and one patient with hypoxic cardiomyopathy died during catheterization. Three patients in critical condition from their congenital heart defects (one with truncus arteriosus with interrupted arch; one with coarctation, ventricular septal defect, atrial septal defect, and patent ductus arteriosus; and one with ventricular septal defect and atrial septal defect) died within 48 hours of catheterization. Nonfatal complications occurred in 31 patients.

The most recent prospective study was from January to December of 1978 and included 155 neonates less than 28 days of age from the New England Regional Infant Cardiac Program.[18] Thirty-eight of the infants weighed less than 2 kg. Among the 155 neonates, there were 10 deaths within 24 hours of the catheterization (6.4 per cent), and a further 9 of the 145 survivors (6.2 per cent) died within 48 hours of the catheterization. Death was associated with catheterization in only one patient who had transposition of the great arteries and who died after an embolus lodged in his left anterior descending coronary artery. The other deaths were due to inoperable lesions such as hypoplastic left-heart syndrome, pulmonary disease, failed medical therapy, or surgical complications. Patients who were judged to be in the high risk group had a mortality rate that was 10 times higher than that for patients in the low risk group.

These studies were from different eras of pediatric cardiology and cannot be directly compared with each other or even with cardiac catheterization techniques and management of neonates in the 1980s.

The first study from 1963 to 1965 was before balloon atrial septostomy, flow-directed balloon catheters, and PGE$_1$ were available. Biplane cineangiography and fluoroscopy were probably not available generally, and all catheterizations were performed via the cutdown technique.

During the second study from 1970 to 1972, the percutaneous technique of vessel entry was only just being introduced, and biplane fluoroscopy and cineangiography were in their infancy. Two-dimensional echocardiography was not yet available.

The last study was completed just after the introduction of PGE$_1$ but probably does not reflect the success of this drug in the management of critically ill neonates with ductal-dependent lesions.

A prospective study performed in the last 5 years would probably show very few catheterizations of patients with inoperable cardiac lesions and few diagnostic catheterizations of patients with pure pulmonary problems.

Morbidity

The major risks of cardiac catheterization in ill premature and newborn infants are probably the same now as they were in the earlier studies:
1. Cardiac perforation and tamponade.
2. Blood loss.
3. Failure to improve progressive hypoxemia, hypoxia, hypotension, acidemia, or depressed myocardial function.
4. Thrombotic or traumatic occlusion of iliofemoral and brachiocephalic arteries.

Perforation of the heart has become less frequent, and this change may be due to the use of balloon tipped catheters. It should be noted that manipulation of these catheters with the balloon deflated is more hazardous than when

it is inflated, since the catheter tip is relatively tapered when the balloon is deflated.

Blood loss represents a more significant problem in neonates and small premature infants than in older infants and children. Blood sampling for arterial blood gases, saturations, and indocyanine green dye curves presents a cumulative blood loss, which may have to be replaced. Using a percutaneous sheath with a bleed-back or hemostasis valve reduces blood loss during catheter exchanges.

Hypotension is common after angiography with ionic contrast material.[21] Both the magnitude and the incidence of hypotension have been reduced in the last few years with the introduction of nonionic contrast material.[9] Subclinical volume depletion may be present in neonates and premature babies owing to diuretic administration, nonhumidified respirators, and blood sampling during the catheterization. The first angiogram may produce profound and progressive hypotension and bradycardia when blood volume is low. Atrial filling pressures should be checked before angiography is performed. Calcium chloride may be required to reverse hypotension and bradycardia in infants who have had large doses of diuretics prior to the catheterization.

ARTERIAL COMPLICATIONS

Since the introduction of the percutaneous sheath technique, major arterial complications have virtually disappeared.[88] Minor complications involving decreased femoral or peripheral pulses with pallor and coolness of the limb still occur, but the incidence of minor arterial complications has also been reduced by systemic heparinization during arterial catheterization.[54] Most of the problems from arterial cannulation improve within 24 hours; rarely does the infant need surgical embolectomy or arterioplasty. Recent reports have shown that the use of streptokinase or urokinase can be helpful in opening occluded femoral arteries if systemic heparinization for 24 hours does not improve the circulation.[101] Femoral pulses may also be compromised if relatively large catheters are introduced via the umbilical artery catheter; trauma to the umbilical artery–iliac artery junction may occur, or thrombi may accumulate at this junction upon catheter withdrawal from the descending aorta.

Embolic phenomena are rare and appear to occur at the same frequency in neonates as in older infants and children. The risk of systemic embolism is higher in children with right-to-left intracardiac shunts and polycythemia. The overall incidence may be as high as 1 to 2 per cent.

ARRHYTHMIAS

Arrhythmias such as transient supraventricular tachycardia, atrial flutter or fibrillation, ventricular tachycardia/fibrillation, and second and third degree heart block are the most common major and minor complications occurring during cardiac catheterization. Catheter-induced arrhythmias are usually transient and resolve spontaneously with withdrawal of the catheter. Except for patients with tetralogy of Fallot (and other similar lesions), who become more cyanotic with tachycardia, very fast ventricular rates are usually well tolerated by neonates and infants. On the other hand, bradycardia is less well tolerated by neonates, for they rely on rapid heart rate for maintenance of cardiac output. Recent digitalis administration is a risk factor for the development of atrial tachycardia, ventricular tachycardia, and third degree heart block during cardiac catheterization. Catheter manipulation usually precipitates such arrhythmias, and use of balloon tipped catheters may reduce their incidence.

INFECTIONS

Systemic infections are rare after cardiac catheterization, and bacterial endocarditis prophylaxis is not recommended in infants undergoing catheterization. Localized wound infections have virtually disappeared since the introduction of the percutaneous sheath technique. We recommend the administration of systemic broad spectrum antibiotics in children receiving PGE_1 for as long as this drug is administered.

SUMMARY

The indications for cardiac catheterization in premature and newborn infants are similar to those in older infants and children with symptomatic congenital cardiovascular disease. All available noninvasive investigative data must be assessed in the context of the patient's problems, and whether any additional information is necessary to manage these problems must be determined. If needed information is not available from noninvasive sources, cardiac catheterization should be performed to obtain the required data.

When the decision is made to catheterize a newborn infant, the choice and sequence of procedures performed on the patient will be dictated by a number of factors, including the nature of the patient's problem and his or her condition, the type of equipment available, the skills of the investigating physicians and technical personnel, the availability of definitive therapy, and the clinical judgment of the clinician conducting the procedure.

References

1. Adams FH, Lind J (1957): Physiologic studies on the cardiovascular status of normal newborn infants. Pediatrics 19:431–437.
2. Baldwin E deF, Moore LV, Noble RP (1946): The demonstration of ventricular septal defect by means of right heart catheterization. Am Heart J 32:152–162.
3. Bernard C (1876): Lecons sur la cheleur animale. Paris, Balliere, pp 42, 78, 80–81.
4. Bing RJ, Vandam LD, Gray FD (1947): Physiological studies in congenital heart disease. I. Procedures. Bull Johns Hopkins 80:107–120.
5. Bradley RD (1964): Right heart catheterization with miniature catheter in severely ill patients. Lancet 2:941–942.
6. Brannon ES, Weens HS, Warren JV (1945): Atrial septal defect; study of hemodynamics by techniques of right heart catheterization. Am J Med Sci 210:480–491.
7. Braunwald E (1968): Cooperative study on cardiac catheterization. Deaths related to cardiac catheterization. Circulation (Suppl III) 37:17–26.
8. Cabal LA, Udayakumar D, Siassi B, Hodgman JE, Emmanouilides G (1980): Cardiogenic shock associated with perinatal asphyxia in preterm neonates. J Pediatr 96:705–710.
9. Carlsson E, Rudolph A, Stanger P, Teitel D, Weber W, Yoshida H (1985): Pediatric angiocardiography with iohexol. Invest Radiol (Suppl) 20:75–78.
10. Carter SA, Bajec SF, Yannicelli E, Wood EH (1960): Estimation of left to right shunts from arterial dilution curves. J Lab Clin Med 55:77–88.
11. Castellanos A, Pereiras R (1939): Counter-current aortography. Riv Cubana Cardiol 2:187–203.
12. Castellanos AR, Pereiras R, Garcia A (1937): La angiocardiografica radio-opaqua. Arch de La Soc de Estudios de la Habana 31:523–596.
13. Castellanos AR, Perieras R, Garcia A (1939): Angiocardiography in the child. Proceedings of 7th Congress of the Pan American Medical Association, Havana, January 1939, pp 75–82, 109–113.
14. Cayler GG, Rudolph AM, Nadas AS (1963): Systemic blood flow in infants and children with and without heart disease. Pediatrics 32:186–201.
15. Chapman DW, Earle DM, Gugle LJ, Huggins RA, Zimdahl WT (1949): Intravenous catheterization of the heart in suspected congenital heart disease; report of 72 cases. Arch Int Med 84:640–659.
16. Chauveau A, Marey J (1863): Cardiographic apparatus and experiments: New demonstrations of the mechanism of the movements of the heart by using continuously recording instruments. Acad Natl Med (Paris) Bull 26:268–319.
17. Chauveau A, Marey J (1861): Determmalis graphique des rapports du choc du coeur avec les movements des oreillettes et des ventricles; enregistreur (sphygmographe). C R Acad Sci (Paris) pp 622–625.
18. Cohn HE, Freed MD, Hellenbrand WE, Fyler DC (1985): Complications and mortality associated with cardiac catheterization in infants under one year. Pediatr Cardiol 6:123–131.
19. Cournand A, Baldwin JS, Hummelstein A (1949): Cardiac catheterization in congenital heart disease. New York, The Commonwealth Fund.
20. Cournand A, Ranges HA (1941): Catheterization of the right ventricle in man. Proc Soc Exp Biol Med 46:452–562.
21. Dawson P (1985): Chemotoxicity of contrast media and clinical adverse effects: A review. Invest Radiol (Suppl) 20:84–91.
22. Desilets DT, Hoffman R (1965): A new method of percutaneous catheterization. Radiology 85:147–148.
23. Dexter L, Haynes FW, Burwell CS, Eppinger EC, Seibel RE, Evans JM (1947): Studies of congenital heart disease. 1. The techniques of venous catheterization as a diagnostic procedure. J Clin Inves 26:547–553.
24. Dieffenbach JR (1832): Physiologico-surgical observations on cholera. Cholera Arch 1:86–105.
25. Downing DF (1959): Cardiac catheterization in congenital heart disease. JAMA 170:770–772.
26. Duff DE, Mullins CE (1978): Transseptal left heart catheterization in infants and children. Cathet Cardiovasc Diagn 4:213–223.
27. Emmanouilides GC, Moss AJ, Duffie ER Jr, Adams FH (1964): Pulmonary arterial pressure changes in human newborn infants from birth to 3 days of age. J Pediatr 65:327–333.
28. Emmanouilides GC, Moss AJ, Monset-Couchard M, Marcano BP, Rzeznic B (1970): Cardiac output in newborn infants. Biol Neonate 15:186–197.
29. Faithfull NS, Harder R (1971): Ketamine for cardiac catheterization. An evaluation of its use in children. Anesthesia 26:318.
30. Falsetti HL, Mates RE, Carrol RJ, Gupta RL, Bell AL (1974): Analysis and correction of pressure wave distortion in fluid filled catheter systems. Circulation 49:165–172.
31. Fegler G (1969): Measurement of cardiac output in anesthetized animals by a thermodilution method. Quart J Exp Physiol 39:153.
32. Fick A (1870): Uber die Messung des Blutquantums in den Herzventrikeln. Sits der Physik-Med ges Wurtzberg, p 16.
33. Forssmann W (1929): Die sondierung des rechten herzens. Klin Wochenschr 8:2085–2087.
34. Forssmann W (1931): Ueber kontrastdarstellung der hohlen des lebenden herzens und der lungenschlagader. Munch Med Wochenschr 78:490–492.

35. Freed MD, Keane JF, Rosenthal A (1974): The effect of heparinization to prevent arterial thrombosis after percutaneous cardiac catheterization in children. Circulation 50:565–569.

36. Garson A, Gillette PC, Porter CJ, Hawkins EP, Titus JL, Cooley DA, McNamara DG (1982): Epicardial tumors undetected by angiography as a cause of ventricular tachycardia in infants: Electrophysiology and surgical cure (abstr). Pediatr Cardiol 3:351.

37. Garson A, Gillette PC, Titus JL, Hawkins EP, Kearney D, Cooley DA, McNamara DG (1984): Surgical treatment of ventricular tachycardia in infants. N Engl J Med 310:1443–1445.

38. Garson A, Gillette PC (1980): Clinical-electrophysiologic correlation in 103 children with supraventricular tachycardia. Circulation 62:III–72.

39. Garson A, Gillette PC (1981): Electrophysiologic studies of supraventricular tachycardia in children. II. Prediction of specific mechanism by noninvasive features. Am Heart J 102:383–388.

40. Garson A, Gillette PC (1980): Prediction of the mechanism of supraventricular tachycardia in children (abstr). Pediatr Cardiol 1:321.

41. Garson A, Smith RT, Moak JP, Kearney DL, Hawkins EP, Titus JL, Cooley DA, Ott DA (1987): Incessant ventricular tachycardia in infants: Myocardial hamartomas and surgical cure. J Am Coll Cardiol 10:619–626.

42. Garson A (1983): The Electrocardiogram in Infants and Children: A Systemic Approach. Philadelphia, Lea & Febiger, pp 170–193.

43. Gay JH (1975): Cardiac catheterization in small infants: The percutaneous approach. Am J Cardiol 36:493–495.

44. Gutgesell HP, Huhta JC, Latson LA, Huffines D, McNamara DG (1985): Accuracy of 2-dimensional echocardiography in the diagnosis of congenital heart disease. Am J Cardiol 55:514–518.

45. Hesslein PS, Mullins CE, Kugler JD, Gillette PC (1980): Percutaneous sheath brachial vein cardiac catheterization in children. Cathet Cardiovasc Diagn 6:197–205.

46. Holling HE, Zak GA (1950): Cardiac catheterization in the diagnosis of congenital heart disease. Br Heart J 12:153–182.

47. Huhta JC, Cohen M, Gutgesell HP (1984): Patency of the ductus arteriosus in normal neonates: Two-dimensional echocardiography versus Doppler assessment. J Am Coll Cardiol 4:561–564.

48. Huhta JC, Glasow P, Murphy DJ, Gutgesell HP, Ott DA, McNamara DG, Smith OE (1987): Surgery without catheterization for congenital heart defects: Management of 100 patients. J Am Cardiol Coll 9:823–829.

49. Huhta JC, Gutgesell HP, Nihill MR (1985): Cross-sectional echocardiographic diagnosis of total anomalous pulmonary venous connexion. Br Heart J 53:525–534.

50. Huhta JC, Moise KJ Jr, Fisher DJ, Sharif DS, Wasserstrum N, Martin C (1987): Detection and quantitation of constriction of the fetal ductus arteriosus by Doppler echocardiography. Circulation 75:406–412.

51. Huhta JC, Smallhorn JF, Macartney FJ (1982): Two-dimensional echocardiographic diagnosis of situs. Br Heart J 48:97–108.

52. Huhta JC, Smallhorn JF, Macartney FJ, Anderson RH, de Leval MR (1982): Cross-sectional echocardiographic diagnosis of systemic venous return. Br Heart J 48:388–403.

53. Huhta JC, Smallhorn JF, Macartney FJ (1984): Cross-sectional echocardiographic diagnosis of azygos continuation of the inferior vena cava. Cathet Cardiovasc Diagn 10:221–232.

54. Hurwitz RA, Franken EA Jr, Girod DA, Smith JA, Smith WL (1977): Angiographic determination of arterial patency after percutaneous catheterization in infants and small children. Circulation 56:102–105.

55. James LS (1959): Biochemical aspects of asphyxia at birth in adaption to extra-uterine life. Proceedings of the 31st Ross Conference on Pediatric Research, Vancouver, British Columbia, pp 66–71.

56. Keane JF, Fellows KE, Lang P, Fyler DC (1982): Pediatric arterial catheterization using a 3.2 French catheter. Cathet Cardiovasc Diagn 8:201–208.

57. Keane JF, Freed MD, Fellows KE, Fyler DC (1979): Pediatric cardiac angiography using a 4 French catheter. Cathet Cardiovasc Diag 3:313–319.

58. Kearney DL, Titus JL, Hawkins EP, Ott DA, Garson A (1987): Pathologic features of myocardial hamartomas causing childhood tachyarrhythmias. Circulation 75:705–710.

59. Kinsman JM, Moore JW, Hamilton WF (1929): Studies on circulation. I. Injection method: Physical and mathematical considerations. Am J Physiol 89:322–339.

60. Kjellberger SR, Mannheimer I, Rudhi U, Jonsson B (1959): Diagnosis of Congenital Heart Disease. Chicago, Year Book Medical Publisher.

61. Komp DM, Sparrow AW (1970): Polycythemia in cyanotic congenital heart disease—a study of altered coagulation. J Pediatr 76:231–236.

62. Krovetz LJ, Shanklin DR, Scheibler GL (1968): Serious and fatal complications of catheterization and angiography in infants and children. Am Heart J 76:39–47.

63. LaFarge CG, Miettinen OS (1970): The estimation of oxygen consumption. Cardiovasc Res 4:23–30.

64. Lategola M, Rahn M (1953): A self-guiding catheter for cardiac and pulmonary arterial catheterization and occlusion. Proc Soc Exp Biol Med 84:667–668.

65. Lillehei CW, Cohen M, Warden HE, Varco RL (1955): The direct-vision intracardiac correction of congenital anomalies by controlled cross circulation: Results in thirty-two patients with ventricular septal defects, tetralogy of Fallot and atrioventricularis communis defects. Surgery 38:11–29.

66. Lister G, Hoffman JIE, Rudolph AM (1974): Oxygen uptake in infants and children: A simple method for measurement. Pediatrics 53:656–662.

67. Lucas RV Jr, St. Geme JW, Anderson RC, Adams P Jr, Ferguson DJ (1961): Maturation of the pulmonary vascular bed: A physiological and anatomic correlation in infants and children. Am J Dis Child 101:467–475.

68. Lurie PR, Armer RM, Klatte EC (1963): Percutaneous guide wire catheterization: Diagnosis and therapy. Am J Dis Child 106:189–196.

69. Mullins CE (1983): Transseptal left heart catheterization: Experience with a new technique in 520 pediatric and adult patients. Pediatric Cardiol 4:239–246.

70. McMichael J, Sharpy-Schafer EP (1944): Cardiac output in man by direct Fick method. Br Heart J 6:33–40.

71. Neches WH, Mullins CE, Williams RL, Vargo TA, McNamara DG (1972): Percutaneous sheath cardiac catheterization. Am J Cardiol 30:378–384.

72. Pavy FW (1860): Certain points connected with diabetes. Lancet 2:555–556.

73. Perry LW, Galioto FM, Blair T, Shapiro SR, Avckman RN, Scott LP (1981): Two-dimensional echocardiography for catheter location and placement in infants and children. Pediatrics 67:541–547.

74. Pollack MM, Reed TP, Holbrook PR, Fields AI (1980): Bedside pulmonary artery catheterization in pediatrics. J Pediatr 96:274–276.

75. Porter CJ, Gillette PC, Mullins CE, McNamara DG (1978): Cardiac catheterization in the neonate. J Pediatr 93:97–101.

76. Rashkind WJ, Miller WW (1966): Creation of an atrial septal defect without thoracotomy: A palliative approach to complete transposition of the great arteries. Am Med Assoc J 196:991–992.

77. Rice MJ, Seward JB, Hayler DJ, Mair DD, Feldt RH, Puga FJ, Danielson GK, Edwards WP, Tajik AJ (1983): Impact of 2-dimensional echocardiography on the management of distressed newborn in whom cardiac disease is suspected. Am J Cardiol 51:288–292.

78. Rios B, Nihill MR, Mullins CE (1984): Left ventricular endomyocardial biopsy in children with the transseptal long sheath technique. Cathet Cardiovasc Diagn 10:417–423.

79. Rosenthal A, Nathan DG, Marty AT, Button LN, Miettinen OS, Nadas AS (1970): Acute hemodynamic effects of red cell volume reduction in polycythemia of cyanotic congenital heart disease. Circulation 42:297–307.

80. Rowe RD, Vlad P, Keith JD (1956): Selective angiocardiography in infants and children. Radiology 66:344.

81. Rowe RD, James LS (1957): The normal pulmonary arterial pressure during the first year of life. J Pediatr 51:1–4.

82. Rowe RD (1960): Cardiac catheterization in the newborn infant. Heart Bull 9:61–68.

83. Rudolph AM, Cayler GG (1958): Cardiac catheterization in infants and children. Pediatr Clin North Am 5:907–943.

84. Rudolph AM, Drorbaugh JE, Auld PAM, Rudolph AJ, Nadas AS, Smith CA, Hubbell JP (1961): Studies on the circulation in the newborn period. The circulation in the respiratory distress syndrome. Pediatrics 27:551–566.

85. Rudolph AM (1968): Cooperative study on cardiac catheterization. Complications occurring in infants and children. Circulation (Suppl III) 37:59–66.

86. Sapin SO, Linde LM, Emmanouilides GC (1963): Umbilical vessel angiography in the newborn infant. Pediatrics 31:946.

87. Schostal SJ, Krovetz LJ, Rowe RD (1972): An analysis of errors in conventional cardiac catheterization data. Am Heart J 83:596–603.

88. Sequeira F, Girod DA, Stacki M, Franken EA, Hurwitz RA (1980): Arterial spasm during and following pediatric cardiac catheterization. Pediatr Cardiol 1:176A.

89. Silove ED, Tynan MJ, Simcha AJ (1972): Thermal dilution measurement of pulmonary and systemic blood flow in secundum atrial septal defect and transposition of great arteries with intact interventricular septum. Br Heart J 34:1142–1146.

90. Sones FM Jr (1955): Heart catheterization in infancy. Physiological studies. Pediatrics 16:544–554.

91. Srouji MN, Rashkind WJ (1969): The effects of cardiac catheterization on the acid-base status of infants with congenital heart disease. Pediatrics 75:943–951.

92. Stanger P, Heymann MA, Tarnoff H, Hoffman JIE, Rudolph AM (1974): Complications of cardiac catheterization of neonates, infants and children. A three year study. Circulation 50:595–608.

93. Stark J, Smallhorn JF, Huhta JC, DeLeval MR, Macartney FJ, Rees PG, Taylor JFN (1983): Surgery for congenital heart defects diagnosed with cross-sectional echocardiography. Circulation (Suppl II) 68:129–138.

94. Swan HJC, Gorry W, Forrester J, Marcus H, Diamond G, Chonett D (1970): Catheterization of the heart in man with use of a flow directed balloon tipped catheter. N Engl J Med 288:447–451.

95. Takahashi M, Petry EL, Lurie PR, Kirkpatrick SE, Stanton RE (1970): Percutaneous heart catheterization in infants and children: Catheter placement and manipulation with guide wires. Circulation 42:1037–1048.

96. Taketa RM, Sahn DJ, Simon AL, Pappelbaum SJ, Friedman WF (1975): Catheter positions in congenital cardiac malformations. Circulation 51:749–757.

97. Vick GW, Huhta JC, Gutgesell HP (1985): Assessment of the ductus arteriosus in preterm infants utilizing suprasternal two-dimensional/Doppler echocardiography. J Am Coll Cardiol 5:973–977.

98. Victorica BE, Gessner IH (1975): A simplified method for quantifying left to right shunts from arterial dilution curves. Circulation 51:530–534.

99. Vlad P, Hohn A, Labert EC (1964): Retrograde arterial catheterization of the left heart. Experience with 500 children. Circulation 29:787–793.

100. Wedemeyer AL, Lewis JH (1973): Improvement in hemostasis following phlebotomy in cyanotic patients with heart disease. J Pediatr 83:46–50.

101. Wessel DL, Keane JF, Fellows KE, Robichaud H, Lock JE (1986): Fibrinolytic therapy for femoral arterial thrombosis following cardiac catheterization in infants and children. Am J Cardiol 58:347–351.

102. Yang SS, Bentivoglio LG, Maranhao V, Goldberg H (1978): Basic measurements and calculations. In Cardiac Catheterization Data to Hemodynamic Parameters. 2nd ed. Philadelphia, FA Davis, pp 1–54; 233–358.

103. Ziegler RF (1954): Clinical cardiac catheterization in infants and children. Pediatr Clin North Am 1:93–113.

28 ANGIOGRAPHY

Havdaya Nath
Benigno Soto

Angiocardiography remains the mainstay of diagnosis in congenital heart disease. Recent advances in echocardiography have significantly contributed to the noninvasive evaluation of patients with cardiac malformations and have decreased the need for cardiac catheterization, particularly in newborn infants. Still, in most older patients and many newborn patients, angiography is required prior to surgery. In this chapter we will describe the principles of angiocardiography, including the equipment, angiographic projections, and approach to the interpretation of the angiogram. The details of angiographic morphology of individual lesions are provided in subsequent chapters.

HISTORICAL PERSPECTIVE

Cardiac catheterization preceded angiocardiography by almost a century. In 1831, Dieffenbach[33] introduced a catheter into the left ventricle through the brachial artery for blood letting in a patient dying of cholera. Following the discovery of x-rays in 1895, Alwens and Frick[2] observed the embolization of bismuth carbonate suspended in oil to the pulmonary arteries in dogs following an intravenous injection. Forssmann[39] is credited with the first right-sided heart catheterization performed on himself in 1929, and in 1931 pulmonary angiography was first performed by Moniz.[72] Castellanos[24] first reported right atrial and ventricular angiography through peripheral venous injection in children and infants in 1937 and countercurrent aortography through brachial and femoral arterial injections in 1939.[23] Although right-sided heart catheterization was perfected by Cournand,[28] it was not until 1946 that Celis[35] performed right-sided heart angiocardiography through a catheter in the right ventricle. This procedure was improved by Chavez and associates in 1947.[27] Jonsson and colleagues[58] injected contrast medium into the aorta and left side of the heart through Cournand-type catheters using a manually operated high-pressure injector in Sweden in 1949. Seldinger[85] introduced percutaneous arterial puncture and guide wire technique in 1953, which has revolutionized angiography in general. This technique was popularized in infants and children by Lurie and associates[68] in the United States.

Angiocardiography would not have reached the modern-day sophistication without the simultaneous innovations in the technology of image recording, catheters, and pressure injectors. The first roll film changer, described by Ruggles[83] in 1925, was capable of a filming rate of 15 exposures per second. A biplane film changer was described by Fredzell and coworkers[40] in 1950. The most popular film changer is made by Elema-Schonander and is an adaptation of a model described by Gidlund[50] in 1949. Although cineradiography was first described by MacIntyre in 1896,[70] it was Janker[56] who revived interest in the procedure in 1936. This technique became more practical with the development of image intensifiers between 1949 and 1952, in both the United States and Holland. The first simultaneous biplane cineangiography was described by Abrams[1] in 1959.

Initial catheters were rubber ureteral catheters. Recent advances in plastic chemistry have made possible catheters made of nylon, Teflon, polyethylene, and polyurethane. In 1959, Odman[76] from Sweden introduced Kifa catheters, which are composed of a polyethylene base made radiopaque with lead oxide. In 1970, Swan and Ganz[96] introduced flow-directed balloon catheters, which were rapidly adapted for pediatric use.

EQUIPMENT

The angiogram can be filmed using either 35-mm cine film or 100-mm spot large-format screen film, and it can be digitized for further electronic image manipulation and storage. A large-format screen film combination provides the best resolution (four to five line pairs per millimeter) but suffers from a limited acquisition rate (six or fewer films per second). Hence, 35-mm cineangiography remains the most widely used imaging technique. Some laboratories supplement usual 35-mm cine film recording with large film recording in selected cases in which anatomic detail is more important, such as imaging the pulmonary arteries.[42]

Biplane angiography is essential for accurate anatomic diagnosis, particularly in neonates. The capability to electronically zoom in the x-ray image intensifier to a 6- or 5-inch field of view is necessary for studying young infants. If a zoom lens is also used, it is possible to magnify a selected portion of the image to fill the 35-mm film format.[8] Availability of C-arm fluoroscopy in both planes is ideal. Minimum requirements are a C-arm in the frontal plane and a fixed tube in the lateral plane. The equipment should be capable of filming at 60 to 90 frames per second with generators of 1000 mA and high heat capacity x-ray tubes. For neonates, the use of a small focal spot of 0.6 mm or less is preferable. Good quality video recording equipment (either tape or disk) is also necessary for immediate review of each angiogram as it is performed, in

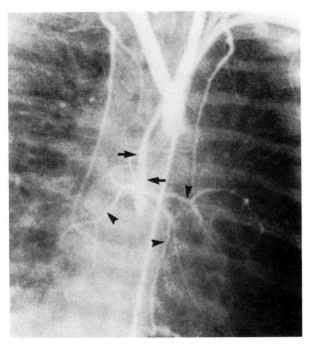

Figure 28–1. Aortic valvular atresia. Single film aortogram. There is excellent opacification of the hypoplastic ascending aorta (arrows) and both coronary arteries (arrowheads).

order to tailor the angiographic examination for each patient.

Proper radiographic technique, cine film, and film processing are key elements in obtaining high-quality cineangiograms. Low kilovolt peak (55 to 60 kVp) should be used to increase the subject contrast. To minimize image noise, it is often advantageous to use a somewhat larger image intensifier input phosphor dose rate (about 45 μR per frame for 9-inch mode) on infants than on adults.[35] A wide latitude (low contrast), fine grain emulsion cine film is preferred. A good, suitable, and consistent film developing technique coupled with a quality control program is also essential.

CONTRAST MATERIALS

A safe contrast medium is an essential requirement in neonatal angiography because many neonates requiring cineangiography are severely compromised hemodynamically. We have come a long way from the first postmortem angiogram performed in 1896 using a solution of calcium oxide.[52] The subsequent inorganic contrast medium was sodium iodide, which was very toxic. The first organic iodides were introduced in 1929. In the mid 1950s, Renografin in Germany and Hypaque in the United States were introduced; both are diatrizoic acid derivatives. To date, these are the most commonly used contrast agents in pediatric angiocardiography.

Renografin and Hypaque are identical in their chemical composition and are sodium meglumine salts of diatrizoic acid. They are triiodinated ionic monomeric compounds with a 3:2 ratio of iodine atoms to free ions in solution.

The toxicity of these compounds is primarily due to their hypertonicity and secondarily to their chemotoxicity.[91] The osmolality of a solution depends on the number of dissolved particles. When these ionic contrast media yield three atoms of iodine in solution, they form two ions, giving two osmotic active particles. Renografin-76 contains 370 mg of iodine per milliliter with an osmolality of 1270 mosm/liter at 37°C and a pH adjusted between 6.0 and 7.7. Hypaque-M 75 per cent contains 385 mg of iodine per milliliter with an osmolality of 2108, and its pH is adjusted between 6.5 and 7.7. These agents cause bradycardia, arrhythmias, reduction in coronary blood flow secondary to a drop in systemic arterial pressure, decreased myocardial contractility, and an immediate and transient rise in peak systolic and diastolic pressures. Increases in pulmonary vascular resistance and pressure are also observed following contrast administration, which are probably due to both acute expansion of intravascular volume and changes in erythrocyte morphology.[91] The hyperosmolality of the contrast medium depletes the water content of the erythrocytes, which may make the red cells incapable of changing shape to negotiate the pulmonary capillary bed. Contrast-induced increases in pulmonary vascular resistance may be of importance in studying infants with severe pulmonary vascular disease, such as total anomalous pulmonary venous drainage (TAPVD) to the portal vein (see Chapter 34). Contrast-induced reductions in left ventricular contractility are similar whether injections are performed in the right or the left side of the heart.

The nonionic contrast media (metrizamide, iohexol) are less hypertonic. These agents have a 3:1 ratio of iodine atoms to the number of particles. Nonionic contrast agents have an osmolality of only 600 mosm/liter, even in concentrations equal to that of Renografin-76. Although the osmolality of these agents is still twice that of human blood, it is less than half that of diatrizoate compounds. Hence, nonionic contrast media present a lower osmotic load to the circulation. In addition, the nonionic contrast agents have been shown to have a slight positive ionotropic effect on the left ventricular myocardium. (A similar effect has also been reported with ionic contrast media containing calcium ions.[54]) As a result of their lower osmolality, nonionic contrast agents produce less sensation of pain and heat during intravascular injection, thus reducing patient discomfort and movement. Metrizamide is not stable in solution and has to be prepared for intravascular injection shortly before the procedure. However, iohexol is stable in solution and less cumbersome to use. A large body of experience is available regarding the use of these nonionic agents in peripheral angiography and angiocardiography in adults, but a limited number of reports is available regarding their use in children for angiocardiography.[7,20,34,53,62] Most of this experience has been in older infants and children. All reports indicate no appreciable difference in radiopacity between ionic and nonionic agents. All authors found less movement or crying of patients following the use of iohexol or metrizamide. Although both types of media caused a mild and transient rise in ventricular systolic and end diastolic pressures, the magnitude of increase in the heart rate was lower with nonionic media.[34,53] There was no appreciable difference in the serum and urine chemistries following the use of either agent, with one exception. Carlsson and coworkers[20] reported a rise in creatine phosphokinase levels as well as serum potassium concentration 24 hours following the use of iohexol. They had no explanation for the elevation of the serum potassium level and believed that the rise in the creatine phosphokinase value was secondary to premedication given through intramuscular injections. Other investigators have not found any elevation of the serum potassium value after the use of either ionic or nonionic agents.

Thus, current evidence suggests that nonionic contrast materials are well tolerated, significantly less painful, and produce equally good angiograms. When nonionic contrast agents are used there is the slight advantage of a positive ionotropic effect as well as lower heart rates, which may be beneficial when studying critically ill infants. At this time, nonionic contrast agents are significantly more expensive than Renografin or Hypaque, which weighs against their relatively minor advantages.[7]

DOSAGE AND RATE OF ADMINISTRATION OF CONTRAST MEDIUM

The total dose of contrast medium used should not exceed 5 to 6 ml/kg. If larger volumes of contrast are needed, we have performed the angiographic examination in more than one sitting, with a period of 1 to 2 days between the examinations. At this time there is no evidence to suggest that use of nonionic contrast agents allows the use of larger volumes of contrast medium, since the concentration of iodine is the same. We use 1.5 to 2 ml/kg for each contrast injection in the newborn. Injections of such large volumes of contrast medium induce a rapid fall in serum pH with acidosis.[65] Rapid reductions in serum pH as a result of contrast injections can be cumulative and particularly detrimental in a newborn with severe cyanosis and metabolic acidosis. Therefore, it is advisable to allow an interval of 10 to 15 minutes between contrast injections to allow serum buffering and lung excretion of the contrast acid load.

The rate of contrast injection is as important as the dose per injection. Cardiac lesions associated with high flow such as ventricular septal defect or truncus arteriosus require injection of large contrast volumes very rapidly. Contrast injections lasting more than two cardiac cycles are usually of no use in neonates because the contrast medium gets diluted and washed away due to the rapid heart rates normally present in these patients.

SINGLE FILM AORTOGRAPHY

Single film aortography is a technique for obtaining a bedside portable aortogram, following injection of contrast medium through an indwelling umbilical artery catheter. This technique was useful in the past for the diagnosis of aortic valvular atresia[46,47] as well as patent ductus arteriosus.[55] The umbilical arterial catheter is positioned at the level of the fifth or sixth thoracic vertebra. For the demonstration of patent ductus arteriosus an angled lateral view is obtained; the procedure is performed using a vertical x-ray tube, and the infant is turned into a lateral position with the head raised about 30 degrees. Alternatively, a lateral x-ray beam may be used; the patient is placed supine on the cassette and turned to 30 to 40 degrees in the sagittal axis. For demonstrating the hypoplastic ascending aorta in aortic atresia, a similar lateral or left anterior oblique view can be used. Then 0.75 to 1.0 ml/kg of Renografin-60 is rapidly injected through the umbilical artery catheter and the exposure is made at the end of the injection (Fig. 28–1). Although single film aortography can be a useful technique in selected patients, it has largely become obsolete in most institutions as a result of advances in two-dimensional and Doppler echocardiography (which can demonstrate the patency of the ductus arteriosus and the presence of aortic valvular atresia). Development of surgical techniques for repair of the hypoplastic left-heart syndrome has mandated a complete cardiac catheterization in that disorder at institutions performing such surgery to demonstrate the intracardiac anatomy.[75]

BALLOON OCCLUSION ANGIOGRAPHY

Sometimes it is difficult to visualize a particular anatomic structure because blood flow to that structure is either diminished or significantly increased. The usual method of circumventing this problem is to place the catheter as close to the area of interest as possible. However, in small infants, placing the catheter in the area of interest may not always be possible. An alternative technique is to occlude either the runoff or the inflow to the area of interest; as a result, more contrast medium can be redirected to the structures one wants to visualize.[21] Obstruction of runoff or inflow can be achieved by the use of occluding balloon catheters, which are available in various French sizes with balloon diameters ranging from 3 mm to 10 mm. Contrast injection can be performed either proximal or distal to the occluding balloon. Such balloon occlusion angiograms are sometimes essential in the demonstration of pathologic anatomy (Fig. 28–2). The balloon occlusion technique provides excellent anatomic detail while requiring injection of only small volumes of contrast medium. However, the size of the balloon must be chosen with care. An undersized balloon will not occlude the vessel, whereas an oversized balloon can lead to vessel rupture.[21] The balloon should be floated to the position of occlusion rather than inflated in situ, in order to minimize the risk of perforating a small vessel. The balloon on the occlusion catheter should be tested several times for prompt deflation before insertion into the patient to prevent inadvertent prolonged occlusion of a crucial vessel such as the aorta. It is advisable to use carbon dioxide for balloon inflation to prevent systemic air embolism should balloon rupture occur.

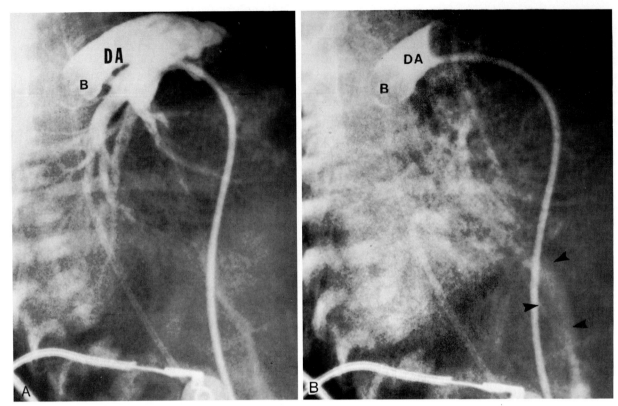

Figure 28–2. Lateral view of a balloon occlusion pulmonary angiogram. This neonate with TAPVD to the portal vein had suprasystemic pressure in the pulmonary artery and a large patent ductus arteriosus. Hence, there was poor opacification of the pulmonary arteries and veins. Because of this, a balloon catheter was passed into the descending aorta through the patent ductus arteriosus. A pulmonary angiogram was obtained during the occlusion of ductus arteriosus. *A,* Arterial phase. *B,* Venous phase. Notice the faint opacification of the common venous channel (arrowheads) as it crosses the diaphragm to join the portal vein. Compare with Figure 28–10*A.* B = balloon; DA = ductus arteriosus.

DIGITAL SUBTRACTION ANGIOGRAPHY

Digital subtraction angiography is a technique in which the video signal from the image intensifier television camera is digitized and scaled logarithmically and the background image is electronically subtracted from the images obtained after contrast injection. The subtracted image is reconverted to analog form, and the angiogram is available for review in real time almost instantaneously.[61] The angiogram can be stored in analog form on a conventional videotape, as hard copy on a copy film, or in digital form on a disk or magnetic tape. The subtraction of the background image as well as window and leveling capabilities increases the contrast resolution severalfold. Digital subtraction permits imaging of the arterial system after intravenous injection of the contrast agent and a reduction of the amount of contrast medium required when the injection is made in the appropriate cardiac chamber or great vessel. As a result, digital subtraction angiography has become an established complementary procedure in peripheral angiography and adult heart disease. However, application of digital subtraction angiography to congenital heart disease has been limited,[32,64,73,99] and the number of

neonates examined has been small. The advantages of digital subtraction angiography are as follows:

1. Adequate visualization can be achieved with smaller contrast volumes in digital subtraction angiography. Current digital subtraction equipment design requires a minimum volume of 3 ml per injection and a contrast concentration of no less than 20 per cent to provide acceptable contrast resolution. Most investigators have used Renografin-76 diluted in half (50 per cent) with sterile water. For intra-arterial injections, even lower concentrations can provide adequate angiograms (Fig. 28–3).

2. Digital angiography permits image acquisition at varying radiation dose levels. The system may be operated at radiation dose levels comparable with those of fluoroscopy[32,64] or cineangiography.[73,99] High radiation doses are usually needed for visualization of the peripheral arterial tree after venous injections of contrast (an input phosphor dose rate of 1 μR/frame in 9-inch mode). Lower radiation doses can be used when contrast is injected directly into an area of interest (such as aortic coarctation). Obviously, the lowest radiation dose necessary to achieve adequate visualization of the area of interest should be used, recognizing that the signal-to-noise ratio goes down as the radiation dose is reduced.

Radiation dose is dependent on frame rate as well as radiation energy setting. Most digital angiography systems cannot record at more than 30 frames per second, whereas most cineangiography systems can record up to 60 frames per second.

3. Digital subtraction angiograms are available for review and analysis almost instantaneously. Although similar results can be achieved by video recording, the contrast resolution of digital subtraction angiography can be superior. Improved resolution may be of significant advantage during interventional procedures such as angioplasty.

4. Digital acquisition of the angiographic information allows computer processing to obtain functional information such as ejection fraction and size of vessels. Such measurements can be valuable during angioplasty (such as choosing the appropriate balloon catheter size for pulmonary or aortic valvuloplasty).

The disadvantages of digital subtraction angiography are as follows:

1. Technical constraints limit frame acquisition rates with digital subtraction angiography. Current commercially available digital subtraction technology allows the following frame rates:
   a. 512 × 512 matrix: 30 frames per second for a maximum of 10 seconds.
   b. 1024 × 1024 matrix: 3 frames per second for a maximum of 10 seconds.

The 30 frames per second acquisition rate with 512 × 512 matrix is more than adequate for most situations. Even small ventricular septal defects can be visualized in oblique projections.[99] However, in neonates with very rapid heart rates, some detail of the atrioventricular valves such as straddling or overriding may not be detected.

2. Biplane imaging during digital subtraction angiography is difficult. Most commercial digital subtraction equipment is only capable of single plane acquisition. Even when biplane acquisition is possible, total acquisition rates cannot exceed those stated previously. Lack of biplane imaging is a significant drawback in the application of digital techniques to congenital heart disease.

3. Spatial resolution of digital subtraction angiography is inferior. When images are obtained using a 512 × 512 matrix and a 6-inch mode, a spatial resolution of two line pairs per millimeter can be obtained, which is lower than the two to three line pairs per millimeter resolution possible with cineangiography. Such reductions in spatial resolution can be a problem in visualizing small vessels in infants.

4. Patient movement can make digital subtraction impossible. Since subtraction is an essential element in this technique, voluntary or involuntary movements during contrast injections can produce misregistration artifacts, which significantly reduce the image quality. Patient movements can be a major problem among neonates. Voluntary movement can be reduced by heavy sedation or general anesthesia and use of nonionic contrast media (which are less painful). Involuntary movements of diaphragmatic and cardiac motion can be reduced by ECG gating and by use of respirators in neonates. However, if ECG gating is used, acquisition rates are significantly reduced.

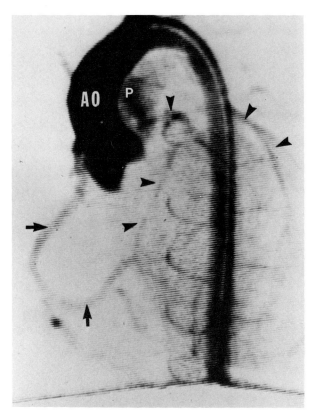

Figure 28–3. Anomalous origin of left coronary artery from pulmonary artery in a 2-month-old infant. Digital subtraction angiography of ascending aorta in left anterior oblique projection. Nine milliliters of 25 per cent Renografin-76 was injected at 10 ml/sec. There is excellent opacification of ascending aorta and right coronary artery (arrows). There is opacification of all the branches of the left coronary artery (arrowheads). There is also opacification of the pulmonary artery from which the left coronary artery arises. AO = aorta; P = pulmonary artery.

5. Digital subtraction image processing can be time consuming. Although instant real time playback of the angiogram is possible, processing the whole examination and storing it on videotape or obtaining hard copy images are time-consuming chores.

ANGIOGRAPHIC PROJECTIONS AND THE ROLE OF AXIAL ANGIOGRAPHY

The initial descriptions of angiocardiography involved the use of frontal and lateral projections. A large body of literature has appeared describing the angiographic morphology of most congenital cardiac malformations.[10–12,30,37,86,94] The major disadvantage of frontal and lateral projections is the superimposition of the cardiac chambers, septa, and valves due to the oblique position of the heart in the thorax and the normal curvilinear contour of the ventricular

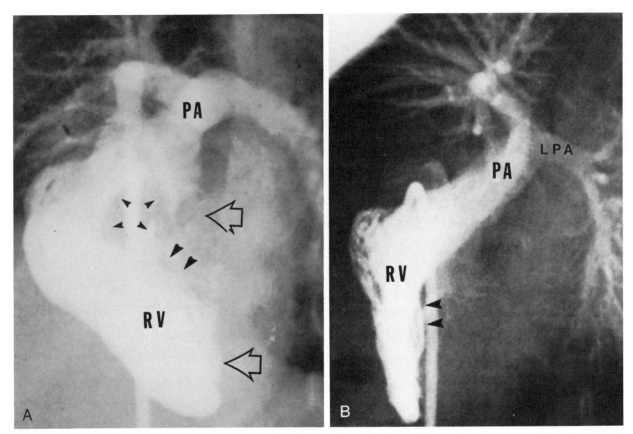

Figure 28–4. Right ventricular angiogram in long-axis view. *A*, Diastolic frame. *B*, Systolic frame. LPA = left pulmonary artery; PA = pulmonary artery; clear arrows = anterior septal contour; large arrowheads = posterior septal contour; small arrowheads = tricuspid annulus; RV = right ventricle. (Reproduced by permission of the American Heart Association, Inc. From Ceballos R, et al [1981]: Angiographic anatomy of the normal heart through axial angiography. Circulation 64:351–359.)

septum. To overcome this problem, right anterior oblique (RAO) and left anterior oblique (LAO) projections were suggested.[60] However, these straight oblique projections also demonstrated overlap of the ventricular structures, since the anterior part of the ventricular septum is situated to the left of the posterior septum. Puyau and Burko[80] first suggested cranial angulation to display the entire ventricular septum without foreshortening. Bargeron and colleagues[9] introduced the concept of modern axial angiography in 1977, and axial angiography is now in widespread use in most pediatric cardiac catheterization laboratories.[38,81,90]

Axial angiography can be defined as a method in which the x-ray beam is oriented perpendicular to the long axis of the heart or its great arteries independent of their position within the thorax. The ventricular septum normally describes an arch of approximately 120 degrees that is open posteriorly and to the left, so that the anterior border of the septum is situated to the left of its posterior margin. Hence, a single x-ray beam angulation will not display the anterior and posterior portions of the septum. To depict the anterior septum a 60-degree LAO orientation with respect to the sagittal plane of the body is needed. However, with this obliquity alone, the apex and base of the heart will be superimposed.[18] To avoid this problem 30 degrees of cranial angulation should be added. Cranial angulation allows the apex of the heart to be seen inferiorly and the

atrioventricular groove and the atria to be seen superiorly. The resulting view is called the long axial oblique view (Figs. 28–4 and 28–5).[9] Such a view can be achieved in several ways, depending on the available design of the x-ray equipment:

1. If anteroposterior and lateral x-ray tubes are fixed, the infant is positioned obliquely across the table such that the long axis of the heart on the video screen is parallel to the long axis of the x-ray table (15 to 20 degrees). The infant's right shoulder is elevated 30 degrees by a radiolucent wedge. The primary imaging for this projection is accomplished by the lateral tube. Thus, careful collimation is necessary.

2. If the lateral tube is mobile (C-arm), the right shoulder of the patient is elevated 30 degrees and the lateral tube is angled cranially 15 to 20 degrees.

The projection orthogonal to the long axial oblique view is a modified RAO projection that is called the elongated RAO view (Figs. 28–6 and 28–7) (RAO 30 degrees + 15 to 20 degrees of cranial angulation).

To profile the most posterior or inferior part of the septum, the x-ray beam should be oriented in a 45-degree LAO direction. The 20-degree cranial angulation should be maintained. The resulting projection is called the four-chamber view since the four cardiac chambers are separated from each other with the atrial chambers and septum su-

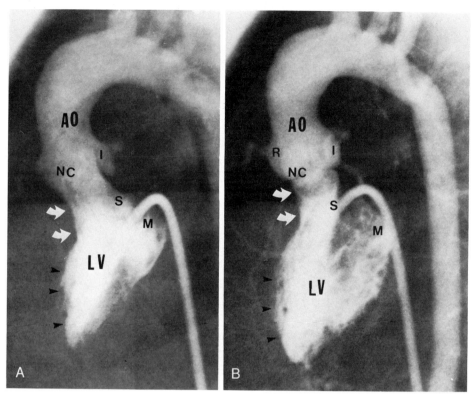

Figure 28–5. Left ventriculogram in the long-axis view. *A*, Systolic phase. *B*, Diastolic phase. AO = aorta; R = right coronary cusp; l = left coronary cusp; LV = left ventricle; m = mural leaflet of mitral valve; NC = noncoronary cusp; S = septal leaflet of mitral valve; white arrows = infundibular septum; arrowheads = trabecular septum. (Reproduced by permission of the American Heart Association, Inc. From Ceballos R, et al [1981]: Angiographic anatomy of the normal heart through axial angiography. Circulation 64:351–359.)

periorly and the ventricles and crux cordis inferiorly. The four-chamber view can be obtained in different ways:

1. When the x-ray tubes are fixed, the patient's thorax is raised 30 degrees from the table and the left shoulder is elevated 45 degrees. The vertical x-ray beam is used to obtain the angiogram.

2. If the anteroposterior tube can be angled, the C-arm is rotated 45 degrees to the patient's left with a cranial angulation of 30 degrees. An additional useful projection is the so-called sitting up view, which is obtained by a 30-degree cranial angulation of the x-ray beam to the sagittal plane of the body. The sitting up view is very useful in demonstrating the pulmonary artery bifurcation (see Fig. 28–28) and certain anomalies of the aortic arch.[9,59]

The heart is a complex three-dimensional structure. The degree of angulation needed in each plane to achieve adequate demonstration of various components of the cardiac anatomy will depend on the orientation of the heart in the thorax as well as on the degree of rotation of the heart around its axis. The angulations described above will be appropriate in the majority of cases. However, modifications to these techniques should be made to suit each particular case. It has been suggested that certain types of muscular ventricular septal defects and overriding or straddling atrioventricular valves are better demonstrated by caudally angulated LAO projections.[16,17]

One can readily appreciate that the principles of axial angiography are based on the presence of a curvilinear ventricular septum. If the septum has a significantly different shape, axial angiography will not provide a true profile or separate the cardiac chambers.[41] The examples in this category include hearts with so-called superoinfer-

ior ventricles. In these hearts, the ventricular septum has a horizontal shape. These patients need ventriculography in the frontal projection to demonstrate the location and size of the ventricular septal defect and axial angiography,

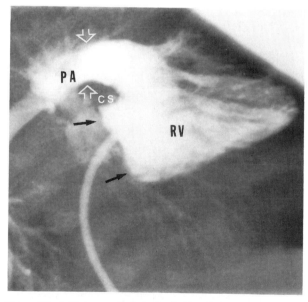

Figure 28–6. Right ventriculography in the elongated right anterior oblique projection. CS = crista supraventricularis; arrows = tricuspid valve; clear arrows = pulmonary valve; PA = pulmonary artery; RV = right ventricle; black arrows = tricuspid annulus. (Reproduced by permission of the American Heart Association, Inc. From Ceballos R, et al [1981]: Angiographic anatomy of the normal heart through axial angiography. Circulation 64:351–359.)

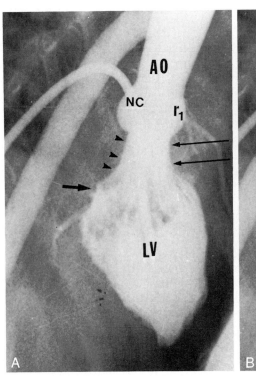

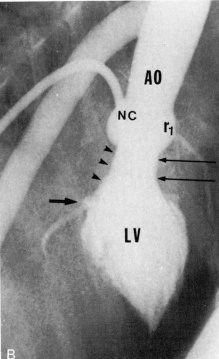

Figure 28–7. Left ventriculogram in the elongated right anterior oblique projection. *A,* Diastolic phase. *B,* Systolic phase. AO = aorta; short arrow = posterior commissure; long arrows = infundibular septum; arrowheads = atrioventricular septum; l = left coronary cusp; LV = left ventricle; NC = noncoronary cusp; r = right coronary cusp. (Reproduced by permission of the American Heart Association, Inc. From Ceballos R, et al [1981]: Angiographic anatomy of the normal heart through axial angiography. Circulation 64:351–359.)

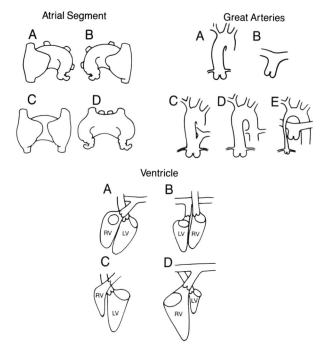

Figure 28–8. A diagrammatic approach to the sequential analysis of congenital heart disease. The three segments of cardiac anatomy are atrial segment, ventricular mass, and great arteries. See text for analysis of their connections and relations. Atrial segment: A = situs solitus; B = situs inversus; C = right atrial isomerism; and D = left atrial isomerism. Ventricles: A = normal. There are two normally related ventricles (*d*-isomer); B = inverted ventricles (*l*-isomer); C = hypoplasia of right ventricle; and D = hypoplasia of left ventricle. While concordant ventriculoarterial connection is shown in A, C, and D, any type of ventriculoarterial connection is possible. Great arteries: A = aorta; B = pulmonary artery; C = truncus arteriosus; D = pulmonary atresia; and E = aortic atresia.

preferably in the four-chamber projection, to demonstrate the atrioventricular connections. In corrected transposition, the septum is usually vertically oriented. In these patients, ventriculography is indicated in frontal or oblique views without angulation. Long axial oblique views may be needed to demonstrate the arterial outflow tract.[44]

ANGIOGRAPHIC ANATOMY, CHAMBER LOCALIZATION, AND SEQUENTIAL ANALYSIS

Precise and complete understanding of the features of complex congenital heart disease has become increasingly necessary, as greater numbers of congenital cardiac defects are currently amenable to palliative or corrective surgery. The ensuing description provides a simplified, practical approach to the interpretation of the angiographic appearances of congenital cardiac lesions. Such analysis is based on the examination of the different cardiac and vascular structures in an orderly sequential manner considering morphology, spatial relations, and connections separately.[6] We distinguish between connections and relations: the former refer to the union of one chamber or vessel to another and hence impose certain physiologic implications on the transport of blood through the heart, whereas the latter refer only to the spatial orientation of one cardiac or vascular structure to another. Accurate analysis of connections and relations is facilitated by the use of the axial views previously described that allow identification of each of the basic components involved in congenital cardiac malformation.

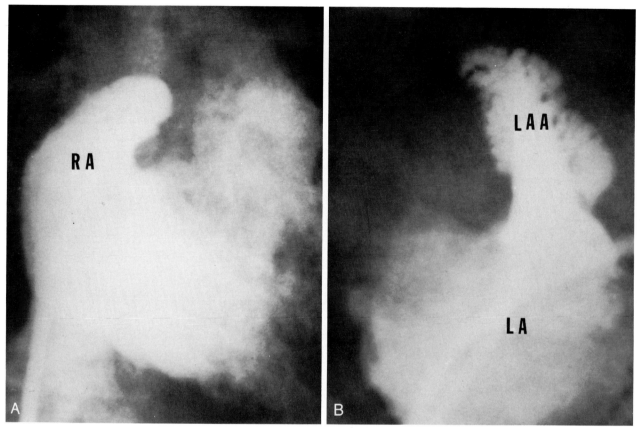

Figure 28–9. *A*, Angiogram of right atrial appendage in elongated right anterior oblique projection. The tip of the appendage is blunt, and it has a broad base. *B*, Left atrial appendage in contrast to its counterpart. This structure is finger-shaped and appears more trabeculated. LA = left atrium; LAA = left atrial appendage; RA = right atrium. (Reproduced by permission of the American Heart Association, Inc. From Ceballos R, et al [1981]: Angiographic anatomy of the normal heart through axial angiography. Circulation 64:351–359.)

The cardiovascular structures have four components: (1) veins, systemic and pulmonary; (2) atria; (3) ventricles; and (4) great arteries. Hence, the segmental approach would systematically evaluate venoatrial connections; atria—their number, morphology, and arrangement; ventricles—their number, morphology, and arrangement; atrioventricular connections; ventriculoarterial connections; great arteries—their number, morphology, and arrangement; and, lastly, associated anomalies such as shunts and stenoses. The schematic representation of segmental analysis is shown in Figure 28–8.

Atria

Morphology

There are always two atrial chambers. These may be morphologically distinct right and left atria as in the normal heart or have similar morphology, either right or left, a condition known as atrial isomerism.[101] Common atrium implies a single atrial chamber, devoid of a septum but possessing two symmetrical or asymmetrical atrial appendages.

Atrial morphology is established by the characteristic angiographic appearance of the right and left atria and their appendages. The morphology of the right atrium is best appreciated in the elongated RAO view. In this view the right atrium is seen as a globe-shaped structure. The superior and inferior venae cavae are in continuity with the posterior border seen on the right. The tricuspid valve is seen in profile. The right atrial appendage is seen superiorly and to the left. This appendage is triangular with a broad base of implantation and a blunt vertex (Fig. 28–9A).

The morphology of the left atrium also is well seen in the RAO view. In this view the left atrium appears as a quadrangular structure. The upper contour is formed by the roof in its continuation to the entrance of the right and left pulmonary veins. The anterolateral border is on the left with the left atrial appendage appearing as a prominent structure. In contrast to the right atrial appendage, this structure is finger shaped and communicates with the main atrial cavity through a narrow orifice (Fig. 28–9B). Thus, the distinct angiographic appearances of the atrial appendages facilitate identification of the morphology of the atria. It is important to emphasize that the venous connections should not be used to define atrial morphology.

Atrial Relations (Situs)

The spatial arrangement of the atria with regard to each other defines the atrial relations, which traditionally have been known as atrial situs. When two morphologically

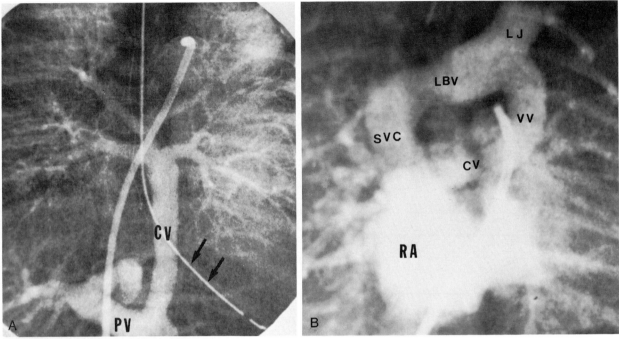

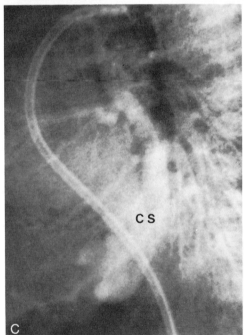

Figure 28–10. Types of total anomalous pulmonary venous connection. All the angiograms are levophase of pulmonary arteriograms. *A*, To the portal vein. AP view. All the pulmonary veins join a common channel, which crosses the diaphragm adjacent to the nasogastric tube (arrows) through the esophageal hiatus to join the portal vein. Notice the small size of the pulmonary veins reflecting decreased pulmonary blood flow. Compare with *B*. *B*, Connection to the left superior vena cava. AP view. All the pulmonary veins join a common channel. This joins the left superior vena cava or the vertical vein, which joins the left internal jugular vein to form the brachiocephalic vein, then drains into the right superior vena cava, which in turn connects to the right atrium. *C*, Connection to the coronary sinus. Lateral view. All the pulmonary veins join a common channel, which in turn connects to the coronary sinus that is draining into the right atrium. CS = coronary sinus; CV = common channel; LBV = left brachiocephalic vein; LJ = left jugular vein; PV = portal vein; RA = right atrium; SVC = superior vena cava; VV = vertical vein.

different atrial chambers are present, relations are either normal (situs solitus) or inverted (situs inversus). When two atria of similar morphology (isomerism) are present, the term right or left atrial isomerism is preferable to situs ambiguous.

Venoatrial Connection

The major systemic veins entering the right atrium are the superior and inferior venae cavae and the coronary sinus. Two sets of pulmonary veins from each lung drain into the left atrium. Anomalies of the systemic venous return are rare, particularly in the neonatal period. Abnormalities of the pulmonary venous return are not infrequent; these should be described as to their extent (partial, hemitotal, or total) and by the chamber or structure to which the abnormal vein(s) is connected.

In the neonatal period TAPVD is more common and important than hemitotal or partial anomalous connection (see Chapter 34). TAPVD is classified according to the site of connection.[31,77] About 37 per cent of TAPVDs are connected to the left superior vena cava. About 14 per cent are connected to the right superior vena cava, 11 per cent to the right atrium, 16 per cent to the coronary sinus, and approximately 15 per cent below the diaphragm, mostly to the portal vein. About 7 per cent of patients have anomalous connections to multiple sites. These groups of patients can be subdivided according to the presence or absence of obstructed pulmonary venous connection. Infants with obstructed TAPVD become symptomatic earlier in life, mostly during the first week. The diagnosis is made through pulmonary angiography (Fig. 28–10A). The angiogram classically demonstrates a common venous channel that passes inferiorly to enter the portal vein. Infants with obstructed TAPVD have severe pulmonary venous and arterial hypertension and exhibit very sluggish flow through the pulmonary vascular bed. These infants also frequently have a right-to-left shunt through the ductus arteriosus, decreasing the amount of contrast medium reaching the pulmonary vascular bed. Consequently, the diagnosis may be missed on angiography.[31,66] It may then be necessary to perform selective right or left pulmonary angiography or pulmonary angiography with balloon occlusion of the ductus arteriosus or descending thoracic aorta (see Fig. 28–2). Another source of misdiagnosis is complicating pulmonary outflow tract obstruction. It is not uncommon for patients with right isomerism and pulmonary atresia to also have TAPVD.[31] In such patients, the pulmonary blood flow is severely diminished, resulting in poor opacification of the pulmonary veins and their anomalous connection.

In contrast, patients with unobstructed TAPVD have increased pulmonary blood flow, requiring rapid, large volume injections to demonstrate the anomalous connection (Fig. 28–10B).

Ventricles

Morphology

Normally, there are two ventricles, one right and the other left, that are morphologically distinct from each other. Each ventricle possesses an inlet and trabecular and outlet portions. In the right ventricle the inlet segment is smooth and supports the tricuspid valve, whereas the trabecular segment is composed of coarse, prominent trabeculations well seen in both systole and diastole (see Figs. 28–4 and 28–28). The outlet or outflow tract is elongated with a prominent muscular ridge (the crista supraventricularis) forming part of its posterior aspect separating the atrioventricular and arterial valves (see Fig. 28–6). These features are best shown in long axial and elongated RAO views. In the long axial view (see Fig. 28–4), the right ventricle is seen as a triangular structure with its base superior and to the right and the apex inferior and to the left. The right ventricular outflow tract or infundibulum is seen as a wide channel formed by the crista supraventricularis on the right side and by part of the trabecula septomarginalis on the left. The pulmonic valve is located on top of the infundibulum (see Fig. 28–4). The tricuspid valve is seen in diastole as a negative shadow overlying the right upper contour of the right ventricle. In the elongated RAO view (see Fig. 28–6), the right ventricle has a slightly similar appearance. The tricuspid valve is seen in profile

along the posterior border. The outflow tract is seen as a channel formed by the crista supraventricularis posteriorly and the free wall of the ventricle anteriorly. The pulmonic valve is separated from the tricuspid valve by the whole length of the crista. The superior border of the ventricle is formed by the free anterior wall of the ventricle with its prominent characteristic trabeculations.

By contrast, in the left ventricle, the inlet or inflow tract is short and smooth walled and supports the mitral valve. The trabecular segment has fine trabeculations (Figs. 28–5 and 28–11) that are better visualized in diastolic images. The outlet or outflow tract is short when compared with that of the right. One of its walls is formed by a continuity between the arterial and atrioventricular valves. In the long axial view of the left ventriculogram, the left ventricle appears as a triangular structure with its base directed superiorly and its apex directed inferiorly (see Fig. 28–5). The right contour of the left ventricle is formed inferiorly by the trabecular septum and only in a short superior segment by the infundibular septum. The clearly defined outflow tract is bounded by the infundibular septum anteriorly and by the septal mitral leaflet posteriorly. The aortic valve is located on top of the left ventricular outflow tract. In the elongated view the posterosuperior contour of the left ventricle, to the right, shows a smooth, straight line that extends from the noncoronary aortic cusp to the crux cordis that does not change during the cardiac cycle (see Fig. 28–7). This line represents contrast material accumulated under the septal leaflet of the mitral valve in its insertion into the muscular atrioventricular septum. From this point downward, the contour of the left ventricle is bound by its inferior free wall. The infundibular septum is represented by the short upper segment of the left anterosuperior contour of the left ventricle related to the right and left cusps of the aortic valve. Thus, in this projection the outflow tract of the left ventricle is bound by the infundibular septum anteriorly and by the atrioventricular septum posteriorly.

In the four-chamber projection the left ventricle appears as an elongated hemicircle with a medial, relatively straight component and a lateral rounded component crowned by the aorta (see Fig. 28–11). Anteriorly, there are two well-defined contours. The superior contour extends from the aortic valve to a point marked by the posterior leaflet of the mitral valve in its proximity to the ventricular septum (crux). This contour is formed by the atrioventricular component of the muscular septum that separates the right atrium from the left ventricle. From this point downward the anterior wall is represented by the most posterior portion of the interventricular septum.

There is a difference of opinion in the literature regarding the number of segments required for a chamber to be called a ventricle. Anderson and coworkers proposed that an inlet segment must be present for a chamber to be called a ventricle.[5] They subsequently modified this concept and suggested that in most situations two ventricles are present.[3] One ventricle may be incomplete, lacking either inlet and/or outlet segments; the incomplete ventricle may be quite rudimentary or hypoplastic. Nonetheless, the incomplete ventricle does constitute a ventricle, and the

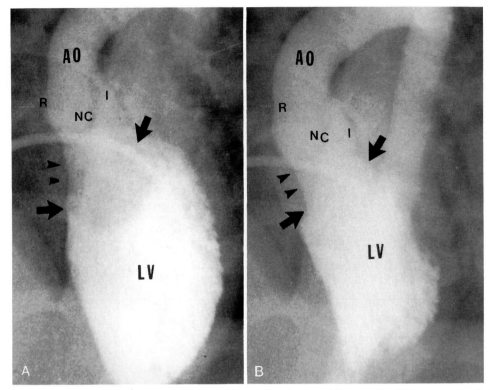

Figure 28–11. Left ventriculogram in the four-chamber view. *A,* Diastolic phase. *B,* Systolic phase. AO = aorta; R = right coronary cusp; l = left coronary cusp; LV = left ventricle; NC = noncoronary cusp; arrows = commissures; arrowheads = atrioventricular septum. (Reproduced by permission of the American Heart Association, Inc. From Ceballos R, et al [1981]: Angiographic anatomy of the normal heart through axial angiography. Circulation 64:351–359.)

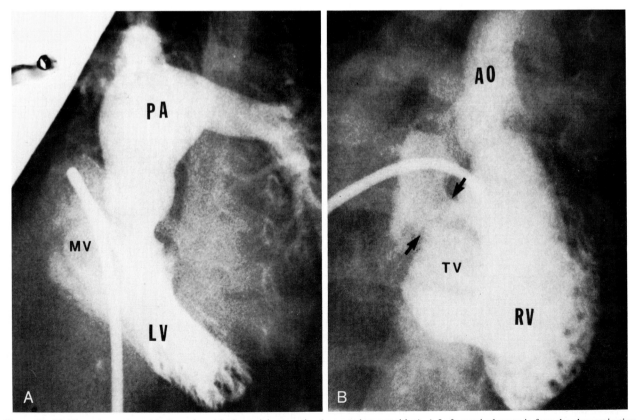

Figure 28–12. Discordant atrioventricular and ventriculoarterial connection (corrected transposition). *A,* Left ventriculogram in four-chamber projection. *B,* Right ventriculogram in a similar view. Ventricular relationship is inverted. The morphologic left ventricle is anterior and to the right. Pulmonary artery arises from this chamber. The morphologic right ventricle is to the left and is connected to the aorta. There is a muscular ventricular septal defect (arrows). AO = aorta; LV = left ventricle; MV = mitral valve; PA = pulmonary artery; RV = right ventricle; TV = tricuspid valve.

incomplete ventricle's trabecular morphology allows it to be characterized as a right or a left ventricle. We prefer not to use the terms outlet chamber or trabecular pouch to describe incomplete ventricles. Very rarely, a true solitary ventricular chamber is present.[63,98] There is a continuous spectrum between the univentricular and biventricular heart; by necessity, arbitrary classifications have to be made in borderline situations. More detailed descriptions on the subject are available.[5,89,100]

Ventricular Relations

The spatial arrangement of one ventricle to the other is used to describe the ventricular relations. Van Praagh and associates[102] suggested that the internal organization of the ventricles is analogous to stereoisomers: (1) the *"d"* isomer is similar to the dorsum of the right hand. In such a ventricle only the palm of the right hand can be applied to the septum such that the dorsum is against the free wall and the thumb is in the inflow tract with the other four fingers in the outflow tract (see Fig. 28–28). (2) An *"l"* isomer is present when the left hand can be applied to the right ventricle with the palm against the septum so that the thumb is in the atrioventricular valve and the fingers are in the outflow tract. The *"l"* isomer is also called ventricular inversion or *"l"* loop (Fig. 28–12). Since the ventricles may rotate in space without altering the relation of the chambers, it is possible to define either normal or inverted ventricles even in the event of unusual cardiac position. In such rotational malformations the inherent relations of the chambers to one another are not affected and the ventricular relations are determined by their respective relations to the ventricular septum.

Atrioventricular Connection

When two atria, two ventricles, and two atrioventricular valves are present, three different types of connection are possible:[4] (1) concordant, when the morphologic right atrium is connected to the right ventricle and the left atrium to the left ventricle (see Fig. 28–20A); (2) discordant, when the right atrium is connected to the left ventricle and the left atrium to the right ventricle (see Fig. 28–12); and (3) ambiguous, when atrial isomerism is present and the atrioventricular connections are neither discordant nor concordant.

In the case of univentricular atrioventricular connection, the following connections are possible: (1) Two atria and two atrioventricular valves are connected to a single ventricle, which has been described by some authors as double inlet[97] (Fig. 28–13). (2) Isolated connection is possible through one atrioventricular valve with atresia of the other valve. The patent atrioventricular valve is termed either right or left according to its spatial location or its attachment to an atrium with definite morphology. (In such situations it is better to avoid the terms tricuspid or mitral valves, since their morphologic distinction by angiography is not possible.) (3) Isolated atrioventricular connection can occur through a common atrioventricular valve.

In the neonatal period, atresia of an atrioventricular valve is more commonly encountered. Right atrioventricular valve atresia (tricuspid atresia) is more common than

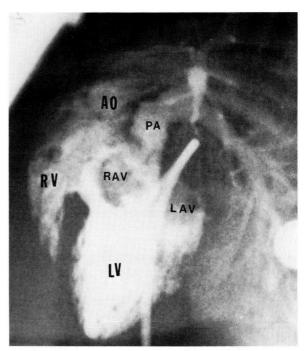

Figure 28–13. Double inlet left ventricle. Left ventriculogram in four-chamber view. Both AV valves enter the morphologic left ventricle. A smaller morphologic right ventricle is identified to the right (normal ventricular relation). This ventricle lacks the inlet segment. There is a muscular ventricular septal defect. Ventriculoarterial connection is discordant. AO = aorta; LAV = left atrioventricular valve; LV = left ventricle; PA = pulmonary artery; RAV = right atrioventricular valve; RV = right ventricle.

left atrioventricular valve (mitral valve) atresia. Tricuspid atresia (see Chapter 43) has been defined as that condition in which there is no direct communication between the right atrium and the right ventricle.[36] In these patients there is obligatory right-to-left shunting at the atrial level. The majority of patients (about 70 per cent) with tricuspid atresia have normal ventriculoarterial connections. The pulmonary artery connects with the small infundibular chamber, and the aorta connects to the left ventricle. The ventriculoarterial connection is discordant in about 20 per cent of patients. When the ventriculoarterial connection is concordant, the majority of such patients have some form of pulmonary outflow tract obstruction.

Angiographically, a right atriogram performed in the frontal or four-chamber projection demonstrates right atrioventricular valve atresia, interatrial communication, and the patent left atrioventricular connection. A selective left ventriculogram performed in the four-chamber projection demonstrates the location and size of the ventricular septal defect, type of ventriculoarterial connection, as well as the presence, extent, and types of pulmonary outflow tract obstruction (Fig. 28–14).

Mitral (left atrioventricular valve) atresia (see Chapter 36) is a rare congenital cardiac anomaly that occurs most frequently in hearts with aortic atresia and the hypoplastic left-heart syndrome.[67] Less commonly, mitral atresia occurs in patients with univentricular atrioventricular connections, transposition of the great arteries, or double-outlet right ventricle. As in tricuspid atresia, selective opacification of the left atrium or pulmonary vein will demonstrate

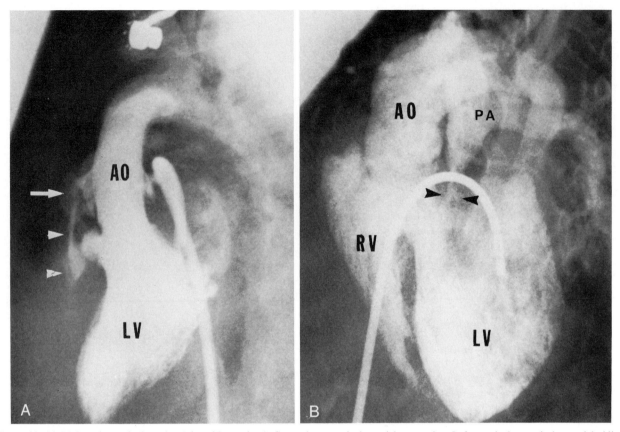

Figure 28–14. Right atrioventricular valve (tricuspid) atresia. *A,* Concordant ventriculoarterial connection. Left ventriculogram in long axial oblique view. Aorta originates from this ventricle. A severely hypoplastic right ventricle (arrowheads) is opacified through a restrictive ventricular septal defect. Pulmonary artery (arrow) arises from the right ventricle. There is severe subvalvular pulmonary stenosis (upper arrowhead). *B,* A different patient with a larger muscular ventricular septal defect and right ventricular chamber. In this patient, the ventriculoarterial connection is discordant. There is valvular and subvalvular pulmonary stenosis (arrowheads), which is partly obscured by the catheter. AO = aorta; LV = left ventricle; PA = pulmonary artery; RV = right ventricle.

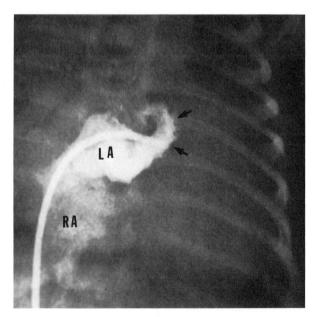

Figure 28–15. Left atrioventricular valve (mitral) atresia. AP view of left atriogram. The tip of the catheter is in the left atrial appendage (arrows). Notice the typical fingerlike shape of the left atrial appendage. Mitral valve is atretic. Right atrium (RA) is opacified through the atrial septal defect. LA = left atrium; RA = right atrium.

the morphology of the atretic left atrioventricular valve (Fig. 28–15).

Patients with a double-inlet atrioventricular connection usually do not present in the neonatal period unless there is associated pulmonary outflow obstruction. As mentioned previously, ventriculography should be performed in these patients not only in axial projections but also in the frontal projection to demonstrate the size of the ventricular septal defect, the nature of pulmonary outflow obstruction, and the size of the pulmonary arteries.

Varying degrees of atrioventricular valvular straddling and/or overriding are sometimes present; such abnormalities should be clearly described in the angiographic analysis. The degree of overriding is particularly important when defining univentricular hearts. Overriding of one atrioventricular valve is present when its annulus is partly committed to the opposite ventricle. Straddling of an atrioventricular valve implies that the tensor apparatus of the valve is partially committed to the opposite ventricle.[71]

Atrioventricular Relation

The spatial arrangement of one atrioventricular connection to the other determines the atrioventricular relation.

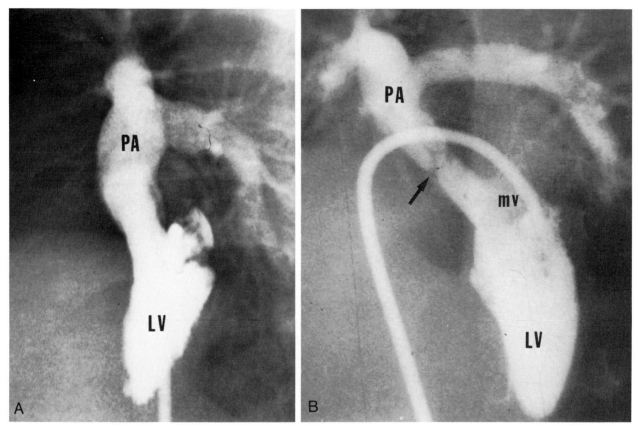

Figure 28–16. *A*, Complete transposition. Left ventriculogram in long axial oblique view. Pulmonary artery arises from the normally related left ventricle. Ventricular septum is intact and pulmonary outflow tract is normal. *B*, A different patient with complete transposition and intact ventricular septum. There is long, tubular fibromuscular tunnel-like stenosis in the left ventricular outflow tract. In addition there is a discrete subvalvular membranous stenosis (arrow). LV = left ventricle; MV = mitral valve; PA = pulmonary artery.

In normal hearts and in most cases with congenital malformations, the atrioventricular connections are aligned side by side in an arrangement described as parallel. There are occasions, however, when the atrioventricular connections cross each other, a feature often reported as criss-cross heart;[48] it is our opinion that this is merely a particular pattern of spatial arrangement. Obviously there is a spectrum of possible spatial arrangements between the parallel and crossed patterns, including what has been called the over-and-under ventricles (which again is only a particular spatial arrangement).

Ventriculoarterial Connections

Four types of ventriculoarterial connections are possible, whether with two ventricles or a solitary ventricular chamber:

1. Concordant connection: The right ventricle is connected to the pulmonary artery and the left ventricle to the aorta (see Figs. 28–4, 28–7, 28–20, and 28–21).

2. Discordant connection: The right ventricle is connected to the aorta and the left ventricle to the pulmonary trunk (see Figs. 28–12 and 28–16). This ventriculoarterial connection is also called complete transposition of the great arteries.

3. Double-outlet: Both great arteries, or one plus more than 90 per cent of the circumference of the other, are

supported by only one ventricle.[95] Double-outlet ventriculoarterial connection is possible with ventricles of either right or left ventricular morphology or with a solitary ventricular chamber.

4. Single-outlet: It is possible that only one great vessel is connected to the ventricular mass. The single vessel of a single outlet ventricle may be the aorta in the case of pulmonary atresia, the pulmonary artery in the case of aortic atresia, or a truncus arteriosus.

All of the above ventriculoarterial connections are encountered in the neonatal period. Complete transposition of the great arteries (concordant atrioventricular and discordant ventriculoarterial connections [see Chapter 46]) is probably the most common abnormal ventriculoarterial connection presenting in the newborn period (Fig. 28–16). About 70 per cent of patients with complete transposition will have an intact ventricular septum and a normal left ventricular outflow tract.[43] The two most common anomalies associated with complete transposition of the great vessels are ventricular septal defect and left ventricular outflow tract obstruction. Obstruction to the pulmonary outflow tract is more common when a ventricular septal defect is present. Selective right and left ventricular angiograms are necessary to define the ventriculoarterial connection and to determine whether ventricular septal defect and/or ventricular outflow tract obstruction are present. Selective left ventriculogram performed in the long axial

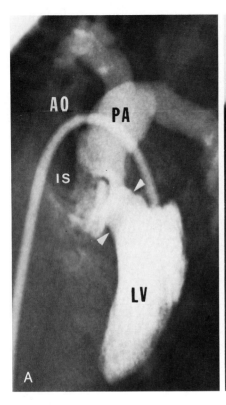 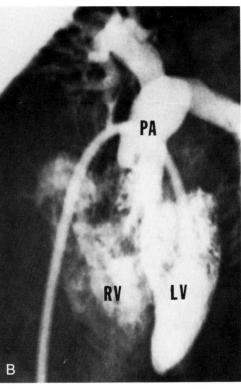

Figure 28–17. Double-outlet right ventricle with a subpulmonary ventricular septal defect (Taussig-Bing complex). Left ventriculogram in four-chamber projection. *A,* An early frame. *B,* A later frame. The only outlet to the left ventricle is a large, perimembranous ventricular septal defect (arrowheads) that is committed to the pulmonary artery. Aorta is faintly visualized. Notice that the infundibular septum is projected anterior and to the right of the left ventricle and lies over the right ventricle. AO = aorta; IS = infundibular septum; LV = left ventricle; RV = right ventricle.

oblique view is usually the best projection to define the nature of the left ventricular outflow tract obstruction (see Fig. 28–16B). An ascending aortogram may be necessary to define the coronary arterial pattern when an "arterial switch" procedure is contemplated.

Patients with a double-outlet right ventricle do not usually present in the newborn period unless they have pulmonary outflow tract obstruction. The physiology in patients with double-outlet right ventricle is determined by the type of the ventricular septal defect and its relation to the great vessels, as well as by the status of the pulmonary outflow tract.[93] When severe obstruction to the pulmonary outflow tract is present, patients with a double-outlet right ventricle physiologically resemble those with tetralogy of Fallot no matter what the position of the great vessels. When pulmonary outflow tract obstruction is absent and a large subpulmonary ventricular septal defect is present, patients with double-outlet right ventricle resemble patients with complete transposition of the great vessels (so-called Taussig-Bing anomaly). When pulmonary outflow tract obstruction is absent and a large subaortic ventricular septal defect is present, patients with double-outlet right ventricle resemble those with simple large ventricular septal defect.

Angiography in patients with double-outlet right ventricle should define ventriculoarterial connections; location and size of ventricular septal defect; status of the pulmonary outflow tract and the size of the pulmonary arteries; and other associated anomalies (e.g., left ventricular hypoplasia, straddling mitral valve, coarctation of the aorta). The most important angiographic view in patients with double-outlet right ventricle is a selective left ventriculogram obtained in the four-chamber projection (Fig. 28–17),

which will clearly demonstrate the atrioventricular and ventriculoarterial connections, the size of the left ventricle, and the size and location of the ventricular septal defect. Selective right ventriculography in the four-chamber projection complements left ventriculography in demonstrating the pulmonary outflow tract as well as the aorta.

Patients with single outlet from the ventricle almost always present in the neonatal period with the possible exception of those with truncus arteriosus. Whereas the atretic aorta almost always is connected to the morphologic left ventricle, the aorta in patients with pulmonary atresia may originate from either the right or the left ventricle. Aortic atresia is most frequently associated with the hypoplastic left-heart syndrome. In these patients, the aorta is of relatively normal caliber up to the origin of the innominate artery and is markedly hypoplastic in its ascending portion. The systemic circulation is perfused by the pulmonary artery through the ductus arteriosus. The ventricular septum is usually intact. Therefore, the morphology of the aortic atresia can be demonstrated either by right ventriculography, by pulmonary arteriography, or by retrograde injection of the descending thoracic aorta through an umbilical arterial catheter (see Fig. 28–1).

In patients with pulmonary atresia, a ventricular septal defect is usually present. In the newborn period, the ductus arteriosus provides perfusion to the pulmonary arteries and large aortopulmonary collaterals are uncommon.[30] Therefore, selective right ventriculography in frontal and lateral projections will usually demonstrate the appropriate anatomy. An aortogram is sometimes required to demonstrate the morphology of the pulmonary arteries as well as the aortic arch branches necessary for the creation of a palliative shunt (Fig. 28–18).

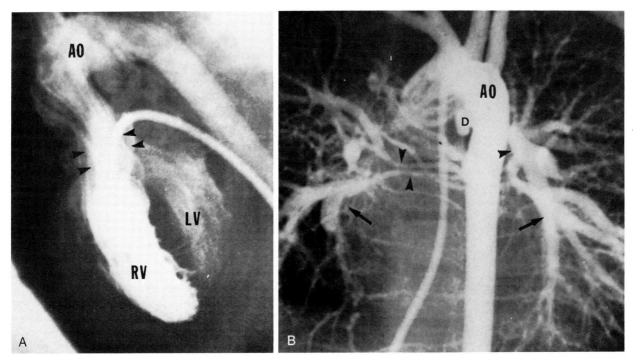

Figure 28–18. Pulmonary atresia with ventricular septal defect. *A,* Right ventriculogram in long axial oblique view. A large perimembranous ventricular septal defect (arrowheads) leads to the overriding aorta and partially opacifies the left ventricle. Pulmonary arteries are poorly visualized. *B,* Same patient. Ascending aortogram. A small patent ductus arteriosus is seen. Numerous systemic pulmonary collaterals (arrowheads) of varying sizes opacify segmental pulmonary arterial branches (arrows). Central pulmonary arteries are not visualized. AO = aorta; D = patent ductus arteriosus; LV = left ventricle; RV = right ventricle.

Truncus arteriosus (see Chapter 46) is an uncommon congenital cardiac malformation in which a single arterial trunk arises from the heart by way of a single arterial valve; the common arterial trunk gives origin directly to the coronary, systemic, and one or both pulmonary arteries.[29] Truncus arteriosus is characterized by a single truncal valve; a subarterial ventricular septal defect; and a deficiency in the aortopulmonary septum, the extent of which determines the size of the main pulmonary artery before its division into right and left branches.[25] These anatomic abnormalities are best shown by the combination of right and/or left ventriculography and truncal angiography. Ventriculography performed in the long axial view demonstrates the subarterial ventricular septal defect, the extent of origin of the truncus arteriosus from each ventricle, and the morphology of the pulmonary arteries (Fig. 28–19). Patients with truncus arteriosus have markedly increased pulmonary blood flow; the anatomy of the pulmonary artery and its branches (in addition to the aortic arch) is better defined with truncal angiography than with ventriculography. Truncal angiograms performed in frontal and lateral projections are usually adequate; supplemental angiograms in an elongated RAO view or four-chamber projection can better demonstrate the origins of the right and left pulmonary arteries.

Great Arteries

Normally there are two great arteries arising from the heart: the aorta and the pulmonary artery. As described previously, there may be a single outlet from the heart.

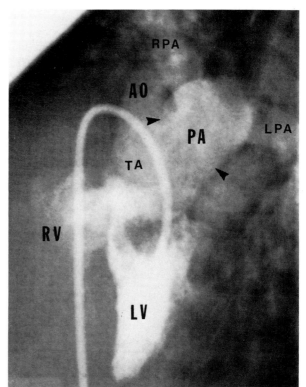

Figure 28–19. Type I truncus arteriosus. Left ventriculogram in four-chamber projection. The truncus arteriosus arises almost equally from both ventricles. There is a large subarterial ventricular septal defect. The short pulmonary trunk (arrowheads) is identified arising posteriorly from the truncus before dividing into right and left pulmonary arteries. AO = aorta; LPA = left pulmonary artery; LV = left ventricle; PA = main pulmonary artery; RPA = right pulmonary artery; RV = right ventricle; TA = truncus arteriosus.

Table 28–1. ASSOCIATED ANOMALIES
IN SEQUENTIAL ANALYSIS

Shunts
  Atrial septal defect
  Ventricular septal defect
  Patent ductus arteriosus
  Atrioventricular septal defect
  Aortopulmonary window
  Arteriovenous malformation
Stenoses
  Right side of heart
    Pulmonary stenosis (subvalvular, valvular)
    Pulmonary artery stenosis
  Left side of heart
    Mitral stenosis
    Aortic stenosis (valvular, subaortic, supravalvular)
    Coarctation of aorta
    Interruption of aortic arch
Combination of lesions

The spatial relations of the great arteries after origin from the heart can be variable. Normally, the aorta is posterior and to the right and the pulmonary trunk is anterior and to the left (see Fig. 28–21). When the ventricles are inverted (as in corrected transposition), the spatial relationship of the great arteries may also be inverted (see Fig. 28–12). However, it is important to appreciate that the relationship of the great arteries has poor correlation with the underlying ventricular anatomy and relationships.

Associated Anomalies

Evaluation of the associated anomalies is as important as the sequential analysis described previously. These anomalies can be primarily characterized as shunts or stenoses (Table 28–1).

Shunts

A shunt implies the presence of abnormal communication between the two sides of the circulation. The direction of the shunt (i.e., right to left or left to right) will depend on the relative resistances imposed by the systemic and pulmonary circulations. Hence, the shunt can occur at the atrial or ventricular level or at the level of the great arteries. Combined shunts can also exist.

VENTRICULAR SEPTAL DEFECT

An isolated ventricular septal defect is uncommonly seen in the neonatal period (see Chapter 35), but the presence of a ventricular septal defect as a part of more complex congenital malformations is very common (see Chapters 48 and 50). Thus, evaluation of the angiographic morphology of a ventricular septal defect is crucial. Over the years, several classifications of ventricular septal defects have been proposed.[12,51,88] At our institution we follow a classification proposed by Soto and associates.[88] The ventricular septal defects are classified as perimembranous, which can extend into either the inlet or infundibular or trabecular portions of the muscular septum; muscular, which can also be in the inlet or infundibular or trabecular portions of the septum; and juxta-arterial. Multiple ventricular septal defects may be present. Axial angiography is ideally suited for precise localization of the ventricular septal defects according to the above classification.[84] Perimembranous ventricular septal defects

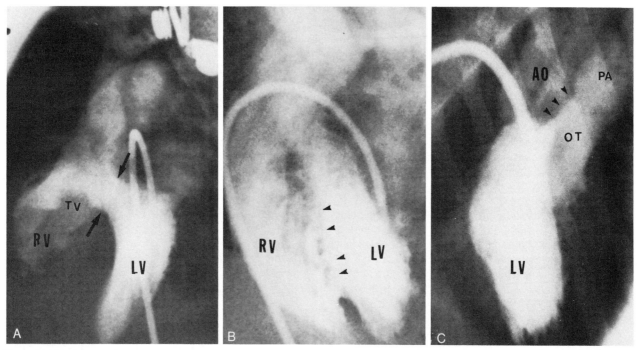

Figure 28–20. *A,* Perimembranous ventricular septal defect. Long axial oblique projection. The relationship of the perimembranous defect (arrows) to the tricuspid valve is clearly identified. *B,* Multiple muscular ventricular septal defects. Long axial oblique view of left ventriculogram. Multiple, small, ventricular septal defects in the trabecular septum (arrowheads) are well seen. *C,* Subarterial defect. An early frame from a left ventriculogram in elongated right anterior oblique view. The contrast material enters the right ventricular outflow tract through a subarterial ventricular septal defect (arrowheads). AO = aorta; LV = left ventricle; OT = right ventricular outflow tract; PA = pulmonary artery; RV = right ventricle; TV = tricuspid valve.

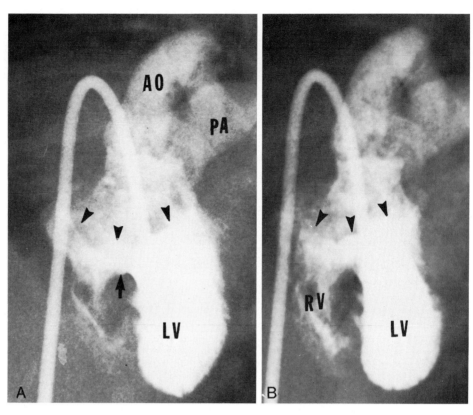

Figure 28–21. Atrioventricular septal defect. Four-chamber view of left ventricle. *A,* Diastolic frame. *B,* Systolic frame. Ventriculoarterial connection is concordant. A common AV orifice and anterior leaflet of common AV valve are seen (arrowheads). There is a large interventricular communication (arrow). The great arteries are normally related, i.e., aorta to the right and posterior and the pulmonary artery anterior and to the left. AO = aorta; LV = left ventricle; PA = pulmonary artery; RV = right ventricle.

are the most common type, either as an isolated entity or when present as a part of a more complex congenital anomaly. Morphologically, perimembranous ventricular septal defects are contiguous with the aortic valve (or pulmonary valve in patients with discordant ventriculoarterial connection) and the mitral-tricuspid fibrous continuity. Perimembranous ventricular septal defects are best demonstrated by selective left ventriculography in the long axial oblique projection (Fig. 28–20*A*).

Muscular ventricular septal defects are remote from both the aorta and tricuspid valve. The separation from the tricuspid valve is an important feature in recognizing the location of muscular ventricular septal defect in patients with double-outlet right ventricle. Muscular ventricular septal defects are also well demonstrated with left ventriculography obtained in the long axial oblique view (see Figs. 28–13 and 28–14). Multiple muscular ventricular septal defects may be present, most of which are in the trabecular septum (Fig. 28–20*B*).

A ventricular septal defect related to both semilunar valves is called juxta-arterial. The roof of the defect is formed by the semilunar valves, and the inferior border is formed by muscular structures. Juxta-arterial defects are best seen in the elongated RAO view, in which the defect appears immediately beneath the right and left coronary cusps over the left contour of the left ventricle (Fig. 28–20*C*). Juxta-arterial defects are not as clearly seen in the long axial oblique view because they are obscured by the ventricular outflow tract.

ATRIOVENTRICULAR SEPTAL DEFECT

Atrioventricular septal defects (see Chapter 35) have had several names in the past, including endocardial cush-

ion defect, ostium primum defect, atrioventricular canal defect, and persistent atrioventricular canal. As shown by Becker and Anderson,[13] the pathognomonic feature of this group of malformations is a defect in the atrioventricular septum. Piccoli and his colleagues[78] have classified atrioventricular septal defects into those with a common atrioventricular orifice (complete defects) and those with partitioned right and left annuli (partial defects). The complete form of atrioventricular septal defect is frequently encountered in the first month of life. It may be present as an isolated entity or coexist with a wide spectrum of other congenital cardiac defects, such as tetralogy of Fallot[74] and double-outlet right ventricle.[92]

There is extensive literature on the angiographic morphology of atrioventricular septal defect.[10,86,87] Selective left ventriculography is essential for accurate diagnosis. Most of the earlier literature referred to the angiographic features apparent in frontal and lateral projections in which a typical elongated, narrowed, left ventricular outflow tract known as the "gooseneck" deformity is demonstrated.[15] However, the morphology and classification of the atrioventricular septal defect into partial and complete forms is more easily accomplished by axial angiography.[87] A selective left ventriculogram obtained in the four-chamber projection demonstrates the deficiency of the atrioventricular septum, the common atrioventricular orifice, the morphology of the common atrioventricular valve, and the extent of the interventricular communication (Fig. 28–21). The deficiency of the atrioventricular septum and the consequent elongation and narrowing of the left ventricular outflow tract (the "gooseneck" deformity as seen in frontal projection) can be observed in the elongated RAO view. The four-chamber projection will also accurately demonstrate

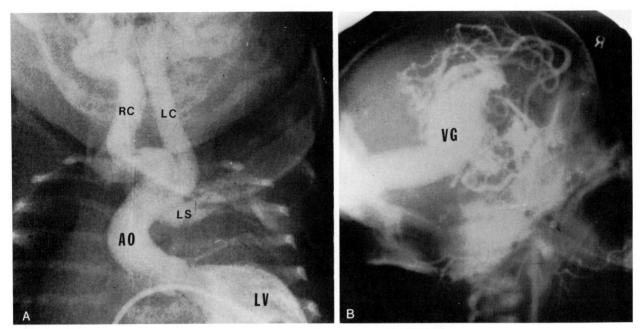

Figure 28-22. Aneurysm of vein of Galen. *A,* Left ventriculogram in AP view. The branches of the aortic arch are huge. *B,* Lateral view of right innominate arteriogram demonstrates opacification of the large aneurysm of vein of Galen. AO = aorta; LC = left carotid artery; LS = left subclavian artery; LV = left ventricle; RC = right carotid artery; VG = vein of Galen.

the presence and severity of atrioventricular valve incompetence and communication from the left ventricle to the right atrium.

The other forms of cardiac shunts include patent ductus arteriosus, atrial septal defect, aortopulmonary window, and arteriovenous malformations such as aneurysm of the vein of Galen. Isolated atrial septal defect rarely presents in neonatal life. Patent ductus arteriosus does not often require angiographic demonstration. An unsuspected aneurysm of the vein of Galen may be recognized during left ventriculography by visualization of enlarged brachiocephalic vessels and rapid opacification of the internal jugular veins as well as the superior vena cava (Fig. 28-22*A*). However, cerebral angiography is required for proper evaluation (Fig. 28-22*B*).

Stenoses

Stenosis of the atrioventricular valves is uncommon. Stenosis of the semilunar valves or the great arteries can occur either on the right or the left side.

PULMONARY VALVULAR STENOSIS

If a newborn presents with pulmonary valvular stenosis (see Chapter 45), the stenosis usually is very severe and critical. The tricuspid valve may or may not be competent. The size of the right ventricular chamber depends on the competency of the tricuspid valve. If the tricuspid valve is incompetent, the ventricular chamber tends to be larger. The lateral view of the selective right ventriculogram is the best projection to demonstrate the morphology of the pulmonic valve (Fig. 28-23). In the newborn period the stenosis is usually secondary to commissural fusion, resulting in a dome-shaped valve. The stenotic valve leaflets

are mildly thickened and smooth and dome with systole but return to normal in diastole. The fused leaflets curl to the apex of the dome in systole, and a jet of contrast material is seen passing across the valve.[22] If the leaflets do not move between systole and diastole, a dysplastic valve should be suspected,[57] but pulmonary valve dysplasia is uncommon in the neonatal period. The main pulmonary artery and the left pulmonary artery may be dilated in critical valvular pulmonary stenosis. However, main pulmonary artery dilatation is less pronounced in severe pulmonary valvular stenosis in the newborn period than in the older child.

PULMONARY VALVULAR ATRESIA WITH INTACT VENTRICULAR SEPTUM

Pulmonary valvular atresia with intact ventricular septum (see Chapter 45) accounts for approximately 30 per cent of all neonates presenting with cyanotic congenital heart disease.[45] As in critical pulmonary stenosis in the newborn period, the extent of right ventricular hypoplasia in pulmonary valvular atresia with intact ventricular septum will depend on competency of the tricuspid valve. A lateral view of the right ventriculogram is again an ideal projection to demonstrate the extent of atresia of the right ventricular outflow tract. If the tricuspid valve is competent, the pressure in the right ventricle can be suprasystemic and persistent fistulous communications between the right ventricular endomyocardium and the coronary arterial circulation can provide a source of egress of blood from the blind right ventricle.[49] Selective right ventriculography elegantly demonstrates opacification of the sinusoids as well as retrograde filling of the coronary arteries (Fig. 28-24). In patients with pulmonary valvular atresia and intact ventricular septum, left ventriculography or aortog-

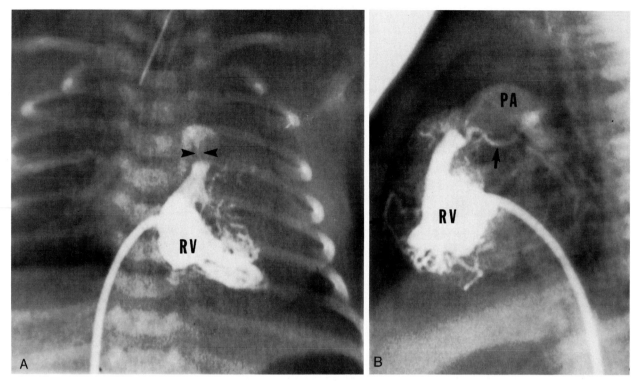

Figure 28–23. Critical pulmonary valvular stenosis. Right ventriculogram. *A*, AP view. *B*, Lateral projection. Right ventricle is small and hypertrophied. A small jet of contrast medium (arrowheads) is identified opacifying the pulmonary artery (compare with Fig. 28–24). The tricuspid valve is competent. There is visualization of myocardial sinusoids (arrows). PA = pulmonary artery; RV = right ventricle.

raphy is necessary to demonstrate the anatomy of the pulmonary arteries, which immediately after birth are perfused by way of the ductus arteriosus.

AORTIC STENOSIS

The stenotic aortic valve (see Chapter 36) may be unicuspid, bicuspid, or tricuspid and associated with varying degrees of commissural fusion. There is an increased incidence of valvular dysplasia when patients with aortic stenosis present in the neonatal period. Selective left ventriculography is the procedure of choice; the aortic valve abnormality can be recognized in any projection. The angiogram in valvular aortic stenosis classically demonstrates doming of the aortic valve with a thin jet of contrast medium entering the aorta (Fig. 28–25). In infants critically ill with aortic stenosis, left ventricular function may be severely depressed, which can result in rather poor opacification of the ascending aorta. An elongated RAO view will demonstrate the left ventricular outflow tract, which is useful in detecting associated subaortic stenosis or ventricular papillary muscle abnormalities, both of which are associated with aortic stenosis if coarctation of the aorta is also present.[69]

COARCTATION OF THE AORTA

Coarctation of the aorta (see Chapter 37) and aortic valvular stenosis can coexist. A bicuspid aortic valve is found in over 70 per cent of patients with aortic coarctation.[14] In a newborn with coarctation of the aorta, there

can be associated hypoplasia of the aortic arch as well as obstructive lesions in the left ventricular outflow tract. Thus, angiographic examination of patients with coarctation should include a left ventriculogram performed in

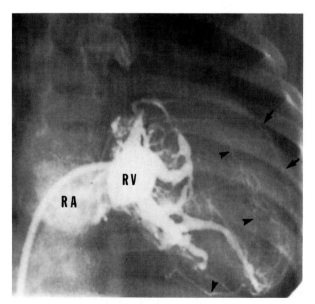

Figure 28–24. Pulmonary atresia with intact ventricular septum. Right ventriculogram in right anterior oblique view. Pulmonary outflow tract and pulmonary valve are atretic. Numerous myocardial sinusoids (arrowheads) are opacified. There is faint visualization of left anterior descending artery (arrows). There is minimal tricuspid regurgitation. RA = right atrium; RV = right ventricle.

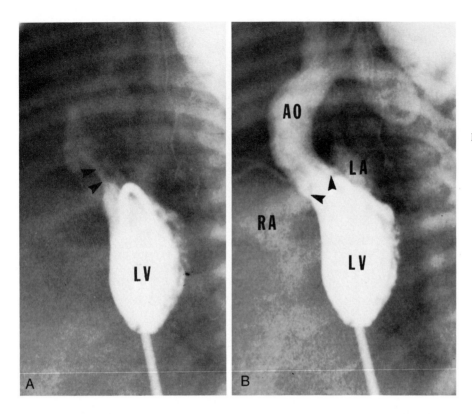

Figure 28–25. Severe aortic valvular stenosis. *A,* Left ventriculogram in long axial oblique view. An early frame. The jet of contrast (arrowheads) through the severely stenotic aortic valve is seen. *B,* Same patient, a later frame from the same angiogram. Thickened aortic valve leaflets are seen (arrowheads). There is mitral regurgitation and opacification of right atrium through the stretched foramen ovale. AO = aorta; LA = left atrium; LV = left ventricle; RA = right atrium.

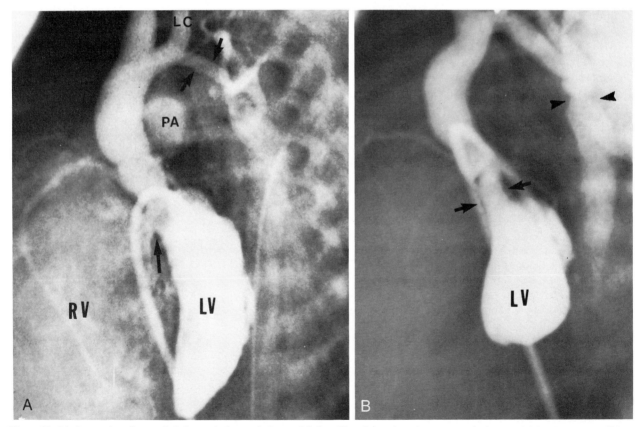

Figure 28–26. Coarctation of aorta. *A,* Left ventriculogram in long axial view. There is a perimembranous ventricular septal defect (arrow) opacifying a large right ventricle. There is severe tubular hypoplasia of aortic arch distal to the left carotid artery (arrows). There is also right-to-left shunt through a patent ductus arteriosus. *B,* Another patient. There is a focal coarctation (arrowheads) distal to left subclavian artery. There is also tunnel-like subaortic stenosis (arrows). LC = left carotid artery; LV = left ventricle; PA = pulmonary artery; RV = right ventricle.

both four-chamber and elongated RAO views. The former will demonstrate the ascending aorta, aortic arch, brachiocephalic vessels, and the extent of the coarctation (Fig. 28–26). The elongated RAO view will demonstrate the left ventricular outflow tract.

INTERRUPTION OF AORTIC ARCH

Interruption of the aortic arch (see Chapter 38) is an uncommon cardiac anomaly. It is rarely present with right aortic arch.[79] It is classified according to the site of interruption.[26] The three types are distal to the left subclavian artery, proximal to the left subclavian artery, and proximal to the left carotid artery. Interruption between the left carotid artery and left subclavian artery is the most common.[82] Aortic arch interruption is frequently associated with ventricular septal defect, patent ductus arteriosus and subaortic stenosis, and aorticopulmonary septal defect.[19]

Angiography in patients with interrupted aortic arch should delineate the anatomy of the aortic arch, the caliber of the brachiocephalic branches, the site of interruption, and the presence of other intracardiac anomalies. Selective left ventriculography performed in the long axial oblique projection will demonstrate the left ventricular outflow tract, the location and size of the ventricular septal defect, and the anatomy of the aortic arch (Fig. 28–27). Supplemental aortography performed in frontal and lateral projections can also be useful.

Combination of Anomalies

Quite frequently in the symptomatic newborn a combination of anomalies exists as a complex congenital malformation. A typical example is severe tetralogy of Fallot (Fig. 28–28) or pulmonary atresia with ventricular septal defect, both of which have large ventricular septal defect, severe obstruction to the right ventricular outflow tract, and biventricular origin of the aorta (see Chapter 46). As a result of right ventricular outflow tract obstruction, such patients present with right-to-left intracardiac shunt and cyanosis.

SUMMARY

Systematic angiographic analysis of the various segments of the heart and its great vessels provides a complete description of the anatomic abnormalities underlying the disrupted physiology with which the symptomatic neonate with congenital heart disease presents. We believe that nomenclature and terminology must be kept as descriptive as possible to help clinicians and angiographers understand and communicate about complex congenital heart disease. With progressive advancements in technology and surgical techniques, complete corrective surgery is becoming possible in a wider variety of complex malformations. Angiography is an important step in completing the assessment of congenital cardiac malformations so that appropriate surgical therapy can be planned.

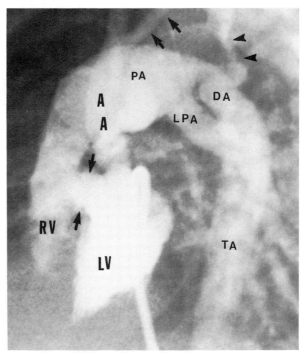

Figure 28–27. Interruption of aortic arch. Left ventriculogram in long axial oblique view. There is a large perimembranous ventricular septal defect (lower arrows). Concordant ventriculoarterial connection is present. Aorta is interrupted after the origin of the left carotid artery (upper arrows). The descending aorta is opacified through the patent ductus arteriosus. The left subclavian artery (arrowheads) arises from descending aorta. Ascending aorta is smaller than pulmonary artery. AA = ascending aorta; DA = patent ductus arteriosus; LPA = left pulmonary artery; LV = left ventricle; PA = pulmonary trunk; RV = right ventricle; TA = descending thoracic aorta.

References

1. Abrams HL (1959): An approach to biplane cineangiocardiography: 3 early clinical observations. Radiology 73:531–538.
2. Alwens W, Frick A (1914): Ueber die Lokalisation von Luftembolien in der Lunge. Frankfurt Z Pathol 15:315:326.
3. Anderson RH, Becker AE, Tynan M, Macartney J, Rigby ML, Wilkinson JL (1984): The univentricular atrioventricular connection: Getting to the root of a thorny problem. Am J Cardiol 54:822–828.
4. Anderson RH, Macartney FJ, Shinebourne EA, Tynan M (1978): Atrioventricular connections. In Anderson RH, Shinebourne EA (eds): Pediatric Cardiology 1977. London, Churchill Livingstone, pp 27–35.
5. Anderson RH, Macartney FJ, Shinebourne EA, Tynan M (1978): Definition of cardiac chambers. In Anderson RH, Shinebourne EA (eds): Pediatric Cardiology 1977. London, Churchill Livingstone, pp 5–15.
6. Arciniegas JG, Soto B, Coghlan HC, Bargeron LM (1981): Congenital heart malformations: Sequential angiographic analysis. AJR 137:673–681.
7. Baltaxe HA, Mooring P, Kugler J, Pinsky W, Chu WK (1983): Comparative hemodynamic effect of metrizamide and Renografin-76 in infants with congenital heart disease. AJR 140:1097–1101.
8. Bargeron LM (1979): Cineangiography in the neonate. In Godman JM, Marquis RM (eds): Paediatric Cardiology. New York, Churchill Livingstone, vol 2, pp 119–133.
9. Bargeron LM, Elliott LP, Soto B, Bream PR, Curry GC (1977): Axial cineangiography in congenital heart disease: I. Concept, technical and anatomic considerations. Radiology 56:1075–1083.

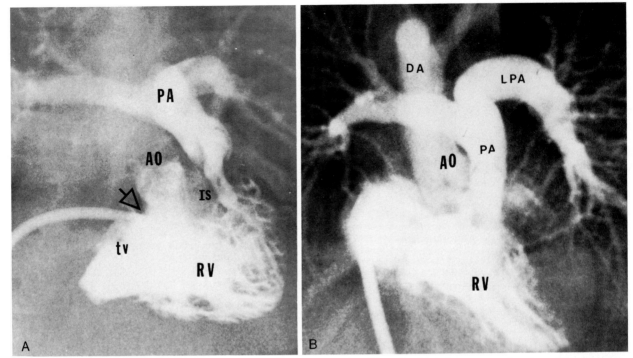

Figure 28–28. Tetralogy of Fallot. *A,* Right ventriculogram in elongated right anterior oblique view. Typical appearance of tetralogy of Fallot. The infundibular septum is deviated anteriorly and to the left, leading to outflow tract obstruction. Pulmonary valve is bicuspid and stenotic. A perimembranous ventricular septal defect (arrow) opacifies the aorta. Notice that in this view the main pulmonary artery and the origin of the left pulmonary artery are superimposed. *B,* Same patient. Right ventriculogram in "sitting-up" view (frontal projection with 20 to 25 degrees cranial angulation). Notice that the origins of right and left pulmonary arteries are clearly displayed. There is a right aortic arch. AO = aorta; DA = descending aorta; IS = infundibular septum; LPA = left pulmonary artery; PA = pulmonary artery; RV = right ventricle; TV = tricuspid valve.

10. Baron MG (1968): Endocardial cushion defect. Radiol Clin North Am 6:343–360.

11. Baron MG (1971): Radiologic notes in cardiology: Angiographic differentiation between tetralogy of Fallot and double-outlet right ventricle: Relationships of the mitral and aortic valves. Circulation 43:451–455.

12. Baron MG, Wolf BS, Steinfeld L, Gordon AJ (1963): Left ventricular angiocardiography in the study of ventricular septal defects. Radiology 81:223–235.

13. Becker AE, Anderson RH (1982): Atrioventricular septal defects: What's in a name? J Thorac Cardiovasc Surg 83:461–469.

14. Becker AE, Becker MJ, Edwards JE (1970): Anomalies associated with coarctation of aorta: Particular reference to infancy. Circulation 41:1067–1074.

15. Bleiden LC, Randall PA, Casteneda AR, Lucas RV Jr, Edwards JE (1974): The "goose neck" of the endocardial cushion defect: Anatomic basis. Chest 65:13–17.

16. Brandt PWT (1984): Axially angled angiocardiography. Cardiovasc Intervent Radiol 7:166–169.

17. Brandt PWT, Calder AL (1977): Cardiac connections: The segmental approach to radiologic diagnosis in congenital heart disease. Curr Probl Diagn Radiol 7(3).

18. Brandt PWT, Clarkson PM, Neutze JM, Barratt-Boyes BG (1972): Left ventricular cineangiocardiography in endocardial cushion defect (persistent common atrioventricular canal). Aust Radiol 16:367–376.

19. Braunlin E, Peoples WM, Freedom RM, Fyler DC, Goldblatt A, Edwards JE (1982): Interruption of the aortic arch with aortico-pulmonary septal defect. Pediatr Cardiol 3:329–335.

20. Carlsson EC, Ruldolph A, Stanger P, Teitel D, Weber W, Yoshida H (1985): Pediatric angiocardiography with iohexol. Invest Radiol 20:S75–S78.

21. Castaneda-Zuniga WR, Bass JL, Lock JE (1981): Selective opacification of arteries with balloon-occlusion angiography. Radiology 138:727–729.

22. Castaneda-Zuniga WR, Formanek A, Amplatz K (1978): Radiologic diagnosis of different types of pulmonary stenoses. Cardiovasc Intervent Radiol 1:45–57.

23. Castellanos A, Pereiras R (1939): Countercurrent aortography. Rev Cubana Cardiol 2:187–203.

24. Castellanos A, Pereiras R, Garcia A (1937): La angiocardiografia radio-opaqua. Arch Soc Habana 31:523–596.

25. Ceballos R, Soto B, Kirklin JW, Bargeron LM (1983): Truncus arteriosus: An anatomical-angiographic study. Br Heart J 49:589–599.

26. Celoria GC, Patton RB (1959): Congenital absence of the aortic arch. Am Heart J 58:407–413.

27. Chavez I, Dorvecker N, Celis A (1947): Direct intracardiac angiography: Its diagnostic value. Am Heart J 33:560–593.

28. Cournand A, Ranges HA (1941): Catheterization of the right auricle in man. Proc Soc Exp Biol Med 46:462.

29. Crupi G, Macartney FJ, Anderson RH (1977): Persistent truncus arteriosus: A study of 66 autopsy cases with special reference to definition and morphogenesis. Am J Cardiol 40:569–578.

30. Davis GD, Fulton RE, Ritter DG, Mair DD, McGoon DC (1978): Congenital pulmonary atresia with ventricular septal defect: Angiographic and surgical correlates. Radiology 128:133–144.

31. Delisle G, Ando M, Calder AL, Zuberbuhler JR, Rochenmacher S, Alday LE, Mangini O, Van Praagh SV, Van Praagh RV (1976): Total anomalous pulmonary venous connection: Report of 93 autopsied cases with emphasis on diagnostic and surgical considerations. Am Heart J 91:99–122.

32. Dickinson DF, Wilson N, Partridge JB (1984): Digital subtraction angiography in infants and children with congenital heart disease. Br Heart J 51:485–491.

33. Dieffenbach J (1832): Physiologisch-Chirurgisch Beobachtigen bie Cholera-Kranken. Cholera Arch 1:86.

34. DiSessa TG, Zednikove M, Hiraishi S, Jarmakani JM, Higgins CB, Friedman WF (1983): The cardiovascular effects of metrizamide in infants. Radiology 148:687–691.

35. Doby T (1976): Development of Angiography and Cardiovascular Catheterization. Littleton, MA, Publishing Sciences Group, p 198.
36. Edwards JE, Burchell HB (1949): Congenital tricuspid atresia: A classification. Med Clin North Am 33:1177–1196.
37. Edwards JE, Carey LS, Neufeld HN, Lester RC (1965): Congenital Heart Disease. Philadelphia, WB Saunders.
38. Fellows KE Jr, Keane JF, Freed MD (1977): Angled views in cineangiocardiography of congenital heart disease. Circulation 56:485–490.
39. Forssmann W (1929): Die Sondierung des rechten Herzens. Klin Wochenschr 32:1503–1505.
40. Fredzell G, Lind J, Ohlson E, Wegelius C (1950): Direct serial roentgenography in two planes simultaneously at 0.09-second intervals: Physiological aspect of roentgen diagnosis; apparatus and its application to angiocardiography. AJR 63:548–558.
41. Freedom RM (1983): Axial angiocardiography in the critically ill infant. Cardiol Clin 1:387–409.
42. Freedom RM, Culham JAG, Moes CAF (1984): Angiocardiography of Congenital Heart Disease. New York, Macmillan, pp 7–9.
43. Freedom RM, Culham JAG, Moes CAF (1984): Complete transposition of great arteries. In Angiocardiography of Congenital Heart Disease. New York, Macmillan, pp 514–532.
44. Freedom RM, Culham JAG, Moes CAF (1984): Congenitally corrected transposition of the great arteries. In Angiocardiography of Congenital Heart Disease. New York, Macmillan, pp 536–552.
45. Freedom RM, Culham JAG, Moes CAF (1984): Pulmonary atresia and intact ventricular septum. In Angiocardiography of Congenital Heart Disease. New York, Macmillan, pp 231–250.
46. Freedom RM, Culham JAG, Rowe RD (1977): Angiocardiography of subaortic obstruction in infancy. AJR 129:813–824.
47. Freedom RM, Culham JAG, Rowe RD (1977): Aortic atresia with normal left ventricle: Distinctive angiocardiographic findings. Cathet Cardiovasc Diagn 3:283–295.
48. Freedom RM, Culham JAG, Rowe RD (1978): The criss-cross and superoinferior ventricular heart: An angiocardiographic study. Am J Cardiol 42:620–628.
49. Freedom RM, Harrington DP (1974): Contribution of intramyocardial sinusoids in pulmonary atresia and intact ventricular septum to a right-sided circular shunt. Br Heart J 36:1061–1065.
50. Gidlund AS (1949): A new apparatus for direct cineroentgenology. Acta Radiol 32:81–88.
51. Goor DA, Lillehei CW, Rees R, Edwards JE (1970): Isolated ventricular septal defect. Developmental basis for various types and presentation of classification. Chest 58:468–482.
52. Haschek E, Lindenthal TO (1896): Ein Beitrag zur praktischen Vorwerthung der photographic nach Rontgen. Wien Klin Wochenschr 9:63–64.
53. Hellstrom M, Jacobsson B, Eriksson BO, Jagenburg R (1983): Nonionic contrast media in cardioangiography in infants. A comparison of iohexol and metrizamide. Acta Radiol 366 (Suppl):126–133.
54. Higgins CB (1984): Overview of cardiovascular effects of contrast media: Comparison of ionic and nonionic media. Invest Radiol 19:S187–S189.
55. Higgins CB, DiSessa T, Kirkpatrick SE, Ti CC, Edwards DK, Friedman WF, Kelley MJ, Kurlinski J (1980): Assessment of patent ductus arteriosus in pre-term infants by single lateral film aortography. Radiology 135:641–646.
56. Janker R (1936): Roentgen cinematography. AJR 36:384–390.
57. Jeffery RF, Moller JH, Amplatz K (1972): The dysplastic pulmonary valve: A new roentgenographic entity. AJR 114:322–338.
58. Jonsson G, Broden B, Karnell J (1949): Selective angiocardiography. Acta Radiol 32:486–497.
59. Kattan K (1970): Angled view in pulmonary angiography. Radiology 94:79–82.
60. Kjellberg SR, Mannheimer E, Rudhe U, Jonsson B (1959): Diagnosis of Congenital Heart Disease, 2nd ed. Chicago, Year Book Medical Publishers.
61. Kruger RA, Riederer SJ (1984): Basic Concepts of Digital Subtraction Angiography. Boston, GK Hall, pp 170–196.
62. Kunnen M, Van Egmond H, VerHarren H, Matthys D, Blanc-Quaert A (1985): Cardioangiography in children with iohexol, ioxaglate and metrizoate. Ann Radiol 28:315–321.
63. Lev M, Liberthson RR, Kirkpatrick JR, Eckner RAO, Arcilla RA (1969): Single (primitive) ventricle. Circulation 39:577–591.
64. Levin AR, Goldberg HL, Borer JS, Rothenberg LN, Nolan FA, Engle MA, Cohen B, Skelly NT, Carter J (1983): Digital angiography in the pediatric patient with congenital heart disease: Comparison with standard methods. Circulation 68:374–383.
65. Levin AR, Grossman H, Schubert ET, Winchester P, Gilladoga A (1969): Effect of angiocardiography on fluid and electrolyte balance. AJR 105:777–783.
66. Long WA, Lawson EE, Harned HS, Henry GW (1984): Infradiaphragmatic total anomalous pulmonary venous drainage: New diagnostic, physiologic and surgical considerations. Am J Perinatol 1:227–234.
67. Lucas RV, Anderson RC, Amplatz K, Adams P, Edwards JE (1963): Congenital causes of pulmonary venous obstruction. Pediatr Clin North Am 10:781–834.
68. Lurie PR, Armer RM, Klatte EC (1963): Percutaneous guide wire catheterization: Diagnosis and therapy. Am J Dis Child 106:103–110.
69. Macartney FM, Bain HH, Ionescu MI, Deverall PB, Olive S (1976): Angiocardiographic/pathologic correlations in congenital mitral valve anomalies. Euro J Cardiol 4:191–211.
70. MacIntyre J (1897): X-ray records for the cinematograph. Arch Clin Skiagraphy 1:37.
71. Milo S, Siew YH, Macartney FJ, Wilkinson JL (1979): Straddling and overriding atrioventricular valves: Morphology and classification. Am J Cardiol 44:1122–1134.
72. Moniz E, Carvalho L, Lima PA (1931): Angiopneumographie. Presse Med 39:996–999.
73. Moodie DS (1985): Assessing cardiac anatomy with digital subtraction angiography. J Am Col Cardiol 5:48S–54S.
74. Nath PH, Soto B, Bini RM, Bargeron LM, Pacifico AD (1984): Tetralogy of Fallot with atrioventricular canal. J Thorac Cardiovasc Surg 87:421–430.
75. Norwood WI, Stellin GJ (1981): Aortic atresia with interrupted aortic arch: Reparative operation. J Thorac Cardiovasc Surg 81:239–244.
76. Odman P (1959): The radiopaque polyethylene catheter. Acta Radiol 52:52–64.
77. Paster SB, Swensson RE, Uabek SM (1977): Total anomalous pulmonary venous connection. Pediatr Radiol 6:132–140.
78. Piccoli GP, Gerlis LM, Wilkinson JL, Lozsadi K, Macartney FJ, Anderson RH (1979): Morphology and classification of atrioventricular defects. Br Heart J 42:621–632.
79. Pierpont MEN, Zollikofer CL, Moller JH, Edwards JE (1982): Interruption of the aortic arch with right descending aorta: A rare condition and a cause of bronchial compression. Pediatr Cardiol 2:153–159.
80. Puyau FA, Burko H (1966): The tilted left anterior oblique position in the study of congenital cardiac anomalies. Radiology 87:1069–1075.
81. Rajani M, Shrivastava S, Tandon R, Bhargava S (1980): Right ventricular cineangiography in tetralogy of Fallot. Cardiovasc Intervent Radiol 3:13–17.
82. Reardon JM, Hallman GL, Cooley DA (1984): Interrupted aortic arch: Brief review and summary of an eighteen year experience. Texas Heart Instit J 11:250–257.
83. Ruggles HE (1925): X-ray motion pictures of the thorax. A motion picture presented at the Eleventh Annual Meeting of the RSNA, Cleveland, Ohio, December 7–11.
84. Santamaria H, Soto B, Ceballos R, Bargeron LM, Coghlan HC, Kirklin JW (1983): Angiographic differentiation of types of ventricular septal defects. AJR 141:273–281.
85. Seldinger SI (1953): Catheter replacement of the needle in percutaneous arteriography: A new technique. Acta Radiol 39:368–376.
86. Somerville J, Jefferson K (1968): Left ventricular angiocardiography in atrioventricular defects. Br Heart J 30:446–457.
87. Soto B, Bargeron LM Jr, Pacifico AD, Vanini V, Kirklin JW (1981): Angiography of atrioventricular canal defects. Am J Cardiol 48:492–499.
88. Soto B, Becker AE, Moulaert AJ, Lie JT, Anderson RH (1980): Classification of ventricular septal defects. Br Heart J 43:332–343.
89. Soto B, Bertranou GE, Souza A, Bargeron LM (1979): Angiographic study of univentricular heart of right ventricular type. Circulation 60:1325–1334.

90. Soto B, Coghlan CH, Bargeron LM (1984): Present status of axially angled angiocardiography. Cardiovasc Intervent Radiol 7:156–165.

91. Sovak M, Ranganathan R, Lang JG, Lasser EC (1978): Concepts in design of improved intravascular contrast agents. Ann Radiol 21:283–289.

92. Sridaromont S, Feldt RH, Ritter DG (1975): Double-outlet right ventricle associated with persistent common atrioventricular canal. Circulation 52:933–942.

93. Sridaromont S, Feldt RH, Ritter DG, Davis GD, Edwards JE (1976): Double outlet right ventricle: Hemodynamic and anatomic correlations. Am J Cardiol 38:85–93.

94. Sridaromont S, Ritter DG, Feldt RH, Davis GD, Edwards JE (1978): Double-outlet right ventricle: Anatomic and angiocardiographic correlations. Mayo Clin Proc 53:555–577.

95. Stewart RW, Kirklin JW, Pacifico AD, Blackstone EH, Bargeron LM (1979): Repair of double-outlet right ventricle. J Thorac Cardiovasc Surg 78:502–514.

96. Swan HJC, Ganz W, Forrester J, Marcus H, Diamond G, Chonette D (1970): Catheterization of the heart in man with use of a flow directed balloon-tipped catheter. New Engl J Med 283:447–451.

97. Tandon R, Becker AE, Moller JH, Edwards JE (1974): Double inlet left ventricle. Br Heart J 36:747–759.

98. Thies WR, Soto B, Diethelm E, Bargeron LM, Pacifico AD (1985): Angiographic anatomy of hearts with one ventricular chamber: The true single ventricle. Am J Cardiol 55:1363–1366.

99. Tonkin ILD (1985): Digital subtraction angiography in congenital heart disease. Semin Roentgenol 20:283–289.

100. Tynan MF, Becker AE, Macartney FJ, Quero-Jimenez M, Shinebourne EA, Anderson RH (1979): Nomenclature and classification of congenital heart disease. Br Heart J 41:544–553.

101. Van Mierop LHS, Wiglesworth FW (1962): Isomerism of the cardiac atria in the asplenia syndrome. Lab Invest 2:1303–1315.

102. Van Praagh R, David I, Gordon D, Wright GB, Van Praagh S (1981): Ventricular diagnosis and designation. In Goodman MJ, Marquis RM (eds): Paediatric Cardiology. Edinburgh, Churchill Livingstone, vol 4.

29 PNEUMOPERICARDIUM

Walker A. Long

Pneumopericardium is the most common cause of cardiac tamponade in the newborn period but remains the least common form of pulmonary air leak. Pneumopericardium occurs in isolation but most frequently in association with other forms of air leak, including pneumothorax, pneumomediastinum, and interstitial emphysema. Neonatal pneumopericardium nearly always occurs as a complication of positive pressure ventilation; most cases occur in premature infants with severe hyaline membrane disease (HMD) who require vigorous mechanical ventilation. Pneumopericardium also occurs in term infants hyperventilated for meconium aspiration and for persistent pulmonary hypertension of the newborn syndrome (PPHNS). Even with prompt diagnosis and appropriate treatment, the outcomes of newborns who develop pneumopericardium are often poor. The purpose of this chapter is to review the diagnosis and management of neonatal pneumopericardium, a rare but life-threatening event, with the hope that the poor outcomes of most infants with this disorder can be improved by earlier recognition and consistent treatment.

HISTORICAL PERSPECTIVE

Pneumopericardium had been recognized at autopsy for many years, but whether air accumulated in the pericardial space during life (rather than as a postmortem artifact) remained unknown until Bricheteau's clinical description of pneumopericardium in 1844.[8] Chest radiographic diagnosis of pneumopericardium was described by Wenckebach in 1910.[82]

Pneumopericardium has been reported to occur in association with a great variety of disorders.[20] A 1980 French review of pneumopericardium in all age groups collected 220 reported cases;[5] a 1984 American review collected 252 reported cases.[20] Some of the more unusual causes of pneumopericardium include anerobic pericardial infection,[7] blunt chest trauma,[56] endotracheal laser surgery,[78] foreign body aspiration,[75] and marihuana smoking.[4] Pediatric pneumopericardium was reported rarely prior to 1969,[19,26,48,59] although neonatal pneumothorax was recognized early.[22,33,49] The advent of mechanical ventilation for treatment of HMD in the late 1960s greatly increased the frequency of neonatal pneumopericardium, and reports on neonatal cases became commonplace after 1968.[2,5,6,10,12,13,15,17,22,24,26,27,32,34–36,40–47,51–54,57,58,63,66,77,80,81,83] A 1985 review of English language reports of neonatal pneumopericardium collected 127 cases.[34]

DIAGNOSIS

Epidemiology

The incidence of pneumopericardium among neonates admitted to intensive care units appears to be approximately 1.3 per cent; Burt and Lester identified 50 cases among 3841 admissions over a 2-year period.[10] Neonatal pneumopericardium appears to be substantially more common in males than in females,[10,30,41] probably because hyaline membrane disease tends to be more severe in males. In the largest series from a single institution, 35 of 50 neonates with pneumopericardium were male;[10] in the second largest series from a single institution, 35 of 47 neonates were male.[27] Rarely, neonatal pneumopericardium occurs spontaneously[36] or during ventilation with continuous positive airway pressure (CPAP),[2] but the overwhelming majority of neonates who develop pneumopericardium are on mechanical ventilation at the time.[34] Glenski and Hall found that 121 of 127 infants with neonatal pneumopericardium reported through 1984 were receiving positive pressure ventilation at the time pneumopericardium occurred.[34] In their own 19 cases, Glenski and Hall found that mean gestational age was 32 weeks, mean birthweight was 1720 g, and mean age at occurrence was 59 hours.[34]

Table 29–1. FACTORS PREDISPOSING TO NEONATAL PNEUMOPERICARDIUM*

Factor	Number	Per Cent
Intubation	50/50	100
Endotracheal tube misplacement	14/50	28
Paracardiac chest tube placement	8/50	16
Pericardial aspiration after clinical diagnosis	7/50	14
CPR with intracardiac drugs	5/50	10
Mediastinal aspiration	1/50	2
Chest surgery	1/50	2

*Adapted from Burt TB, Lester PD (1982): Neonatal pneumopericardium. Radiology 142:81–84.

Table 29–2. SIGNS OF NEONATAL PNEUMOPERICARDIUM

Sign	Burt and Lester*		Emery et al†	
	Number	Per Cent	Number	Per Cent
Bradycardia	26/50	52	35/47	74
Cyanosis	21/50	42	36/47	76
Asymptomatic or not recorded	11/50	22	5/47	11
Muffled heart sounds	10/50	20	18/24‡	75
Hypotension	5/50	10	41/47	88
Cardiac collapse	4/50	8	42/47	89
Apnea	1/50	2	0/47	0

*Adapted from Burt TB, Lester PD (1982): Neonatal pneumopericardium. Radiology 142:81–84.
†Adapted from Emery RW, Foker J, Thompson TR (1984): Neonatal pneumopericardium: A surgical emergency. Ann Thorac Surg 37:128–132.
‡Heart sounds at the time of pneumopericardium were recorded in only 24 of 47 patients.

History

Pneumopericardium should be suspected in any neonate whose condition suddenly deteriorates. Although sudden cardiovascular collapse in the neonatal intensive care unit most commonly follows intraventricular hemorrhage or pneumothorax, pneumopericardium should always be considered, particularly during vigorous mechanical ventilation of premature infants. Glenski and Hall found that mean airway pressure (17 cm), peak inspiratory pressure (32 cm), and inspiratory time (0.74 second) just before the occurrence of pneumopericardium were significantly elevated compared with values 6 hours previously.[34] Except for intubation, the most common factor predisposing to neonatal pneumopericardium in Hall and Lester's study was abnormal endotracheal tube placement (Table 29–1). The diagnosis of symptomatic neonatal pneumopericardium is usually made only after chest radiography but really should be made at the bedside in most cases. Asymptomatic neonatal pneumopericardium is likely to be diagnosed only by incidental chest radiography.

Physical Examination

Symptomatic isolated neonatal pneumopericardium is readily diagnosed clinically. The findings are those of cardiac tamponade. Initially, the neonate with symptomatic pneumoperiardium has an elevated pulse and respiratory rate, and his or her blood pressure is low. Pulses are weak, and despite assertions to the contrary,[67] pulsus paradoxus is sometimes observed.[46] As pericardial distention progresses, tachycardia quickly changes to bradycardia. As demonstrated in Table 29–2, typically neonates with tension pneumopericardium exhibit hypotension, cyanosis, and bradycardia. Of more importance diagnostically, heart sounds are diminished in intensity in many patients.

Heart Rate

As demonstrated by the observations of both Emery et al[27] and Burt and Lester,[10] many neonates with pneumopericardium exhibit bradycardia by the time they are recognized clinically (Table 29–2). However despite assertions by two different groups[27,41] that tachycardia indicates pneumothorax and bradycardia indicates pneumopericardium, heart rate is not useful in differentiating pneumopericardium from pneumothorax. Tachycardia is apparently rare by the time neonatal pneumopericardium and neonatal pneumothorax become symptomatic and are recognized clinically, but tachycardia has been reported in both.[46,60] More commonly, bradycardia is reported during both neonatal pneumopericardium[27,41] and pneumothorax.[60] Ogatta et al studied 46 infants with pneumothorax, and in only two infants was heart rate increased; 44 infants exhibited reductions in heart rate.[60] Thus, bradycardia is not useful in distinguishing pneumopericardium from pneumothorax.

Heart Sounds and Breath Sounds

The key to bedside recognition of pneumopericardium is conscious comparison of breath sounds and heart sounds. In pneumopericardium, unlike pneumothorax, *breath sounds are normal*, and *heart sounds are either muffled or distant*,[10,11,27,46] or *quite commonly absent*.[52,83] Hamman sign (a pericardial crunch or knock)[38] can sometimes be detected, as can precordial tympany.[52]

A characteristic murmur coincident with heartbeat was described by Bricheteau in the original description of pneumopericardium;[8] in the review of 252 patients by Cummings et al,[20] this murmur (termed *bruit de moulin* or noise of the millwheel) was found in 52 of 159 patients in whom auscultatory findings were recorded. Bruit de moulin has been observed in neonates with pneumopericardium.[35] However, the bruit de moulin is uncommon unless both fluid and air are present in the pericardium.[20]

Chest Radiograph

As mentioned earlier, Wenckebach described radiographic recognition of pneumopericardium in 1910.[82]

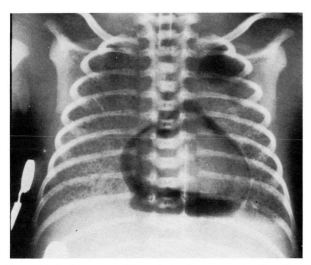

Figure 29–1. Demonstrated is an isolated pneumopericardium in an intubated infant mechanically ventilated for hyaline membrane disease. The endotracheal tube and umbilical arterial catheter are seen.

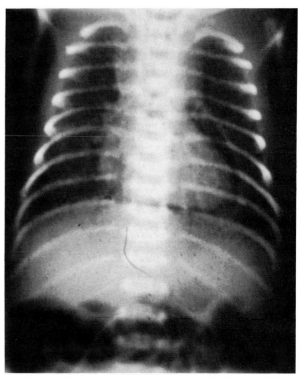

Figure 29–2. Demonstrated is left paracardiac air in an intubated infant mechanically ventilated for hyaline membrane disease. The left paracardiac air could be either a pneumomediastinum, a medial pneumothorax, or a pneumopericardium. The endotracheal tube and umbilical arterial catheter are seen.

Recognition of neonatal pneumopericardium on chest radiograph is usually straightforward; when air surrounds the entire heart, the diagnosis of pneumopericardium is easy (Fig. 29–1). Even when air does not surround the entire heart, the presence of air beneath the heart is virtually diagnostic of pneumopericardium, for pneumomediastinum and pneumothorax cause air beneath the heart only when bilateral tension or central pneumothoraces are present.[10,77] However, when only paracardiac air is present (Fig. 29–2), as is common when the pneumopericardium is small and as yet asymptomatic, distinguishing pneumopericardium from pneumomediastinum or medial pneumothorax can be more difficult.[21] Decubitus views can be quite helpful, for mediastinal air does not move with changes in patient position, while both pleural[21] and pericardial[10,21] air do. Thus a collection of left-sided paracardiac air that is a left pneumomediastinum will not move in any position (Fig. 29–3A), but a collection of left-sided paracardiac air that is a left medial pneumothorax will move to the left lateral chest wall when the patient is placed in the right decubitus position (Fig. 29–3B), and a collection of left-sided paracardiac air that is a left pneumopericardium will move to the right pericardium when the patient is placed in the left decubitus position (Fig. 29–3C).

In the majority of infants with pneumopericardium, other types of pulmonary air leak are also present. Pneumothorax is most common, followed by pulmonary interstitial emphysema, pneumomediastinum, and pneumoperitoneum (Table 29–3). Even when more than one type of air leak is present, differentiation of pneumopericardium from pneumomediastinum and medial pneumothorax is usually possible with decubitus views.

Postmortem Radiography

Radiographs taken after death have demonstrated unsuspected pneumopericardium.[35,71,83] In one study 13 of 29 cases of neonatal pneumopericardium were recognized after death.[67] Prompt postmortem radiography is probably indicated in any neonate who dies suddenly to identify either pneumopericardium,[35,71,83] gas embolism,[35,61] or both.[35]

Electrocardiogram

Maurer et al[55] and Reed and Thomas[64] have documented electrocardiographic changes during progressive tension pneumopericardium in dogs. Reductions in electrocardiographic voltages during tension pneumopericardium have been observed clinically in adults[79] and, despite assertions to the contrary,[52] also in neonates.[67,83] In the review by Cummings et al,[20] the electrocardiogram was described in 29 of 252 patients with pneumopericardium. Tension pneumopericardium was commonly accompanied by low voltages and bradycardia.[20] Obviously, it would be rare for a neonate with cardiovascular collapse to happen to be connected to a 12-lead ECG machine; however, all mechanically ventilated neonates are monitored electrocardiographically. A quick glance at the QRS amplitude on the ECG monitor can indicate whether low voltages are present.

Transillumination

Transillumination is a well-established diagnostic tool in pneumothorax and pneumomediastinum.[43] The diagnosis

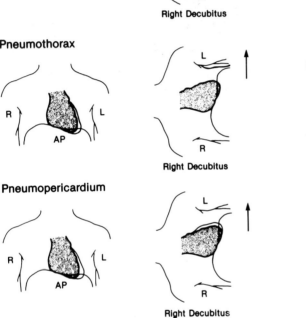

Left Paracardiac Air

Pneumomediastinum

A.

Right Decubitus

Left Decubitus

Pneumothorax

B.

Right Decubitus

Left Decubitus

Pneumopericardium

C.

Right Decubitus

Left Decubitus

Figure 29–3. Schematic representations of the effects of decubitus positioning on left paracardiac air are shown. In *A*, the location of pneumomediastinum does not change with decubitus positioning. In *B*, medial pneumothorax moves to the left lateral chest wall in the right decubitus position. In *C*, pneumopericardium moves to the right heart border in the left decubitus position.

of pneumopericardium can also be made with fiberoptic light.[11,46] Characteristic findings include the presence of transillumination that is limited to the substernal area and that flickers with each heartbeat.

Echocardiogram

Pneumopericardium can also be diagnosed by echocardiography.[25,75] Because air interferes with ultrasound imaging, pericardial air can either interfere with[75] or prevent[25] echocardiographic visualization of the heart. A small pneumopericardium causes heavy echoes in the pericardial space but does permit some ultrasound transmission into the heart.[75] A large pneumopericardium can totally block ultrasound visualization of the heart.[25] If pericardial air is moved into and out of a given echocardiographic

window by cardiac contraction or lung inflation, an "on again, off again" echo picture of the heart is generated in time with the ECG or ventilator.[25] This echo alternans phenomenon is nicely recorded on M-mode echocardiography.[25]

PATHOGENESIS

The mechanisms by which extra-alveolar air enters the pericardium have been the subject of debate since the 1940s. In several experimental studies,[22,40,50,55,62,64] increasing airway pressures have resulted in alveolar rupture and either pneumothorax (if air ruptures through the visceral pleura) or interstitial emphysema and pneumomediastinum (if air ruptures into the pericapillary interstitial space), but pneumopericardium has been observed in only one study.[37] The route by which extra-alveolar air enters the pericardium remains unknown; the pericardial reflections of the pulmonary veins are suspected by some authors.[6,27,28,52] Congenital pericardial defects are rare but can predispose to pneumopericardium in both adults[39] and neonates.[74]

As stated earlier, the great majority of neonatal pneumopericardium occurs as a complication of vigorous mechanical ventilation. Whether inspiratory or expiratory pressures are more important in the pathogenesis has been subject to debate.[17,28,34,52,77,83] However, both Cohen et al[17] and Glenski and Hall[34] have presented convincing evidence that high peak inspiratory pressures (PIP) rather than high positive end-expiratory pressures (PEEP) are the major factor in the pathogenesis of neonatal pneumopericardium. In support of this contention, only two examples of neonatal pneumopericardium during CPAP have been reported.[2,6]

In considering the pathogenesis of neonatal pneumopericardium, it is useful to contrast the pressures in the right and left atria and in the airways in the normal spontaneously breathing premature infant on the one hand (Fig. 29–4A) and in the ill premature infant being mechanically ventilated for respiratory distress syndrome on the other (Fig. 29–4B). Central venous pressures and airway pressures are usually expressed in cm of water (cm H_2O) whereas atrial, ventricular, pulmonary, and systemic arterial pressures are expressed in mm mercury (mmHg).

$$1 \text{ mmHg} = 1.36 \text{ cm } H_2O$$
$$1 \text{ cm } H_2O = 0.74 \text{ mm Hg}$$

Pericardial pressures and pleural pressures remain negative throughout the normal respiratory cycle (−7 cm H_2O inspiration, −2 cm H_2O expiration). During mechanical ventilation, pericardial and pleural pressures can become slightly positive but seldom exceed 1 to 2 cm H_2O. As is evident in Figure 29–4B, both peak inspiratory pressures (PIP) and mean airway pressures (MAP) during vigorous mechanical ventilation markedly exceed cardiac filling pressures (atrial pressures). However, positive end-expiratory pressures (PEEP) during mechanical ventilation rarely exceed cardiac filling pressures. Thus, positive end-expiratory pressures are unlikely to contribute to pneumopericardium-induced cardiac tamponade. On the other hand, even relatively low peak inspiratory pressures are likely to result in catastrophic pneumopericardium if a ball valve communication between the airways and the pericardial space exists (Fig. 29–4B). The majority of cases of neonatal pneumopericardium are associated with very high peak inspiratory pressures because high pressures are required to force the initial rupture of air into the extra-alveolar spaces. High inspiratory pressures may also be required for secondary rupture of extra-alveolar air into the pericardial space, but whether this thesis is correct or not remains unknown. In adult dogs, Decosta has shown that airway pressures of 24.5 to 27.2 cm H_2O (18 to 20 mmHg) are required for air to rupture into the mediastinum.[22] In newborns it appears that there is a correlation between airway pressures required for alveolar rupture

Table 29–3. OTHER FORMS OF AIR LEAK ACCOMPANYING NEONATAL PNEUMOPERICARDIUM

Sign	Burt and Lester*	Per Cent	Emery et al†	Per Cent
Isolated pneumo-pericardium	4/50	8	1/47	2
Pneumothorax	‡		38/47	81
Pulmonary interstitial emphysema	27/50	54	29/47	62
Pneumo-mediastinum	33/50	66	21/47	45
Pneumo-peritoneum	‡		6/47	13

*Adapted from Burt TB, Lester PD (1982): Neonatal pneumopericardium. Radiology 142:81–84.
†Adapted from Emery RW, Foker J, Thompson TR (1984): Neonatal pneumopericardium: A surgical emergency. Ann Thorac Surg 37:128–132.
‡Incidence not provided.

and gestational age: More immature infants require less airway pressure for alveolar rupture to occur.[33]

PHYSIOLOGIC EFFECTS

The physiologic effects of pericardial air, like pericardial fluid, depend on the amount present in the pericardial space[64] and the time course of its accumulation.[55] Since air is compressible, greater volumes of air than liquid can be accommodated in the pericardial space without ill effects. The magnitude of hemodynamic embarrassment caused by progressive pericardial distention (whether by air or fluid) is determined by several factors, including the distensibility of the pericardium, ventricular filling pressures, and cardiac reserve.

Early Tamponade

In essence, few hemodynamic or clinical consequences are found during progressive pericardial distention until pericardial pressure approaches central venous or pulmonary venous pressure, after which ventricular filling is impeded, and stroke volume begins to fall. During the early phases of progressive cardiac tamponade, heart rate increases and pulse pressure narrows as stroke volume falls. As pericardial pressures increase further, diastolic pressures in the four cardiac chambers and pulmonary artery progressively increase. Cardiac output can be maintained only so long as ventricular filling pressures exceed pericardial pressures and heart rate can increase.

Late Tamponade

Further increases in pericardial pressures compress the heart and reduce cardiac volumes. Reduction in cardiac size during tension pneumopericardium is well documented radiographically in neonatal pneumopericardium[10,30,58,81] because progressive distention of the pericardium with air still permits radiographic visualization of actual cardiac

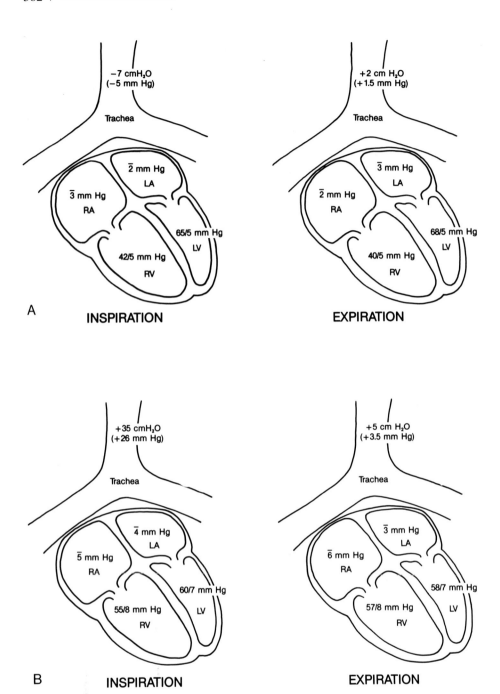

A   INSPIRATION   EXPIRATION

B   INSPIRATION   EXPIRATION

Figure 29–4. *A*, Normal airway and cardiac pressures in a hypothetical spontaneously breathing premature infant are depicted. Note that positive airway pressure occurs only during expiration, and never exceeds ventricular filling pressures. The modest changes in cardiac pressures during the respiratory cycle are due to changes in venous filling or preload. Note that right and left atrial pressures remain approximately equal in both inspiration and expiration; as a result, significant right-to-left atrial shunting does not occur. *B*, Airway and cardiac pressures in a hypothetical premature infant being mechanically ventilated for severe hyaline membrane disease (HMD) are depicted. Note that during mechanical ventilation positive airway pressure exceeds ventricular filling pressures during each inspiration. As in normal breathing, right-sided cardiac pressures rise, and left-sided cardiac pressures fall during mechanical inspiration; and the converse happens during expiration. However, the respiratory changes in right-sided cardiac pressures during mechanical ventilation are due to the direct effects of positive airway pressure rather than indirect effects of changes in preload. Note that during mechanical ventilation for severe HMD right atrial pressures remain slightly higher than left atrial pressures during both inspiration and expiration, promoting right-to-left atrial shunting. Any communication between the airway and the pericardial space during vigorous mechanical ventilation would permit pericardial pressure to rise to inspiratory pressures (which far exceed ventricular filling pressures); cardiac tamponade would result.

size. Marked cardiac compression by pericardial air has also been documented at autopsy.[48] In contrast, when cardiac tamponade is caused by pericardial fluid or blood, all that can be detected radiographically is enlargement of the cardiac silhouette, and cardiac compression cannot be observed. However, the advent of two-dimensional echocardiography now permits accurate determination of cardiac size during fluid-induced cardiac tamponade, and similar reductions in cardiac volumes are present no matter what the cause of the tamponade. Eventually, diastolic pressures in the four cardiac chambers and pulmonary artery equalize, and cardiac output falls. Reductions in cardiac output caused by progressive pericardial distention are

greatly exacerbated if reflex slowing of the heart occurs, because during tamponade cardiac output is virtually entirely heart rate dependent. Reflex bradycardia during cardiac tamponade, blockable by atropine, is well documented in newborn animals,[30] and is present in the great majority of neonates with tension pneumopericardium. In the series of Emery et al,[27] bradycardia was present in 35 of 47 (74 per cent) neonates with pneumopericardium; in the report of Mansfield et al,[52] bradycardia was present in 7 of 8 (87 per cent) infants; in Burt and Lester's series, bradycardia was present in 26 of 50 (52 per cent). However, bradycardia is a relatively late finding in neonatal pneumopericardium.

Rate of Progression

Pericardial distention that develops slowly is better tolerated for two reasons. First, gradual pericardial distention permits more stretching of pericardial tissue; as a result, relatively large air volumes can be accommodated within the pericardial space without large increases in pericardial pressure. Second, gradual pericardial distention permits compensatory increases in intravascular volume; higher ventricular filling pressures raise the threshold pericardial pressure required for cardiac tamponade.[23,64,65]

Neonatal Effects

Pericardial distention is tolerated less well in the newborn period because the newborn has a relatively small cardiac reserve (see Chapter 2). Small pneumopericardiums may have no detectable effects, modest to large pneumopericardiums may be well tolerated if they develop slowly, and sudden large pneumopericardiums may cause immediately fatal cardiac tamponade.

Animal Models of Pneumopericardium

Beck and Isaac[3a] sutured the pericardium to the left thoracic wall in adult dogs and 2 weeks later opened the pericardial space without entering the pleural space. Simply exposing the pericardium to atmospheric pressure reduced cardiac output 36 per cent; thereafter applying −8 cm H_2O pressure restored only 25 per cent of the cardiac output reduction caused by atmospheric pressure.[3a] Application of +8 cm H_2O reduced cardiac output 64 per cent.[3a] Grosfeld et al[37] placed a Foley cather in the right lower lobe bronchus of 15 anesthetized adult cats, and applied 2-minute periods of increasing airway pressure. Pulmonary interstitial emphysema was observed at airway pressures greater than 40 cm H_2O. Pneumomediastinum and pneumothorax were observed at airway pressures greater than 50 cm H_2O. Subcutaneous emphysema and pneumoretroperitoneum were observed at airway pressures greater than 60 cm H_2O. At airway pressures greater than 70 cm H_2O, the animals rapidly deteriorated; pneumopericardium and gas embolism occurred in one third of the animals. Higgins et al[40] injected progressively larger quantities of air (10 to 60 ml) into the pericardiums of five anesthetized puppies 2 days after subxiphoid (extrapleural) placement of pericardial catheters and observed that 20-ml air injections (10 ml/kg) reduced cardiac size on chest radiographs, that 40-ml air injections (20 ml/kg) decreased mean arterial pressure 22 per cent, and that 60-cc air injections (30 ml/kg) caused cardiovascular collapse. Reed and Thomas[64] injected progressively larger quantities of air into the pericardiums of six intact chest anesthetized dogs after placing pericardial catheters percutaneously using a transthoracic approach and observed that critical cardiac tamponade occurred after injection of a mean of 8.7 ± 1.9 ml/kg of air; mean pericardial pressure at the time of critical cardiac tamponade was 12.2 ± 2.8 mmHg.

Clinical Measurements

Adcock et al studied the hemodynamic effects of progressive pneumopericardium in a patient who required pericardiocentesis[1] and found no effects on hemodynamics until a mean pericardial pressure of 14.5 cm H_2O (10.8 mmHg) was reached. Frank tamponade was observed at a mean pericardial pressure of 26.6 cm H_2O (19.6 mmHg). In this patient, filling pressures had to exceed pericardial pressure by 3.5 cm H_2O (2.6 mmHg) for hemodynamics to remain adequate.[1]

Similar observations in human newborns are not available. However, in view of the puppy experiments of Higgins et al[40] as well as the normally lower filling pressures and reduced cardiac reserve of the neonate, one can speculate that pericardial pressures above 8 to 10 cm H_2O (6.0 to 7.5 mmHg) would be very poorly tolerated in the premature newborn.

NATURAL HISTORY

Although both spontaneous[31,36,53] and isolated[26,31,36,53,68] pneumopericardiums appear to be more benign, the natural history of neonatal pneumopericardium is characterized by both exacerbation and recurrence.[35] Spontaneous resolution of neonatal pneumopericardium has been reported,[31,76,83] but such outcomes are the rare exception rather than the rule. Typically, untreated neonatal pneumopericardium runs a rapid downhill course to tension pneumopericardium and death. The latter course for tension neonatal pneumopericardium is almost inevitable if the pneumopericardium remains untreated during mechanical ventilation.

Exacerbation

Several reports[27–29] have demonstrated that most infants with pneumopericardium identified in the asymptomatic stage subsequently develop symptoms; in fact 40 per cent of initially asymptomatic infants with pneumopericardium eventually die of tension pneumopericardium.[27]

Recurrence

Pneumopericardium recurs in the majority of infants treated with pericardiocentesis alone.[18,27–29,46,52,63,67,69,72,83] The recurrence rate is highest in those infants who remain on vigorous mechanical ventilation, in whom it approaches 100 per cent. Recurrences have been documented up to 3 days after what appeared to be total resolution of neonatal pneumopericardium.[10]

Intraventricular Hemorrhage

The patient population at risk for developing pneumopericardium is also at risk for developing intraventricular hemorrhage: Male premature infants with severe respiratory distress syndrome who require vigorous mechanical ventilation are at high risk for many complications. Nevertheless the incidence of intraventricular hemorrhage appears to be extraordinarily high in infants with pneumopericardium;[32,34,40,46,63] usually, either intraventricular hemorrhage is found at postmortem examination if pneumopericardium kills the patient,[34] or kills the patient later if he survives the pneumopericardium.

Air Embolism

Systemic air embolism, which occurs in association with neonatal pneumopericardium,[35,61] is a catastrophic complication of vigorous mechanical ventilation that very frequently proves fatal. Air embolism should always be considered when critically ill infants suddenly deteriorate.

Death

Although neonatal pneumopericardium is not always the immediate cause of death, few patients who develop it survive. Mortality is in excess of 70 per cent.[10,27–29,34,67]

TREATMENT

Approaches to management of pneumopericardium have varied widely, partly because the clinical effects of pneumopericardium can be so variable. Obviously, there is agreement that infants in cardiovascular collapse must have immediate pericardiocentesis to relieve tension pneumopericardium, but controversy exists in regard to subsequent management in even those infants. In essence, there are several forms of therapy, many of which may be appropriate in a given patient at one time or another.

Asymptomatic Patients Not Receiving Positive Airway Pressure Ventilation

Although some authors have argued that every pneumopericardium should be drained continuously,[6] there is probably a consensus that the neonates with pneumopericardium who are asymptomatic and who are not on CPAP or intermittent mechanical ventilation (IMV) can be observed. However, as considered further in the following sections, very close observation is warranted, for such infants are at substantial risk of developing symptomatic pneumopericardium, a disorder which is rapidly fatal unless it is immediately recognized and treated.

Asymptomatic Patients Receiving Positive Airway Pressure Ventilation

Some authors have argued that asymptomatic infants with pneumopericardium should also be observed, even if

they are on mechanical ventilation;[31,63,83] others have argued that every pneumopericardium observed in neonates on any form of positive airway pressure ventilation should be drained continuously.[27–29] The latter approach is far better, for there is a 40 per cent incidence of tension pneumopericardium and a 60 per cent overall mortality rate for pneumopericardium among neonates who are initially asymptomatic,[27] and the risk of developing symptoms is much higher if the asymptomatic infant with pneumopericardium is on positive airway pressure ventilation.

Symptomatic Patients

In symptomatic neonates with pneumopericardium, there is agreement that air must be evacuated from the pericardium immediately, but there has been disagreement about whether subsequent continuous pericardial drainage is required. Some authors have argued that only recurrent pneumopericardium should be drained continuously.[32,46,54] However, Emery et al point out that recurrences occur in more than 80 per cent of neonates in whom symptomatic pneumopericardium is treated by aspiration alone,[28] and that repeated pericardial taps carry substantial risk of myocardial or coronary laceration. After emergency pericardiocentesis, continuous drainage should be established in any neonate with symptomatic pneumopericardium,[27–29] for recurrence is the rule rather than the exception, even among patients not on positive airway pressure ventilation.

Observation

In some cases, even mechanically ventilated infants with pneumopericardium have survived without pericardial evacuation.[10,24,30,42,63] As considered previously, simply observing the infant with pneumopericardium may be appropriate therapy if the infant is entirely asymptomatic, the pneumopericardium is small, and the infant is not on any form of positive airway pressure ventilation. All other pneumopericardiums should be continuously drained. However, is it critical that all infants managed only with observation be observed on a monitor in an intensive care unit until the pneumopericardium has resolved, and that all equipment for emergency pericardiocentesis be present at the bedside in a ready-to-use state. It is a good idea for each nursing shift to run a monitor ECG rhythym strip and tape it to the bedside for ready comparison in detection of pneumopericardium-induced ECG changes. Chest radiographs should be repeated at least daily until complete resolution of the pneumopericardium and at any sign of deterioration.

Nitrogen Washout

Use of 100 per cent oxygen to speed resolution of neonatal pneumothorax was suggested in 1963 by Chernick and Avery.[14] Absence of nitrogen in inspired gas prompts rapid exit of nitrogen dissolved in the blood through the lungs; as a result, nitrogen in the pneumothorax moves to the blood and is also eventually exhaled. This same principle applies equally well to pneumopericardium.[83] However, use of 100 per cent oxygen to hasten resolution of pneumopericardium should only be done in infants weighing more than 1500 g, i.e., those with no risk of retrolental fibroplasia. Further, high oxygen concentrations (> 50 per cent) should not be used for more than a few hours even in infants weighing more than 1500 g unless lung disease demands it, because high oxygen concentrations are toxic to the lung.

Reduction in Mean Airway Pressure

Since neonatal pneumopericardium is clearly related to positive pressure mechanical ventilation, reducing mean airway pressure would appear to be logical treatment and has in fact been suggested by several groups.[6,28,77,83] However Glenski and Hall have presented evidence that those infants with pneumopericardium in whom mean airway pressures are reduced do less well.[34] Thus, it would appear that attempting to minimize continued or recurrent pericardial air leak by underventilating the lungs during severe respiratory distress syndrome is a poor trade. A better approach to management of pneumopericardium complicating severe respiratory distress syndrome is to establish adequate continuous pericardial drainage and to manage the respiratory distress syndrome as dictated by its severity and clinical course.

Atropine

Experiments in puppies have demonstrated that bradycardia in cardiac tamponade is reflexively mediated.[30] Slowing of the heart rate during pericardial distention appears to be particularly common in newborns. As considered in Chapters 2 and 68, cardiac output in newborns is uniquely heart rate dependent because the neonatal myocardium is operating near its maximum potential on the Starling curve and on the sympathetic neuraxis. Thus, sudden reductions in heart rate can be disastrous in any newborn. In neonates with tension pneumopericardium, reflex reductions in heart rate are catastrophic because stroke volume is already severely compromised and cannot increase. Atropine would appear to be indicated in any neonate with symptomatic pneumopericardium, but its administration should not delay emergency pericardial drainage.

Volume Loading

As is the case for atropine, volume loading has not been described as a therapeutic approach in neonatal pneumopericardium. However experimental data clearly demonstrate that those animals with higher cardiac filling pressures tolerate larger increases in pericardial pressures than those with lower cardiac filling pressures.[23,64,65] Thus, it would appear that in neonates with pneumopericardium there could be much gained (if tension pneumopericardium should develop later or recur) and presumably little lost by restoring vascular volumes to at least normal with red blood cells; the advantage of red cell transfusion is that volume *useful* in oxygen transport is provided to the infant. If tension pneumopericardium should develop or recur after transfusion, having higher cardiac filling pressures and greater red cell mass could only be beneficial, and it might improve outcome.

Emergency Pericardiocentesis

Inserting a needle into the pericardial space and draining pericardial air during neonatal tension pneumopericardium is a life-saving maneuver, but complications are not uncommon. Hemopericardium[10] and fatal lacerations of the right ventricle and left anterior descending coronary artery have been reported.[27] Nevertheless, there is no alternative when neonates with pneumopericardium become symptomatic because unrecognized or untreated tension pneumopericardium is universally fatal. If symptomatic neonatal pneumopericardium develops, and emergency pericardiocentesis proves successful, the most important decision to be made has to do with subsequent management.

Repeated Pericardial Aspiration

Some authors have used repeated pericardial aspiration in management of recurrent pneumopericardium.[52,58,83] However, given the facts that neonatal pneumopericardium typically worsens or recurs[27] and that each aspiration carries with it substantial risk of myocardial or coronary laceration,[10,27] managing neonatal pneumopericardium with repeated pericardial aspiration whenever symptoms recur is a temporizing and dangerous approach to a chronic problem. In infants with pneumopericardium who remain on positive airway pressure, recurrence and exacerbation are the rule rather than the exception, and continuous pericardial drainage should be established in all cases.[27–29]

Continuous Pericardial Drainage

Matthieu et al first described continuous pericardial drainage for neonatal pneumopericardium in 1970.[54] In the ensuing two decades, neonatology has been slow to recognize the importance of continuous pericardial drainage in neonatal pneumopericardium. Despite assertions to the contrary,[31,63,76,83] there is little doubt that continuous pericardial drainage should be instituted in virtually every case of symptomatic neonatal pneumopericardium.[6,17,27–29] *Not* inserting a pericardial catheter in neonates with pneumopericardium should be a rare occurrence for the following reasons. First, in the great majority of cases, the cause of the pneumopericardium—mechanical ventilation with very high airway pressures—continues whether the patient remains as yet asymptomatic or has responded favorably to emergency pericardiocentesis. In Glenski and Hall's 1985 review, 121 of 127 reported cases of neonatal pneumopericardium occurred during positive pressure mechanical ventilation, and those infants in whom attempts to reduce airway pressures were made after recognition and treatment of pneumopericardium did worse. Second, in the great majority of cases, neonatal pneumopericardium recognized in the asymptomatic stage becomes symptomatic later.[27] Delaying institution of proper therapy until the patient develops symptoms does nothing but expose the infant to increased risk of catastrophic collapse. Third, neonatal pneumopericardium carries a very high mortality—84 per cent in Glenski and Hall's 19 patients,[34] 74 per cent in Emery et al's 47 patients,[27] and 72 per cent in Burt and Lester's 50 patients.[10] More effective therapy is needed to combat this excessive mortality. In the short run, establishing effective continuous drainage of the pericardial space is the single intervention most likely to make a significant difference in the outcome of neonatal pneumopericardium.[27–29] The long-term answer to neonatal pneumopericardium will come from the advent of surfactant replacement therapy, which should greatly reduce the incidence and severity of respiratory distress syndrome.[48a]

Continous Pericardial versus Continuous Pleural Drainage

Just as very few clinicians would perform an emergency evacuation of tension pneumothorax and not follow up that procedure with chest tube insertion, so too should emergency pericardiocentesis virtually always be followed by placement of a pericardial catheter for continuous drainage of the pericardial space. The only question remaining is what type of continuous pericardial drainage should be employed.

Complications of Continuous Pericardial Drainage

Pericardial tubes placed to drain neonatal pneumopericardium have been responsible for hemopericardium[10] and pneumothorax.[27] However, the risks of not establishing continuous pericardial drainage far exceed the hazards of doing so, for exacerbation and recurrence of pneumopericardium are common among infants who do not receive continuous drainage, and hemopericardium and pneumothorax are rare among infants who do receive continuous pericardial drainage.

Percutaneous Subxiphoid Insertion of an End Hole Catheter

End hole Teflon intravenous catheters have commonly been used to establish continuous pericardial drainage,[2,6,10,32,46,54] largely because such catheters are readily available in neonatal intensive care units. However, end hole pericar-

dial catheters attached to negative suction are quite likely to become obstructed;[27] obstruction commonly results either from myocardial or pericardial tissue occlusion of the end hole or from secretions. For these reasons it is preferable to insert multiple hole catheters for continuous pericardial drainage.[27–29,32,67]

Surgical Placement

Emery et al[27–29] and others[32,67] have made a strong case for inserting multiple hole pericardial catheters. Emery et al[27–29] place pericardial catheters under direct vision via a small subxiphoid incision. Using direct vision for pericardial tube placement prevents lacerations of the coronary arteries or right ventricle, which can complicate blind insertions of pericardial catheters, and permits placement of a catheter that is less likely to become occluded by either positioning or pericardial debris. One disadvantage of the approach of Emery et al is that a surgeon is required, and not all neonatal intensive care units have immediate surgical access.

Percutaneous Subxiphoid Insertion of Multiple Hole Catheters

In 1966 Nordstrom described an adaptation of the Seldinger technique,* in which pericardial catheters are inserted percutaneously to drain pericardial effusion.[59a] Advantages of placing pericardial catheters percutaneously by the Seldinger technique include (1) multiple hole catheters can be inserted, (2) catheter positions can be better controlled (because the wire can be safely maneuvered to the desired position in the pericardium [anterior in pneumopericardium, posterior in pericardial effusion], and then the catheter can be advanced over the wire), and (3) no incisions are necessary.

Catheter Patency

Even multiple hole indwelling pericardial catheters cannot prevent recurrence of pneumopericardium if catheter occlusions occur, and secretions can plug pericardial catheters.[17,27,66] Emery et al, who place multihole 10 French catheters in the pericardial space under direct vision using the subxiphoid approach, recommend stripping pericardial tubes in a manner analogous to postoperative handling of chest tubes.[27] Reiffel and Priebe suggest reinjecting air to clear obstructed pericardial tubes.[66] Both approaches are worthwhile.

OUTCOME

Although some authors have not been able to document whether evacuation of neonatal pneumopericardium makes

---

*The Seldinger technique is a percutaneous technique for cardiac catheterization in which a needle is inserted into the vessel, a wire is passed through the needle, and a catheter is passes over the wire.

a difference in survival,[10] Emery et al found that substitution of direct vision pericardial drainage for percutaneous pericardial drainage not only markedly reduced death from tension pneumopericardium but also markedly improved overall survival among infants with pneumopericardium.[27] It would seem that establishing early and effective pericardial drainage with a multiple hole catheter, whether that drainage is established under direct vision or by percutaneous techniques, is likely to reduce the morbibity and mortality of neonatal pneumopericardium.

References

1. Adcock JD, Lyons RH, Barnwell JB (1940): The circulatory effects produced in a patient with pneumopericardium by artificially varying the intrapericardial pressure. Am Heart J 19:283–296.

2. Alpan G, Goder K, Glick B, Peleg O, Avital A, Eyal F (1984): Pneumopericardium during continuous positive airway pressure in respiratory distress syndrome. Crit Care Med 12:1080–1081.

3. Astapov BM (1969): Artificial pneumopericardium (clinico-roentgenological and experimental investigations). Kardiologiia 9:126–130.

3a. Beck CS, Isaac L (1931): Pneumopericardiac tamponade: A study of the effects of atmospheric pressure, negative pressure, and positive pressure upon the heart. J Thor Surg 1:124–148.

4. Birrer RB, Calderon J (1984): Pneumothorax, pneumomediastinum, and pneumopericardium following Valsalva's maneuver during marajuana smoking. NY State J Med 84:619–620.

5. Bouillet P (1980): Les pneumopericardes spontanes. Paris, Thes Med, VI.

6. Brans YW, Pitts M, Cassady G (1976): Neonatal pneumopericardium. Am J Dis Child 130:393–396.

7. Brenner JI, Warren JW, Shayne RS, Berman MA, McLaughin JS, Young LW (1984): Anerobic pyopneumopericardium. Am J Dis Child 138:791–792.

8. Bricheteau I (1844): Observation d'hydropneumopericarde accompagnee d'un bruit de fluctuation perceptible à l'oreille. Arch Gen Med 4:334–339.

9. Brown ZA, Clark JM, Jung AL (1977): Systemic gas embolism. Am J Dis Child 131:984–985.

10. Burt TB, Lester PD (1982): Neonatal pneumopericardium. Radiology 142:81–84.

11. Cabatu EE, Brown EG (1979): Thoracic transillumination: Aid in the diagnosis and treatment of pneumopericardium in the neonate. Pediatrics 64:958–960.

12. Campbell RE (1970): Intrapulmonary interstitial emphysema—a complication of hyaline membrane disease. Am J Roentgenol Radium Ther Nucl Med 110:449–456.

13. Cegrell L, Svenningsen NW (1975): Successfully treated pneumopericardium in a newborn infant during IPPV. Acta Paediatr Scand 64:135–137.

14. Chernick V, Avery ME (1963): Spontaneous alveolar rupture at birth. Pediatr 32:816–824.

15. Cimmino CV (1967): Some radiodiagnostic notes on pneumomediastinum, pneumothorax, and pneumopericardium. Va Med Mon 94:205–212.

16. Cizek TA, Modanlon HD, Owings D, Nelson P (1981): Mean airway pressure—significance during mechanical ventilation in neonates. J Pediatr 99:121–126.

17. Cohen DJ, Baumgart S, Stephenson LW (1983): Pneumopericardium in neonates—is it PEEP or is it PIP? Ann Thorac Surg 35:179–183.

18. Cohen S, Lockhart CH (1981): Pneumopericardium—a complication of prolonged ventilation. Anesthesiology 32:465–467.

19. Cooperstock M (1944): Purulent pericarditis complicating pneumonia: Recovery in an infant following therapeutic aspiration and development of pneumonia. J Pediatr 24:656–661.

20. Cummings RG, Wesley RLR, Adams DH, Lowe JE (1984): Pneumopericardium resulting in cardiac tamponade. Ann Thorac Surg 37:511–518.

21. Cyrlak D, Milne ENC, Imray TJ (1984): Pneumomediastinum: A diagnostic problem. CRC Crit Rev Diagn Imaging 23:75–117.

22. Decosta EJ (1940): Spontaneous pneumothorax in the newborn infant. Am J Obstet Gyncol 39:578–592.

23. DeCristofaro D, Liu CK (1969): The haemodynamics of cardiac tamponade and blood volume overload in dogs. Cardiovasc Res 3:292–298.

24. Douglas-Jones J, Bustamente S, Mirza, M (1981): Pneumopericardium in a newborn infant. J Pediatr Surg 16:75–76.

25. Dupont T, Sauget Y, Cuvillier P, Moulront S, Gomez J, Lescut J, Peltier, JM (1984): L'echographie dans le pneumopericarde: Interet de la voie sous-xyphoidienne. Ann Cardiol Angeiol 33:83–85.

26. Durward PC (1966): Pneumopericardium in a neonate. Australas Radiol 10:229–230.

27. Emery RW, Foker J, Thompson TR (1984): Neonatal pneumopericardium: a surgical emergency. Ann Thorac Surg 37:128–132.

28. Emery RW, Laudes RG, Lindsay WG, Thompson T, Nicoff DM (1978): Surgical treatment of pneumopericardium in the neonate. World J Surg 2:631–637.

29. Emery RW, Lindsay WG, Nicoloff DM (1978): Placement of pericardial drainage tube for treatment of pneumopericardium in the neonate. Ann Thorac Surg 26:84–85.

30. Fletcher BD, Outerbridge EW. Youssef S, Boulande RP (1974): Pulmonary interstitial emphysema in a newborn infant treated by lobectomy. Pediatr 54:808–810.

31. Gershanik JJ (1971): Neonatal pneumopericardium. Am J Dis Child 121:438–439.

32. Gil-Rodriguez JA, Lewis BW, Savege TM, Sykes EE, Walling PT (1972): Pneumopericardium complicating the treatment of respiratory distress syndrome in the newborn. Br J Anaesth 44:1219–1221.

33. Glaser J, Landau DB (1935): Pneumothorax in the newborn. Am J Dis Child 50:786–997.

34. Glenski JA, Hall RT (1984): Neonatal pneumopericardium: Analysis of ventilatory variables. Crit Care Med 12:439–442.

35. Gregory GA, Tooley WH (1970): Gas embolism in hyaline membrane diease. N Engl J Med 282:1141–1142.

36. Grosfeld JL, Kilman JW, Frye TR (1970): Spontaneous pneumopericardium in a newborn infant. J Pediatr 76:614–616.

37. Grosfeld JL, Boyer D, Clatworthy HW Jr (1971): Hemodynamic and manometric observations in experimental air-block syndrome. J Pediatr Surg 6:339–334.

38. Hamman L (1945): Mediastinal emphysema. JAMA 128:1–6.

39. Hayashi Y, Araki H, Yamada A, Tomoike H, Nakamura M (1985): A peculiar extra heart sound after artificial pneumothorax in congenital pericardial defect: A diagnostic clue. Clin Cardiol 8:311–313.

40. Higgins CB, Broderick TW, Edwards DK, Shumaker A (1979): The hemodynamic significance of massive pneumopericardium in preterm infants with respiratory distress syndrome. Radiology 133:363–368.

40a. Holt JP, Rhode, EA, Kine, H (1960): Pericardial and ventricular pressures. Circ Res 8:1171–1181.

41. Hurd TE, Nova R, Gallagher TJ (1984): Tension pneumopericardium: A complication of mechanical ventilation. Crit Care Med 12:200–201.

42. Kirkpatrick BV, Felman AH, Eitzman DV (1974): Complications of ventilation therapy in respiratory distress syndrome: Recognition and management of acute air leaks. Am J Dis Child 128:496–502.

43. Kuhns LR, Bednarek FJ, Wyman MD, Roloff DW, Borer RC (1975): Diagnosis of pneumothorax or pneumomediastinum in the neonate by transillumination. Pediatr 56:355–360.

44. Kunze J (1970): Pneumoperikard nach spontanpneumothorax in der neugeborenenperiode. Padiat Prax 9:377–379.

45. Lange H, Kemperdick H, Gauchel FD (1974): Spontanes pneumoperikard beim neugeborenen. Klin Paediatr 86:264–267.

46. Lawson EE, Gould J, Taeusch HW (1980): Neonatal pneumopericardium: Current management. J Pediatr Surg 15:181–185.

47. Lohrer A (1972): Zur Pathogenese des pneumoperikards beim neugeborenen. Schweiz Med Wschr 102:1248–1251.

48. Loftis JW, Susen AF, Marcy JH, Sherman FE (1962): Pneumopericardium in infancy. Am J Dis Child 103:61–65.

48a. Long WA, Sanders RL (1988): New treatment methods in idiopathic respiratory distress syndrome: Replacement of surface active material. Clin Crit Care Med 13:21–56.

49. Lubchenco LO (1959): Recognition of spontaneous pneumothorax in premature infants. Pediatr 24:996–1004.

50. Macklin CC (1939): Transport of air along sheaths of pulmonic vessels from alveoli to mediastinum. Arch Int Med 64:913–926.

51. MacPherson RI, Chernick V, Reed M (1972): The complications of respiratory therapy in the newborn. J Can Assoc Radiol 23:91–102.

52. Mansfield PB, Graham CB, Beckwith JB, Hall DG, Sauvage LR (1973): Pneumopericardium and pneumomediastinum in infants and children. J Pediatr Surg 8:691–699.

53. Markarian M, Abelow RC (1971): Neonatal pneumopericardium (letter). Pediatr 47:634–635.

54. Matthieu JM, Nussle D, Torrado A, Sadeghi H (1970): Pneumopericardium in the newborn. Pediatr 46:117–119.

55. Maurer ER, Mendez FL Jr, Finkelstein M, Lewis R (1958): Cardiovascular dynamics in pneumopericardium and hydropericardium. Angiology 9:176–179.

56. McDouglad CB, Mulder GA, Hoffman JR (1985): Tension pneumopericardium following blunt chest trauma. Ann Emer Med 14:167–170.

57. Mikity VG, Taber P (1973): Complications in the treatment of respiratory distress syndrome. Pediatr Clin North Am 20:419–431.

58. Moodie DS, Kleinberg F, Hattery RR, Feldt RH (1976): Neonatal pneumopericardium. Mayo Clin Proc 51:101–106.

59. Netto DJL (1944): Pneumopericardium in a 42 day old infant. Am J Dis Child 67:288–289.

59a. Nordstrom B (1966): Percutaneous catheterization of the pericardium. Acta Radiol Diagnosis 4:662–670.

60. Ogatta ES, Gregory GA, Kitterman JA, Phibbs RH, Tooley WH (1976): Pneumothorax in respiratory distress syndrome: Incidence and effects on vital signs, blood gases, and pH. Pediatr 56:177–183.

61. Oppermann HC, Ille L, Obladen M, Richter E (1979): Systemic air embolism in the respiratory distress syndrome of the newborn. Pediatr Radiol 8:139–145.

62. Ovenfors CO (1964): Pulmonary interstitial emphysema: Experimental roentgen diagnostic study. Acta Radiol (Suppl) 224:1–131.

63. Pomerance JJ, Weller MH, Richardson CJ, Soule JA, Cato A (1974): Pneumopericardium complicating respiratory distress syndrome: Role of conservative management. J Pediatr 84:883–886.

64. Reed JR, Thomas WP (1984): Hemodynamics of progressive pneumopericardium in the dog. Am J Vet Res 45:301–307.

65. Refsum H, Junemann M, Lipton MJ, Skioldebrand C, Carlsson E, Tyberg JV (1981): Ventricular diastolic pressure-volume relations and the pericardium. Effects of changes in blood volume and pericardial effusion in dogs. Circulation 64:997–1004.

66. Reiffel RS, Priebe CJ Jr (1977): Evacuation of pericardial, anterior mediastinal, and peripleural air collections in neonatal respiratory distress. J Thorac Cardiovasc Surg 73:868–871.

67. Reppert SM, Ment LR, Todres ID (1977): The treatment of pneumopericardium in the newborn. J Pediatr 90:115–117.

68. Rhodes PG, Berry DL, Goodwin CC (1980): Pneumopericardium in a neonate not artificially ventilated (letter). Arch Dis Child 55:164–165.

69. Sagel SS, Wimbush P, Goldenberg DD (1973): Tension pneumopericardium following assisted ventilation for hyaline membrane disease. Radiology 106:175–178.

70. Schuhfried G (1979): Pneumopericard bei maschinell beatmeten Neugeborenen. Padiatr Padol 14:135.

71. Seppanen U (1985): The value of perinatal post-mortem radiography: Experience with 514 cases. Ann Clin Res 17 (Suppl 44): 5–58.

71a. Sharp JT, Bunnell IL, Holland JF, Griffith GT, Greene DG (1960): Hemodynamics during induced cardiac tamponade in man. Am J Med 29:640–646.

72. Shawker TH, Dennis JM, Gareis JW (1972): Pneumopericardium in the newborn. Am J Roent Radium Ther Nucl Med 116:514–518.

73. Singh KR, Wiglesworth FW, Stern L (1972): Pneumopericardium in the neonate—a complication of respirator management. Can Med Assoc J 106:1195–1196.

74. Siplovich L, Bar-Ziv J, Karplus M, Mres AJ (1979): The pericardial "window": A rare etiologic factor in neonatal pneumopericardium. J Pediatr 94:975–976.

75. Tijhen Y, Schmaltz AA, Ibrahim Z, Nolte K (1978): Pneumopericardium as a complication of foreign body aspiration. Pediatr Radiol 7:121–123.

76. Van Nostrand C, Beamish WE, Schiff D (1975): Neonatal pneumopericardium. Canad Med Assoc J 112:186–189.

77. Varano LA, Maisels MJ (1974): Pneumopericardium in the newborn: diagnosis and pathogenesis. Pediatr 53:941–945.

78. Vourc'h G, Le Gall R, Colchen A (1985): Pneumopericardium: An unusual complication of endotracheal laser surgery. Br J Anaesth 57:451–452.

79. Wegryn RL, Zarnoff LJ, Weiner RS (1969): Spontaneous tension pneumopericardium. N Engl J Med 279:1440–1441.

80. Weingartner L (1969): Pneumoperikard in neuborenenalter. Padiatr Padol 5:212–216.

81. Weller MH (1973): The roentgenographic course and complications of hyaline membrane disease. Pediatr Clin North Am 20:381–431.

82. Wenckebach KF (1910): Beobachtungen bei exsudativer und adhasiver Perikarditis. Z Kiln Med 69:402.

83. Yeh TF, Vidyasagar D, Pildes RS (1974): Neonatal pneumopericardium. Pediatr 54:429–433.

30 PATENT DUCTUS ARTERIOSUS IN THE PRETERM NEONATE

James C. Huhta

Persistence of a patent ductus arteriosus (PDA) is a common, sometimes remitting clinical problem in the management of the preterm neonate. The pathogenesis of ductal patency after birth is not well understood, but it appears to be closely related to the prostaglandin environment and its production by the lungs and ductus arteriosus. The incidence of PDA in preterm infants with respiratory distress appears to be related, in part, to the levels of circulating prostaglandin.[14]

HISTORICAL PERSPECTIVE

The ductus arteriosus and its closure has been a subject of interest since Galen wrote, "the connecting vessel between the aorta and the vena arterialis, while all other parts of the body increase in size, not only stops growing but actually diminishes, becoming after a time completely shriveled and solidified (the ligamentum arteriosum)."[24] Fallopius, in 1561, noted the ductus was of large size.[23] An account of fetal channels and their variable times of closure is found in the writings of Carcano (1574).[11] Harvey stated that "this canal gradually shrinks after birth and is finally obliterated like the umbilical vessels."[29] The physiology of the fetal circulation was studied by Pohlman[48] using starch granules and direct pressure measurements, by Everett and Johnson[22] using radioactive phosphorus, and by Barclay and Barcroft[4-6] using angiocardiography. Dye dilution curves in human newborns[50] showed bidirectional ductal shunting early after birth.

Burnard[10] and Powell[49] noted delayed closure of the ductus in preterm infants, and Danilowicz et al[19] pointed out that patency in this group could persist until 4 to 6 months of age. Rudolph et al described abnormalities in the circulation of preterm infants with the respiratory distress syndrome.[51] The report of Danilowicz[19] using serial catheterization techniques in three premature infants of 36, 32, and 30 weeks' gestation, respectively, showed sequential decrease of the pulmonary-to-systemic flow ratio from as high as 4 to 8:1 to 1.4 to 1.8:1 and a parallel decrease in the pulmonary artery pressure. Danilowicz et al also speculated that delayed ductal closure may be related to other complications that are more common in preterm infants. Kitterman and colleagues[32] found an incidence of PDA of 15 per cent in preterm infants of 1750 g or less, and recommended cardiac catheterization and operative closure when heart failure cannot be controlled in infants with respiratory distress syndrome. Since these observations, the diagnostic criteria and the medical and surgical management of the ductus in preterm infants have been areas of active investigation.

PHYSIOLOGY

The three general aspects of an aortic-pulmonary communication through a PDA are (1) left-to-right shunt to the pulmonary circulation, (2) increased flow through the lungs with diastolic volume overload, and (3) increased flow through the left atrium, left ventricle, and aorta. Using aortic isthmus and descending aortic electromagnetic flow probes during surgery, Cassels[12] showed the diastolic steal of blood flow from the upper and lower aortic circulations with a large ductus and the normalization of flow after ductal closure. Spach and coworkers demonstrated these findings angiographically[58] in a variety of hemodynamic settings.

Immediately after birth, the presence of left-to-right shunt from the aorta to the pulmonary artery through the ductus arteriosus is a normal phenomenon in the normal, term neonate.[31] The ductus arteriosus normally constricts and closes within 18 to 24 hours without causing recognizable difficulty. When Doppler techniques are used, the magnitude of left-to-right shunt in such normal circumstances has been estimated to be as high as 1.8:1.[21] The factors that determine the magnitude of left-to-right shunt are many, but the principal ones are the pulmonary artery/systemic/arterial resistance ratio and the size of the ductus arteriosus. As pulmonary artery pressure drops after birth, there is a higher potential pressure gradient between the aorta and the pulmonary artery; the larger the ductus, the more flow (and pressure) will be transmitted to the pulmonary bed. Any factor that increases the ratio of pulmonary vascular resistance to systemic resistance will tend to decrease ductal shunt. If pulmonary vascular resistance rises more than pulmonary blood flow falls, pulmonary artery pressure will also rise. The effects of an independent increase in pressure in the pulmonary arterial bed on the immature pulmonary parenchyma are not known. Therefore, any hemodynamic assessment of the ductus in the preterm infant must take into account (1) the magnitude of the shunt (Qp:Qs), (2) the size of the ductus, and (3) the pulmonary artery pressure.

PATHOPHYSIOLOGY

The physiologic effects of a PDA in preterm human infants are complex and not well understood today. Our knowledge is limited because of the multiorgan effects of ductal patency and the limitations of available techniques in accurately assessing ductal hemodynamics.

Pulmonary Effects

The preterm infant is born with less pulmonary arterial muscle and an immature pulmonary parenchyma. The mechanism of pulmonary difficulty associated with ductal patency is interstitial edema and decreased compliance of the lung due to pulmonary edema. The preterm lung may be more susceptible to fluid shifts because of altered tissue characteristics of the preterm pulmonary interstitium and underdevelopment of the vascular-alveolar integrity. The pulmonary effects of PDA can be difficult to separate from those of parenchymal disease, particularly clinical hyaline membrane disease, which is a process associated with decreased lung compliance and decreased functional residual capacity leading to increased work of breathing. When the hemodynamic effects of ductal patency are contributing to hyaline membrane disease, experienced clinicians often can separate these two processes by the evolving picture on the chest radiograph and the altered clinical course of respiratory distress. However, progress in this area has been hampered by the difficulty in clinical diagnosis of ductal patency and clinically significant shunt.

The pure pulmonary effects of a PDA are best demonstrated by the clinical effect of surgical ductal ligation on the pulmonary dynamics. Griffin and associates studied the pulmonary compliance of 14 infants before and after surgical closure of a PDA.[28] There was improvement and normalization of compliance after surgery. Most preterm infants with a significant PDA and assisted ventilation receive positive end-expiratory pressure therapy. If the pulmonary problem is due primarily to the PDA, then ventilation following surgery should be altered by decreasing the end-expiratory pressure to physiologic levels. Soon after surgery for PDA dramatic improvement in pulmonary compliance has been observed; life-threatening hypotension from iatrogenic "tamponade" has resulted from previously well-tolerated end-expiratory pressures of 5 to 6 cm H_2O. The systemic hypotension resolved immediately after decreasing the end-pressure to 2 to 3 cm H_2O. Intraoperative tension pneumopericardium with tamponade after ligation of a PDA in a premature infant has been described.[30]

Bronchopulmonary dysplasia may complicate the course of respiratory distress syndrome with PDA.[45] There is no evidence that PDA directly causes this transition; however, when prolonged ventilator therapy is needed, in part due to the PDA, the risk of bronchopulmonary dysplasia is increased. Delay in ligation of a large PDA will result in more survivors with bronchopulmonary dysplasia.[42]

Renal and Gastrointestinal Effects

Organ perfusion is related to systolic and diastolic flow; the presence of the low resistance pulmonary vascular bed in parallel with the lower body (as occurs with a PDA)

compromises systemic diastolic arterial flow.[1] With a large pulmonary blood flow, reversal of flow in diastole in the descending aorta can occur.[31,44,62] Studies using continuous wave Doppler ultrasonography in the descending aorta[31,44,62] and pulsed Doppler ultrasonography in the lower extremities confirm the diastolic abnormality induced by ductal patency.

Decreased renal perfusion with a PDA can aggravate the volume retention associated with congestive heart failure. There is evidence that efforts to increase urine output with furosemide in this situation may actually promote patency of the ductus arteriosus by effects on prostaglandin metabolism.[27]

Intestinal ischemia is believed to be one of the necessary factors in the development of necrotizing enterocolitis. PDA had been implicated in the pathogenesis of this feared complication of the care of preterm infants because of its effect on bowel perfusion. The importance of a PDA in this disease cannot be overestimated because the currently accepted prevention for necrotizing enterocolitis, namely, restriction of enteral feeding, may not be the key factor in this disease.[46] Treatment with prostaglandin inhibitors such as indomethacin may also induce intestinal perforation.

Cerebral Effects

There is accumulating evidence that a PDA is related, in some patients, to the development of intracranial hemorrhage and ischemia due to diastolic "cerebral steal." The pathophysiology of cerebral steal can be surmised by examining the blood velocity pattern in the aortic isthmus above the ductus in infants with a PDA. Diastolic flow toward the ductus must come from the upper body, including the cerebral circulation. Direct measurements of carotid[21,36,63] or middle cerebral[40] Doppler ultrasound flow velocity show diastolic changes with a significant PDA. The occurrence of intraventricular hemorrhage appears to correlate with cerebral blood flow changes.[38,41]

Cardiac Effects

A large left-to-right shunt through a PDA will lead to enlargement of the left atrium and left ventricle; these findings on M-mode echocardiography may contribute to the diagnosis of a significant PDA, but the effects of fluid restriction on the degree of left atrial enlargement make this criterion less reliable.[56,59] Increased left ventricular dimension increases the myocardial wall stress and this effect, in combination with possible coronary artery steal, could lead to myocardial ischemia in preterm infants. In general, myocardial function is normal in infants with PDA, but I have encountered several critically ill preterm infants who did not have increased left ventricular output despite a large left-to-right shunt. Thus, one of the most important uses of new Doppler ultrasound methods may be in measurements of cardiac output in preterm infants.[2,3] Infants with PDA with compromises in ventricular func-

Table 30–1. DUCTAL PATENCY IN 257 STUDIES WITHIN THE FIRST 2 WEEKS AFTER BIRTH (156 INFANTS)

	Birthweight (g)	No. Infants	Patency Rate
Group I	500–700	20	16/41 (39%)
Group II	700–1000	47	40/90 (44%)
Group III	1000–1250	41	38/63 (60%)
Group IV	1250–1500	19	14/24 (58%)
Group V	1500–2000	19	14/29 (48%)
Group VI	2000–2500	10	6/10 (60%)

Table 30–2. CARDIOVASCULAR SCORE IN PREMATURE INFANTS WITH PDA

Variable	0	1	2
Heart rate/minute	<160	160–180	>180
Heart murmur	None	Systolic murmur	Murmur extending into diastole
Peripheral pulse	Normal	Bounding brachial	Bounding brachial and dorsalis pedis
Precordial pulsation	None	Palpable	Visible
Cardiothoracic ratio	<0.6	0.6–0.65	>0.65

A score of 3 or greater correlated with a left atrial to aortic ratio of 1.3:1 or greater in 107 of 117 observations (91%).

Adapted from Yeh TF, et al. (1981): Clinical evaluation of premature infants with patent ductus arteriosus: A scoring system with echocardiogram, acid–base, and blood gas correlations. Crit Care Med 9:655–657.

tion and cardiac output may need inotropic support in addition to urgent closure of their PDA.[37]

DIAGNOSTIC CRITERIA

Physical Examination

Physical examination is the mainstay of diagnosis of persistent PDA. The pathognomonic murmur of PDA was described by Gibson[26] as a nearly continuous machinery murmur at the upper sternal border starting early in systole, but not holosystolic, with variable radiation (and a decrescendo quality) into diastole. Other cardiovascular findings include increased peripheral pulses of a bounding or collapsing quality and often palpable palmar pulses in the very low birthweight infant, a prominent precordial impulse, and sometimes an ejection murmur at the aortic valve. A correlation of the murmur intensity and mean pulmonary artery pressure was found by Krovetz and Warden.[33] However, the presence of a heart murmur is not a reliable criterion for detection of a PDA in a preterm infant. Further, either increased pulmonary vascular resistance or mechanical ventilation may totally obscure the murmur in preterm infants who have wide-open PDA.

Two-dimensional Doppler Echocardiography

In a review of 257 two-dimensional Doppler echocardiographic examinations in 156 preterm infants at Texas Children's Hospital[44] in whom PDA was suspected on clinical grounds, the diagnosis was confirmed in 39 to 58 per cent depending on the birthweight (Table 30–1). Such a high prevalence, even in a selected population, has been suspected clinically for many years. The most common murmur simulating a PDA was mild peripheral left pulmonary stenosis; a two-fold increase in blood velocity as measured by pulsed Doppler ultrasound was detected in the left main pulmonary artery in infants with PDA. The most important finding of the preliminary data is how frequently the ductus is closed even in very premature infants (see Table 30–1).

However, detecting patency is a very different question from determining whether a hemodynamically significant patent ductus is present. In the National Collaborative Study, approximately 12 per cent of preterm infants with a birthweight of 1750 g or less had a "significant" PDA.[25] Clinical criteria for hemodynamic significance include need for ventilatory support for at least 48 hours; tachycardia (heart rate > 170 beats per minute); tachypnea (respiratory rate > 70 breaths per minute); hepatomegaly (> 3 cm below the right costal margin); echocardiographic left atrial to aortic ratio greater than 1.15; and cardiomegaly (cardiothoracic ratio > 0.65) evident on the chest radiograph. The clinical scoring system of Yeh and associates (Table 30–2) formalizes this process, and a score of 3 or greater was associated with a left atrial to aortic ratio of 1.3:1 in 91 per cent of cases.[64]

Electrocardiography

Electrocardiography has been studied in infants with a PDA. An upward concavity in the R-ST segment is associated with diastolic overload, and inverted left precordial T waves suggest left ventricular myocardial ischemia.[33]

DIAGNOSTIC TESTS

Cardiac Catheterization

The "gold standard" for diagnosis of PDA is cardiac catheterization with angiography. If angiography is performed at the bedside, it is necessary to time the injection with the radiographic exposure in order to assess the aortic arch. Variations in this technique may require multiple injections, and experience is necessary for interpretation (Fig. 30–1). Nonionic contrast media should be safer due to their lower osmolarity. Because contrast injections are relatively hazardous in preterm infants and because each change in the premature infant's condition may either be due to or cause a change in ductal patency (thus necessitating another angiogram), other noninvasive tests have been substituted for angiography. However, no organized evaluation of their accuracy has been conducted.[20] Often a test such as Doppler echocardiography can be used for the diagnosis of ductal patency, but Doppler echocardiographic studies do not provide all the information that a heart catheterization would provide.

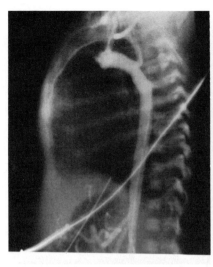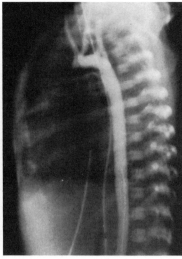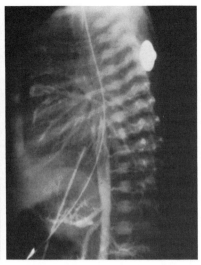

Figure 30–1. Umbilical angiograms in three preterm infants. A hand injection of nonionic radiographic contrast medium is performed through an umbilical arterial catheter. An infant with a closed ductus (left panel) may have a heart murmur with no evidence of ductal shunt. A small shunt through a ductus may cause a significant murmur but no clinical problem (middle panel). A large ductus will cause significant opacification of the lung (right panel) and shunting of blood from the descending aorta. In such a case it may be difficult to time the injection to visualize the ductus itself because of the large shunt.

Echocardiographic Contrast Aortography

One of the most reliable tests for ductal patency is echocardiographic contrast aortography.[54] This technique requires an umbilical arterial catheter and should be extremely sensitive to the presence of left-to-right ductal shunt, but it has not been compared systematically with angiography.

Radionuclide Angiography

Radionuclide angiography was studied in preterm infants by Vick and coworkers[61] and is useful in the quantitation of a large left-to-right shunt rather than in detection of patency. Prospective comparisons of early surgical closure versus conventional therapy using a radionuclide-determined Qp:Qs ratio of greater than 4 at 1 day of age are currently underway. In the future, shorter half-life radionuclides will dramatically reduce the radiation exposure for this test (see Chapter 26).

Two-dimensional Doppler Echocardiography

Two-dimensional echocardiography has been used for visualization of the ductus arteriosus[53,62] for several years and can be useful in identifying a widely patent ductus (Figs. 30–2 to 30–4). The detection of a ductus that is constricted and small requires Doppler ultrasound techniques, ideally, a two-dimensional, directed pulsed Doppler procedure.[18,35,57,59,62] Imaging from the suprasternal notch (Fig. 30–5) can be performed in even the critically ill infant, and the pulsed Doppler sample volume can be placed in the pulmonary end of the ductus in search of abnormal diastolic velocity (Fig. 30–6). A qualitative application of pulsed Doppler findings can be used to identify the infant

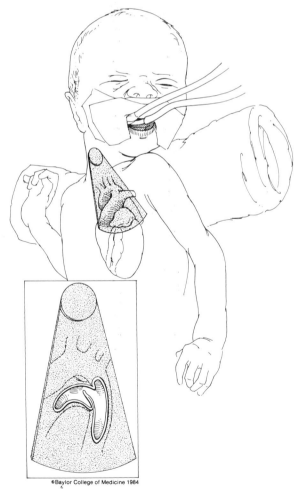

©Baylor College of Medicine 1984

Figure 30–2. Position of a preterm infant for ductal imaging by echocardiography and the appearance of the image containing the left pulmonary artery, the ductus, and the descending aorta (insert). Note the small roll placed behind the shoulders to extend the neck a small amount and gain access to the suprasternal notch.

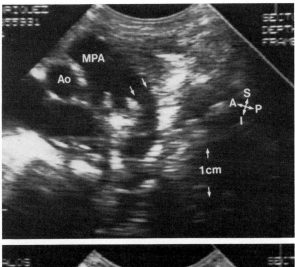

Figure 30–3. Two-dimensional echocardiographic 7.5 MHz imaging of a large unconstricted ductus in two different very low birthweight infants. The "straight through" aspect of the ductus from the main pulmonary artery (MPA) to the descending aorta can be appreciated (white arrows in the upper panel). Ao = aorta; A = anterior; cm = centimeter; I = inferior; P = posterior; S = superior.

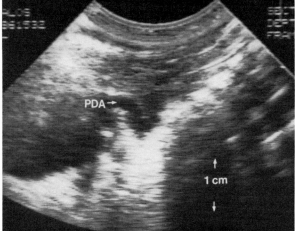

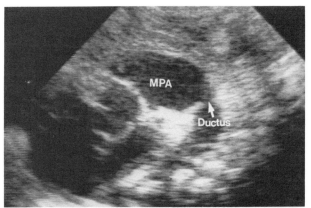

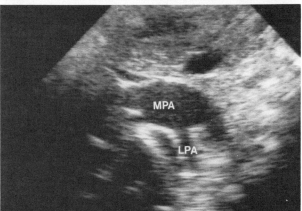

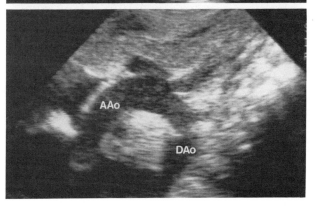

Figure 30–4. A widely patent ductus arteriosus in a preterm infant with severe persistent pulmonary hypertension. Note the relative underdevelopment of the left pulmonary artery (LPA) compared with the ductus, which can cause a functional peripheral pulmonary artery stenosis murmur. The ascending aorta (AAo) and descending aorta (DAo) are normal.

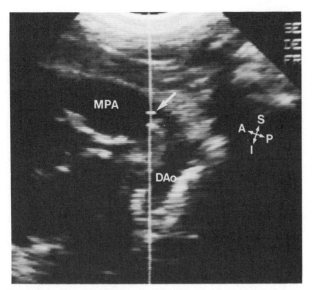

Figure 30–5. The location of the pulsed Doppler sample volume (white arrow) in the pulmonary end of the ductus. A = anterior; DAo = descending aorta; I = inferior; MPA = main pulmonary artery; P = posterior; S = superior.

with a large shunt (Fig. 30–7). In a series of 18 consecutive premature infants having angiography via an umbilical artery catheter, the presence of ductal patency was correctly predicted in eight (no false positives). In the three infants with a large shunt shown angiographically, the pulsed Doppler picture was one of diastolic reversal of blood velocity in the descending aorta below the ductus, diastolic runoff in the left pulmonary artery and aortic isthmus, and increased aortic valve blood velocity. The presence of left-to-right interatrial shunting in the preterm infant suggests that the left atrial pressure is elevated because of ductal shunt (Fig. 30–8). Therefore, the pulsed Doppler study is useful in grading the severity of shunt, as well as in detecting patency and separating the large, straight-through ductus with hemodynamic significance from one that is constricted and of little clinical importance.[52] Because the presence of a large ductus does not, per se, indicate a large left-to-right shunt, depending on the pulmonary vascular resistance, both anatomic and hemodynamic assessments are necessary. The flow through a cardiac valve can be estimated by integrating the Doppler velocity through it (the time-velocity integral).[60] Increased aortic flow has been found by this technique when a large shunt is suspected (Figs. 30–9 and 30–10).[37] Continuous wave Doppler techniques can be used with good accuracy in the follow-up of such patients for the detection of patency (Fig. 30–11).[44] In addition, the aortic to pulmonary artery pressure gradient can be measured with accuracy[55] and the pulmonary artery pressure can be estimated (Figs. 30–12 and 30–13). A useful way to present such data in a premature infant with a PDA is to use pulse Doppler techniques 1) to estimate the ratio of the pulmonary to the systemic flows (Qp:Qs) by comparing mitral/tricuspid valve or aortic/pulmonary valve time-velocity integrals, 2) to estimate the pulmonary artery to aortic systolic pressure ratio, and 3) to compare the two ratios (Fig. 30–14). A combined ratio of approximately 1.4 or greater after heart

rate correction and without including the measurements of the valve annuli (which add a large error factor) can be used to differentiate a large shunt from a small shunt. In this way, it has been learned that many premature infants with a PDA change their hemodynamic situation, which is not at all surprising. In serial follow-up of 25 infants (70 echocardiographic studies) who were critically ill with a PDA, my colleagues and I confirmed our suspicions that even a constricted ductus may have a large shunt and that a large ductus may have minimal shunt. Researchers have used these techniques to document serially the variability of response to indomethacin; even indomethacin levels greater than 200 ng/ml are not adequate to ensure closure.[52]

The physician caring for the preterm infant must make the judgment about treatment. It appears that the liberal use of noninvasive tests such as echocardiography will become more common in this decision-making process.

MANAGEMENT

There is controversy about the best treatment for a symptomatic preterm infant with PDA.[45] The ideal management of PDA in the preterm infant would be prevention.

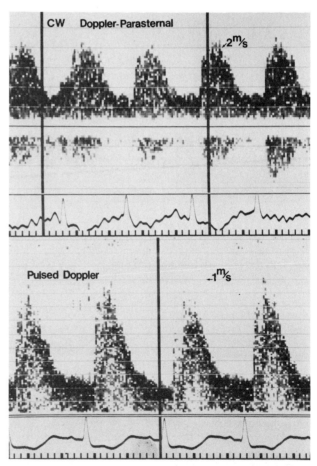

Figure 30–6. Continuous wave (CW) and pulsed Doppler tracings in a preterm infant with a large patent ductus arteriosus. Note the sampling in the ductus (lower panel) with a late systolic and diastolic velocity directed into the pulmonary artery (upper deflection). m/s = meters per second.

Figure 30–7. Typical pulsed Doppler findings in a preterm infant with a patent ductus arteriosus and a large left-to-right shunt. *A,* Doppler in the ductus with systolic and diastolic velocity toward the transducer (upper deflection) in systole and diastole (open arrow). *B,* Diastolic run-off (open arrow) into the left pulmonary artery (LPA) indicative of large shunt. *C,* Descending aorta (DAo) above the ductus (isthmus), with systolic flow inferiorly followed by diastolic flow toward the ductus (open arrow). *D,* Reversal of diastolic flow in the descending aorta (open arrow) below the ductus. m/s = meters per second.

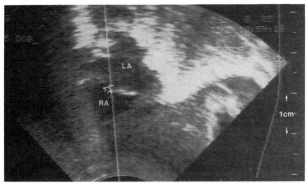
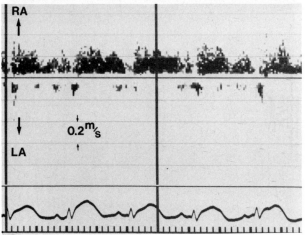

Figure 30–8. Pulsed Doppler sampling at the fossa ovalis in a preterm infant with a patent ductus arteriosus. There is flow from the left atrium (LA) to the right atrium (RA) (upward deflection). m/s = meters per second.

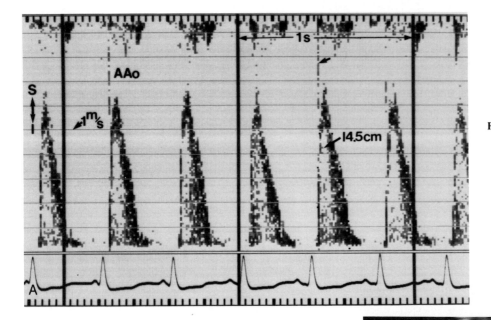

Figure 30–9. Doppler tracing of the ascending aorta to calculate the time-velocity integral (TVI) to estimate aortic valve flow. *A,* Ascending aortic velocity with a peak velocity of 1.3 meters per second (m/s) taken from suprasternal notch.

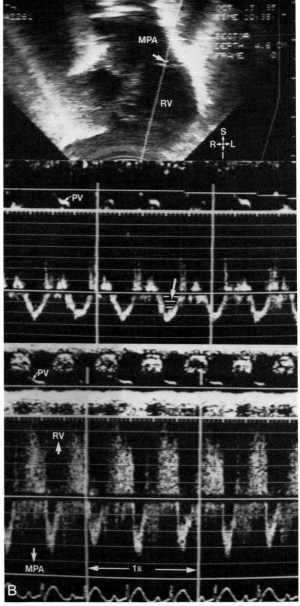

Figure 30–9 *Continued. B,* Pulmonary valve (PV) TVI obtained from the subcostal approach. Note that the evidence of diastolic turbulence in the main pulmonary artery is seen as the Doppler sample volume (white arrow) is advanced from the right ventricle (RV) into the main pulmonary artery (MPA). AAo = ascending aorta; A = anterior; cm = centimeter; I = inferior; P = posterior; S = superior.

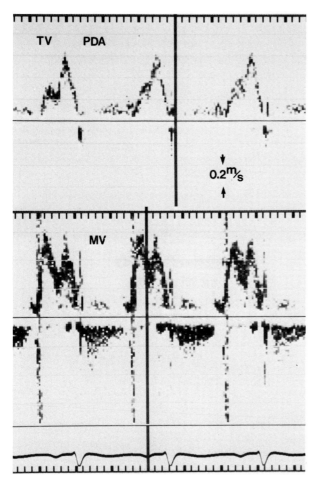

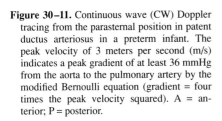

Figure 30–10. Pulsed Doppler tracing of the tricuspid valve (TV) (upper panel) and mitral valve (MV) (lower panel) for the calculation of Qp:Qs in patent ductus arteriosus using the area under the diastolic velocity tracings. Note the greater area under the mitral tracing and, assuming equal valve areas, this means a Qp:Qs greater than 1 with a magnitude proportional to the area ratio.

Most neonatal units now restrict the parenteral water intake to levels that are not associated with an increased incidence of ductal patency.[8] Identification of infants at high risk would facilitate preventive possibilities. Cotton and colleagues[16] developed a profile of factors associated with symptomatic PDA using discriminate analysis. Variables associated with PDA included birthweight less than 1250 g, hyaline membrane disease, intrauterine growth retardation, positive end-expiratory pressure, and acute prenatal distress. Early prophylactic pharmacologic (indomethacin)[39] or surgical closure of the ductus appears to be associated with a decreased rate of later complications. Studies going on at this time should help to clarify this important question. Such a dramatic step as wholesale treatment of all or even selected infants is far from being widely accepted. Preterm infants treated with corticosteroids for more than 24 hours prior to birth may have a decreased incidence of PDA, and further work is needed to confirm this observation.[13]

Indomethacin was effective in the treatment of PDA in a multicenter collaborative double-blind study with a "closure" rate of 79 per cent for indomethacin and 28 per cent for placebo.[25] Reopening occurred in 26 per cent of the indomethacin-treated group whereas only in 12 per cent of the placebo group. Both parenteral and oral indomethacin are equally distributed, and there is a longer half-life for infants of less than 32 weeks' gestation. There are several relevant contraindications for the use of indomethacin that would favor a surgical approach. Further, indomethacin does cause a 50 per cent reduction in creatinine clearance in preterm infants.[34] The medical management of PDA is discussed in more detail in Chapter 54.

Surgical treatment requires a highly skilled team to achieve a low operative mortality and morbidity. Many groups now perform the surgery in the neonatal intensive care unit.[47] Patients with respiratory disease appear to have a higher mortality in surgical series,[9] which is probably

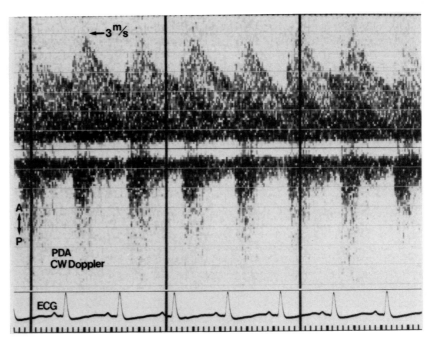

Figure 30–11. Continuous wave (CW) Doppler tracing from the parasternal position in patent ductus arteriosus in a preterm infant. The peak velocity of 3 meters per second (m/s) indicates a peak gradient of at least 36 mmHg from the aorta to the pulmonary artery by the modified Bernoulli equation (gradient = four times the peak velocity squared). A = anterior; P = posterior.

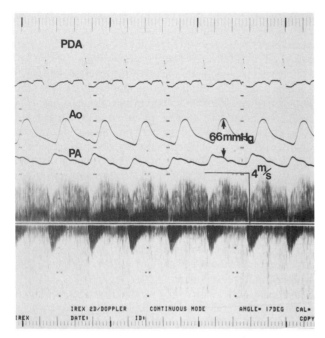

Figure 30–12. Simultaneous aortic and pulmonary artery pressure tracings in the catheterization laboratory in a child with patent ductus arteriosus, with parasternal continuous wave Doppler performed simultaneously. The 4 meter per second jet estimates accurately the 66 mmHg gradient.

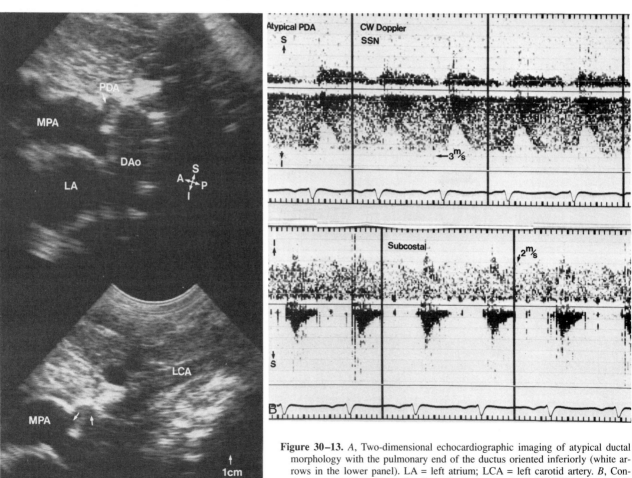

Figure 30–13. *A,* Two-dimensional echocardiographic imaging of atypical ductal morphology with the pulmonary end of the ductus oriented inferiorly (white arrows in the lower panel). LA = left atrium; LCA = left carotid artery. *B,* Continuous wave Doppler tracing from the suprasternal notch (SSN—upper panel) and the subcostal position (lower panel) in the same preterm infant with an inferiorly oriented jet from the patent ductus arteriosus. A = anterior; cm = centimeter; DAo = descending aorta; I = inferior; MPA = main pulmonary artery; P = posterior; S = superior.

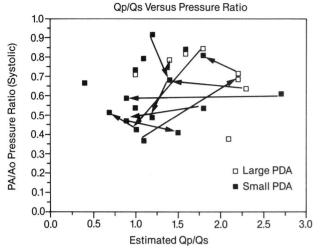

Figure 30–14. A plot of estimated pulmonary to aortic systolic pressure ratio (ordinate) and estimated pulmonary to systemic flow ratio (abscissa) in the presence of patent ductus arteriosus (data from 25 infants). The lines connect the sequential chronological studies in individual preterm infants. Note the changes in individual infants at different times (arrows), signifying significant changes in hemodynamic status.

because of a later time of treatment compared with medically managed infants. Early ductal ligation may offer the advantages of improved outcome and the relative certainty that the ductus is no longer influencing the clinical course.[17] The surgical management of PDA is presented in Chapter 61.

References

1. Alverson DC, Eldridge M, Aldrich M, Werner SB, Angelus P, Berman W Jr (1984): Effect of patent ductus arteriosus on lower extremity blood flow velocity patterns in preterm infants. Am J Perinatol 1:216–222.
2. Alverson DC, Eldridge MW, Johnson JD, Aldrich M, Angelus P, Berman W Jr (1984): Noninvasive measurement of cardiac output in healthy preterm and term newborn infants. Am J Perinatol 1:148–151.
3. Alverson DC, Eldridge MW, Johnson JD, Burstein R, Papile L, Dillon T, Yabek S, Berman W Jr (1983): Effect of patent ductus arteriosus on left ventricular output in premature infants. J Pediatr 102:754–757.
4. Barclay AE, Barcroft J, Barron DH, Franklin KJ (1939): A radiographic demonstration of the circulation through the heart in the adult and in the foetus and the identification of the ductus arteriosus. Br J Radiol 12:505–517.
5. Barclay AE, Franklin KJ, Pritchard MML (1944): The Foetal Circulation. Oxford, Blackwell Scientific Publications.
6. Barcroft J (1947): Researches on Prenatal Life. Springfield, Charles C Thomas.
7. Baylen BG, Ogata H, Ikegami M, Jacobs HC, Jobe AH, Emmanouilides GC (1983): Left ventricular performance and regional blood flows before and after ductus arteriosus occlusion in premature lambs treated with surfactant. Circulation 67:837–843.
8. Bell EF, Warburton D, Stonestreet B, Oh W (1980): Effect of fluid administration on the development of symptomatic patent ductus arteriosus and congestive heart failure in premature infants. N Engl J Med 302:598–604.
9. Bhat R, Fisher E, Raju TNK, Vidyasagar D (1982): Patent ductus arteriosus: Recent advances in diagnosis and management. Pediatr Clin North Am 29:1117–1136.
10. Burnard ED (1959): Discussion on the significance of continuous murmur in the first few days of life. Proc R Soc Med 52:77–78.
11. Carcano LG (1574): Anatomici Libra II.
12. Cassels DE (1973): Hemodynamics. In: Cassels DE (ed): The Ductus Arteriosus. Springfield, Charles C Thomas, p. 143.
13. Clyman RI, Ballard PL, Sniderman S, Ballard RA, Roth R, Heymann MA, Granberg JP (1981): Prenatal administration of betamethasone for prevention of patent ductus arteriosus. J Pediatr 98:123–126.
14. Clyman RI, Brett C, Mauray F (1980): Circulating prostaglandin E2 concentrations and incidence of patent ductus arteriosus in preterm infants with respiratory distress syndrome. Pediatrics 66:725–729.
15. Collins C, Koren G, Crean P, Klein J, Roy WL, MacLeod SM (1985): Fentanyl pharmacokinetics and hemodynamic effects in preterm infants during ligation of patent ductus arteriosus. Anesth Analg 64:1078–1080.
16. Cotton RB, Lindstrom DP, Stahlman MT (1981): Early prediction of symptomatic patent ductus arteriosus from perinatal risk factors: A discriminant analysis model. Acta Paediatr Scand 70:723–727.
17. Cotton RB, Stahlman MT, Bender HW, Graham TP, Catterton WZ, Kovar I (1978): Randomized trial of early closure of symptomatic patent ductus arteriosus in small preterm infants. J Pediatr 93:647–651.
18. Daniels O, Hopman JCW, Stoelinga GBA, Busch HJ, Peer PGM (1981): A combined Doppler echocardiographic investigation in premature infants with and without respiratory distress syndrome. In Rijsterborgh H (ed): Echocardiology. The Hague, Martinus Nijhoff, pp 409–415.
19. Danilowicz D, Rudolph AM, Hoffman JIE (1966): Delayed closure of the ductus arteriosus in premature infants. Pediatrics 37:74–78.
20. Dooley KJ (1984): Management of the premature infant with a patent ductus arteriosus. Pediatr Clin North Am 31:1159–1174.
21. Ellison P, Eichorst D, Rouse M, Heimler R, Denny J (1983): Changes in cerebral hemodynamics in preterm infants with and without patent ductus arteriosus. Acta Paediatr Scand 311(Suppl):23–27.
22. Everett NB, Johnson RT (1950): A study of the time of closure of the ductus arteriosus utilizing radio phosphorus (abstract). Anat Rec 106:194.
23. Fallopius G (1600): Observationes Anatomicae. In Idem Opera omnia, in unum congesta, and in medicinae studiosorum gratiam excusa. Francofurti apud haeredes Andreae Wecheli, Claud. 1561. Marnium and Jo. Aubrium.
24. Galen (1968): Opera Omnia IV:243. Kuhn Edition. A. Translation from Dalton JC: Doctrines of the Circulation. Philadelphia, Lea's Son & Co, p 68, 1884. B Galen: On the Usefulness of the Parts of the Body. Translated from the Greek with an introduction and commentary by Mary Tallmadge May. Vol 1. Ithaca, Cornell University Press, 1968, p 333.
25. Gersony WM, Peckham GJ, Ellison RC, Miettinen OS, Nadas AS (1983): Effects of indomethacin in premature infants with patent ductus arteriosus: Results of a national collaborative study. J Pediatr 102:895–906.
26. Gibson GA (1900): Persistence of the arterial duct and its diagnosis. Edinburgh Med 8:1–10.
27. Green TP, Thompson TR, Johnson DE, Lock JE (1983): Furosemide promotes patent ductus arteriosus in premature infants with the respiratory distress syndrome. N Engl J Med 308:743–748.
28. Griffin AJ, Ferrara JD, Lax JO, Cassels DE (1972): Pulmonary compliance: An index of cardiovascular status in infancy. Am J Dis Child 123:89–95.
29. Harvey W (translated by Chauncey Leake) (1941): Anatomical Studies on the Motion of the Heart and Blood. 3rd ed. Springfield, Charles C Thomas.
30. Hickey PR (1986): Intraoperative tension pneumopericardium with tamponade after ligation of patent ductus arteriosus in a premature neonate. Anesthesiology 64:641–643.
31. Huhta JC, Cohen M, Gutgesell HP (1984): Patency of the ductus arteriosus in normal neonates: Two-dimensional echocardiography versus Doppler assessment. J Am Coll Cardiol 4:561–564.
32. Kitterman JA, Edmunds H, Gregory GA, Heymann MA, Tooley WH, Rudolph AM (1972): Patent ductus arteriosus in premature

infants: Incidence, relation to pulmonary disease and management. N Engl J Med 287:473–477.

33. Krovetz LJ, Warden HE (1962): Patent ductus arteriosus: An analysis of 515 surgically proven cases. Dis Chest 42:46–57.

34. Kuhl PG, Soeding K, Seyberth HW (1985): Aminoglycoside treatment and renal prostaglandin excretion in premature infants. Dev Pharmacol Ther 8:61–67.

35. Lichey C, Ursinus W, Dippmann G, Linke M (1985): Patent ductus arteriosus in premature infants with respiratory distress syndrome. Zentralbl Chir 110:992–997.

36. Lipman B, Serwer GA, Brazy JE (1982): Abnormal cerebral hemodynamics in preterm infants with patent ductus arteriosus. Pediatrics 69:778–781.

37. Lundell BP, Boreus LO (1983): Digoxin therapy and left ventricular performance in premature infants with patent ductus arteriosus. Acta Paediatr Scand 72:339–343.

38. Maher P, Lane B, Ballard R, Piecuch R, Clyman RI (1985): Does indomethacin cause extension of intracranial hemorrhages: A preliminary study. Pediatrics 75:973–977.

39. Mahoney L, Carnuo V, Brett C, Heymann MA, Clyman RI (1982): Prophylactic indomethacin therapy for patent ductus arteriosus in very low birth weight infants. N Engl J Med 306:506–510.

40. Martin CG, Snider AR, Katz SM, Peabody JL, Brady JP (1982): Abnormal cerebral blood flow patterns in preterm infants with a large patent ductus arteriosus. J Pediatr 101:587–593.

41. Ment LR, Duncan CC, Ehrenkranz RA, Lange RC, Taylor KJ, Kleinman CS, Scott DT, Sivo J, Gettner P (1984): Intraventricular hemorrhage in the preterm neonate: Timing and cerebral blood flow changes. J Pediatr 104:419–425.

42. Mikhail M, Lee W, Toews W, Synhorst DP, Hawes CR, Hernandez J, Lockhart C, Whitfield J, Pappas G (1982): Surgical and medical experience with 734 premature infants with patent ductus arteriosus. J Thorac Cardiovasc Surg 83:349–357.

43. Montanes P, Vick GW, Huhta JC, Murphy DJ (1985): Clinical criteria for diagnosis of patent ductus arteriosus in premature infants—are they reliable? Unpublished observations.

44. Murphy DJ, Vick GW, Ramsay JM, Danford DA, Huhta JC (1987): Continuous wave Doppler echocardiography in patent ductus arteriosus. J Cardiovasc Ultrason 6:273–278.

45. Nickerson BG (1985): Bronchopulmonary dysplasia: Chronic pulmonary disease following neonatal respiratory failure. Chest 87:528–535.

46. Ostertag SG, LaGamma EF, Reisen CE, Ferrentino FL (1986): Early enteral feeding does not affect the incidence of necrotizing enterocolitis. Pediatrics 77:274–280.

47. Oxnard SC, McGough EC, Jung AL, Ruttenberg HD (1977): Ligation of the patent ductus arteriosus in the newborn intensive care unit. Ann Thorac Surg 23:564–567.

48. Pohlman A (1909): The course of the blood flow to the heart of the fetal mammal with a note on the reptilian and amphibian circulations. Anat Rec 3:75–109.

49. Powell M (1963): Patent ductus arteriosus in premature infants. Med J Aust 2:58–60.

50. Prec KJ, Cassels DE (1955): Dye dilution curves and cardiac output in newborn infants. Circulation 11:789–798.

51. Rudolph AM, Drorbaugh JE, Auld PAM, Rudolph AJ, Nadas AS, Smith CA, Hubbell JP (1961): Studies on the circulation in the neonatal period: The circulation in the respiratory distress syndrome. Pediatrics 27:551–566.

52. Ramsay JM, Murphy DJ Jr, Vick GW, Garcia-Prats JA, Huhta JC (1987): Response of the patent ductus arteriosus to indomethacin treatment. Am J Dis Child 141:294–297.

53. Rigby ML, Pickering D, Wilkinson A (1984): Cross-sectional echocardiography in determining persistent patency of the ductus arteriosus. Arch Dis Child 59:341–345.

54. Sahn DJ, Allen HD, George W (1977): The utility of contrast echocardiographic techniques in the case of critically ill infants with cardiac and pulmonary disease. Circulation 56:959–968.

55. Sharif DS, Huhta JC, Mullins CE, Murphy DJ (1987): Simultaneous catheter and CW Doppler pressure gradients with patent ductus arteriosus: PA pressure prediction (abstr). American College of Cardiology, March 1987, New Orleans, Vol 9, No. 2 (suppl A), 128A.

56. Silverman NH, Lewis AB, Heyman MA, Rudolph AM (1974): Echocardiographic assessment of ductus arteriosus shunt in premature infants. Circulation 50:821–825.

57. Smallhorn JF, Anderson RH, Macartney FJ (1982): Suprasternal cross-sectional echocardiography in assessment of patent ductus arteriosus. Br Heart J 48:449–458.

58. Spach MS, Serwer GA, Anderson PAW, Canent RV, Levin AR (1980): Pulsatile aortopulmonary pressure-flow dynamics of patent ductus arteriosus in patients with various hemodynamic states. Circulation 61:110–122.

59. Valdes-Cruz LM, Dudell GG (1981): Specificity and accuracy of echocardiographic and clinical criteria for diagnosis of patent ductus arteriosus in fluid-restricted infants. J Pediatr 98:298–305.

60. Valdes-Cruz LM, Horowitz S, Mesel E, Sahn DJ, Fisher DC, Larson D (1984): A pulsed Doppler echocardiographic method for calculating pulmonary and systemic blood flow in atrial level shunts: Validation studies in animal and initial human experience. Circulation 69:80–86.

61. Vick GW, Satterwhite C, Cassady G, Philips J, Yester MV, Logic JR (1982): Radionuclide angiography in the evaluation of ductal shunts in preterm infants. J Pediatr 101:264–267.

62. Vick GW, Huhta JC, Gutgesell HP (1985): Assessment of the ductus arteriosus in preterm infants utilizing suprasternal two-dimensional/Doppler echocardiography. J Am Coll Cardiol 5:973–977.

63. Wilcox WD, Carrigan TA, Dooley KJ, Giddens DP, Dykes FD, Lazzara A, Ray JL, Ahmann PA (1983): Range-gated pulsed Doppler ultrasonographic evaluation of carotid arterial blood flow in small preterm infants with patent ductus arteriosus. J Pediatr 102:294–298.

64. Yeh, TF, Ravol D, Luken J, Thalji A, Lilien L, Pildes RS (1981): Clinical evaluation of premature infants with patent ductus arteriosus: A scoring system with echocardiogram, acid-base, and blood gas correlations. Crit Care Med 9:655–657.

31 BRONCHOPULMONARY DYSPLASIA AND THE HEART

Andrew Bush

Elliot A. Shinebourne

DEFINITION

Bronchopulmonary dysplasia (BPD) is now diagnosed[155] in infants who meet the following criteria:

1. A respiratory disorder that began with acute lung injury during the first 2 weeks of life.
2. At least 28 days of postnatal age.
3. Significant clinical, radiographic, and functional abnormalities, namely physical signs such as tachypnea and retraction; hyperinflation or obvious cystic areas with fibrotic strands on the chest radiograph; arterial $PO_2 < 60$ mmHg or $PCO_2 > 45$ mmHg while breathing ambient air at sea level.

HISTORICAL PERSPECTIVE

In the early 1970s, aggressive treatment of low birthweight premature infants with respiratory distress using positive pressure ventilation and oxygen-enriched mixtures resulted in dramatically better survival rates.[77,117] However, it gradually became apparent that some babies who survived acute respiratory distress in the first postnatal days went on to develop chronic lung disease. In 1967 Northway and colleagues published the first description of this syndrome and gave it the name bronchopulmonary dysplasia.[151] Their retrospective survey of 32 patients, of whom nine had persistent pulmonary disease beyond the twenty-eighth postnatal day, described four radiologic stages of BPD.[115] Stage 1 (2 to 3 days) was indistinguishable from hyaline membrane disease (HMD). Stage 2 (4 to 10 days) was characterized radiologically by bilateral nearly complete opacification of the lung fields and pathologically by alveolar necrosis and repair of alveolar epithelium, with persisting hyaline membranes and emphysematous coalescence of alveoli. There was also focal thickening of capillary basement membranes. Survivors entered the stage of transition, stage 3 (10 to 20 days), with radiographs showing a spongy appearance, cystic areas alternating with radiodense bands. The pathologic findings were emphysema, surrounding atelectasis, persisting alveolar epithelial injury, and interstitial edema. Stage 4 showed larger cystic areas, fewer bands, and cardiomegaly. Postmortem examination showed emphysema, early fibrosis, bronchial muscle hypertrophy, and pulmonary vascular disease. However, even severe radiologic stage 4 disease could be reversed. Functionally, the lungs went from being very stiff in severe HMD to hyperinflated and floppy in stage 4 BPD.

Even in this first description, the importance of the cardiovascular system was recognized.[115] Five of nine patients who entered stage 4 died; all had right ventricular hypertrophy, three at least had a patent arterial duct, one had a patent foramen ovale, and one had multiple pulmonary thromboses. The four survivors did not have clinical evidence of severe pulmonary vascular disease. In their discussion on etiology, Northway and colleagues considered the role of prolonged intermittent positive pressure ventilation (IPPV) and FiO_2 greater than 0.8, together with mucosal injury, but no clear conclusions were possible.[115]

Other descriptions soon followed,[9,17,21] and Northway's initial views were modified as the syndrome became better categorized. Although it was clear that severe HMD was the most common precursor of BPD,[150] other preceding insults were recognized, including the aspiration of meconium,[176] congenital heart disease,[17] immature lung with apnea,[66] tracheoesophageal fistula with recurrent aspiration pneumonia,[168] neonatal tetanus,[227] and congenital myopathy.[158] BPD was described in babies who had not required artificial ventilatory support[150] and in full-term infants.[8,176] The important role of the arterial duct[72] and fluid overload,[22] both resulting in increased lung water, became appreciated. The radiologic descriptions were also modified,[150] and it was realized that a steady progression from stage 1 to stage 4 was unusual.[58] Stages 1 and 2 were acknowledged to be indistinguishable from the changes of hyaline membrane disease, and stage 4 was not necessarily preceded by stage 3 disease.[14]

Neonatal practice was modified in the light of fears of pulmonary barotrauma and oxygen toxicity.[150] Airway pressures used were as low as possible, and less ambitious, though physiologically adequate, targets for blood gas parameters were set.[175] However, chronic lung disease as a late sequela to HMD remains a problem; 36 out of 210 infants ventilated for HMD in Cambridge, England, in the 3-year period of August 1980 to July 1983 went on to develop BPD, and three died.[76] It has been estimated that 1300 infants will develop BPD in the United States each year.[15] There has not been a prospective study of an entire at-risk population with defined diagnostic criteria,[155] but it is clear that there is still a high incidence of BPD in low birthweight babies.[186,223]

There have been many studies of airway function and lung mechanics in chronic BPD,[30,107–109,231,241] but relatively little work has been done on pulmonary circulatory physiology in this condition, despite the recognition of the prognostic importance of cor pulmonale from the earliest descriptions.[151] The purpose of this chapter is to review the problems of BPD with particular emphasis on the cardiovascular manifestations of the disease.

PATHOPHYSIOLOGY

The thorax is a flexible compartment containing two air pumps and two blood pumps; the two blood pumps are enclosed in a much more rigid bag, the pericardium. It is rarely realistic to consider any disease as affecting one component of the thorax in isolation. Similarly, therapeutic maneuvers designed to support the function of one component without consideration of their effect on other components may have disastrous consequences. The introductory sections below will first consider cardiopulmonary interactions in infants with BPD, and then possible etiologic factors in the pathogenesis of BPD.

How the Heart Affects the Lungs

Large airway resistance may be increased due to bronchial compression by enlargement of the pulmonary arteries or left atrium[93,206] and may be diagnosed by ventilation-perfusion scanning.[42] Left atrial pressure increases are transmitted to the pulmonary circulation and may increase lung water,[204] resulting in interstitial and alveolar edema. Interstitial and alveolar edema cause a fall in small airway caliber and compress small blood vessels, increasing bronchial[93,140] and pulmonary vascular[234] resistance, respectively, and reducing dynamic lung compliance;[95] diuresis may improve oxygenation.[121] Pulmonary vascular occlusion as a consequence of severe pulmonary hypertension or vasoconstriction or reduced pulmonary blood flow due to low output cardiac failure may increase wasted ventilation by increasing the parallel dead space.[64,153] Left-to-right shunt has been shown to cause carbon dioxide retention[93] as well as to increase the alveolar-arterial oxygen tension gradient and to decrease lung compliance.[125] However, the decrease in lung compliance seen in left-to-right shunts appears to be due to associated pulmonary hypertension rather than to excessive pulmonary blood flow.[15a]

How the Lungs Affect the Heart

Any cause of increased pulmonary vascular resistance will increase right ventricular afterload and, hence, right ventricular work. Pulmonary hypertension ultimately affects both right and left ventricular function, becoming self-perpetuating.[163] Increases in pulmonary artery pressure may be associated with increased right ventricular end-diastolic pressure;[194] as a result, coronary blood flow to the subendocardial region of the right ventricular free wall may be impaired[123] at a time when increased wall

stress results in increased myocardial oxygen requirements. The consequences are myocardial ischemia, tricuspid valve insufficiency, and arrhythmias due to sinoatrial and atrioventricular node damage.[56]

Gas exchange may be improved in patients with pulmonary disease by adding positive end-expiratory pressure (PEEP), but the cardiac effects of PEEP necessitate caution in its use. High airway pressures may raise the pulmonary vascular resistance.[84] PEEP can also reduce venous return[43] and thus cardiac output, so oxygen despatch (cardiac output multiplied by pulmonary venous blood oxygen content) from the lungs may fall despite improved gas exchange. Volume loading may counteract the reductions in cardiac output caused by PEEP,[230] but volume loading has detrimental effects on the lungs in BPD. PEEP may also increase right-to-left shunting through the arterial duct and the foramen ovale.[60] Further, PEEP may also cause cardiac dysfunction by the production of negative inotropic humoral agents,[78] which suggests that inflammatory mediators may spill over from the lung into the peripheral circulation and produce other cardiovascular effects. Optimum PEEP is the best compromise between pulmonary and cardiac effects,[211] and optimum PEEP is often the airway pressure at which pulmonary compliance is maximal.[85]

How the Heart Chambers Affect Each Other

Both right ventricular pressure and volume overload may affect the left heart by distorting the interventricular septum (Fig. 31–1). Such alterations in left ventricular geometry reduce its compliance and thereby increase left ventricular end-diastolic pressure for any given end-diastolic volume.[123] As a result, left ventricular filling may decrease and cause reductions in cardiac output and increases in left atrial pressure. The left ventricle is responsible for coronary blood flow, and impaired left ventricular function may lead to decreases in myocardial perfusion. The resulting inadequate cardiac output eventually causes metabolic acidosis, which exacerbates pulmonary hypertension.[163,182]

The Pathogenesis of Pulmonary Edema

The balance of forces keeping the lung dry can be perturbed by major changes in one factor or relatively minor changes in several. For example, small changes in microvascular pressures may lead to large changes in lung water if pulmonary capillary permeability is increased. Pulmonary edema results if the microvascular pressures are high, lung tissue pressure is low, plasma colloid osmotic pressure is low, pulmonary capillary permeability is increased, or lung lymphatics are obstructed.

Pulmonary artery pressure may be elevated in BPD, although few measurements have been published.[2,23,34] Left ventricular hypertrophy, which may result in decreased left ventricular diastolic compliance and possibly left atrial hypertension, has been described in BPD[136] and may con-

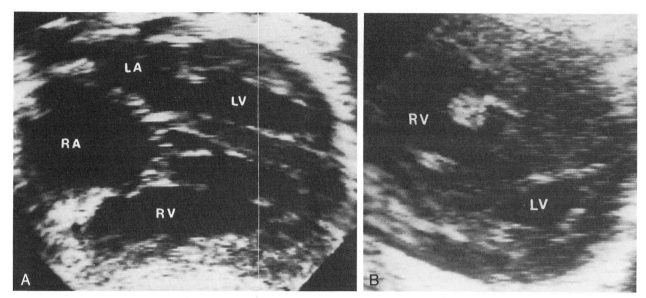

Figure 31–1. Cross-sectional echocardiograms from an infant with bronchopulmonary dysplasia and very elevated pulmonary vascular resistance. *A*, Subcostal four-chamber view. There is an increased right ventricular cavity dimension, with right-to-left bulging of both the atrial and ventricular septa (into the left atrium and left ventricle, respectively). *B*, Parasternal short axis view. There is loss of the normal convexity of the interventricular septum, with increased right ventricular cavity size and increased echodensity of tricuspid papillary muscles, consistent with marked fibrosis. LA = left atrium; LV = left ventricle; RA = right atrium; RV = right ventricle.

tribute to edema formation by elevating microvascular pressures. However, left atrial pressure is usually normal in BPD.[23]

The perivascular tissue pressure may be abnormally low in pulmonary edema, at least in part related to surface tension effects.[6,20,103] Colloid osmotic pressure is reduced in premature infants,[130] especially at the lower gestational ages particularly predisposed to HMD and BPD, and low colloid osmotic pressure may contribute to pulmonary edema.[24] Endothelial permeability is increased in HMD,[102] but the mechanism is obscure;[155] possible explanations include neutrophil-mediated damage,[137] immaturity[10] or imbalance[154] of protease-antiprotease systems, toxic oxygen radicals,[50,152] activation of the complement cascade,[160] vasoactive mediators such as the leukotrienes,[207] and thromboembolism.[204] Potential mechanisms by which endothelial permeability may be increased have been reviewed recently.[205]

An increased pulmonary blood flow can itself increase lung water and protein content,[40] and infants with HMD or BPD may have increased pulmonary blood flow as a result of hypoxemia-induced increases in cardiac output or as a result of patency of the arterial duct. Further, lung lymphatic drainage may be impaired in BPD by involvement of lymphatic channels in the fibrotic process and by any elevation of central venous pressure once cor pulmonale occurs.[15] Renal factors may also be important in pulmonary edema and in HMD and BPD[202] because glomerular and tubular function may be impaired by perinatal asphyxia in premature infants. Asphyxia[92] and mechanical ventilation[89] may cause elevation in antidiuretic hormone levels. Aldosterone secretion may also be increased by mechanical ventilation,[44] leading to sodium retention.

Whether pulmonary edema develops is important in HMD and BPD not only because of the physiologic and

mechanical effects of pulmonary edema on gas exchange and cardiac function, but also because pulmonary edema fluid may contain inhibitors of surfactant function.[98,99,189] Lack of functional surfactant may exacerbate pulmonary dysfunction in both HMD and BPD. Further, edema formation may be an important prerequisite for later fibrosis in BPD.[8]

Summary of Pathophysiology

Derangements in heart or lung function caused by either disease or medical intervention cannot be considered in isolation because the cardiopulmonary system is so tightly integrated that any change in cardiac function has effects on pulmonary function, and vice versa. Keeping heart-lung interactions in mind is important in considering not only pathogenesis but also the therapy for BPD.

ETIOLOGY

No single factor can be said to "cause" BPD. In a major workshop[14,59,150,172,180,220] on the subject, the etiologic factors in order of importance were stated to be immaturity, hyaline membrane disease, oxygen toxicity, prolonged positive pressure ventilation, patency of the arterial duct, and pulmonary air leak. Clearly, these are not independent variables, but for convenience each will be considered separately.

Immaturity

Premature babies are more likely to develop HMD, more likely to be ventilated for this disorder, more likely to have a patent arterial duct, and more likely to develop BPD.[76] Improvement in obstetric care may have contributed to the decline in incidence of HMD.[216] Immaturity per se does not impair alveolar development[91] but may result in differences in development of small airways.[39] Other factors, such as oxygen-enriched mixtures and artificial ventilation, are known to be disruptive of lung growth. BPD has rarely been described in full-term infants.[8,176]

Hyaline Membrane Disease

BPD was first described as a sequel to HMD,[151] and HMD is still the most important preceding insult.[76,150] However, any acute lung injury in the neonatal period may be followed by BPD.[17,66,158,168,227] Most infants recover from acute lung injury with few or no sequelae. It is not known which factors result in the development of chronic lung disease in a minority of infants.

Oxygen Toxicity

Assessment of the specific roles of oxygen and barotrauma in the pathogenesis of BPD is fraught with difficulty. It is virtually impossible to design a feasible and ethical study to determine how much these two factors are injurious in their own right and how much they are merely prolonging life while underlying factors produce chronic pulmonary damage. The fundamental factors influencing oxygen toxicity are concentration of oxygen used, length of exposure, and subject susceptibility.[151] The use of oxygen-enriched mixtures to ventilate premature babies is a necessary and life-saving measure. Thus, although it is true that BPD has never been reported in children not exposed to such mixtures, there is no immediate prospect for the elimination of oxygen-enriched mixtures in the management of premature infants with respiratory distress.

Modern neonatal intensive care uses the lowest FiO_2 possible, since it has been realized that it is not necessary to raise arterial PO_2 to adult levels to ensure adequate tissue oxygenation.[175] The duration of oxygen therapy, rather than the concentration used, may be important in determining long-term outcome.[86,203,209,210] Coincidental with this trend to use lower oxygen concentrations in neonatal practice, there has been a fall in the incidence of BPD, but so many other factors have changed in the same time period that no conclusions can be drawn.

The positive evidence that oxygen is wholly or partly responsible for the development of BPD is not conclusive, but there is little evidence to suggest that oxygen is without blame. Prolonged exposure to an FiO_2 greater than 0.6 is associated with the development of BPD, whereas prolonged artificial ventilation is not a prerequisite.[16,176] Even an FiO_2 of 0.4 may be unsafe.[26,86] Oxygen has long been known to be toxic to the lungs and to impair ciliary motility and mucociliary transport.[122] Although oxygen damages capillaries,[157] bronchial[27,28] and alveolar[116] epithelium, and type 2 pneumocytes,[243] the endothelial cell is the primary target.[110,153] In adult volunteers, administration

for 16 hours of greater than 95 per cent oxygen leads to alveolar capillary leaking, with the release of fibronectin and fibroblast growth factor.[50] Twenty-four hours of 100 per cent oxygen causes reduction in vital capacity[41] and carbon monoxide transfer.[35,169] High concentrations of oxygen may close small bronchi and bronchioles.[31] Oxygen breathing decreases lung volume and compliance in neonates[147] and increases lung lymph flow in newborn lambs.[82] The most important mediator of oxygen lung damage may be the generation of free radicals, damaging alveolar macrophages and resulting in chemotaxis and mediator release.[50,152] Impaired lung growth may be due to inhibition of endothelial and epithelial proliferation rather than cell destruction.[213] Fibrosis is a well-recognized sequel of oxygen toxicity.[9,27,28,110,151] The lesions of BPD are different from those of oxygen toxicity, but the differences are quantitative, not qualitative.[27,28,220] Changes very similar to BPD can be produced in animal models with oxygen.[52,110,219]

It therefore seems likely but is not proven that oxygen toxicity is important in the pathogenesis of BPD. It is prudent to minimize the use of oxygen-enriched mixtures in view of the known pulmonary toxicity of oxygen. Paradoxically, it has been suggested that too rapid weaning from oxygen may worsen oxygen toxicity, but the mechanism is unknown.[37]

Artificial Ventilation

Although BPD usually follows prolonged periods of intermittent positive pressure ventilation (IPPV) or PEEP, it has rarely been reported in children who have never been ventilated.[16,119] BPD is rarely seen in children who have received negative pressure ventilation.[168,208] Residual pulmonary changes have certainly been described after negative pressure ventilation; these have been attributed to the reparative changes of the acute injury.[193] Such residual pulmonary changes after negative pressure ventilation may in fact represent mild BPD.[15] The apparently low incidence of BPD after negative pressure ventilation has been interpreted as merely showing that very sick neonates at risk for BPD cannot be kept alive on such ventilators.[150] Increased airway resistance has been demonstrated in those survivors of HMD who received IPPV but not in those who required oxygen alone or continuous positive airway pressure (CPAP) ventilation.[209] The endotracheal tube itself may be an important cause of late morbidity after mechanical ventilation if tracheal stenosis results, but intubation per se does not appear to cause BPD.[52,118,176]

High airway pressures certainly compromise cardiac function and may cause elevations in pulmonary vascular resistance.[84] Irrespective of the role of artificial ventilation in the etiology of BPD, it would seem reasonable to minimize airway pressures and the duration of intubation and ventilation. A PaO_2 between 50 and 70 mmHg and a $PaCO_2$ between 40 and 60 mmHg would be acceptable,[242] although a high parallel deadspace may make control of $PaCO_2$ difficult or impossible.[167] The ventilator settings should be chosen to minimize airway pressures;[215] for example, in severe HMD a low respiratory rate (30 to 40 cycles per minute) with a prolonged inspiratory time was associated with reduced mortality and subsequent lower incidence of development of chronic lung disease.[174] Others have disputed the importance of high airway pressures.[15] Less aggressive ventilation, with the acceptance of more severe blood gas abnormalities, has also been shown to improve the prognosis in persistent pulmonary hypertension of the newborn syndrome, with fewer infants going on to develop chronic lung disease (one of 15 severely affected cases[242] instead of up to 25 per cent of survivors who were treated conventionally[69]). However, avoidance of high airway pressures during standard mechanical ventilation probably does not totally prevent BPD.[62,185] It is possible that high frequency mechanical ventilation may have a role in the future; the reduction in peak airway pressures possible with high frequency mechanical ventilation might be beneficial, but present data are only preliminary.[71,129]

Patency of the Arterial Duct

Left-to-right and right-to-left shunting of any cause will increase the difficulties of managing sick neonates. However, in 1973 the first suggestion that arterial duct patency was important in the pathogenesis of BPD was put forth.[72] In one pathologic study, all patients who succumbed to BPD had patency of the arterial duct at postmortem examination;[215] other studies have found a lower but still substantial incidence of ductal patency in infants dying of BPD.[23,126] The duct normally closes within 15 hours of birth, but many open and close repeatedly in the first days of life. Patency of the duct is associated with an increased requirement for oxygen-enriched mixtures, an increased duration of ventilatory support,[76] and an increased incidence of BPD.[101] Ductal patency is encouraged by hypoxia[73] and overuse of fluids.[22] The diagnosis of a patent arterial duct during HMD may be very difficult for there may be few or no clinical signs,[57] and no highly sensitive and specific noninvasive laboratory method of diagnosis is in general use. Doppler echocardiography in combination with cross-sectional echocardiography appears promising, but the highly reactive arterial duct of premature infants ill with HMD or BPD necessitates a diagnostic tool that can be applied continuously. In any case, early diagnosis and closure of a patent arterial duct during HMD is important because ductal closure has been shown to increase lung compliance[144,244] and because early closure may help prevent BPD. Some authors suggest that prophylactic indomethacin should be administered to infants under 1000 g weight who develop a systolic murmur,[127] but this approach has not been generally adopted yet, perhaps because of the nephrotoxicity of the drug.[138]

Airleaks

Air dissection related to the use of high airway pressure has been reported. Some have suggested that air dissection may contribute to the development of a large parallel deadspace and the cystic air-filled spaces of late stage BPD.[231] It is certain that these airleaks may result in tension pneumothorax, but in a recent larger series[76] there was no association between pneumothorax and subsequent chronic lung disease. As discussed, high airway pressures should be avoided not only because of their relationship to pneumothorax and their possible role in the development of chronic lung disease but also because of their adverse affects on pulmonary vascular resistance and systemic venous return.

Summary of Etiology

The main etiologic factors in the pathogenesis of BPD are likely to be HMD, oxygen toxicity, patency of the arterial duct, and barotrauma, but BPD may develop in the absence of any of these, with the possible exception of oxygen toxicity. Any factor increasing pulmonary edema makes HMD management more difficult and the development of BPD more likely.

HOW BPD AFFECTS THE PULMONARY CIRCULATION

The neonatal pulmonary circulation contains more smooth muscle than that of adults[88,172] and consequently is much more reactive; relatively trivial stimuli can result in intense pulmonary vasoconstriction. Such stimuli include hypercapnia, acidemia,[182] alveolar hypoxia[67,74,142] and low mixed venous oxygen tension,[67] all of which can cause pulmonary vasoconstriction. Some of these factors may interact,[67] and all are common in BPD. It is also important to maintain body temperature because there is indirect evidence that a decrease in the temperature of blood in the pulmonary artery may increase pulmonary artery pressure.[225]

Pulmonary vascular resistance varies with lung volume;[32,236] the two-compartment model of alveolar and extra-alveolar vessels[94] best accounts for this observation. At low lung volumes, the extra-alveolar vessels (small arterioles and venules) have a reduced caliber and thus higher resistance. At high lung volumes, stretching of the alveolar capillary sheet increases its resistance. In a lung containing areas of both collapse and overinflation (such as in stage 4 BPD), both collapse of extra-alveolar vessels and stretching of alveolar capillary beds are likely to be present. Further, scarring and areas of fibrosis may involve arteries, narrowing the pulmonary vascular bed's cross-sectional area independently of lung volume effects. Pulmonary edema in BPD can further elevate pulmonary vascular resistance by compromising gas exchange and by predisposing to fibrosis. Increased numbers of pulmonary neuroendocrine cells, which contain vasoactive mediators such as serotonin, bombesin, and calcitonin, have been found in BPD and HMD.[104] The importance of this finding remains speculative, but neuroendocrine cells could contribute to pulmonary vasoconstriction in BPD. Organizing mural thrombi have been found at autopsy in the hearts of infants dying after prolonged mechanical ventilation;[54] microembolization from mural thrombi could contribute to pulmonary hypertension in BPD. Finally and speculatively, the relatively fewer vessels in the normal neonatal pulmonary circulation may impair the ability to compensate for pressure and flow challenges in BPD. Degrees of pulmonary vasoconstriction that may be well tolerated in the adult can lead to a self-perpetuating spiral of worsening hypoxemia in the newborn. Elevations in pulmonary vascular resistance in neonates may result in right-to-left shunting through the arterial duct and foramen ovale, which can in itself worsen hypoxemia and respiratory acidosis, thereby further elevating pulmonary vascular resistance.

HOW BPD AFFECTS THE HEART

Some cardiopulmonary interactions have been discussed already. Elevations in pulmonary vascular resistance necessitate increased right ventricular work. The more muscular neonatal right ventricle may cope better with a pressure challenge than the thin-walled adult right ventricle, which copes better with a volume load. However, arterial hypoxemia in BPD may compromise oxygen supply to the myocardium. A postmortem study showed that 11 of 14 infants undergoing prolonged mechanical ventilation had severe cardiac hypertrophy, which was positively correlated with age at death.[54] Fascicles of hypertrophied fibers were found within both ventricles, with swollen, bizarre nuclei in all three layers of the heart. The subendocardium appears to be particularly vulnerable.[54] There were areas of patchy necrosis with large subendocardial scars in the older infants; and in one infant the subendocardial scars were calcified.[54] The papillary muscles were often involved (Fig. 31–1B), and it was suggested that atrioventricular valve dysfunction might result.[54] The main coronary arteries were normal, but the intramural coronary arteries showed intimal proliferation with microscopic thrombi.[54] Some of the damage might have resulted from the combination of increased right ventricular work and arterial hypoxemia, but the author suggested that some damage might have occurred at the time of delivery.[54] Left ventricular dysfunction leading to severe heart failure has also been described in association with perinatal hypoxia.[178] Hypoxia-induced cardiac dysfunction may be suspected in infants with heart failure, the murmur of atrioventricular valve incompetence, or an elevation of the creatine phosphokinase-2 level,[146] but many cases are not recognized until postmortem examination. Systematic examination of the heart at autopsy is necessary, or areas of myocardial damage will be missed.[54] Melnick et al[136] found echocardiographic evidence of left ventricular hypertrophy in eight of nine infants with BPD, and in a subsequent retrospective review of autopsy material they found an increase in left ventricular wall thickness; the right ventricle was normal. The explanation for left ventricular hypertrophy in BPD is obscure,[136] but it could be due to persistent patency of the arterial duct and left-to-right shunt[54] or to systemic hypertension, which is sometimes associated

with BPD.[4] However, other echocardiographic studies have not found evidence of left ventricular dysfunction in BPD.[23,68]

Furthermore, indirect evidence of cardiac involvement in BPD came from a study of α-natriuretic polypeptide in infants and children with various heart and lung diseases.[120] All four infants with BPD (stage 4) had increased levels of this peptide; three of the five highest levels found were in BPD patients. α-Natriuretic peptide is a 28 amino acid polypeptide that causes natriuresis, diuresis, and hypotension;[177,221] its role in the circulatory response to BPD is not known.

CLINICAL FINDINGS

BPD typically occurs in premature infants who have a stormy neonatal course characterized by hyaline membrane disease or other acute lung injury necessitating prolonged ventilatory support and high oxygen concentrations. The course may have been complicated by patency of the arterial duct, airleaks, or both.[133] The acute pulmonary disease progresses to a chronic injury. The child with BPD may need inpatient care for many months. Respiratory infections or anesthesia may cause considerable temporary deterioration in lung function in BPD patients.[133] In this chronic phase somatic growth rate is reduced,[133] although there is usually a later phase of catch-up growth if the infant recovers.[131] BPD survivors are often left with mild chronic airflow limitation, increased functional residual capacity, decreased static[217] and dynamic[30] compliance, abnormal blood gases,[86] and bronchial hyperreactivity,[86,197] although full recovery is possible.[105] Hypoxemia in BPD may be due to ventilation-perfusion mismatch[5,231] as well as anatomic shunting.[23] The chest radiograph may remain abnormal in BPD survivors,[197] but radiographic abnormalities correlate poorly with symptoms.[133] Similarly, the electrocardiogram in BPD survivors may show evidence of persistent right ventricular hypertrophy.[86,105,197] Most important, however, the child with BPD may be left with a neurodevelopmental handicap.[86,133,190,245]

RADIOGRAPHIC FINDINGS

The radiographic descriptions of BPD by Northway et al[151] have been modified in the light of subsequent studies. An abnormal chest radiograph is found in 68 per cent of BPD survivors.[86] The commonest abnormalities seen in chronic BPD are those of hyperinflation with multiple fine lung densities;[58] these abnormalities may be seen particularly in the lower zones,[134] although this lower lung preponderance has been denied by others.[197] The typical cysts of stage 4 BPD are not necessary to establish the diagnosis.[58] Radiologic manifestations of cor pulmonale in BPD are very variable; enlargement of the right ventricular shadow or the right and left pulmonary arteries is unusual. Figure 31–2 shows the chest radiograph of one of the BPD infants we catheterized. Her pulmonary vascular resistance was markedly elevated; she subsequently died of cardiorespiratory failure.[34] A method of scoring radiographic and clinical abnormalities more objectively in BPD has been proposed.[222] Other radiographic findings in BPD include coincidental pneumonia or atelectasis, signs of airleak in the ventilated infant (pneumothorax, pneumomediastinum, surgical emphysema), and rib fractures. Fractured ribs in BPD may be related to overvigorous physiotherapy, osteopenia from furosemide-induced calciuresis,[228] or vitamin D deficiency as a consequence of prolonged parenteral hyperalimentation.[148]

Correlations with autopsy findings have shown that chest radiography in BPD underestimates the extent of lung tissue damage in 63 per cent of cases.[59] The radiograph may also be insensitive to deteriorating cardiovascular function in BPD.[68] Better assessments of both tissue damage and cardiovascular function in BPD may be possible in the future with newer imaging techniques such as nuclear magnetic resonance echoplanar imaging.[184]

THE ELECTROCARDIOGRAM

The electrocardiogram in BPD commonly reflects right ventricular hypertrophy, and the diagnosis can be made by standard criteria.[86,190] Improvement in right ventricular hypertrophy can often be documented by serial tracings, and absence of electrocardiographic improvement in BPD may be an indication for more invasive investigation.[2] Some investigators[136] but not others[190] have reported the presence of left ventricular hypertrophy on the electrocardiograms of infants with BPD.

THE ECHOCARDIOGRAM

The two main indications for echocardiography in BPD are to rule out associated congenital heart disease and to attempt to assess pulmonary hemodynamics noninvasively. Congenital heart disease may mimic or worsen BPD and may be particularly difficult to diagnose. Intracardiac right-to-left shunts may be detected more easily if a peripheral injection of contrast material is given. Various echocardiographic indices have been proposed as markers of increased pulmonary vascular resistance, and some have been thought to be particularly useful in assessing responses to therapeutic intervention.[113] Halliday et al[80] and Fouron et al[68] both used the ratio of right ventricular preejection period to right ventricular ejection time (RPEP/RVET) as a gauge of pulmonary arterial pressures in BPD. Neither correlated their findings with concurrent hemodynamic data, but both groups reached the conclusion that echocardiography would be useful in following treatment and progress. However, the ratio of isovolumic contraction time to ejection time depends on myocardial contractility and ventricular conduction as well as the impedance to ventricular outflow.[68] As already discussed, there is good evidence of impaired myocardial function in BPD,[54] so it is no surprise that Berman et al[23] failed to show any useful correlation between cardiac

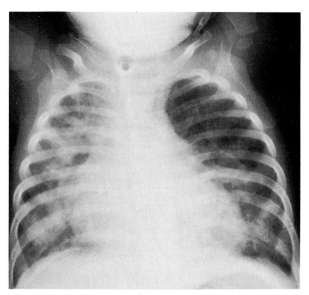

Figure 31–2. Chest radiograph of an infant with advanced bronchopulmonary dysplasia. There are typical lucent areas, with patchy shadowing and cardiomegaly. This infant had marked elevation in pulmonary vascular resistance and subsequently died of cardiorespiratory failure.

catheterization and echocardiographic findings in BPD. The poor predictive value of echocardiography in assessment of pulmonary vascular disease is discussed in detail elsewhere.[87,113,159,195]

PERIPHERAL DOPPLER ULTRASONOGRAPHY

The identification of retrograde diastolic flow in the descending aorta[201] and other large systemic arteries using Doppler ultrasound techniques[124,239] has been shown to be useful in the diagnosis of systemic-to-pulmonary shunts such as a patent arterial duct. Wheller and Menke[235] used this technique on two infants with BPD and demonstrated multiple systemic-to-pulmonary artery fistulas; these fistulas were confirmed at cardiac catheterization in both infants. However, Wheller and Menke[235] warn that detection of retrograde diastolic arterial flow may be difficult in the presence of an umbilical artery catheter or severe systemic vasoconstriction, either of which can significantly increase the small degree of early diastolic retrograde flow that can normally occur.[161] The use of carotid artery flow patterns may obviate some of these problems.[239]

DIFFERENTIAL DIAGNOSIS

BPD can be mimicked or worsened by any form of congenital heart disease in the newborn that causes increased pulmonary blood flow.[58] Overhydration, alone or in combination with cardiac or pulmonary disease, can also mimic or worsen BPD.[22] Primary pulmonary diseases which enter the differential diagnosis of BPD include Wilson-Mikity syndrome,[139] meconium aspiration syndrome,[152] pulmonary interstitial emphysema,[212] viral pneumonia (particularly cytomegalovirus),[238] pulmonary lymphangiectasia.[218] any cause of recurrent pneumonia or aspiration (e.g., immune deficiency, gastroesophageal reflux, tracheoesophageal fistula), cystic fibrosis, and cryptogenic fibrosing alveolitis. Primary pulmonary hypertension tends to be a disease of older children or adults.[58] Cystic fibrosis may present early on, but pulmonary manifestations precede the use of IPPV.[15]

CARDIAC CATHETERIZATION FINDINGS

Despite many attempts to find accurate and reliable noninvasive methods of assessing the heart and pulmonary circulation, the definitive investigation is still cardiac catheterization. We consider that cardiac catheterization is indicated in BPD to rule out associated congenital heart disease, to measure pulmonary vascular resistance, to assess possible prognosis, and to assess the effects of therapeutic interventions such as vasodilator administration or alterations in ventilator settings.

Methods

Assessment of the pulmonary circulation in BPD requires accurate measurements of pressure and flow. The most accurate method of measuring flow is still by the direct Fick principle,[65] which requires measurement of oxygen consumption and pulmonary artery and pulmonary venous blood oxygen contents. Assuming that no extrapulmonary shunts exist, the Fick equation for calculation of cardiac output can be represented by the following:

$$CO = \dot{V}O_2/(10 \times [PVO_2C - PAO_2C])$$

where:

CO	= cardiac output (liters/min/m^2),
$\dot{V}O_2$	= measured oxygen consumption (ml O_2/min/m^2),
PVO_2C	= pulmonary venous blood oxygen content (ml O_2/100 ml),
PAO_2C	= pulmonary arterial blood oxygen content (ml O_2/100 ml).

Unfortunately, there have been very few pulmonary hemodynamic investigations in BPD that have included oxygen consumption measurements, which are necessary for accurate determinations of cardiac output.

We use respiratory mass spectrometry to measure oxygen consumption with an argon dilution technique.[47,48] The mass spectrometry method we use has been compared with standard Douglas bag collections of expired gas and found to be accurate to within ± 0.6 per cent and has been successfully applied to the whole physiologic range of oxygen consumption, from 15 ml/min in premature infants to 6500 ml/min in endurance athletes at maximal exercise.

The method can be applied conveniently in the cardiac catheterization laboratory. The patient is anesthetized by an infusional agent (usually etomidate), paralyzed, and ventilated. A tight-fitting or cuffed endotracheal tube is required. Any air leak around the endotracheal tube is signaled by phasic alterations in CO_2 around the mouth and nose, which can be detected easily with the mass spectrometer. The expired gases are collected and mixed with argon, which is injected into the expiratory circuit at a known flow rate. After complete mixing of expirate and argon, the mass spectrometer is used to measure partial pressures of oxygen, nitrogen, carbon dioxide, and argon. The mass spectrometer can also be used to measure inspired gas tensions and monitor end-tidal gases. The technique has allowed the measurement of oxygen consumption even when 100 per cent oxygen is breathed.[49]

It is important to measure oxygen consumption directly, rather than rely on tables of assumed values. Oxygen consumption tables are usually based on measurements in normal children under normal circumstances, often relying on extrapolation to small babies rather than direct measurement. Reliance on tables can lead to serious errors. Oxygen consumption is altered by environmental temperature,[111] by the presence of congenital heart lesions,[112] and by general[100] and cardiac surgery.[1] Infants with BPD are known to have a much higher oxygen consumption than normal,[232] possibly related in part to increased rate and work of breathing.[241]

As evident in the preceding discussion, the denominator of the Fick equation is the arteriovenous oxygen content difference. Although instruments that measure blood oxygen contents directly can be used, they are less suitable if many samples are to be taken over a short time.[49] We calculate blood oxygen contents using Kelman's subroutine,[115] the blood having been analyzed on an automatic pH and blood gas electrode unit measuring pH, PO_2, and PCO_2 (Corning 165). Other authors have instead relied on oxygen saturations measured spectrophotometrically to calculate oxygen contents, unfortunately usually omitting all reference to calibration of the equipment. Further, oxygen saturations do not account for dissolved oxygen, an error which can be particularly important when oxygen-enriched mixtures are breathed. Thus, the accuracy of oxygen saturation measurements in calculations of blood oxygen contents may be questionable.

Results

The first cardiac catheterization report in BPD was by Harrod et al[86] who studied six infants with BPD on seven occasions; unfortunately, cardiac output was determined in their study using predicted rather than measured oxygen consumptions on all but one occasion. Elevations in pulmonary artery pressure were documented at each study. In the subject studied twice, the pulmonary arterial pressure did not change over a 20-month period.

In 1982 Berman et al reported cardiac catheterization findings in nine subjects with BPD.[23] Cardiac output was determined by the direct Fick method, and oxygen consumption was measured by the flow-through technique.[126] Patients were studied while breathing ambient air and 40 and 80 per cent oxygen. For oxygen-enriched mixtures, it is unclear whether the authors assumed that oxygen consumption was unchanged (which may not be the case) or whether they remeasured oxygen consumptions. Pulmonary vascular resistance was elevated in all nine cases (mean 8.6, range 3.5 to 16.9 Wood units/m[2]). Supplemental oxygen reduced pulmonary vascular resistance by 25 per cent or more in the three most clinically compromised patients. Pulmonary vasodilation was seen with 40 per cent oxygen in patients who vasodilated the lung circuit; 80 per cent oxygen did not cause further vasodilation. Berman et al also found large intrapulmonary right-to-left shunts in six patients (mean 22 per cent, range 3 to 54 per cent). There was close agreement between invasive and noninvasive measurements of preejection period to right ventricular ejection time ratios, but neither measurement correlated well with either pulmonary arterial pressure or pulmonary vascular resistance, nor was either measurement useful in picking out responders to oxygen. Left ventricular function and pressures (as judged by left-sided systolic time intervals) were normal in all cases. Qualitative assessment of wedge angiograms[149] was also normal.

Abman and colleagues have published two reports of invasive studies in BPD.[2,3] In one study, cardiac catheterization was performed in four infants with BPD in whom little improvement in cardiopulmonary status was seen over time.[2] Two of these children proved to have unsuspected congenital cardiac lesions. One infant had an atrial septal defect and a patent arterial duct, the other had an atrial septal defect, ventricular septal defect, patent ar-

terial duct, and interrupted aortic arch. This second infant had severe pulmonary vascular disease that was not diagnosed preoperatively and died after cardiac surgery. The other two children with refractory BPD had unsuspected upper airway obstruction. In the other study, Abman and colleagues looked at the effects of oxygen in infants with BPD.[3] Unfortunately, assumed oxygen consumptions were used for cardiac output calculations from the Fick equation. All six infants had pulmonary hypertension while breathing room air, and high levels of inspired oxygen ($FiO_2 > 0.8$) reduced pulmonary arterial pressure by at least 10 mmHg in each child. The pulmonary vasodilatory response to oxygen was positively correlated with pulmonary arterial pressure on room air. These infants were also studied on supplemental oxygen delivered via nasal cannulas, and reductions in pulmonary arterial pressure on nasal oxygen were nearly as large as those found when the higher oxygen concentrations were used. However, other workers have not found reductions in pulmonary arterial pressure with supplemental oxygen, only reductions in calculated pulmonary vascular resistance.[23,24]

We have reported cardiac catheterization findings in six patients with BPD who were studied while breathing air and 100 per cent oxygen.[34] In four of these infants we also measured the effects of epoprostenol (prostacyclin, PGI_2) given by continuous infusion (5 to 20 ng/kg/min) on the pulmonary circulation.[34] We chose PGI_2 as a blood-borne vasodilator because any acute adverse effects such as systemic hypotension are rapidly reversible by stopping the infusion,[156] but there are theoretical risks that PGI_2 might increase pulmonary capillary permeability and inhibit diuresis.[63] In any case, PGI_2 vasodilated the pulmonary circulation as shown by increased pulmonary blood flow with no change in pulmonary arterial pressure (Fig. 31–3). A similar lung circulation response to PGI_2

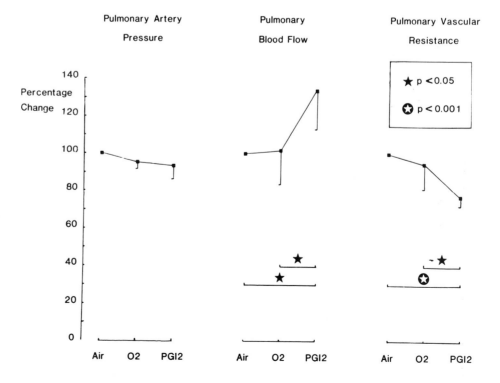

Figure 31–3. Comparison of oxygen and prostacyclin as pulmonary vasodilators in four infants with bronchopulmonary dysplasia, expressed as percentage change over measurements made while the infants were ventilated with air. There was no response to 100 per cent oxygen (O_2), but titrating the optimum dose of prostacyclin (PGI_2) produced a rise in pulmonary blood flow and a fall in pulmonary vascular resistance.[34]

was seen in our studies in children with pulmonary vascular disease secondary to congenital heart disease.[33] In the BPD group we studied, PGI_2 was a more effective pulmonary vasodilator than oxygen. We also found that both elevations in pulmonary vascular resistance and large intrapulmonary right-to-left shunts were associated with a poor prognosis.

Conclusions

There are very few reports containing cardiac catheterization data in patients with BPD; as a result, it is difficult to draw any but preliminary conclusions. It does appear that up to 40 per cent oxygen provides useful pulmonary vasodilation in some cases. It is possible that blood-borne vasodiltors such as prostacyclin may also be useful in reducing pulmonary hypertension in BPD, particularly since reductions in pulmonary arterial pressures could be achieved without additional oxygen toxicity. There is evidence that elevations in pulmonary vascular resistance and large intrapulmonary right-to-left shunts may indicate a poor prognosis, but additional data are needed on a large number of patients with a wide spectrum of BPD severity. It is essential that future hemodynamic studies not rely on assumed rather than measured oxygen consumptions if the direct Fick principle is to be used for calculations of cardiac output.

MEDICAL MANAGEMENT

Infection

In infants undergoing prolonged mechanical ventilation, bacterial cultures of tracheal aspirates usually reveal colonization by flora from the upper airways. Lower respiratory gram-negative or fungal infections[133] may play a role in the pathogenesis of BPD, if only by prolonging the duration of mechanical ventilation. The infant or child with chronic BPD is prone to respiratory infections and has little respiratory reserve; as a result, even trivial infections may precipitate serious acute respiratory failure.[30,133,190,245] Recurrent aspiration may be a factor in repeated infection in BPD patients[192] and may be treatable.[148] Attention to physiotherapy, the early use of antibiotics, and the cessation of smoking by parents (preferably permanently, but minimally at least near the child) should be mandatory.

Corticosteroids

A retrospective review of 23 infants with chronic ventilator lung disease showed that some responded to steroids.[188] The maximum response was achieved with 10 days of therapy, and those who responded once to steroids usually would do so again.[188] There have been two prospective trials of high dose corticosteroids in ventilator-dependent infants, both seriously flawed.[12,128] The number of experimental subjects was small in both studies; one study used six infants in a crossover design,[128] and the other used seven matched pairs.[12] Both studies appeared to show that

dexamethasone hastened weaning from the ventilator, but each used sequential analysis, that is, the trial was stopped as soon as a statistically significant change was shown. Lung compliance was also improved by at least 30 per cent.[12] However, sepsis, systemic hypertension, and prolonged steroid dependency were common in infants receiving steroids. Possible mechanisms by which steroids may be beneficial in BPD include stabilization of cell and lysosomal membranes,[240] increases in surfactant synthesis,[51] reduction in synthesis of leukotrienes and prostaglandins,[79] reduction in neutrophil recruitment to the lung,[81] breakdown of white cell microaggregates,[196] enhancement of β-adrenergic activity,[18] reduction in pulmonary edema,[191] and relaxation of bronchospasm.[12] However, steroids may also potentiate the toxic effects of oxygen[38] and may actually worsen lung damage under certain conditions.[114]

The results of these two prospective steroid trials in BPD[12,128] have been unfortunate. Despite the fact that patient numbers were small and the methodology flawed, some neonatologists seem to believe that a properly controlled clinical trial is now "unethical." It appears that steroid treatment for BPD, with all its attendant dangers, has become standard practice in some centers without any firm scientific basis.[187]

Nutrition

It seems likely that premature infants with BPD, who are known to have a high oxygen consumption,[232] would benefit from a high caloric intake. However, many BPD infants cannot tolerate enteral feeding and must be given parenteral nutrition, which causes problems. First, the immature kidney copes poorly with large fluid and osmotic loads, particularly in the face of hypoxemia.[224] Second, intravenous fat emulsions can themselves cause pulmonary hypertension;[46] fat-laden macrophages in the tracheal aspirate may suggest such overload of the pulmonary circulation with lipid.[171] Third, the prolonged use of intravascular catheters is associated with septic and thromboembolic complications.

On the other hand, poor nutrition may adversely affect prognosis in chronic lung injury and has been related to impaired tolerance of hyperoxia[70] and growth retardation.[190] Poor nutrition may result in lowered plasma colloid osmotic pressure, predisposing to pulmonary edema.[15] Further, it is important to pay special attention to electrolyte and calcium balance during parenteral nutrition in BPD patients, particularly if loop diuretics are used. Finally, low vitamin A levels have been reported in infants with BPD despite appropriate supplementation, and there has been speculation about a possible etiologic role for vitamin A deficiency in BPD,[97] but the evidence for this association is weak at the moment.

Upper Airway Management

Prolonged tracheal intubation may be associated with tracheal necrosis and scarring[170] with subsequent stricture formation leading to upper airway narrowing. Tracheal stenosis delays weaning from the ventilator in BPD, and should be excluded in slowly resolving cases.[2]

Superoxide Dismutase

Oxygen exerts toxic effects via free radicals.[45] If the FiO_2 is very high, free radical generation may overwhelm normal protective mechanisms such as superoxide dismutase (SOD). SOD protects rats against the effects of hyperoxia, and rats made tolerant to hyperoxia have raised SOD levels.[45] It would seem rational to prevent free radical formation from causing continuing lung damage, which was the idea behind the early trials of vitamin E in BPD. However, after early encouraging reports,[62] further work found vitamin E to be quite useless[45,61] (a lesson for the advocates for corticosteroid therapy in BPD). A recent approach, which appears to hold promise, is the use of subcutaneous injections of SOD.[181] Forty-five patients were enrolled in the study of SOD administration during HMD; survivors in the treated group showed fewer clinical and radiologic signs of BPD and required fewer days of CPAP. However, survival was not improved.[181] Theoretical objections to the use of SOD in HMD to prevent BPD include the facts that oxygen radicals are part of the normal body defense against infection[13,106] and that SOD may increase pulmonary edema.[226] Clearly, more studies are needed before SOD can be recommended as effective prophylaxis against BPD. A similar approach is the use of allopurinol to reduce superoxide generation, and this approach too shows promise in infants with respiratory distress.[26a]

Diuretics

In a study of 10 infants with BPD, Kao et al showed that oral chlorothiazide and spironolactone increased airway conductance and dynamic pulmonary compliance but caused increased urinary losses of sodium, potassium, and phosphate.[107] Unfortunately, sequential statistical analysis was used, and the study was terminated early. Kao et al reported similar findings in 10 infants with BPD after intravenous furosemide; maximal improvement in pulmonary mechanics coincided with the onset of diuresis.[109] Diuretic treatment seems rational in BPD, since lung water is increased in BPD and fluid overload undoubtedly worsens the condition.[29] Beneficial effects of diuretic agents in BPD may be related in part to nondiuretic actions, such as an increase in thoracic duct lymph flow[135,214] and, in the case of furosemide, reduced transvascular pulmonary filtration,[25] diminished intrapulmonary shunting and capillary leaking,[7] increased size of pulmonary and systemic capacitance vessels,[53] and increased plasma colloid osmotic pressure.[25] Unlike the thiazides, furosemide causes calciuresis, which may progress to renal calcification and urinary sepsis.[96] The benefits of furosemide in BPD may be short lived and outweighed by the potential for electrolyte disturbances.[162] Additionally, furosemide may increase the incidence of arterial duct patency[75] and may

cause gallstones,[237] bone disease,[228] and ototoxicity.[164] Oral furosemide may be poorly absorbed and show great variation in bioavailability.[164]

Theophyllines

A study of intravenous theophylline in 11 ventilator-dependent infants with BPD showed improved dynamic compliance and pulmonary resistance; five infants were weaned from the ventilator within 72 hours.[180] Theophyllines may also expedite weaning from the ventilator in infants with respiratory distress.[83] Possible beneficial therapeutic effects of theophyllines include bronchodilation, diuresis, increased respiratory muscle strength, and stimulation of breathing.[143] The diaphragm in the preterm infant may be particularly prone to fatigue,[71] which may be a factor in ventilator weaning.[141] It is not yet clear whether theophyllines increase respiratory muscle strength in premature infants, as they may do in adults.[11] However, theophyllines are potentially toxic, particularly in children in whom lower doses are required because of reduced protein binding.[143] Theophyllines also have many potentially hazardous interactions with other drugs and are gastric irritants.

Bronchodilators

Although there is dispute as to the quantity of airway smooth muscle and its response to bronchodilators in normal neonates,[183] there is no doubt that children with BPD have increased airway smooth muscle.[16,151] Inhaled isoproterenol decreased airway resistance and increased specific conductance in nonventilator-dependent children with BPD,[108] the latter presumably related to its effects on small airways. Similar benefits were reported with terbutaline in ventilated infants with BPD.[199] Older BPD infants may not respond to bronchodilators because of extensive fibrosis and fixed airway obstruction.[108] The role of long-term bronchodilator therapy in the management of BPD remains unclear.[108]

Long-term Oxygen Administration

The mainstay of long-term BPD treatment has been low flow continuous oxygen therapy, usually via nasal prongs.[36, 165,166] The aims of oxygen therapy are to abolish alveolar hypoxia, to improve tissue oxygenation, and to reduce right ventricular afterload. The few invasive studies of oxygen therapy in BPD that have been done certainly suggest that low flow oxygen is as effective a pulmonary vasodilator as high flow oxygen. Improvements in oxygenation in patients with BPD are best shown by transcutaneous monitoring, which, nevertheless, may underestimate oxygen's therapeutic benefit.[179] Direct arterial puncture is unsatisfactory in monitoring oxygen therapy in BPD, because the procedure itself may alter the blood gas status of the infant.[165] Many unanswered questions about oxygen therapy in BPD remain because no good controlled trial has shown reduction in mortality or improvements in lung or cardiovascular function among BPD survivors as a result of oxygen therapy. It is not known whether vasodilators other than oxygen might produce sustained reductions in right ventricular work to the same or a greater extent. A further worry is that continued exposure to oxygen may in fact worsen pulmonary damage in BPD,[26,213] particularly since BPD is probably in part related to exposures to high oxygen concentrations in the first place. If oxygen-free radicals are important causes of lung damage, the evidence that their production is directly related to the partial pressure of oxygen[152] is disturbing. Similarly disturbing is the fact that hyperoxia increases somatic growth but markedly inhibits pulmonary development in rats.[19]

PROGNOSIS

Many infants survive the chronic phase of BPD and show improvement in lung function, although subtle abnormalities may remain. However, BPD survivors are at increased risk for systemic hypertension, sudden infant death syndrome, and cor pulmonale, each of which is discussed below.

Systemic Hypertension

Using Doppler technique to determine systemic arterial pressure along with the reference standards of de Swiet et al,[55] Abman et al found systemic hypertension in 13 of 30 BPD survivors.[4] The onset of hypertension in the BPD infants affected was delayed (mean age of onset at age 4.8 months, range 15 days to 15 months); three infants developed left ventricular hypertrophy and one had a cerebrovascular accident.[4] Six of the 13 hypertensive BPD patients required pharmacologic treatment, and all responded well.[4] In 11 of the 13 hypertensive BPD infants, the cause of the blood pressure elevation was not clear; the other two had renal disease.[4] Perhaps significantly, all 13 hypertensive BPD patients had been treated with furosemide, although no renal calcifications were detected in the four infants who had renal ultrasonography performed. Possible etiologic factors in systemic hypertension associated with BPD include thrombosis of renal arteries or arterioles related to umbilical artery catheterization,[145] intermittent hypoxemia elevating systemic vascular resistance, and increased pulmonary angiotensin converting enzyme activity as a consequence of hypoxia.[132] It is therefore important to check arterial blood pressure in all survivors of BPD, but the cause of systemic hypertension found in association with BPD remains speculative.

Sudden Infant Death Syndrome

A recent study of BPD survivors suggested that there may be a sevenfold increase in incidence of sudden death.[233] The study was controlled for prematurity, male sex, low socioeconomic status, maternal age and parity, apnea, multiple birth, Apgar scores at birth, and season of the year, yet a significant difference still emerged. Six out of 53 (11 per cent) BPD survivors died suddenly, compared with a 1.5 per cent incidence of sudden death in the control group. Whether the infants with BPD who died suddenly can be said to have had true sudden infant death syndrome is a matter of definition. The possible mechanisms of sudden death in BPD infants are not clear but may include intermittent and chronic hypoxemia in severely compromised children with immature respiratory control mechanisms, intermittent upper airway obstruction (related to prolonged intubation), and left recurrent laryngeal nerve paralysis secondary to stretching from pulmonary artery trunk enlargement.[229] Sudden death has been reported in BPD infants even when receiving continuous low flow oxygen therapy.[36] The newly described entity of prolonged expiratory apnea could play a role.[200]

Cor Pulmonale

There is considerable pathologic evidence for the involvement of the pulmonary circulation in chronic neonatal hyoxemia,[142] although there are few reports of detailed morphometric studies in BPD similar to those performed in infants with congenital heart disease. Organizing thrombi and an increase in medial muscle[215] are common pulmonary circulatory findings at autopsy in BPD; thromboembolism could be related to sepsis, blood transfusion, or intravenous hyperalimentation.[173] Of 142 BPD subjects, 46 per cent had abnormal thickening of pulmonary arterial walls.[59] Right ventricular hypertrophy is also common.[8] In seven of 12 subjects with BPD who were studied at autopsy,[8] cor pulmonale was considered to be the major factor leading to death, and pulmonary circulatory pathology (medial hyperplasia and adventitial thickening in small pulmonary arteries and arterioles) appeared to be far more important than the airway changes, which had largely regressed.

Detailed morphometric studies of a single premature infant have been reported.[173] The infant had required 3 days of therapy with an oxygen-enriched mixture, without ventilatory support. She had had recurrent pulmonary infections and died within hours of cardiac catheterization, which had shown suprasystemic pressure in the pulmonary artery. At postmortem examination, extreme hypoplasia of the pulmonary circulation was demonstrated. All generations of pulmonary arteries were reduced in number and external diameter and had increased wall thickness. Old thromboembolism and gross right ventricular hypertrophy were present. The authors suggested that lung growth and remodeling may have been disturbed by a series of perinatal and neonatal insults, resulting in such scanty growth of the pulmonary circulation that extreme hypoplasia resulted, determining the outcome. However, these findings should only be extrapolated very cautiously to infants with BPD. Similar measurements are needed on children with BPD dying of nonrespiratory causes such as trauma.[155] Decreased alveolar growth was reported in a detailed study of another child with BPD who died with severe cor pulmonale.[198] Reductions in alveolar growth may be a nonspecific response to pulmonary vascular injury.

It is well known that some children with congenital heart disease eventually develop irreversible changes in the pulmonary circulation, such that even anatomically feasible corrective surgery is contraindicated. We speculate that infants with BPD may also develop severe pulmonary vascular disease that becomes irreversible and may determine the outcome. The rapid development of pulmonary vascular disease complicating congenital heart disease is unusual but well described. Infants with BPD are more likely to have recurrent infections and hypoxic challenges to their compromised pulmonary circulations than most infants with congenital heart disease. Additionally, the major lung injury in BPD occurs in the very immature lung, at a time of rapid growth of the pulmonary circulation[172,173] and may therefore have more potential for reducing vessel numbers.[88] Our own preliminary studies suggest that a high pulmonary vascular resistance may carry a poor prognosis,[34] but clearly more data are needed before firm conclusions can be drawn.

SUMMARY AND CONCLUSIONS

We have reviewed the cardiopulmonary features of BPD, with special emphasis on how the disease and its treatment affect the heart and pulmonary circulation. The incidence of the disease is happily falling, as standards of obstetric, perinatal, and neonatal care rise.[76] However, the treatment of the established case of BPD is still very unsatisfactory, and infants with BPD make great demands on hospital and parental resources.[190] There is a clear need to define the effects of corticosteroids and bronchodilators on airway function in BPD and to delineate their roles in management. We also feel that BPD research should focus much more on the role of the pulmonary circulation. The following important questions are unanswered:

1. To what extent does pulmonary circulatory disease determine prognosis?

2. What (if any) pulmonary vasodilators, alone or in combination with oxygen, are beneficial?

3. What quantitative histologic abnormalities are found in the pulmonary circulation, and what is their significance?

We suggest that detailed hemodynamic assessment should be an early part of the management of children with BPD to rule out unsuspected congenital heart disease, to study the reactivity of the pulmonary circulation, and possibly to determine prognosis. Much more hemodynamic data will be needed, together with properly controlled trials of treatment in large numbers of children, before the specifically cardiovascular problems of BPD can be correctly understood and rationally managed.

References

1. Abdul-Rasool IH, Chamberlain JH (1983): Respiratory gas exchange before and after cardiac operations. J Thorac Cardiovasc Surg 85:856–863.
2. Abman SH, Accurso FJ, Bowman CM (1984): Unsuspected cardiopulmonary abnormalities complicating bronchopulmonary dysplasia. Arch Dis Child 59:966–970.
3. Abman SH, Wolfe RR, Accurso FJ, Koops BL, Bowman CM, Wiggins JW (1985): Pulmonary vascular response to oxygen in infants with severe bronchopulmonary dysplasia. Pediatrics 75:80–84.
4. Abman SH, Warady BA, Lum GM, Koops BL (1984): Systemic hypertension in infants with bronchopulmonary dysplasia. J Pediatr 104:929–931.
5. Adamson TM, Hawker JM, Reynolds EOR, Shaw JL (1969): Hypoxemia during recovery from severe hyaline membrane disease. Pediatrics 44:168–178.
6. Albert RK, Lakshminarayon S, Hildebrandt J, Kirk W, Butler J (1979): Increased surface tension favours pulmonary edema formation in anesthetized dogs' lungs. J Clin Invest 63:1015–1018.
7. Ali J, Chernicki W, Wood LDH (1979): Effect of furosemide in canine low pressure pulmonary edema. J Clin Invest 64:1494–1504.
8. Anderson WR, Engel RR (1983): Cardiopulmonary sequelae of reparative stages of bronchopulmonary dysplasia. Arch Pathol Lab Med 107:603–608.
9. Anderson WR, Strickland MB (1971): Pulmonary complications of oxygen therapy in the neonate. Arch Pathol 91:506–514.
10. Andrew M, Massicote-Nolan PM, Karpatkin M (1983): Plasma protease inhibitors in premature infants: Influence of gestational age, postnatal age, and health status. Proc Soc Exp Med 173:495–500.
11. Aubier M, de Troyer AD, Sampson M, Macklem PT, Roussos C (1982): Aminophylline improves diaphragmatic contractility. N Engl J Med 305:240–246.
12. Avery GB, Fletcher AB, Kaplan M, Brudno DS (1985): Controlled trial of dexamethasone in respirator-dependent infants with bronchopulmonary dysplasia. Pediatrics 75:106–111.
13. Babior BM, Kipnes RS, Curnutte JT (1973): The production by leukocytes of superoxide, a potential bactericidal agent. J Clin Invest 52:741–744.
14. Bancalari E, Abdenour GE, Feller R, Gannon J (1979): Bronchopulmonary dysplasia: Clinical presentation. J Pediatr 95:819–823.
15. Bancalari E, Gerhardt T (1986): Bronchopulmonary dysplasia. Pediatr Clin North Am 33:1–23.
15a. Bancalari E, Jesse MJ, Gelband H, Garcia O (1977): Lung mechanics in congenital heart disease with increased and decreased pulmonary blood flow. J Pediatr 90:192–195.
16. Banerjee CK, Girling DJ, Wigglesworth JS (1972): Pulmonary fibroplasia in newborn babies treated with oxygen and artificial ventilation. Arch Dis Child 47:509–518.
17. Barnes ND, Glover WJ, Hull D, Milner AD (1969): Effects of prolonged positive pressure ventilation in infancy. Lancet 2:1096–1099.
18. Barnes P, Jacobs M, Roberts J (1983): Glucocorticoids preferentially increase fetal alveolar B–receptors: Autoradiographic evidence (abstr). Clin Res 31:70A.
19. Bartlett D (1970): Postnatal growth of the mammalian lung: Influence of low and high oxygen tensions. Respir Physiol 9:58–64.
20. Beck KC, Lai-Fook SJ (1983): Alveolar liquid pressure in excised edematous dog lung with increased static recoil. J Appl Physiol 55:1277–1283.
21. Becker MJ, Koppe JG (1969): Pulmonary structural changes in neonatal hyaline membrane disease treated with high pressure artificial respiration. Thorax 24:689–694.
22. Bell EF, Warburton D, Stonestreet BS, Oh W (1980): Effect of fluid administration on the development of symptomatic patent ductus arteriosus and congestive heart failure in premature infants. N Engl J Med 302:598–604.
23. Berman W, Yabek SM, Dillon T, Burstein R, Corlew S (1982): Evaluation of infants with bronchopulmonary dysplasia using cardiac catheterization. Pediatrics 70:708–712.
24. Bland RD (1972): Cord-blood total protein level as a screening aid for the idiopathic respiratory distress syndrome. N Engl J Med 298:9–13.
25. Bland RD, McMillan DD, Bressack MA (1978): Decreased pulmonary transvascular fluid filtration in awake newborn lambs after intravenous furosemide. J Clin Invest 62:601–609.

26. Boat TH, Kleinerman JI, Fanaroff AA, Matthews LW (1973): Toxic effects of oxygen on cultured human neonatal respiratory epithelium. Pediatr Res 7:607–615.

26a. Boda D, Nemeth I, Hencz P, Denes K (1984): Effect of allopurinol treatment in premature infants with idiopathic respiratory distress syndrome. Dev Pharmacol Ther 7:357–367.

27. Bonikos DS, Bensch KG, Ludwin SK, Northway WH (1975): Oxygen toxicity in the newborn: The effect of prolonged 100% O_2 exposure on the lungs of newborn mice. Lab Invest 32:619–635.

28. Bonikos DS, Bensch KG, Northway WH (1976): Oxygen toxicity in the newborn: The effect of chronic continuous 100 per cent oxygen exposure on the lungs of newborn mice. Am J Pathol 85:623–650.

29. Brown ER, Stark A, Sosenko I, Lawson EE, Avery ME (1978): Bronchopulmonary dysplasia; possible relationship to pulmonary edema. J Pediatr 92:982–984.

30. Bryan MH, Hardie MJ, Reilly BJ, Swyer PR (1973): Pulmonary function studies during the first year of life in infants recovering from respiratory distress syndrome. Pediatrics 52:169–178.

31. Burger EJ, Macklem P (1966): Effect on lungs of breathing 100% oxygen near residual volume. Fed Proc 25:566.

32. Burton AC, Patel DJ (1958): Effect on pulmonary vascular resistance of inflation of the rabbit lungs. J Appl Physiol 12:239–246.

33. Bush A, Busst CM, Booth K, Knight WB, Shinebourne EA (1986): Does prostacyclin enhance the selective pulmonary vasodilator effect of oxygen in children with congenital heart disease? Circulation 74:135–144.

34. Bush A, Busst CM, Knight WB, Shinebourne EA (1986): Pulmonary haemodynamics in bronchopulmonary dysplasia: Response to oxygen and prostacyclin (abstr). Proc Br Paed Assoc 58:104.

35. Caldwell PRB, Lee WL, Schildkraut HS, Archibald ER (1966): Changes in lung volume diffusing capacity and blood gases in men breathing oxygen. J Appl Physiol 21:1477–1483.

36. Campbell AN, Zarfin Y, Groenveld M, Bryan MH (1983): Low flow oxygen therapy in infants. Arch Dis Child 458:795–798.

37. Cedergren B, Gyllensten I, Wersall J (1959): Pulmonary damage caused by oxygen poisoning. Acta Paediatr 48:477–494.

38. Clark JM, Lambertson CJ (1971): Pulmonary oxygen toxicity. Pharmacol Rev 23:37–133.

39. Coates AC, Bergsteinsson H, Desmond K, Outerbridge EW, Beaudry PH (1977): Long term pulmonary sequelae of premature birth with and without idiopathic respiratory distress syndrome. J Pediatr 90:611–616.

40. Coates G, O'Brodovich H, Jeffries AL, Gray GW (1984): Effects of exercise on lung lymph flow in sheep and goats during normoxia and hypoxia. J Clin Invest 74:133–141.

41. Comroe JH, Dripps RD, Dumke PR, Denning M (1945): Oxygen toxicity: The effect of inhalation of high concentrations of oxygen for twenty-four hours on normal men at sea level and at a simulated altitude of 18,000 feet. JAMA 128:710–717.

42. Corr L, McCarthy P, Lavender JB (1986): Investigation of bronchial compression in infants with congenital heart disease using radionuclide scanning (abstr). Proc Br Paed Assoc 58:74.

43. Cournand A, Motley HL, Werko L, Richards DW (1948): Physiologic studies of the effects of intermittent positive pressure breathing on cardiac output in man. Am J Physiol 192:162–174.

44. Cox JR, Davies-Jones AB, Leonard PJ, Singer B (1963): The effects of positive pressure respiration on urinary aldosterone excretion. Clin Sci 24:1–5.

45. Crapo JD, Tierney DF (1974): Superoxide dismutase and pulmonary toxicity. Am J Physiol 226:1401–1407.

46. Dahms BB, Halpin TC (1980): Pulmonary arterial lipid deposit in newborn infants receiving intravenous lipid infusion. J Pediatr 97:800–805.

47. Davies NJH, Denison DM (1979a): The measurement of metabolic gas exchange by mass spectrometry alone. Respir Physiol 36:261–267.

48. Davies NJH, Denison DM (1979b): The uses of long sampling probes in respiratory mass spectrometry. Respir Physiol 36:335–346.

49. Davies NJH, Shinebourne EA, Scallan MJ, Sopwith TA, Denison DM (1984): Pulmonary vascular resistance in children with congenital heart disease. Thorax 39:895–900.

50. Davis WB, Rennard SI, Bitterman PB, Crystal RG (1983): Pulmonary oxygen toxicity. N Engl J Med 309:878–883.

51. de Lemos RA, Shermeta DW, Knelson JH, Kotas R, Avery ME (1970): Acceleration of appearance of pulmonary surfactant in the fetal lamb by administration of corticosteroids. Am Rev Respir Dis 102:459–461.

52. de Lemos R, Wolsdorf J, Nachman R, Block AJ, Leiby G, Wolkinson HA, Allen T, Haller A, Morgan W, Avery ME (1969): Lung injury from oxygen in lambs: The role of artificial ventilation. Anaesthesiology 30:609–618.

53. Demling RH, Will JA (1978): The effect of furosemide on the pulmonary transvascular fluid filtration rate. Crit Care Med 6:317–319.

54. deSa DJ (1977): Myocardial changes in immature infants requiring prolonged ventilation. Arch Dis Child 52:138–147.

55. de Swiet M, Fayers P, Shinebourne EA (1980): Systolic blood pressure in a population of infants in the first year of life: The Brompton study. Pediatrics 65:1028–1035.

56. Donnelly WH, Bucciarelli RL, Nelson RM (1980): Ischemic papillary muscle necrosis in stressed newborn infants. J Pediatr 96:295–300.

57. Dudell GG, Gersony WM (1984): Patent ductus arteriosus in neonates with severe respiratory distress. J Pediatr 104:915–920.

58. Edwards DK (1979): Radiographic aspects of bronchopulmonary dysplasia. J Pediatr 95:823–829.

59. Edwards DK, Colby TV, Northway WH (1979): Radiographic-pathologic correlation in bronchopulmonary dysplasia. J Pediatr 95:834–836.

60. Egan EA, Hessler JR (1976): Positive end-expiratory pressure (PEEP) and right to left shunting in immature goats. Pediatr Res 10:932–937.

61. Ehrenkranz R, Ablow RC, Warshaw J (1979): Prevention of bronchopulmonary dysplasia with vitamin E administration during the acute stages of respiratory distress syndrome. J Pediatr 95:873–878.

62. Ehrenkranz R, Bonta BW, Ablow RC, Warshaw J (1978): Amelioration of bronchopulmonary dysplasia after vitamin E administration. N Engl J Med 299:564–569.

63. Engle WD, Arant BS, Wiriyattian S, Rosenfeld CR (1983): Diuresis and respiratory distress syndrome: Physiologic mechanisms and therapeutic implications. J Pediatr 102:912–917.

64. Fernandez-Bonetti P, Lupi-Herrera E, Martinez-Guerra ML, Barrios R, Seoane M, Sandoval J (1983): Peripheral airways obstruction in idiopathic pulmonary artery hypertension. Chest 83:732–738.

65. Fick A (1870): Veber die Messung des Blutquantums in der herzventikein. Verb Phys Med Ges Wurzb 2:169.

66. Fitzhardinge PM, Pape K, Arstikaitis M, Boyle M, Ashby S, Rowley C, Netley C, Swyer PR (1976): Mechanical ventilation of infants of less than 1501 gm birth weight: Health, growth and neurological sequelae. J Pediatr 88:531–541.

67. Fishman AP (1976): Hypoxia on the pulmonary circulation: How and where it acts. Circ Res 38:221–231.

68. Fouron J-C, Le Guennec J-C, Villemont D, Bard H, Pareault G, Davignon A (1980): Value of echocardiography in assessing the outcome of bronchopulmonary dysplasia of the newborn. Pediatrics 65:529–535.

69. Fox WW, Duara S (1985): Persistent pulmonary hypertension in the neonate: Diagnosis and management. J Pediatr 103:505–514.

70. Frank L, Groseclose E (1982): Oxygen toxicity in newborn rats: The adverse effects of undernutrition. J Appl Physiol 53:1248–1255.

71. Frantz ID, Werthammer J, Stark AR (1983): High-frequency ventilation in premature infants with lung disease: Adequate gas exchange at low tracheal pressure. Pediatrics 71:483–488.

72. Gay JH, Daily WJR, Meyer BHP, Trumps DS, Cloud DT, Moltham MD (1973): Ligation of the patent ductus arteriosus in premature infants: Report of 45 cases. J Pediatr Surg 8:677–683.

73. Gersony WM, Morishima HO, Daniel SS, Kohl S, Cohen H, Brown W, James LS (1976): The hemodynamic effects of intrauterine hypoxia: An experimental model in newborn lambs. J Paediatr 89:631–635.

74. Goldberg SJ, Levy RA, Siassi B, Betten J (1971): The effects of maternal hypoxia and hyperoxia upon the neonatal pulmonary vasculature. Pediatrics 48:528–533.

75. Green TP, Thompson TR, Johnson D, Lock JE (1982): Furosemide enhances the incidence of PDA in infants with RDS (abstr). Pediatr Res 16:288A.

76. Greenough A, Roberton NRC (1985): Morbidity and survival in neonates ventilated for the respiratory distress syndrome. Br Med J 290:597–600.

77. Gregory GA, Kitterman JA, Phibbs RH, Tooley WH, Hamilton WK (1971): Treatment of the idiopathic respiratory distress syndrome with continuous positive airway pressure. N Engl J Med 284:1333–1340.

78. Grindlinger EA, Manny J, Justice R, Dunham B, Shepro D, Hechtman HB (1979): Presence of negative inotropic agents in canine plasma during positive end-expiratory pressure. Circ Res 45:460–467.

79. Gryglewski RJ, Pmozenko B, Korbut R, Grodzinska L, Ocepkiewicza A (1975): Corticosteroids inhibit prostaglandin release from perfused lungs of sensitised guinea pig. Prostaglandins 10:343–355.

80. Halliday HL, Dumpit FM, Brady JP (1980): Effects of inspired oxygen on echocardiographic assessment of pulmonary vascular resistance and myocardial contractility in bronchopulmonary dysplasia. Pediatrics 65:536–540.

81. Hammerschmidt DE, White JG, Craddock PR, Jacob HS (1979): Corticosteroids inhibit complement-mediated granulocyte aggregation: A possible mechanism for their efficiency in shock states. J Clin Invest 63:798–803.

82. Hansen TN, Hazinski TA, Bland RD (1982): Vitamin E does not prevent oxygen-induced lung injury in newborn lambs. Pediatr Res 16:583–587.

83. Harris MC, Baumgart S, Rooklin AR, Fox WW (1983): Successful extubation of infants with respiratory distress syndrome using aminophylline. J Pediatr 103:303–305.

84. Harris P, Segel N, Green I, Housley E (1968): The influence of the airway's resistance and alveolar pressure on the pulmonary vascular resistance in chronic bronchitis. Cardiovasc Res 2:84–92.

85. Harrison MJ (1986): PEEP and CPAP. Br Med J 292:643–644.

86. Harrod JR, L'Heureux P, Wangensteen OD, Hunt CE (1974): Long-term follow-up of severe respiratory distress syndrome treated with IPPB. J Pediatr 84:277–286.

87. Hassan S, Turner P (1983): Systolic time intervals: A review of the method in the non-invasive investigation of cardiac function in health, disease and clinical pharmacology. Postgrad Med J 59:423–434.

88. Haworth SG, Hislop AA (1983): Pulmonary vascular development: Normal values of peripheral vascular structure. Am J Cardiol 52:578–583.

89. Hemmer M, Vequerat CE, Suter PM (1980): Urinary antidiuretic hormone excretion during mechanical ventilation and weaning in man. Anesthesiology 52:395–400.

90. Hirschfield S, Meyer R, Schwartz DC, Korfhagen J, Kaplan S (1975): The echocardiographic assessment of pulmonary artery pressure and pulmonary vascular resistance. Circulation 52:642–649.

91. Hislop A, Wigglesworth JS, Desai R (1986): Influence of mechanical ventilation on lung development (abstr). Proc Br Paed Assoc 58:105.

92. Hopperstein JM, Miltenberger MD, Moran WH (1965): The increase in blood levels of vasopressin in infants during birth and surgical procedures. Surg Gynecol Obstet 127:966–974.

93. Hordof AJ, Mellins RB, Gersory WM, Steeg CN (1977): Reversibility of chronic obstructive lung disease in infants following repair of ventricular septal defect. J Pediatr 90:187–191.

94. Howell JBL, Permutt S, Proctor DF, Riley RL (1961): Effect of inflation of the lung on different parts of pulmonary vascular bed. J Appl Physiol 16:71–76.

95. Howlett G (1972): Lung mechanics in normal infants and infants with congenital heart disease. Arch Dis Child 47:707–715.

96. Hufnagle KG, Khan SN, Penn D, Cacciarelli A, Williams P (1982): Renal calcifications: A complication of long-term furosemide therapy in preterm infants. Pediatrics 70:360–363.

97. Hustead VA, Gutcher GR, Anderson SA, Zachman RD (1984): Relationship of Vitamin A (retinol) status to lung disease in the preterm infant. J Pediatr 105:610–615.

98. Ikegami M, Jacobs H, Jobe A (1983): Surfactant function in respiratory distress syndrome. J Pediatr 102:443–447.

99. Ikegami M, Jobe A, Jacobs H, Lam R (1984): A protein from airways of premature lambs that inhibits surfactant function. J Appl Physiol 54:1134–1142.

100. Ito T, Iyomasa Y, Inoue T (1976): Changes of the postoperative minimal oxygen consumption of the newborn. J Pediatr Surg 11:495–503.

101. Jacob J, Gluck L, Diserra T, Edwards D, Kulovich M, Kuslinsky J, Merritt TA, Friedman WI (1980): The contribution of the PDA in the neonate with severe RDS. J Pediatr 96:79–87.

102. Jeffries AL, Coates G, O'Brodovich H (1984): Pulmonary epithelial permeability in hyaline membrane disease. N Engl J Med 311:1075–1080.

103. Jobe A, Ikegami M, Jacobs H, Jones S, Conaway D (1983): Permeability of premature lamb lungs to protein and the effect of surfactant on that permeability. J Appl Physiol 55:169–176.

104. Johnson DE, Lock JE, Elde RP, Thompson TR (1982): Pulmonary neuroendocrine cells in hyaline membrane disease and bronchopulmonary dysplasia. Pediatr Res 16:446–454.

105. Johnson JD, Malachowski NC, Grobstein R, Welsh D, Daily WJR, Sunshine P (1974): Prognosis of children surviving with the aid of mechanical ventilation in the newborn period. J Pediatr 84:272–276.

106. Johnson L, Bowen FW, Abbasi S, Herrmann N, Weston M, Sacks L, Porat R, Stahl G, Peckham G, Delivoria-Papadopoulos M, Quinn G, Schaffer D (1985): Relationship of prolonged pharmacologic serum levels of vitamin E to incidence of sepsis and necrotizing enterocolitis in infants with birth weight 1,500 grams or less. Pediatrics 75:619–638.

107. Kao LC, Warburton D, Cheng MH, Cedeno C, Platzker ACG, Keens TG (1984): Effect of oral diuretics on pulmonary mechanics in infants with chronic bronchopulmonary dysplasia: Results of a double-blind crossover sequential trial. Pediatrics 74:37–44.

108. Kao LC, Warburton D, Platzker ACG, Keens TG (1984): Effect of isoproterenol inhalation on airway resistance in chronic bronchopulmonary dysplasia. Pediatrics 73:509–514.

109. Kao LC, Warburton D, Sargent CW, Platzker ACG, Keens TG (1983): Furosemide acutely decreases airways resistance in chronic bronchopulmonary dysplasia. J Pediatr 103:624–629.

110. Kaplan HP, Robinson FR, Kapanci Y, Weibel ER (1969): Pathogenesis and reversibility of the pulmonary lesions of oxygen toxicity in monkeys. 1. Clinical and light microscopic studies. Lab Invest 20:94–100.

111. Kappagoda CT, Macartney FJ (1976): Effects of environmental temperature on oxygen consumption in infants with congenital disease of the heart. Br Heart J 38:1–4.

112. Kappagoda CT, Greenwood P, Macartney FJ, Linden RJ (1973): Oxygen consumption in children with congenital diseases of the heart. Clin Sci 45:107–114.

113. Kerber RE, Martins JB, Barnes R, Manuel WJ, Maximov M (1979): Effects of acute hemodynamic alterations on pulmonic valve motion. Circulation 60:1074–1081.

114. Kehrer JP, Klein-Szanto AJP, Sorensen EMB, Pearlman R, Rosner MH (1984): Enhanced acute lung damage following corticosteroid treatment. Am Rev Respir Dis 130:256–261.

115. Kelman GR (1966): Digital computer subroutine for the conversion of oxygen tension into oxygen saturation. J Appl Physiol 21:1375–1376.

116. Kistler GS, Caldwell PRB, Weibel ER (1967): Development of fine structural damage to alveolar and capillary lining cell in oxygen-poisoned rat lungs. J Cell Biol 32:605–628.

117. Koops BL, Morgan LJ, Battaglin FC (1982): Neonatal mortality risk in relation to birthweight and gestational age: Update. J Pediatr 101:969–977.

118. Lalande J (1973): Pulmonary sequelae of neonatal respiratory distress: Evolution during the first years of life. Ann Radiol 16:74–77.

119. Lamarre A, Linsao L, Reilly BJ, Swyer PR, Levison H (1973): Residual pulmonary abnormalities in survivors of idiopathic respiratory distress syndrome. Am Rev Respir Dis 108:56–61.

120. Lang RE, Unger T, Ganten D, Weil J, Bidlingmaier F, Dohleman D (1985): Alpha atrial natriuretic peptide concentrations in plasma of children with congenital heart and pulmonary disease. Br Med J 291:1241.

121. Langman CB, Engle WD, Baumgart S, Fox WW, Polin RA (1981): The diuretic phase of respiratory distress syndrome and its relationship to oxygenation. J Pediatr 98:462–466.

122. Laurenzi GA, Yin S, Guarneri JJ (1968): Adverse effect of oxygen on tracheal mucus flow. N Engl J Med 279:333–339.

123. Laver MB, Strauss W, Pohost GM (1979): Right and left ventricular geometry: Adjustments during acute respiratory failure. Crit Care Med 7:509–519.

124. Lees MH, Newcomb BA, Sunderland CO, Droukas P, Reynolds JW (1981): Doppler ultrasonography in evaluation of PDA shunting (letter). J Pediatr 98:852–853.

125. Lees MH, Way C, Ross BB (1967): Ventilation and respiratory gas transfer of infants with increased pulmonary blood flow. Pediatrics 40:259–271.

126. Lister G, Hoffman JIE, Rudolph AM (1974): Oxygen uptake in infants and children: A simple method for measurement. Pediatrics 53:656–662.

127. Mahony L, Carnero V, Brett C, Heymann MA, Clyman RI (1982): Prophylactic indomethacin therapy for patent ductus arteriosus in very low birthweight infants. N Engl J Med 305:501–510.

128. Mammel MC, Green TP, Johnson D, Thompson TR (1983): Controlled trial of dexamethasone therapy in infants with bronchopulmonary dysplasia. Lancet 1:1356–1358.

129. Marchak BE, Thompson WK, Duffty P, Miyaki T, Bryan MH, Bryan AC, Froese AB (1981): Treatment of RDS by high frequency oscillatory ventilation: A preliminary report. J Pediatr 99:287–292.

130. Markarian M, Jackson JJ, Bannon AE (1966): Serial serum total protein values in premature infants with and without the respiratory distress syndrome. J Pediatr 69:1046–1053.

131. Markestad T, Fitzhardinge AM (1981): Growth and development in children recovering from bronchopulmonary dysplasia. J Pediatr 98:597–602.

132. Mattioli L, Zakheim RM, Mullis K, Molteni A (1975): Angiotensin 1–converting enzyme activity in idiopathic respiratory distress of the newborn infant and in experimental alveolar hypoxia in mice. J Pediatr 87:97–101.

133. Mayes L, Perkett E, Shahlman MT (1983): Severe bronchopulmonary dysplasia: A retrospective review. Acta Paediatr Scand 72:225–229.

134. Maylan FMB, Shannon DC (1979): Preferential distribution of lobar emphysema and atelectasis in bronchopulmonary dysplasia. Pediatrics 63:130–134.

135. McCaffrey C, Levy M (1980): Effect of furosemide on thoracic duct lymph flow in the dog. Am J Physiol 238:F363–F371.

136. Melnick G, Pickoff AS, Ferrer PL, Peyser J, Bancalari E, Gelband H (1980): Normal pulmonary vascular resistance and left ventricular hypertrophy in young infants with bronchopulmonary dysplasia: An echocardiographic and pathologic study. Pediatrics 66:589–596.

137. Merritt TA, Stuard ID, Puccia J, Wood B, Edwards DK, Finkelstein J, Shapiro DL (1981): Newborn tracheal aspirate cytology: Classification during respiratory distress syndrome and bronchopulmonary dysplasia. J Pediatr 98:949–956.

138. Modi N, Sodha N, Cooke RWI (1986): A prospective survey of acute intrinsic renal failure in a neonatal intensive care unit (abstr). Proc Br Paed Assoc 58:104.

139. Mikity VG, Taber P (1973): Complications in the treatment of the respiratory distress syndrome: Bronchopulmonary dysplasia, oxygen toxicity and the Wilson-Mikity syndrome. Pediatr Clin North Am 20:419–431.

140. Motoyama EK, Laks H, Oh T, Rothstein P, Hellenbrand WE, Gewitz GH (1978): Deflation flow volume (DFV) curves in infants with congenital heart disease (CHD): Evidence for lower airway obstruction (abstr). Circulation (Suppl 2)58:107.

141. Muller N, Gulston G, Cade D, Whitton J, Froese AB, Bryan MH, Bryan AC (1979): Diaphragmatic muscle fatigue in the newborn. J Appl Physiol 46:688–695.

142. Naeye RL, Letts HW (1962): The effects of prolonged neonatal hypoxemia on the pulmonary vascular bed and heart. Pediatrics 30:902–908.

143. Nassif EG, Weinberger MM, Shannon D, Guiang SF, Hendeles L, Jimenez D, Ekwo E (1981): Theophylline disposition in infancy. J Pediatr 98:158–161.

144. Naulty CM, Horn S, Conry J, Avery GB (1978): Improved lung compliance after ligation of patent ductus arteriosus in hyaline membrane disease. J Pediatr 93:682–684.

145. Neal WA, Reynolds JW, Jarvis CW, Williams HJ (1972): Umbilical artery catheterization: Demonstration of arterial thrombosis by aortography. Pediatrics 50:6–13.

146. Nelson RM, Bucciarelli RL, Eitzman D, Egan EA II, Gessner IH (1978): Serum creatinine phosphokinase MB fraction in newborns with transient tricuspid insufficiency. N Engl J Med 298:146–149.

147. Nelson RM, Prod'hom LS, Cherry RB, Lipsitz PJ, Smith CA (1963): Pulmonary function in newborn infants: Alveolar-arterial oxygen gradient. J Appl Physiol 18:534–538.

148. Nickerson BG (1985): Bronchopulmonary dysplasia. Chest 87:528–535.

149. Nihill MR, McNamara DG (1978): Magnification pulmonary wedge angiography in the evaluation of children with congenital heart disease and pulmonary hypertension. Circulation 58:1094–1106.

150. Northway WH (1979): Observations on bronchopulmonary dysplasia. J Pediatr 95:815–818.

151. Northway WH, Rosan RC, Porter DY (1967): Pulmonary disease following respiratory therapy of hyaline-membrane disease. N Engl J Med 276:357–368.

152. Nunn JF (1985): Oxygen—friend and foe. J Royal Soc Med 78:618–622.

153. Nussbaum E (1983): Adult-type respiratory distress syndrome in children. Clin Pediatr 22:401–406.

154. Ogden BE, Murphy SA, Saunders GC, Pathak D, Johnson JD (1984): Neonatal lung neutrophils and elastase/proteinase inhibitor imbalance. Am Rev Respir Dis 130:817–821.

155. O'Brodovich HM, Mellins RB (1985): Bronchopulmonary dysplasia. Am Rev Respir Dis 132:694–709.

156. O'Grady J, Warrington S, Moh MJ (1980): Effects of intravenous infusions of prostacyclin (PGI$_2$) in man. Prostaglandins 19:319–333.

157. Ohlsson WTL (1947): A study of oxygen toxicity at atmospheric pressure with special reference to pathogenesis of pulmonary damage and clinical oxygen therapy. Acta Med Scand (Suppl)190:1–93.

158. Oppermann HC, Wille L, Bleyl U, Obladen M (1977): Bronchopulmonary dysplasia in premature infants: A radiological and pathological correlation. Pediatr Radiol 5:137–141.

159. Park SC, Steinfeld L, Dimich I (1973): Systolic time intervals in infants with congestive heart failure. Circulation 47:1281–1288.

160. Parrish DA, Mitchell BC, Henson PM, Larsen GL (1984): Pulmonary response of fifth component of complement-sufficient and -deficient mice to hyperoxia. J Clin Invest 74:956–965.

161. Patel DJ, Greenfield JC, Austen GW, Morrow AG, Fry DL (1965): Pressure-flow relationships in the ascending aorta and femoral artery of man. J Appl Physiol 20:459–463.

162. Patel H, Yeh T-F, Jain R, Pildes R (1985): Pulmonary and renal responses to furosemide in infants with stage III–IV bronchopulmonary dysplasia. Am J Dis Child 139:917–919.

163. Perkin RM, Arias NG (1984): Pulmonary hypertension in pediatric patients. J Pediatr 105:511–522.

164. Peterson RG, Simmons MA, Rumack BH, Levine RL, Brooks JG (1980): Pharmacology of furosemide in the premature newborn infant. J Pediatr 97:139–143.

165. Philip AG, Peabody JL, Lucey JF (1978): Transcutaneous PO$_2$ monitoring in the home management of bronchopulmonary dysplasia. Pediatrics 61:655–657.

166. Pinney MA, Cotton EK (1976): Home management of bronchopulmonary dysplasia. Pediatrics 58:856–859.

167. Pontoppidan H, Hedley-Whyte J, Bendixen HH, Laver MB, Radford EP (1965): Ventilation and oxygen requirements during prolonged artificial ventilation in patients with respiratory failure. N Engl J Med 273:401–409.

168. Pusey VA, MacPherson RI, Chernick V (1969): Pulmonary fibroplasia following prolonged artificial ventilation of newborn infants. Can Med Assoc J 100:451–457.

169. Puy RJM, Hyde RW, Fisher AB, Clark JM, Dickson J, Lambertsan CJ (1968): Alterations in the pulmonary capillary bed during early O$_2$ toxicity in man. J Appl Physiol 24:537–543.

170. Rasche RFH, Kutins LR (1972): Histopathologic changes in airway mucosa of infants after endotracheal intubation. Pediatrics 50:632–637.

171. Recalde AL, Nickerson BG, Vegas M, Scott CB, Landing BH, Warburton D (1984): Lipid-laden macrophages in tracheal aspirates of newborn infants receiving intravenous lipid infusions: A cytologic study. Pediatr Pathol 2:25–34.

172. Reid L (1970): Bronchopulmonary dysplasia—pathology. J Pediatr 95:836–841.

173. Rendas A, Brown ER, Avery ME, Reid LM (1980): Prematurity, hypoplasia of the pulmonary vascular bed, and hypertension: Fatal outcome in a ten month old infant. Am Rev Respir Dis 121:873–880.

174. Reynolds EOR, Taghizadeh A (1974): Improved prognosis of infants mechanically ventilated for hyaline membrane disease. Arch Dis Child 49:505–515.

175. Rhodes PG, Graves GR, Patel DM, Campbell SB, Blumenthal BI (1983): Minimizing pneumothorax and bronchopulmonary dysplasia in ventilated infants with hyaline membrane disease. J Pediatr 103:634–637.

176. Rhodes PG, Hall RT, Leonidas JL (1975): Chronic pulmonary disease in neonates with assisted ventilation. Pediatrics 55:788–796.

177. Richards AM, Ikram H, Yandle TG, Nicholls MG, Webster I, Espiner EA (1985): Renal, haemodynamic and hormonal effects of human alpha atrial natriuretic peptide in healthy volunteers. Lancet 1:545–549.

178. Riemenschneider TA, Nielsen HC, Ruttenberg HD, Jaffe RB (1976): Disturbances of the transitional circulation: Spectrum of pulmonary hypertension and myocardial dysfunction. J Pediatr 89:622–625.

179. Rome ES, Stork EK, Carlo WA, Martin RJ (1984): Limitations of transcutaneous PO_2 and PCO_2 monitoring in infants with bronchopulmonary dysplasia. Pediatrics 74:217–220.

180. Rooklin AR, Moomjian AS, Shutack JG, Schwartz JG, Fox WW (1979): Theophylline therapy in bronchopulmonary dysplasia. J Pediatr 95:882–885.

181. Rosenfeld W, Evans H, Concepcion L, Jhaveri R, Schaeffer H, Friedman A (1984): Prevention of bronchopulmonary dysplasia by administration of bovine superoxide dismutase in preterm infants with respiratory distress syndrome. J Pediatr 105:781–785.

182. Rudolph AM, Yuan S (1966): Response of the pulmonary vasculature to hypoxia and H ion concentration changes. J Clin Invest 45:399–411.

183. Rutter N, Milner AD, Hiller EJ (1975): Effect of bronchodilators on respiratory resistance in infants and young children with bronchiolitis and wheezy bronchitis. Arch Dis Child 50:719–722.

184. Rzedzian B, Chapman B, Mansfield P, Coupland RE, Doyle M, Chrispin A, Guilfoyle D, Small P (1983): Real-time nuclear magnetic resonance clinical imaging in paediatrics. Lancet 2:1281–1282.

185. Saldanha R, Cepeda E, Poland R (1982): The effect of vitamin E prophylaxis on the incidence and severity of bronchopulmonary dysplasia. J Pediatr 101:89–93.

186. Sangal S, Rosenbaum P, Stoskopf P, Sinclair JC (1984): Outcome in infants 501 to 1000 gm birth weight delivered to residents of the McMaster Health Region. J Pediatr 105:969–976.

187. Schick JB, Goetzman BW (1985): Chronic lung disease of prematurity (letter). Pediatrics 76:652.

188. Schick JB, Goetzman BW (1983): Corticosteroid response in chronic lung disease of prematurity. Am J Perinatol 1:23–27.

189. Seeger W, Stohr G, Wolf HRD, Newhof H (1984): Alteration of surfactant function due to protein leakage: Special interaction with fibrin monomer. J Appl Physiol 58:326–338.

190. Shankaran M, Szego E, Eizert D, Siegel P (1984): Severe bronchopulmonary dysplasia: Predictors of survival and outcome. Chest 86:607–610.

191. Shasby DM, Fox RB, Harada RN, Repine JE (1982): Reduction of the edema of acute hyperoxic lung injury by granulocyte depletion. J Appl Physiol 52:1237–1244.

192. Sheagren TG, Mangurten HH, Brea F, Lutostanki S (1980): Rumination: A new complication of neonatal intensive care. Pediatrics 66:551–555.

193. Shepard FM, Johnston RB, Klatte FC, Burke H, Stahlman M (1968): Residual pulmonary findings in clinical hyaline membrane disease. N Engl J Med 279:1063–1071.

194. Sibbald WJ, Driedger AA (1983): Right ventricular function in acute disease states: Pathophysiologic considerations. Crit Care Med 11:339–345.

195. Silverman NH, Snider AR, Rudolph AM (1980): Evaluation of pulmonary hypertension by M-mode echocardiography in children with ventricular septal defect. Circulation 61:1125–1132.

196. Skubitz KM, Craddock PR, Hammerschmidt DG, August JT (1981): Corticosteroids block binding of chemotactic peptide to its receptor on granulocytes and cause disaggregation of granulocyte aggregates in vitro. J Clin Invest 68:13–20.

197. Smyth JA, Tabachnik E, Duncan WJ, Reilly BJ, Levison H (1981): Pulmonary function and bronchial hyperactivity in long-term survivors of bronchopulmonary dysplasia. Pediatrics 68:336–340.

198. Sobonya RE, Logvinoff MM, Taussig LM, Theriault A (1982): Morphometric analysis of the lung in prolonged bronchopulmonary dysplasia. Pediatr Res 16:969–972.

199. Sosulzki R, Abbasi S, Fox WW (1982): Therapeutic value of terbutaline in bronchopulmonary dysplasia (abstr). Pediatr Res 16:309A.

200. Southall DP, Talbert DG, Johnson P, Morley CJ, Salmons S, Miller J, Helms PJ (1985): Prolonged expiratory apnoea: A disorder resulting in severe arterial hypoxaemia in infants and young children. Lancet 2:571–577.

201. Spach MS, Serwer GA, Anderson PAW, Canent RV, Levin AR (1980): Pulsatile aortopulmonary pressure-flow dynamics of patent ductus arteriosus in patients with various haemodynamic states. Circulation 61:110–122.

202. Spitzer AR, Fox WW, Delivoria-Papadopoulos M (1981): Maximum diuresis—a factor in predicting recovery from respiratory distress syndrome and the development of bronchopulmonary dysplasia. J Pediatr 98:476–479.

203. Stahlman M, Hedwall G, Lindstrom D, Snell J (1982): Role of hyaline membrane disease in production of later childhood lung abnormalities. Pediatrics 69:572–576.

204. Staub NC (1974): Pathogenesis of pulmonary edema. Am Rev Respir Dis 109:358–372.

205. Staub NC (1981): Pulmonary edema due to increased microvascular permeability. Ann Rev Med 32:291–312.

206. Stanger P, Lucas RV, Edwards JE (1969): Anatomic factors causing respiratory distress in acyanotic congenital cardiac disease. Pediatrics 43:760–769.

207. Stenmark KR, James SL, Voelkel NF, Toews WH, Reeves JT, Murphy RC (1983): Leukotriene C4 and D4 in neonates with hypoxemia and pulmonary hypertension. N Engl J Med 309:77–80.

208. Stern L, Ramos AD, Outerbridge EW, Beaudry PH (1970): Negative pressure artificial respiration: Use in treatment of respiratory failure of the newborn. Can Med Assoc J 102:595–601.

209. Stocks J, Godfrey S (1976): The role of artificial ventilation, oxygen and CPAP in the pathogenesis of lung damage in neonates: Assessment by serial measurements of lung function. Pediatrics 57:352–362.

210. Stocks J, Godfrey S, Reynolds EOR (1978): Airway resistance in infants after various treatments for hyaline membrane disease: Special emphasis on prolonged high levels of inspired oxygen. Pediatrics 61:178–183.

211. Suter PM, Fairley HB, Isenberg MD (1975): Optimum end-expiratory airway pressure in patients with acute pulmonary failure. N Engl J Med 292:284–289.

212. Swischuk LE (1977): Bubbles in hyaline membrane disease. Differentiation of three types. Radiology 122:417–426.

213. Szoke E, Thet LA (1985): Effects of 100% oxygen exposure on the neonatal lung: Comparison of recovery in air and 60% O_2 (abstr). Am Rev Respir Dis 131:A249.

214. Szwed JJ, Kleit SA, Hamburger RJ (1972): Effect of furosemide on thoracic duct lymph flow in the dog. J Lab Clin Med 79:693–700.

215. Taghizadeh A, Reynolds EOR (1976): Pathogenesis of bronchopulmonary dysplasia following hyaline membrane disease. Am J Pathol 82:241–258.

216. Tarnow-Mordi W, Wilkinson A (1986): Mechanical ventilation of the newborn. Br Med J 292:575–576.

217. Tepper RS, Pagtakhan RD, Taussig LM (1984): Noninvasive determination of total respiratory system compliance in infants by the weighted-spirometer method. Am Rev Respir Dis 130:461–466.

218. Theros EG (1967): Case of the month from the AFIP. Radiology 89:524.

219. Thomas AN, Hall AD (1970): Mechanism of pulmonary injury after oxygen therapy. Am J Surg 120:255–263.

220. Thurlbeck WM (1979): Morphologic aspects of bronchopulmonary dysplasia. J Pediatr 95:842–843.

221. Tikkanen I, Fyhrquist F, Metsarinne K, Leidenius R (1985): Plasma atrial natriuretic peptide in cardiac disease and during infusion in healthy volunteers. Lancet 2:66–69.

222. Toce SS, Farrell PM, Leavitt LA, Samuels DP, Edwards DK (1984): Clinical and roentgenographic scoring systems for assessing bronchopulmonary dysplasia. Am J Dis Child 138:581–585.

223. Tooley WH (1979): Epidemiology of bronchopulmonary dysplasia. J Pediatr 95:851–858.

224. Torrado A, Guignard JP, Prod'hom LS, Gautier E (1977): Hypoxaemia and renal function in newborns with respiratory distress syndrome (RDS). Helv Paediatr Acta 29:399–405.

225. Toubas PL, Hof RP, Heymann MA, Rudolph AM (1974): Effects of hypothermia and rewarming on neonatal circulation (abstr). Pediatr Res 8:451.

226. Turrens JF, Crapo JD, Freeman BA (1984): Protection against oxygen toxicity by intravenous injection of liposome-entrapped catalase and superoxide dismutase. J Clin Inivest 73:87–95.

227. Tsai SH, Anderson WR, Strickland MB, Pliego M (1972): Bronchopulmonary dysplasia associated with oxygen therapy in infants with respiratory distress syndrome. Radiology 105:107–112.

228. Venkataraman PS, Han BK, Tsang RC, Daugherty CC (1983): Secondary hyperparathyroidism and bone disease in infants receiving long-term furosemide therapy. Am J Dis Child 137:1158–1181.

229. Vesselinova-Jenkins CK (1980): Model of persistent foetal circulation and sudden infant death syndrome (SIDS). Lancet 2:831–833.

230. Walkinshaw M, Shoemaker WC (1980): Use of volume loading to obtain preferred levels of PEEP: A preliminary study. Crit Care Med 8:81–86.

231. Watts JL, Ariagno RL, Brady JP (1977): Chronic pulmonary disease in neonates after artificial ventilation: Distribution of ventilation and pulmonary interstitial emphysema. Pediatrics 60:273–281.

232. Weinstein MR, Oh W (1981): Oxygen consumption in infants with bronchopulmonary dysplasia. J Pediatr 99:958–961.

233. Werthammer J, Brown ER, Neff RK, Taeusch HW (1982): Sudden infant death syndrome in infants with bronchopulmonary dysplasia. Pediatrics 69:301–304.

234. West JB, Dollery CT, Heard BE (1965): Increased pulmonary vascular resistance in the dependent zone of the isolated dog lung caused by perivascular edema. Circ Res 17:191–206.

235. Wheller JJ, Menke JA (1985): Continuous wave Doppler ultrasound in the detection of abnormal arterial flow in patients with unusual defects. J Pediatr 107:569–572.

236. Whittenberger JL, McGregor M, Berglund EW, Borst HG (1960): Influence of state of inflation of the lung on pulmonary vascular resistance. J Appl Physiol 15:878–882.

237. Whitington PF, Black DD (1980): Cholelithiasis in premature infants treated with parenteral nutrition and furosemide. J Pediatr 97:647–649.

238. Whitley RJ, Brasfield D, Reynold DW, Stagno S, Tiller RE, Alford CA (1976): Protracted pneumonitis in young infants associated with perinatally acquired cytomegaloviral infection. J Pediatr 89:16–22.

239. Wilcox WD, Corrigan TA, Dooley KJ, Giddens DP, Dykes FD, Lazzara A, Ray JL, Ahmann PA (1983): Range-gated pulsed Doppler ultrasonographic evaluation of carotid arterial blood flow in small preterm infants with patent ductus arteriosus. J Pediatr 102:294–298.

240. Wilson JW (1972): Treatment or prevention of pulmonary cellular damage with pharmacologic doses of corticosteroid. Surg Gynecol Obstet 134:675–681.

241. Wolfson MR, Bhutani VK, Shaffer TH, Bowen FW (1984): Mechanics and energetics of breathing helium in infants with bronchopulmonary dysplasia. J Pediatr 104:752–757.

242. Wong J-T, James LS, Kilchevsky E, James E (1985): Management of infants with severe respiratory failure and persistence of the fetal circulation without hyperventilation. Pediatrics 79:488–494.

243. Yamamoto E, Wittner M, Rosenbaum RM (1970): Resistance and susceptibility to oxygen toxicity in cell types of the gas-blood barrier of the rat lung. Am J Pathol 59:409–436.

244. Yeh TF, Thalji A, Luken L, Lilien L, Carr I, Pildes RS (1981): Improved lung compliance following indomethacin therapy in premature infants with persistent ductus arteriosus. Chest 80:698–700.

245. Yu VYH, Orgill AA, Lim SB, Bajuk B, Astbury J (1983): Growth and development of very low birthweight infants recovering from bronchopulmonary dysplasia. Arch Dis Child 58:791–794.

32 STRUCTURAL HEART DISEASE IN THE LOW BIRTHWEIGHT NEONATE

James C. Huhta

The combination of congenital heart disease and low birthweight or prematurity is uncommon, and the presence of a cardiac defect alone is not thought to result in the premature onset of labor or in growth retardation. Nonetheless, the diagnosis and management of such infants is becoming a well-recognized problem. In the National Collaborative Study on indomethacin treatment of patent ductus arteriosus, some premature infants were excluded because they were found to have a ventricular septal defect.[5] If unrecognized, such an infant might have a thoracotomy for patent ductus arteriosus (PDA) ligation or for another reason without performing a needed pulmonary arterial banding. The experience of the New England Regional Infant Cardiac Program showed that low birthweight was a risk factor for mortality and found that 18.6 per cent of the total of 2137 infants with congenital heart disease who were detected had a birthweight less than 2.5 kg.[4] Fleming et al[3] described the risk of ligation of patent ductus arteriosus in infants in whom the anatomic definition was not optimal; wholesale treatment of all premature infants with indomethacin[8] or other prostaglandin inhibitors to close the ductus could have a disastrous result when ductus-dependent congenital heart disease is unrecognized. Strauss et al reported the reversal of indomethacin closure of a patent ductus arteriosus in such a situation.[12]

The presence of hydrops fetalis or polyhydramnios can precipitate preterm labor. Severe congenital heart defects with either very poor ventricular function or valve regurgitation might be associated with either miscarriage or early labor if hydrops fetalis develops because of the heart disease. Another possibility is low birthweight without prematurity (growth retardation) due to either fetal malnutrition or congenital abnormalities such as those found with genetic defects. It is possible that fetuses with the most severe cardiac defects are lost early in gestation, so that neonates presenting with congenital heart disease and prematurity at a viable gestation are a selected group unrepresentative of the entire population. Until fetal echocardiographic techniques are more advanced (see Chapters 14 and 15) or until we have better markers for congenital heart disorders, an analysis of the neonates presenting with both a heart defect and low birthweight must suffice.

HEART DISEASE AND LOW BIRTHWEIGHT

Several important considerations affect the management of a low birthweight neonate with congenital heart disease: (1) the diagnosis of a cardiac defect may be difficult without a high index of suspicion, especially in the presence of pulmonary disease, (2) cardiac catheterization with angiography and interventional procedures such as balloon atrial septostomy may be technically very difficult or sometimes impossible, (3) options for surgical treatment may be limited by the critical condition of the neonate or the short period of effectiveness of palliative surgery, given the relatively rapid doubling or tripling of birthweight in such small infants, (4) little is known about the natural history of the development of the heart and lungs in the presence of prematurity and heart disease, and (5) therapeutic misadventure will result if the ductus arteriosus is ligated in a congenital cardiac lesion in which ductal patency is providing palliation.

In order to investigate these possibilities, the clinical features of a group of 77 neonates with structural heart disease and low birthweight were examined at birth at either Texas Children's Hospital or Jefferson Davis Hospital, Houston, Texas, from July 1982 to October 1986. Low birthweight was defined as less than 2500 g, and a gestational age determined by examination after birth of less than 37 weeks was defined as prematurity. The records of this group of neonates were examined with particular attention to associated congenital defects, types of congenital heart disease, and outcome. Follow-up status was aimed at determining mortality only. The presence of a ductus arteriosus was determined by two-dimensionally directed pulsed Doppler echocardiography, and the initial anatomic diagnosis was made by real time echocardiographic imaging in all cases. The frequency of the imaging instrument was 5 MHz initially, and later 7.5 MHz, and in the last year of the study 10 MHz imaging (Advanced Technology Laboratories) was used. A complete examination included the usual parasternal, apical, and subcostal echocardiographic views plus a careful suprasternal examination of extracardiac anatomy (Figs. 32–1 and 32–2).[6] Imaging-directed pulsed and blind continuous wave Doppler echocardiography supplemented the examination after 1983. The diagnosis of patent ductus arteriosus and the technique of examination by image-directed pulsed Doppler

Grace Y. Yoon aided in data analysis, and Dr. Victoria E. Judd collated the clinical data.

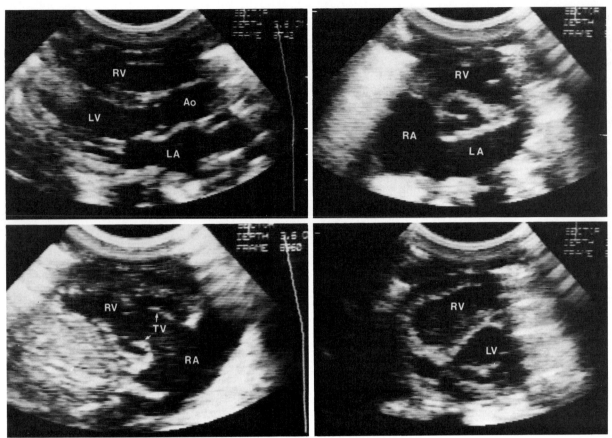

Figure 32–1. Two-dimensional echocardiogram in a normal low birthweight neonate without congenital heart disease. A normal long axis scan (left upper panel) shows the normal left ventricle (LV), right ventricle (RV), left atrium (LA), and aorta (Ao), and a scan of the right ventricular inlet (left lower panel) shows the tricuspid valve (TV) to be normal. Short axis scans show normal aortic and pulmonary valves and ventricular septum (VS) (right panels).

Table 32–1. STRUCTURAL CONGENITAL HEART DISEASE
IN THE LOW BIRTHWEIGHT INFANT: COMPARISON OF DATA
FROM TEXAS CHILDREN'S HOSPITAL (TCH) AND THE
NEW ENGLAND REGIONAL INFANT CARDIAC PROGRAM (NERICP)

Diagnosis*	TCH † Total = 77		NERICP‡ Total = 344
	Per Cent	*Number*	*Per Cent*
Ventricular septal defect	35	27	28
D-Transposition	3	2	4
Tetralogy of Fallot	12	9	9
Coarctation/IAA	5	4	10
Hypoplastic left-heart syndrome	6	5	5
Atrioventricular septal defect	1	1	6
Heterotaxias	4	3	5
Pulmonary stenosis	5	4	3
Pulmonary atresia	4	3	4
Atrial septal defect	5	4	5
TAPVC	3	2	3
Cardiomyopathy	3	2	3
Tricuspid atresia	4	3	3
Single ventricle	—	0	3
Aortic stenosis	1	1	1
Double-outlet right ventricle	4	3	2
Truncus arteriosus	3	2	2
Corrected transposition	3	2	1
Other	—	0	4

*Patent ductus arteriosus excluded.
†Expressed as nearest whole per cent of the total number of infants born with a birth weight less than 2.5 kg.
‡Adapted from Fyler DC (1980): Report of the New England Regional Infant Cardiac Program. Pediatrics (Suppl)65:377–461.

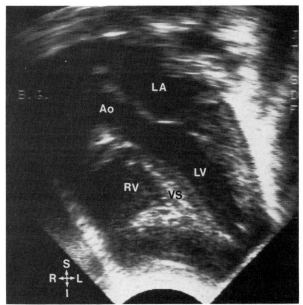

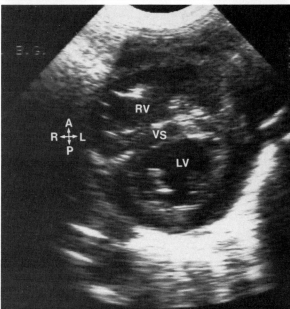

Figure 32–2. Apical and short axis scans (upper and lower panels, respectively) further examine the ventricular septum (VS). A = anterior; Ao = aorta; I = inferior; L = left; LA = left atrium; LV = left ventricle; R = right; RV = right ventricle.

echocardiography have been previously described (see Chapter 30).[7,13]

RESULTS

In the 77 neonates presenting with congenital heart disease (excluding patent ductus arteriosus) and low birthweight, the gestational age by Dubowitz examination immediately after birth ranged from 26 to 42 weeks (mean 34.8), the weight ranged from 820 to 2500 g (mean 1878 g) and the follow-up period has ranged from 2 months to 4 years.

The mortality has been 34 of 77 (44 per cent), and autopsy was obtained to confirm the diagnosis in 19 infants. Major congenital anomalies (MCA) were present in 32 of 77 (42 per cent), including multiple combinations of cleft palate, cerebral or spinal defects, tracheal or esophageal atresia, choanal atresia, and trisomy 18 or 21. Nineteen neonates with a gestational age greater than 36 weeks with obvious growth retardation (birthweight 1580 to 2400 g) were included.

CONGENITAL HEART DISEASE (TABLE 32–1)

The most common defect was ventricular septal defect in 27 of 77 neonates (35 per cent). Gestational ages in these 27 ranged from 28 to 40 weeks. Twenty-one of 27 were premature with clinical respiratory distress syndrome, and six were growth retarded. Twelve of 27 had other major congenital anomalies, including four with a genetic syndrome.

The next most common uncomplicated defects were tetralogy of Fallot in nine (MCA in five), double outlet right ventricle in three, valvular pulmonary stenosis in four, cardiomyopathy in two (dilated in one), coarctation of the aorta (or interruption) in four, and atrial septal defect in four. Twenty-four (31 per cent) had complex congenital heart disease, including two with transposition of the great arteries, five with hypoplastic left-heart syndrome, three with heterotaxy (atrial isomerism), two with corrected transposition, four with pulmonary atresia (intact septum in two), three with tricuspid atresia, two with total anomalous pulmonary venous drainage, two with truncus arteriosus (one with interrupted aortic arch), and one with AV septal defect.

Clinical respiratory distress syndrome developed in 28 (36 per cent) in their first week after birth. Inadvertent ligation of the ductus arteriosus would have definitely harmed those neonates with ductus-dependent congenital heart defects (17 of 77, or 22 per cent), and a total of 25 (32 per cent) may have been affected adversely.

DIAGNOSIS

The presence of other anomalies often led to the diagnosis of congenital heart disease prior to the manifestation of clinical symptoms from the heart problem. The presence of such obvious findings as dextrocardia or trisomy 18 led to echocardiography. Much more often the congenital defect was recognized during echocardiography for evaluation of a suspected patent ductus arteriosus. Pieroni et al[11] reported echocardiographic recognition of aortopulmonary septal defect in a premature infant, a defect that could simulate the hemodynamics of patent ductus arteriosus. Even in patients with severe cyanosis refractory to oxygen therapy, there appeared to have been a tendency, from our retrospective review, to delayed diagnosis due either to failure to suspect congenital heart disease in this population or to a reluctance to proceed

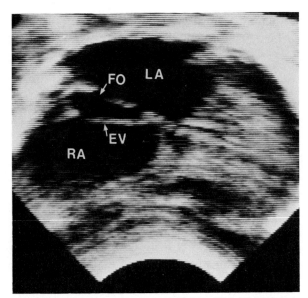

Figure 32–3. Possible false-positive diagnosis of an atrial septal defect at the fossa ovalis (FO) by echocardiography in a premature infant with dropout in a subcostal scan. A prominent eustachian valve (EV) may also cause confusion. LA = left atrium; RA = right atrium.

with further work-up in a critically ill neonate with apparent respiratory difficulties. One patient in this series, an infant weighing 1110 g at 30 weeks' gestation with tricuspid and pulmonary atresia, presented immediately after birth in critical condition with very poor oxygenation, which led to treatment with mechanical ventilation and high concentrations of oxygen. The infant developed severe oxygen toxicity, which appeared to be the cause of fatal respiratory disease.

The detection of congenital heart disease in the low birthweight neonate with respiratory distress syndrome can be challenging. The physical examination may not be helpful because a heart murmur is uncommon in most lesions with pulmonary hypertension and left-to-right shunt as well as left ventricular outflow tract obstruction. Ventricular septal defect causes left atrial and left ventricular enlargement simulating a patent ductus arteriosus and may have negligible murmur. In severe aortic arch obstruction, such as coarctation or interrupted arch, the ductus supplies the lower extremities, so there is no difference in the pulses, and obvious differential cyanosis is unusual. Failure to increase the arterial oxygenation with 100 per cent oxygen *and* positive end-expiratory pressure should be a strong clue to the presence of cyanotic disease. The chest radiograph may show obvious cardiomegaly; however, it is usual to take the first film of a critically ill neonate at peak inspiratory pressure, which may obscure the presence of cardiac enlargement and palliate large left-to-right shunt. Markedly increased pulmonary vascular markings are much more common as an aid in the diagnosis of total anomalous pulmonary venous drainage (two cases in this series) (see Table 32–1) than in neonates with ventricular septal defect, for example. If the patient has dextrocardia, it is possible for the film to be incorrectly labeled, leading to delay in diagnosis if the

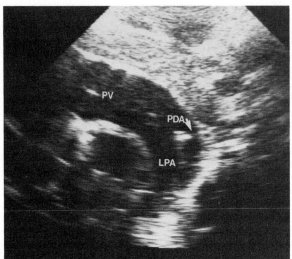

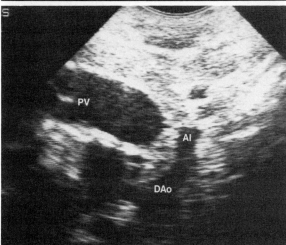

Figure 32–4. High parasternal scan by 7.5 MHz imaging. Normal aortic isthmus (AI) in a preterm infant with a patent ductus arteriosus (PDA). The scan should include the left pulmonary artery (LPA) and the descending aorta (DAo). PV = pulmonary valve.

apex is not palpated routinely. The electrocardiogram may be very useful in identifying complex intracardiac anatomy such as atrioventricular septal defect (in which left axis deviation with a qR pattern in lead aVL is found) or right ventricular hypoplasia (in which left ventricular hypertrophy may be present). Rhythm abnormalities are not much help in the diagnosis with the exception of complete atrioventricular block, which is associated with corrected transposition (one case in this series) or left atrial isomerism with AV septal defect (one case).

Anatomic diagnosis is traditionally performed by cardiac catheterization and angiography. In the low birthweight neonate, such procedures may be dangerous as well as technically difficult; obtaining vascular access in neonates with a birthweight under 2000 g is not simple. Therefore, echocardiography has become the mainstay of anatomic diagnosis in this group of patients. However, there is little or no information concerning the accuracy of echocardiographic diagnosis of congenital heart defects in premature infants. My colleagues and I found that signifi-

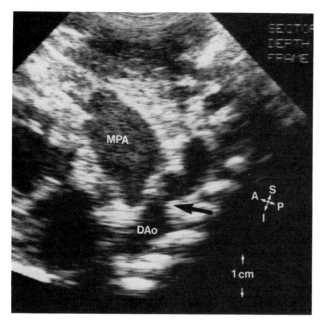

Figure 32–5. Coarctation of the aorta in a preterm infant without a patent ductus arteriosus. The posterior ledge and typical arch appearance aided the diagnosis. A = anterior; cm = centimeter; DAo = descending aorta; I = inferior; MPA = main pulmonary artery; P = posterior; S = superior. (Reprinted with permission of Huhta JC [1986]: Pediatric Imaging/Doppler Ultrasound of the Chest. Philadelphia, Lea and Febiger.)

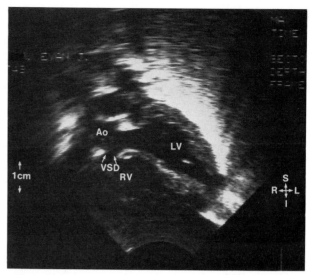

Figure 32–6. Subcostal scan showing a perimembranous ventricular septal defect (VSD) between the left (LV) and right (RV) ventricles. Ao = aorta; cm = centimeter; I = inferior; L = left; R = right; S = superior.

cant errors or omissions in diagnosis were relatively common. A common error by inexperienced examiners was a false-positive diagnosis of atrial septal defect (Fig. 32–3). A more significant error was an overlooked defect in the case of two of three patients with coarctation of the aorta (Figs. 32–4 and 32–5) and patent ductus arteriosus. In both cases, ligation of the ductus resulted in an emergency situation requiring immediate reoperation. In the examination of preterm infants with PDA, it is important to examine the aortic arch to look for signs of transverse arch hypoplasia or pulmonary artery enlargement.[9] Examination of the aortic isthmus will aid in identifying the posterior ledge of coarctation (Fig. 32–5). Detection of ventricular septal defects in the preterm infant remains a problem owing to the difficulty in obtaining high quality images of all portions of the septum (Figs. 32–6 and 32–7). In a very low birthweight neonate with two ventricular septal defects, both were overlooked on the first echocardiographic study, and only the muscular one was seen on several studies over the first 2 months of medical management.

Limited information was available to us about the false-negative rate in our entire population of low birthweight neonates. It is well recognized that careful autopsy information will increase the incidence of cardiac defects in a study population.[1]

EQUIPMENT

We observed that studies with either 7.5 or 10 MHz imaging were superior to those performed with a 5 MHz transducer. Until now there has not been a phased-array transducer that has been been able to match the image quality of high frequency, mechanical transducers in the near-field imaging situation like that found in very small babies. In the last 3 years of the study period, high quality Doppler ultrasound equipment was available and it was possible to obtain useful hemodynamic information. We applied information collected previously in the catheterization laboratory in older patients using continuous wave Doppler ultrasonography to estimate pressure gradients across a ventricular septal defect[10] or a patent ductus arteriosus in order to predict pulmonary artery pressures in premature infants with structural congenital heart disease (see Chapter 30).

MANAGEMENT

In general, those defects that are difficult to treat surgically in the otherwise normal neonate were also difficult to treat in the low birthweight neonate and were associated with a high mortality. The most difficult defects were those with increased pulmonary blood flow. It is known that the pulmonary vasculature undergoes rapid development in the last trimester of normal gestation; most of the arteriolar muscle development occurs during this period.[11] Because the pulmonary bed is relatively unable to protect itself from pulmonary hypertension and high pulmonary blood flow prior to arteriolar development, it is likely that in the presence of left-to-right shunt, more symptoms and pulmonary/interstitial edema result in premature infants than in older neonates. There is little or no information about the level of pulmonary-to-systemic flow ratio, which causes tachypnea in premature infants, and no data about the development of the pulmonary vascular bed in premature infants in the presence of high

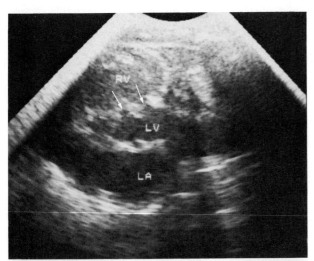

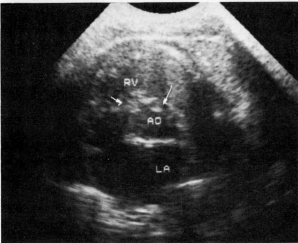

Figure 32–7. Parasternal scans with 10 MHz imaging of a preterm neonate with two ventricular septal defects (white arrows). Ao = aorta; LA = left atrium; LV = left ventricle; RV = right ventricle.

atresia and ventricular septal defect who outgrows a palliative shunt at 1700 g still presents a difficult surgical decision.

SUMMARY

Prematurity and/or low birthweight is a significant factor in the mortality and morbidity of congenital heart disease in the neonate. The most useful strategy for detection of congenital heart disease in the low birthweight neonate was compulsive echocardiographic examination by an experienced person at the first sign of heart disease and in *every* patient being considered for patent ductus arteriosus ligation or pharmacologic closure. Future progress in imaging technology should be aimed at even further improvement in the image quality because echocardiographic techniques provide much of the information that is necessary for the difficult decisions necessary in these babies.

blood flow or pulmonary hypertension. For example, if it were shown that pulmonary vascular disease were to develop more rapidly in this group, then there would be more emphasis on early, corrective surgery, even when the risk would be high.

Technical limitations in surgical technique become a factor as birthweight and body size drop. Palliative procedures such as a subclavian artery to pulmonary artery anastomosis may not be good choices if the likelihood of successful palliation is low. In one cyanotic infant with tetralogy of Fallot, a palliative shunt caused excessive pulmonary blood flow and the infant had successful corrective surgery at a weight of 2100 g. Although it is true that the age at which corrective surgery can be performed is dropping, an 800 g premature infant with pulmonary

References

1. Craft H, Brazy JE (1986): Autopsy: High yield in neonatal population. Am J Dis Child 140:1260–1262.
2. Dooley KJ (1984): Management of the premature infant with a patent ductus arteriosus. Pediatr Clin North Am 31:1159–1174.
3. Fleming WH, Sarafian LB, Kugler JD, Nelson RM Jr (1983): Ligation of patent ductus arteriosus in premature infants: Importance of accurate anatomic definition. Pediatrics 71:373–375.
4. Fyler D (1980): Report of the New England Regional Infant Cardiac Program. Pediatrics (Suppl)65:377–461.
5. Gersony WM (1987): Personal communication.
6. Huhta JC (1986): Pediatric Imaging/Doppler: Ultrasound of the Chest. Philadelphia, Lea & Febiger.
7. Huhta JC, Cohen M, Gutgesell HP (1984): Patency of the ductus arteriosus in normal neonates: Two-dimensional echocardiography versus Doppler assessment. J Am Coll Cardiol 4:561–564.
8. Mahony L, Heyman MA, Carnero V, Brett C, Clyman RI (1983): When to treat the patent ductus arteriosus with indomethacin in very low birth weight infants. Adv Prostaglandin Thromboxane Leukotriene Res 12:491–494.
9. Morrow R, Huhta JC, Murphy DJ, McNamara DG (1986): Quantitative morphology of the aortic arch in neonatal coarctation. J Am Coll Cardiol 8:616–620.
10. Murphy DJ Jr, Ludomirsky A, Huhta JC (1985): Continuous wave Doppler in children with ventricular septal defect: Noninvasive estimation of interventricular pressure gradient. Am J Cardiol 57:428.
11. Pieroni DR, Gingell RL, Roland JM, Chung CY, Broda JJ, Subramanian S (1982): Two-dimensional echocardiographic recognition and surgical management of aortopulmonary septal defect in the premature infant. Thorac Cardiovasc Surg 30:180–183.
12. Strauss A, Modanlou HD, Gyepes M, Wittner R (1982): Congenital heart disease and respiratory distress syndrome. Reversal of indomethacin closure of patent ductus arteriosus by prostaglandin therapy in a preterm infant. Am J Dis Child 136:934–936.
13. Vick GW, Huhta JC, Gutgesell HP (1985): Assessment of the ductus arteriosus in preterm infants utilizing suprasternal two-dimensional/Doppler echocardiography. J Am Coll Cardiol 5:973–977.

SECTION 3
CARDIOVASCULAR DISORDERS OF THE TERM NEONATE

33 EPIDEMIOLOGY

Stephen R. Daniels

At the turn of the century Sir William Osler noted that congenital heart diseases had "only a limited clinical interest, as in a large proportion of the cases the anomaly is not compatible with life, and in others, nothing can be done to remedy the defect or even relieve the symptoms."[53] In the twentieth century there have been many advances in medical and surgical therapy, and the scope of management of these problems continues to broaden. These advances have markedly improved both the survival and the quality of life of children with congenital heart diseases.[26] However, in spite of these improved outcomes, the epidemiology of heart disease presenting in the newborn period remains poorly defined. In the industrialized nations it is known that congenital heart disease is the most common cardiac condition in childhood. It has been estimated that the relative frequency of congenital heart disease compared with acquired heart disease presenting to a tertiary referral center for children is approximately 100:1 today.[45] The relative occurrence of individual heart lesions is speculative. In the past 2 decades, a number of attempts have been made to estimate the frequency of congenital heart disease, but the validity of these estimates has been questioned. Even less is known about the underlying etiologies of the various congenital heart defects. In this chapter current knowledge about the frequency of occurrence of congenital heart disease is reviewed. Thereafter, the utility of studies of the occurrence of congenital heart disease in elucidation of etiologic hypotheses is discussed. Finally, potential etiologic mechanisms for the development of congenital heart disease are presented.

OCCURRENCE OF CONGENITAL HEART DISEASE

In epidemiologic investigation, measures of disease frequency are used to characterize the occurrence of disease and are fundamental to both descriptive and etiologic investigations. Measures of disease frequency describe how common a particular illness is in reference to a population at risk of developing the disease. Measures of disease frequency must be chosen and applied properly if meaningful inferences about the disease being studied are to be made.

Measures of Frequency

In general, two types of disease frequency measures are used (Table 33–1). The first is incidence, which reflects the number of new (incident) cases that develop within a population over a given period of time. The second is prevalence, which reflects the number of existing (prevalent) cases in a population at a given point in time or at a given developmental stage. The timing of observation in incidence and prevalence studies of congenital heart disease is illustrated in Figure 33–1. Incidence is often expressed as a rate, whereas prevalence is a proportion. Incidence measures are usually estimated from cohort studies that follow populations over time. Prevalence is estimated from cross-sectional studies. Both incidence and prevalence measures depend on the current state of medical technology and the ability to detect persons with the disease in question. Prevalent cases represent the survivors of a disease and are not as well suited as incident cases for the study of etiology or the identification of risk factors of a disease.[30] On other hand, it is often easier and less expensive to study prevalent cases, and knowledge of the prevalence is often quite useful for clinical decision making and planning the delivery of health care services.

Incidence

There are two distinct measures of disease incidence: risk and rate.[43] Risk is defined as the probability of a person developing a given disease during a specified period.

Table 33–1. CHARACTERISTICS OF FREQUENCY MEASURES

Measure	Numerator	Denominator	Time	Type of Measure	Units
Incidence	New cases that occur over time in a population at risk	Susceptible persons without the disease at the beginning of the study	Duration of follow-up period (cohort study)	Risk over a period of time or rate	0–1 dimensionless; 1/time
Prevalence	All cases of a disease counted at one survey	All persons in the population of interest with and without the disease	Single point in time (cross-sectional study)	Proportion	0–1 dimensionless

Risk is a probability that can vary between zero and one and is dimensionless. Rate can be defined as the instantaneous potential for the occurrence of disease per unit of time, relative to the size of the population at risk.[11] An incidence rate is expressed in the units of 1/time. However, it is usually not possible to calculate instantaneous rates of incidence. Instead, it is more common to determine an average rate over a given period of time to estimate the instantaneous incidence. This average rate has been called the incidence density.[39]

Prevalence

Two types of measures can be used to quantify the prevalence of a disease. These measures are called point prevalence and period prevalence.[38] Point prevalence is defined as the probability that a person in a population will have the disease at the time of observation. Period prevalence, which is used less frequently, is the probability that a person in a population will be a case any time during a given period. Both measures are expressed as a proportion. A proportion is a fraction in which the numerator is contained in the denominator. It is dimensionless and must range between zero and one.[11] A proportion is often expressed as a percentage. Prevalence can also be determined for a population when the members of that population reach a certain developmental stage. The latter approach contains elements of a period prevalence (in that the population is observed over time) and elements of point prevalence (in that prevalent [as opposed to incident] cases are recorded at a single point of development, such as live birth). Prevalence at a given stage of development is estimated by the same method as for point prevalence.

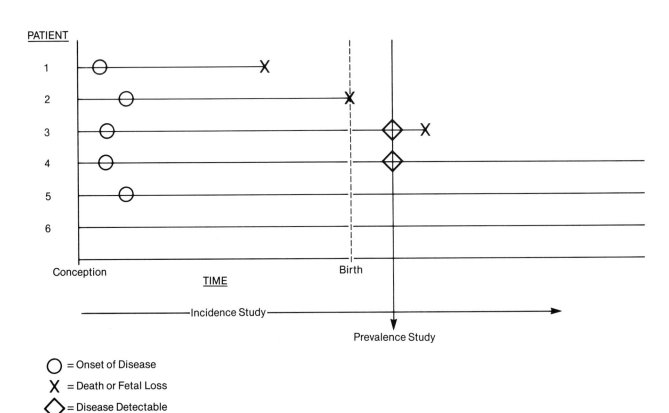

Figure 33–1. Diagram depicting the occurrence of congenital heart disease.

Point prevalence can be estimated as the proportion of persons in the study population who have the disease at the time of observation. The point prevalence depends in part on the incidence rate of the disease. The relationship is complex, however, and point prevalence depends on other factors, such as the duration of the disease.[15] In general, the period prevalence depends on both the point prevalence and the average incidence rate of the disease.[43]

Study Design Considerations

A number of factors make it difficult to achieve an accurate appraisal of the occurrence of congenital heart disease; some of these problems are depicted in Figure 33–1. Most investigators have studied the frequency of congenital heart disease by studying infants who are born alive, which may cause underestimates, because fetuses who undergo spontaneous abortion or stillbirth are not included (patients 1 and 2 in Fig. 33–1). Richards and associates[58] and Mitchell and coworkers[40] have estimated that including stillbirths alone would increase the occurrence of congenital heart defects 0.05 to 0.13 per cent above the frequency found in live births. Until recently, noninvasive techniques for investigating the structure and function of the heart in fetuses have been unavailable.[23] As a result, it has not been possible to study the earliest stages of congenital heart disease. Thus, a true incidence study of congenital heart disease has not yet been done, and a valid estimate of the incidence rate is not available. However, such an incidence study in the population at large would be quite difficult, given the time and effort required to study a single fetus reliably. Allan and colleagues have used fetal echocardiography to study the recurrence of congenital heart disease in mothers with a family history of heart defects.[1]

Accurate incidence studies of congenital heart disease would be useful in determining etiology and identifying risk factors, but prevalence studies might be more relevant in answering clinical questions and allocating resources. Most published reports have attempted to estimate the prevalence of congenital heart disease at live birth. Difficulties in estimating the prevalence can occur in determining both the numerator (cases) and the denominator (reference population).

Estimating the Number of Cases

In estimating the prevalence of congenital heart lesions, problems can arise in accurately determining the number of cases observed. It is necessary to define carefully what constitutes a case, because the criteria used to define a case affect the estimate of prevalence. Furthermore, the means chosen to detect a case also affect the estimate of prevalence. For example, according "case" status only to those infants who came to medical attention (whether because of symptoms or murmur or some laboratory test, such as a chest radiograph showing cardiomegaly) does not provide an accurate depiction of the prevalence of all congenital heart disease. Some defects, which uniformly

cause symptoms, would be completely represented in the study (see patient 3 in Fig. 33–1). Other defects, which have a range of presentation, would only be partially detected; mild forms of heart disease that rarely cause symptoms or present later in life would be excluded (see patient 5 in Fig. 33–1).

To determine the prevalence of congenital heart disease accurately, it would be necessary to study thoroughly every child in a large population. Most congenital heart disease prevalence studies have depended on children who have been referred during the first year of life to one or more tertiary care centers for the evaluation of potential heart disease. However, the patterns of referral to the tertiary care centers clearly affect prevalence estimates derived in this manner. For example, some congenital defects, such as atrial and ventricular septal defects, may close spontaneously. If children with these problems are not referred prior to closure, then they cannot be counted as cases and their prevalence would be underestimated. Other congenital defects, such as mild pulmonic stenosis or bicuspid aortic valve, may not be recognized or considered serious enough for referral.

Once children are referred for suspected cardiac disease, the presence or absence of disease must be determined. Case confirmation has been made easier with the use of noninvasive techniques, such as echocardiography. Of course, other means of confirming cardiac disease include cardiac catheterization, cardiac surgery, and autopsy.

Further difficulty may arise in classifying congenital heart disease. Classification can be especially difficult when an infant is found to have more than one congenital defect. Studies have employed different schemes of classification. One study[14] has used the congenital heart disease coding system developed by the International Society of Cardiology,[24] which provides a unique code for every cardiac malformation and for complexes of lesions. In this scheme, each case is assigned one or more codes based on clinical and diagnostic investigation. The principal diagnosis is then arrived at through a hierarchical system that gives priority to the malformation component with the earliest time of embryologic dysmorphism. Other systems of classification are available: anomalies of the heart can be related to one another in an anatomic or functional sense, as well as an embryologic sense.[70] The selection of a classification scheme should depend on the ultimate purpose for which it is to be used. It may also be useful to include a coding system for associated extracardiac anomalies to aid in the investigation of patterns of teratogenesis.

Reference Population

The other major factor in estimating prevalence is the population at risk of developing the disease. The reference population is represented by all six patients in Figure 33–1. Ideally, the denominator for prevalence would include all persons who could have the condition. However, studying all such persons is rarely feasible. Usually, investigators attempt to select a representative sample of this larger group. A representative sample is a subgroup of a larger

Table 33–2. SELECTION OF CASES IN STUDIES OF THE PREVALENCE OF CONGENITAL HEART DISEASE

	Mitchell et al[40]	Hoffman and Christianson[22]	Keith[27]	NERICP[17] 1969–1977	Ferencz et al[14]
Identification of cases	Inpatient and outpatient records plus interval histories by telephone	Inpatient and outpatient records from Kaiser Foundation Health Plan plus further examination of suspected heart disease by a pediatric cardiologist	Cases followed at Hospital for Sick Children, Toronto	Inpatient, outpatient, and private office records from New England hospitals and pediatric cardiologists	Inpatient and outpatient records from five Washington DC, area pediatric cardiology centers
Number of congenital heart disease cases	420	194	215	3357	664
Confirmation of cases	Cl, C, S, A	Cl, C, S, A	Cl, C, S, A,	Cl, C, S, A	E, C, S, A
Per cent of cases confirmed by clinical examination only	48%	52%	Not stated	0.8%	0%

A = autopsy; C = cardiac catheterization; Cl = clinical; E = echocardiography; S = cardiac surgery.

group selected by some procedure. However, the process of selection introduces the possibility of bias. Selection bias can be minimized by randomly selecting persons for study so that everyone has the same chance of inclusion. Only when such a random selection process is used can the study findings be legitimately generalized to persons in the larger population of interest. In many instances, the research question will help the investigator to select the appropriate reference population. For example, one may want to discover the proportion of distressed infants admitted to a newborn intensive care unit who have structural heart disease. A second area of interest might be to determine what percentage of premature infants have congenital heart disease.

Investigators have attempted to determine the prevalence of congenital heart disease in the population at large. There are a number of possibilities for defining a study sample population more or less representative of this population. Some sample populations have the benefit of being easier to study; others are more difficult to study but are more representative of the general population. For example, one could study all infants referred to a pediatric cardiologist. Using the sample population of patients referred to a pediatric cardiologist would be convenient and would help to ensure consistency in the use of diagnostic techniques among subjects. However, such a sample population would not be representative of the population at large and would be likely to introduce bias into the study. Alternatively, one could choose all the liveborn infants in a particular geographic region as the sample population. Such a geographic approach would be more likely to be representative, but it would be quite difficult to examine each member of the population completely and uniformly. In reality, compromises often have to be made.

Congenital heart disease is relatively rare. Therefore, it is necessary to study large numbers of persons to be sure that all types of defects are represented and that stable estimates of frequency are obtained. One approach to defining the sample population has been to use vital statistics data on live births from a group of counties or states. In this type of study, it is important to employ vigorous methods of case finding, because it is not practical to examine every person. It is also important to link the records of the cases with the data from the population at risk to be sure that the case has indeed emerged from that population. Patterns of referral and of migration into and from the population must also be examined, since these factors may all serve to alter estimates of prevalence artificially. The procedures used to define the cases and the sample population in selected studies on the prevalence of congenital heart disease are shown in Tables 33–2 and 33–3.

Other Measures of Frequency and Association

Another measure that may be of interest in studies of congenital heart disease is the measure of mortality. Frequency measures based on mortality are primarily obtained from the same types of studies used to obtain incidence data. However, mortality data may also be incorporated in proportional studies. Mortality is dependent on the incidence rate of a disease. As with incidence, there are two ways of expressing the frequency of death due to a disease in a population: the first is as the risk or probability of dying, and the second is the mortality rate.[30]

It may also be of interest to compare measures of the frequency of congenital heart disease for different populations. Such comparisons often involve a situation in which one population is exposed to a certain factor while another group remains unexposed. For example, the effect of accidental radiation exposure at a nuclear reactor on the occurrence of congenital heart defects in workers' offspring could be studied. Such a comparison is often referred to as a measure of association, because it reflects the relationship between the study factor (radiation) and the disease (congenital heart defects). The methodology used to select the exposed and nonexposed workers and to determine the disease frequency in their offspring can be quite important for the appropriate interpretation of the results.

Table 33–3. REFERENCE POPULATION IN STUDIES OF THE PREVALENCE OF CONGENITAL HEART DISEASE

	Mitchell et al[40]	Hoffman and Christianson[22]	Keith[27]	NERICP[17] 1969–1977	Ferencz et al[14]
Source of reference population	Offspring of mothers selected from 12 obstetric US clinic populations	Offspring of selected members of the Kaiser Foundation Health Plan	Vital statistics on live births in Toronto	Vital statistics on live births in New England states	Vital statistics data from live births, Washington/Baltimore study area
Number of live births	54,765	19,044	28,698	1,528,686	179,697
Length of follow-up					
Shortest	Birth to 1 month	Birth to 5 years	Not stated	Birth to 1 year	Birth to 1 year
Longest	Birth to 9 years	Birth to 13 years			

In prevalence studies, frequently used measures of association are the prevalence ratio and the prevalence difference.[30] The prevalence ratio is the prevalence for an exposed group divided by the prevalence from a comparable reference, or unexposed, group. The prevalence difference is calculated by subtracting the prevalence for the reference group from the prevalence estimate for the group that has been exposed. The prevalence ratio is dimensionless and depends on the relationship of prevalence in the two groups rather than the absolute frequency of disease occurrence. For this reason, the prevalence ratio is useful in etiologic investigation. The prevalence difference is more useful as a measure of public health impact or for individual health decisions, because it retains the element of disease frequency. By way of illustration, exposure to a factor may increase the occurrence of a rare disease by four times, giving a prevalence ratio of 4 and suggesting an important potential etiologic relationship. However, because of the disease's rarity, the prevalence difference would be low and the number of cases of the disease that could be eliminated by removing the factor might still remain quite small. Such measures of association derived from observational studies[30] can provide valid etiologic clues to disease and valid public health information.

Finally, the change in occurrence of congenital heart disease over calendar time may be of interest. Change in occurrence with time is sometimes referred to as a secular trend or a period effect. These changes can be analyzed by a longitudinal methodologic strategy referred to as cohort analysis.[30] The interpretation of an apparent secular change can be difficult. The first question is whether the apparent change is due to variation in the diagnosis, reporting, case-fatality ratio, or some factor other than a true change in frequency. Several procedures may help to indicate whether a true change is occurring over time.[37] The trend for the congenital heart defect in question should be compared with trends for other congenital defects. It may also be helpful to compare the frequency with which the disorder in question is present during autopsies performed at different periods during the observed secular change. Finally, it may be helpful to determine to what extent there may be trends in the ability to identify and classify the defect. Such observations will help to determine if the frequency has actually remained the same, but because of

previous diagnostic inaccuracy, cases were previously assigned to other diagnostic categories. By way of illustration, Layde and coworkers[33] attempted to verify a suspected increase in the occurrence of ventricular septal defects in the United States by investigating changes in the frequency of spontaneous closure from two different periods. They found that the rate of spontaneous closure was similar in 1970 to 1972 and 1975 to 1976. The unchanged rate of spontaneous closure suggested that an observed increase in the occurrence of ventricular septal defect was probably not due to improved clinical diagnosis of more minor ventricular septal defects (which would be more likely to close spontaneously).

ESTIMATES OF THE FREQUENCY OF CONGENITAL HEART DISEASE

A number of studies have been published over the past 25 years that provide estimates of the prevalence (some reports mistakenly claim to estimate the incidence) of congenital heart disease.[4,7,10,13,14,17,21,27,32,40] The estimates range from 2.08 to 10.19 cases of congenital heart disease per 1000 live births in the 10 studies presented in Table 33–4. It is likely that many of the differences in the estimates of prevalence are due to differences in methodology (see Tables 33–2 and 33–3). However, the studies were done at different times and in different locations, so it is not possible to exclude the possibility that true differences in prevalence existed. Mitchell and colleagues[40] have demonstrated that there are no substantial differences in prevalence of congenital heart disease between black and white children.

These studies have also attempted to estimate the prevalence of individual heart defects at live birth. These prevalences are presented in Table 33–5, which lists the defects in the order of decreasing frequency found in the New England Regional Infant Cardiac Program,[17] the largest study published to date.

In some reports, prevalence figures for individual lesions were not published. The figures in Table 33–5 are those calculated from the data presented in the original reports and published by Ferencz and associates.[14] In most studies, the definition of congenital heart disease was similar to that used by Mitchell and coworkers.[40]

Table 33–4. PREVALENCE OF CONGENITAL HEART DISEASE AT LIVE BIRTH FROM 10 STUDIES

Study (Location) (Years of Study)	Number of Live Births	Number with Congenital Heart Disease	Prevalence Per 1000 Live Births
Carlgren[7] (Sweden) (1941–1950)	58,105	369	6.35
Mitchell et al[40] (USA) (1956–1965)	Live births: 54,765 Still births: 1344 Total: 56,109	Live births: 420 Still births: 37 Total: 457	Live births: 7.67 Still births: 27.53 Total: 8.14
Hoffman and Christianson[22] (USA) (1959–1969)	19,044	Definite: 163 Possible: 31 Total: 194	Definite: 8.56 Possible: 1.63 Total: 10.19
Feldt et al[13] (USA) 1950–1969	32,393	186	5.74
Dickinson et al[10] (England) (1960–1969)	160,480	884	5.51
Bound and Logan[4] (England) (1957–1971)	56,982	338	5.93
Keith[27] (Canada)	28,698	215	7.49
Laurson[32] (Denmark) (1963–1973)	Approx. 855,000	5,249	6.14
NERICP[17] (USA) (1969–1977)	1969–1974: 1,083,083 1975–1977: 445,603 Total: 1,528,686	1969–1974: 2251 1975–1977: 1106 Total: 3,357	1969–1974: 2.08 1975–1977: 2.48 Total: 2.20
Ferencz et al[14] (USA) (1969–1977)	179,697	664	3.70

Congenital heart disease is defined as a gross structural abnormality of the heart or intrathoracic great vessels that is actually or potentially of functional importance. Thus, persistent left superior vena cava or arrhythmia unassociated with a structural malformation was not classified as congenital heart disease. One structural abnormality not well covered by any of the studies is bicuspid aortic valve, which is often difficult to diagnose clinically. Roberts has estimated that the prevalence of bicuspid aortic valve in an autopsy series in adults was 0.9 per cent.[59] As noted in Table 33–2, the study of Ferencz and

associates[14] was the only one to employ systematically the use of echocardiography for diagnostic purposes.

There are numerous differences between studies in the estimates of prevalence for individual heart lesions. Again, some of these differences are likely due to variations in study methodology, such as different lengths of follow-up of study subjects (see Table 33–3) and different methods used for case finding and confirmation (see Table 33–2). It is, however, interesting to note that the prevalence estimates from the two most recent studies[14,17] are similar.

Table 33–5. REPORTED ESTIMATES OF PREVALENCE PER 1000 LIVE BIRTHS FOR SPECIFIC CONGENITAL HEART DEFECTS

Defect	Carlgren[7]	Mitchell et al[40]	Hoffman and Christianson[22]	Feldt et al[13]	Dickinson et al[10]	Bound and Logan[4]	Keith[27]	Laurson[32]	NERICP[17] (1969–1974)	Ferencz et al[14]
Ventricular septal defect	1.70	2.26	2.68	1.91	1.80	1.67	1.89	1.48	0.38	0.86
D-transposition	0.38	0.20	0.31	0.43	0.27	0.33	0.30	0.29	0.21	0.21
Tetralogy of Fallot	0.31	0.29	0.31	0.28	0.32	0.51	0.54	0.36	0.21	0.26
Coarctation of aorta	0.62	0.51	0.47	0.31	0.35	0.33	0.43	0.43	0.18	0.24
Hypoplastic left-heart syndrome	0.10	0.24	0.05	0.25	0.16	0.19	0.20	0.18	0.16	0.27
Patent ductus arteriosus	0.60	0.64	0.47	0.59	0.65	0.39	0.74	0.77	0.14	0.09
Atrioventricular septal defect	0.17	0.27	0.31	0.25	0.13	0.44	0.28	0.15	0.12	0.36
Pulmonary stenosis	0.27	0.66	1.15		0.42	0.16	0.61	0.36	7	0.19
Pulmonary atresia	0.07	0.09	0.05		0.04			0.04	0.07	0.08
Secundum atrial septal defect	0.24	0.57	0.52	0.40	0.32	0.49	0.36	0.58	0.07	0.32
Total anomalous pulmonary venous drainage	0.05		0.05		0.07	0.12	0.09		0.06	0.08
Tricuspid atresia	0.09	0.90		0.18	0.09	0.09		0.05	0.06	0.04
Aortic stenosis	0.34	0.29	0.31	0.34	0.28	0.25	0.36	0.29	0.04	0.11
Double-outlet right ventricle		0.07	0.05						0.03	0.06
Truncus arteriosus	0.07	0.13	0.21		0.06	0.07	0.09	0.09	0.03	0.06
Other	1.36	1.35	1.57	0.59	0.53	0.89	1.60	1.07	0.18	0.49

Estimates of Prevalence in Clinically Defined Subgroups

While the estimates of prevalence demonstrated in Table 33–5 are of academic and some clinical interest, they may not answer the questions most commonly faced by clinicians who care for sick newborn infants. Clinicians are often more interested in the prevalence of a disorder in a reference population or sub-population which is similar to the patients they see on a daily basis. So, for example, the clinician might wonder about the prevalence of congenital heart disease among infants seen in a neonatal intensive care unit. It may also be of interest to know the prevalence of structural heart disease in premature infants and the relative frequency of hemodynamically significant patent ductus arteriosus compared to other heart defects in this population. Finally, one might want an estimate of the frequency of congenital heart disease among infants presenting with other specific problems, such as infants of diabetic mothers or infants with chromosomal abnormalities.

Studies yielding this sort of information have been published, but it is important to use caution in interpreting the results. The most difficult aspect of these studies is the question of whether the results and conclusions can be generalized to a clinical setting other than the one in which the data were collected (external validity). Many factors play a role in determining whether results can be extrapolated to other populations, including the spectrum of disease observed in the study group, the setting for the study, the referral pattern, and the completeness of follow-up and assessment of the outcome.

In the seriously ill newborn, a number of findings, including cyanosis, tachypnea, heart murmurs, and abnormal laboratory findings, may suggest the presence of congenital heart disease. However, it may be difficult to distinguish heart disease from the other causes of distress in neonates on clinical features alone. Murphy and colleagues[44] used echocardiography to study 104 distressed infants in a newborn intensive care unit who were younger than 7 days of age and in whom congenital heart disease other than an isolated patent ductus arteriosus was clinically suspected. They determined that 40 infants did not have structural heart disease, although 3 (7.5 per cent) were subsequently found to have incidental cardiac lesions. Sixty-four infants (61 per cent) had structural heart disease.

Premature infants may have a different prevalence of structural congenital heart disease than full-term infants. Richards and coworkers[58] found a prevalence of 1.73 per cent in premature infants compared with 0.49 per cent in full-term newborns. Hoffman and Rudolph[21] report a fourfold increase in the prevalence of ventricular septal defects detected by clinical examination and cardiac catheterization in premature infants compared with full-term infants. They also point out, however, that this increase may be illusory because premature infants receive more intensive care than term infants, so there may be increased detection of defects in that group, depending on the criteria for diagnosis. It is also important to know whether prematurity was diagnosed on birthweight alone, as in the study of Hoffman and Rudolph,[21] or if other measures of prematurity were used. When birthweight is the sole criterion, some infants who are small for dates may be mistakenly classified as premature, or infants of diabetic mothers who may be premature but large for dates may be mistakenly excluded.

Levy and associates reviewed the association of low birthweight, young gestational age, and small size for dates with congenital heart disease in the New England Regional Infant Cardiac Program.[34] They found that low birthweight and small for gestational age infants are significantly more likely to have congenital heart disease than are normal infants. The small for gestational age infants also had a significantly higher number of extracardiac anomalies. Patent ductus arteriosus and secundum atrial septal defects were associated with low birthweight, whereas ventricular septal defect, patent ductus arteriosus and tetralogy of Fallot were most common in small for dates infants.[34] They note, however, that the use of nonmatched retrospective controls and lack of information on socioeconomic status may have biased their results.

Of particular interest in the premature infant is the frequency of occurrence of patent ductus arteriosus. In premature infants, failure of closure of the ductus arteriosus is due to developmental immaturity and, as such, is probably not related to significant structural abnormality as it would be in a full-term infant. Nevertheless, it may be a significant cause of morbidity and mortality in premature infants. Kitterman and colleagues[29] reported that between 1967 and 1970, 15 per cent of infants with birthweight less than 1750 g had patent ductus arteriosus. The prevalence rose to 35 per cent in 1971. They found an association of low birthweight and young gestational age with patent ductus arteriosus. Other authors have demonstrated the relationship of patent ductus arteriosus to respiratory distress syndrome.[68] The findings of selected studies on the prevalence of patent ductus arteriosus are presented in Table 33–6.[6,20,29,57,68,75] Reller and coworkers[57] investigated the prevalence of hemodynamically significant patent ductus arteriosus in infants of 27 to 33 weeks' gestational age. They found that two fluid balance regimens

Table 33–6. RESULTS OF SELECTED STUDIES ON THE PREVALENCE OF PATENT DUCTUS ARTERIOSUS IN PREMATURE INFANTS

Author	Year	Prevalence of Patent Ductus Arteriosus (%)	Birthweight or Gestational Age
Burnard[6]	1959	10	Not stated
Kitterman et al[29]	1967–1970	15	< 1750 g
	1971	35	
Zachman[75]	1974	23	< 1500 g
Siassi et al[68]	1976	21	< 2500 g
		36	< 2000 g
		77	28–30 weeks
Heymann[20]	1983	45	< 1750 g
		75–80	< 1200 g
Reller et al[57]	1985	64 during first week of life; 76 total	27–33 weeks

did not affect the prevalence of patent ductus arteriosus which was 64 per cent in the two groups combined during the first week of life. The prevalence for the entire study was 76 per cent. These investigators used both clinical examination and echocardiography to determine the presence of a patent ductus arteriosus and they found that the clinical findings of a murmur and a hyperdynamic precordial impulse were very specific for the presence of patent ductus arteriosus but were not very sensitive. Patent ductus arteriosus in the majority of the infants (66 per cent) was clinically silent and was picked up by echocardiographic criteria alone.[57] The common occurrence of clinically silent ductus may mean that the presence of a patent ductus arteriosus was underestimated in some of the earlier studies.

Congenital cardiac malformations are more common among infants of diabetic mothers than in the normal population.[41,66,69] It has been estimated that the prevalence of heart defects in these infants is from three to ten times greater than in the general population. Most reviewers have found no relationship between gestational factors, age at onset, and severity of diabetes and the risk for cardiac defects. Ventricular septal defects are the most commonly found defects, but an increased prevalence of transposition of the great arteries and malformations of the aorta has also been reported.[69]

Another situation in which the prevalence of congenital heart disease may be increased is the infant born with abnormal chromosomes. Congenital heart disease is frequently a constituent of the syndromes characteristic of trisomy 13, 18, and 21. Most cases of trisomy 13 and 18 are lethal within a few months after birth, which allows autopsy confirmation of congenital heart disease in liveborn infants with the disorders. Warkany and associates reported a prevalence of congenital heart lesions of 84 per cent for trisomy 13 and 99 per cent for trisomy 18 among autopsied cases described in the literature.[71] The most common lesions in trisomy 13 patients were ventricular septal defects, patent ductus arteriosus, and atrial septal defect. The most common heart defects for patients with trisomy 18 were ventricular septal defects, patent ductus arteriosus, and pulmonary valve stenosis.

The situation is different for patients with trisomy 21, which is compatible with survival. The prevalence of congenital heart disease must be determined in a way similar to that for the general population. It is well known that congenital heart disease is an important feature of Down syndrome, but valid estimates of the frequency are difficult to find. Berg and coworkers reviewed the literature and found estimates of the prevalence of congenital heart defects in patients with trisomy 21 varied from 7 to 70 per cent.[3] A more recent estimate of the prevalence of congenital heart disease in hospitalized patients with Down syndrome was 62 per cent.[18] It was also estimated that 4 per cent of critical heart disease in the first year of life was associated with trisomy 21. The variation in frequency is due to a number of factors, including differences in diagnostic methods, the source of patient populations, and the age of patients included in the study. In a review of autopsy series, Warkany and associates[71] reported the presence of structural abnormalities of the heart in 52 per cent of patients with Down syndrome. Rowe and Uchida[65] studied the population of patients followed with trisomy 21 at the Hospital for Sick Children in Toronto. Of 184 patients, 38 per cent had definite cardiac defects while 5.4 per cent were uncertain. The most common defects in children with Down syndrome appear to be ventricular septal defect, atrial septal defect, patent ductus arteriosus, and atrioventricular septal defects.[71]

The New England Regional Infant Cardiac Program found somewhat different results with respect to Down syndrome.[17] The cardiac defects associated with trisomy 21 were atrioventricular septal defects (63 per cent), ventricular septal defects (16 per cent), tetralogy of Fallot (8 per cent), patent ductus arteriosus (4 per cent), and double-outlet right ventricle (2 per cent). This difference in frequency probably reflects the fact that the New England Regional Program was concerned mainly with cardiac problems that cause trouble in infancy.

Mortality in Congenital Heart Disease

It is well recognized that despite modern therapeutic intervention, congenital heart disease can cause mortality. Many children with congenital heart defects die in the first few weeks of life, whereas others survive for varying lengths of time. Keith studied 10,535 cases of cardiac defects seen at the Hospital for Sick Children, Toronto, Canada, over a 20-year period from 1950 to 1970.[27] Twenty-seven per cent of the patients died during the period of observation. Of the patients who died, 34 per cent died during the first month of life.

The investigators in the New England Regional Infant Cardiac Program used a multivariable analysis to investigate a series of factors that might influence the survival of children with congenital heart disease.[17] The variables that were determinants of survival included the anatomic diagnosis, age at admission, birthweight, presence and severity of extracardiac anomalies, sex, need for surgery, age at surgery, and the calendar year of presentation. However, this investigation used survival as a dichotomous (yes, no) type of variable. Such dichotomous analysis does not allow the analysis of factors that might be related to increased time of survival. Further research is needed that employs the methods of survival analysis to determine the factors that are related to the time of survival, particularly within specific diagnostic categories. Such research could give insights into strategies for improving survival in infants with congenital heart disease.

ETIOLOGY OF CONGENITAL HEART DISEASE

Epidemiologic research can be useful in studying the etiology of congenital heart disease. However, despite considerable research effort, the underlying causal mechanisms of congenital heart disease remain poorly defined.

It should be stressed that "malformations of the heart" is a classification that includes a wide range of heterogeneous disorders. It is unlikely that all heart defects have a common etiology. It is equally unlikely that individual defects have a single cause. Nevertheless, it is important to examine studies on the patterns of occurrence of congenital heart defects, because they may yield clues to potential causal associations.

As discussed previously, studies of incidence are better suited for investigating etiologic inferences than are studies of prevalence. However, despite their limitations, prevalence studies can be useful for investigating etiologic hypotheses and, in the case of congenital heart disease, their feasibility makes them an attractive alternative.

Hypotheses of etiology may be generated by the observed clustering of disease by time, space, race, gender, or family. For example, Rothman and Fyler[62] investigated the seasonal distribution of births of infants with congenital heart disease. They also studied the relationship of such births with population density. They found seasonal peaks for complex ventricular septal defects, malposition defects, and transposition of the great arteries. In addition, an increased occurrence of pulmonary atresia with ventricular septal defects and tricuspid atresia was found to be associated with increased population density. These findings in conjunction with the results from other studies may lead to testable etiologic hypotheses.

Nora has suggested that it is necessary to consider genetic epidemiology in the etiology of congenital heart disease, thereby stressing the importance of both heredity and environment.[48] He has further suggested that etiologic mechanisms of congenital heart disease can be divided into three major categories: (1) primary genetic factors, which account for about 8 per cent, (2) primary environmental factors, which account for approximately 2 per cent, and (3) multifactorial inheritance (genetic-environmental interaction), which accounts for 90 per cent of congenital heart disease. In the multifactorial (also called polygenic) group, many genes act in concert with various (usually unknown) environmental triggers to produce structural abnormalities during embryogenesis. If this model is correct, then the vast majority of congenital heart defects could be prevented by the dissociation of hereditary and environmental components. In this model, although the genetic predisposition is inevitable, the expression of these genes depends on the environmental exposure of the fetus. Although all aspects of the prenatal environment may not be subject to modification, certain factors, if known, could be subject to intervention.

Genetic Factors

There are three main lines of evidence that help to support the hypothesis that congenital heart disease is, at least in part, genetically determined. First is the fact that congenital defects of the heart are common in some forms of chromosomal aberration. Second is the presence of heart diseases, such as hypertrophic cardiomyopathy, which appear to be due to single gene mutations and are inherited

Table 33–7. ASSOCIATION OF CONGENITAL HEART DEFECTS WITH SELECTED CHROMOSOMAL ABNORMALITIES

Chromosomal Defect	Estimated Prevalence of CHD (%)	Associated Heart Defects
Autosomal		
Trisomy		
13	84	VSD, PDA, ASD
18	99	VSD, PDA, PS
21	52	VSD, ASD, ECD
Deletion		
4p-	40	VSD, ASD, PDA
5p-	25	VSD, ASD, PDA
13q-	50	VSD
18q-	50	VSD
Sex		
XO (Turner)	44	CA, PS, AS
XXY (Kleinfelter)	?	TF, Ebstein
XXXXY	15	PDA, ASD

AS = aortic stenosis; ASD = atrial septal defect; CA = coarctation of the aorta; CHD = congenital heart disease; ECD = endocardial cushion defect; PDA = patent ductus arteriosus; PS = pulmonic stenosis; TF = tetralogy of Fallot; VSD = ventricular septal defect.

following a mendelian pattern. Finally, there is the knowledge that cardiovascular diseases tend to cluster in families.

As discussed previously, congenital heart defects are common in patients with trisomy 13, 18, or 21. Heart disease can also be observed in other forms of chromosomal abnormality. Selected chromosomal abnormalities that have been associated with congenital heart defects are presented in Table 33–7. It is important to remember that this relationship remains one of association only. A true causal mechanism linking abnormal chromosomes to specific heart defects has yet to be discovered. In instances in which the association is less regular, the relationship may be one of coincidence rather than cause and effect. It is also possible that a third (unknown) factor is responsible for independently causing both the chromosomal aberration and the heart problem. Chromosomal abnormalities and neonatal congenital heart disease are further considered in Chapter 48.

A number of syndromes that include heart disease appear to be the result of genetic abnormalities that are inherited in a mendelian pattern. Examples of autosomal dominant cardiovascular abnormalities include hypertrophic cardiomyopathy and Romano-Ward (prolonged QT interval, sudden death) and Noonan syndromes (associated with pulmonic stenosis and other defects). Examples of syndromes that are inherited in a pattern consistent with an autosomal recessive gene include the Jervell-Lange-Nielsen syndrome (deafness, prolonged QT interval) and Friedreich ataxia (cardiomyopathy). Syndromes that include neonatal congenital heart disease are further considered in Chapter 50.

As in chromosomal abnormalities, no direct relationship between a single gene and a cardiac anomaly has been discovered. It is suspected that the gene for hypertrophic cardiomyopathy is located on chromosome 6.[48]

Table 33–8. ASSOCIATION OF CONGENITAL HEART DISEASE WITH SELECTED ENVIRONMENTAL FACTORS

	Estimate of Prevalence of CHD (%)	Associated Heart Defects
Maternal Illness		
Infection		
Rubella	7 (prospective)	PDA, PAS, PS
Coxsackie B	2	PDA, VSD
Other		
Diabetes	2–5	VSD, TGA, CA
Systemic lupus	?	Heart block
Gestational Factors		
Birth order	?	PS, TGA, PDA
Maternal age	?	Down syndrome, other defects?
Extrinsic Factors		
Drugs		
Thalidomide	39 (autopsy)	TF, VSD, ASD
Hydantoin	2–10	PS, AS, CA
Trimethadione	15–50	TGA, TF
Lithium	10	Ebstein
Personal habits		
Alcohol	25–40	VSD, ASD, PDA
Smoking	?	PS, AS, VSD
Other (environmental)		
Hypoxia?	?	PDA
Population density?	?	PA, TA, VSD

AS = aortic stenosis; ASD = atrial septal defect; CA = coarctation of aorta; CHD = congenital heart disease; PA = pulmonary atresia; PAS = pulmonary artery stenosis; PDA = patent ductus arteriosus; PS = pulmonary stenosis; TA = tricuspid atresia; TF = tetralogy of Fallot; TGA = transposition of great arteries; VSD = ventricular septal defect.

However, the metabolic deficiency caused by the abnormal gene remains unknown. It is likely that with the development of new molecular genetic techniques, genetically induced heart lesions that are the direct result of metabolic abnormalities caused by minor chromosomal aberrations will be discovered.

The familial clustering of congenital heart disease has long been recognized. In the 1950s several publications suggested that after one case of a congenital heart defect has occurred in a family there is approximately a 2 per cent chance of a similar event in subsequent pregnancies.[2] Nora has since demonstrated that the risk of recurrence of a congenital heart defect in a subsequent child varies with the type of lesion and the frequency with which the lesion is found in the general population.[47,51] Some more recent studies have suggested that the frequency of recurrence may be even higher than that previously published. Whittemore and coworkers reported a 16.1 per cent recurrence for congenital heart defects in a prospective study of 428 pregnancies over a 15-year period in a cohort of 233 mothers with congenital heart disease.[74] Rose and colleagues retrospectively determined the recurrence of congenital heart disease in the children of 219 probands with atrial septal defect, coarctation of the aorta, aortic valve stenosis, or complex dextrocardia.[60] They found that 8.8 per cent of children in this group had substantial cardiac defects. Allan and associates used fetal echocardiography

to ascertain the presence of congenital heart defects in the offspring of 1021 mothers referred because of a family history of congenital heart disease.[1] They found a recurrence of 2 per cent with one previously affected child, 10 per cent with two previously affected children, and 0 per cent in the 41 cases in which a parent had congenital heart disease. However, certain heart defects, such as coarctation of the aorta, were associated with a much higher (6.6 per cent) frequency of recurrence. The issue of recurrence risk is further considered in Chapter 10.

Environmental Factors

Although the familial clustering of congenital heart disease may be due to shared genes, it may also be due to shared environment. The observation that monozygotic twins are more often discordant than concordant for the presence of congenital heart disease supports the concept of environmental causality.[61] There is also experimental evidence that implicates environmental factors in the production of congenital heart disease. Studies in mammals have shown that maternal vitamin A deficiency, hypervitaminosis A, folic acid deficiency, hypoxia, salicylate ingestion, and other manipulations can all cause abnormalities in the development of the heart.[72] The evidence for environmental factors producing congenital heart defects in humans can be divided into three categories: (1) maternal illness, (2) gestational properties, and (3) extrinsic factors, including medication use. Some suspected environmental teratogens and the congenital heart defects that have been associated with them are listed in Table 33–8.

A number of maternal conditions have been linked to structural heart disease. Maternal rubella infection during the first trimester of pregnancy can lead to a constellation of congenital anomalies, including congenital heart defects.[73] The initial case reports of congenital rubella syndrome led to a number of retrospective studies on the frequency of congenital heart defects in children of mothers who had suffered rubella.[73] These studies estimated a prevalence of congenital heart disease of around 35 per cent in exposed infants. However, since retrospective estimates start with abnormal infants and work back in time to a history of maternal rubella, it is likely that there was selection bias, and the estimates of prevalence were probably too high. A subsequent prospective study estimated that congenital heart defects occurred in 7 per cent of children whose mothers had rubella in early pregnancy;[67] this occurrence was 14 times more common than for controls. Reexamination of the surviving children at ages 8 to 11 demonstrated a definite diagnosis of congenital heart disease in 6 per cent, but murmurs were heard in another 8 per cent.[67] The congenital heart disease caused by maternal rubella infection, as demonstrated by cardiac catheterization, includes patent ductus arteriosus, pulmonary artery stenosis, and valvular pulmonary stenosis.[9]

The recognition of congenital rubella syndrome stimulated interest in other potential viral etiologies. Brown and Evans reported that intrauterine exposure to coxsackieviruses B_3 and B_4, measured by seroconversion, resulted in an increased frequency of congenital heart disease.[5] Other possible infectious causes include maternal infection with herpes simplex and toxoplasmosis.[31] The topic of neonatal cardiac infections is considered in Chapter 47.

Other maternal disorders that may cause congenital heart disease include diabetes,[31] systemic lupus erythematosus,[8] and nutritional deficiencies.[56]

Gestational factors that may be associated with congenital heart disease include maternal age and parity. Other factors such as maternal nausea, intrauterine growth retardation, threatened spontaneous abortion and prematurity have also been linked with congenital heart defects, but it is difficult to determine if these factors could cause defects, if they are merely present because the fetus has a heart abnormality, or whether both the heart defect and the gestational factor are related to some unknown third causal factor.

It is well known that increased maternal age is associated with an increase in the frequency of trisomy 21 and its associated congenital heart heart defects in offspring.[55] Rothman and Fyler[63] used multiple linear regression to investigate the influence of maternal age and parity on the occurrence of congenital heart disease. Infants with Down syndrome were excluded from their analysis. They found that infants experienced increasing risk of transposition of the great arteries with increasing birth order. For patent ductus arteriosus, there was a decrease in risk with increasing birth order. There was a higher risk of atrial septal defect for first-born infants, but no consistent trend for later born children. There was no significant association between the risk of tetralogy of Fallot and order of birth. In their study, typically the birth order effect was found to outweigh the impact of maternal age on the occurrence of congenital heart disease.

The experience with thalidomide suggested the possibility of drug-induced teratogenesis. Although thalidomide is best known as a teratogen that causes limb deformities, it also may cause cardiac deformities. Kajii reported malformations of the heart in 39 per cent of necropsies performed in children with thalidomide syndrome.[25]

In recent years the search for other pharmacologic teratogens has intensified. Characteristic syndromes, including congenital heart defects, have been described for phenytoin[36] and trimethadione,[76] two anticonvulsant drugs. However, when drug induced malformations are suspected, it may be difficult to separate the effect of the medication from the effect of the underlying indication for treatment. Thus, epilepsy itself could account for some or all of the observed association. Monson and colleagues evaluated an untreated epileptic population for comparison.[42] They found that while untreated women with epilepsy gave birth to more children with congenital malformations than nonepileptic women, anticonvulsant-treated women had an even greater proportion of abnormal offspring. In studies of this type, it may still be difficult to separate the degree of severity of the underlying condition from the effect of medication use. One approach, when there is more than one acceptable treatment, is to compare the prevalence of malformations in groups of similar severity using the different treatments.

The use of insulin during pregnancy has been associated with an increase in congenital heart disease in the offspring.[64] However, again the underlying disease (maternal diabetes) must be considered and probably accounts for much of this association. Further research is needed to determine which factors in women with diabetes are responsible for the development of congenital malformations. Hypoglycemia, hyperglycemia, rapid shifts in glucose level, vascular abnormalities, and exogenous insulin use are all possible candidates for this causal role.

A number of other medications, including exogenous hormones,[19,64] lithium,[52] aspirin,[64,77] and antibiotics,[64,77] have been suggested as potential causes of cardiovascular birth defects. Others, such as the anti-nausea drug Bendectin (doxylamine and pyridoxine) have been suggested,[64] but later found probably not to be associated with congenital heart disease.[77]

Two personal habits have been associated with an increased prevalence of congenital heart disease. Maternal alcohol use during pregnancy may lead to multiple congenital anomalies. The fetal alcohol syndrome includes such cardiac defects as ventricular and atrial septal defects and patent ductus arteriosus.[35] Maternal cigarette smoking has been associated with intrauterine growth retardation and an increased prevalence of valvular heart defects.[28]

Other environmental exposures have been associated with congenital heart disease. For example, hypoxia has been investigated as a teratogen. Penaloza and colleagues[54] have shown that patent ductus arteriosus is more frequent among schoolchildren in Peru at high altitudes than at sea level. The prevalence was shown to increase gradually as the altitude increased, suggesting a dose-response relationship. Rothman and Fyler reported an association between population density and certain heart defects that appeared greater than could be explained by differential case ascertainment.[62]

Finally, paternal environmental exposure may be a cause of congenital heart disease. Such exposures in fathers could cause birth defects in one of three ways: (1) gene mutation, (2) chromosomal damage, or (3) by acting as a teratogen carried in the semen.[16] Erickson and colleagues investigated the potential association between paternal exposure to agent orange and congenital defects, including cardiovascular defects.[12] They found no evidence to support an association. Further research on other potential paternal teratogens is needed. Teratogens and neonatal heart disease are futher considered in Chapter 49.

Genetic-Environmental Interaction

Nora has proposed a model of multifactorial or polygenic inheritance to explain the majority of cases of congenital heart disease.[47] As he points out, this model should not be taken as a vague category, meaning only that many factors are involved.[48] Instead, it represents a group of mathematical models of inheritance that can vary from simple to complex. The model requires a person who is genetically predisposed to have cardiovascular anomalies and to react adversely to specific teratogens. This person must then be exposed in utero to a particular environmental factor during a vulnerable period in embryogenesis.[48] Thus, in this model there is interaction between a large number of genes and specific environmental triggers.

Because multifactorial inheritance, such as mendelian inheritance, is based on mathematical models, it should predict the expected outcome with respect to cardiovascular disease in first-degree relatives. A knowledge of the incidence of a given disorder both in the general population and in the first-degree relatives of those affected with it offers evidence as to whether a disease is or is not polygenic. The theoretical mathematics of the multifactorial model also predict that if a given polygenic disease occurs more frequently in one sex than the other, then children are more likely to inherit the disease from a parent of the less frequently affected sex. This phenomenon, known as the Carter effect, is explained by the assumption that the genes causing the disease are more readily expressed in the sex that is more frequently affected. The less frequently afflicted sex must then be more richly endowed with the genes that cause it for the disease to be expressed. Therefore, when a person of the less frequently affected sex has the disease, it should confer an increased risk to the offspring of that person.[60] Finally, the polygenic model predicts that cardiac defects that are common in the population, such as ventricular septal defect, should recur more frequently than rare defects such as truncus arteriosus. These theoretical predictions allow the model to be tested against what is observed in nature.

Nora and colleagues first attempted to test the model in family studies and found results that were consistent with it.[49] They reported a recurrence of 1 to 5 per cent which, given the population prevalence, supports the model. The sex distribution for some types of congenital heart disease has also been found to conform to that which would be predicted by the model in some studies.[60] Based on these lines of evidence, the theory of multifactorial inheritance of congenital heart disease has gained wide acceptance.

Recently, however, new evidence has been produced that calls this model into question. First, it has been reported that the recurrence risk is somewhat higher for children of affected probands than for siblings.[50] The polygenic model predicts that the recurrence should be the same for these groups. Also, several groups of investigators using different methodology have detected a higher frequency of recurrence than would be predicted by the multifactorial model. Whittemore and coworkers reported a 16 per cent recurrence for congenital heart defects in a prospective study of affected mothers.[74] Rose and associates detected a recurrence of approximately 9 per cent in a retrospective study of probands of either sex with one of four selected congenital heart defects.[60] It should be remembered that the mathematical model for multifactorial inheritance should predict the incidence of congenital heart disease. Published studies have all determined the prevalence in liveborn infants and used that as an approximation of the incidence. In an attempt to obtain improved ascertainment and a better estimate of incidence, Allan and colleagues used fetal echocardiography to detect recurrence of cardiovascular defects in the offspring

of mothers with a family history of heart disease.[1] Their overall recurrence of 2 per cent was consistent with the polygenic model, but they had a pattern of recurrence that was different from expected. They found that rare anomalies, such as truncus arteriosus and complex congenital heart defects, recurred much more commonly than would be predicted by the polygenic model. Finally, Rose and associates[60] did not find the sex distribution predicted by the model. In probands with atrial septal defects, 70 per cent were female. One would therefore expect, under the multifactorial model, that the incidence of heart disease in the offspring of males with atrial septal defect would be higher than that of females with the defect. In fact, using the prevalence as an approximation for incidence, they found that the reverse was true. Only 14 per cent of the offspring with congenital heart disease and only 9.1 per cent of those with atrial septal defect had fathers who had an atrial septal defect.

At present, there is no model that accurately predicts the occurrence or recurrence of congenital heart disease. Newman has used an epidemiologic approach in an attempt to determine the etiology of ventricular septal defects.[46] He has suggested that the consistency of occurrence among persons with widely differing genetic makeup and environment, and the frequency of discordance in identical twins, indicates that ventricular septal defects often occur as random errors in development, at a frequency determined by the complexity of normal cardiac morphogenesis. Further research is clearly needed to elucidate the specific etiologic mechanisms that produce particular congenital heart defects.

References

1. Allan LD, Crawford DC, Chita SK, Anderson RH, Tynan MJ (1986): Familial recurrence of congenital heart disease in a prospective series of mothers referred for fetal echocardiography. Am J Cardiol 58:334–337.
2. Anderson RC (1954): Causative factors underlying congenital heart malformations. Pediatrics 14:143–152.
3. Berg JM, Crome L, France NE (1960): Congenital cardiac malformations in mongolism. Br Heart J 22:331–346.
4. Bound JP, Logan WFWE (1977): Incidence of congenital heart disease in Blackpool 1951–1971. Br Heart J 39:445–450.
5. Brown GC, Evans TN (1967): Serologic evidence of coxsackie virus etiology of congenital heart disease. JAMA 199:183–187.
6. Burnard ED (1959): Discussion on the significance of continuous murmurs in the first few days of life. Proc R Soc Med 52:77–78.
7. Carlgren LE (1959): The incidence of congenital heart disease in children born in Gothenburg 1941–1950. Br Heart J 21:40–50.
8. Chameides L, Truex RC, Vetter V (1977): Association of maternal lupus erythematosus with congenital complete heart block. N Engl J Med 297:1204–1207.
9. Cooper LZ, Ziring PR, Ockerse AB, Fedun BA, Keily B, Krugman S (1969): Rubella: Clinical manifestations and management. Am J Dis Child 118:18–29.
10. Dickinson DF, Arnold R, Wilkinson JL (1981): Congenital heart disease among 160,480 liveborn children in Liverpool, 1960 to 1969: Implications for treatment. Br Heart J 46:55–62.
11. Elandt-Johnson RC (1975): Definition of rates: Some remarks on their use and misuse. Am J Epidemiol 102:267–271.
12. Erickson JD, Mulinare J, McClain PW, Fitch TG, James LM, McClearon AB, Adams MJ (1984): Vietnam veterans' risk for fathering babies with birth defects. JAMA 252:903–912.

13. Feldt RH, Avasthey P, Yoshimasu F, Kurland LT, Titus JL (1971): Incidence of congenital heart disease in children born to residents of Olmstead County, Minnesota, 1950–1969. Mayo Clin Proc 46:794–799.

14. Ferencz C, Rubin JD, McCarter RJ, Brenner JI, Neill CA, Perry LW, Hepner SI, Downing JW (1985): Congenital heart disease: Prevalence at livebirth: The Washington-Baltimore Infant Study. Am J Epidemiol 121:31–36.

15. Fletcher RH, Fletcher SW, Wagner EH (1982): Clinical Epidemiology: The Essentials. Baltimore, Williams & Williams, pp 75–90.

16. Friedman JM (1984): Does agent orange cause birth defects? Teratology 29:193–221.

17. Fyler DC (1980): Report of the New England Regional Cardiac Program. Pediatrics (Suppl)65:375–461.

18. Greenwood RD, Nadas AS (1976): The clinical course of cardiac disease in Down syndrome. Pediatrics 58:893–897.

19. Heinonen OP, Slone D, Monson RR, Hook EB, Shapiro S (1977): Cardiovascular birth defects and antenatal exposure to female sex hormones. N Engl J Med 296:67–70.

20. Heymann MA (1983): Patent ductus arteriosus. In Adams FH, Emmanouilides GC (eds): Heart Disease in Infants and Children and Adolescents. Baltimore, Williams & Wilkins, pp 158–177.

21. Hoffman JIE, Rudolph AM (1965): The natural history of ventricular septal defects in infancy. Am J Cardiol 16:634–653.

22. Hoffman JIE, Christianson R (1978): Congenital heart disease in a cohort of 19,502 births with long-term follow-up. Am J Cardiol 42:641–647.

23. Huhta JC (1986): Uses and abuses of fetal echocardiography: A pediatric cardiologist's view. J Am Coll Cardiol 8:451–458.

24. International Society of Cardiology (1970): Classification of Heart Disease in Childhood. Groningen, VRB Offsetdrukerij.

25. Kajii T (1965): Thalidomide experience in Japan. Ann Paediatr 205:341–354.

26. Kaplan S (1977): Long term results after surgical treatment of congenital heart disease. Mod Concepts Cardiovasc Dis 46:1–6.

27. Keith JD (1978): Prevalence, incidence and epidemiology. In Keith JD, Rowe RD, Vlad P (eds): Heart Disease in Infancy and Childhood. New York, Macmillan, pp 3–13.

28. Kelsey JL, Dwyer T, Holford TR, Bracken MB (1978): Maternal smoking and congenital malformations: An epidemiologic study. J Epidemiol Community Health 32:102–107.

29. Kitterman JA, Edmunds LH, Gregory GA, Heymann MA, Tooley WH, Rudolph AM (1972): Patent ductus arteriosus in premature infants: Incidence, relation to pulmonary disease and management. N Engl J Med 287:473–477.

30. Kleinbaum DG, Kupper LL, Morgenstern H (1982): Epidemiologic Research: Principles and Quantitative Methods. Belmont, Lifetime Learning Publications, pp 96–157.

31. Koskimies O, Lapinleimu K, Saxen L (1978): Infections and other maternal factors as risk indicators for congenital malformations: A case-control study with paired serum samples. Pediatrics 61:832–837.

32. Laursen HB (1980): Some epidemiological aspects of congenital heart disease in Denmark. Acta Paediatr Scand 69:619–624.

33. Layde PM, Dooley K, Erickson JD, Edmonds LD (1980): Is there an epidemic of ventricular septal defects in the U.S.A.? Lancet 1:407–408.

34. Levy RJ, Rosenthal A, Fyler DC, Nadas AS (1978): Birthweight of infants with congenital heart disease. Am J Dis Child 132:249–254.

35. Loser H, Majewski F (1977): Type and frequency of cardiac defects in embryo-fetal alcohol syndrome: Report of 16 cases. Br Heart J 39:1374–1379.

36. Loughnan PM, Gold H, Vance JC (1973): Phenytoin teratogenicity in man. Lancet 1:70–72.

37. MacMahon B, Pugh TF (1970): Epidemiology: Principles and Methods. Boston, Little, Brown & Company, pp 157–174.

38. Mausner JS, Bahn AK (1974): Epidemiology: An Introductory Text. Philadelphia, WB Saunders, pp 206–212.

39. Miettinen OS (1976): Estimability and estimation in case-referent studies. Am J Epidemiol 103:226–235.

40. Mitchell SC, Korones SB, Berendes HW (1971): Congenital heart disease in 56,109 births. Circulation 43:323–332.

41. Mitchell SC, Sellman AH, Westphal MC, Park J (1971): Etiologic correlates in a study of congenital heart disease in 56,109 births. Am J Cardiol 28:653–657.

42. Monson RR, Rosenberg L, Hartz SC, Shapiro S, Heinonen OP, Slone D (1973): Diphenylhydantoin and selected congenital malformations. N Engl J Med 289:1049–1052.

43. Morgenstern H, Kleinbaum DG, Kupper LL (1980): Measures of disease incidence used in epidemiologic research. Int J Epidemiol 9:97–104.

44. Murphy DJ, Meyer RA, Kaplan S (1985): Noninvasive evaluation of newborns with suspected congenital heart disease. Am J Dis Child 139:589–594.

45. Nadas AS (1986): Congenital heart disease. In Gellis SS, Kagan BJ (eds): Current Pediatric Therapy. Philadelphia, WB Saunders, p 135.

46. Newman TB (1985): Etiology of ventricular septal defects: An epidemiologic approach. Pediatrics 76:741–749.

47. Nora JJ (1968): Multifactorial inheritance hypothesis for the etiology of congenital heart diseases: The genetic environmental interaction. Circulation 38:604–617.

48. Nora JJ (1983): Etiologic aspects of heart disease. In Adams FH, Emmanouilides GC (eds): Heart Disease in Infants, Children and Adolescents. Baltimore, Williams & Wilkins, pp 2–10.

49. Nora JJ, McGill CW, McNamara DG (1970): Empiric recurrence risks in common and uncommon heart lesions. Teratology 3:325–330.

50. Nora JJ, Nora AH (1978): The evolution of specific genetic and environmental counseling in congenital heart disease. Circulation 57:205–213.

51. Nora JJ, Nora AH (1978): Genetics and Counseling in Cardiovascular Diseases. Springfield, IL, Charles C Thomas.

52. Nora JJ, Nora AH, Toews WH (1974): Lithium, Ebsteins anomaly and other congenital heart defects. Lancet 2:594–595.

53. Osler W (1900): The Principles and Practice of Medicine. New York, D Appleton Co, p 765.

54. Penaloza D, Arias-Stella J, Sime F, Marticorena E (1964): The heart and pulmonary circulation in children at high altitudes: Physiological, anatomical and clinical observations. Pediatrics 34:568–582.

55. Penrose LS (1954): Observations on the etiology of mongolism. Lancet 2:505–509.

56. Pitt DB, Samson PE (1961): Congenital malformations and maternal diet. Aust Ann Med 10:268–274.

57. Reller MD, Lorenz JM, Kotagal UR, Meyer RA, Kaplan S (1985): Hemodynamically significant PDA: An echocardiographic and clinical assessment of incidence, natural history and outcome in very low birth weight infants maintained in negative fluid balance. Pediatr Cardiol 6:17–24.

58. Richards MR, Merritt KK, Samuels MH, Langman AG (1955): Congenital malformations of the cardiovascular system in a series of 6,053 infants. Pediatrics 15:12–32.

59. Roberts WC (1970): The congenital bicuspid aortic valve: A study of 85 autopsy patients. Am J Cardiol 26:72–83.

60. Rose V, Gold RJM, Lindsay G, Allen M (1985): A possible increase in the incidence of congenital heart defects among the offspring of affected parents. J Am Coll Cardiol 6:376–382.

61. Ross LJ (1959): Congenital cardiovascular anomalies in twins. Circulation 20:327–342.

62. Rothman KJ, Fyler DC (1976): Association of congenital heart defects with season and population density. Teratology 13:29–34.

63. Rothman KJ, Fyler DC (1976): Sex, birth order, and maternal age characteristics of infants with congenital heart defects. Am J Epidemiol 104:527–534.

64. Rothman KJ, Fyler DC, Goldblatt A, Kreidberg M (1979): Exogenous hormones and other drug exposures of children with congenital heart disease. Am J Epidemiol 109:433–439.

65. Rowe RD, Uchida IA (1961): Cardiac malformation in mongolism: A prospective study of 184 mongoloid children. Am J Med 31:726–735.

66. Rowland TW, Hubbell JP, Nadas AS (1973): Congenital heart disease in infants of diabetic mothers. J Pediatr 83:815–820.

67. Sheridan MD (1964): Final report of a prospective study of children whose mothers had rubella in early pregnancy. Br Med J 2:536–539.

68. Siassi B, Blanco C, Cabal LA, Goran AG (1976): Incidence and clinical features of patent ductus arteriosus in low birthweight infants: A prospective analysis of 150 consecutively born infants. Pediatrics 57:347–351.

69. Soler NG, Walsh CH, Malins JM (1976): Congenital malformations in infants of diabetic mothers. Q J Med 178:303–313.

70. Van Mierop LHS (1984): Diagnostic code for congenital heart disease. Pediatr Cardiol 5:331–362.

71. Warkany J, Passarge E, Smith LB (1966): Congenital malformations in autosomal trisomy syndromes. Am J Dis Child 112:502–517.

72. Warkany J (1971): Congenital malformations. Chicago, Year Book Medical Publishers, pp 470–472.

73. Wesselhoeft C (1947): Rubella (German measles). N Engl J Med 236:943–950, 978–988.

74. Whittemore R, Hobbins JC, Engle MA (1982): Pregnancy and its outcome in women with and without surgical treatment of congenital heart disease. Am J Cardiol 50:641–651.

75. Zachman RD, Steinmetz GP, Botham RJ, Graven SN, Ledbetter MK (1974): Incidence and treatment of the patent ductus arteriosus in the ill premature neonate. Am Heart J 87:697–703.

76. Zackai EH, Mallman WJ, Niederer B, Hanson JW (1975): The fetal trimethadione syndrome. J Pedia284.

77. Zierler S, Rothman KJ (1985): Congenital heart disease in relation to maternal use of Bendectin and other drugs in early pregnancy. N Engl J Med 313:347–352.

34 TOTAL ANOMALOUS PULMONARY VENOUS DRAINAGE

Catherine Bull

Of all the causes of cardiorespiratory distress in the neonate, total anomalous pulmonary venous drainage (TAPVD) is perhaps the diagnosis most often missed. Unrecognized, the condition carries a high mortality, and when the diagnosis is delayed, the sequelae of long-term ventilation or pulmonary infection in the affected infant can prejudice the outcome of surgical repair. Conversely, when promptly diagnosed, effectively managed, and surgically corrected, the condition is among the most satisfying of congenital cardiac conditions to treat, since survivors of neonatal surgery thrive so well.

HISTORICAL PERSPECTIVE

TAPVD in a neonate was first described by Wilson[21] in 1793. Reporting a series of cases in 1952, Snellen and Albers[17] first suggested that TAPVD might prove a relatively common anomaly in clinical practice. Muller,[14] calling the condition "transposition of the pulmonary veins," first attempted to repair the TAPVD surgically in 1951.

EMBRYOLOGY

At 25 to 27 days' gestation the embryo is about 4 mm long, and the heart is just beginning to beat. The septum primum is beginning to separate the two atria, which drain through an atrioventricular canal to the ventricle. It is at this stage that the lung buds begin to grow out from the foregut, with angioblasts developing in parallel. Thus, the primordial pulmonary vascular plexus is scarcely differentiated from the splanchnic plexus, and since the pulmonary artery has not yet connected to the sixth arch, no separate pulmonary circulation is established.

The common pulmonary vein develops as an endothelial sprout from the superior wall of the left atrium and grows toward the lung bud. By 30 days' gestation, the pulmonary artery has connected to the sixth arch, and the common pulmonary vein has connected to the pulmonary venous plexus and has canalized, and the connections between pulmonary and splanchnic plexuses are involuting. Later, the common pulmonary vein is annexed into the left atrium.[15]

If the left atrial outgrowth fails to make appropriate connection to the pulmonary plexus, alternative routes of venous drainage must develop as the differentiating pulmonary arterial circulation evolves. These various alternative routes presumably account for the development of TAPVD and some allied conditions listed in Table 34-1.

Figure 34-1 shows diagramatically the heart of a 6-mm embryo. If the septum primum grew abnormally far to the left, the common pulmonary vein might arise from the right side of the septum and join the pulmonary plexus normally but later be incorporated into the roof of the right atrium. The resulting anomaly would be called TAPVD to right atrium.

If the common pulmonary vein fails to develop or to canalize, adjacent systemic venous sytems may accommodate the increasing pulmonary blood flow. The right common cardinal vein (continuous with the sinus venosus) destined to be the right superior vena cava (SVC) is nearby. Its connection with the pulmonary venous plexus will result in TAPVD to the right SVC. The pulmonary plexus may instead connect to the left common cardinal vein. Normally, part of this structure involutes, leaving only a segment to form the coronary sinus. If the vein atrophies above its connection to the pulmonary veins, the latter will drain to the right atrium via the coronary sinus, termed TAPVD to coronary sinus. If, on the other hand, the atrophic segment is below the connection to the pulmonary veins, a connection by a vertical vein to the innominate vein and right SVC will persist, the pulmonary venous blood being carried superiorly. This anomaly is called TAPVD to left vertical vein.

A final alternative pathway for pulmonary venous return is to maintain the primitive connections with the splanchnic plexus. The pulmonary plexus can drain into a common channel closely related to the esophagus and pierce the diaphragm with the esophagus or the vagus nerve, coming to communicate with either the portal system or the ductus venosus. This anomaly is called infra-diaphragmatic TAPVD. Pulmonary venous drainage from different areas may drain to different veins, which is termed mixed TAPVD.

ANATOMY

TAPVD is thus described according to the main channel by which pulmonary venous return to the heart occurs

Table 34–1. MALFORMATIONS RELATED TO TAPVD

PAPVD
The pulmonary veins of one lung or part of one lung drain anomalously.

PULMONARY VEIN ATRESIA
The pulmonary venous connection to the left atrium fails to canalize or becomes atretic secondarily. Any pulmonary venous return depends on connection with bronchial veins.

PULMONARY VEIN STENOSIS
The pulmonary venous connection to the heart is normal, but the orifice of each vein entering the left atrium is stenosed. The condition may be unilateral.

SCIMITAR SYNDROME
Unilateral PAPVD. Typically, the pulmonary venous return from the right lung descends, meeting the inferior vena cava at or below the inferior vena cava–right atrium junction.

COR TRIATRIATRUM
The absorption of the pulmonary veins into the left atrium is disturbed, so that a fibrous wall separates the pulmonary venous confluence from the mitral valve.

PULMONARY SEQUESTRATION
A segment of pulmonary parenchyma is sequestered from the bronchial tree. Such segments often drain anomalously to the systemic venous system. They may also have a systemic arterial supply.

PAPVD = Partial anomalous pulmonary venous drainage.

Table 34–2. SITES OF ANOMALOUS PULMONARY VENOUS CONNECTIONS

Site	Per Cent
Supracardiac	50
Left superior vena cava	40
Right superior vena cava	10
Cardiac	25
Coronary sinus	20
Right atrium	5
Infracardiac	20
Mixed	5

Adapted from Gersony WM (1979): Presentation, diagnosis and natural history of total anomalous pulmonary venous drainage. In Godman MJ, Marquis RM. (eds): Paediatric Cardiology, vol. 2. London, Churchill Livingstone.

(Table 34–2). All hearts with TAPVD have a patent foramen ovale or secundum atrial septal defect allowing blood to reach the left side of the heart. Absence of direct pulmonary venous drainage to the left atrium may account for the left atrial underdevelopment that can be quite striking in TAPVD. The smallness of the chamber may also be related to the absence of the left atrial elements formed by incorporation of the pulmonary veins. In utero, the small capacity and low compliance of the left atrium may interfere with forward flow of blood across the foramen ovale; such inadequate intrauterine left ventricular flow may explain the finding of marginal left ventricular hypoplasia in many neonates with TAPVD.[6]

Obstruction to pulmonary venous return along its abnormal pathway back to the heart heavily influences the presentation and physiology of TAPVD. The approximate prevalence and commonest site of obstruction in the different types of TAPVD are shown in Table 34–3.

Additional Anomalies

Although it is usually seen in the absence of other cardiac malformations, persistent patent ductus arteriosus and ventricular septal defect sometimes complicate TAPVD. The condition can also occur in the context of complex congenital heart disease. In particular, fetuses with anomalies of lateralization (heterotaxia)—bilateral left or right sidedness—very frequently have anomalies of pulmonary venous drainage. So-called right isomerism implies the presence of two right atria and so (almost by definition)

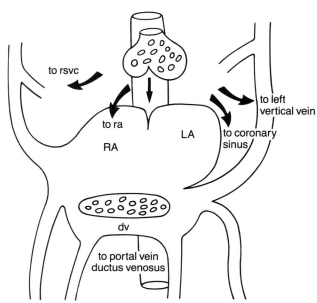

Figure 34–1. Diagram of the heart of a 6-mm embryo. The lung bud is growing from the foregut. Developing venous channels failing to connect appropriately to the left atrium may return to right or left cardinal veins or to the right atrium or may pass infradiaphragmatically to join the ductus venosus or portal vein. dv = ductus venosus; LA = left atrium; RA = right atrium; rsvc = right superior vena cava.

Table 34–3. PREVALENCE AND SITE OF OBSTRUCTION

Connection	Severe Obstruction (Per Cent)	Site of Obstruction
Left superior vena cava (LSVC)	40	LSVC impinges on left main bronchus or stenosis at LSVC–innominate junction
Right superior vena cava (RSVC)	75	Pulmonary venous trunk–RSVC junction
Coronary sinus	10	Coronary sinus ostia
Right atrium	5	Pulmonary venous–right atrium junction
Infracardiac	95 to 100	At diaphragm, entrance to portal vein or ductus venosus
All occasionally have obstruction at PFO		

Adapted from Gersony WM (1979): Presentation, diagnosis and natural history of total anomalous pulmonary venous drainage. In Godman MJ, Marquis RM. (eds): Paediatric Cardiology, vol. 2. London, Churchill Livingstone.

Table 34–4. SYNDROMES ASSOCIATED WITH TAPVD

Syndromes	Associated Abnormalities
Chromosomal Anomalies	
Cat eye (partial trisomy 22)	Skin tags, ears, eyes, rectal agenesis
Dysmorphic Syndromes	
Marden, Walker[11]	Facies, contractures, hypotonia
D'Ercole[3]	Short stature, retardation, late puberty
Knobloch, Layer[9]	Encephalocoele, lung hypoplasia, eyes
Mardini, Nyhan[12]	Lung agenesis, thumbs
Piepkorn et al[16]	Facies, short stature, palate urogenital
Wiedemann et al[20]	Facies, skeletal
VATER	Rectal agenesis, arms, vertebrae

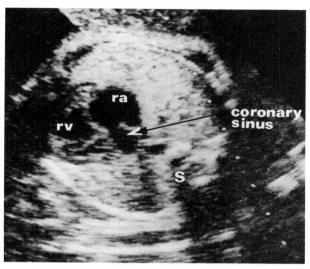

Figure 34–2. Antenatal ultrasound examination at 24 weeks' gestation showing fetus with TAPVD to coronary sinus (arrow). (Courtesy of Dr. L. Allan.) ra = right atrium; rv = right ventricle.

anomalous pulmonary venous return. By contrast, hearts with left isomerism (two left atria) have, by definition, anomalous systemic venous return, but frequently the pulmonary veins also drain in an unusual manner to the heart or to large extracardiac systemic veins. Children with right or left isomerism also have right or left lungs bilaterally, often recognizable by the bronchial anatomy on chest radiograph or bronchial tomography.[2] The diagnosis of TAPVD should then be considered. Although typically occurring as an isolated cardiac malformation, TAPVD can constitute part of a dysmorphic syndrome. Syndromes associated with TAPVD are shown in Table 34–4.

The Lungs

The pulmonary vascular tree of some babies with TAPVD is abnormal at birth.[7] Obstruction to pulmonary venous return can certainly be present even in utero, and muscularization of the intra- and extrapulmonary veins of neonates dying very early of infradiaphragmatic TAPVD has been blamed on long-standing intrauterine pulmonary venous obstruction. Such prenatal pulmonary vascular changes must militate against later successful repair of the defect.

PHYSIOLOGY

Fetal Circulation

In utero, the ductus arteriosus is patent, and the pulmonary vascular resistance is high. Hence, the pulmonary blood flow is low, so the sequelae of anomalous pulmonary venous return are well tolerated by the fetus. Figure 34–2 shows a fetus of 24 weeks' gestation with TAPVD to the coronary sinus. She was eventually born at term weighing 2.9 kg.

Postnatal Hemodynamics

All anatomic types of TAPVD have some features in common. All have "complete mixing" of pulmonary and systemic venous return in the right atrium, much of which crosses the tricuspid valve as usual. However, since there

is no pulmonary venous return to the left atrium, the right atrial pressure tends to exceed the left, and a mixture of oxygenated and desaturated blood also shunts from the right to left atrium and is ejected from the left ventricle into the systemic circuit. The circulatory adjustments and clinical features are influenced by several factors, principally the level of the pulmonary vascular resistance and the presence of obstruction to pulmonary venous drainage.

Pulmonary Vascular Resistance

In the absence of pulmonary venous obstruction, pulmonary vascular resistance in TAPVD falls sharply from the time of the first breath. At birth, because left and right ventricles are equally thick, the systemic and pulmonary venous return mixing in the right atrium will be distributed approximately equally to the left and right ventricles, provided the foramen ovale is widely patent. However, with time the pulmonary vascular resistance falls substantially relative to systemic vascular resistance, and the right ventricle ejects against a smaller afterload, thins, and becomes more compliant. As a result, the right ventricle is able to accommodate more and more blood in diastole, which it ejects into the pulmonary artery. Pulmonary flow thus increases (and hence pulmonary venous return), so that while left ventricular output is maintained at low to normal levels, pulmonary blood flow may be three or more times greater than systemic blood flow. With a large total cardiac output and dilated right atrium and ventricle, the heart enlarges as the lungs become plethoric.

As the pulmonary blood flow increases, the proportion of oxygenated blood in the right atrium, and hence blood oxygenation in the systemic circuit, increases. When arterial oxygen saturations exceed 85 per cent, cyanosis may not be noted. Conversely, when pulmonary blood

Table 34–5. DETERMINANTS OF DEGREE OF CYANOSIS

Pulmonary blood flow Qp (determined by pulmonary vascular resistance)
Pulmonary venous desaturation (pulmonary edema worsens)
Cardiac output (determines arteriovenous oxygen difference and hence systemic venous oxygen saturation)

flow is low, most right atrial blood will consist of desaturated systemic venous return, and cyanosis will be striking (Table 34–5 and Fig. 34–3).

Obstruction to Pulmonary Venous Return

After birth, increases in pulmonary blood flow cause increases in pressure when venous obstruction is present. Once the pressure in the capillary vasculature exceeds plasma oncotic pressure, transudation of fluid into the pulmonary alveoli occurs. If the rate of accumulation of fluid exceeds the capacity of the lymphatics to clear it, pulmonary edema results. The pulmonary edema will exacerbate the child's hypoxia, and the very stiff lungs increase the work of breathing, accounting for respiratory distress. High pulmonary venous pressure also results in pulmonary arterial hypertension, which serves to limit pulmonary flow, and since the pulmonary venous return is thus low, the heart remains small although the lungs are edematous.

Patency of the Ductus Arteriosus

The ductus arteriosus may remain patent for days or weeks after birth, particularly in infants hypoxic with pulmonary venous obstruction. If the pulmonary vascular resistance is very high, blood will shunt from the pulmonary artery to the aorta. If resistances reverse, the direction of flow will reverse.

Ductal right-to-left shunting in conditions of high pulmonary vascular resistance may occasionally be important

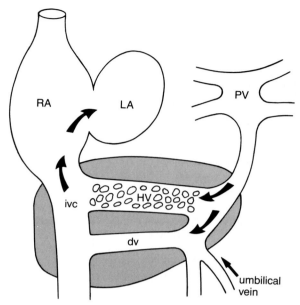

Figure 34–4. Infracardiac TAPVD with patent ductus venosus. As in the fetus, inferior vena caval blood may stream preferentially to the left atrium and account for a false-negative hyperoxia test. When the ductus venosus closes, pulmonary venous return is forced through the high resistance hepatic bed, and pulmonary edema ensues. This diagram also shows how infradiaphragmatic TAPVD may be suspected if unexpectedly red blood is withdrawn on insertion of an umbilical venous catheter. dv = ductus venosus; HV = hepatic vein; ivc = inferior vena cava; LA = left atrium; PV = pulmonary venous confluence; RA = right atrium.

in maintaining systemic blood flow, particularly when the left atrium and left ventricle are hypoplastic or the foramen ovale restrictive. Under these circumstances, the neonate may present with persistent pulmonary hypertension of the newborn syndrome, with little evidence of pulmonary edema because of diversion of blood flow from the lungs to the systemic circuit. The heart remains small and pulmonary vascularity reduced.

Patency of the Ductus Venosus

During fetal life, a proportion of umbilical venous blood bypasses the hepatic capillary circulation via the ductus venosus. After birth, the umbilical flow is eliminated, but infradiaphragmatic anomalous pulmonary venous drainage to the ductus venosus can bypass the hepatic circulation (Fig. 34–4). As long as the channel remains patent, the pulmonary venous pressure stays low and the child presents with features of unobstructed TAPVD. Pulmonary edema ensues when the ductus venosus closes and the pulmonary venous return is forced through the hepatic capillaries. Infradiaphragmatic TAPVD is virtually the only congenital malformation in which closure of the ductus venosus is of hemodynamic significance.

The Foramen Ovale

In the absence of a ventricular septal defect or patent ductus arteriosus, the foramen ovale is the only means by

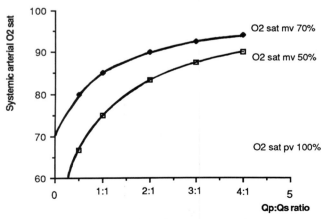

Figure 34–3. Relationship of arterial oxygen saturation to pulmonary blood flow in conditions with complete intracardiac mixing of systemic and pulmonary venous return. Calculations assume that the pulmonary venous blood is fully saturated. Qp:Qs ratio = ratio of pulmonary blood flow to systemic blood flow.

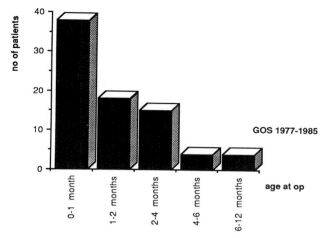

Figure 34–5. Age distribution of patients undergoing surgery for TAPVD at the Hospital For Sick Children, Great Ormond Street, 1977 to 1985. GOS = Great Ormond Street.

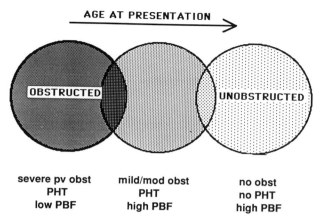

Figure 34–6. Physiology related to age at presentation. obst = obstruction; pv = pulmonary venous; PBF = pulmonary blood flow; PHT = pulmonary hypertension.

which blood can reach the systemic circuit. Obstruction to this obligatory right-to-left atrial shunt would result in low left ventricular output and systemic hypotension. Severe restriction is unusual, but lesser degrees of obstruction may account for elevation of right atrial pressure and liver enlargement in patients with TAPVD and high pulmonary blood flow—a picture of cardiac failure.

PRESENTATION

The age at presentation depends largely on the presence of obstruction to the pulmonary venous return. Infants with obstructed TAPVD become symptomatic very early in the neonatal period; children born with completely unobstructed anomalous pulmonary venous return may occasionally not come to medical attention until much later in childhood. However, for most neonates, the combined stresses of an increased pulmonary arterial pressure and a high pulmonary blood flow soon precipitate symptoms of heart failure (Figs. 34–5 and 34–6) whether or not frank pulmonary venous obstruction is present.

Thus, neonates with TAPVD can present with the signs and symptoms of pulmonary venous obstruction, excessive pulmonary blood flow, or both. They may be breathless or cyanotic, or both. Dyspnea is prominent when pulmonary blood flow is very high (gross plethora) or in the presence of interstitial edema related to pulmonary venous obstruction.

DIAGNOSIS

Differential Diagnosis

Identifying the child with TAPVD from neonates cyanotic and breathless from other causes is by no means easy. Conditions easily confused with TAPVD in the neonatal period include all patients with persistent right-to-left

atrial and ductal shunting, those with primary pulmonary disease, and those with other forms of congenital heart disease (Table 34–6). Differential diagnosis requires clinical examination and special investigations.

Examination of the Neonate with TAPVD

Clinical findings in neonates with TAPVD are variable and depend on the infant's underlying physiology. Cyanosis may be mild or severe (see Table 34–5). Depending on the pulmonary blood flow and degree of pulmonary venous obstruction, breathlessness may also be mild or very severe. Confusingly, the degree of respiratory distress of an individual patient can wax and wane. The liver may be enlarged in the presence of a huge pulmonary blood flow, a restrictive atrial septal defect, or hyperinflated lungs. Tachycardia, weak pulses, and cool extremities may be present, indicating low cardiac output related to low left ventricular output secondary to hypoxia, acidosis, or severe obstruction to left ventricular filling.

Table 34–6. DIFFERENTIAL DIAGNOSIS OF TAPVD IN THE NEONATE

Persistent pulmonary hypertension of the newborn syndrome
Idiopathic
Meconium aspiration
Group B streptococcal infection
Congenital heart disease
Other
Pulmonary disease
Respiratory distress syndrome
Lymphangiectasia
Other
Cardiac disease
Severe left heart disease: hypoplastic left-heart syndrome, left ventricular outflow tract obstruction, left ventricular dysfunction
Other

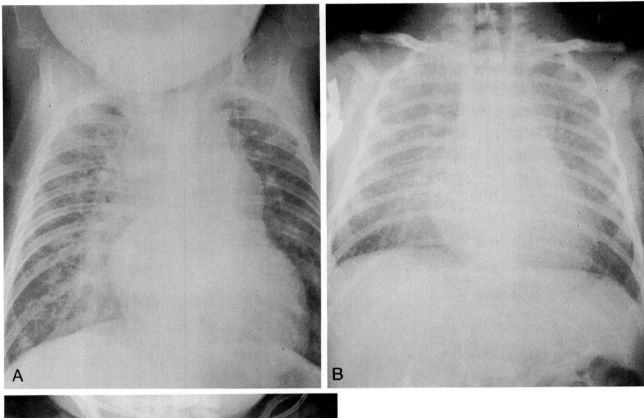

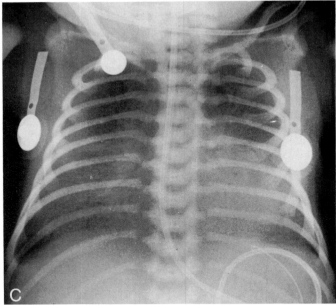

Figure 34–7. Chest radiographs of neonates with TAPVD and respiratory distress syndrome (RDS). *A,* Unobstructed TAPVD to left vertical vein. Note the large heart, plethoric lung fields, and the shadow corresponding to the dilated left vertical vein. *B,* Obstructed infracardiac TAPVD. Note the small heart, upper lobe blood diversion, fluid in the fissures, and Kerly B-lines. *C,* RDS showing a different reticular pattern and air bronchograms.

Murmurs may *not* be present, particularly if pulmonary blood flow is low because of persistently elevated pulmonary vascular resistance. Once the pulmonary resistance has dropped, there is often a systolic murmur corresponding to the excessive blood flow across the pulmonary valve and later a diastolic murmur of flow across the tricuspid valve. The second heart sound is split, in contrast to many cyanotic cardiac lesions presenting early, such as transposition of the great arteries or pulmonary atresia.

Radiology

Figure 34–7 shows chest radiographs of two children with TAPVD. These radiographs compare the appearances of cases with unobstructed (Fig. 34–7*A*) and obstructed (Fig. 34–7*B*) pulmonary venous return. Also shown is the radiograph of a child with respiratory distress syndrome (Fig. 34–7*C*) to contrast the reticular pattern of this condition with the appearance of pulmonary edema due to

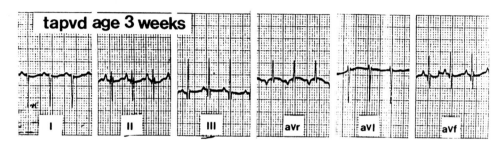

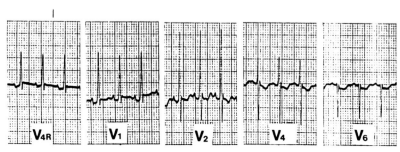

Figure 34–8. ECG of neonate with TAPVD. The dominant R wave in lead V_1 is normal for age.

obstructed pulmonary venous return. Unfortunately, these "typical" features are soon complicated by the changes of infection or ventilation damage to the neonatal lung if the diagnosis of TAPVD is delayed.

Electrocardiography

In the first week of life, the normal neonatal ECG shows right ventricular dominance similar to that seen in infants with TAPVD. Though electrocardiographic features of right ventricular hypertrophy persist beyond the first week of life in infants with TAPVD (Fig. 34–8), this is rarely helpful diagnostically, as persistent right ventricular hypertrophy is seen in many of the pulmonary and cardiac diseases with which TAPVD can be confused.

Oximetry

Even if not clinically cyanotic, children with TAPVD are at least mildly desaturated and typically demonstrate an inadequate rise in arterial oxygen saturation when breathing 100 per cent O_2 (hyperoxia test). Although an arterial PO_2 (with the sample taken from the right arm with the baby breathing 100 per cent oxygen for 5 minutes) of over 150 mmHg is said virtually to exclude cyanotic congenital heart disease,[18] such rises can occur in TAPVD if blood returning to the right atrium streams rather than mixes (see Fig. 34–4).[4,10] Infradiaphragmatic TAPVD may be diagnosed by umbilical venous catheterization, which can demonstrate a higher venous than arterial saturation.[10]

Two-Dimensional Echocardiography

Ultrasonographic examination of the heart of a child in whom the possibility of TAPVD has been raised is enor-

mously helpful, since with sufficient expertise, the diagnosis can almost always be proved or excluded. Some echocardiographic features are easy to appreciate, while others require greater experience with neonatal cardiac ultrasonography (Fig. 34–9). Although spectacular echocardiographic pictures of the pulmonary venous return in TAPVD can sometimes be obtained, the difficulties of achieving diagnostic echocardiograms should not be underestimated, particularly in a ventilated neonate. Thus, if diagnostic doubt remains for a child with unexplained respiratory distress, it is often necessary to transfer the baby to a cardiac center for assessment. There, if the child proves to have TAPVD, cross-sectional echocardiography is also important in ruling out significant associated anomalies, especially persistent ductus arteriosus and ventricular septal defect.

The presence of a normally connected heart with a *small* left atrium (Fig. 34–9A) excludes many forms of cyanotic congenital heart disease and those left-heart syndromes with left atrial hypertension due to left ventricular dysfunction. However, this scenario is common to many causes of neonatal pulmonary hypertension, including primary pulmonary parenchymal and vascular pathology. To diagnose TAPVD definitively, the anomalous connections of all pulmonary veins to a confluence and thence to the systemic venous system must be visualized (Fig. 34–9B to D).

While a view of the four chambers of the heart is held, a sharp injection of saline into a large vein can be seen as a stream of bright bubbles (contrast echo). Shunting of these bubbles from the right to left atrium occurs in TAPVD but also in other cardiac and pulmonary conditions with right-to-left atrial shunting. However, failure of such bubbles to cross the atrial septum excludes TAPVD.[10] Most patients can be adequately diagnosed with the above investigations, that is, *without* invasive studies. However, sometimes cardiac catheterization and angiography are indicated.

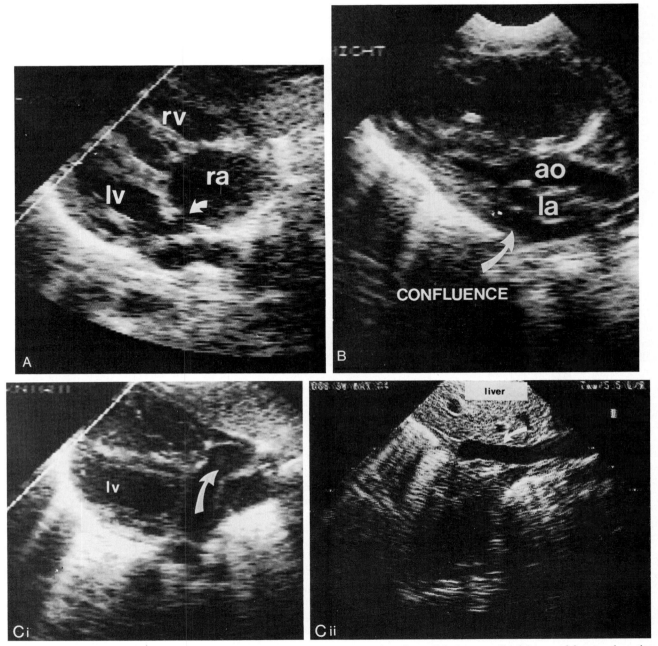

Figure 34–9. Ultrasound diagnosis of TAPVD. *A,* "Scenario." Normal cardiac connections. Large right heart, small left heart, atrial septum bows into left atrium. Arrow shows a small atrial septal defect. lv = left ventricle; ra = right atrium; rv = right ventricle. *B,* The abnormal "space" behind the left atrium suggests TAPVD, but, particularly when pulmonary flow is low, this confluence of the anomalous veins may not be conspicuously dilated. ao = ascending aorta; la = left atrium. *C,* Dilated systemic veins also suggest anomalous pulmonary venous return, e.g., (i) arrow in a dilated coronary sinus and (ii) arrow points out a channel descending through the diaphragm but distinguishable from the aorta and inferior vena cava. (Because they do not all run in the same plane, the long axes of these vessels cannot be imaged together.) IVC = inferior vena cava; lv = left ventricle.

Cardiac Catheterization and Angiography

Cardiac catheterization in these sick infants is not without risk; there is morbidity associated with the investigation itself, and the child may approach subsequent surgery in poor condition. In most surgical series, the preoperative condition of the baby has an important influence on postoperative mortality.[8] Moreover, diagnostic accuracy is less than 100 per cent, particularly when the index of suspicion of the condition is low.[10] We do not embark on cardiac catheterization unless the diagnosis or some aspect of it is uncertain or complicating anomalies need assessment.

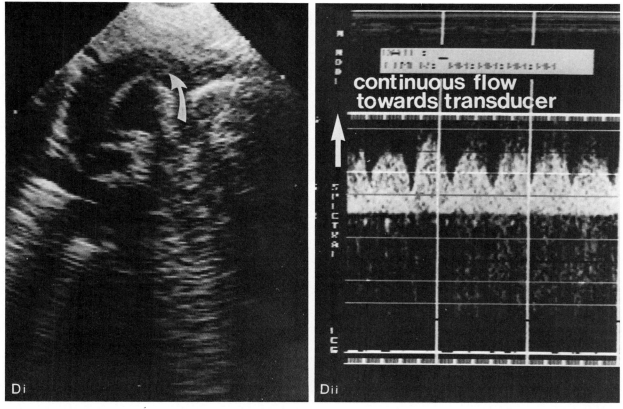

Figure 34–9. *Continued. D*, (i) Connection of the pulmonary veins to the systemic venous channel, e.g., TAPVD to the left vertical vein. The Doppler ultrasound signal (ii) within the channel shows blood flowing toward the greatly dilated innominate vein.

We have once performed catheterization only to perform balloon atrial septostomy.

Hemodynamics

Typically, pressures in the right heart are elevated, often to suprasystemic levels, when the pulmonary venous return is obstructed. Elevated pulmonary arterial wedge pressures may give evidence of pulmonary venous obstruction. If a pulmonary vein is entered from the systemic venous system, a gradient across a site of obstruction may be registered (Fig. 34–10). Measured oxygen saturations in the venous system will usually show a "step up" in saturation just beyond the connection of the anomalous pulmonary vein (Fig. 34–11), but complete admixture of systemic and pulmonary venous return can render oxygen saturations in all cardiac chambers and both great arteries similar. Streaming of inferior vena caval blood to the left atrium and superior vena caval blood to the right ventricle may lead to higher left heart than right heart saturations in infradiaphragmatic TAPVD, so the diagnosis of TAPVD should not be easily discarded on account of evidence from oxygen saturations alone. Because it is usually impossible to obtain a genuine mixed venous oxygen saturation, it is often difficult to estimate the pulmonary-systemic flow ratio by the Fick method in TAPVD.

Angiography

It is often possible to enter the common trunk or individual pulmonary veins from the systemic venous system, and angiograms may be taken in the anomalous vein if this is entered. Direct injection of the anomalous veins has the advantage of delineating the anatomy, including sites of obstruction, better than injection of a large dose of contrast material into the pulmonary artery to watch the late, often extremely faint pathway of the anomalous pulmonary venous return (Fig. 34–12). Pulmonary arterial injections are particularly disappointing in the presence of a persistent patent ductus arteriosus, pulmonary hypertension, and pulmonary venous obstruction, because the descending aorta opacifies preferentially.

NATURAL HISTORY

Left alone, patients with obstructed TAPVD rarely survive more than a few weeks. Those with unobstructed return may survive longer but at best fail to thrive, experiencing tachypnea and poor feeding and often succumbing to chest infections in the first year of life (Fig. 34–13). The results of medical management are necessarily limited in a condition in which the underlying

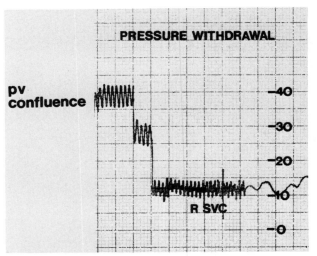

Figure 34–10. Withdrawal across the site of obstruction in the case of obstructed TAPVD to RSVC demonstrated in Figure 34–12A. pv = pulmonary vein; RSVC = right superior vena cava.

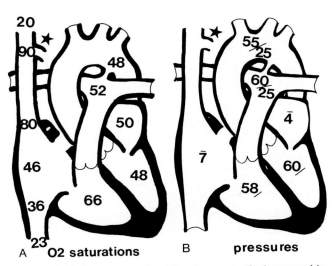

Figure 34–11. Oxygen saturation (A) and pressures (B) documented in the case of obstructed TAPVD to RSVC demonstrated in Figure 34–12A. RSVC = right superior vena cava.

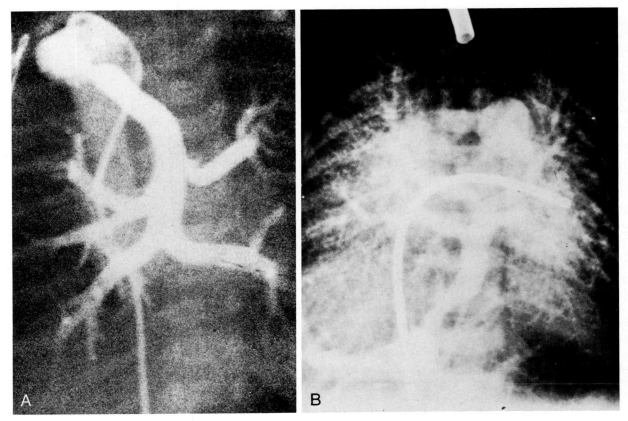

Figure 34–12. Angiography. A, Injection directly into the pulmonary vein showing obstructed TAPVD to right superior vena cava. B, Late phase of pulmonary arterial injection showing obstructed infradiaphragmatic TAPVD. SVC = superior vena cava.

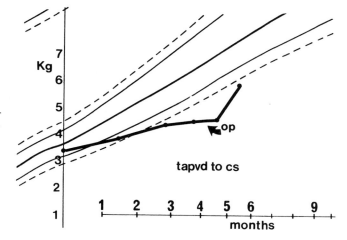

Figure 34–13. Weight Centile plot (solid dark line) of a child with unobstructed TAPVD to the coronary sinus. cs = coronary sinus; op = operation.

problem is of "plumbing." Thus, once the diagnosis is established, all patients need surgery, usually urgently.

MANAGEMENT

Medical Management

Medical therapy is usually aimed at optimizing the infant's condition in the hours before planned surgery. The child is usually helped by correction of acidosis and attention to fluid balance, generally with fluid restriction. Elective ventilation treats pulmonary edema and takes over the considerable work of breathing. Administration of prostaglandin E_1 (0.01 µg/kg/min) may effectively open the ductus venosus, which can be helpful in

infradiaphragmatic TAPVD[1] as well as the ductus arteriosus, which can be helpful when left ventricular output is poor, since it may allow the right ventricle to contribute to systemic circulation. Both maneuvers serve also to decompress a pulmonary circulation operating at suprasystemic pressures.

Balloon Atrial Septostomy

Some authors[10,13] advocate performing balloon atrial septostomy in at least some patients with TAPVD. If the foramen ovale was even marginally obstructive, the procedure may improve left ventricular filling, ameliorate features of low cardiac output and decrease the pulmonary venous pressure (Fig. 34–14).

Figure 34–14. Balloon atrial septostomy was performed as an emergency procedure at the bedside under ultrasound control in this patient with TAPVD. Views of left ventricular volume in end-diastole before and after septostomy (not shown) showed immediate improvement in left ventricular filling. The arrowheads point out the balloon tearing the foramen ovale (A) and then repositioned in the left atrium with no obstruction (B). LA = left atrium; RA = right atrium; RV = right ventricle.

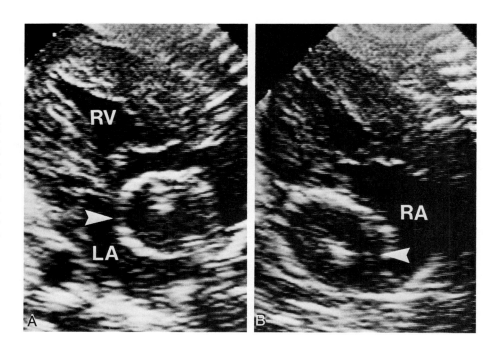

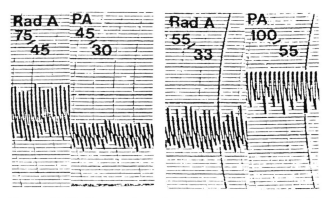

Figure 34–15. Postoperative pulmonary hypertensive crisis after TAPVD repair. The pulmonary arterial pressure can fluctuate from almost normal to suprasystemic levels, causing acute right ventricular strain once the intra- and extracardiac shunts have been closed at operation. PA = pulmonary artery; Rad A = radial artery.

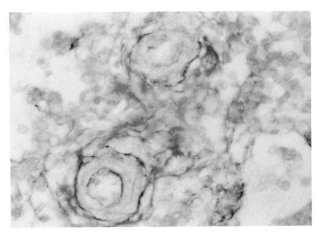

Figure 34–16. Photomicrograph of thick-walled muscular alveolar wall arteries (Magnification: × 540). Mean percentage arterial medial thickness of arteries of all sizes was significantly greater than normal at 5 hours of age. (Reproduced with permission of Haworth SG [1982]: Total anomalous pulmonary venous return. Prenatal damage to pulmonary vascular bed and extrapulmonary veins. Br Heart J 48:513–524.)

Surgical Management

Surgery is mandatory for this condition and the timing of operation is usually dictated by the child's condition. If venous return is obstructed, there is no advantage in delay, and operation should be arranged as soon as the diagnosis is confirmed. For an occasional unobstructed patient in good condition, the risk of operating early may be greater than the risks of delaying operation until the child is a few months old. This balance will depend largely on local surgical and postoperative expertise.

SURGERY

No extracardiac or palliative procedure is appropriate to the management of this lesion; intracardiac repair using cardiopulmonary bypass with or without circulatory arrest is needed regardless of the young age and small size of most patients. While primary definitive repair is conceptually appealing, the operation still carries a significant mortality, which is frustrating, as the repair itself almost always looks technically satisfactory even in infants who die early postoperatively. Many of the postoperative difficulties encountered are explicable as complications common to all neonates approaching surgery in poor preoperative condition. Such infants tolerate cardiopulmonary bypass poorly. However, some problems that are a frequent feature of the postoperative course following the repair of TAPVD are almost certainly related to the pulmonary vascular bed in this particular condition.

Pulmonary Hypertensive Crises

If the pulmonary artery pressure is monitored postoperatively, large fluctuations in pressure (and presumptively in pulmonary vascular resistance) are recorded in the very early postoperative phase of some patients. The pulmonary pressure can rise from almost normal to suprasystemic levels within minutes (Fig. 34–15), sometimes triggered by stimuli such as suction. Death due to acute right heart failure may occur during these episodes.[19] The substrate for such pulmonary vascular reactivity is presumably the thick-walled intrapulmonary arteries present even at birth in this condition (Fig. 34–16), which may respond vigorously to many of the physiologic stimuli known to constrict the neonatal pulmonary circulation, including upper airway stimulation (see Chapter 7).

LONG-TERM PROGNOSIS

Pulmonary vascular disease, a concern in patients operated late in childhood, should be avoided in those repaired in the neonatal period or in early infancy, provided no technical problems give rise to long-standing pulmonary venous obstruction. Thus, for survivors of neonatal surgery, the outlook is usually excellent because TAPVD is nearer to a surgically "curable" condition than most congenital cardiac defects.

References

1. Bullaboy CA, Johnson DH, Azar H, Jennings RB (1984): Total anomalous pulmonary venous connection to portal system: A new therapeutic role for prostaglandin E_1? Pediatr Cardiol 5:115–116.
2. Deanfield JE, Leanage R, Stroobant J, Chrispin AR, Taylor JFN, Macartney FJ (1980): Use of high kilovoltage filtered beam radiographs for detection of bronchial situs in infants and young children. Br Heart J 44:577–583.
3. D'Ercole A (1976): Case report. Synd Indent 4:5–8.
4. Enriques AMC, McKay R, Arnold RM, Wilkinson JL (1986): Misleading hyperoxia test. Arch Dis Child 61:604–606.

5. Gersony WM (1979): Presentation, diagnosis and natural history of total anomalous pulmonary venous drainage. In Godman MJ, Marquis RM (eds): Paediatric Cardiology. Vol 2. London, Churchill Livingstone.
6. Graham TP, Jarmakani JM, Canent RV (1972): Left heart volume characteristics with a right ventricular volume overload. Total anomalous pulmonary venous return and large atrial septal defect. Circulation 45:389–396.
7. Haworth SG (1982): Total anomalous pulmonary venous return. Prenatal damage to pulmonary vascular bed and extrapulmonary veins. Br Heart J 48:513–524.
8. Katz NM, Kirklin JW, Pacifico AD (1978): Concepts and practices in surgery for total anomalous pulmonary venous connection. Ann Thorac Surg 25:479–487.
9. Knobloch WH, Layer JM (1971): Retinal detachment and encephalocele. J Pediatr Ophthal 8:181–184.
10. Long WA, Lawson EE, Harned HS, Henry GW (1984): Infradiaphragmatic total anomalous pulmonary venous drainage: New diagnostic, physiologic and surgical considerations. Am J Perinatol 1:227–235.
11. Marden PM, Walker WA (1966): A new generalized connective tissue syndrome. Am J Dis Child 112:225–228.
12. Mardini MK, Nyhan WL (1985): Agenesis of the lung. Report of four patients with unusual anomalies. Chest 87:522–527.
13. Mullins CE, ElSaid GM, Neches WH, Williams RL, Vargo TA, Nihill MR, McNamara DG (1973): Balloon atrial septostomy for total anomalous pulmonary venous return. Br Heart J 35:752–757.
14. Muller WH (1951): The surgical treatment of transposition of the pulmonary veins. Ann Surg 134:683–693.
15. Neill CA (1956): Development of the pulmonary veins—with reference to the embryology of anomalies of pulmonary venous return. Pediatrics 18:880–887.
16. Piepkorn M, Karp LE, Hickok D, et al (1977): Lethal neonatal dwarfing condition with short ribs, polysyndactyly, cranial synostosis, cleft palate, cardiovascular and urinogenital anomalies and severe ossification defect. Teratology 16:345–350.
17. Snellen HA, Albers FH (1952): The clinical diagnosis of anomalous pulmonary venous drainage. Circulation 6:801–805.
18. Warburton D, Rehan M, Shinebourne EA (1981): Selective criteria for differential diagnosis of infants with symptoms of congenital heart disease. Arch Dis Child 56:94–100.
19. Wheeler J, George BL, Mulder DG, Jarmakani JM (1979): Diagnosis and management of postoperative pulmonary hypertensive crisis. Circulation 60:1640–1646.
20. Wiedemann HR, Grosse KR, Dibbern H (1985): Dysplasia syndrome of unusual appearance and cardiovascular anomalies. In Atlas of Characteristic Syndromes. London, Wolfe Medical Pub, pp 368–369.
21. Wilson J (1793): A description of a very unusual formation of the human heart. Philos Trans R Soc Lond 88:346.

35 VOLUME LOADS EXCEPT TAPVD

Gerald Barber

Alvin J. Chin

There are relatively few lesions in the newborn that produce a pure volume overload. These lesions can be either extracardiac, as in arteriovenous malformations or truncus arteriosus (with truncal valve insufficiency), or intracardiac, as in complete atrioventricular septal defect (common atrioventricular canal), or both, as in aortico–left ventricular tunnel. When a pressure overload lesion coexists with a left-to-right shunt, it increases the volume overload. Ventricular septal defect with coarctation of the aorta and conotruncal anomalies with coarctation of the aorta are examples of combined pressure-volume overloads. Isolated ventricular septal defects seldom present in the first month of life as a volume overload, although this presentation is common thereafter. This chapter will discuss arteriovenous malformations, complete atrioventricular septal defect, aortico–left ventricular tunnel, and combined pressure and volume overloads. Truncus arteriosus is discussed in Chapter 46.

ARTERIOVENOUS MALFORMATION

An arteriovenous malformation is an abnormal vascular connection in which blood can pass from artery to vein without passing through a capillary network. This anomalous connection can occur in either the systemic or pulmonary circulation. While arteriovenous malformations may be either congenital or acquired, the majority presenting as a volume overload in the neonate are congenital.

History

An arteriovenous fistula resulting in congestive heart failure in the neonate was first described by Silverman et al[43] in 1955. They reported two cases. The first was a 4-hour-old male who was dyspneic without cyanosis. While his liver was not palpable on admission, he developed hepatomegaly over the first 12 hours of life. Digitalization was started, but the patient died shortly thereafter. An autopsy revealed a massive vascular network that almost entirely replaced the right cerebral hemisphere. The second case described by Silverman et al was a 3-day-old male infant who developed tachypnea, cyanosis, and a heart murmur on the first day of life. By day 3, hepatomegaly and cardiomegaly had developed; the child died shortly thereafter. His autopsy revealed an arteriovenous fistula between the middle cerebral artery and the sagittal sinus. A third

case was added to the literature by Pollock and Laslett[35] in 1958. Their patient appeared normal shortly after birth except for a disproportionately large head. The child became tachypneic and lethargic at 51 hours of age. Hepatomegaly was noted, and digitalization was begun. The child died at 83 hours of age. Autopsy revealed a connection between the posterior cerebral and superior cerebellar arteries and the internal cerebral veins. Since these first two reports, many other cases have been described with similar findings.

Epidemiology

The majority of arteriovenous malformations do not cause heart failure in the neonate. Those that do are usually of cerebral or hepatic origin. Other possible fistulous connections are between the subclavian artery and the innominate vein, and between the internal mammary artery and the ductus venosus. Hemangiomas are also a source of possible fistulous connections.

Clinical Findings

Physical Examination

When an arteriovenous malformation causes symptoms in the neonate, they usually begin in the first few days of life. The child is tachypneic and tachycardic. Central cyanosis is present in 70 per cent of the patients.[36] Peripheral pulses may be bounding. The skin may show signs of coexistent cutaneous hemangiomas. A continuous murmur may be present over the site of the fistula. Head circumference may be enlarged in infants with cerebral arteriovenous fistulas. Cardiac examination reveals an active precordium. The heart is enlarged on palpation or percussion. Murmurs of increased aortic or pulmonary flow may be present, as may be a third heart sound or gallop. Abdominal examination frequently reveals hepatomegaly.

Chest Radiograph

The chest radiograph frequently shows evidence of cardiomegaly and increased pulmonary vascular markings (Fig. 35–1).

Electrocardiogram

The electrocardiogram shows evidence of right or biventricular hypertrophy (Fig. 35–2).

Echocardiogram

Two-dimensional echocardiography reveals dilation of both left and right ventricular chambers.[45] There may be evidence of tricuspid regurgitation by pulsed Doppler ultrasound examination. If there is right-to-left shunting at the foramen ovale, a microbubble contrast study will reveal rapid return to the superior vena cava in cases of cerebral fistulas.[45] An enlarged superior or inferior vena cava may be an indirect sign of an arteriovenous fistula; occasionally, the fistula may be visualized directly.[3,45] Color Doppler should greatly facilitate accurate diagnosis.

Computed Tomography

The site and size of the fistulous connection can be detected by computed tomography with contrast enhancement (Fig. 35–3).

Cardiac Catheterization

Cardiac catheterization reveals a step-up in oxygen saturation either in the superior vena cava for cerebral fistulas or in the hepatic region of the inferior vena cava for fistulas located in the liver or lower extremities. Pulmonary artery pressure is usually elevated, and there may be systemic desaturation secondary to a right-to-left shunt at the foramen ovale. Angiography near the arterial site of the fistula reveals the nature and extent of the fistula (Fig. 35–4).

Differential Diagnosis

The main differential diagnosis of a neonate with a continuous murmur and bounding pulses is patent ductus arteriosus. This diagnosis can be made by two-dimensional

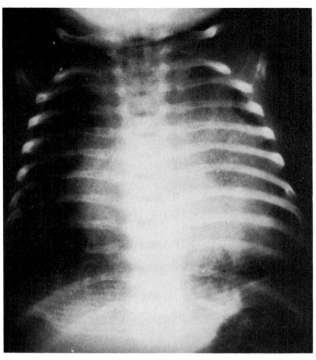

Figure 35–1. Chest radiograph of a newborn with a right subclavian artery–to–innominate vein arteriovenous malformation. Marked cardiomegaly is seen. This patient had no appreciable increase in pulmonary vascular markings.

and color Doppler echocardiography. Other causes of cardiomegaly, such as myocarditis, do not have the other features of an arteriovenous malformation such as a continuous murmur with bounding pulses.

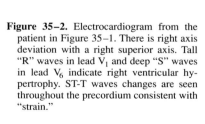

Figure 35–2. Electrocardiogram from the patient in Figure 35–1. There is right axis deviation with a right superior axis. Tall "R" waves in lead V_1 and deep "S" waves in lead V_6 indicate right ventricular hypertrophy. ST-T waves changes are seen throughout the precordium consistent with "strain."

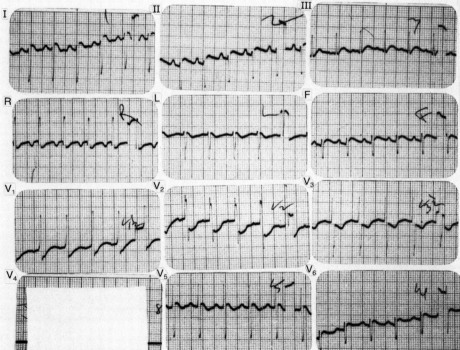

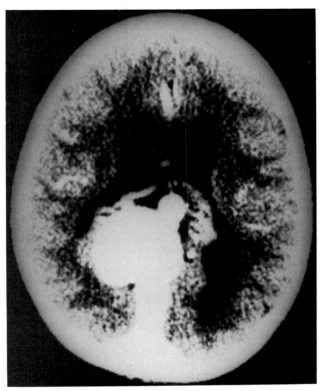

Figure 35–3. Contrast-enhanced cerebral CT scan of an infant with an arteriovenous malformation. The aneurysm of the vein of Galen is easily detected. (Photograph courtesy of Dr. Ortega, Department of Radiology, Children's Hospital of Philadelphia.)

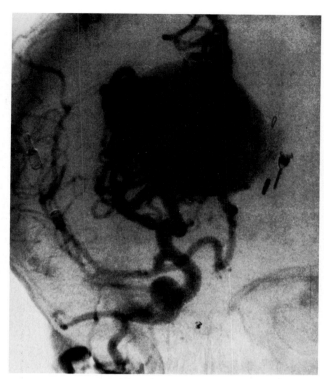

Figure 35–4. Postoperative cerebral angiogram of the child with an arteriovenous malformation involving the vein of Galen. The aneurysm seen in Figure 35–3 is again easily outlined. Surgical clips and a ventriculoperitoneal shunt are apparent. (Photograph courtesy of Dr. Ortega, Department of Radiology, Children's Hospital of Philadelphia.)

Medical Management

The medical management of arteriovenous malformations presenting in the newborn is the same as that in any volume overload cardiac lesion, namely digoxin and diuretics. These patients frequently succumb secondary to the severe cardiac failure or to the complications of the fistula, such as hemorrhage. Embolization of the feeding arteries has been attempted[14] with occasional success, as has radiotherapy[27] and corticosteroid therapy.[19,47]

COMPLETE ATRIOVENTRICULAR SEPTAL DEFECT

Complete atrioventricular septal defect (common atrioventricular canal) results from a deficiency of the endocardial cushion tissue in the developing heart. This abnormality leads to absence of the anterior portion of the atrial septum, absence of the inlet septum of the ventricles, and failure of fusion of the superior and inferior components of the anterior leaflets of the mitral valve. There is thus an unrestrictive atrial septal defect, an unrestrictive ventricular septal defect, and a common atrioventricular valve. This defect can be classified based on the morphology and attachments of the common atrioventricular valve leaflets.[33,34,37] Only when there is common atrioventricular valve regurgitation, as there is in 15 per cent of the pa-

tients with the complete form of atrioventricular septal defect, does this lesion present in the neonate.[8] If this situation does not occur, volume overload secondary to left-to-right shunting across the septal defects frequently does not occur until after the first month of life when pulmonary vascular resistance falls.

History

Complete atrioventricular septal defect has long been a recognized clinical entity. In 1909 Keith[23] reported the pathologic findings in 14 cases. Rogers and Edwards[39] in 1948 published a report of five cases and a review of the 50 cases previously reported in the literature. With recognition of the limited life expectancy in unoperated patients, surgical techniques for correction of complete atrioventricular septal defects were described as early as 1956.[9]

Epidemiology

The prevalence of complete atrioventricular septal defect has been reported as 1 per cent,[40] 1.3 per cent,[40] 2.8 per cent,[16] 5 per cent,[40] and 7 per cent[42] of patients with congenital heart disease. Familial cases of atrioventricular septal defect have been reported.[12]

Clinical Findings

Physical Examination

Infants with complete atrioventricular septal defect are frequently small and appear undernourished. They frequently fail to gain weight despite caloric intake in excess of 125 kcal/kg/day. The infant is tachypneic and tachycardic. Auscultation of the lungs may be normal. S_1 is normal, and S_2 is narrowly split. Accentuation of the pulmonic component of the second heart sound may be heard. A holosystolic murmur at the left lower sternal border or the apex is heard in cases with insufficiency of the common atrioventricular valve. After the immediate postnatal period, there is also an ejection type (crescendo-decrescendo) murmur at the left upper sternal border secondary to increased flow across the pulmonic valve. There is frequently a mid-diastolic murmur at the left lower sternal border and apex as a result of the increased flow across the common atrioventricular valve. Abdominal palpation almost invariably reveals hepatomegaly. The major exceptions to liver enlargement are patients with heterotaxia syndrome, in whom a midline liver may remain normal despite severe congestive heart failure. Femoral pulsations are usually normal. With severe failure the infant may have peripheral edema.

Chest Radiograph

The chest radiograph in complete atrioventricular septal defect frequently reveals marked cardiomegaly involving all the cardiac chambers. The main pulmonary artery is prominent; pulmonary vascularity is increased. Frequently, as is true with most cases of increased pulmonary blood flow, hyperinflation is present (Fig. 35–5).

Electrocardiogram

Over 95 per cent of patients with complete atrioventricular septal defect have a left axis deviation with a

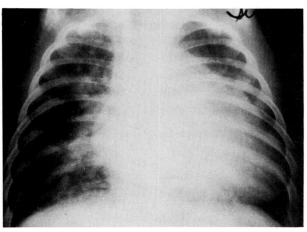

Figure 35–5. Chest radiograph of a neonate with complete atrioventricular septal defect. Marked cardiomegaly is apparent as well as increased pulmonary vascularity.

counterclockwise frontal plane loop. There is frequently evidence of right ventricular hypertrophy with tall R waves in leads V_4R and V_1 and deep S waves in lead V_6 (Fig. 35–6).

Echocardiogram

The echocardiogram is diagnostic in complete atrioventricular septal defect. The deficiency of the central core structures of the heart is readily apparent on subcostal, apical, and parasternal two-dimensional views (Fig. 35–7). Alignment of the common atrioventricular valve vis-à-vis the atria and the ventricles is important to assess preoperatively (Fig. 35–8). The morphology and attachment sites (Fig. 35–9) of the common atrioventricular valve leaflets, typically five in number, are easier to evaluate from the subcostal approach. Other anomalies, such as double-orifice mitral valve (Fig. 35–10), solitary left ventricular papillary muscle, and malalignment ventricular septal defects

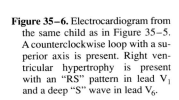

Figure 35–6. Electrocardiogram from the same child as in Figure 35–5. A counterclockwise loop with a superior axis is present. Right ventricular hypertrophy is present with an "RS" pattern in lead V_1 and a deep "S" wave in lead V_6.

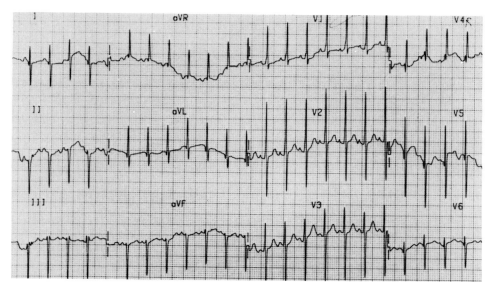

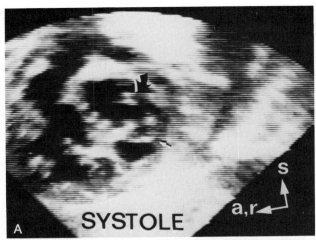

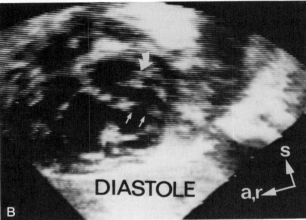

Figure 35–9. Atrioventricular (AV) valve in a child with an atrioventricular septal defect. *A*, Systole. Both papillary muscles are visible in the left ventricle (arrows). *B*, Diastole. The common AV valve can be seen to attach to only one of the two papillary muscles (small arrows). a = anterior; r = right; s = superior.

Figure 35–7. Subcostal four-chamber echocardiogram of a child with an atrioventricular (AV) septal defect. Both ventricles can be seen as well as the common AV valve. The defect in the inferior portion of the atrial septum is apparent. LA = left atrium; LV = left ventricle; RA = right atrium; RV = right ventricle; S = superior; L = left.

(in cases with coexisting tetralogy of Fallot) are frequently seen in patients with atrioventricular septal defect.[8,24,46,50] These lesions are easily detected by echocardiography. The atria may be dilated as a result of the common atrioventricular valve regurgitation. Pulsed Doppler echocardiographic interrogation can be used to detect turbulent systolic flow on the atrial side of the valve secondary to the regurgitation. The turbulent regurgitant flow can be mapped in the atrium by sampling at multiple sites, and the severity of the regurgitation can thus be graded. Color Doppler echocardiography can also be used to map the common atrioventricular valve regurgitation and to grade its severity.[38]

Cardiac Catheterization

In patients with complete atrioventricular septal defect there is a step-up in oxygen saturation in the right atrium secondary to left-to-right shunting at the level of the atrial septal defect. In patients with common atrioventricular valve regurgitation, the jet may be from left ventricle to right atrium, further contributing to the step-up in the right atrium. There is often a further step-up in the right ventricle. Saturation in the pulmonary veins is frequently reduced secondary to ventilation-perfusion mismatching often seen in patients with markedly increased pulmonary blood flow. Pressure tracings in the atria may reveal a large v wave in cases of severe common atrioventricular

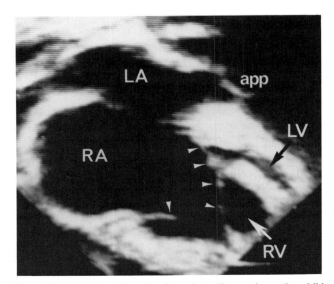

Figure 35–8. Subcostal four-chamber echocardiogram in another child with an atrioventricular (AV) septal defect. The atrioventricular valve is malaligned with respect to the ventricular septum. The right ventricle is larger than normal, and the left ventricle is hypoplastic secondary to this malalignment. The small white arrows point to the common AV valve. app = left atrial appendage; LA = left atrium; LV = left ventricle; RA = right atrium; RV = right ventricle.

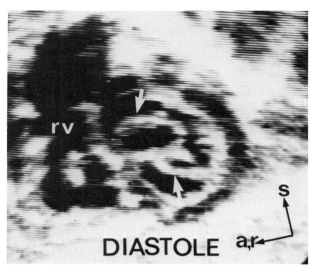

Figure 35–10. Atrioventricular (AV) valve in another child with an atrioventricular septal defect. A double orifice is visualized emptying into the left ventricular chamber (arrows). a = anterior; r = right; rv = right ventricle; s = superior.

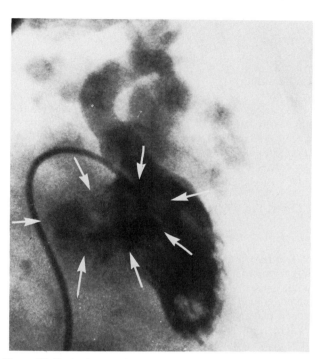

Figure 35–11. Angiogram of the neonate in Figures 35–5 and 35–6. The catheter was passed from the inferior vena cava through the right and left atria to the left ventricle. The patient was positioned in a hepatoclavicular projection. No additional muscular ventricular septal defects were appreciated. Arrows outline the common atrioventricular valve orifice.

valve insufficiency. Pressures are elevated in the right ventricle and pulmonary artery to systemic or near-systemic levels secondary to the unrestrictive ventricular septal defect. Macartney et al[28] reviewed the angiographic features of atrioventricular septal defect. They found that the discriminating features were (1) immediate right ventricular outflow tract opacification, (2) identification of the anterior attachment of the mitral component, (3) recognition of a single straddling atrioventricular orifice, and (4) passage of contrast medium above or below the anterior or posterior bridging leaflets. Angiography (Fig. 35–11) in the left ventricle should be performed in the hepatoclavicular projection to optimize detection of additional small muscular ventricular septal defects, which occur in 15 per cent of cases.[8,15,44]

Differential Diagnosis

The differential diagnosis of complete atrioventricular septal defect includes a large atrial septal defect or common atrium, a large ventricular septal defect, a single ventricle, or total anomalous pulmonary venous return. These lesions typically have a right axis on ECG with a clockwise frontal plane loop, whereas complete atrioventricular septal defect has a left axis with a counterclockwise frontal plane. Echocardiography can easily differentiate complete atrioventricular septal defect from these other lesions.

Medical Management

The medical management of complete atrioventricular septal defect is similar to that of any volume overload lesion. Myocardial contractility is enhanced through the use of digoxin, and preload can be adjusted with diuretics.

Caloric intake needs to be maintained at a higher than normal level because these patients frequently have a high metabolic state secondary to their intracardiac shunt and pulmonary edema. Because of severe tachypnea, however, caloric intake may be difficult to maintain. Frequently, one has to resort to nasogastric feedings to achieve adequate caloric intake. Reparative surgery is performed at 6 months of age or earlier in those infants who fail to thrive despite adequate digoxin and diuretics.

AORTICO–LEFT VENTRICULAR TUNNEL

Aortico–left ventricular tunnel is a rare disorder in which there is an anomalous communication between the ascending aorta and the outflow portion of the left ventricle that bypasses the aortic valve. Unlike a ruptured sinus of Valsalva aneurysm, the origin of aortico–left ventricular tunnel is distal to the aortic sinuses.

History

Aortico–left ventricular tunnel was first reported by Edwards in 1961.[13] He believed this lesion to be acquired rather than congenital. In 1963, Levy et al[25] added three more cases to the literature. They defined the clinical profile and suggested the congenital nature of this lesion.

Since that time approximately 48 cases have been described.

Epidemiology

The exact incidence of aortico–left ventricular tunnel is unknown. Two out of 1754 cases of congenital heart disease reviewed by Okoroma et al[31] had an aortico–left ventricular tunnel. Males outnumber females with this lesion by three to one.[26]

Clinical Findings

Physical Examination

The physical examination of patients with an aortico–left ventricular tunnel is typical. The majority of the patients present in the first month of life with evidence of severe congestive heart failure. Examination reveals tachypnea and tachycardia. A widened pulse pressure is invariably detected. Cyanosis is present in less than 5 per cent of the patients.[26] Palpation of the precordium reveals an increased ventricular impulse.[4,11] A to-and-fro murmur is present over the precordium. The diastolic component is usually louder than the systolic component; a diastolic thrill may be palpated.

Chest Radiograph

The chest radiograph in aortico–left ventricular tunnel reveals marked cardiomegaly with a dilated ascending aorta.[4,11,17,26] An indentation in the anterior esophagus from severe left ventricular enlargement has been described.[5,31]

Electrocardiogram

The electrocardiogram reveals severe left ventricular hypertrophy (85 per cent of cases) and left ventricular strain and/or left axis deviation (30 per cent of cases).[26] Biventricular hypertrophy may be present,[11] but rarely the ECG may be normal.[17]

Echocardiogram

Perry et al[32] first retrospectively described the echocardiographic appearance of an aortico–left ventricular tunnel in 1983; subsequently, prospective echocardiographic recognition has been described.[4,11,17,22] The left ventricle is typically dilated. Ventricular septal dropout is detected immediately below the aortic valve as well as in the aortic root just distal to the right coronary artery. With careful imaging, the tunnel connecting these dropouts can be visualized. Pulsed Doppler examination of the ascending aorta reveals retrograde diastolic flow consistent with aortic run-off. When the sample volume is placed in the suspected tunnel, turbulent diastolic flow toward the left ventricle is detected; systolic flow is toward the ascending aorta. This Doppler pattern confirms the diagnosis of an aortico–left ventricular tunnel. Recently, color Doppler echocardiographic imaging of an aortico–left ventricular tunnel has been described; the diagnosis was verified by magnetic resonance imaging.[22]

Cardiac Catheterization

Cardiac catheterization in aortico–left ventricular tunnel frequently reveals normal right-sided hemodynamics. Occasionally, there is a gradient across the right ventricular outflow tract caused by "bulging of the posterolateral wall of the right ventricular infundibulum by the tunnel as it passed through the septum."[26] Left-sided hemodynamics reveal a markedly widened aortic pulse pressure. Angiography may reveal a round double density anterior and superior to the aortic sinuses, with immediate reflux of contrast material from the aorta to the left ventricle.[25] Occasionally, the tip of the catheter may enter the tunnel and allow clearer visualization of the tunnel itself.[26]

Differential Diagnosis

Other causes of a to-and-fro murmur, such as tetralogy of Fallot with absent pulmonary valve, ruptured sinus of Valsalva aneurysm, coronary arteriocameral fistula, and coronary arteriovenous fistula, rarely present with severe congestive heart failure in the neonatal period.[26] Two-dimensional echocardiography can readily differentiate these lesions.

Medical Management

There has been no successful survivor of long-term medical management of aortico–left ventricular tunnel.[26] Since as many as two thirds of the survivors of surgery eventually develop pronounced aortic regurgitation,[41] surgery should be done as early as possible to minimize dilation of the ascending aorta and aortic annulus.

COMBINED PRESSURE-VOLUME OVERLOAD

The magnitude of left-to-right shunting from even a large (non-restrictive) ventricular septal defect is usually small in the first few weeks of life because of high pulmonary vascular resistance in the neonate. Only when a pressure-overload lesion such as coarctation coexists does the left-to-right shunt become hemodynamically significant in the first few days.

Any conotruncal anomaly can be associated with coarctation; relatively common examples include transposition with single ventricle and the Taussig-Bing form of double-outlet right ventricle. The reader is referred to more extensive reviews[1,10,48,49] for detailed description of these lesions. In this chapter, we will discuss coarctation with ventricular septal defect in the setting of normally aligned great arteries.

History

In 1950 Calodney and Carson[6] reported their autopsy findings in 22 cases of coarctation of the aorta presenting in infancy. In 19 of the 22 cases, the cause of death was congestive heart failure. Nine of the 22 cases had a ventricular septal defect, and 6 of the 22 had a bicuspid aortic valve. They advised digoxin, diuretics, and oxygen therapy for the infant with congestive heart failure secondary to coarctation of the aorta with or without associated lesions. Once the infant was medically stabilized, they recommended surgical relief of the coarctation.

Epidemiology

Of the patients with coarctation of the aorta who present with congestive heart failure during the neonatal period, 80 to 85 per cent have another lesion complicating their coarctation,[20] the most common of which is a bicuspid aortic valve. The second most common is ventricular septal defect, which occurs in 30 to 35 per cent of all patients with coarctation.[18]

Clinical Findings

Physical Examination

Patients with a ventricular septal defect complicating coarctation of the aorta have tachypnea and tachycardia. If the ductus is restrictive or closed, blood pressure is decreased in the lower extremity, and femoral pulses are weak to absent. Examination of the lungs may reveal rales. A nonspecific systolic murmur may be heard along the precordium as well as in the back along the left scapula. A holosystolic murmur may be detected at the left lower

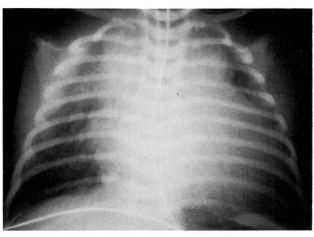

Figure 35–12. Chest radiograph from a neonate with coarctation of the aorta and multiple ventricular septal defects. Cardiomegaly with some increase in pulmonary vascularity is apparent.

sternal border in cases with a restrictive ventricular septal defect. Abdominal examination reveals hepatomegaly.

Chest Radiograph

The chest radiograph frequently shows cardiomegaly with increased pulmonary vascular markings (Fig. 35–12). A "3" sign may be seen at the area of the coarctation.

Electrocardiogram

The electrocardiogram of patients with coarctation of the aorta reveals right ventricular hypertrophy whether or nor a ventricular septal defect is present (Fig. 35–13). Right ventricular strain may be present in ductus-dependent cases.

Figure 35–13. Electrocardiogram from the same child as in Figure 35–12. An "rSR'" pattern is seen in lead V_1, with a deep "S" wave in lead V_6 diagnostic of severe right ventricular hypertrophy. The axis is indeterminate.

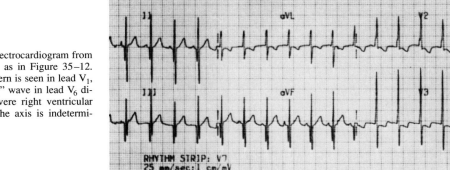

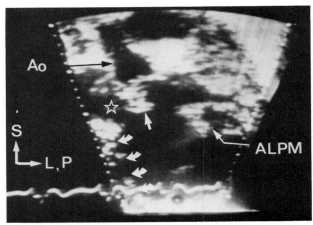

Figure 35–14. Subcostal echocardiogram of a malalignment ventricular septal defect (star). The arrows point to the two parts of the ventricular septum. The left ventricular outflow tract is significantly narrowed by the posterior malalignment of the infundibular septum. Ao = aorta; ALPM = anterolateral papillary muscle; L = left; P = posterior; S = superior.

Echocardiogram

Two-dimensional echocardiography reveals the size and anatomic type of ventricular septal defect. Subcostal sweeps are also useful in characterizing the severity of infundibular septal malalignment (Fig. 35–14) in cases of coarctation with a "malalignment-type" ventricular septal defect.[2] Marked infundibular septal deviation causes important subaortic stenosis, which frequently requires early surgical palliation with a "Norwood-type" procedure.[30] Suprasternal imaging of the aortic arch reveals the co-

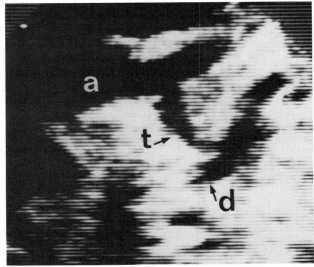

Figure 35–15. Suprasternal echocardiogram of coarctation of the aorta. While the most common location of the coarctation is distal to the left subclavian artery in the juxtaductal region, this coarctation is proximal to the left subclavian artery. Recognition of this variant is important preoperatively, as it requires a reverse subclavian flap to repair the coarctation. a = ascending aorta; d = descending aorta; t = transverse arch.

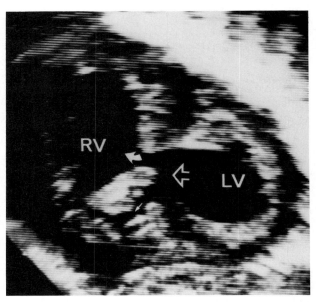

Figure 35–16. Echocardiogram of a muscular septal defect in a child who also had coarctation of the aorta. There appears to be a single defect on the left ventricular side (hollow arrow). Multiple defects (solid arrows) are seen from the right ventricular side, however. LV = left ventricle; RV = right ventricle.

arctation and allows differentiation of this anomaly from interruption of the aortic arch.[21] It is important to determine whether the narrowest portion of the arch is distal to the left subclavian artery, as is typically the case, or between the left common carotid artery and the left subclavian artery origins (Fig. 35–15); approximately 75 per cent of patients with large muscular ventricular septal defects (Fig. 35–16) have some degree of aortic arch hypoplasia at autopsy.[29] Pulsed Doppler evaluation reveals continuous laminar flow immediately proximal to the narrowing (Fig. 35–17). Continuous turbulent flow is seen im-

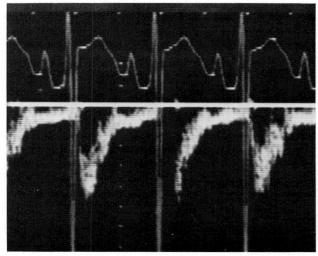

Figure 35–17. Laminar flow in the distal aortic arch proximal to a coarctation of the aorta. Note that the flow is continuous in the upper descending aorta proximal to a coarctation.

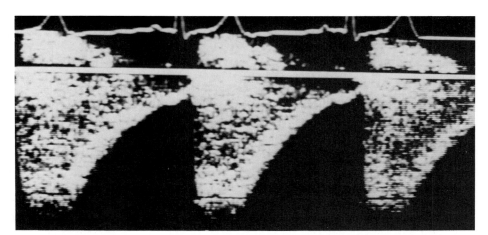

Figure 35–18. Turbulent flow distal to the narrowing in a patient with coarctation of the aorta without a patent ductus arteriosus.

mediately distal to the narrowing in cases without a patent ductus and in cases with a left-to-right systolic ductal flow (Fig. 35–18). Systolic ductal flow can also be right to left (Fig. 35–19); in such cases, if the systolic flow in the upper descending aorta is laminar (Fig. 35–20), the ductus is nonrestrictive.[7] In cases without a patent ductus, continuous wave Doppler echocardiography accurately measures peak instantaneous gradient across the coarctation.[51]

Cardiac Catheterization

If coarctation repair alone is contemplated, as in cases with a small ventricular septal defect, catheterization is unnecessary. When repair of both lesions is preferable, as in the case of a large ventricular septal defect, left ventricular angiography is helpful in detecting additional small

muscular ventricular septal defects.[15] Data obtained from oximetry in patients with a ventricular septal defect and coarctation often reveal a step-up in oxygen saturation from the superior vena cava to the right atrium (from left-to-right shunting across the foramen ovale). Additional step-ups in the right ventricle and pulmonary artery are secondary to left-to-right flow across the ventricular septal defect. Subaortic obstruction is difficult to diagnose by pressure measurements, since flow across this area is typically low before the coarctation is repaired and the

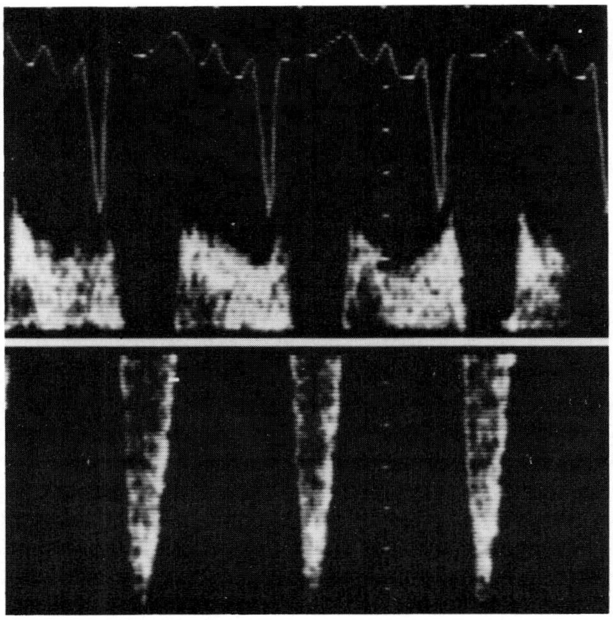

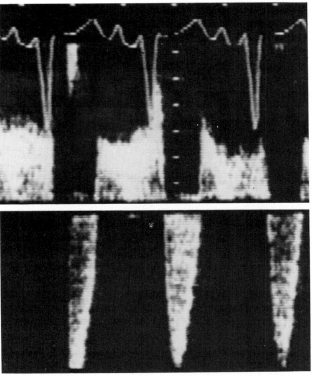

Figure 35–20. Laminar flow in the descending aorta distal to the narrowing in a neonate with coarctation of the aorta and an unrestrictive ductus arteriosus.

Figure 35–19. Laminar right-to-left systolic ductal flow in a neonate with a ductal dependent coarctation of the aorta.

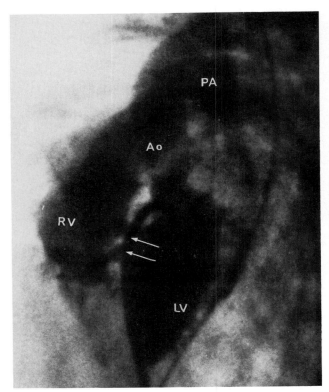

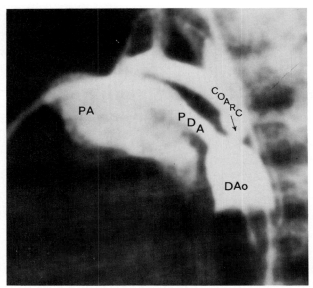

Figure 35–23. Antegrade aortogram in a child with coarctation of the aorta. The balloon catheter is passed from the inferior vena cava through the right atrium, right ventricle, pulmonary artery, and ductus arteriosus into the descending aorta. The side holes on the catheter are proximal to the balloon. The balloon is then inflated, occluding the descending aorta and forcing injected contrast to move retrogradely as the injection is made. COARC = coarctation; DAo = descending aorta; PA = pulmonary artery; PDA = patent ductus arteriosus.

Figure 35–21. Left ventricular angiogram of the patient in Figures 35–12 and 35–13. A long axial oblique projection is used to profile the majority of the ventricular septum. Multiple muscular ventricular septal defects (arrows) are visualized with opacification of the right ventricle and pulmonary artery on the left ventriculogram. The membranous septum is intact. Ao = ascending aorta; LV = left ventricle; PA = pulmonary artery; RV = right ventricle.

ventricular septal defect closed. Angiography (Fig. 35–21) should be performed in the long axial oblique projection to profile optimally the ventricular septum and the subaortic region.[15] An aortic injection should be performed in a 30-degree left anterior oblique and a 60-degree right anterior oblique projection to visualize the coarctation if it is not seen on the ventriculogram. This injection can be made either retrograde (Fig. 35–22) through the aorta or antegrade using a balloon catheter passed through the ductus arteriosus (Fig. 35–23).

Differential Diagnosis

The differential diagnosis of the neonate with a normal or increased right brachial pulse and decreased femoral pulses is not difficult. The challenge is to distinguish aortic coarctation from interruption of the aortic arch; this differentiation is easily made with two-dimensional echocardiography. When both the right brachial and the femoral pulses are weak, as occurs both in cases of coarctation and of interruption when an aberrant right subclavian artery is present, the clinical diagnosis is more complicated. Occasionally, infants with coarctation (with a normal right subclavian artery origin) may present in shock with markedly impaired left ventricular performance and weak pulses in all extremities. Myocarditis or anomalous left coronary artery (arising from the pulmonary artery) must be considered in these cases. Echocardiography, by demonstrating the aortic arch anatomy, can distinguish between coarc-

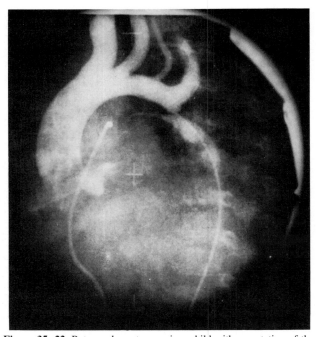

Figure 35–22. Retrograde aortogram in a child with coarctation of the aorta.

tation and these other causes of impaired left ventricular performance.

Medical Management

If the ductus is restrictive and the patient is ductal dependent, prostaglandin E_1 should be administered immediately. Such patients require surgical intervention in the neonatal period. If the patient is not ductal dependent, an inotropic agent such as digoxin may be necessary if left ventricular performance is diminished. With modern surgical techniques for repair of coarctation, there is no indication for continued medical management of infants with the combination of coarctation and ventricular septal defect. If the ventricular septal defect is large (nonrestrictive) and is of an anatomic type that never closes spontaneously, it should be surgically closed at the same time the coarctation is repaired. A malalignment-type ventricular septal defect associated with an infundibular septum that is deviated posteriorly or leftwardly from its normal position between the limbs of the septal band (septomarginal trabecula) is an example of a defect that never undergoes spontaneous closure. If the ventricular septal defect is restrictive, it need not be closed at the time the coarctation is repaired. Such ventricular septal defects may either close spontaneously or become hemodynamically insignificant after coarctation repair.

References

1. Anderson RH, Becker AE, Wilcox BR, Macartney FJ, Wilkinson JL (1983): Surgical anatomy of double-outlet right ventricle—a reappraisal. Am J Cardiol 52:555–559.
2. Anderson RH, Lenox CC, Zuberbuhler JR (1983): Morphology of ventricular septal defect associated with coarctation of aorta. Br Heart J 50:176–181.
3. Bhat AM, Meny RG, Ormond RS (1984): Sonography in cranial arteriovenous malformation presenting with cardiac failure. Clin Pediatr 23:248.
4. Bjork VO, Hongo T, Aberg B, Bjarke B (1983): Surgical repair of aortico-left ventricular tunnel in a 7 day old child. Scand J Thorac Cardiovasc Surg 17:185–189.
5. Bove KB, Schwartz DC (1967): Aortico-left ventricular tunnel. A new concept. Am J Cardiol 19:691–696.
6. Calodney MM, Carson MJ (1950): Coarctation of the aorta in early infancy. J Pediatr 37:46–77.
7. Chin AJ, Helton JG, Barber G, Aglira BA, Alston A, Sands B (1986): Pulsed Doppler characterization of neonatal coarctation with or without ductus arteriosus (abstr). Am Heart J 112:649.
8. Chin AJ, Keane JF, Norwood WI, Castaneda AR (1982): Repair of complete common atrioventricular canal in infancy. J Thorac Cardiovasc Surg 84:437–445.
9. Cooley JC, Kirklin JW (1956): The surgical treatment of persistent common atrioventricular canal: Report of 12 cases. Proc Staff Meetings Mayo Clin 31:523–527.
10. Corno A, Becker AE, Bulterijs AH, Lam J, Nijveld A, Schuller JL, Marcelletti C (1982): Univentricular heart: Can we alter the natural history? Ann Thorac Surg 34:716–727.
11. Diamant S, Luber JM, Gootman N (1985): Successful repair of aortico-left ventricular tunnel associated with severe aortic stenosis in a newborn. Pediatr Cardiol 6:171–173.
12. Disegni E, Pierpont ME, Bass JL, Kaplinsky E (1985): Two-dimensional echocardiography in detection of endocardial cushion defect in families. Am J Cardiol 55:1649–1652.
13. Edwards JE (1961): Atlas of Acquired Diseases of the Heart and Great Vessels. Vol 3. Philadelphia, WB Saunders, p 1142.
14. Fabiani JN, Mercier JN, Ribierre M (1979): Traitement pour embolization d'une fistule arterioveineuse vertebrale congenitale. Arch Fr Pediatr 36:34.
15. Fellows KE, Westerman GR, Keane JF (1982): Angiocardiography of multiple ventricular septal defects in infancy. Circulation 66:1094–1099.
16. Fontana RS, Edwards JE (1962): Congenital Cardiac Disease: A Review of 357 Cases Studied Pathologically. Philadelphia, WB Saunders, pp 109–110.
17. Fripp RR, Werner JC, Whitman V, Nordenberg A, Waldhausen JA (1984): Pulsed Doppler and two-dimensional echocardiographic findings in aortico-left ventricular tunnel. J Am Coll Cardiol 4:1012–1014.
18. Gersony WM (1983): Coarctation of the aorta. In Adams FH, Emmanouilides GC (eds): Heart Diseases in Infants, Children and Adolescents. 3rd ed. Baltimore, Williams & Wilkins, pp 188–199.
19. Goldberg SJ, Fonkalsrud E (1969): Successful treatment of hepatic hemangioma with corticosteriods. JAMA 208:2473.
20. Hesslein PS, Gutgesell HP, McNamara DG (1983): Prognosis of symptomatic coarctation of the aorta in infancy. Am J Cardiol 51:299–303.
21. Huhta JC, Gutgesell HP, Latson LA, Huffines FD (1984): Two-dimensional echocardiographic assessment of the aorta in infants and children with congenital heart disease. Circulation 70:417–424.
22. Humes RA, Hagler DJ, Julsrud PR, Levy JM, Feldt RH, Schaff HV (1986): Aortico-left ventricular tunnel: Diagnosis based on two-dimensional echocardiographic, color flow Doppler imaging, and magnetic resonance imaging. Mayo Clin Proc 61:901–907.
23. Keith A (1909): Malformations of the Heart. Lancet 2:433.
24. Lee CN, Danielson GK, Schaff HV, Puga FJ, Mair DD (1985): Surgical treatment of double-orifice mitral valve in atrioventricular canal defects. Experience in 25 patients. J Thorac Cardiovasc Surg 90:700–705.
25. Levy MJ, Lillehei CW, Anderson RH, Amplatz K, Edwards JE (1963): Aortico-left ventricular tunnel. Circulation 27:841–853.
26. Levy MJ, Schachner A, Blieden LC (1982): Aortico-left ventricular tunnel collective review. J Thorac Cardiovasc Surg 84:102–109.
27. Lucet PH (1973): Fistules arterio-veineuses systemiques. In Gerard R, Louchet E (eds): Precis de Cardiologie de l'Enfant. Paris, Masson et Cie, p 428.
28. Macartney FJ, Rees PG, Daly K, Piccoli GP, Taylor JF, de Leval MR, Stark J, Anderson RH (1979): Angiocardiographic appearances of atrioventricular defects with particular reference to distinction of ostium primum atrial septal defect from common atrioventricular orifice. Br Heart J 42:640–656.
29. Moene RJ, Oppenheimer-Dekker A, Wenink AC (1981): Relation between aortic arch hypoplasia of variable severity and central muscular ventricular septal defects: Emphasis on associated left ventricular abnormalities. Am J Cardiol 48:111–116.
30. Norwood WI, Lang P, Hansen DD (1983): Physiologic repair of aortic atresia-hypoplastic left heart syndrome. N Engl J Med 308:23–26.
31. Okoroma EO, Perry LW, Scott LP, McClenathan EM (1976): Aortico-left ventricular tunnel. J Thorac Cardiovasc Surg 71:238–244.
32. Perry JC, Nanda NC, Hicks D, Harris JP (1983): Two-dimensional echocardiographic identification of aortico-left ventricular tunnel. Am J Cardiol 52:913–914.
33. Piccoli GP, Gerlis LM, Wilkinson JL, Lozsadi K, Macartney FJ, Anderson RH (1979): Morphology and classification of atrioventricular defects. Br Heart J 42:621–632.
34. Piccoli GP, Wilkinson JL, Macartney FJ, Gerlis LM, Anderson RH (1979): Morphology and classification of complete atrioventricular defects. Br Heart J 42:633–639.
35. Pollock AQ, Laslett PA (1958): Cerebral arteriovenous fistula producing cardiac failure in the newborn infant. J Pediatr 53:731–736.
36. Quero Jimenez M, Acerete Guillen G (1983): Arteriovenous fistulas. In Adams FH, Emmanouilides GC (eds): Heart Diseases in Infants, Children and Adolescents. 3rd ed. Baltimore, Williams & Wilkins, pp 491–500.
37. Rastelli GC, Kirklin JW, Titus JL (1966): Anatomic observations on complete forms of persistent common atrioventricular canal

with special reference to atrioventricular valves. Mayo Clin Proc 41:296.

38. Reeder GS, Currie PJ, Hagler DJ, Tajik AJ, Seward JB (1986): Use of Doppler techniques (continuous-wave, pulsed-wave, and color flow imaging) in the noninvasive hemodynamic assessment of congenital heart disease. Mayo Clin Proc 61:725–744.

39. Rogers HM, Edwards JE (1948): Incomplete division of the atrioventricular canal with patent interatrial foramen primum (persistent common atrioventricular ostium): Report of 5 cases and review of literature. Am Heart J 36:28.

40. Rowe RW, Freedom RM, Mehrizi A, Bloom KR (eds) (1981): The Neonate with Congenital Heart Disease. Philadelphia, WB Saunders, pp 373–396.

41. Serino W, Andrade JL, Ross D, de Leval M, Somerville J (1983): Aortico-left ventricular communication after closure: Late postoperative problems. Br Heart J 49:501–506.

42. Sherman FE (1963): An Atlas of Congenital Heart Disease. Philadelphia, Lea & Febiger, pp 123–131.

43. Silverman BK, Breckx T, Craig J, Nadas AS (1955): Congestive failure in the newborn caused by cerebral A-V fistula. Am J Dis Child 89:539–543.

44. Soto B, Bargeron LM, Pacifico AD, Vanini V, Kirklin JW (1981): Angiography of atrioventricular canal defects. Am J Cardiol 48:492–499.

45. Stanbridge RDL, Westaby S, Smallhorn J, Taylor JFN (1983): Intracranial arteriovenous malformation with aneurysm of the vein of Galen as cause of heart failure in infancy: Echocardiographic diagnosis and results of treatment. Br Heart J 49:157–162.

46. Studer M, Blackstone EH, Kirklin JW, Pacifico AD, Soto B, Chung GK, Kirklin JK, Bargeron LM (1982): Determinants of early and late results of repair of atrioventricular septal (canal) defects. J Thorac Cardiovasc Surg 84:523–542.

47. Toulokian RJ (1970): Hepatic hemangioendothelioma during infancy: Pathology, diagnosis and treatment with prednisone. Pediatrics 45:71.

48. Van Praagh R, Plett JA, Van Praagh S (1979): Single ventricle. Pathology, embryology, terminology and classification. Herz. 4:113–150.

49. Van Praagh S, Davidoff A, Chin AJ, Shiel F, Reynolds J, Van Praagh R (1982): Double outlet right ventricle: Anatomic types and developmental implications based on a study of 101 autopsied cases. Coeur 13 (numero special):389–440.

50. Warnes C, Somerville J (1983): Double mitral valve orifice in atrioventricular defects. Br Heart J 49:59–64.

51. Wyse RK, Robinson PJ, Deanfield JE, Tunstall PDS, Macartney FJ (1984): Use of continuous wave Doppler ultrasound velocimetry to assess the severity of coarctation of the aorta by measurement of aortic flow velocities. Br Heart J 52:278–283.

36 AORTIC VALVE OBSTRUCTION

Ernest A. Kiel

INTRODUCTION

Perhaps the most striking clinical presentation in pediatric cardiology is that of a newborn infant with sudden onset of shock and poor cardiac output. In 1814, J. R. Farre described such a presentation of a newborn with aortic atresia.[19]

During the first forty-eight hours, he seemed to enjoy the most perfect health: his countenance was lively and ruddy, his skin warm, the meconium and urine were properly evacuated, he took the breast eagerly, and slept easily.... He slept quietly the greater part of the night, but at an early hour the following morning, I was called to him. His cries expressed the distress he then suffered. The diaphragm labored excessively, and the whole line of its attachment was marked by its vehement action; the heart thumped against the ribs, the pulse at the wrist could not be felt, the skin was pallid and cold.... The labor of the diaphragm ceased, his respiration became more and more feeble, his sensorium during the last few hours was torpid, but he died without convulsion. His death happened seventy-nine hours after birth, and about thirty hours after the respiration was affected.

This description of a neonate with severe left heart outflow obstruction could easily apply to the common clinical picture seen today. In addition to newborns with severe cyanosis, newborns with shock from severe left heart outflow obstruction are among the most distressing to physicians and parents, particularly because most are initially thought to be healthy.

Lambert et al[43] reviewed the clinical presentation and autopsy data of 165 infants dying from cardiac disease in the first month of life. Over one half of these infants died in the first week of life, indicating that severe congenital cardiac lesions need to be detected and managed very early if survival is to be expected. The most common cardiac defect causing death at this age was hypoplastic left-heart syndrome, comprising 22 per cent of the deaths. Complete transposition of the great arteries and complex congenital cardiac anomalies were the two next most common cardiac causes of neonatal death. From this information, one can easily realize that severe obstruction to systemic blood flow plays a major role in neonatal morbidity and mortality.

Outflow obstruction of the left heart can occur at one or several levels. Aortic stenosis can be subvalvular (either discrete subvalvular obstruction or idiopathic hypertrophic cardiomyopathy), valvular, or supravalvular. Obstruction to systemic flow can occur distally in the form of coarctation of the aorta or complete interruption of the aortic arch. A combination of obstruction at several levels may be present as hypoplasia of the aortic arch complex. The most severe form of outlet obstruction is represented by

aortic valve atresia with hypoplasia of the aortic arch and left ventricle. The following discussion will be limited to obstructive lesions of the aortic valve, including severe valvular stenosis and aortic atresia, and their clinical presentation in the newborn and infant.

When considering the clinical presentation of severe left ventricular outflow obstruction in the newborn, one must take into account the important relationship of intrauterine cardiac physiology and perinatal hemodynamic changes. Theoretical changes in cardiac flow patterns in utero may contribute to formation of these lesions and may be important considerations in management of the infant after birth. Normal intrauterine anatomic shunts across the ductus arteriosus and foramen ovale should be remembered as well as abnormal, alternative flow patterns that may develop in response to the defects.[7]

Normally, the ascending aorta receives approximately 50 per cent of the combined ventricular output of the fetal heart.[35] One half of this flow is delivered to the coronary and brachiocephalic circulation, while 25 per cent of combined output traverses the aortic isthmus. Aortic isthmus flow is combined with the 40 to 45 per cent of combined ventricular output that crosses the ductus arteriosus to supply the descending aorta. Thus, approximately two thirds of combined ventricular output will enter the descending aorta, while only one fourth crosses the transverse aorta.

Cardiac lesions that present significant or complete barriers to fetal left heart blood flow must rely entirely or in part on maintenance of circulation through the right ventricle and pulmonary artery. Therefore, in the presence of severe aortic valve obstruction, the 25 per cent of combined fetal ventricular output supplying the aortic isthmus and brachiocephalic and coronary artery flow must be delivered retrogradely from flow across the ductus arteriosus.[35] While this volume of flow is sufficient to supply needs to the upper circulation during fetal life, the diminished volume of ascending aortic and left ventricular flow may importantly affect development of normal aortic size and result in aortic and ventricular hypoplasia and possible coarctation.[68] Once one understands these concepts, the necessity of maintaining ductal patency postnatally to provide ongoing systemic cardiac output and perfusion becomes obvious. In addition, the abruptness of cardiac decompensation that occurs postnatally with ductal constriction becomes clear.

When barriers to inflow and outflow of the left ventricle are present, the usual alternative pathway of blood flow is the foramen ovale. Normally, the foramen ovale allows uninhibited flow of blood from the right atrium to the left atrium. If significant obstruction to fetal left heart flow is present, left atrial pressure may rise abnormally, leading to herniation of foramenal tissue into the right atrium. Left-to-right foramenal flow can subsequently develop and allow a volume and pressure release for the left atrium.[7] Other uncommon alternative routes that decompress the left atrium and bypass the left heart postnatally are also seen.[7,57] These include anomalous pulmonary venous drainage to systemic veins and anomalous drainage to the coronary sinus, either directly or via left ventricular myocardial sinusoids. Premature closure of the foramen ovale has been implicated in formation of hypoplasia of the left heart.[51]

Disturbances in left heart flow patterns and hemodynamics may also have an important role in the development of endocardial fibroelastosis (EFE). EFE is commonly associated with aortic atresia and severe aortic stenosis, particularly in the presence of a small left ventricular chamber. Anderson and Kelly[3] reviewed the findings of EFE in association with congenital cardiac anomalies and commented on its frequent occurrence in aortic stenosis and atresia. They hypothesized that a combination of high intrauterine blood pressures and myocardial ischemia or anoxia contributed to the development of EFE in various congenital cardiac defects. The exact causes of EFE remain unclear. The degree of EFE and the severity of left ventricular pathology may vary, depending upon the severity of fetal aortic obstruction as well as the time of onset in utero. Clinically, the severity of in utero left ventricular hypoplasia and fibroelastosis correlates with morbidity and mortality after birth. Mocellin et al[49] have related neonatal death in severe aortic stenosis with left ventricular hypoplasia and the presence of EFE. Indeed, newborns with aortic stenosis who exhibit left ventricular hypoplasia and EFE respond poorly to medical and surgical intervention.

VALVULAR AORTIC STENOSIS IN THE NEWBORN INFANT

Historical Perspective

As early as 1761, Giovanni Battista Morgagni described the findings of aortic stenosis in the human. Alexander[2] translated his early description of a young man who "happening to take a long journey from Trent to Padua; which he performed, partly on foot and partly on horseback, within the space of two days; immediately after coming off his journey, and while he was stooping to his portmanteau, which was laid on the ground, he fell down dead." Morgagni observed that "the semilunar valves...were not bony, indeed, but hard, and what immediately occurred to the eyes, very small; for they were contracted and corrugated."

Helen Taussig in her classic text in 1947[74] described anomalies of the aortic valve in infants, children, and adults. She attempted to differentiate congenital aortic stenosis from acquired diseases but indicated that the etiology often remained obscure. Edwards[16] and later Roberts[63] described the pathology of valvular aortic stenosis. Although various degrees of stenosis and numbers of valve leaflets are seen, bicuspid and tricuspid stenotic valves predominate in children and adults. Subsequently, in the 1960s and early 1970s, several reports of aortic valvular stenosis in infancy were published.[9,20,33,37,42,50,52,59] Often, the valve is described as unicuspid or very thick and nodular with distortion of the cusp margins, leaflets, and valve ring. Well-formed but thickened valve leaflets with small annular size are occasionally described. The surgical approaches to critical aortic stenosis are described in Chapter 62.

Epidemiology

Aortic valvular stenosis accounts for 3 to 6 per cent of congenital cardiovascular malformations.[27,36] However, symptomatic aortic stenosis in the neonate or infant is relatively uncommon, accounting for only 10 per cent or less of aortic stenosis as a whole.[33] Of infants presenting with significant congenital cardiac defects in the newborn period, aortic stenosis makes up 1 to 3 per cent of all cardiac lesions.[43,66] Aortic stenosis occurs more often in males than in females, with a sex ratio as high as four to one. In neonates this male predominance persists but to a lesser degree, with occasional female predominance.[52]

Although aortic stenosis in infancy usually occurs as an isolated lesion, it frequently is associated with coexisting cardiovascular anomalies such as ventricular septal defect, patent ductus arteriosus, coarctation of the aorta and mitral valve anomalies.[33,42] The common occurrence of coexisting endocardial fibroelastosis has been well described.[9,20,33,37,42,49,50,52,59] Associated genetic syndromes rarely are present, although aortic stenosis is seen in conjunction with Turner (XO) syndrome.[10] The recurrence risk appears to be higher in offspring of patients than in siblings.[54]

Experimental Pathology

Experimental models of left ventricular outflow obstruction[21] and aortic stenosis[47] have been created in laboratory settings. These studies have been helpful in understanding hemodynamic and pathologic changes, which probably develop in utero. In experimental models of aortic outflow obstruction in lambs, significant reductions in left ventricular output, thickening of left ventricular free walls, and reductions in chamber volume are seen; the latter reductions in chamber volume are similar to those seen clinically in severe aortic stenosis. Morphometric studies of lung preparations in experimental aortic stenosis reveal findings similar to those detected in lungs of infants dying of severe aortic stenosis, including an increased number of resistance vessels and muscularization. Additional studies in such models may yield answers to questions on the etiology and pathogenesis of these lesions.

Clinical Profile

The presence of aortic valve stenosis in the infant, older child, and adult often produces no clinical symptoms

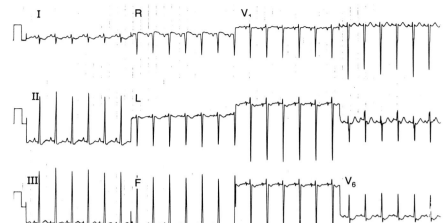

Figure 36–1. Twelve-lead electrocardiogram revealing left ventricular hypertrophy and ST segment changes of "strain" in a 2-month-old with severe aortic stenosis.

whatsoever. Absence of clinical symptoms in the newborn with severe aortic stenosis is infrequent. In contrast to the older child, the newborn often presents with early, rapidly progressing symptomatology and a more malignant clinical profile. In fact, the newborn with critical aortic stenosis can be considered to represent a different disease spectrum than the aortic stenosis found in the older infant or child.

Age at Presentation

The newborn infant with valvular aortic stenosis generally appears healthy at birth and is normal in size and weight. Although the initial signs and symptoms of the defect may be seen shortly after delivery,[14,33] there is usually a delay before cardiac disease is apparent. Over one half of infants with severe aortic stenosis are discovered prior to 3 months of age, with the majority of these presenting in the neonatal period.[9,14,15,20,33,37,42,50,52,59,71] Mocellin[49] suggests that those patients presenting at birth or shortly thereafter are more likely to have reduced left ventricular size or extensive endocardial fibroelastosis.

Physical Examination

The findings of congestive heart failure and low cardiac output at initial presentation are often striking. The infant commonly evolves signs and symptoms of respiratory difficulty, and a referral diagnosis of suspected pneumonia and sepsis is encountered. Tachypnea and dyspnea are seen in over two thirds of patients. At times, rales and abnormal respiratory sounds are present. Respiratory symptoms may impair the ability of the infant to take the breast or bottle, and consequently feeding difficulties and failure to thrive are seen.[50] There are signs of systemic venous congestion with hepatosplenomegaly, but peripheral or facial edema is uncommon. Cyanosis is clinically present in one fourth to one half of infants and may be secondary to pulmonary congestion and edema or may be evidence of poor cardiac output. Findings that are more indicative of aortic obstruction and diminished cardiac output include

pallor, tachycardia, diminished peripheral pulses or blood pressure, and delayed or decreased perfusion with cool extremities. A history of colic or excessive irritability may indicate anginal pain similar to that described in patients with anomalous origin of the coronary arteries. The significance of this historical clue may not be appreciated until the severity of aortic stenosis is confirmed.

Physical examination almost invariably reveals a cardiac murmur. This murmur is most often grade 2 or 3, but a systolic thrill is found in approximately one third of patients. The murmur may be audible at either the right upper sternal margin or at the mid-to-lower left sternal border. A systolic ejection click is common (at least 50 per cent in all series) and was found in all cases in one series.[66] A diastolic rumble or filling sound can be present. The apical impulse is almost always hyperactive and has been localized to the right, left, or both ventricles.[42,50]

Electrocardiography

A variety of electrocardiographic patterns can be seen. Left ventricular hypertrophy is most commonly seen (Fig. 36–1).[14,15,33,39,50,52,71] Biventricular or right ventricular hypertrophy may be present,[42] with a right ventricular hypertrophy pattern more prominent in early presentation (Fig. 36–2). The QRS axis ranges from 0 degrees to +150 degrees. Right, left, or combined atrial enlargement can be seen. ST segment and T wave changes are the rule, and a strain pattern is described in over three fourths of patients. A right ventricular hypertrophy pattern suggests an increase in right ventricular volume load because of left-to-right atrial shunting across the foramen ovale or because of pulmonary hypertension secondary to poor left ventricular compliance and elevated left atrial pressure.

Chest Radiography

Unlike the radiologic findings of aortic stenosis in older infants and children, in which cardiac size is often normal, the chest radiograph in affected neonates almost always reveals moderate to severe cardiac enlargement.

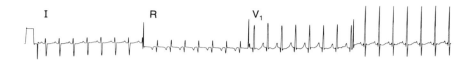

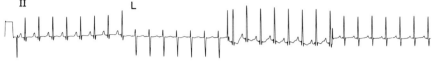

Figure 36–2. Twelve-lead electrocardiogram in a 4-day-old with aortic stenosis, revealing a pattern of right ventricular hypertrophy.

Only in rare instances is little or no cardiomegaly seen. Specific chamber enlargement may be difficult to detect, although left atrial enlargement is common, and the older infant may have a left ventricular configuration. Post-stenotic aortic dilation is not seen as a rule. Pulmonary vascular markings may be normal or increased owing to left-to-right atrial shunting (Fig. 36–3). Pulmonary venous congestion is frequent, and at times a pattern of pulmonary venous obstruction is evident.[17]

Echocardiograpy

The evolution of echocardiographic techniques in the evaluation of congenital cardiac defects in critically ill newborns has done much to alleviate difficulties in diagnosis and in guiding early management. Huhta et al[38] found that echocardiography combined with Doppler evaluation was comparable to catheterization and angiography in diagnosing and assessing cardiovascular anatomy and hemodynamics in infants with severe aortic stenosis. Two-dimensional echocardiographic evaluation can determine valve anatomy (including number and deformity of valve cusps and degree of valve motion), presence of poststenotic aortic dilation, and status of the left ventricle. The ventricle may be fairly normal in size, with evidence of concentric hypertrophy (Fig. 36–4) or may show severe dilation and dysfunction (Fig. 36–5). Increased echogenicity of papillary muscle and endocardial reflections might suggest the presence of fibroelastosis.

The concomitant use of Doppler ultrasound techniques can produce an accurate noninvasive assessment of the degree of obstruction and cardiac hemodynamics, avoiding the need for cardiac catheterization. Continuous wave Doppler ultrasound evaluation has been shown to provide

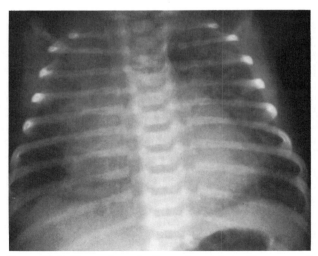

Figure 36–3. Chest radiograph of a newborn infant with severe aortic stenosis, showing cardiomegaly and a redistribution of pulmonary flow to the apex of the lung fields, suggesting pulmonary venous obstruction.

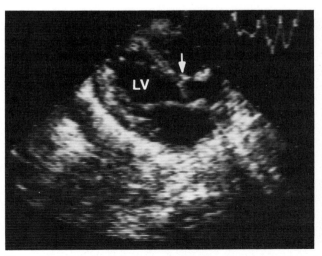

Figure 36–4. Parasternal long axis two-dimensional echo projection of a 6-week-old infant with thickened, bicuspid aortic valve (arrow) and normal left ventricular (LV) cavity size with concentric hypertrophy. The left atrium is enlarged.

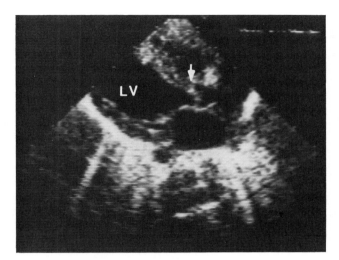

Figure 36–5. Parasternal long axis projection of a 6-day-old infant with abnormal, stenotic aortic valve (arrow) and dilated, myopathic left ventricle. The left atrium is also enlarged. LV = left ventricle.

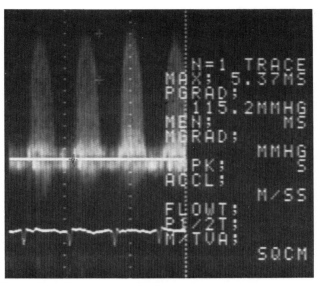

Figure 36–6. Continuous wave Doppler tracing across the stenotic aortic valve in a 6-week-old infant. The Doppler velocity is increased at 5.37 M/sec, yielding a transvalvar gradient estimate of 115 mmHg (confirmed at catheterization).

accurate estimation of transvalvular pressure gradients in aortic stenosis in older patients[8] as well as in early infancy[31] (Fig. 36–6). There may be pitfalls, however, in Doppler ultrasound assessment in newborns with profoundly diminished left ventricular function. When cardiac output is low, Doppler velocity measurements may not accurately reflect the severity of obstruction, and caution must be used in these instances.

Cardiac Catheterization

Cardiac catheterization can provide hemodynamic and anatomic detail of the degree of aortic stenosis and status of the left ventricle. However, in the critically ill neonate, catheterization has significant risks; many centers consider noninvasive evaluation adequate to direct surgical and management decisions. Aortic valve pressure gradients can be determined by entering the left ventricle via the foramen ovale or retrogradely across the aortic valve. It is not unusual for the foramen ovale to be functionally or anatomically closed in the older infant, necessitating retrograde or transseptal puncture catheterization to measure left ventricular pressure. Sometimes, obtaining left ventricular pressures is not possible. Aortic valve systolic pressure gradients vary between 40 and 130 mmHg when aortic stenosis presents in infancy.[9,20,33,42,50,52] Left ventricular end-diastolic pressure is abnormally elevated in over half of the patients, indicating significant ventricular dysfunction. Right heart pressures may also be elevated if left atrial hypertension is present or if foramenal obstruction was present in utero. Oximetry usually demonstrates left-to-right atrial shunting; right-to-left ductal shunting may also be demonstrated by oximetry if the ductus arteriosus is patent and aortic obstruction is severe.

Left ventricular angiography can reveal a small, restrictive chamber (Fig. 36–7) or, alternatively, a dilated, myopathic left ventricle (Fig. 36–8).[24] The functional state and degree of ventricular hypertrophy can be evaluated by

angiography. The aortic valve apparatus generally is deformed and immobile, or it may be noted to have good excursion and dome during systole. Often, the aortic annulus is diminutive. Orifice size and eccentricity can be subjectively evaluated angiographically. It is also important to determine competence of the mitral apparatus and to detect the presence of associated cardiac anomalies.

Differential Diagnosis

Severe aortic stenosis presenting in infancy must be differentiated from other entities that present with respiratory symptoms and signs of a low cardiac output. Neonatal sepsis and pneumonia are commonly the initial diagnoses in these infants. The presence of cardiomegaly, poor pulses, and a murmur may be found in neonatal sepsis with shock, but these findings should arouse suspicion of a cardiac etiology. Other causes of severe left ventricular outlet obstruction must be ruled out, particularly hypoplastic left-heart syndrome or severe coarctation of the aorta. Complex cardiac anomalies with ventricular septal defect and outflow obstruction must be considered. The differential diagnosis also includes primary cardiomyopathies that present acutely in the infant—primary endocardial fibroelastosis, viral or bacterial myocarditis, and glycogen storage disease involving the heart. Large peripheral arteriovenous malformations are usually obvious on examination, but intracerebral or intrahepatic arteriovenous malformations causing congestive heart failure may be missed unless specifically sought. Tachyarrhythmias also cause heart failure, but usually present at several weeks or months of age. Finally, anomalous origin of the coronary artery from the pulmonary artery can present in an identical manner and must be excluded.

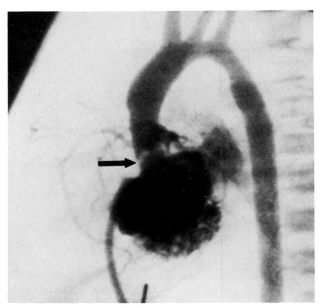

Figure 36–7. Long axial oblique left ventriculogram in a neonate with critical aortic stenosis. The aortic valve leaflets (arrow) are thickened and dome in systole. The left ventricle is small and irregular. Autopsy revealed marked fibroelastosis and hypertrophy of the chamber.

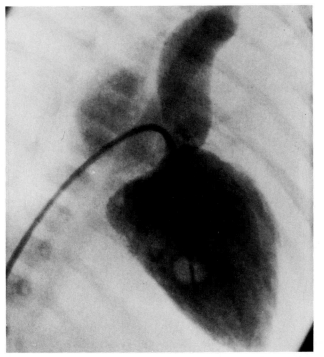

Figure 36–8. End-systolic frame of patient with severe aortic valve stenosis and dilated, myopathic left ventricle.

Treatment

Once a diagnosis of significant aortic valve stenosis is made, whether to proceed to surgical therapy must be decided.[14,15,39,71] With severe aortic obstruction, surgical valvotomy is mandatory if there is any hope of improving cardiac function. At best, operative intervention in this lesion should be considered a palliative measure, with a high likelihood of future operative therapy being required. Surgical techniques for relief of aortic valve stenosis are considered in Chapter 62 and will not be discussed here. Significant operative mortality and morbidity may be expected, depending on the degree of left ventricular dysfunction and damage or on the extent of associated cardiac anomalies.

Medical management of these severely ill infants is based on improving cardiac function and output while preparations for surgical intervention are made. The importance of basic care, such as supplemental oxygen and mechanical ventilation (if needed), correction of acidosis, normalization of hemoglobin, provision of carbohydrate substrate, and sedation, cannot be overemphasized.[73] Inotropic support with digoxin or rapidly acting intravenous agents (dopamine, dobutamine, epinephrine, or isoproterenol) should be instituted.[28] When using digitalis preparations, one should keep in mind that reductions in renal perfusion and drug clearance may necessitate alterations in dosage. Diuretic therapy may relieve pulmonary edema and respiratory distress as well as decrease preload and improve cardiac performance. However, excessive intravascular volume reduction with diuretics can result in inadequate ventricular filling and worsening of cardiac output. There is probably little place for afterload reduction in unoperated acutely decompensated critical aortic stenosis.

Two specific measures for nonoperative management should be considered in more detail. In the newborn with critical aortic stenosis, marked improvement in systemic cardiac output can be achieved with the use of prostaglandin E_1 (PGE_1) infusion. Reopening the ductus arteriosus allows a right-to-left ductal shunt and increased systemic blood flow, which is analogous to the fetal hemodynamic situation. In addition, a right-to-left ductal shunt diverts blood flow from the pulmonary vascular bed and therefore from the left ventricle, thereby relieving left ventricular overload. PGE_1 is routinely used to palliate and to manage a number of critical cardiac lesions in the newborn period and may be the most beneficial mode of acute medical therapy.[22,58] Apnea and central nervous system depression are common side effects and may require the use of mechanical ventilatory support.

The second specific modality to be considered by the pediatric cardiologist is the potential application of aortic balloon valvuloplasty to relieve aortic valve obstruction. Balloon dilation of aortic stenosis has been applied to older children and adults with reasonably low risk and good results.[41] Reports have now indicated reasonable success of aortic balloon valvuloplasty in infants and newborns.[69,70] The technique can potentially be applied using umbilical arterial placement of catheters to reduce arterial risk in the small infant. This concept in interventional therapy may become a standard form of treatment in selected cases in the future, replacing surgical valvotomy in a number of patients (see Chapter 56).

AORTIC ATRESIA (HYPOPLASTIC LEFT-HEART SYNDROME)

Definition

The hypoplastic left-heart (HLH) syndrome is a term that has been used to describe a variety of cardiac lesions having as a common denominator both obstruction and degrees of underdevelopment of the left ventricle, left heart valves, and aortic arch.[53] A variation frequently encountered by the pediatric cardiologist consists of aortic valve atresia with hypoplasia or atresia of the left ventricle and mitral valve. Aortic valve atresia will be the anomaly primarily discussed in this chapter. Mitral valve atresia can be considered a separate entity, but atresia or degrees of mitral valve hypoplasia and stenosis are consistently seen in the HLH with aortic atresia. Mitral atresia and HLH occur without aortic atresia but are a relatively rare anomaly. A ventricular septal defect is invariably present in mitral atresia and allows a right-to-left ventricular shunt into a dextroposed aorta. Clinical differentiation from HLH with aortic atresia is difficult, although a later onset of symptoms and a longer life span are generally seen.

Historical Perspective

Aortic atresia was recognized to result in severe distress and death in the newborn as early as the beginning of the ninteenth century (see Introduction).[19] Probably the first comprehensive description of the pathology of HLH was published by Lev[45] in 1952, although earlier descriptions of this entity were detailed by Taussig[75] and by Abbott.[1] The largest series reviewing the clinical facets of aortic atresia and HLH is that of Noonan and Nadas,[53] which was reported in 1958. The inadequacy of therapy was recognized from the beginning and remained unchanged for many years. However, surgical considerations emerged as a potential for treatment in the 1970s,[13,26] and successful palliation became a reality in the 1980s, as reported by Norwood et al.[55,56] Recently, controversial surgical approaches have aroused great debate and set this disease into the public limelight.[4]

Epidemiology

The hypoplastic left-heart syndrome comprises 7 to 9 per cent of congenital cardiac lesions presenting in the first year of life[23] but up to 22 per cent of infants dying in the neonatal period of cardiac disease.[43] The lesion appears one to two times out of 10,000 live births.[29] Male predominance is seen, with a male to female ratio of between 3:2 and 2:1.[23,53] There is most likely a multifactorial inheritance pattern, with a recurrence risk in siblings of 2.2 per cent for congenital heart defects (one fourth of which are HLH).[54] Familial clustering of aortic atresia has been reported,[61] although aortic atresia is not strongly related to any genetic syndrome.

Pathogenesis

The etiology of aortic atresia remains unknown. Some investigators[46,51] have suggested that premature closure of the foramen ovale may lead to the development of hypoplastic left-heart syndrome. This theory is difficult to accept, as only 10 to 15 per cent of patients with aortic atresia have a sealed foramen ovale. Other speculations have suggested abnormal left-sided inflow differentiation resulting in mitral atresia or abnormal outflow formation.[12] Experimental production of the syndrome[32] tends to support abnormal intracardiac streaming and flow patterns as a basis for pathogenesis. Associated cardiac anomalies most commonly include ventricular septal defect,[64,76] coarctation of the aorta,[77] interruption of the aortic arch,[65] and rarely transposition of the great arteries.[48] The frequent presence of a discrete coarctation may be of surgical importance in approaching palliative operation.

Clinical Profile

History and Physical Examination

The typical scenario of aortic atresia begins with an infant who is apparently healthy at birth.[11,23,26,53,67] The newborn often remains healthy appearing until onset of ductal closure, when an acute shocklike state begins. Seventy-five per cent of patients come to medical attention within the first week of life.[23] The ductus arteriosus becomes the focal point in allowing even transient survival in these patients.[79] The clinical picture is very similar to that of the newborn with critical aortic stenosis (see preceding discussion). Dyspnea and respiratory symptoms are generally apparent, although significant cyanosis is not obvious. Tachycardia, cardiomegaly and cardiac hyperactivity, a gallop rhythm, and hepatomegaly are present. Cardiac output is markedly diminished, with weak or absent pulses in all extremities, delayed perfusion and capillary refill, and diminished blood pressure. Auscultation of the heart is usually unrewarding in determining a specific diagnosis. The second heart sound is loud and single. A nonspecific systolic ejection murmur may be audible, or occasionally a murmur of tricuspid valve regurgitation may also be heard. A prominent diastolic ventricular filling sound or tricuspid flow murmur may also be heard.

Electrocardiography

The electrocardiogram in aortic atresia most often reveals a pattern of right ventricular hypertrophy with ST and T wave changes (Fig. 36–9).[23,53,78] Frequently, a qR pattern is seen. Atrial enlargement is common. However, the presence of left ventricular hypertrophy or a normal electrocardiogram has been described,[72] and these features should not lead one to exclude aortic atresia from a diagnostic consideration.

Chest Radiography

The typical findings on chest radiograph in aortic atresia are moderate to marked cardiomegaly with global cardiac

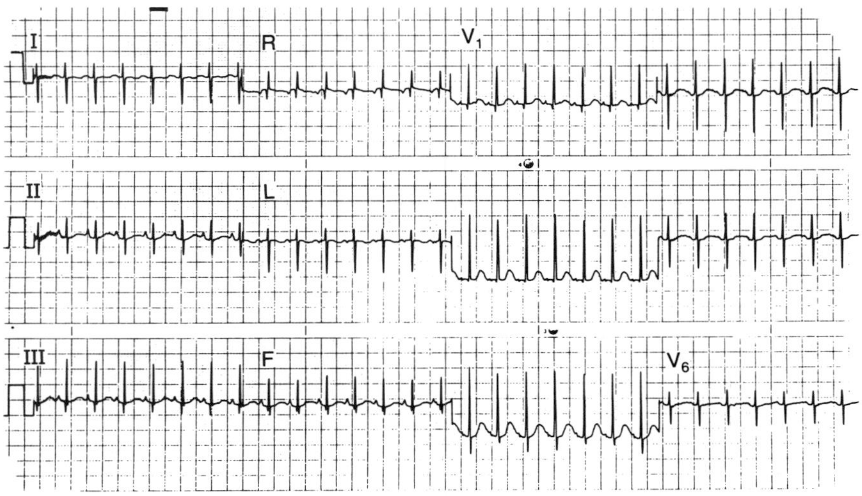

Figure 36–9. Electrocardiogram in a newborn infant with aortic valve atresia. There is evidence of right ventricular hypertrophy and a qR pattern in V_1. Note that left ventricular voltages are unremarkable.

enlargement. Because of the obligatory left-to-right foramen shunt seen in these patients, there is marked increase in pulmonary blood flow and arterial markings (Fig. 36–10). If significant restriction in foramenal flow or closure of the foramen ovale is present, then a picture of pulmonary venous obstruction may be seen on the chest radiograph and may suggest obstructed total anomalous pulmonary venous return.

Echocardiography

Echocardiography in the newborn with aortic atresia has become both sensitive and specific in detailing the anatomy of the lesion.[6,18,44] The dilated right ventricular chamber and pulmonary artery are apparent, while the very hypoplastic left ventricular chamber is usually seen (Fig. 36–11). Atresia of the aortic valve is evident. The tiny ascending aorta and arch are frequently visualized (Fig. 36–12). An atrial septal communication should be searched for, as infants do poorly with restrictive atrial defects, and balloon septostomy may be necessary. Concurrent use of Doppler echocardiography can enhance the noninvasive evaluation. Patency of the ductus arteriosus can be determined with pulsed or continuous wave Doppler ultrasonography. The direction of flow in the aortic arch can also be assessed. Retrograde flow would indicate atresia rather than severe stenosis of the aortic valve. Doppler studies can be used to determine flow velocity at the foramen ovale and the presence of restriction. Current technology and skill in echocardiographic assessment of aortic atresia should allow restriction of cardiac catheterization for palliative management (balloon septostomy) in selected cases.[5]

Cardiac Catheterization

Hemodynamic findings at cardiac catheterization in aortic atresia vary depending on the status of the foramen ovale, ductus arteriosus, and pulmonary vascular bed.[40] Right ventricular and pulmonary artery pressures are significantly elevated and may be suprasystemic if the ductus arteriosus is constricted to any extent. Atrial pressures are generally elevated also, but left atrial hypertension and differences in right and left atrial pressures may indicate inadequacy of the foramenal communication. Oxygen saturations reflect the obligatory left-to-right atrial shunt and complete admixture of saturated and desaturated blood through the right heart. Systemic arterial oxygen saturation and PO_2 reflect those of the pulmonary artery, as systemic flow is supplied across the ductus arteriosus. The resulting saturation correlates with the amount of pulmonary blood flow. Krovetz et al[40] indicated that lower saturations result from elevated pulmonary vascular resistance secondary to restricted flow at the foramen ovale.

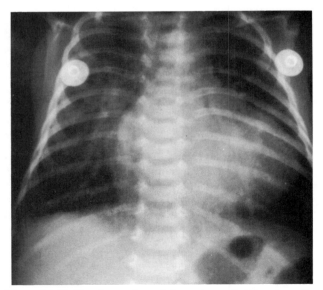

Figure 36–10. The chest radiograph in aortic atresia. There is cardiomegaly, suggesting right heart enlargement as well as increased pulmonary vascular markings.

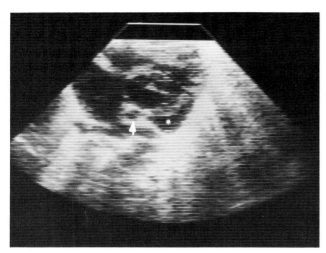

Figure 36–11. Subcostal echocardiogram depicting a large right ventricle and tricuspid valve as well as tiny left ventricular chamber (*) and aortic root (arrow).

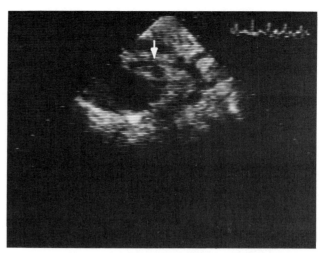

Figure 36–12. Aortic arch echocardiographic projection in aortic atresia shows the very hypoplastic aortic arch. Note comparative size of the ascending aorta (arrow) and the right pulmonary artery posterior to the ascending aorta.

Cardiac angiography in aortic atresia reveals a variety of aortic sizes and anatomy.[25] The classic picture is one of retrograde visualization of a hypoplastic ascending aorta with no evidence of antegrade flow. The diminutive aorta may be no more than 2 or 3 mm in diameter (Fig. 36–13), or it may be near normal caliber. The coronary circulation is usually seen, and its distribution may indicate relative ventricular chamber size and the degree of left ventricular hypoplasia. The presence of discrete coarctation may not be apparent angiographically but is usually present at the time of surgery. Biplane angiography of the right ventricle determines its size and function, the presence of tricuspid regurgitation, and patency of the ductus arteriosus. Retrograde flow into the aortic arch is frequently seen without selective arch injections (Fig. 36–14). The left ventricle can vary in size to a great degree. Often, the chamber cannot be entered with the cardiac catheter. Angiography of the left atrium or direct injection in the left ventricle can indicate chamber size as well as the presence of ventricular septal communications or coronary sinusoids.

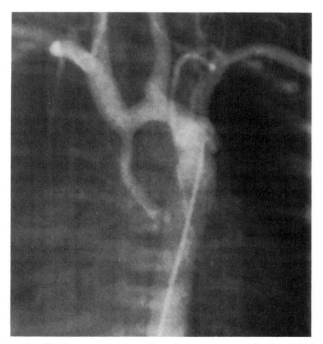
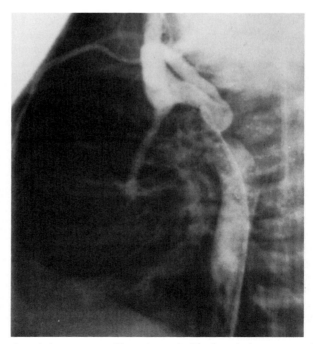

Figure 36–13. Anteroposterior and lateral cineangiogram of a hypoplastic aortic arch in a neonate with aortic atresia. The lateral view suggests the presence of an associated coarctation of the descending aorta.

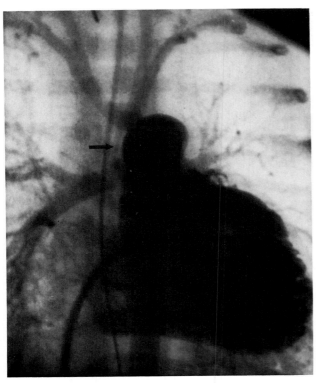

Figure 36–14. Right ventricular angiogram in aortic atresia reveals filling of the aorta from contrast flow across the ductus arteriosus. The tiny ascending aorta (arrow) fills retrogradely and can be compared with pulmonary artery size.

Differential Diagnosis

The differential diagnosis for aortic atresia is essentially the same as that for severe aortic stenosis in the newborn (see preceding discussion). Medical management is often unrewarding as these patients generally have a poor prognosis,[30] even despite aggressive medical attention. With the evolution of surgical palliation, medical support has taken a supportive and temporizing role in hopes of improving hemodynamics and clinical status, to gain time for discussion of the defect and its implications with family members. Important decisions concerning surgical palliation can then be made.

Treatment

Basic supportive measures are no different from those previously discussed for severe aortic stenosis.[22,28,58,73] Knowledge of perinatal hemodynamics illustrates the important role of the ductus arteriosus and its patency in ensuring even temporary survival. Specific therapy in the form of balloon[62] or blade[60] atrial septostomy may be required if an inadequate atrial communication is present. Even after complete cardiologic evaluation and stabilization has been performed, evidence suggests that variations in anatomy or ventricular function have little effect on surgical outcome.[34]

The surgery for hypoplastic left-heart syndrome is covered in Chapter 62. Two considerations may arise: staged surgical palliation and repair,[56] or possible cardiac transplantation, through either xenograft[4] or allograft methods. The ethical dilemmas involved may present the family and physician with many emotional and personal conflicts that make management decisions difficult. However, continued surgical advances may alleviate some of these pains and allow this previously untreatable lesion to be overcome.

References

1. Abbott ME (1936): Atlas of Congenital Cardiac Disease. New York, American Heart Association, pp 60–64.
2. Alexander B (1769): The seats and causes of diseases investigated by anatomy. In Rashkind WJ (ed): Congenital Heart Disease. Stroudsburg, Hutchison Ross Publishing Co, 1982, pp 115–116.
3. Anderson DH, Kelly J (1956): Endocardial fibro-elastosis. I. Endocardial fibro-elastosis associated with congenital malformations of the heart. Pediatrics 18:513–538.
4. Bailey LL, Nehlsen-Cannarella SL, Concepcion W, Jolley WB (1985): Baboon-to-human cardiac xenotransplantation in a neonate. JAMA 254:3321–3329.
5. Bash SE, Huhta JC, Vick GW III, Gutgesell HP, Ott DA (1986): Hypoplastic left heart syndrome: Is echocardiography accurate enough to guide surgical palliation? J Am Coll Cardiol 7:610–615.
6. Bass JL, Ben-Shacher G, Edwards JE (1980): Comparison of M-mode echocardiography and pathologic findings in the hypoplastic left heart syndrome. Am J Cardiol 45: 79–86.
7. Beckman CB, Moller JH, Edwards JE (1975): Alternate pathways to pulmonary venous flow in left-sided obstructive anomalies. Circulation 52:509–516.
8. Berger M, Berdoff RL, Gallerstein PE, Goldberg E (1984): Evaluation of aortic stenosis by continuous wave Doppler ultrasound. J Am Coll Cardiol 3:150–156.
9. Bicoff JP, Thompson W, Arbeiter HI, Weinberg M, Agustsson MH (1963): Severe aortic stenosis in infancy. J Pediatr 63:161–164.
10. Char F (1973): Tables of heritable cardiovascular conditions and associated syndromes. In Bergsma D (ed): The Fourth Conference on the Clinical Delineation of Birth Defects. Part XV. Baltimore, Williams & Wilkins, pp 313–322.
11. Deely WJ, Ehlers KH, Levin AR, Engle MA (1971): Hypoplastic left heart syndrome. Anatomic, physiologic, and theraputic considerations. Am J Dis Child 121:168–175.
12. De La Cruz MV, Munoz-Castellanos L, Nadal-Ginard B (1971): Extrinsic factors in the genesis of congenital heart disease. Br Heart J 33:203–213.
13. Doty DB, Marvin WJ Jr, Schieken RM, Lauer RM (1980): Hypoplastic left heart syndrome. Successful palliation with a new operation. J Thorac Cardiovasc Surg 80:148–152.
14. Downing DF (1956): Congenital aortic stenosis. Clinical aspects and surgical treatment. Circulation 14:188–199.
15. Edmunds LH, Wagner HR, Heymann MA (1980): Aortic valvulotomy in neonates. Circulation 61:421–427.
16. Edwards JE (1958): Pathologic aspects of cardiac valvular insufficiencies. Arch Surg 77:634–640.
17. Elliott LP, Schiebler GL (1979): The X-ray Diagnosis of Congenital Heart Disease in Infants, Children and Adults. Springfield, Charles C Thomas Publisher, pp 206–211.
18. Farooki ZQ, Henry JG, Green EW (1976): Echocardiographic spectrum of the hypoplastic left heart syndrome. Am J Cardiol 38:337–343.
19. Farre JR (1814): On malformations of the human heart. In Rashkind WJ (ed): Congenital Heart Disease. Stroudsburg, Hutchinson Ross Publishing Co, 1982, pp 152–160.
20. Feldman BH, Scott LP (1964): Aortic stenosis in infancy. Pediatrics 33:931–936.
21. Fishman NH, Hof RB, Rudolph AM, Heymann MA (1978):

Models of congenital heart disease in fetal lambs. Circulation 53:1138–1143.

22. Freed MD, Heymann MA, Lewis AB, Roehl SL, Kensey RC (1981): Prostaglandin E₁ in infants with ductus arteriousus-dependent congenital heart disease. Circulation 64:899–905.

23. Freedom RM (1983): Hypoplastic left heart syndrome. In Adams FH, Emmanouilides GC (eds): Moss' Heart Disease in Infants, Children, and Adolescents. 3rd ed. Baltimore, Williams & Wilkins, p 415.

24. Freedom RM, Culham JAG, Moes CAF (1984): Angiocardiography of Congenital Heart Disease. New York, Macmillan, pp 372–375.

25. Ibid, pp 339–357.

26. Freedom RM, Williams WG, Dische MR, Rowe RD (1976): Anatomic variants in aortic atresia: Potential candidates for ventriculo-aortic reconstruction. Br Heart J 38:821–826.

27. Friedman WF, Benson LN (1983): Aortic stenosis. In Adams FH, Emmanouilides GC (eds): Moss' Heart Disease in Infants, Children and Adolescents, 3rd ed. Baltimore, Williams & Wilkins, p 171.

28. Friedman WF, George BL (1984): New concepts in drugs in the treatment of congestive heart failure. Pediatr Clin North Am 31:1197–1227.

29. Fyler DC (1980): Report of the New England regional cardiac program. Pediatrics 65(Part 2, Suppl):436–439.

30. Fyler DC, Rothman KJ, Buckley LP, Cohn HE, Hellenbrand WE, Castaneda AR (1981): The determinants of 5 year survival of infants with critical congenital heart disease. In Engle MA (ed): Pediatric Cardiovascular Disease. Philadelphia, FA Davis Co, pp 393–405.

31. Hagler DJ, Tajik AJ, Seward JB, Ritter DG (1986): Non-invasive assessment of pulmonary valve stenosis, aortic valve stenosis, and coarctation of the aorta in critically ill neonates. Am J Cardiol 57:369–372.

32. Harh JY, Paul MH, Gallen WJ, Friedberg DZ, Kaplan S (1973): Experimental production of hypoplastic left heart syndrome in the chick embryo. Am J Cardiol 31:51–56.

33. Hastreiter AR, Oshima M, Miller RA, Lev M, Paul MH (1963): Congenital aortic stenosis syndrome in infancy. Circulation 28:1084–1095.

34. Helton JG, Aglira BA, Chin AJ, Murphy JD, Pigott JD, Norwood WI (1986): Analysis of potential anatomic or physiologic determinants of outcome of palliative surgery for hypoplastic left heart syndrome. Circulation 74(Suppl I):70–76.

35. Heymann MA, Rudolph AM (1973): Effects of congenital heart disease on fetal and neonatal circulations. In Friedman WF, Lesch M, Sonnenblick EH (eds): Neonatal Heart Disease. New York, Grune & Stratton, pp 53–67.

36. Hoffman JIE (1969): The natural history of congenital isolated pulmonic and aortic stenosis. Ann Rev Med 20:15–28.

37. Hohn AR, Van Praagh S, Moore AAD, Vlad P, Lambert EC (1965): Aortic stenosis. Circulation 31(Suppl III):4–12.

38. Huhta JC, Latson LA, Gutgesell HP, Cooley DA, Kearney DL (1984): Echocardiography in diagnosis and management in symptomatic aortic stenosis in infants. Circulation 70:438–444.

39. Keane JF, Bernhard WF, Nadas AS (1975): Aortic stenosis surgery in infancy. Circulation 52:1138–1143.

40. Krovetz LJ, Rowe RD, Schiebler GL (1970): Hemodynamics of aortic valve atresia. Circulation 42:953–959.

41. Lababidi Z, Jiunn-Ren WU, Walls JT (1984): Percutaneous balloon aortic valvuloplasty: Results in 23 patients. Am J Cardiol 53:194–197.

42. Lakier JB, Lewis AB, Heymann MA, Stanger P, Hoffman JIE, Rudolph AM (1974): Isolated aortic stenosis in the neonate. Natural history and hemodynamic considerations. Circulation 50:801–808.

43. Lambert EC, Canent RV, Hohn AR (1966): Congenital cardiac anomalies in the newborn. A review of conditions causing death or severe distress in the first month of life. Pediatrics 37:343–351.

44. Lange LW, Sahn DJ, Allen HD, Ovitt TW, Goldberg SJ (1980): Cross-sectional echocardiography in hypoplastic left ventricle: Echocardiographic-angiographic-anatomic correlations. Pediatr Cardiol 1:287–299.

45. Lev M (1952): Pathologic anatomy and interrelationship of hypoplasia of the aortic tract complexes. Lab Invest 1:61–70.

46. Lev M, Arcilla R, Rimoldi HJA, Licata RH, Gasul BM (1963): Premature narrowing or closure of the foramen ovale. Am Heart J 65:638–647.

47. Levin DL, Perkin RM, Parkey M, Mayhew E, Hartwig R (1980): Experimental aortic stenosis in fetal lambs. Circulation 62:1159–1164.

48. McGarry KM, Taylor JFN, Macartney FJ (1980): Aortic atresia occurring with complete transposition of the great arteries. Br Heart J 44:711–713.

49. Mocellin R, Sauer U, Simon B, Comazzi M, Sebening F, Buhlmeyer K (1983): Reduced left ventricular size and endocardial fibroelastosis as correlates of mortality in newborns and young infants with severe aortic valve stenosis. Pediatr Cardiol 4:265–272.

50. Mody MR, Nadas AS, Bernhard WF (1967): Aortic stenosis in infants. New Eng J Med 276:832–838.

51. Moerman PL, Van Dijck H, Lauweryns JM, Eggermont E, Van Der Hauwaert LG (1986): Premature closure of the foramen ovale and congenital pulmonary cystic lymphangiectasis in aortic valve atresia or severe aortic valve stenosis. Am J Cardiol 57:703–705.

52. Moller JH, Nakib A, Eliot RS, Edwards JE (1966): Symptomatic congenital aortic stenosis in the first year of life. J Pediatr 69:728–734.

53. Noonan JA, Nadas AS (1958): The hypoplastic left heart syndrome. Pediatr Clin North Am 5:1029–1056.

54. Nora JJ (1980): Update on the etiology of congenital heart disease and genetic counseling. In Van Praagh R, Takao A (eds): Etiology and Morphogenesis of Congenital Heart Disease. New York, Futura Publishing Co, pp 21–39.

55. Norwood WI, Kirklin JK, Sanders SP (1980): Hypoplastic left heart syndrome: Experience with palliative surgery. Am J Cardiol 45:87–91.

56. Norwood WI, Lang P, Hansen DD (1983): Physiologic repair of aortic atresia–hypoplastic left heart syndrome. N Engl J Med 308:23–26.

57. O'Connor WM, Cash JB, Cottrill CM, Johnson GL, Noonan JA (1982): Ventriculocoronary connections in hypoplastic left hearts: An autopsy microscopic study. Circulation 66:1078–1086.

58. Olley PM, Coceani F, Bodach E (1976): E-type prostaglandins. A new emergency therapy for certain cyanotic congenital heart malformations. Circulation 53:728–731.

59. Ongley PA, Nadas AS, Paul MH, Rudolph AM, Starkey GWB (1958): Aortic stenosis in infants and children. Pediatrics 21:207–221.

60. Park SC, Neches WH, Zuberbuhler JR, Lenox CC, Mathews RA, Fricker FJ, Zoltun RA (1978): Clinical use of blade atrial septostomy. Circulation 58:600–606.

61. Rao SS, Gootman N, Platt N (1967): Familial aortic atresia. Am J Dis Child 118:919–922.

62. Rashking WJ, Miller WW (1966): Creation of an atrial septal defect without thoracotomy. Am Med Assoc J 196:991–992.

63. Roberts WC (1973): Valvular, subvalvular and supravalvular aortic stenosis: Morphologic features. In Edward JE (ed): Cardiovascular Clinics. Clinical-Pathologic Correlations 2. Philadelphia, FA Davis Co, pp 97–111.

64. Roberts WC, Perry LW, Chandra RS, Myers GE, Shapiro SR, Scott LP (1976): Aortic valve atresia: A new classification based on necropsy study of 73 cases. Am J Cardiol 37:753–756.

65. Rosenquist GC, Taylor JFN, Stark J (1974): Aortopulmonary fenestration and aortic atresia. Report of an infant with ventricular septal defect, persistent ductus arteriosus, and interrupted aortic arch. Br Heart J 36:1146–1149.

66. Rowe RD, Freedom RM, Mehrizi A, Bloom KR (1981): The Neonate with Congenital Heart Disease. Philadelphia, WB Saunders Co, pp 564–565.

67. Ibid, pp 209–211.

68. Rudolph AM, Heymann MA, Spitznas U (1972): Hemodynamic considerations in the development of narrowing of the aorta. Am J Cardiol 30:514–525.

69. Rupprath G, Neuhaus K (1985): Percutaneous balloon valvuloplasty for aortic valve stenosis in infancy. Am J Cardiol 55:1655–1656.

70. Sanchez GR, Mehta AV, Ewing LL, Brickley SE, Anderson TM, Black IFS (1985): Successful percutaneous balloon valvuloplasty of the aortic valve in an infant. Pediatr Cardiol 6:103–106.

71. Sink JD, Smallhorn JF, Macartney FJ, Taylor JFN, Stark J, deLeval MR (1984): Management of critical aortic stenosis in infancy. J Thorac Cardiovasc Surg 87:82–86.

72. Strong WB, Liebman J, Perrin E (1970): Hypoplastic left ventricle syndrome. Electrocardiographic evidence of left ventricular hypertrophy. Am J Dis Child 120:511–514.

73. Talner NS, Campbell AGM (1973): Recognition and management of cardiologic problems in the newborn infant. In Friedman WF, Lesch M, Sonnenblick EH (eds): Neonatal Heart Disease. New York, Grune & Stratton, pp 115–119.

74. Taussig HB (1947): Congenital Malformations of the Heart. New York, The Commonwealth Fund, pp 428–439.

75. Taussig HB (1947): Congenital Malformations of the Heart. New York, The Commonwealth Fund, pp 177–189.

76. Thien G, Gallucci V, Macartney FJ, Del Torso S, Pellegrino PA, Anderson RH (1979): Anatomy of aortic atresia. Cases presenting with a ventricular septal defect. Circulation 59:173–178.

77. Von Rueden TJ, Knight L, Moller JH, Edwards JE (1975): Coarctation of the aorta associated with aortic valvular atresia. Circulation 52:951–954.

78. Von Rueden TJ, Moller JH (1978): The electrocardiogram in aortic valvular atresia. Chest 73:66–70.

79. Watson DG, Rowe RD (1962): Aortic valve atresia. Report of 43 cases. JAMA 179:14–18.

37 COARCTATION

Herbert G. Whitley
Lowell W. Perry

The prevalence of coarctation of the aorta is 0.2 in 1000 live births.[16,21] Although it is the eighth most common defect (5.1 per cent) among congenital defects in all age groups,[33] coarctation constitutes a much higher percentage of lesions presenting in infancy. In the New England Infant Cardiac Program, a regional study of cardiac defects in infants under 1 year of age, coarctation of the aorta was fourth in diagnostic frequency, accounting for 7.5 per cent of all congenital cardiovascular defects.[21] In the Baltimore-Washington Infant Study, coarctation was sixth in diagnostic frequency in the same age group.[16] Infancy is the most common period of presentation of coarctation, with one half of all cases being diagnosed in this age group.[9,55,67,75] Coarctation of the aorta is the second leading cardiovascular cause of death in the first month of life,[33] with an attrition rate of up to 50 per cent by 1 year of age.[21]

HISTORICAL PERSPECTIVE AND DEFINITION

First described by Morgagani in 1760 as a simple constriction of the thoracic aorta opposite the ligamentum arteriosum, coarctation of the aorta is a considerably more complex lesion. Bonnet, in 1903, first noted fundamental differences in the pathology and clinical presentation between coarctation diagnosed in infancy ("infantile") and in adulthood ("adult"). Infantile coarctation was commonly associated with intracardiac lesions, a patent ductus arteriosus, preductal location of the localized constriction, and a uniformly dismal prognosis. In contrast, adult coarctation was associated with a closed ductus arteriosus, a juxtaligamental or postligamental thoracic constriction, and a generally benign clinical course. This tidy generalization began to unravel in the 1950s with the realization that isolated coarctation can present in infancy and lead to death.[23] Indeed, it is now appreciated that 15 to 20 per cent of patients presenting in infancy have isolated coarctations.[51] In addition, older children may present with infantile coarctation and major associated cardiac lesions.[51]

At present, coarctation of the aorta is defined as a congenital narrowing of the aorta, either localized or of significant length, most commonly in the region of the insertion of the ductus arteriosus (or ligamentum arteriosum) into the upper descending thoracic aorta. The position of the localized lesion can be described as preductal,

postductal, or juxtaductal, but the location of the coarctation has little relevance to clinical presentation. The true determinants of clinical severity are presence and extent of transverse aortic narrowing, presence and severity of associated intracardiac lesions, and degree of constriction of the localized site.

SEX AND INHERITANCE

Coarctation of the aorta in all age groups has a male predominance of almost 2:1,[6] but in infancy the male predominance is negligible.[20,21] The prevalence is about 0.2 in 1000 live births,[16,21] and in autopsy series, 1 in 1540 cases.[33]

The recurrence risk for children having one parent with coarctation is approximately 2.7 per cent, which is consistent with the expected rate for multifactorial inheritance.[53] However, Rose and coworkers[61] noted a recurrence risk of 4.4 per cent, which was attributed to unknown environmental factors. The recurrence risk for siblings is lower at 2 per cent.[54] A seasonal variation in incidence has been noted, with the most pronounced excess in male births from October to December.[6]

PATHOLOGY

The localized lesion of coarctation is caused by a thickening of media of the superior, anterior, and posterior portions of the aortic wall.[15] This diaphragm-like structure, resembling a "curtain" in longitudinal sections, makes the lumen narrow and eccentric. Usually, the outer wall of the aorta demonstrates concavity or "waisting" at the site of the localized medial thickening.[56] The aorta above and below the medial thickening is dilated. In children and adults, intimal thickening develops as a progressive lesion at the coarctation site as a result of turbulent blood flow, but intimal thickening is absent in infants.[34]

Tubular hypoplasia of the aorta is commonly present with coarctation in infancy.[4,68] Although tubular hypoplasia occasionally may occur as the sole lesion, it nearly always is associated with medial thickening.[4,56,68] Indeed, the majority of infants presenting in congestive heart failure have both tubular hypoplasia of the aorta and medial thickening.[68]

The tubular hypoplasia of the aorta may involve only the isthmus (i.e., that segment between the left subclavian artery and the insertion of the ductus) or may extend more proximally to the left common carotid artery or the innominate artery.[64] The extent of narrowing is variable. The isthmus may be short, with a correspondingly longer segment between the left common carotid artery and the left subclavian artery.[64]

The origin and involvement of the subclavian arteries in coarctation vary and can be suspected from clinical examination. The orifice of the left subclavian artery may be stenotic when proximal to the coarctation site; clinically, this additional stenosis would produce differential upper extremity pulsations. Occasionally, the right subclavian artery arises anomalously distal to the coarctation site, causing decreased right brachial pulses. When both subclavian arteries arise distal to the coarctation site, pulses are decreased throughout the body except in the temporal and carotid arteries.[70]

Coarctation of the aorta associated with right aortic arch is unusual.[28]

ASSOCIATED ANOMALIES

In infancy, coarctation of the aorta commonly is associated with other cardiac anomalies. Becker and colleagues,[4] in a classic autopsy study of 100 infants with coarctation, helped to define the nature and extent of these associated defects. They divided the anomalies into five broad categories: (1) tubular hypoplasia of the aortic arch, (2) abnormal communications (exclusive of cases with positional anomalies of the great vessels), (3) left ventricular outflow obstructive lesions, (4) left ventricular inflow obstructive lesions, and (5) positional anomalies of the great vessels.

Becker and colleagues found tubular hypoplasia of the aortic arch (exclusive of seven cases with aortic atresia) in 49 of 93 patients, and in 63 per cent of patients under 6 months of age. The common occurrence of tubular hypoplasia with coarctation in infancy, especially in neonates and small infants, has been corroborated by others.[21,56,63,68] Tubular hypoplasia of the aorta is peculiar to infancy, is considered part of the coarctation complex in infancy rather than a separate entity, and is usually associated with additional intracardiac anomalies leading to congestive heart failure.[4]

Associated abnormal communications include, most commonly, patent ductus arteriosus (PDA) and ventricular septal defect (VSD), with a much smaller prevalence of atrial septal defect, atrioventricular septal defect, and single ventricle. Of infants with coarctation of the aorta and shunting lesions, about two thirds have PDA and about one third have VSD (with or without PDA).[21,23,26,31,33,40,55,68,75,77,82] The severity of the lesions associated with coarctation is a major determinant of the clinical symptomatology and of medical and surgical management. Left-to-right intraatrial shunting is a frequent finding at cardiac catheterization, but the prevalence of true atrial septal defect is only about 6 per cent.[23,33]

Left ventricular outflow obstruction, defined as subaortic stenosis, valvular aortic stenosis, or aortic atresia, occurs in 37 per cent of infants with coarctation at au-

topsy.[4] It is now appreciated that of all lesions, aortic atresia has the highest association with coarctation, with 75 per cent of cases having an associated coarctation.[43] Bicuspid aortic valve occurs in 27 to 47 per cent of patients,[4,62,76,77] but the incidence of true valvular stenosis is much less, usually about 10 per cent.[21,55,76,77] Subaortic stenosis is present in a few infants with coarctation but is much more prevalent in infants with complete interruption of the aortic arch.[48]

Left ventricular inflow obstruction, due to mitral valve anomalies, is common in autopsy studies, being present in from 26 to 58 per cent of cases.[4,62] Parachute mitral valve is present in 7.5 to 10 per cent of autopsy cases.[4,62] However, clinical studies have shown only 2 to 8 per cent of infants with coarctations have associated congenital mitral valve disease,[14,18,21] and only a few require mitral valve replacement.[14,18] Early death with coarctation may be associated with significant mitral valve disease.[14]

Five per cent of patients with transposition of the great arteries and biventricular heart have associated coarctation of the aorta.[47,79] Double-outlet right ventricle, a less common lesion, has a much higher association with coarctation. In general, about 10 per cent of patients with coarctation will have an associated positional anomaly of the great vessels, most frequently transposition.[4,23,33]

ETIOLOGY

The etiology of the coarctation lesion appears to be intimately related to the cardiac flow patterns in utero. In a series of fetal lambs, Rudolph determined that, of the combined ventricular output of both ventricles, 25 per cent traverses the aortic isthmus and 42 per cent traverses the ductus arteriosus.[63] Although no comparable flow data are available on human fetuses, it is known that the diameter of the aortic isthmus is 25 per cent less than that of ascending or descending aorta in normal premature and term newborns.[63] This decreased diameter would correspond to decreased flow through the aortic isthmus.

Coarctation is rare in lesions with decreased pulmonary blood flow and correspondingly increased aortic isthmus flow. Coarctation was not present in 330 pathologic specimens of tetralogy of Fallot[30] or in a large series of patients with pulmonary atresia and intact ventricular septum, pulmonary atresia and VSD, tricuspid atresia with normally related great vessels, and truncus arteriosus with decreased pulmonary blood flow.[66]

In contrast, in lesions in which there is obviously decreased aortic isthmus flow (e.g., left ventricular inflow and outflow tract obstructive lesions), there is a very high prevalence of coarctation. Up to 75 per cent of cases of aortic atresia have associated coarctation of the aorta.[43,80]

The association of coarctation of the aorta with anomalies with intracardiac communications such as VSD, atrial septal defect, atrioventricular septal defect, and transposition of the great arteries is well known. An unusual type of VSD, so-called malalignment VSD, has a high association with aortic arch anomalies.[44,49,78] As the name implies, there is a malalignment between the conus septum and septal band. The septal insertion of the conus septum extends along the posterior edge of the defect into the left ventricle[49] where it functionally obstructs the anterior portion of the left ventricular outflow tract and thus may decrease antegrade aortic flow. The malaligned VSD is in a subpulmonic location, and pulmonary artery ductal flow is increased. This type of VSD is more frequently associated with interrupted aortic arch, especially type B, than with coarctation.[77] The malaligned VSD is the mirror image of that seen in tetralogy of Fallot, in which the infundibular septum is to the right and anterior, the VSD is in a subaortic position, blood flow to the aorta during fetal life is increased, and aortic coarctation does not occur.[44]

Atrioventricular septal defects may produce decreased antegrade aortic flow by functionally obstructing the subaortic area[20] or by obligatory left ventricular to right atrial shunting in fetal life.[63] In one study, all hearts with narrowing of the aorta and transposition of the great vessels had right ventricular inflow tract obstruction, represented by tricuspid valve hypoplasia, or right ventricular outflow tract obstruction, represented by malaligned VSD or redundant muscle tissue.[47] These defects presumably caused decreased aortic flow during morphogenesis.

Decreased antegrade aortic flow, with increased pulmonary artery and ductal flow, is the essential prerequisite to the hemodynamic theory of coarctation. Hutchins first noted that the coarctation shelf resembled a branch point of the normal aorta with the apex of the infolding dorsal aortic wall opposite the aortic end of the ductus.[30] He theorized that this apex was created by division of the ductal blood flow into the proximal and distal aorta. For retrograde perfusion of the ascending aorta via the ductus to be possible, ductal flow must be greater than ascending aortic flow.

A spectrum of abnormalities can occur as a result of decreased antegrade aortic flow, depending on the relative proportions of aortic and ductal blood flow.[22] On one end of the spectrum is aortic atresia, in which there is essentially no antegrade aortic flow and all segments of the arch are supplied by retrograde flow through the ductus. When the lesion obstructing antegrade arch flow is not so severe, the brachiocephalic and left common carotid arteries are supplied by antegrade flow. The aortic isthmus and left subclavian artery are supplied by retrograde flow from the ductus. The area between the left common carotid artery and left subclavian artery carries little blood flow and may be hypoplastic or even atretic. Occasionally, the aortic isthmus area may be hypoplastic or atretic. When antegrade aortic flow is only mildly compromised, a juxtaductal shelf may develop without any significant tubular hypoplasia.

The hemodynamic theory of reduced antegrade aortic flow is the most unifying theory proposed to explain the three essential features of the coarctation syndrome, that is, the localized shelf, associated intracardiac defects, and tubular hypoplasia.[22] However, the idea that ectopic ductal tissue is present in the aorta and its constriction produces the localized lesion has persisted through the years (Skodaic theory). The latter explanation has not gained wide acceptance because of several factors[15,33]: (1)

the area of medial thickening is opposite the ductal insertion site, not adjacent to it; (2) the ductus frequently is patent in the presence of a clear localized obstruction; (3) the theory does not explain the frequent occurrence of transverse arch hypoplasia; and (4) many investigators cannot find ductal tissue histologically in the coarctation area.[30] However, other investigators have found a sling of ductal tissue around the aortic isthmus orifice.[27]

PATHOPHYSIOLOGY

Isolated Coarctation of the Aorta

Isolated coarctation of the aorta may be associated with a patent foramen ovale and/or patent ductus arteriosus (PDA). Significant preductal coarctations, with the right ventricle supplying a substantial portion of distal systemic blood flow through the PDA, will have a pathophysiology similar to that of complex coarctations. The following discussion applies to isolated coarctation with postductal physiology in which the left ventricle becomes the main systemic pumping chamber shortly after birth.

The pathophysiology will depend on four factors: (1) the severity of the constriction, (2) the presence and extent of collateral circulation, (3) the rapidity of closure of the ductus, and (4) the location of coarctation.

In utero, both the right ventricle and left ventricle are exposed to the high afterload imposed by the constrictive lesion. The right ventricle, since it is the dominant pumping chamber in utero, will hypertrophy in response to the increased afterload, which accounts for the right ventricular hypertrophy present initially in young infants with isolated coarctation of the aorta. If the coarctation is not severe, this compensatory mechanism should ensure adequate distal perfusion in utero. If the constrictive lesion is severe and located distal to the insertion of the ductus arteriosus, collateral circulation must develop in utero to enable survival of the fetus. Collateral circulation has been demonstrated in the first few weeks of life in infants with severe isolated coarctation of the aorta,[25,33] presumably reflecting in utero development of collateral vessels. Matthew and colleagues showed well-developed collateral circulation on angiography in 89 per cent of a small series of children under 2 years of age with isolated coarctation of the aorta.[45] Poor collateral circulation undoubtedly contributes to the death of infants with isolated coarctation of the aorta.[3]

After birth, the left ventricle assumes the burden of the increased afterload imposed by the coarctation. Several compensatory mechanisms come into play to ensure adequate perfusion to the lower half of the body.[51] These include elevation of the systolic pressure in the proximal aortic segment, vasoconstriction of systemic arterioles to maintain a high diastolic pressure, and bypassing the obstruction by means of collateral vessels. The ductus plays an important role in the sequence of pathophysiologic events. Closure of the ductus proceeds progressively from the pulmonary to the aortic end during the first 1 to 2 weeks of life.[63] As the aortic end of the ductus closes, blood can no longer bypass the coarctation by traversing the distal lumen of the ductus to reach the descending aorta.[74] If the constrictive lesion is severe and the compensatory mechanisms are not adequate, sudden left ventricular failure may follow closure of the aortic end of the ductus.

Graham and colleagues[24] have studied by angiography and echocardiography the hemodynamic events leading to congestive heart failure in infants with isolated coarctation of the aorta. In infants presenting with heart failure in the first 2 weeks of life, all had a normal-sized left ventricle, but decreased left ventriclular systolic output and diminished ejection fraction. Cardiomegaly was due to right-sided heart enlargement secondary to left-to-right atrial shunting, pulmonary hypertension, or possibly a more distensible right ventricle. Thus, the constrictive lesion, suddenly exacerbated by a closing ductus, imposes an afterload increase on an inadequately prepared left ventricle, resulting in biventricular failure. Echocardiographic measurements of left ventricular pump function became normal in all postoperative patients, indicating that the afterload-related decrease in pump function was not permanent.

In contrast, in older infants, 1 to 7 months of age, there was much less impairment of left-sided heart function and left ventricular muscle mass was increased. These infants develop heart failure with right-sided heart enlargement and, to a lesser degree, left-sided heart enlargement. In these infants, the elevated afterload had been overcome by the left ventricular hypertrophy.[24]

Complex Coarctation of the Aorta

Associated lesions play a major role in the pathophysiology of complex coarctations and often are the major determinants of the natural history. In contrast to isolated coarctation of the aorta, in complex coarctations the right ventricle is the pumping chamber responsible for providing blood flow to the lower body, both prenatally and postnatally. The right ventricular pressure is near or at systemic levels and pulmonary hypertension is invariably present. Shunting of blood will occur through great vessel communications (e.g., PDA) or intracardiac communications (e.g., VSD, atrial septal defect).

Again, the ductus arteriosus plays a pivotal role in the pathophysiology of complex coarctations. When the ductus is patent, blood flows to the lower extremities. The direction of blood flow through the ductus, however, depends on the respective pressures and resistances in the pulmonary and systemic circuits. The pressure and peripheral resistance in the descending aorta are usually higher than that in the pulmonary artery.[33] Thus, during catheterization and angiography, the most common pattern of blood flow is antegrade through the coarctation and then left-to-right from aorta to pulmonary artery through the ductus.[33] However, right-to-left blood flow from the pulmonary artery to the aorta through the ductus may occur when pulmonary vascular resistance exceeds systemic vascular resistance.

The direction of ductal flow in patients with coarctation has been studied using Doppler echocardiography. Cloez

and colleagues[10] evaluated 58 patients with preductal coarctation of the aorta, interrupted aortic arch, and aortic valve atresia. They found two major ductal flow patterns, distinguished by the size of the ductus arteriosus. With a large patent ductus arteriosus, bidirectional flow was present, with right-to-left shunting occurring in early systole and left-to-right shunting beginning in late systole and extending into late diastole. The ductal shunting pattern corresponded to the variation in pressure gradient between the descending aorta and the pulmonary artery. The right-to-left pattern of shunt flow always corresponded to systemic right ventricular pressures and severe pulmonary hypertension.

However, when the ductus was nearly closed, as shown by echocardiography and diminished femoral pulses, only a small, turbulent, continuous flow directed toward the descending aorta was found. As the ductus closes, the infant may be in extremis and will need ductal reopening with prostaglandins or immediate surgery.[10]

Associated lesions add to the hemodynamic burden of coarctation. Intracardiac communications (most commonly VSD) will add a volume and pressure overload to the right ventricle. Reductions in left ventricular output as a result of left ventricular outflow obstructions and mitral regurgitation will require increased pressure work by the right ventricle to provide flow distal to the coarctation. A long segment of tubular hypoplasia produces additional hemodynamic burden and is always associated with an additional intracardiac communication or obstructive lesion.[4] The presence or absence of a collateral circulation probably has little influence on the pathophysiology of complex coarctations. It was assumed at one time that collateral circulation did not develop in infants with complex coarctations, since the impetus to develop such a circulation (i.e., upper body hypertension) would not be present in the fetus. Consequently, with closure of the ductus, an inadequate collateral circulation would result in the infant's death. However, most cases of heart failure and many deaths in infancy occur while the ductus is still patent.[33] Hypertension in the upper extremities is present in the majority of infants with coarctation of the aorta in the first week of life, regardless of location.[11,33] Collateral circulation has been demonstrated in the majority of infants with preductal coarctation.[33,45]

CLINICAL FEATURES

The majority of infants with coarctation of the aorta who present for medical attention in the first year of life will have signs and symptoms of congestive heart failure. Most infants will have complex coarctations, but 15 to 20 per cent of cases with isolated coarctation of the aorta will present in this manner.[51] Although a few infants may be diagnosed because of an asymptomatic murmur or upper body hypertension, their subsequent clinical course will not be discussed in this section.

Dyspnea, irritability, failure to thrive, and feeding difficulties are the hallmarks of presentation. In general, those infants with tubular hypoplasia of the aorta and associated severe anomalies tend to present the earliest.

With isolated coarctation, the time of presentation frequently is related to the time of closure of the aortic end of the ductus, which is usually within 7 to 14 days. The infant will appear tachypneic and may have an ashen gray color related to low cardiac output.[11] Cyanosis may be present in up to one half of these infants,[9] either due to a common mixing lesion or low cardiac output. Differential cyanosis (i.e., cyanosis of the toes and left hand with pink right hand and mucous membranes) may occur with complex coarctation and right-to-left shunt via the ductus arteriosus. However, differential cyanosis is uncommon because of the following: (1) complex coarctations frequently have additional intracardiac anomalies with bidirectional shunting that will increase the saturation of blood in the right ventricle and minimize any saturation difference between preductal and postductal locations; (2) in preductal coarctation with widely patent ductus, the ductal flow is either predominantly left-to-right or bidirectional, which again should minimize saturation differences.

DIAGNOSIS

Physical Examination

On palpation, a right ventricular impulse is apparent in coarctation due to right ventricular hypertrophy. Auscultation usually reveals a nonspecific systolic ejection murmur along the left sternal border.[11] Continuous murmurs are uncommon,[33] even though the vast majority of these infants have a patent ductus at the time of presentation. The second heart sound is usually loud and only narrowly split. When cardiac output is low, no murmurs are present. A gallop rhythm, pulmonary rales, and hepatomegaly are usually present. Mild edema of the eyelids and dorsum of the hands and feet is sometimes seen.[11]

Careful palpation of the pulses and blood pressure determinations by Doppler ultrasound techniques in both arms and one leg are essential to the diagnosis of coarctation. Variations in the position of the subclavian arteries in relation to the coarctation account for differences in upper extremity blood pressure. When the origin of the left subclavian artery is involved in the coarctation lesion, right arm pressure will be higher. The reverse situation occurs when the right subclavian artery arises aberrantly distal to the coarctation of the aorta site.

In most cases of coarctation, both complex and isolated, the upper extremities will have elevated blood pressures, with corresponding hypotension in the legs.[11] The differences are found in the systolic pressures with gradients ranging from 20 to 140 mmHg.[22] In general, the higher gradients are found with isolated coarctation of the aorta.

The arterial pulsations and blood pressures in coarctation will be similar in all four extremities in at least three different situations: (1) In preductal coarctation with marked tubular hypoplasia and intracardiac communications, the right ventricular pressure will be systemic since it provides blood flow to the lower extremities via the ductus; there will be low, but equal, systolic pressures in the left ventricle, right ventricle, ascending aorta, descending aorta, and ductus. (2) The infant with isolated coarctation of the aorta may present in a low-output state secondary to biventricular failure; pressures in all four extremities will be low and only following inotropic support does left ventricular output increase enough to produce a pressure gradient between upper and lower extremities. (3) In rare cases, when the coarctation of the aorta is proximal to the left subclavian artery with aberrant origin of the right subclavian artery distal to the coarctation of the aorta, both brachial and femoral pulsations will be weak and equal and the carotid and temporal pulsations are correspondingly stronger.[70]

Echocardiography

Echocardiography has proved useful in the diagnosis and management of patients with coarctation of the aorta.[13,29,65,70,81] This procedure is helpful especially in complex cases, when associated defects (e.g., transposition of great arteries or single ventricle) assume major importance or when heart failure obscures the usual clinical signs. Doppler echocardiography has added to the reliability of noninvasive studies by confirming the diagnosis made by two-dimensional echocardiography and even suggesting the diagnosis when cross-sectional echocardiography is inconclusive.[59]

Two-dimensional echocardiography has been especially useful in defining associated anomalies in coarctation of the aorta. Smallhorn and coworkers have been able to define the type and position of ventricular septal defects.[69] They have shown that large perimembranous defects frequently are associated with aortic override and abnormally high insertion of the tricuspid valve. This high insertion of the tricuspid valve, along with high right ventricular pressure, allows tricuspid valve tissue to be forced through the defect during systole, obscuring the defect and narrowing the left ventricular outflow tract. Malalignment defects, which are less common than perimembranous defects,[69] also consistently narrow the left ventricular outflow tract by posterior displacement of the infundibular septum.

Left ventricular inflow tract abnormalities are difficult to assess at catheterization but may be seen on echocardiography. Using two-dimensional echocardiography, Celano[8] noted a high prevalence of mitral valve anomalies that had previously been documented only on autopsy studies.[62] Although there was excellent correlation of two-dimensional echocardiography with angiography for major mitral valve abnormalities, the technique was more sensitive than angiography in identifying minor mitral valve anomalies (e.g., anomalous chordae, papillary muscle abnormalities, and eccentric valve position).

In infants with coarctation of the aorta, an associated patent ductus arteriosus cannot be readily detected clinically; however, in some instances associated patent ductus arteriosus can be imaged by two-dimensional echocardiography from the suprasternal notch.[71] Doppler studies have proved useful in detecting patterns of blood flow in the patent ductus.[10]

Latson and associates have noted that the echocardiographic estimate of left ventricular size has accurately predicted mortality in infants with severe left ventricular outflow

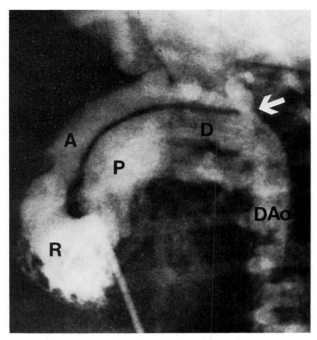

Figure 37–1. Right ventriculogram in a patient with transposition of the great arteries and ventricular septal defect. The narrow aorta comes off the right ventricle anterior to a large dilated pulmonary artery. Note the aortic arch hypoplasia proximal to a discrete coarctation lesion (arrow). A large patent ductus arteriosus continues directly into the descending aorta. A = ascending aorta; D = ductus arteriosus; DAo = descending aorta; P = pulmonary artery; R = right ventricle.

obstruction.[37] Wing and colleagues followed medically managed infants with isolated coarctation of the aorta using serial M-mode echocardiography; left ventricular function appeared to improve as the left ventricle grew and hypertrophied, and right ventricular size diminished toward normal.[83]

Cardiac Catheterization

Physiology of Postductal Coarctation

In the absence of heart failure, a gradient of varying degrees will be present across the site of coarctation. Left ventricular and ascending aortic systolic pressures will be elevated. Although a bicuspid aortic valve is a frequent finding, a significant gradient across the valve is rarely present. With increasing degrees of afterload imposed on the left ventricle, left ventricular end-diastolic and left atrial pressures will rise; frequently a left-to-right atrial shunt through a stretched foramen ovale is present. Right-sided pressures will depend on several factors, including the degree of left-to-right shunting at both the ductal and atrial levels and the magnitude of pulmonary vascular resistance. The combination of pressure and volume overload may produce marked dilatation, mainly of the right-sided chambers.

With severe coarctation and rapid closure of the ductus, biventricular failure will quickly ensue; in such cases, a

gradient may not be present across the coarcted area, and left ventricular, ascending aortic, and descending aortic systolic pressures will be similar and low.

In the absence of heart failure or significant intrapulmonary shunting, left-sided heart and aortic saturations are normal. Right-sided heart saturations are elevated secondary to left-to-right shunting at the atrial or ductal levels.

Physiology of Preductal Coarctation

With the right ventricle supplying at least a portion of blood to the lower body through the ductus, much will depend on the status of the ductus. With a widely patent ductus, the systolic pressures in the right ventricle, main pulmonary artery, ascending aorta, descending aorta, and left ventricle are similar. With gradual closure of the ductus, a gradient will develop between the main pulmonary artery and descending aorta. With ductal closure, both ventricles will experience increased pressure work as well as volume overload via intracardiac communications (i.e., VSD, stetched foramen ovale) and cardiac failure supervenes.

Saturations throughout the heart will reflect bidirectional shunting through intracardiac and/or ductal communications. Differential cyanosis (i.e., lower saturations in the lower body as compared with the upper) may occur secondary to desaturated blood supplied to the lower body from the right ventricle. In the case of transposition of the great arteries associated with coarctation of the aorta, the reverse situation may occur, with upper body saturations lower than those of the lower body. Clinically, this phenomenon is rarely observed, either because a substantial portion of deoxygenated blood from the higher aorta does cross the coarcted area to reach the descending aorta or because of intracardiac communications that decrease the partial pressure of oxygen (PO_2) of pulmonary blood supplied to the descending aorta.

Angiography

Left ventricular angiography in oblique views is the most useful injection in infancy to demonstrate both the coarctation of the aorta and the associated lesions (Figs. 37–1 and 37–2). The papillary muscles and chordae tendinae can be examined. The left ventricular outflow tract, a common site of narrowing, frequently is shown to advantage in this view. The size, location, and number of VSDs must be determined. The size and function of the left ventricle can be examined. A bicuspid aortic valve may be demonstrated. With sufficient amounts of contrast material, the coarctation site is well delineated. If the PDA, pulmonary artery, and descending aorta fill from the left ventricular injection only after contrast medium has traversed the aortic arch and no VSD is present, the left ventricle is probably supplying lower body blood flow in a postductal arrangement.[22] However, a preductal location of the coarctation is implied when the right ventricular injection opacifies the descending aorta from the patent ductus arteriosus. Left ventricular contrast injection will usually demonstrate the anatomy of the aortic arch.

Collateral vessels may be demonstrated even in infancy, being more prevalent with isolated postductal coarctation than with complex coarctations.[46]

DIFFERENTIAL DIAGNOSIS

The diagnosis of coarctation usually is not difficult when one diligently palpates pulses and measures blood pressures in upper and lower extremities. The diagnosis should always be expected and excluded in infants presenting in heart failure, whether they are acyanotic or cyanotic.

Diagnosis of coarctation is most difficult when congestive heart failure has developed because arterial pressure gradients between the upper and lower extremities are often reduced or absent. Additionally, associated lesions (e.g., double-outlet right ventricle or transposition of the great arteries) or cyanosis may dominate the clinical picture, leading one away from considering the presence of coarctation of the aorta.

Although most infants with coarctation of the aorta and no major associated defects do not become symptomatic until the second postnatal week, occasionally they may present within the first several days of life with signs and symptoms consistent with persistent pulmonary hypertension of the newborn syndrome (PPHNS). Cyanosis, heart failure, lack of differential blood pressures, and marked differences in PO_2 between the umbilical and the right radial artery secondary to desaturated right ventricular blood perfusing the lower body via the PDA may be present.[41] The diagnosis of coarctation should be suspected on two-dimensional echocardiography in infants with PPHNS if left-to-right bulging of the atrial septum (secondary to elevated left atrial pressures in coarctation) is present; in infants with idiopathic PPHNS and PPHNS secondary to lung disease, the atrial septum bulges right to left.[41] In most cases, the coarctation of the aorta is demonstrated with two-dimensional echocardiography, but in a few cases, accurate diagnosis requires cardiac catheterization.

Interrupted aortic arch, especially type A, can be difficult to distinguish from preductal coarctation echocardiographically,[13] but the differentiation may not be clinically important since both will require early surgical exploration and relief of the aortic arch obstruction.

Hypoplastic left-heart syndrome generally presents earlier as severe heart failure. Pulses tend to be weak in all four extremities. Electrocardiograms and chest radiographs may be similar to those of preductal coarctation of the aorta. Two-dimensional echocardiography will demonstrate the mitral and/or aortic valvular abnormalities and frequently an associated coarctation.

Aortic stenosis is a rare cause of heart failure in the newborn. Left ventricular hypertrophy on electrocardiography is consistent with aortic stenosis and rare with isolated coarctation. Doppler echocardiography has been used to distinguish the two lesions.[59]

Primary endocardial and myocardial diseases may present with signs and symptoms similar to coarctation of the

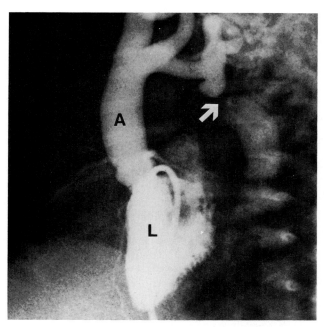

Figure 37–2. Left ventriculogram. The ventricular septum is intact. The transverse aortic arch is mildly hypoplastic. There is a severe discrete coarctation (arrow) distal to the left subclavian artery. Multiple collateral vessels are present. A = ascending aorta; L = left ventricle.

aorta.[22] Careful echocardiographic evaluation of the aortic arch should lead to the correct diagnosis.

MANAGEMENT

Infants with coarctation of the aorta may require general supportive measures and intravenous therapy, depending on the severity of the coarctation. Digoxin may be used to treat mild heart failure, but infants in severe heart failure are better managed using diuretics and intravenous inotropic agents such as dobutamine or dopamine, which can be titrated to the clinical response. Endotracheal intubation frequently is required.

Prostaglandin E_1 (PGE_1) opens the ductus arteriosus and allows the infant to reach a referral hospital.[58] The effects of PGE_1 in a group of 107 acyanotic ductal-dependent lesions, 80 of whom had coarctations or interrupted aortic arch, have been reported.[19] Seventy per cent of these infants were under 10 days of age. Neither pre-infusion PO_2 nor age is critical for response to PGE_1 in acyanotic patients. The maximal response to PGE_1 in acyanotic patients is 1½ hours, with a range of 15 minutes to 4 hours. Favorable responses to PGE_1 include an increase in lower body perfusion, an increase in urine output, a decrease in the amount of base needed to correct metabolic acidosis, and a decrease in pressure gradients between the main pulmonary artery and the descending aorta.[19]

Leoni and associates[39] have documented how the salutary effects of PGE_1 have affected subsequent outcome in critically ill neonates with coarctation of the aorta. In a group of 52 neonates, all 14 infants who received preoperative PGE$_1$ survived surgical correction. On the other hand, only 71 per cent (27/38) who did not receive preoperative PGE$_1$ survived surgery. The two groups were comparable with respect to coagulopathy, urgency of operation, associated anomalies, and other medical treatment.

Another advance in the management of critically ill neonates is the diagnostic reliability of echocardiography, which may obviate the need for cardiac catheterization. Echocardiography has a high sensitivity and specificity in diagnosing aortic arch anomalies.[13,29,70] Combined clinical and echocardiographic assessment allows selected infants and neonates with coarctation to have surgery without prior invasive studies.[42]

In recent years, balloon angioplasty has been advocated as an alternative to surgical repair in some infants. The initial enthusiasm for percutaneous transluminal angioplasty (PTA) was tempered by a knowledge of the high rate of recurrence of coarctation of the aorta after surgical repair. PTA was considered for initial treatment and also for restenosis after surgery. However, despite some initial improvement in infantile coarctations after PTA,[12,17,36,72] most studies have shown no lasting benefit.[60] Deaths related to perforation of the aorta in infants after PTA have been reported.[12,17] Because of the lack of lasting benefit and risk of mortality associated with this procedure, PTA has been abandoned by many as a primary therapeutic option in neonates.[60] Others have found PTA in symptomatic neonatal coarctation to be safe and effective palliation (see Chapter 56). PTA has been more impressive in patients with recoarctation.[1,32] The periaortic scarring at the restenosed coarctation site provides a limiting factor to contain bleeding from disruption of the aortic wall.[32]

MEDICAL OUTCOME

Despite substantial improvement in medical management, the treatment is primarily surgical. The major impetus to surgical correction came from the poor prognosis with medical management, with 85 to 90 per cent mortality in those under 4 weeks of age presenting in congestive heart failure.[23,67] In the neonatal period, the majority of patients have complex coarctation with extensive aortic arch hypoplasia.

The natural history of isolated coarctation of the aorta is better than that of coarctation of the aorta with associated lesions.[7] Approximately 5 per cent of patients with isolated coarctation will develop intractable congestive heart failure within the first weeks of life and will certainly die without surgical intervention.[35] Another 10 per cent present in less severe congestive heart failure between 1 and 6 months of age, and a few of these might survive into early childhood without operation.[35] Eighty-five per cent of patients with isolated coarctation of the aorta should live to adulthood.[35]

SURGICAL OUTCOME

At present, the most widely used operation for infantile coarctation of the aorta has been the subclavian flap aortoplasty technique. In some cases unsuitable for this technique, patch aortoplasty has been used. These two techniques have substantially lower rates of recoarctation, which is a significant problem with end-to-end anastomosis.[2,46,50,57]

Besides the technical considerations of the type of coarctation repair and subsequent end result, other surgical management issues revolve around how to deal with the associated anomalies at the time of initial surgery. With the most common intracardiac problem (i.e., VSD) it must be decided whether to band the pulmonary artery at the time of surgery, repair the VSD along with the coarctation, or repair the coarctation and observe closely for improvement or persistent congestive heart failure. Most centers now use the latter option and will repair the VSD promptly if symptoms do not improve after coarctation repair.[52] Regardless of initial size, the VSD tends to decrease in size or to disappear.[52]

Hospital mortality for repair of isolated coarctation is 3 to 4 per cent,[35,82] whereas hospital mortality for coarctation with associated defects ranges from 24 to 32 per cent.[35,82] Incremental risk factors for hospital mortality include (1) associated cardiac anomalies other than VSD; (2) age (small size), especially with major anomalies; and (3) preoperative functional status.[35] Some groups have noted an increased risk of mortality with VSDs, with mortality rates of 22 to 25 per cent.[26,82] Factors associated with significantly increased mortality in patients with VSDs include young age, elevated atrial and ventricular end-diastolic pressures, low weight, high admission blood urea nitrogen, preoperative ventilation, and large VSDs.[38] The most common causes of hospital death are postoperative cardiac failure and respiratory complications.[35]

Of all hospital survivors, 83 per cent are alive at 15-year follow-up. The survival rate is best for primary coarctation (92 per cent), less for coarctation with VSD (81 per cent), and poor for those with coarctation and major lesions (41 per cent at 3 years).[35] In one study dealing with coarctation of the aorta and transposition of the great arteries, it is clear that the presence of coarctation adversely affects the survival.[79] A 5-year survival rate of 57 per cent was noted for transposition of the great arteries and coarctation, whereas during the same time period at the same institution the 5-year survival rate for uncomplicated transposition of the great arteries was 89 per cent.[79]

Long-term morbidity includes recoarctation, which occurs in from 16 to 54 per cent of cases, including all types of repairs.[5] The subclavian flap technique and patch aortoplasty have improved the prognosis but not alleviated the problem of recoarctation. The restenosis rate is much higher when the initial operation is performed in infancy, regardless of the type of repair.[35,40,55]

Other morbidity includes the development of aortic or mitral valve disease. In Kirklin's series,[35] 7 per cent of patients with coarctation repaired in infancy have required surgery for subvalvular or valvular aortic stenosis at 3 to 7 years of age. The majority of patients with associated congenital mitral valve disease have not required mitral valve replacement during childhood.[14,18]

The prognosis has improved markedly with the advances in medical and surgical treatment. However, significant morbidity and mortality remain and these patients will require lifelong medical surveillance.

Surgery for neonatal coarctation is considered more fully in Chapter 62.

References

1. Allen HD, Marx GR, Ovitt TW (1985): Balloon angioplasty for coarctation: Serial evaluation. J Am Coll Cardiol 5:405(abstract).
2. Allen RG, Maria-Garcia J, Nayek G (1980): Methods of management and results following surgery for coarctation of the aorta in infancy. J Pediatr Surg 15:953–960.
3. Bahn RC, Edwards JE, DuShane JW (1951): Coarctation of the aorta as a cause of death in early infancy. Pediatrics 8:192–203.
4. Becker AE, Becker MJ, Edwards JE (1970): Anomalies associated with coarctation of the aorta (particular reference to infancy). Circulation 41:1067–1075.
5. Beekman RH, Rocchini AP, Behrendt DM, Rosenthal A (1981): Reoperation for coarctation of the aorta. Am J Cardiol 48:1108–1114.
6. Boon AR, Roberts DF (1976): A family study of coarctation of the aorta. J Med Genet 13:420–433.
7. Campbell M (1970): Natural history of coarctation of the aorta. Br Heart J 32:633–640.
8. Celano V, Pieroni DR, Morera JA, Roland JMA, Gingell RL (1984): Two-dimensional echocardiographic examination of mitral valve abnormalities associated with coarctation of the aorta. Circulation 69:924–932.
9. Chang JHT, Burrington JD (1972): Coarctation of the aorta in infants and children. J Pediatr Surg 7:127–135.
10. Cloez JL, Isaaz K, Pernot C (1986): Pulsed Doppler flow characteristics of ductus arteriosus in infants with associated congenital anomalies of the heart or great arteries. Am J Cardiol 57:845–851.
11. Colodney NM, Carson MJ (1950): Coarctation of the aorta in early infancy. J Pediatr 37:46–77.
12. deLezo JS, Fernandez R, Sancho M, Concha M, Arizon J, Franco M, Alemany F, Barcones F, Lopez-Rubio F, Valles F (1984): Percutaneous transluminal angioplasty for aortic isthmus coarctation in infancy. Am J Cardiol 54:1147–1149.
13. Duncan WJ, Ninomiya K, Cook DH, Rowe RD (1983): Noninvasive diagnosis of neonatal coarctation and associated anomalies using two-dimensional echocardiography. Am Heart J 106:63–69.
14. Easthope RN, Tawes RL, Bonham-Carter RE, Aberdeen E, Waterston DJ (1969): Congenital mitral valve disease associated with coarctation of the aorta. Am Heart J 77:743–754.
15. Edwards JE, Christensen NA, Clagett OT, McDonald JR (1984): Pathologic considerations in coarctation of the aorta. Proc Staff Meet Mayo Clin 23:324–332.
16. Ferencz C, Rubin JD, McCarter RJ, Brenner JI, Neill CA, Perry LW, Hepner SI, Downing JW (1985): Congenital heart disease: Prevalence at live birth. Am J Epidemiol 121:31–36.
17. Finley JP, Beauliea RG, Nanton MA, Roy DL (1983): Balloon catheter dilatation of coarctation of the aorta in young infants. Br Heart J 50:411–415.
18. Freed MD, Keane JF, Van Praagh R, Castenada AR, Bernhard WF, Nadas AS (1974): Coarctation of the aorta with congenital mitral regurgitation. Circulation 49:1175–1184.
19. Freed MD, Heymann MA, Lewis AB, Roehl SL, Kensey RC (1981): Prostaglandin E₁ in infants with ductus arteriosus–dependent congenital heart disese. Circulation 64:899–905.
20. Freedom RM, Dische MR, Rowe RD (1977): Pathologic anatomy of subaortic stenosis and atresia in the first year of life. Am J Cardiol 39:1035–1044.
21. Fyler DC (1980): Report of the New England regional infant cardiac program. Pediatrics 64(suppl):376–461.
22. Gersony WM (1983): Coarctation of the aorta. In Adams FH, Emmanouilides GC (eds): Heart Disease in Infants, Children, and Adolescents. 3rd ed. Baltimore, Williams & Wilkins, pp 190–193.
23. Glass IH, Mustard WT, Keith JD (1960): Coarctation of the aorta in infants: A review of twelve years' experience. Pediatrics 26:109–121.
24. Graham TP, Atwood GF, Boerth RC, Boucek RJ, Smith CW (1977): Right and left heart size and function in infants with symptomatic coarctation. Circulation 56:641–647.
25. Hallidie-Smith KA (1972): Postductal coarctation of aorta causing myocardial ischemia and heart failure in first week of life. Arch Dis Child 47:719–724.
26. Hammon JW, Graham TP, Boucek RJ, Bender HW (1985): Operative repair of coarctation of the aorta in infancy: Results with and without ventricular septal defect. Am J Cardiol 55:1555–1559.
27. Ho SY, Anderson RH (1979): Coarctation, tubular hypoplasia, and the ductus arteriosus: Histological study of 35 specimens. Br Heart J 41:268–274.
28. Honey M, Lincoln JCR, Osborne MP, DeBono DP (1975): Coarctation of aorta with right aortic arch: Report of surgical correction in two cases: one with associated anomalous origin of left circumflex coronary artery from the right pulmonary artery. Br Heart J 37:937–945.
29. Huhta JC, Gutgesell HP, Latson LA, Huffines FD (1984): Two-dimensional echocardiographic assessment of the aorta in infants and children with congenital heart disease. Circulation 70:417–424.
30. Hutchins GM (1971): Coarctation of the aorta explained as a branch point of the ductus arteriosus. Am J Pathol 63:203–209.
31. Kamau P, Miles V, Toews W, Kelminson L, Friesen R, Lockhart C, Butterfield J, Hernandez J, Hawes CR, Pappas G (1981): Surgical repair of coarctation of the aorta in infants less than six months of age: Including the question of pulmonary artery banding. J Thorac Cardiovasc Surg 81:171–179.
32. Kan JS, White RI, Mitchell SE, Farmlett EJ, Donahoo JS, Gardner TJ (1983): Treatment of restenosis of coarctation by percutaneous transluminal angioplasty. Circulation 68:1087–1094.
33. Keith JD (1978): Coarctation of the aorta. In Keith JD, Rowe JD, Vlad P (eds): Heart Disease in Infancy and Childhood. New York, Macmillan, pp 6–8, 736–754.
34. Kennedy A, Taylor DG, Durrant TE (1979): Pathology of the intima in coarctation of the aorta: A study using light and scanning electron microscopy. Thorax 34:366–374.
35. Kirklin JW, Barratt-Boyes BG: Cardiac Surgery. New York, John Wiley & Sons, pp 1036–1070.
36. Lababidi ZA, Daskalopoulos DA, Stoeckle H (1984): Transluminal balloon coarctation angioplasty: Experience with 27 patients. Am J Cardiol 54:1288–1291.
37. Latson LA, Cheatham JP, Gutgesell HP (1981): Relation of the echocardiographic estimate of left ventricular size to mortality in infants with severe left ventricular outflow obstruction. Am J Cardiol 48:887–891.
38. Leanage R, Taylor JFN, DeLeval MR, Stark J, Macartney FJ (1981): Surgical management of coarctation of aorta with ventricular septal defect. Br Heart J 46:269–277.
39. Leoni F, Huhta JC, Douglas J, MacKay R, DeLeval MR, Macartney FJ, Stark J (1984): Effect of prostaglandin on early surgical mortality in obstructive lesions of the systemic circulation. Br Heart J 52:654–659.
40. Liberthson RR, Pennington DG, Jacobs ML, Daggett WM (1979): Coarctation of the aorta: Review of 234 patients and clarification of management problems. Am J Cardiol 43:835–840.
41. Long WA (1984): Structural cardiovascular abnormalities presenting as persistent pulmonary hypertension of the newborn. In Philips JB (ed): Symposium on neonatal pulmonary hypertension. Clin Perinatol 11:601–626.
42. Macartney F, Douglas J. Spiegelhalter D (1984): To catheterise or not to catheterise? An approach based on decision theory. Br Heart J 51:330–338.
43. Mahowald JM, Lucas RV, Edwards JE (1982): Aortic valvular atresia: Associated cardiovascular anomalies. Pediatr Cardiol 2:99–105.
44. Marino B, Chiariello L, Mercanti C, Bosman C, Colloridi V, Reale A, Marino B (1981): Morphology of aortic arch obstruction with patent ductus arteriosus. Cardiovasc Dis Bull Texas Heart Inst 8:238–249.

45. Matthew R, Simon G, Joseph M (1972): Collateral circulation in coarctation of the aorta in infancy and childhood. Arch Dis Child 47:950–953.

46. Midgley FM, Scott LP, Perry LW, Shapiro SR, McClenathan JE (1978): Subclavian flap aortoplasty for treatment of coarctation in early infancy. J Pediatr Surg 13:265–268.

47. Moene RJ, Ottenkamp J, Oppenheimer-Dekker A, Bartelings MM (1985): Transposition of the great arteries and narrowing of the aortic arch: Emphasis on right ventricular characteristics. Br Heart J 53:58–63.

48. Moerman P, Goddeeris P, Lauwerijns J, Van Der Hauwaert LG (1980): Cardiovascular malformations in DiGeorge syndrome (congenital absence or hypoplasia of the thymus). Br Heart J 44:452–459.

49. Moulaert AJ, Bruins CC, Oppenheimer-Dekker A (1976): Anomalies of the aortic arch and ventricular septal defects. Circulation 53:1011–1015.

50. Moulton AL, Brenner JI, Roberts G, Tavares S, Ali S, Nordenberg A, Burns JE, Ringel R, Berman MA (1984): Subclavian flap repair of coarctation of the aorta in neonates. J Thorac Cardiovasc Surg 87:220–235.

51. Nadas AS, Fyler DC (1972): Pediatric Cardiology. 3rd ed. Philadelphia, WB Saunders, pp 452–474.

52. Neches WH, Park SC, Lenox CC, Zuberbuhler JR, Siewers RO, Hardesty RL (1977): Coarctation of the aorta with ventricular septal defect. Circulation 55:189–194.

53. Nora JJ, Nora AH (1976): Recurrence risks in children having one parent with a congenital heart disease. Circulation 53:701–702.

54. Nora JJ, Nora AH (1978): The evolution of specific genetic and environmental counseling in congenital heart diseases. Circulation 57:205–213.

55. Patel R, Singh SP, Abrams L, Roberts KD (1977): Coarctation of aorta with special reference to infants. Br Heart J 39:1246–1253.

56. Pellegrino A, Deverall PB, Anderson RH, Smith A, Wilkinson JL, Russo P, Tynan M (1985): Aortic coarctation in the first three months of life: An anatomopathological study with respect to treatment. J Thorac Cardiovasc Surg 89:121–126.

57. Penkoske PA, Williams WG, Olley PM, LeBlanc J, Trusler GA, Moes CAF, Judakin R, Rowe RD (1984): Subclavian arterioplasty: Repair of coarctation of the aorta in the first year of life. J Thorac Cardiovasc Surg 87:894–900.

58. Radford DT, Bloom KR, Coceani F, Fariello R, Olley PM (1976): Prostaglandin E_1 for interrupted aortic arch in the neonate. Lancet 2:95.

59. Robinson PJ, Wyse RKH, Deafield JE, Franklin R, Macartney FJ (1984): Continuous wave Doppler velocimetry as an adjunct to cross-sectional echocardiography in the diagnosis of critical left heart obstruction in neonates. Br Heart J 52:552–556.

60. Rocchini AP, Kveselis D (1984): The use of balloon angioplasty in the pediatric patient. In Rosenthal A (ed): Symposium on Pediatric Cardiology. Pediatr Clin North Am 31:1293–1305.

61. Rose V, Gold RJM, Lindsay G, Allen M (1985): Possible increase in the incidence of congenital heart defects among the offspring of affected parents. J Am Coll Cardiol 6:376–382.

62. Rosenquist GC (1974): Congenital mitral valve disease associated with coarctation of the aorta: A spectrum that includes parachute deformity of the mitral valve. Circulation 49:985–993.

63. Rudolph AM, Heymann MA, Spitznas V (1972): Hemodynamic considerations in the development of narrowing of the aorta. Am J Cardiol 30:514–525.

64. Rowe RD, Freedom RM, Mehrizi A, Bloom KR (1981): The Neonate with Congenital Heart Disease. 2nd ed. Philadelphia, WB Saunders, pp 166–192.

65. Sahn DJ, Allen HD, McDonald G, Goldberg SJ (1977): Real-time cross-sectional echocardiographic diagnosis of coarctation of the aorta: A prospective study of echocardiographic-angiographic correlations. Circulation 56:762.

66. Shinebourne EA, Elseed AM (1974): Relation between fetal flow patterns, coarctation of the aorta, and pulmonary blood flow. Br Heart J 36:492–498.

67. Shinebourne EA, Tam ASY, Elseed AM, Paneth M, Lennox SC, Cleland WP, Lincoln C, Joseph MC, Anderson RH (1976): Coarctation of the aorta in infancy and childhood. Br Heart J 38:375–380.

68. Sinha SN, Kardatzke ML, Cole RB, Muster AJ, Wessel HU, Paul MH (1969): Coarctation of the aorta in infancy. Circulation 40:385–398.

69. Smallhorn JF, Anderson RH, Macartney FJ (1983): Morphological characterization of ventricular septal defects associated with coarctation of the aorta by cross-sectional echocardiography. Br Heart J 49:485–494.

70. Smallhorn JF, Huhta JC, Adams PA, Anderson RH, Wilkinson JL, Macartney FJ (1983): Cross-sectional echocardiographic assessment of coarctation in the sick neonate and infant. Br Heart J 50:349–361.

71. Smallhorn JF, Huhta JC, Anderson RH, McCartney FJ (1982): Suprasternal cross-sectional echocardiography in assessment of patent ductus arteriosus. Br Heart J 48:321–330.

72. Sperling DR, Dorsey TJ, Rowen M, Gazzaniga AB (1983): Percutaneous transluminal angioplasty of congenital coarctation of the aorta. Am J Cardiol 51:562–564.

73. Subramanian AR (1972): Coarctation or interruption of aorta proximal to origin of both subclavian arteries: Report of three cases presenting in infancy. Br Heart J 34:1225–1226.

74. Talner NS, Berman MA (1974): Postnatal development of obstruction in coarctation of the aorta: Role of the ductus arteriosus. Pediatrics 56:562–569.

75. Tawes RL, Aberdeen E, Waterson DJ, Bonham-Carter RE (1969): Coarctation of the aorta in infants and children: A review of 333 operative cases including 179 infants. Circulation 39–40 (suppl): 173–184.

76. Tawes RL, Berry CL, Aberdeen E (1969): Congenital bicuspid aortic valves associated with coarctation of the aorta in children. Br Heart J 31:127–128.

77. Van Mierop LHS, Kutsche LM (1984): Interruption of the aortic arch and coarctation of the aorta: Pathogenetic relations. Am J Cardiol 54:829–834.

78. VanPraagh R, Bernhard WJ, Rosenthal A, Parisi LF, Fyler DC (1971): Interrupted aortic arch: Surgical treatment. Am J Cardiol 27:200–211.

79. Vogel M, Freedom RM, Smallhorn JF, Williams WG, Trusler GA, Rowe RD (1984): Complete transposition of the great arteries and coarctation of the aorta. Am J Cardiol 53:1627–1632.

80. Von Rueden TJ, Knight L, Moller JH, Edwards JE (1975): Coarctation of the aorta associated with aortic valvular atresia. Circulation 52:951–954.

81. Weyman AE, Caldwell RL, Hurwitz RA, Girod DA, Dillon JC, Feigenbaum H, Green D (1978): Cross-sectional echocardiographic detection of aortic obstruction: II. Coarctation of the aorta. Circulation 67:498–502.

82. Williams WG, Shindo G, Trusler GA, Dische MR, Olley PM (1980): Results of repair of coarctation of the aorta during infancy. J Thorac Cardiovasc Surg 79:603–608.

83. Wing JP, Findlay WA, Sahn DJ, McDonald G, Allen HD, Goldberg SV (1978): Serial echocardiographic profiles in infants with coarctation of the aorta. Am J Cardiol 41:1270–1276.

38 INTERRUPTED AORTIC ARCH

Herbert G. Whitley
Lowell W. Perry

Complete interruption of the aortic arch (IAA) is an uncommon congenital malformation, occurring in 0.003 per 1000 births.[4] IAA is present in 0.175 per cent of clinical cardiac cases in the pediatric age group.[16] However, among infants and autopsy cases, IAA accounts for 1.3 per cent of critical infant cardiac disease and 1.4 per cent of all autopsy cases.[40] There is no sexual predominance.[38] IAA is an absence of anatomic continuity between two segments of the aortic arch. Also included are cases with a fibrous strand connecting two widely separated ends of the aortic arch.[17]

The first case of IAA in which the aortic isthmus portion of the arch was absent was described by Steidele in 1778.[33] In subsequent years, more proximal areas of IAA were described. In 1959, Celoria and Patton classified 28 cases of IAA according to site of obstruction into types A, B, and C.[3]

PATHOLOGY

Type A in Celoria and Patton's classification is interruption of the arch distal to the left subclavian artery and accounts for 42 per cent of all cases.[40] The most common type (53 per cent of all cases[40]) is type B in which the interruption is between the left common carotid artery (LCCA) and left subclavian artery (LSCA). Type C (less than 5 per cent of all cases[40]) occurs between the LCCA and innominate artery. Most are characterized by flow from the ductus arteriosus into the descending aorta except for rare instances in which the ductus closes during fetal life; these latter defects have extensive collateral circulation and frequently are discovered in late childhood or adulthood with clinical signs and symptoms similar to coarctation.[7]

COEXISTING CARDIAC ANOMALIES

A large ventricular septal defect (VSD) is nearly always present in IAA. In 60 per cent of cases, the VSD involves the conal septum and produces conoventricular malalignment resulting in a subpulmonary VSD.[9] The malalignment is in a leftward direction and is the most common mechanism of subaortic stenosis in these patients.[10] Since the VSD is larger than the aortic orifice, the potential for preferential flow to the right ventricle and pulmonary artery is established.[25]

Infracristal defects, atrioventricular septal defects, and muscular defects account for the remaining cases of VSD, and some of these have the potential for subaortic narrowing.[9] Rare cases of IAA with intact ventricular septum nearly always are associated with aortopulmonary window.[9,28]

Numerous other complex cardiac anomalies, including total anomalous pulmonary venous drainage[1] but not tetralogy of Fallot and not pulmonary stenosis, may be associated with IAA. Of particular note is the strong association of IAA with persistent truncus arteriosus and aortopulmonary window.[17] IAA is rare in situs inversus or with l-ventricular loop.[9]

LEFT VENTRICULAR OUTFLOW ANOMALIES

Subaortic stenosis is commonly associated with IAA and usually is secondary to conoventricular malalignment, but sometimes it is due to an adherent mitral valve or accessory endocardial cushion tissue.[10] Subaortic stenosis may not be significant at birth but can become severe after surgical repair and require repeat surgical intervention.[27]

Bicuspid aortic valve occurs in association with IAA with about the same frequency as in coarctation, 30 to 50 per cent,[16,38] although aortic valve stenosis is uncommon (about 12 per cent).[9]

AORTIC ARCH

The ascending aorta is about half its usual diameter in IAA. The main pulmonary artery is dilated. As in the fetus, the descending aorta is a direct continuation of the widely patent ductus arteriosus.

Anomalous origins of the brachiocephalic vessels are common in IAA. Anomalous origin of the right subclavian artery occurs in about half of patients with IAA type B, but in less than 5 per cent of patients with IAA type A or coarctation of the aorta.[18,38] The anomalous right subclavian artery usually arises from the descending aorta. Rarely, the right subclavian artery arises from the right pulmonary artery as a continuation of a right-sided ductus.[18] Recently, origin of the right subclavian artery from the right common carotid artery as a trifurcation, with the internal and external carotid arteries, has been noted.[18] The association of anomalous right subclavian artery with IAA type B may have pathogenetic significance.[18]

DiGEORGE SYNDROME

Up to 68 per cent of cases with IAA, almost invariably type B, may have associated absence or hypoplasia of thymic tissue and parathyroid glands (DiGeorge syndrome).[4-6,38,39] These patients have depressed cellular immunity and are prone to serious infections.[21] Because of diminished parathyroid hormone, hypocalcemia with seizures and/or arrhythmias may occur.[5] DiGeorge syndrome is present in 68 per cent of patients with IAA (usually type B), in 33 per cent of patients with truncus arteriosus, in less than 2 per cent of patients with tetralogy of Fallot, and in less than 1 per cent of patients with VSD or transposition of the great vessels.[38,39] Only about 3 per cent of patients with DiGeorge syndrome have no heart disease. One half of the cases of DiGeorge syndrome have heart defects that are rare (i.e., IAA, truncus arteriosus).[39]

ETIOLOGY AND EMBRYOLOGY

Analogous to the situation with coarctation, the hemodynamic theory most clearly explains the etiology of IAA. Reduced blood flow into the arch results in lack of development of a certain portion of the arch. This theory derives from the strong association of IAA with intracardiac malformations such as subpulmonary VSD and subaortic stenosis, which reduce aortic blood flow during fetal life.[10,11,20,24,25,27,38]

Recently, the pathogenesis of IAA type B has been proposed to be distinct from that of type A or coarctation.[38,39] Several lines of evidence support this hypothesis. It is known that the left fourth embryonic arch forms that portion of the aortic arch between the left common carotid artery and left subclavian artery (the deficient portion in IAA type B). The right fourth arch develops into the proximal portion of the right subclavian artery. In an extensive review of autopsy cases from other institutions as well as their own, Van Mierop and Kutsche have observed that anomalous origin of the right subclavian artery is much more common in IAA type B (42 per cent) than in IAA type A (2 per cent) or in coarctation of the aorta (5 per cent).[38] These observations have led Van Mierop and Kutsche to suggest that involution of the left fourth arch will result in IAA type B and involution of both right and left fourth arches will result in IAA type B and anomalous right subclavian artery. Involution of the right fourth arch prior to 7 weeks of gestation would result in three alternate routes for formation of the right subclavian artery, all of which have been observed in autopsy studies.[18]

Although the exact pathologic mechanism for involution of the fourth aortic arches is unknown, a developmental error in neural crest tissue may be causally related.[38,39] Two lines of evidence support the role of neural crest cells in aortic arch anomalies. First, studies of chimaeric quail and chick embryos have shown that mesoectodermal cells from the neural crest form the walls of large arteries derived from the embryonic aortic arches, including the fourth arches.[19] Second, neural crest cells also participate in the formation of the parathyroid and thymus glands.[19]

Van Mierop and Kutsche have noted that DiGeorge syndrome, which is associated with a defect in development of the parathyroids and thymus, is much more prevalent in IAA type B than in type A or coarctation.[38,39] A developmental error in neural crest tissue may result in involution of the left fourth arch, resulting in IAA type B. More extensive embryonic error would result in associated anomalous right subclavian artery and DiGeorge syndrome with associated anomalies of the face, ears, and palate.[11,39]

Neural crest cells also contribute to the development of the aortopulmonary and truncoconal septa, and the relationship of these cells to IAA with associated VSD, truncus arteriosus, and tetralogy of Fallot requires further investigation.[39]

HEMODYNAMICS

Hemodynamics of IAA are similar to those of preductal coarctation. As long as the ductus remains widely patent, blood flow to the lower portions of the body is adequate. Gradual closure of the ductus initiates a series of physiologic events that result in rapid cardiac failure. The increased afterload on both ventricles imposed by the closing ductus will elevate left ventricular end-diastolic and left atrial pressures and increase left-to-right shunting via the foramen ovale. Volume overload of the left ventricle (from right-to-left ventricular shunt) and pressure overload of the right ventricle lead to biventricular failure. The metabolic acidosis induced by inadequate lower body perfusion produces decreased myocardial function.

As in preductal coarctation, differential cyanosis is infrequent secondary to significant intracardiac mixing and pulmonary venous desaturation.[22]

CLINICAL FEATURES

Nearly all infants with IAA will present in the first week of life with severe congestive heart failure, cyanosis, and respiratory distress.[4] The median age of death is 4 to 10 days without surgical intervention.[4,40]

Auscultation of the heart is of little help in IAA. The second heart sound is single or narrowly split. Murmurs are present in the majority of patients but are variable and may be holosystolic or ejection systolic in timing.[30]

Upper extremity pulses and systolic blood pressures usually will be greater than those in the lower extremities in IAA but may be equal and low with a widely patent ductus arteriosus or severe congestive heart failure. Differences in upper extremity pulse volume will correlate with the position of the subclavian arteries in relation to the interrupted segment. Right brachial pulsations greater than left brachial pulsations would suggest interruption proximal to the left subclavian artery (type B). Left brachial pulsations greater than right brachial pulsations would suggest interruption distal to the left subclavian artery (type A) with aberrant origin of the right subclavian artery. Strong carotid pulsations with correspondingly weaker brachial and femoral pulsations suggest IAA type B with aberrant origin of the right subclavian artery.[34]

Patients with DiGeorge syndrome may have peculiar facies consisting of mild hypertelorism, slight antimongoloid slant eyes, low-set malformed ears, a short philtrum, a fish-mouth appearance, and palatal anomalies.[6,11]

DIAGNOSIS

The diagnosis of IAA should be suspected in any critically ill neonate with congestive heart failure and signs of inadequate systemic cardiac output. Differential upper and lower extremity blood pressure and pulses would suggest either coarctation or IAA.

Radiographic Features

Chest radiographs usually reveal moderate to marked cardiomegaly in IAA. Increased pulmonary vascular markings may be obscured by pulmonary venous congestion. Although nonspecific, the absence of a thymic shadow on the chest radiograph should suggest DiGeorge syndrome.[21]

Electrocardiogram

Commonly, right ventricular hypertrophy and right or biatrial enlargement are present on the ECG in IAA. However, the ECG may be normal or even show left or combined ventricular hypertrophy.

Echocardiography

Echocardiography is useful in the detection of IAA. The initial clues are a large pulmonary trunk and a small ascending aorta.[32] The suprasternal notch view will demonstrate the small ascending aorta with a straight course to its branches and direct continuity between the ductus arteriosus and descending aorta (Fig. 38–1).[29,35] The characteristic V sign on angiography of IAA type B is not well seen on echocardiography because the brachiocephalic and carotid arteries are in different planes.[32] The apical four-chamber view or subcostal sagittal plane views are best for viewing the conoventricular septal defect.[29] The frequently associated subaortic stenosis due to leftward displacement of the infundibular septum is also best demonstrated in these views.[32]

If intact ventricular septum is noted in IAA, one should think of other diagnoses, such as proximal or distal aortopulmonary window or anomalous origin of one pulmonary artery from the ascending aorta.[29]

Catheterization and Angiography

The hemodynamic data in IAA reflect complex circulatory adjustments and are comparable to those for preductal coarctation. With a widely patent ductus, right ventricular

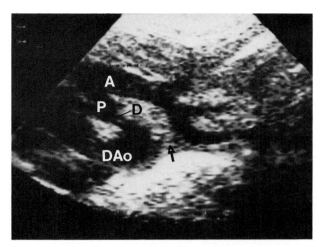

Figure 38–1. Two-dimensional echocardiogram from suprasternal notch demonstrates interrupted aortic arch (arrow) distal to the left subclavian artery. Descending aorta fills via patent ductus arteriosus from the pulmonary artery. A = ascending aorta; D = ductus arteriosus; DAo = descending aorta; P = pulmonary artery.

pressures are at systemic levels. With ductal closure, a gradient will develop between the main pulmonary artery and descending aorta. Atrial and ventricular end-diastolic pressures are elevated in the presence of significant congestive heart failure.

Although anatomic narrowing in the subaortic region is present in IAA, it is rare to have a gradient in that region at catheterization because of left-to-right shunt through the VSD and inadequate forward flow through the aortic valve.[32] Significant gradients often develop postoperatively secondary to increased flow across the left ventricular outflow tract.[27]

Saturation data in IAA generally reflect bidirectional shunting at both the atrial and the ventricular level. Pulmonary venous blood may be desaturated secondary to severe pulmonary edema. Significant saturation differences between preductal and postductal blood are rare because of significant intracardiac mixing and desaturation of pulmonary venous blood.[14,30]

Angiography in IAA demonstrates the hypoplastic ascending aorta that ascends almost vertically into the neck in both frontal and lateral views and divides into two branches of about equal size (the V sign).[38] It is of paramount importance to accurately delineate the aortic arch, usually with a left ventricular injection. If ventricular left-to-right shunt obscures the aortic arch anatomy, then aortography is necessary. The catheter may be placed in the aorta via the VSD or the left ventricle (Fig. 38–2).

The position of the right subclavian artery is important to delineate on angiography. Frequently, retrograde flow in brachiocephalic vessels arising from the descending aorta distal to the interruption may be present.[12,15] Vertebral-subclavian steal is common with a closed or closing ductus.[9] Although central nervous system symptoms are absent in infants, they have been reported in older children with similar physiology after coarctation repair.[31]

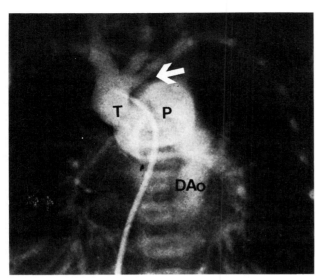

Figure 38–2. The catheter is in the truncal root in this posteroanterior cineangiogram from a patient with truncus arteriosus and IAA, type A. Note the interrupted arch distal to the left subclavian artery (arrow). The ductus arteriosus continues into the descending aorta. The ascending aorta (truncus) divides into branches of about equal size. DAo = descending aorta; P = pulmonary root; T = truncal root.

MANAGEMENT

Management of IAA requires vigorous medical supportive measures with intravenous fluids, correction of acidosis, inotropic agents, diuretics, and respiratory support. Dopamine may be used to improve urine output, but PGE$_1$ will be far more beneficial in improving lower body perfusion and urine output.[2,13] Generally, these infants will respond dramatically to PGE$_1$ infusions within 30 minutes, with return of palpable femoral pulses and blood pressure in lower extremities and lessening of metabolic acidosis.[4]

The presumptive diagnosis of DiGeorge syndrome will require additional therapeutic steps. These infants should receive calcium and vitamin D supplementation. To prevent serious infections, they should be managed in reverse isolation, receive prophylactic antibodies, and receive only irradiated blood products.[21,39]

A variety of surgical procedures have been attempted on infants with IAA.[8,23,26,27,36,37] At the present, primary repair of the arch defect, along with closure of the VSD, appears to be the preferred treatment.[26,27] Significant residual postoperative problems have included residual narrowing at the aortic anastomotic site and subvalvular aortic stenosis.[26,27] In Norwood's series, six of nine (67 per cent) children studied 1 to 3 years after primary or staged repair had developed significant subaortic stenosis and four (44 per cent) required additional surgical intervention.[27] Surgery for IAA is more fully considered in Chapter 62.

OUTCOME

Without surgical intervention, 75 per cent of infants with IAA are dead by 1 month of age and 90 per cent by 1 year of age.[9,22,30,40] Over 50 per cent will not survive the operative or immediate postoperative period.[4] However, surgical results in recent years have been promising and allow for guarded optimism for long-term survival (see Chapter 62).

References

1. Barratt-Boyes BG, Nicholls TT, Brandt PWP, Neutze JM (1972): Aortic arch interruption association with patent ductus arteriosus, ventricular septal defect, and total anomalous pulmonary venous connection: Total correction in an 8-day-old infant by means of profound hypothermia and limited cardiopulmonary bypass. J Thorac Cardiovasc Surg 63:367–373.
2. Campbell DB, Waldhausen JA, Pierce WS, Fripp R, Whitman V (1984): Should elective repair of coarctation of the aorta be done in infancy? J Thorac Cardiovasc Surg 88:929–938.
3. Celoria GC, Patton RB (1959): Congenital absence of the aortic arch. Am Heart J 58:407. Cited in Kirklin JW, Barratt-Boyes BG (1985): Cardiac Surgery. New York, John Wiley & Sons.
4. Collins-Nakai RL, Dick M, Parisi-Buckely L, Fyler D, Castenada AR (1976): Interrupted aortic arch in infancy. J Pediatr 88:959–962.
5. Conley ME, Beckwith JB, Mancer JFK, Tenckhoff L (1979): The spectrum of the DiGeorge syndrome. J Pediatr 94:883–890.
6. DiGeorge AM (1965): Discussion of paper by Cooper MD, Peterson RDA, Good RA: A new concept of the cellular base of immunology. J Pediatr 67:907–908.
7. Dische RM, Tsai M, Baltaxe HA (1974): Solitary interruption of the arch of the aorta. Am J Cardiol 35:271–277.
8. Fowler BN, Lucas SK, Razook JD, Thompson WM, Williams GR, Elkins RL (1984): Interruption of the aortic arch: Experience in 17 infants. Ann Thorac Surg 37:25–32.
9. Freedom RM, Bain HH, Esplugas E, Dische R, Rowe RD (1977): Ventricular septal defect in interruption of the aortic arch. Am J Cardiol 39:572–582.
10. Freedom RM, Dische MR, Rowe RD (1977): Pathologic anatomy of subaortic stenosis and atresia in the first year of life. Am J Cardiol 39:1035–1044.
11. Freedom RM, Rosen FS, Nadas AS (1972): Congenital cardiovascular disease and anomalies of the third and fourth pharyngeal pouch. Circulation 46:167–172.
12. Garcia OL, Hernandez FA, Tamer D, Poole C, Gelband H, Castellanos AW (1979): Congenital bilateral subclavian steal: Ductus-dependent symptoms in interrupted aortic arch associated with ventricular septal defect. Am J Cardiol 44:101–104.
13. Heymann MA, Berman W, Rudolph AM, Whitman V (1979): Dilatation of the ductus arteriosus by prostaglandin E$_1$ in aortic arch abnormalities. Circulation 59:169–173.
14. Higgins CB, French JW, Silverman JF, Wexler D (1977): Interruption of the aortic arch: Preoperative and postoperative clinical, hemodynamic and angiographic features. Am J Cardiol 39:563–571.
15. Jaffe RB (1976): Complete interruption of the aortic arch: Characteristic angiographic features with emphasis on collateral circulation to the descending aorta. Circulation 53:161–168.
16. Keith JD (1978): Prevalence, incidence and epidemiology. In Keith JD, Rowe RD, Vlad P (eds): Heart Disease in Infancy and Childhood. New York, Macmillan, pp 4–8.
17. Kirklin JW, Barratt-Boyes BG (1985): Cardiac Surgery. New York, John Wiley & Sons, pp 1070–1080.
18. Kutsche LM, Van Mierop LHS (1984): Cervical origin of the right subclavian artery in aortic arch interruption: Pathogenesis and significance. Am J Cardiol 53:892–895.
19. LeLievre CS, LeDouarin NM (1975): Mesenchymal derivatives of neural crest: Analysis of chimaeric quail and chick embryos. J Embryol Exp Morphol 34:125–154. Cited in Van Mierop LHS, Kutsche LM (1984): Interruption of the aortic arch and coarctation of the aorta: Pathogenetic relations. Am J Cardiol 54:829–834.
20. Marino B, Chiariello L, Mercanti C, Bosman C, Colloridi V, Reale A, Marino B (1981): Morphology of aortic arch obstruction with patent ductus arteriosus. Cardiovasc Dis Bull Texas Heart Inst 8:238–249.

21. Marmon LM, Balsara RK, Chen R, Dunn JM (1984): Congenital cardiac anomalies associated with the DiGeorge syndrome: A neonatal experience. Ann Thorac Surg 38:146–150.

22. McNamara DG, Rosenburg HS (1968): Interruption of the aortic arch. In Watson H (ed): Pediatric Cardiology. St Louis, CV Mosby, pp 224–232.

23. Monro JL, Brawn W, Conway N (1977): Correction of type B interrupted aortic arch with ventricular septal defect in infancy. J Thorac Cardiovasc Surg 74:618–623.

24. Moore GW, Hutchings GM (1978): Association of interrupted aortic arch with malformations producing reduced blood flow to the fourth aortic arches. Am J Cardiol 42:467–472.

25. Moulaert AJ, Bruins CC, Oppenheimer-Dekker A (1976): Anomalies of the aortic arch and ventricular septal defects. Circulation 53:1011–1015.

26. Moulton AL, Bowman FO (1981): Primary definitive repair of type B interrupted aortic arch, ventricular septal defect, and patent ductus arteriosus: Early and late results. J Thorac Cardiovasc Surg 82:501–510.

27. Norwood WI, Lang P, Castaneda AR, Hougen TJ (1983): Reparative operations for interrupted aortic arch with ventricular septal defect. J Thorac Cardiovasc Surg 86:832–837.

28. Oppenheimer-Dekker A, Gittenberger-deGroot AC, Roosendaal H (1982): The ductus arteriosus and associated cardiac anomalies in interruption of the aortic arch. Pediatr Cardiol 2:185–193.

29. Riggs TW, Berry TE, Aziz KY, Paul MH (1982): Two-dimensional echocardiographic features of interruption of the aortic arch. Am J Cardiol 50:1385–1390.

30. Roberts WC, Morrow AG, Braunwald E (1962): Complete interruption of the aortic arch. Circulation 26:39–59.

31. Saalouke MG, Perry LW, Breckbill DL, Shapiro SR, Scott LP (1978): Cerebrovascular abnormalities in postoperative coarctation of the aorta. Am J Cardiol 42:97–101.

32. Smallhorn JF, Anderson RH, McCartney FJ (1982): Cross-sectional echocardiographic recognition of interruption of aortic arch between left carotid and subclavian arteries. Br Heart J 48:229–235.

33. Steidele RJ (1778): Sammi Chir Med Beob Vienna, vol 2, p 114. Cited in Kirklin JW, Barratt-Boyes BG (1985): Cardiac Surgery. New York, John Wiley & Sons.

34. Subramanian AR (1972): Coarctation or interruption of aorta proximal to origin of both subclavian arteries: Report of three cases presenting in infancy. Br Heart J 34:1225–1226.

35. Tibbits PA, Oetgen WJ, Potter BM, Chandra RS, Avery GB, Perry LW, Scott LP (1981): Interruption of aortic arch masquerading as persistent fetal circulation with definitive diagnosis by two-dimensional echocardiography. Am Heart J 102:936–938.

36. Trusler GA, Izukawa T (1975): Interrupted aortic arch and ventricular septal defect: Direct repair through a median sternotomy incision in a 13-day-old infant. J Thorac Cardiovasc Surg 69:126–131.

37. Turley K, Yee ES, Ebert PA (1984): The total repair of interrupted aortic arch complex in infants: The anterior approach. Circulation 70:I16–I20

38. Van Mierop LHS, Kutsche LM (1984): Interruption of the aortic arch and coarctation of the aorta: Pathogenetic relations. Am J Cardiol 54:829–834.

39. Van Mierop LHS, Kutsche LM (1986): Cardiovascular anomalies in DiGeorge syndrome and importance of neural crest as a possible pathologic factor. Am J Cardiol 58:133–137.

40. Van Praagh R, Bernhard WF, Rosenthal A, Parisi LF, Fyler DC (1971): Interrupted aortic arch: Surgical treatment. Am J Cardiol 27:200–211.

41. Zaka KG, Roland JMA, Cutilleta AF, Gardner TJ, Donahoo JS, Kidd L (1980): Management of aortic arch interruption with prostaglandin E$_1$ infusion and microporous expanded polytetrafluorethylene grafts. Am J Cardiol 46:1001–1005.

39 NEONATAL HYPERTENSION

Stephen J. Elliott

Thomas N. Hansen

In the past, neonatal hypertension was considered to be a rare event and received little attention in most reviews of pediatric hypertension.[37,43,47] Recently, however, with the advent of neonatal intensive care, hypertension has been recognized as a significant problem for the newborn. Several different phenomena are responsible for this increased recognition. First, our ability to measure the arterial blood pressure in the newborn has improved dramatically. We can easily measure arterial blood pressure noninvasively using either the Doppler technique or oscillometry or invasively using indwelling arterial catheters connected to strain gauge manometers. Second, the use of umbilical arterial catheters has increased the occurrence of renovascular hypertension.[2] Third, circulatory support of the critically ill neonate frequently involves use of pharmacologic agents that may elevate blood pressure.

The literature on neonatal hypertension is sparse. There are no large epidemiologic studies that examine blood pressure measurements in the newborn, and there are few attempts comparing values between healthy and sick infants.[30,32,55,59]

The purpose of this chapter is to review the history of blood pressure measurements in the neonate, and then review the etiologies, clinical presentations, and therapies of the various causes of neonatal hypertension.

HISTORICAL PERSPECTIVE

Measurements of blood pressure in newborns were recorded as early as 1879.[64] Until recent times, the presence of hypertension in the neonate could only be inferred from premortem descriptions consistent with heart failure in association with postmortem findings of ductal thrombosis and embolic renal artery occlusion.[29,41,63,76]

In 1959, however, Ashworth and colleagues developed a sphygmomanometer for recording blood pressures in newborns.[8] The instrument overcame the difficulties of pulse detection in the neonate[67] by connecting a forearm cuff to a column of xylol that oscillated when arterial pulsations were detected. Using this technique, Ashworth and Neligan[9] measured blood pressures in normal neonates in the first 24 hours of life whereas Neligan and Smith studied similarly aged sick newborns.[59] Since that time, the literature concerning blood pressure in the neonate has consisted primarily of studies attempting to establish normal values for blood pressure in the neonate, and of case reports of neonatal hypertension.

MEASUREMENT TECHNIQUES

In the neonate, traditional, clinical methods of blood pressure measurement are often inaccurate and may lack reproducibility among observers.[67] The sounds of Korotkoff are barely audible in neonates, making auscultation techniques impractical. The palpation method remains popular in many nurseries but is also subject to observer error and may give estimates of systolic blood pressure that are 5 to 10 mmHg below the actual value.[3] The flush technique correlates well with mean arterial pressure in normal infants, but the value attained may be influenced by anemia, hypothermia, or peripheral edema.

By contrast, newer, more sophisticated techniques have allowed measurement of blood pressure with minimal handling of the infant. Direct intravascular recordings using indwelling arterial catheters and strain gauge manometers provide continuous pressure wave tracings and digital display of systolic, mean, and diastolic blood pressures. This method has become the standard by which all others are evaluated.[27]

Both Doppler technique and Dinamap oscillometry are simple, noninvasive techniques that are widely used in level II nurseries where infants do not have indwelling arterial catheters.[38] Several studies have shown that the systolic blood pressure measured using Doppler ultrasound, and the systolic and diastolic pressures obtained using the Dinamap oscillometer, correlate well with direct intravascular measurements.[22,25,27,48] One study does suggest, however, that in low birthweight infants with systemic hypotension the Dinamap oscillometer may overestimate both systolic and diastolic blood pressures.[21]

Although most of the current noninvasive techniques for measuring blood pressure in the neonate allow the infant to remain relatively undisturbed, the values obtained by all of these techniques are still affected by the infant's wakefulness. De Swiet[72] found that the systolic blood pressure measured using the Doppler technique was significantly higher in awake infants compared with sleeping infants (5.1 mmHg and 7.0 mmHg higher at 4 days and 6 weeks of age, respectively). Further subdivision of the level of consciousness did not reduce the variability, but values obtained on infants who were sucking or feeding had greater variance. In light of these data it appears that using an average of several repeated measurements of blood pressure over time, with the infant asleep or in the quiet awake state, should provide the most reproducible and accurate estimate of the systemic blood pressure.

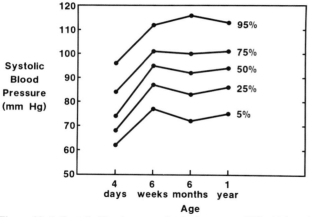

Figure 39–1. Systolic blood pressure in the first year of life. (Adapted from de Swiet M, Fayers P, Shinebourne EA [1980]: Systolic blood pressure in a population of infants in the first year of life: The Brompton Study. Pediatr 65:1028–1035.)

NORMAL VALUES

In her original studies, Ashworth showed that in the normal newborn, arterial blood pressure decreased in the first few hours after birth and then rose steadily through day 7. Using similar techniques, Contis and Lind[17] found that the highest systolic blood pressure occurred within the first 15 minutes of delivery. In their study, systolic blood pressures measured at 30 minutes after birth ranged from 70 to 122 mmHg, whereas those measured at 7 days ranged from 72 to 120 mmHg.

In a study of both normal and sick newborns, Neligan and Smith[59] found that systolic blood pressure in normal infants peaked within 5 minutes of delivery and subsequently decreased, reaching its nadir within 1 hour. In addition, they found that asphyxiated infants had a mean initial systolic blood pressure that was significantly higher than that of normal newborns (99.1 mmHg versus 84.0 mmHg). Finally, they found that premature infants with hyaline membrane disease had lower systolic blood pressures than premature infants without lung disease.

Levison[44] and coworkers used a mercury-silicone strain gauge to obtain repeated measurements of systolic blood pressure in term and preterm infants. They found that normal term infants had mean systolic pressures of 62 mmHg at 12 to 24 hours and of 76 mmHg by the fifth day. By comparison, preterm infants (27 to 34 weeks, 960 to 1984 g) had mean systolic pressures of 36 mmHg on the first day after birth, 53 mmHg by the seventh day, and 76 mmHg by the seventh week.

The most comprehensive study on the normal blood pressure of term infants was carried out by de Swiet and coworkers in Brompton, England, using the Doppler technique.[72] In their study, they found that systolic arterial pressure rose from a mean of 76 mmHg at 4 days, to 96 mmHg at 6 weeks, and then remained unchanged at 6 months and 1 year (Fig. 39–1). Subsequent data[23] showed that most of the increase between 4 days and 6 weeks of age occurred during the first 2 weeks. In 99 term infants

Table 39–1. AORTIC BLOOD PRESSURES IN HEALTHY NEWBORNS DURING FIRST 12 HOURS AFTER BIRTH

Birthweight (g)	Measurement	Blood Pressure (mmHg)		
		1 Hour	*6 Hours*	*12 Hours*
1001 – 2000	Systolic	49	52	50
	Diastolic	26	31	30
	Mean	35	40	38
2001 – 3000	Systolic	59	58	59
	Diastolic	32	34	35
	Mean	43	43	42
> 3000	Systolic	70	66	66
	Diastolic	44	41	41
	Mean	53	50	50

Adapted from Kitterman JA, et al (1969): Aortic blood pressure in normal newborn infants during the first 12 hours of life. Pediatrics 44:959–968.

the mean systolic blood pressure was 70 mmHg at 2 days, 84 mmHg at 2 weeks, and 93 mmHg at 6 weeks.

In preterm infants the most comprehensive measurements of blood pressure were made by Kitterman and associates in San Francisco using indwelling umbilical artery catheters and strain gauge manometry to provide direct, intravascular measurements of systolic, diastolic, and mean aortic blood pressure.[39] Forty-five infants of gestational age 26 to 41 weeks, and birthweight 1050 to 4220 g were studied, and average values for systolic, diastolic, and mean blood pressure for each of the first 12 hours of life were reported. Average mean blood pressure ranged from 35 to 40 mmHg in the lowest weight group and from 50 to 54 mmHg in the highest weight group (Table 39–1). In a follow-up report from the same investigators,[74] data from 16 infants with birthweight less than 1000 g were combined with the original measurements to provide blood pressure nomograms that included very low birthweight infants (Fig. 39–2).

Several studies including the one from San Francisco[17,44,74] have shown a direct linear relationship between birthweight

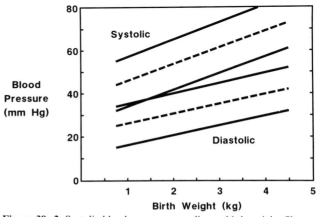

Figure 39–2. Systolic blood pressure according to birth weight. Shown are linear regressions (interrupted lines) and 95 per cent confidence limits (continuous lines) for systolic (r = 0.79) and diastolic (r = 0.71) pressures. (Adapted from Versmold HT et al [1981]: Aortic blood pressure during the first 12 hours of life in infants with birth weight 610 to 4220 grams. Pediatr 67:607–613.)

Table 39–2. AORTIC BLOOD PRESSURES IN
HEALTHY PREMATURE NEWBORNS
DURING FIRST 12 HOURS AFTER BIRTH

Birthweight (g)	Measurement	Blood Pressure (mmHg)		
		2–3 Hours	7–8 Hours	11–12 Hours
< 1000	Systolic	35	41	40
	Diastolic	22	26	25
	Mean	26	31	30
1000 – 1250	Systolic	35	43	43
	Diastolic	21	25	27
	Mean	26	31	33

Adapted from Moscoso P, et al (1983): Spontaneous elevation in arterial blood pressure during the first hours of life in the very low birth weight infant. J. Pediatr 103: 114–117.

and blood pressure. In addition, others have shown that gestational age is also positively correlated with blood pressure.[32,44,74] Finally, Moscoso and colleagues[57] used direct intravascular measurements and found that systolic, diastolic, and mean arterial blood pressure spontaneously increase over time during the first 8 hours after birth in infants weighing less than 1250 g (Table 39–2). Beyond the first 12 hours, little is known about the normal blood pressure in the preterm infant.

In the absence of large population-based studies of neonatal systemic blood pressure, especially in preterm infants, many clinicians rely on Lieberman's arbitrary criteria, which defines neonatal hypertension as systolic pressure greater than 90 mmHg or diastolic pressure greater than 65 mmHg in term infants and systolic pressure greater than 80 mmHg or diastolic pressure greater than 45 mmHg in preterm infants.[45]

ETIOLOGY

Essential Hypertension

Hennekens and associates have shown that systolic blood pressure may be similar among siblings and that this similarity may be statistically evident by 1 month of age.[34] However, most investigators imply that the entity of essential hypertension does not exist in the newborn period.[3,37]

Renovascular Hypertension

Renovascular hypertension has emerged as the single most common cause of systemic hypertension in the newborn period.[2] Early case reports[29,76] of fatal renal artery thromboembolism included descriptions consistent with heart failure induced by systemic hypertension. Since that time, congenital lesions of the renal artery, including stenosis,[46] hypoplasia,[7] intimal hyperplasia,[26] and idiopathic arterial calcification[53] have been associated with hypertension.

In recent years, the use of umbilical arterial catheters has been associated with an increased occurrence of renal

thromboembolism and subsequent renovascular hypertension. The incidence of thrombosis complicating umbilical artery catheters has been reported to range from 4.6 to 95 per cent.[16,28,31,56,58,73] Using clinical criteria, Gupta and colleagues[31] reported a 5 per cent incidence of thrombotic complications following umbilical artery catheterization. In postmortem studies of infants with umbilical catheters, thrombosis has been noted in 21 per cent,[16,28] 58 per cent,[58] and 59 per cent.[73] Finally, investigators using aortography have recorded incidences of thrombosis of 24 per cent,[28] 91 per cent,[56] and 95 per cent.[58] Nearly all thromboses have been found in the aorta and iliac vessels; the true incidence of renal artery occlusion is unknown.

Of 17 infants with renovascular hypertension, 15 (88 per cent) had umbilical artery catheters.[2] In the most comprehensive, prospective study to date,[56] hypertension was a complication in 2 of 73 (2.7 per cent) umbilical arterial catheterizations. Agreement does not exist regarding the relative safety of various catheter positions. Although several investigators[28,58] have advocated positioning of the catheter tip below the level of the renal arteries, Mokrohisky and coworkers[56] have shown no difference in the incidence of hypertension between catheters placed above the tenth thoracic vertebra (high placement) and those placed below the the third lumbar vertebra (low placement). Furthermore, in the evaluation of all catheter-associated complications, including thrombosis and hypertension, there was no correlation between complication occurrence and sex, birthweight, gestational age, Apgar score, size of catheter, rate of fluid infusion, or amount of blood sampling. Duration of catheterization does not seem to increase the risk of thrombotic complications.[28,58] Administration of antibiotics through the catheter has been associated with an increased rate of complications, but cause and effect have not been proven.[56]

In conclusion, although umbilical arterial catheterization appears to be a risk factor for renal artery occlusion and subsequent development of renovascular hypertension, the relative degree of risk posed by the catheter and the role of contributing factors remain to be elucidated.

Renal Parenchymal Disease

A variety of congenital renal diseases may present as hypertension in the neonate. Infantile polycystic kidney disease,[62] renal dysplasia, renal hypoplasia, renal cortical necrosis,[6,13] and obstructive uropathy have all been associated with elevated systemic blood pressure.

Endocrinologic Hypertension

Infants with congenital adrenal hyperplasia secondary to 11-hydroxylase deficiency may develop systemic hypertension.[24] Hypertension has also been reported in infants with bronchopulmonary dysplasia treated with corticosteroids and in those infants treated with vitamin D derivatives.[19] Pheochromocytoma is very rare in the newborn period.[65]

Abdominal Wall Defect

Adelman and Sherman[5] have reported four infants with systemic hypertension following closure of abdominal wall defects. The pathogenesis of this form of hypertension is uncertain, since in the infants described there was no evidence of volume overload or reduced blood pressure in the lower extremities. Possible etiologies include compression of the renal vasculature, sympathetic stimulation of the splanchnic bed, or mechanical distortion of nerves within the abdominal wall.

Infection

Congenital rubella may cause obliterative vasculitis with subsequent hypertension, especially if the renal arterial supply is compromised.[51]

Systemic candidiasis has become a more commonly recognized infection in neonatal intensive care units.[11] This organism may lead to invasion of the renal parenchyma and produce hypertension by compression of the arterial circulation or of the urinary outflow tract.

Cardiac Disease

Coarctation of the aorta produces hypertension limited to the upper extremities in association with hypotension and diminished pulses in the lower extremities. During the first 3 days of life, a patent ductus arteriosus may obscure clinical signs of a coarctation.[68]

Iatrogenic

Administration of eye drops containing phenylephrine has been well documented to induce systemic hypertension.[71] Since mydriasis is necessary for adequate funduscopy in small premature infants, hypertension of this origin may be commonly seen in a neonatal intensive care unit.

Pressor agents such as dopamine are frequently used to maintain normotension in sick newborns and yet are among the most common causes of elevated blood pressure. Infusion rates and dosage must be carefully monitored, as should a continuous display of systemic blood pressure in those infants receiving pressor support.

Data[60] obtained from studies in rats suggests that chronic caffeine administration may exacerbate renovascular hypertension by antagonizing adenosine receptors and preventing any adenosine mediated attenuation of renin release.[20] Caffeine is commonly used to prevent apnea in preterm infants and may indeed play a role in exacerbating hypertension in those with some compromise in renal perfusion.

Bronchopulmonary Dysplasia

Two previous studies have shown that the incidence of systemic hypertension in graduates of neonatal intensive care units ranges between 1 and 8.9 per cent.[37,69] More recently, however, Abman and associates[1] have shown that in infants with bronchopulmonary dysplasia (chronic lung disease following recovery from hyaline membrane disease) the incidence of systemic hypertension is much greater (43 per cent). In this study, definitive conclusions regarding etiology could not be made since comprehensive diagnostic evaluations were not performed. However, in comparison to normotensive infants with bronchopulmonary dysplasia, there were no significant differences in duration of umbilical catheterization or incidence of thrombotic complications. The suggested mechanisms responsible for hypertension in infants with bronchopulmonary dysplasia have included hypoxia-induced elevation of systemic vascular resistance[1] or alterations in the activity of angiotensin converting enzyme[50] or release of vasoactive substances from the injured lung.[33]

CLINICAL FINDINGS

Symptoms and Signs

The most extensive review of the clinical features of hypertension in the neonate was published by Adelman[2] in 1978. In his review of 17 newborns with hypertension, he found that 53 per cent had tachypnea, cyanosis, or signs of heart failure, whereas 29 per cent had neurologic symptoms that included lethargy, coma, tremors, apnea, opisthotonus, seizures, and hemiparesis. Interestingly, nearly 25 per cent of the infants had no symptoms referable to systemic hypertension.

In another report of nine neonates with hypertension published by Adelman and associates,[4] eight had respiratory symptoms, five had neurologic symptoms, and seven had evidence of congestive heart failure.

Finally, in Zuelzer and colleagues' original description of four infants with renal artery occlusion, three had symptoms suggestive of congestive heart failure.[76]

Laboratory Data

Hematuria and proteinuria are usually present in those infants with renovascular hypertension.[4] In addition, elevation of blood urea nitrogen and serum creatinine values may be detected if renal failure has occurred. Diagnostic confirmation of renovascular hypertension requires demonstration of a renal vascular lesion and an increased plasma renin activity. Renin is produced by the juxtaglomerular apparatus of the kidney and catalyzes the conversion of angiotensinogen to angiotensin I. Quantitation of its enzymatic activity is achieved by incubating plasma with inhibitors that block removal of the reaction product, angiotensin I. Since the reaction is enzyme limited, production of angiotensin I reflects renin activity and is reported in units of nanograms per milliliter of plasma per hour. Some laboratories report results for the total 3-hour incubation, in which case the units are measured every 3 hours.

Interpretation of plasma renin activity in the neonate is difficult, however, because the newborn has a relatively high plasma renin activity when compared with the adult[40] and data are scarce comparing plasma renin activity in hypertensive newborns with normal infants. The higher baseline renin activity in the neonate may result from extrarenal production of renin in the placenta or salivary gland or from enhanced renal production. The juxtaglomerular apparatus of the neonatal kidney may be appropriately responding to perceived diminished renal blood flow or may be up-regulated to produce more renin than the adult for any given stimulus. Increased renin activity has been described in normotensive newborns with respiratory distress syndrome or severe lung disease and in hypotensive infants,[2] whereas normal renin activities have been reported in infants with renovascular hypertension.[5] Adelman et al report normal values for supine neonates to be 81 ± 18 ng/ml/3 hr (mean $\pm$ SEM),[4] but norms may vary from one laboratory to another. If a lesion has been localized radiographically, plasma renin activity obtained from the ipsilateral renal vein should be higher than that of the contralateral renal vein and activity in the inferior vena cava would be expected to have an intermediate value. Although selective sampling from each renal vein may be very helpful in the interpretation of renin activity results, it remains an invasive procedure that may be difficult to justify unless surgical intervention is seriously being considered.

Radiologic Evaluation

Since hypertension in the neonate is predominantly of renovascular origin, arteriographic and radioisotopic studies of the kidney may be very helpful in establishing the etiology. Several studies[28,56,58] have shown that aortography via the indwelling umbilical artery catheter is more sensitive than either clinical findings alone or postmortem examination in the detection of catheter-associated thromboses. In one series,[2] 9 of 13 hypertensive neonates had arteriographic evidence of renal artery occlusion. In the absence of an indwelling umbilical artery catheter arteriography may be performed via percutaneous femoral artery puncture.

One alternative to arteriography, especially if no umbilical artery catheter is in place, is the radioisotopic renal scan. Scintigraphy has the added advantage of providing information regarding the renal parenchyma. Rosen and coworkers[66] reported that in hypertensive pediatric patients renal abnormalities were identified using ^{99m}Tc succimer with 92 per cent sensitivity and 97 per cent specificity. Although only 4 of the 80 patients in this series were neonates, all had abnormal scans, as evidenced by focal abnormalities, asymmetrical renal size, or asymmetrical distribution of the radioactive tracer.

On the other hand, sequential images obtained after injecting ^{131}I iodohippurate sodium can be used to calculate effective renal plasma flow, urine flow fraction, and urinary ^{131}I iodohippurate sodium concentration for each kidney.[52] Neonates with renovascular hypertension typically have asymmetrical technetium scans with delayed clearance of ^{131}I iodohippurate sodium in the involved kidney.

If obstructive uropathy is suspected, ultrasound evaluation of the kidneys should be performed.

MANAGEMENT

Management of the neonate with hypertension should be directed at correcting the underlying etiology. In cases of iatrogenic hypertension, simply discontinuing the offending medication may alleviate the problem; in patients with renal candidiasis, antifungal therapy will usually reduce the blood pressure. Infants with hypertension resulting from coarctation of the aorta eventually require surgical correction, whereas those with hypertension complicating repair of abdominal wall defects usually spontaneously improve over time.

Although hypertension associated with bronchopulmonary dysplasia is usually self-limited, in the study of Abman and associates 6 of the 13 infants required therapy.[1] All infants were treated with hydrochlorothiazide (4 mg/kg/day). Four required hydrochlorothiazide and propranolol (6 mg/kg/day), and three others also required hydralazine (6 mg/kg/day) for adequate control. All 6 infants received furosemide, but for variable durations and without a clear relationship to the presence or resolution of the hypertension. The mean duration of therapy was 7.7 months.[1]

There is still considerable controversy over the appropriate management of renovascular hypertension. In light of earlier reports suggesting that the response to medical therapy was poor and that the outcome was often fatal,[12,18] some authors[42,61,75] have advocated an aggressive surgical approach. Although this approach has traditionally been nephrectomy,[10] several other options including thrombectomy,[35,42] endarterectomy, and aortorenal graft revascularization[15] may allow salvage of the involved kidney.

Recently, aggressive medical therapy has been proposed as a viable alternative to surgical intervention.[4,49,70] In 1978, Adelman and coworkers[4] reported nine infants with renovascular hypertension who were successfully managed with medical therapy alone. In these infants, mild hypertension was managed with diuretics alone, whereas more severe hypertension was treated with hydralazine (0.2 to 1.0 mg/kg/dose). Methyldopa (10 to 50 mg/kg/day) or propranolol (0.5 to 2.0 mg/kg/day) was added if hydralazine alone failed to achieve adequate control. Extreme elevations of blood pressure were treated with diazoxide or nitroprusside.

Captopril, a peptidyl dipeptidase inhibitor that blocks conversion of the relatively inactive angiotensin I to the more active angiotensin II, has been used in the management of hypertension in children[36,54] and to a lesser extent in neonates.[14] It has its maximal effect in those hypertensive states in which the renin-angiotensin system is most active, but it will also be effective if endogenous angiotensin is contributing to hypertension in sodium-depleted, normoreninemic patients. Bifano and colleagues[14] achieved control of refractory neonatal hypertension using captopril in dosages of 0.6 to 2.6 mg/kg/day for a period

Table 39–3. PHARMACOLOGIC THERAPY FOR NEONATAL HYPERTENSION

Agent	Dosage
Furosemide	1.0 – 5.0 mg/kg/day
Hydrochlorothiazide	4.0 mg/kg/day
Chlorothiazide	25 – 50 mg/kg/day
Hydralazine	1.0 – 9.0 mg/kg/day
Propranolol	0.5 – 6.0 mg/kg/day
Methyldopa	5.0 – 50 mg/kg/day
Captopril	0.6 – 2.6 mg/kg/day
Diazoxide	2.0 – 5.0 mg/kg/dose
Nitroprusside	0.5 – 3.0 µg/kg/min

cially in cases of documented renovascular hypertension. Obviously, severe hypertension will still require emergency therapy with diazoxide or nitroprusside.

SUMMARY

Systemic hypertension is a serious, potentially fatal condition that is being recognized with increasing frequency in the neonate. The majority of cases have some well-defined etiology, and all neonates presenting with hypertension merit a careful diagnostic workup. Once the diagnosis is clear a consistent approach to management should be instituted, with aggressive medical therapy and surgical intervention if indicated.

of 12 to 50 days, whereas Hymes and Warshaw[36] successfully treated a 1-month-old infant delivered at 33 weeks' gestation with a dosage of 0.6 to 1.8 mg/kg/day over a 2-month period. Mirkin and Newman[54] reported on 73 pediatric patients treated with captopril (0.3 to 6.0 mg/kg/day), but only 4 were under 6 months of age. For infants under 2 months of age, the International Collaborative Study Group has recommended initial dosing of 0.05 to 0.1 mg/kg/dose.[54]

In some patients captopril may increase the serum creatinine and blood urea nitrogen concentrations and decrease the glomerular filtration rate[36,54] by decreasing renal perfusion pressure. In fact, hypotension and postural syncope may be seen in as many as 10 per cent of recipients.[54] Hyperkalemia has also been described[36] and may be explained by either inhibition of aldosterone secretion or by a direct tubular effect. If renal function has been compromised, captopril may induce hyperkalemia to a degree necessitating withdrawal of the drug.

In many instances, pharmacologic therapy of neonatal hypertension has been adapted from studies performed in older children and adults. Those drugs that have been reported to be effective in the newborn period are listed in Table 39–3. Although the traditional approach to the medical management of hypertension in the adult is administration of a diuretic, followed by a β-adrenergic blocker and then a vasodilator, this approach has not been as useful in treating hypertension in neonates. Diuretics alone are seldom effective in the treatment of hypertension in the neonate. (Only 4 of 17 of Adelman's patients responded to diuretics alone.[2]) Clinicians have been unwilling to risk the use of β-adrenergic blockers (especially those administered parenterally) in infants with compromised cardiopulmonary function, thus limiting the usefulness of propranolol in this group of infants. As a result, hydralazine, a vasodilator agent, has become one of the mainstays in the therapy of the neonate with hypertension, especially during the early stages when parenteral administration is required. Later when drugs may be administered orally, propranolol may be added to the regimen to ensure adequate control of the blood pressure. Captopril is still considered a second-line drug in the therapy for hypertension in the neonate, but as more experience is accumulated it may become useful earlier in therapy, espe-

References

1. Abman SH, Warady BA, Lum GM, Koops BL (1984): Systemic hypertension in infants with bronchopulmonary dysplasia. J Pediatr 104:928–931.
2. Adelman RD (1978): Neonatal hypertension. Pediatr Clin North Am 25:99–110.
3. Adelman RD (1984): Neonatal hypertension. Annales Nestlé 42:32–42.
4. Adelman RD, Merten D, Vogel J, Goetzman BW, Wennberg RP (1978): Nonsurgical management of renovascular hypertension in the neonate. Pediatrics 62:71–76.
5. Adelman RD, Sherman MP (1980): Hypertension in the neonate following closure of abdominal wall defects. J Pediatr 97:642–644.
6. Anand SK, Northway JD, Smith JA (1977): Neonatal renal papillary and cortical necrosis. Am J Dis Child 131:773–777.
7. Angella JJ, Sommer LS, Poole C, Fogel BJ (1968): Neonatal hypertension associated with renal artery hypoplasia. Pediatrics 41:524–526.
8. Ashworth AM, Neligan GA, Rogers JE (1959): Sphygmomanometer for the newborn. Lancet 1:801–804.
9. Ashworth AM, Neligan GA (1959): Changes in the systolic blood pressure of normal babies during the first twenty-four hours of life. Lancet 1:804–807.
10. Baldwin CE, Holder TM, Ashcraft KW, Amoury RA (1981): Neonatal renovascular hypertension—a complication of aortic monitoring catheters. J Pediatr Surg 16:820–821.
11. Baley JE, Kliegman RM, Fanaroff AA (1984): Disseminated fungal infections in very low birth weight infants: Clinical manifestations and epidemiology. Pediatrics 73:144–152.
12. Bauer SB, Feldman SM, Gellis SS, Retik AB (1985): Neonatal hypertension. N Engl J Med 293:1032–1033.
13. Bernstein J, Meyer R (1961): Congenital abnormalities of the urinary system. J Pediatr 59:657–668.
14. Bifano E, Post EM, Springer J, Williams ML, Streeten DH (1982): Treatment of neonatal hypertension with captopril. J Pediatr 100:143–146.
15. Burdick JF, Helikson MA, Hudak ML, Williams GM (1982): Revascularization for bilateral renal artery occlusion after umbilical artery catheterization. Surgery 91:650–655.
16. Cochran WD, Davis HT, Smith CA (1968): Advantages and complications of umbilical artery catheterization in the newborn. Pediatics 42:769–777.
17. Contis G, Lind J (1963): Study of systolic blood pressure, heart rate, body temperature of normal newborn infants through the first week of life. Acta Paediatr Scand [Suppl] 146:41–47.
18. Cook GT, Marshall VF, Todd JE (1966): Malignant renovascular hypertension in a newborn. J Urol 96:863–866.
19. Curcic VG, Curcic B (1975): Effect of vitamin D on serum cholesterol and arterial pressure in infants. Nutr Metab 18:57–61.
20. Deray G, Jackson EK, Herzer WA, Branch RA (1985): Inhibition of prostaglandin-mediated renin release by adenosine. Clin Res 33:282A.
21. Diprose GK, Evans DH, Archer LN, Levene MI (1986): Dinamap

fails to detect hypotension in very low birthweight infants. Arch Dis Child 61:771–773.

22. Dweck HS, Reynolds DW, Cassady G (1974): Indirect blood pressure measurement in newborns. Am J Dis Child 127:492–494.

23. Earley A, Fayers P, Ng S, Shinebourne EA, de Swiet M (1980): Blood pressure in the first six weeks of life. Arch Dis Child 55:755–757.

24. Edwards RW, Harvey DR, Knight-Jones E (1968): Hypertension and excretion of 11-oxygenated steroids. Arch Dis Child 43:611–615.

25. Elseed AM, Shinebourne EA, Joseph MC (1973): Assessments of techniques for measurement of blood pressure in infants and children. Arch Dis Child 48:932–936.

26. Formby D, Emery JL (1969): Intimal hyperplasia of the aorta and renal vessels in an infant with hypertension. J Pathol 98:205–208.

27. Frieson RH, Lichtor JL (1981): Indirect measurement of blood pressure in neonates and infants utilizing an automatic non-invasive oscillometric monitor. Anesth Analg 60:742.

28. Goetzman BW, Stadalnik RC, Bogren HG, Blankenship WJ, Ikeda RM, Thayer J (1975): Thrombotic complications of umbilical artery catheters: A clinical and radiographic study. Pediatrics 56:374–379.

29. Gross RE (1945): Arterial embolism and thrombosis in infancy. Am J Dis Child 70:61–73.

30. Gupta JM, Scopes JW (1965): Observations on blood pressure in newborn infants. Arch Dis Child 40:637–644.

31. Gupta JM, Roberton NR, Wigglesworth JS (1968): Umbilical artery catheterization in the newborn. Arch Dis Child 43:382–387.

32. Hall RT, Oliver TK (1971): Aortic blood pressure in infants admitted to a neonatal intensive care unit. Am J Dis Child 121:145–147.

33. Hazinski TA, Blalock WA, Engelhardt B (1986): Vasopressin excess in infants with bronchopulmonary dysplasia (abstr). Pediatr Res 20:431A.

34. Hennekens CH, Jesse MJ, Klein BE, Gourley JE, Blumenthal S (1976): Aggregation of blood pressure in infants and their siblings. Am J Epidemiol 103:457–463.

35. Henry CG, Gutierrez F, Lee JT, Hartmann AF, Bell MJ, Bower RJ, Strauss AW (1981): Aortic thrombosis presenting as congestive heart failure: An umbilical artery catheter complication. J Pediatr 98:820–822.

36. Hymes LC, Washaw BL (1983): Captopril: Long term treatment of hypertension in a preterm infant and in older children. Am J Dis Child 137:263–266.

37. Ingelfinger J (1982): Pediatric Hypertension. Philadelphia, WB Saunders, pp 229–240.

38. Kirkland RT, Kirkland JL (1972): Systolic blood pressure measurements in the newborn infant with the transcutaneous Doppler method. J Pediatr 80:52–56.

39. Kitterman JA, Phibbs RH, Tooley WH (1969): Aortic blood pressure in normal newborn infants during the first 12 hours of life. Pediatrics 44:959–968.

40. Kotchen TA, Strickland AL, Rice TW, Walters DR (1972): A study of the renin-angiotensin system in newborn infants. J Pediatr 80:938–946.

41. Kowalski W (1921): Ueber thrombose des Ductus arteriosus bei Neugeborener. Virchow's Arch 233:191.

42. Krueger TC, Neblett WW, O'Neill JA, MacDonell RC, Dean RH, Thieme GA (1985): Management of aortic thrombosis secondary to umbilical artery catheters in neonates. J Pediatr Surg 20:328–332.

43. Lawson JD, Boerth R, Foster JH, Dean RH (1977): Diagnosis and management of renovascular hypertension in children. Arch Surg 112:1307–1316.

44. Levison H, Kidd BS, Gemmell PA, Swyer PR (1966): Blood pressure in normal full-term and premature infants. Am J Dis Child 111:374–379.

45. Lieberman J (1976): Clinical Pediatric Nephrology. Philadelphia, JB Lippincott, p 2.

46. Ljunquist A, Wallgren G (1962): Unilateral renal artery stenosis and fatal arterial hypertension in a newborn infant. Acta Paediatr Scand 51:575–584.

47. Loggie JM (1979): Juvenile hypertension. In Moss AJ (ed): Pediatrics Update. New York, Elsevier, pp 237–249.

48. Lui K, Doyle PE, Buchanan N (1982): Oscillometric and intra-arterial blood pressure measurements in the neonate: A comparison of methods. Aust Paediatr J 18:32–34.

49. Malin SW, Baumgart S, Rosenberg HK, Foreman J (1985): Non-surgical management of obstructive aortic thrombosis complicated by renovascular hypertension in the neonate. J Pediatr 106:630–634.

50. Mattioli L, Zakheim RM, Mullis K, Molteni A (1975): Angiotensin I converting enzyme activity in idiopathic respiratory distress of the newborn infant and in experimental alveoloar hypoxia in mice. J Pediatr 87:97–101.

51. Menser MA, Dorman DC, Reye RD (1966): Renal artery stenosis in the rubella syndrome. Lancet 1:790–792.

52. Merten DF, Vogel JM, Adelman RD, Goetzman BW, Bogren HG (1978): Renovascular hypertension as a complication of umbilical arterial catheterization. Pediatr Radiol 126:751–757.

53. Milner LS, Heitner R, Thomson PD, Levin SE, Rothberg AD, Beale P, Ninin DT (1984): Hypertension as the major problem of idiopathic arterial calcification of infancy. J Pediatr 105:934–938.

54. Mirkin BL, Newman TJ (1985): Efficiency and safety of captopril in the treatment of severe childhood hypertension: Report of the International Collaborative Study Group. Pediatrics 75:1091–1100.

55. Modanlou H, Yeh S, Siassi B, Hon EH (1974): Direct monitoring of arterial blood pressure in depressed and normal newborn infants during the first hour of life. J Pediatr 85:553–559.

56. Mokrohisky ST, Levine RL, Blumhagen JD, Wesenberg RL, Simmons MA (1978): Low positioning of umbilical artery catheters increases associated complications in newborn infants. N Engl J Med 299:561–564.

57. Moscoso P, Goldberg RN, Jamieson J, Bancalari E (1983): Spontaneous elevation in arterial blood pressure during the first hours of life in the very low birth weight infant. J Pediatr 103:114–117.

58. Neal WA, Reynolds JW, Jarvis CW, Williams HJ (1972): Umbilical artery catheterization: Demonstration of arterial thrombosis by aortography. Pediatrics 50:6–13.

59. Neligan GA, Smith CA (1960): The blood pressure of newborn infants in asphyxial states and in hyaline membrane disease. Pediatrics 26:735–744.

60. Ohnishi A, Branch RA, Jackson K, Hamilton R, Biaggioni I, Deray G, Jackson EK (1986): Chronic caffeine administration exacerbates renovascular, but not genetic, hypertension in rats. J Clin Invest 78:1045–1050.

61. Plumer LB, Mendoza SA, Kaplan GW (1976): Hypertension in infancy: The case for aggressive management. J Urol 113:555–557.

62. Rahill WJ, Rubin MI (1972): Hypertension in infantile polycystic renal disease. Clin Pediatr 11:232–235.

63. Rauchfuss C (1859): Ueber Thrombose des Ductus arteriosus botalli. Virchow's Arch 17:376.

64. Ribemont A (1879): Recherches sur la tension du sang dans les vaisseaux du foetus et du nouveau-né à propos du moment ou l'on doit lier le cordon ombilical. Arch Tocol 6:577.

65. Robinson MJ, Kent M, Stocks J (1973): Phaeochromocytoma in childhood. Arch Dis Child 48:137–142.

66. Rosen PR, Treves S, Ingelfinger J (1985): Hypertension in children. Am J Dis Child 139:173–177.

67. Rucker MP, Connel JW (1924): Blood pressure in the newborn. Am J Dis Child 27:6–24.

68. Rudolph AM (1974): Congenital Diseases of the Heart. Chicago, Year Book Medical Publishers, pp 338–340.

69. Sheftel DN, Hustead V, Friedman A (1983): Hypertension screening in the followup of premature infants. Pediatrics 71:763–766.

70. Siegler RL (1976): Conservative management of neonatal renal artery embolism. Urology 8:484–487.

71. Solosko D, Smith RB (1972): Hypertension following 10 percent phenylephrine ophthalmic. Anesthesiology 36:187–189.

72. de Swiet M, Fayers P, Shinebourne EA (1980): Systolic blood pressure in a population of infants in the first year of life: The Brompton Study. Pediatrics 65:1028–1035.

73. Tyson JE, de Sa DJ, Moore S (1976): Thromboatheromatous complications of umbilical arterial catheterization in the newborn period. Arch Dis Child 51:744–754.

74. Versmold HT, Kitterman JA, Phibbs RH, Gregory GA, Tooley WH (1981): Aortic blood pressure during the first 12 hours of life in infants with birth weight 610 to 4220 grams. Pediatrics 67:607–613.

75. Woodard JR, Patterson JH, Brinsfield D (1967): Renal artery thrombosis in newborn infants. Am J Dis Child 114:191–194.

76. Zuelzer WW, Kurnetz R, Newton WA (1951): Occlusion of the renal artery: IV. Am J Dis Child 81:21–25.

40 CARDIOMYOPATHIES

David J. Fisher

This chapter will discuss the cardiomyopathies that may be encountered in fetuses and in newborn and young infants. Although most of the available information regarding cardiomyopathies in fetuses is from necropsy data, this information has been included because the advent of fetal echocardiography should increase the frequency of the diagnosis of fetal cardiomyopathy in vivo. Cardiomyopathy is defined by abnormally reduced systolic contractile function or abnormal diastolic function rather than by abnormal pump function (cardiac output). Although the pediatric cardiologist generally is called on to evaluate patients with symptoms and signs of congestive cardiac failure, patients with conditions such as fluid overload should not be included in the group of cardiomyopathies unless there is also evidence of systolic and/or diastolic muscle dysfunction. Thus, this chapter will attempt to identify the evidence for muscle dysfunction for each cardiomyopathy. The cardiomyopathies reviewed in this chapter include those associated with birth asphyxia, maternal diabetes mellitus, Pompe disease, endocardial fibroelastosis, myocarditis, coronary arterial occlusion, and anomalous left coronary artery. The chest radiograph frequently demonstrates cardiomegaly with pulmonary edema in these diseases and will not be discussed further.

BIRTH ASPHYXIA

Several clinical studies have demonstrated that severe birth asphyxia (Fig. 40–1) may result in a cardiomyopathy.[12,77] An ischemic basis for the dysfunction has been postulated based on electrocardiographic ST segment and T wave changes (Fig. 40–2), reduced myocardial thallium uptake (Fig. 40–3), increased serum creatinine kinase MB activity, and necropsy evidence of subendocardial and papillary muscle necrosis.[11,22,30,66,77] The physical examination may be normal, a S_3 gallop may be heard, or there may be a tricuspid insufficiency murmur.[11,77] Affected patients are characterized by left and/or right ventricular dilation, normal myocardial thickness, and reduced shortening fraction.[21,77] As asphyxia has been associated with hypoxemia, acidemia, hypoglycemia, hypocalcemia, polycythemia, and/or pulmonary arterial hypertension, it has been suggested that one or more of these metabolic or hemodynamic alterations may be fundamental in producing

the cardiomyopathy.[11,73,77] Experimental data supporting a link between these abnormalities and myocardial ischemia and/or cardiomyopathy remain elusive.

Hypoxemia and Hypoxia

Although clinical studies have demonstrated that hypoxemia occurs frequently in patients who developed asphyxial cardiomyopathy, data from animal experiments suggest that hypoxemia alone (reduced blood oxygen tension, saturation, and content) is unlikely to produce myocardial hypoxia in vivo. Fetal lambs are normally hypoxemic (PaO_2 = 20 to 25 mmHg) compared with adult sheep, but left ventricular myocardial oxygen consumption per gram of myocardium is similar in fetuses and adults.[35] Furthermore, reducing arterial PaO_2's to the range of 12 to 14 mmHg was associated with a four- to sevenfold increase in coronary blood flow, so that hypoxemia per se did not produce subendocardial or papillary muscle ischemia, and myocardial oxygen consumption was not diminished in fetal or newborn lambs.[31,32,36,37] Indeed, myocardial contractility and pump function during hypoxemia were increased through augmented β-sympathetic function in neonatal lambs.[31] Although hypoxemia did not produce tissue hypoxia, similar levels of hypoxemia did produce tissue hypoxia in the liver, gastrointestinal tract, and kidneys in lambs.[24,25,56] These organs apparently released metabolic acids into the systemic circulation during severe hypoxemia, and metabolic acidemia occurred when the buffering capacity was exceeded.

Acidemia and Acidosis

Acidemia has also been noted to occur frequently in newborns with asphyxial cardiomyopathy. The reduction in intracellular pH that occurs during severe coronary ischemia does depress contractility,[15] and severe near total coronary occlusion produced a greater pH reduction in the subendocardium than in the subepicardium.[95] The excess hydrogen ions apparently interfere with the interaction between calcium and troponin.[82,95] However, models of metabolic acidemia in mature dogs and newborn lambs produced only a 30 to 40 per cent reduction in coronary blood flow, which is unlikely to produce tissue ischemia and/or acidosis.[33,34,46,54] Thus, it appears that systemic metabolic acidemia is unlikely to produce a significant enough reduction in coronary blood flow to account for the signs of myocardial ischemia and cardiomyopathy that can occur after birth asphyxia.

The author greatfully acknowledges the constructive review of this manuscript by Dr. Michael R. Nihill as well as the secretarial assistance of Ms. Cheryl Robideau.

499

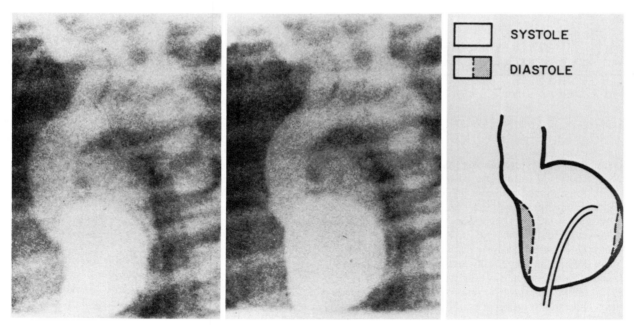

Figure 40–1. A left ventricular angiogram from an asphyxiated newborn infant. Systolic excursion is greatly diminished and mitral insufficiency is also demonstrated. (Reproduced with permission from Rowe RD, Hoffman T [1972]: Transient myocardial ischemia of the newborn infant: A form of severe cardiorespiratory distress in full-term infants. J Pediatr 81:243–250.)

There are several flow-independent factors that have been proposed as mechanisms by which acidemia may reduce contractility. Acidemia could reduce intracellular pH by direct equilibration across the sarcolemma, but the data are conflicting, and the degree of intracellular pH reduction that is necessary to reduce contractility in the absence of ischemia is unknown.[75,102] Alternatively, acidemia interferes with adrenergic receptor binding and di-

minishes the response to endogenous catecholamines.[4,61] Reductions in the myocardial response to endogenous catecholamines may account for some of the reduction in contractility and pump performance during asphyxia, but they would not account for the necropsy evidence of selective subendocardial and/or papillary muscle ischemia.[22] Nonetheless, it is important for clinicians to note that acidemia reduces the inotropic and chronotropic responses

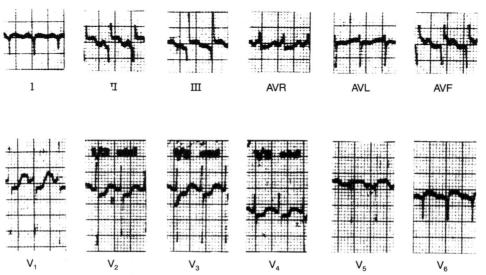

Figure 40–2. An electrocardiogram performed 6 hours after birth in an asphyxiated full-term newborn infant. Prominent Q waves are demonstrated in leads I, II, III, aV$_f$, and V$_6$, and ST elevation is demonstrated in leads II and V$_6$, consistent with inferolateral myocardial infarction. (Reproduced with permission from Kilbride H, Fulginiti VA [1980]: Myocardial infarction in the neonate with normal heart and coronary arteries. Am J Dis Child 134:759–762.)

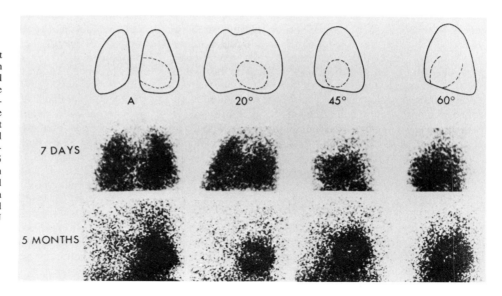

Figure 40–3. Thallium-201 images at 7 days and at 5 months after birth in a patient with transient myocardial ischemia. The different views are depicted above the images. Decreased myocardial thallium uptake is present on this study performed at 7 days after birth, whereas normal myocardial thallium uptake is present on the study performed at 5 months after birth. (Reproduced with permission from Finley JP et al [1979]: Transient myocardial ischemia of the newborn infant demonstrated by thallium myocardial imaging. J Pediatr 94:263–270.)

to endogenous and exogenously administered catecholamines.[4] Thus, the importance of a normal pH for maximizing cardiac output must be kept in mind.

Hypoglycemia

Early studies in cultured cells and isolated hearts had supported the concept that the fetal and newborn myocardium depended exclusively on glucose for an energy substrate. Although circulating free fatty acids were demonstrated to be the predominant energy substrate in adult hearts of several species, little myocardial free fatty acid uptake occurred in newborn dogs, cows, rats, and mice.[9,10,18,91,93,94,101,105] Thus, it was intriguing that data from clinical studies suggested an association between hypoglycemia and asphyxial cardiomyopathy.[1,11,73,104]

There is little information available regarding myocardial substrate utilization in normal human fetuses or newborns. However, recent studies have shown that glucose could supply no more than one third of the myocardial energy requirements in chronically catheterized fetal and newborn lambs.[35,38] Lactate appears to be the major myocardial energy substrate for fetal lambs in utero.[35] Previous work had demonstrated the occurrence of an important postnatal rise in circulating free fatty acid concentrations in lambs.[90] More recently, we have determined that free fatty acids appear to be an important energy substrate in lambs as early as 5 to 6 days after birth.[34] Werner et al have demonstrated that free fatty acid uptake accounts for 95 per cent of myocardial energy demands as early as 1 to 2 days after birth in the newborn pig heart in vitro.[98,99] Thus, there may be considerable species variability regarding neonatal myocardial energy substrate utilization, but it is unlikely that glucose supplies all of the energy demands of the perinatal heart. As an alternative, there is some evidence to suggest that some glucose may be critical for certain perinatal (and/or adult) myocardial metabolic pathways, but this hypothesis has not been addressed directly.[99]

Another mechanism by which the circulating glucose concentrations may affect myocardial function is through their influence on myocardial glycogen content. The increased resistance to myocardial hypoxia in the developing organism is based at least in part on its greater myocardial glycogen stores as well as its greater ability to sustain myocardial function through increased glycolytic rates during periods of anerobic metabolism.[19,59,75,87] It is possible that if birth asphyxia is severe enough to cause myocardial hypoxia (through an unknown mechanism), then the simultaneous occurrence of hypoglycemia could inhibit the glycogen-dependent protective mechanisms by limiting the source for myocardial glycogen stores.[44] Thus, although the mechanism(s) by which hypoglycemia may acutely influence myocardial function remain unknown, a relationship between low circulating glucose concentrations and cardiac dysfunction has been observed repeatedly in the neonatal period. Consequently, it appears that myocardial function may be dependent on normal circulating glucose concentrations in newborns even though we do not understand why. However, there does not appear to be any known mechanism that could link hypoglycemia and the subendocardial ischemia of birth asphyxia.

Hypocalcemia

The positive inotropic effect of calcium in the mature heart is tightly regulated through calcium binding and release at the sarcoplasmic reticulum.[14,29] Fetal and young newborn dog hearts have very limited sacroplasmic reticulum.[62] In amphibian hearts, which also have very little sarcoplasmic reticulum, myofibrillar calcium content appears to be a function of transsarcolemonal calcium flux and extracellular calcium concentration rather than a function of release of calcium from the sarcoplasmic reticulum.[14,29] These differences may form some of the basis of the greater sensitivity of the newborn rabbit heart to changes in extracellular calcium concentrations.[58] If these principles are applicable to human newborns, one may conceptualize how contractile function may be reduced during periods of hypocalcemia, but it is more difficult to understand how hypocalcemia alone could have resulted in congestive heart failure that persisted for several days after the serum concentration was restored to normal.[89] Thus, it is probably important to normalize a low serum calcium concentration in the asphyxiated newborn with congestive heart failure and diminished contractility, but it is difficult to implicate hypocalcemia as a cause of congestive heart failure that persists even when the calcium concentration is restored to normal.

Polycythemia

Polycythemia has been associated with asphyxia and congestive heart failure.[43] There are several mechanisms by which polycythemia could contribute to asphyxial myocardial ischemia. Although resting coronary blood flow was normal in mature polycythemic dogs, the higher viscosity of polycythemic blood–increased coronary vascular resistance and reduced subendocardial coronary vasodilator reserve capacity.[88] As subendocardial supply-demand mismatches are avoided during severe hypoxemia by the profound neonatal coronary vasodilator reserve capacity,[32] it is possible that the reduced vasodilator reserve of polycythemia may result in subendocardial ischemia when polycythemia occurs in association with hypoxemia. This potential interaction of hypoxemia and polycythemia on the subendocardium has not been validated experimentally.

Studies in mature dogs have demonstrated that polycythemia also causes several hemodynamic alterations that may be relevant to the development of myocardial ischemia, including increases in pulmonary and systemic vascular resistance as well as reductions in cardiac output. The increases in resistances should increase right- and left-sided myocardial demands, whereas severe reductions in cardiac output could reduce coronary filling pressures. Although these hemodynamic alternations are unlikely to produce ischemic cardiomyopathy by themselves, myocardial ischemia could take place when they occur in the presence of additional stresses such as hypoxemia. It is noteworthy that the increase in pulmonary vascular resistance during polycythemia with hypoxemia is greater than the increases in resistance from each stress alone.

These hemodynamic effects of polycythemia offer some support for the therapeutic normalization of the hematocrit in certain affected patients. The subsequent normalization of systemic and pulmonary vascular resistances may ease loading conditions in the ischemic heart. However, it is important to know whether or not hypervolemia is also present. In the absence of hypervolemia, exchange transfusion should be safer than phlebotomy because the latter may reduce an already low cardiac output.[41]

Pulmonary Arterial Hypertension

A severely elevated pulmonary vascular resistance could produce a subendocardial supply-demand mismatch that could account for some of the cases of right ventricular subendocardial and papillary muscle ischemia in newborns.[11,22,73,76] Acute experiments in mature dogs have demonstrated that progressive pulmonary arterial constriction produced congestive heart failure when the stenosis was great enough to produce a right ventricular myocardial supply-demand mismatch.[92] The heart failure caused by progressive elevation in right ventricular afterload apparently was mediated by diminished right ventricular high energy phosphate stores that occurred during subendocardial ischemia.[92]

There were no significant changes in left ventricular subendocardial energy stores or blood flow, as right ventricular afterload was elevated, and it was postulated that the reductions in cardiac output resulted from reduced left-sided filling from poor right heart function.[92] Although this mechanism may account for some of the cases of right ventricular myocardial ischemia in asphyxiated newborns, it could not account for the documented cases of left ventricular subendocardial and papillary muscle ischemia.[11,73,77] If right ventricular myocardial ischemia is to be implicated, it should be recognized that the perfusion pressure to all areas of the myocardium is generated in the aorta.[92] Thus, the maintenance of at least a normal aortic pressure may be very important in minimizing the extension of right ventricular myocardial ischemia during resuscitation of asphyxiated newborns.

MATERNAL DIABETES MELLITUS

Older reports regarding infants of diabetic mothers had described a dilated cardiomyopathy with congestive heart failure, but there is little information on this entity.[70,96] In contrast, a hypertrophic cardiomyopathy with congestive heart failure has been described in detail more recently in newborns of diabetic mothers.[49,96] The hemodynamic, echocardiographic, and histologic characteristics of the hypertrophic cardiomyopathy in the newborn of a diabetic mother are similar to those of familial hypertrophic cardiomyopathy.[55] These similarities include asymmetrical septal hypertrophy, dynamic subaortic stenosis, and myofibrillar disarray.[8,49,63,96] The hypertrophic cardiomyopathy is different in the newborn of a diabetic mother in that it is not familial, it generally regresses over 6 to 12 months after birth, and it may involve the right ventricular outflow tract as well as the left.[50] It has been estimated that 30 per cent of newborns of diabetic mothers have cardiomegaly, that 5 to 10 per cent have congestive heart failure, and that diabetic hypertrophic cardiomyopathy does seem to be more commonly associated with poor maternal glucose regulation.[8,63,68]

A systolic ejection murmur in a newborn of a diabetic mother should raise the suspicion of hypertrophic obstructive cardiomyopathy. The ECG is not specific. A full evaluation, including echocardiography and Doppler examination, is necessary because of the apparently increased incidence of congenital heart defects in newborns of diabetic mothers.[74] Echocardiography in infants affected by hypertrophic cardiomyopathy should rule out structural con-

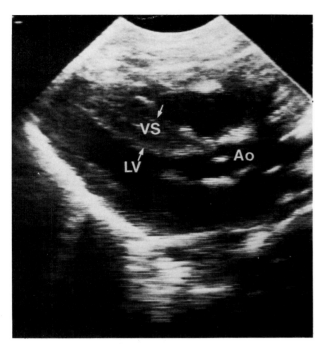

Figure 40–4. Parasternal long axis view of a two-dimensional echocardiogram from a newborn of a diabetic mother. The image demonstrates increased thickness of the ventricular septum consistent with asymmetric septal hypertrophy. The arrows depict the edges of ventricular septum. Ao = aortic root; LV = left ventricle; VS = ventricular septum.

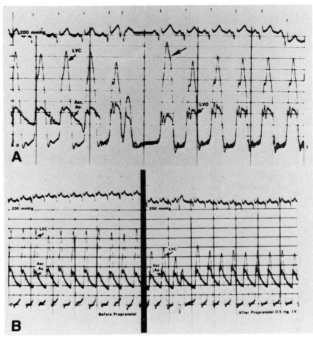

Figure 40–5. Hemodynamic tracings from a 3-week-old infant of a diabetic mother. *A*, Demonstration of subaortic stenosis. Asc Ao = ascending aorta; LVC = left ventricular cavity; LVO = left ventricular outflow tract. *B*, The significant reduction in pressure gradient after 0.5 mg IV propranolol administration demonstrates the dynamic nature of this subaortic obstruction. (Reproduced with permission from Way GL et al [1979]: The natural history of hypertrophic cardiomyopathy in infants of diabetic mothers. J Pediatr 95:1020–1025.)

genital heart defects and demonstrate septal hypertrophy (Fig. 40–4) as well as outflow tract obstruction.[63,96,97] The shortening fraction was typically normal in asymptomatic patients but may be increased in those with congestive heart failure.[49,63] Thus, the cardiomyopathy does not appear to be primarily systolic in nature but may be due to other factors such as diastolic restriction.[63] Doppler examination may demonstrate the dynamic nature of any hemodynamically significant obstruction. In the setting of an appropriate history and noninvasive evaluation, there does not appear to be any need for cardiac catheterization in most cases.

The management of asymptomatic newborns with this cardiomyopathy is purely supportive.[63,96] However, patients with severe congestive heart failure present more of a management problem. Digitalis glycosides are contraindicated;[63,96] they appear to make symptoms worse, perhaps by reducing left ventricular chamber volume and by increasing the dynamic outflow obstruction. In contrast, early experience with propranolol suggests a beneficial effect (Fig. 40–5), perhaps through increasing chamber volume.[63,96] Treatment with calcium channel blockers has resulted in some successes in children with hypertrophic cardiomyopathy, but they should not be used in newborns of diabetic mothers because of the great sensitivity during the neonatal period to the functional effects of calcium channel blockers.[6,28,86] Cardiovascular collapse has been reported in otherwise normal newborns after calcium channel blockers were administered to control supraventricular tachycardia.[28]

POMPE DISEASE

Pompe disease is an autosomal recessive disorder that is biochemically characterized by the absence of lysosomal acid α-1,4 glucosidase (acid maltase). Absence of acid maltase results in excessive glycogen storage in most tissues. The clinical manifestations include a large tongue, generalized muscle weakness, a poor ability to suck, and somatic wasting. Systemic symptoms often appear within 1 to 3 months after birth and progress rapidly so that death occurs most often before 1 year of age.

Cardiac manifestations occasionally are present at birth but more commonly begin in the 2- to 4-month-old infant with the onset of of congestive heart failure. A subaortic outflow murmur may be present. The electrocardiogram (Fig. 40–6) typically shows a short PR interval without preexcitation, very tall and often wide left precordial QRS complexes, and T wave changes.[27] The echocardiogram (Fig. 40–7) shows severe hypertrophy of the septum, free wall, posterior wall, and papillary muscles of the left ventricle.[72,83,84] The combination of severe hypertrophy and hyperdynamic systolic function produces near cavity obliteration during contraction. There is no evidence of diminished systolic contractile function early in Pompe disease. Instead, the cardiac dysfunction may result from dynamic outflow obstruction[72,84] or diastolic dysfunction, although the latter has not been defined in detail. Later in

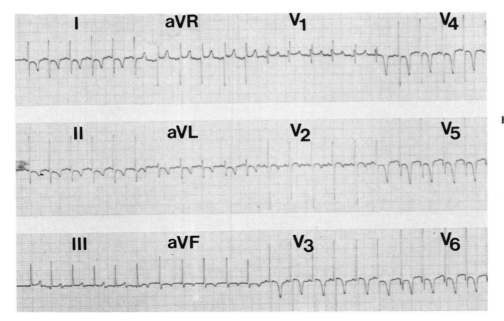

Figure 40–6. A typical electrocardiogram from a 1-month-old patient with Pompe disease, demonstrating the short PR interval, left ventricular hypertrophy, right ventricular hypertrophy, and inverted left precordial T waves. (The tracing was kindly furnished by Dr. Donald M. Gross.)

the course of Pompe disease there may be systolic dysfunction and cavity dilation. Cardiac catheterization does not appear to provide any additional diagnostic information, unless a myocardial biopsy is necessary for diagnosis.

The diagnosis of Pompe disease is generally established by demonstration of absent α-1,4 glycosidase in skeletal muscle, lymphocytes, or cultured skin fibroblasts. There is no primary treatment. Attempts at enzyme replacement have not been successful to date. Most patients die before 1 year of age in spite of conventional treatment for congestive heart failure. As in the case of newborns of diabetic mothers, digitalis is contraindicated in Pompe disease when there is dynamic subaortic obstruction secondary to hypertrophy and hyperdynamic systolic function.

ENDOCARDIAL FIBROELASTOSIS

Endocardial fibroelastosis is characterized by the presence of a white, glistening fibroelastic membrane over the left ventricular inner surface.[20] Left atrial, right ventricular, and valvular fibroelastosis also may occur.[20,60] Endocardial fibroelastosis may be primary and isolated, or it may occur secondary to left-sided obstructive lesions such as aortic stenosis or coarctation of the aorta. The primary form will be discussed in this section. Infectious, hypoxic, genetic, and hemodynamic theories have been put forward to explain the primary form, but they remain unconfirmed.

Symptoms of congestive heart failure may be present at birth but most often occur during the first year of life. Presentation is often prompted by an infection. An S_3 gal-

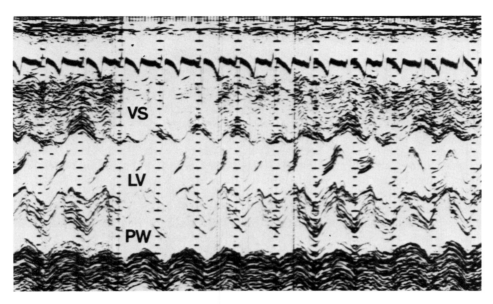

Figure 40–7. A typical M-mode echocardiogram in Pompe disease, demonstrating severe thickening of the ventricular septum and the left ventricular posterior wall. There is also some encroachment of the left ventricular cavity dimension. LV = left ventricle; PW = left ventricular posterior wall; VS = ventricular septum. (This tracing was kindly supplied by Dr. Donald M. Gross.)

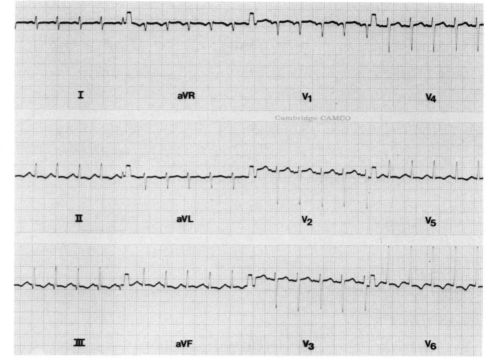

Figure 40–8. A typical electrocardiogram in a 5-month-old patient with primary endocardial fibroelastosis, demonstrating left ventricular hypertrophy with left lateral T wave inversion.

lop is common and prominent, and the murmur of mitral regurgitation may be present. The typical ECG (Fig. 40–8) shows left ventricular hypertrophy with inverted left precordial T waves.[81,91] The PR interval is normal. The ECG may progress to signs of myocardial ischemia. The echocardiogram (Fig. 40–9) demonstrates an extremely dilated but only mildly or moderately thickened left ventricle with a particularly bright (echo dense) endocardium. The shortening fraction is diminished. Mitral regurgitation is frequently present. Cardiac catheterization may be necessary to rule out origination of an anomalous left coronary artery from the pulmonary artery, or a biopsy may be necessary to exclude the rare cases of myocarditis that present with left ventricular hypertrophy.[48]

There is no primary therapy. Management is directed at the symptoms of congestive heart failure. Digitalis therapy has been shown to prolong survival and perhaps to produce long-term survival.[52,64] Diuretics and afterload reduction also appear to be beneficial. Medical therapy should be maintained at least until there are no symptoms of congestive heart failure and the ECG and heart size are normal, which generally would be at least 2 to 3 years after presentation. The prognosis is particularly poor for patients who present in the first weeks or months after birth, in whom the course is almost universally fatal. Patients who present later in the first year of life or after 1 year of age have a better prognosis, although the mortality is in the range of 25 to 40 per cent. It is interesting that survival time has been related to the number of cardiac chambers that are involved.[40] The average survival time was 120 days with one fibroelastic chamber and 300 days with three affected chambers.

MYOCARDITIS

Myocarditis may be associated with an acute cardiac dysfunction, or a chronic cardiomyopathy may develop. The diagnostic features and management of myocarditis in newborns are similar to those in infants and older children, and the details can be found in Chapter 47. Low

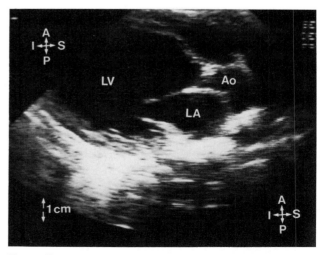

Figure 40–9. Parasternal long axis view of a two-dimensional echocardiogram from a 5-month-old female with primary endocardial fibroelastosis. The image demonstrates severe left ventricular cavity dilation with normal left ventricular and septal wall thickness. A = anterior; Ao = aortic root; I = inferior; LA = left atrium; LV = left ventricle; P = posterior; S = superior.

QRS voltage and inverted left precordial T waves are commonly seen on the ECG. Left ventricular hypertrophy is rare in myocarditis.[48] The acute myocardial dysfunction of myocarditis is characterized by left ventricular dilation, reduced shortening fraction, and normal wall thickness. Digitalis and diuretics should be administered for congestive heart failure when acute myocardial dysfunction occurs during myocarditis. Although the efficacy and timing of anti-inflammatory agents in myocarditis remains controversial, catheterization for biopsy may be performed before and after therapy to provide histologic confirmation of efficacy as well as guidance regarding the duration of therapy. As is the case in treatment of endocardial fibroelastosis, digitalis and diuretics should be administered in chronic myocardial dysfunction due to myocarditis until there are no signs of cardiac failure and the heart size and the ECG are normal.

ANOMALOUS ORIGIN OF THE LEFT CORONARY ARTERY

Pathophysiology

This rare lesion is characterized by the anomalous origin of the left main coronary artery (ALCA) from the pulmonary artery, most often from its left sinus. ALCA generally occurs as an isolated lesion, but infrequently it is accompanied by a patent ductus arteriosus or a ventricular septal defect. Collateral vessels connecting the two coronary arteries are very important in the development of myocardial ischemia. As the pulmonary vascular resistance decreases postnatally, the pulmonary arterial contribution to left coronary arterial perfusion pressure and flow diminishes. By 6 weeks of age, pulmonary arterial pressures fall below levels necessary for adequate perfusion of the left ventricle, which must work against systemic afterload. As patients with single coronary arteries generally do not develop myocardial ischemia as infants, the development of myocardial ischemia in infants with ALCA appears to result from inadequate left coronary perfusion pressure from the pulmonary artery in conjunction with inadequate collateral blood flow from the right coronary artery. The concept that symptoms in ALCA are a function of both pulmonary arterial pressure and the extent of collateral circulation is supported by the findings from case reports of ALCA in association with a ventricular septal defect.[69,71] The ALCA was well tolerated until surgical closure of the ventricular septal defect reduced pulmonary arterial pressure and thus, perfusion to the left ventricular myocardium from the anomalous left coronary artery. Although coronary perfusion pressure and blood flow appear to be closely linked in ALCA, experimental data in mature dogs indicate that coronary perfusion pressure per se is not an independent determinant of myocardial function.[85] Therefore, the main problem at initial presentation appears to be reduced perfusion pressure without adequate collateral coronary flow. The pathophysiology that has been outlined for isolated ALCA accounts for the majority of patients, the so-called infantile

variety.[2,23,100] A smaller group of patients present as asymptomatic older children or adults, or they present with a continuous murmur. These patients would appear to have developed adequate collateral flow in early infancy. One possible explanation of why some infants with ALCA remain asymptomatic while others develop myocardial dysfunction and even infarction may be differences in the rate at which pulmonary vascular resistance drops postnatally. Infants with ALCA in whom pulmonary vascular resistance drops rapidly are more likely to develop myocardial ischemia and infarction; infants with ALCA in whom pulmonary vascular resistance drops more slowly would have time to develop life saving collateral vessels between the normally perfused right and the anomalous left coronary arteries.

The diminished pulmonary arterial blood oxygen content perfusing the anomalous left coronary artery should not by itself produce myocardial hypoxia. Although in ALCA the left coronary artery presumably derives its blood flow from the pulmonary artery in utero, only a 5 to 10 per cent reduction in the (in utero) left coronary oxygen saturation should result, and fetal myocardial hypoxia should not be present.[37,38] Similarly, when the very young newborn with ALCA derives its left coronary arterial blood flow from the pulmonary artery, postnatal left coronary blood oxygen content should also be well tolerated because it is higher than normal fetal aortic blood oxygen content. As long as cardiac output is adequate, the blood oxygen content in the pulmonary artery and therefore the left coronary artery in ALCA is higher than that in many cyanotic congenital heart defects. These considerations suggest that the development of myocardial ischemia in ALCA occurs postnatally and is dependent on factors other than reduced left coronary blood oxygen content.

Clinical Presentation

Most newborns with ALCA are asymptomatic initially but develop episodic tachypnea, crying, anxiety, pneumonia and/or congestive heart failure between 3 to 4 weeks and 4 months after birth.[100] Most infants with ALCA do not have a murmur, but 10 to 15 per cent demonstrate mitral insufficiency.[100] Less frequently, a systolic murmur may be heard at the left lower sternal border, or a continuous murmur may be heard higher along the left sternal border.[100] Diastolic murmurs are uncommon. A third heart sound may be present but is not prominent, as in endocardial fibroelastosis and myocarditis. The typical ECG (Fig. 40–10) demonstrates anterolateral ischemia, with deep Q waves and tall R waves, ST segment depression, and T wave inversion in the I, AVL and left precordial leads.[5] ST segment elevation, a sign of acute infarction (or pericarditis), is a rare but virtually pathognomonic sign of ALCA in infants beyond the immediate newborn period with cardiomyopathy. Echocardiography demonstrates left ventricular dilation, diminished contraction and normal wall thickness of the posterior wall, exaggerated septal motion, and left atrial dilation.[39,45,84] Regional dyskinesis may be demonstrated. Aneurysmal dilation of the left ventricle

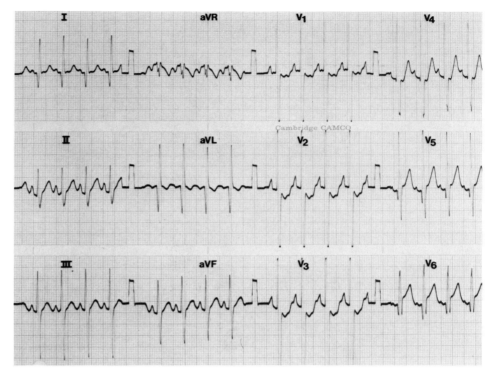

Figure 40–10. A typical electrocardiogram from a 6-week-old male with an anomalous left coronary artery originating from the pulmonary artery. The tracing demonstrates deep Q waves in I, aV_L, and the lateral precordial leads, consistent with either severe hypertrophy or infarction. ST elevation in V_5 and V_6 indicates lateral wall infarction.

and direct origin of the left coronary artery from the pulmonary artery also have been shown noninvasively.[36,45] Alternatively, the defect may be demonstrated by myocardial imaging with thallium-201.[49] One cannot rely on echocardiographic demonstration of what appears to be normal origin of the left coronary artery from the ascending aorta to rule out ALCA; angiography is necessary if this infrequently encountered lesion is to be demonstrated in all cases. Collateral coronary flow may occur by different pathways; the left anterior descending coronary artery may receive collateral flow from a right conal branch, a marginal branch, or septal branches. Alternatively, the left circumflex coronary artery may receive collateral flow from apical or posterior terminal branches of the right coronary artery.[53]

Surgery

Surgical approaches to ALCA have varied. Early attempts at pulmonary artery banding, aorticopulmonary anastomosis, and pericardial or epicardial abrasion were unsuccessful.[3,13,42] Ligation of the pulmonary arterial origin of the left coronary artery has been utilized to terminate the left-to-right shunt.[76,78,79] Ligation of the anomalous coronary artery may be helpful when collaterals are large and there is a significant steal of right coronary blood to the pulmonary artery, but this procedure would appear to be potentially harmful at the initial presentation if collateral flow and perfusion pressure to the left coronary artery are restricted. In a number of older infants and children, aortocoronary anastomosis has been performed with both arterial and saphenous vein grafts as well as

by direct reimplantation; success has been variable.[17,26,47] Although aortic reimplantation and transpulmonary left subclavian arterial grafting have been performed in a few patients with ALCA and congestive heart failure as early as 3 months after birth,[2,51,65,103] no series has been reported in which surgery was performed at the time of presentation. As a result, it is difficult to judge the effect of early surgery on either surgical morbidity and mortality or the functional and biochemical recovery of the affected myocardium. The earliest series of surgical anastomosis was performed an average of 2 weeks after presentation, and the results were disappointing;[23] these authors suggested delaying surgery until 18 months of age.[23]

Thus, the need for surgery in ALCA, the type of procedure to be performed, and its timing remain controversial. If the pathophysiology of the myocardial ischemia of the infantile form is dependent on inadequate left coronary blood flow secondary to reduced pulmonary perfusion pressure in the absence of adequate collateral vessels, then early surgical therapy should be useful if left coronary flow can be restored before the biochemical effects of ischemia produce irreversible myocardial dysfunction. Although complete arterial occlusion must be reversed within the first few hours in order to produce significant functional recovery, the coronary ischemia of ALCA initially may be more like the subtotal occlusion of chronic ischemia.[7] Unfortunately, the period of time that is available to prevent a completed infarct remains unknown. We also do not know if the infarcts in infants with ALCA have been completed by the time of initial presentation. Surgical restoration of left coronary flow in infants with ALCA will not provide functional correction for a completed infarct.

Additional important questions remain unanswered. The importance of coronary artery steal in the pathophysiology of the ischemia in ALCA remains unknown. Although several retrospective series have addressed the question of whether morbidity and mortality in ALCA are greater with medical or surgical therapy, no prospective randomized trial has been published. Mortality of medical therapy alone in ALCA has ranged from as little as 13 per cent to as much as 93 to 100 per cent for young infants with congestive heart failure secondary to ALCA.[2,23,100] As a result, no firm recommendation for early surgical therapy in symptomatic infants seems justified, even though logically establishing normal left coronary perfusion should be beneficial. Further, the timing of early surgical intervention (if surgery is to be performed) and the procedure of choice remain unknown. Because these questions remain unanswered, the management of ALCA remains controversial in this era when early coronary arterial reperfusion has become standard therapy in arteriosclerotic myocardial ischemia and infarction.

CORONARY ARTERIAL OCCLUSION

Coronary arterial occlusion from embolus or thrombus is even less common than birth asphyxia or anomalous left coronary artery as a cause of coronary ischemia and infarction. Both coronary emboli and thrombi have been reported in fetuses and in newborns in the absence of birth asphyxia or structural heart defects.[16,57,67,80] The necropsy reports are consistent with ischemic cardiomyopathy. The causes were unknown. Therapy has not been reported.

DIFFERENTIAL DIAGNOSIS

The differential diagnosis of the newborn or young infant with congestive heart failure and cardiomyopathy should prompt an orderly review of the data available from history, physical examination, ECG, echocardiography, and Doppler studies. In addition to the entities described in this chapter, the differential diagnosis includes polyarteritis nodosa, idiopathic calcification and medial necrosis of the coronary arteries, hydrops fetalis, tachyarrhythmias and bradyarrhythmias.

The cardiomyopathies of birth asphyxia and gestational diabetes are distinguished by their histories. The physical examination suggests dynamic subaortic stenosis in newborns of diabetic mothers and in some cases of Pompe disease. Prominent third heart sounds are typical in endocardial fibroelastosis and ALCA. The ECG typically shows left ventricular hypertrophy in endocardial fibroelastosis and in anomalous origin of the left coronary artery from the pulmonary artery but not in birth asphyxia or in myocarditis. Infants with Pompe disease often demonstrate biventricular hypertrophy and a short PR interval; ST elevation is very suggestive of ALCA. In newborns of diabetic mothers, half of the patients demonstrate left ventricular hypertrophy on ECG and half demonstrate right ventricular hypertrophy. T wave changes are usually present in asphyxia, Pompe disease, endocardial fibroelastosis, myocarditis, and ALCA. Echocardiography shows left ventricular cavity dilation in asphyxia, endocardial fibroelastosis, myocarditis (when there is cardiac dysfunction), and ALCA. Initially, left ventricular cavity size is reduced in newborns of diabetic mothers, and dynamic subaortic obstruction can be present in both disorders. The left ventricular free wall is greatly thickened in newborns of diabetic mothers and in cases of Pompe disease, but it is only moderately thickened in endocardial fibroelastosis. Systolic contractile function is diminished in asphyxia, endocardial fibroelastosis, and ALCA. Systolic function is normal or is increased early in the course of newborns of diabetic mothers and in cases of Pompe disease, but diastolic function may be depressed.

An accurate diagnosis and hemodynamic assessment can be made in many infants with symptomatic cardiomyopathies without cardiac catheterization if characteristic findings such as macroglossia, woody muscles, and a short PR interval (Pompe disease) are found. However, cardiac catheterization is necessary to differentiate between endocardial fibroelastosis and ALCA. Cardiac catheterization to perform myocardial biopsy may also be useful in infants with myocarditis to confirm the diagnosis and to evaluate the effects of any anti-inflammatory therapy.

References

1. Amatayakul O, Cumming GR, Haworth JC (1970): Association of hypoglycaemia with cardiac enlargement and heart failure in newborn infants. Arch Dis Child 45:717–720.
2. Arciniegas E, Farook ZQ, Hakimi M, Green EW (1980): Management of anomalous left coronary artery from the pulmonary artery. Circulation 62(Suppl 1):180–189.
3. Baisch BF, Giknis FL (1965): Rare anomalies of coronary circulation amenable to surgical correction: Left coronary to left pulmonary artery fistula and supranummerary coronary artery. Ann Thorac Surg 1:170–178.
4. Beierholm EA, Grantham RN, O'Keefe DD, Laver MB, Daggett WM (1975): Effects of acid–base changes, hypoxia, and catecholamines on ventricular performance. Am J Physiol 228:1555–1561.
5. Bland EF, White PD, Garland J (1933): Congenital anomalies of the coronary arteries: Report of an unusual case associated with cardiac hypertrophy. Am Heart J 8:787–801.
6. Boucek RJ Jr, Shelton N, Artman M, Mushlin PS, Stranes VA, Olson RD (1984): Comparative effects of verapamil, nifedipine and diltiazem on contractile function in the isolated immature and adult rabbit heart. Pediatr Res 18:948–952.
7. Braunwald E, Kloner RA (1982): The stunned myocardium: Prolonged postischemic ventricular dysfunction. Circulation 66:1146–1149.
8. Breitweser JA, Meyer RA, Sperling MA, Tsang RC, Kaplan S (1980): Cardiac septal hypertrophy in hyperinsulinemic infants. J Pediatr 96:535–539.
9. Breuer E, Barta E, Pappova E, Zlatos L (1967): Developmental changes of myocardial metabolism. I. Peculiarities of cardiac carbohydrate metabolism in the early postnatal period in dogs. Biol Neonate 11:367–377.
10. Breuer E, Barta E, Zlatos L, Pappova E (1968): Developmental changes of myocardial metabolism. II. Myocardial metabolism of fatty acids in the early postnatal period in dogs. Biol Neonate 12:54–64.
11. Bucciarelli RL, Nelson RM, Egan EA, Eitzman DV, Gessner IH (1977): Transient tricuspid insufficiency of the newborn: A form of myocardial dysfunction in stressed newborns. Pediatrics 59:330–337.

12. Burnard ED, James LS (1961): Failure of the heart after undue asphyxia at birth. Pediatrics 28:545–565.
13. Case RB, Morrow AG, Stainsby W, Nestor JO (1958): Anomalous origin of the left coronary artery: Physiologic defect and suggested surgical treatment. Circulation 17:1062–1068.
14. Chapman RA (1983): Control of cardiac contractility at the cellular level. Am J Physiol 245:H535–H552.
15. Cobbe SM, Pole–Rosen PA (1980): The time of onset and severity of acidosis in myocardial ischaemia. J Mol Cell Cardiol 12:745–760.
16. Cochrane WA, Bowden DH (1954): Calcification of the arteries in infancy and childhood. Pediatrics 14:222–231.
17. Cooley DA, Hallman GL, Bloodwell RD (1966): Definitive surgical treatment of anomalous origin of the left coronary artery from pulmonary artery: Indications and results. J Thorac Cardiovasc Surg 52:798–808.
18. Cox SJ, Gunberg DL (1972): Metabolite utilization by isolated embryonic rat hearts in vitro. Embryo Exp Morph 28:235–245.
19. Dawes GS, Mott JC, Shelley HJ (1959): The importance of cardiac glycogen for the maintenance of life in fetal lambs and new-born animals during anoxia. J Physiol (Lond): 146:516–538.
20. Dennis JL, Hansen AE, Corpening TN (1953): Endocardial fibroelastosis. Pediatrics 12:130–140.
21. DiSessa TG, Leitner M, Ti CC, Gluck L, Coen R, Friedman WF (1981): The cardiovascular effects of dopamine in the severely asphyxiated neonate. J Pediatr 99:772–776.
22. Donnelly WH, Bucciarelli RL, Nelson RM (1980): Ischemic papillary muscle necrosis in stressed newborn infants. J Pediatr 96:295–300.
23. Driscoll DJ, Nihill MR, Mullins CE, Cooley DA, McNamara DG (1981): Management of symptomatic infants with anomalous origin of the left coronary artery from the pulmonary artery. Am J Cardiol 47:642–648.
24. Edelstone DI, Lattanzi DR, Paulone ME, Holzman IR (1983): Neonatal intestinal oxygen consumption during arterial hypoxemia. Am J Physiol 244:G278–G283.
25. Edelstone DI, Paulone ME, Holzman IR (1984): Hepatic oxygenation during arterial hypoxemia in neonatal lambs. Am J Obstet Gynecol 150:513–518.
26. El–Said GM, Ruzyllo W, Williams RL, Mullins CE, Hallman GL, Cooley DA, McNamara DG (1979): Early and late results of saphenous vein graft for anomalous origin of the left coronary artery from pulmonary artery. Circulation 48(Suppl III):2–6.
27. Elhers KH, Hagstrom JWC, Lukas DS, Redo SF, Engle MA (1962): Glycogen storage disease of the myocardium with destruction to left ventricular outflow. Circulation 25:96–109.
28. Epstein ML, Kiel EA, Victorica BE (1985): Cardiac decompensation following verapamil therapy in infants with supraventricular tachycardia. Pediatrics 75:737–740.
29. Fabiato A (1983): Calcium-induced release of calcium from the cardiac sacroplasmic reticulum. Am J Physiol 245(1):C1–C14.
30. Finley JP, Howman-Giles RB, Gilday DL, Bloom KR, Rowe RD (1979): Transient myocardial ischemia of the newborn infant demonstrated by thallium myocardial imaging. J Pediatr 94:263–270.
31. Fisher DJ (1983): Left ventricular oxygen consumption and function in hypoxemia in conscious lambs. Am J Physiol 244:H664–H671.
32. Fisher DJ (1984): Increased regional myocardial blood flows and oxygen deliveries during hypoxemia in lambs. Pediatr Res 18:602–606.
33. Fisher DJ (1986): Acidaemia reduces cardiac output and left ventricular contractility in conscious lambs. J Devel Physiol 8:23–31.
34. Fisher DJ (1986): Myocardial uptake of free fatty acids in unanesthetized newborn and adult sheep. Unpublished data.
35. Fisher DJ, Heymann MA, Rudolph AM (1980): Myocardial oxygen and carbohydrate consumption in fetal lambs in utero and in adult sheep. Am J Physiol 238:H399–H405.
36. Fisher DJ, Heymann MA, Rudolph AM (1981): Myocardial consumption of oxygen and carbohydrates in newborn sheep. Pediatr Res 15:843–846.
37. Fisher DJ, Heymann MA, Rudolph AM (1982): Fetal myocardial oxygen and carbohydrate consumption during acutely induced hypoxemia. Am J Physiol 242:H657–H661.
38. Fisher DJ, Heymann MA, Rudolph AM (1982): Fetal myocardial oxygen and carbohydrate metabolism in sustained hypoxemia in utero. Am J Physiol 243:H959–H963.
39. Fisher EA, Sepehri B, Lendrum B, Luken J, Levitsky S (1981): Two-dimensional echocardiographic visualization of the left coronary artery in anomalous origin of the left coronary artery from the pulmonary artery. Circulation 63:698–704.
40. Forfar JO, Miller RA, Bain AD, MacLeod W (1964): Endocardial fibroelastosis. Br Med J 2:7–12.
41. Fouron JC, Hebert F (1973): The circulatory effects of hematocrit variations in normovolemic newborn lambs. J Pediatr 82:995–1003.
42. Gasul BM, Loeffler E (1949): Anomalous origin of the left coronary artery from the pulmonary artery. Report of four cases. Pediatrics 4:498–507.
43. Gatti RA, Muster AJ, Cole RB, Paul MH (1966): Neonatal polycythemia with transient cyanosis and cardiorespiratory abnormalities. J Pediatr 69:1063–1072.
44. Gelli MG, Enhorning G, Hultman E, Bergstrom J (1968): Glucose infusion in the pregnant rabbit and its effect on glycogen content and activity of the fetal heart under anoxia. Acta Pediatr Scand 57:209–214.
45. Glaser J, Bharati S, Whitman V, Liebman J (1973): Echocardiographic findings in patients with anomalous origin of the left coronary artery (abstr). Circulation (Suppl 4):63.
46. Goodyer AVN, Eckhardt WF, Ostberg RH, Goodkind MJ (1961): Effects of metabolic acidosis and alkalosis on coronary blood flow and myocardial metabolism in the intact dog. Am J Physiol 200:628–632.
47. Grace RR, Angelini P, Cooley DA (1977): Aortic implantation of an anomalous left coronary artery arising from pulmonary artery. Am J Cardiol 39:608–613.
48. Greenwood RD, Nadas AS, Fyler DC (1976): The clinical course of primary myocardial disease in infants and children. Am Heart J 92:549–560.
49. Gutgesell HP, Pinsky WW, DePuey EG (1980): Thallium-201 myocardial perfusion imaging in infants and children: Value in distinguishing anomalous left coronary artery from gestive cardiomyopathy. Circulation 61:596–599.
50. Gutgesell HP, Speer ME, Rosenberg HS (1980): Characterization of the cardiomyopathy in infants of diabetic mothers. Circulation 61:441–450.
51. Hamilton JRL, Mulholland HC, O'Kane HOJ (1986): Origin of the left coronary artery from the right pulmonary artery: A report of successful surgery in a 3-month-old child. Ann Thorac Surg 41:446–448.
52. Hastreiter AR, Miller RA Management of primary endomyocardial disease: The myocarditis-endocardial fibroelastosis syndrome. Pediatr Clin North Am 11:401–430.
53. Hawker RR (1976): Angiographic assessment of anomalous origin of the left coronary artery from the pulmonary artery in infancy and childhood. Pediatr Radiology 5:69–74.
54. Hearse DJ, Crome R, Yellon DM, Wyse R (1983): Metabolic and flow correlates of myocardial ischaemia. Cardiovas Res 17:452–458.
55. Henry WL, Clark CE, Epstein SE (1973): Asymmetric septal hypertrophy: Echocardiographic identification of the pathognomonic anatomic abnormality of IHSS. Circulation 47:225–233.
56. Iwamoto HS, Rudolph AM (1985): Metabolic responses of the kidney in fetal sheep: Effect of acute and spontaneous hypoxemia. Am J Physiol 249(6P+2):F836–841.
57. James TN, Froggatt P, Marshall TK (1973): De Subitaneis mortibus. II. Coronary embolism in the fetus. Circulation 48:890–896.
58. Jarmakani JM, Nakanishi T, George BL, Bers D (1982): Effect of extracellular calcium on myocardial mechanical function in the neonatal rabbit. Dev Pharmacol Ther 5:1–13.
59. Jarmakani JM, Nakazawa M, Nagatoma T, Langer GA (1978): Effect of hypoxia on mechanical function in the neonatal mammalian heart. Am J Physiol 235:H469–H474.
60. Lambert EC, Shumway CN, Terplan K (1953): Clinical diagnosis of endocardial fibrosis. Analysis of literature with report of four new cases. Pediatrics 11:255–269.
61. Lefkowitz RJ, Sharp GWG, Haber E (1973): Specific binding of

beta-adrenergic catecholamines to a subcellular fraction from cardiac muscle. J Biol Chem 248:342–349.

62. Legato M (1979): Cellular mechanisms of normal growth in the mammalian heart. II. A quantitative and qualitative comparison between the right ventricular and left ventricular myocytes in the dog from birth to five months of age. Circ Res 44:263–279.

63. Mace S, Hirschfeld SS, Riggs T, Fanaroff AA, Merkatz R (1979): Echocardiographic abnormalities in infants of diabetic mothers. J Pediatr 95:1013–1019.

64. Manning JA, Sellers FJ, Bynum RS, Keith JD (1964): The medical management of clinical endocardial fibroelastosis. Circulation 29:60–65.

65. Matsumoto A, Sato S, Kondo J, Kumada J, Goto H, Kohno M, Matsumura H, Niimura I (1976): Definitive surgical treatment of anomalous origin of the left coronary artery. A new technical approach used successfully in a seven-month-old male infant. Gen Thorac Cardiovasc Surg 72:249–255.

66. Nelson RM, Bucciarelli RL, Eitzman EM, Egan EA Jr, Gessner IH (1978): Serum creatine phosphokinase MB fraction in newborns with transient tricuspid insufficiency. N Engl J Med 298:146–149.

67. Oppenheimer EH, Esterley JR (1967): Some aspects of cardiac pathology in infancy and childhood. III. Coronary embolism. Johns Hopkins Med J 120:317–325.

68. Pildes RS (1973): Infants of diabetic mothers. N Engl J Med 289:902–904.

69. Pinsky WW, Gillette PC, Duff DF, Wanderman N, Morriss JH, Mullins CE, McNamara DG (1978): Anomalous origin of the left coronary artery from the pulmonary artery with ventricular septal defect. Circulation 57:1026–1030.

70. Poland RL, Walther LJ, Chang C (1975): Hypertrophic cardiomyopathy in infants of diabetic mothers (abstr). Pediatr Res 9:269.

71. Rao BNS, Lucas RV Jr, Edwards JE (1970): Anomalous origin of the left coronary artery from the right pulmonary artery associated with ventricular septal defect. Chest 59:616–620.

72. Rees A, Elbl F, Minhas K, Solinger R (1976): Echocardiographic evidence of outflow tract obstruction in Pompe's disease (glycogen storage disease of the heart). Am J Cardiol 37:1103–1106.

73. Riemenschneider TA, Nielson HC, Ruttenberg HD, Jaffe RB (1976): Disturbances of the transitional circulation: Spectrum of pulmonary hypertension and myocardial dysfunction. J Pediatr 89:622–625.

74. Roland TW, Hubbell JP Jr, Nadas AS (1973): Congenital heart disease in infants of diabetic mothers. J Pediatr 83:815–820.

75. Rovetto MJ, Lamberton WF, Neely JR (1975): Mechanisms of glycolytic inhibition in ischemic rat hearts. Circ Res 37:742–751.

76. Rowe CG, Young WP (1960): Anomalous origin of the coronary arteries with special reference to surgical treatment. J Thorac Cardiovasc Surg 39:777–780.

77. Rowe RD, Hoffman T (1972): Transient myocardial ischemia of the newborn infant: A form of severe cardiorespiratory distress in full-term infants. J Pediatr 81:243–250.

78. Rudolph AM, Gootman NL, Kaplan N, Rohman M (1963): Anomalous left coronary artery arising from the pulmonary artery with large left–to–right shunt in infancy. J Pediatr 63:543–549.

79. Sabiston DC, Ross RS, Criley JM, Gaertner RA, Neill CA, Taussig HB (1963): Surgical management of congenital lesions of the coronary circulation. Ann Surg 157:908–924.

80. Sapire DW, Markowitz R, Valdes–Dapena M, Engel S (1977): Thrombosis of the left coronary artery in a newborn infant. J Pediatr 90:957–959.

81. Sellars FJ, Keith JD, Manning JA (1964): The diagnosis of primary endocardial fibroelastosis. Circulation 29:49–59.

82. Serur JR, Skelton CL, Boden R, Sonnenblick EH (1976): Respiratory acid-base changes and myocardial contractility: Interaction between calcium and hydrogen ions. Mol Cell Cardiol 8:823–836.

83. Shapir Y, Roguin N (1985): Echocardiographic findings in Pompe's disease with left ventricular obstruction. Clin Cardiol 8:181–185.

84. Shapiro J, Boxer R, Krongrad E (1979): Echocardiography in infants with anomalous origin of the left coronary artery. Pediatr Cardiol 1:23.

85. Smalling RW, Kelley K, Kirkeeide RL, Fisher DJ (1985): Regional myocardial function is not affected by severe coronary depressurization provided coronary blood flow is maintained. J Am Coll Cardiol 5:948–955.

86. Spicer RL, Rocchini AP, Crowley DC, Vasiliades J, Rosenthal A (1983): Hemodynamic effects of verapamil in children and adolescents with hypertrophic cardiomyopathy. Circulation 67:413–420.

87. Su JY, Friedman WF (1973): Comparison of the responses to fetal and adult cardiac muscle to hypoxia. Am J Physiol 224:1249–1253.

88. Surjadhana A, Rouleau J, Boerboom L, Hoffman JIE (1978): Myocardial blood flow and its distribution in anesthetized polycythemic dogs. Circ Res 43:619–631.

89. Troughton O, Singh SP (1972): Heart failure and neonatal hypocalcaemia. Br Med J 4:76–79.

90. Van Duyne CM, Parker HR, Havel RF, Holm LW (1960): Free fatty acid metabolism in fetal and newborn sheep. Am J Physiol 199:987–990.

91. Vlad P, Rowe RD, Keith JD (1955): The electrocardiogram in primary endocardial fibroelastosis. Br Heart J 17:189–197.

92. Vlahakes GJ, Turley K, Hoffman JIE (1981): The pathophysiology of failure in acute right ventricular hypertension: Hemodynamic and biochemical correlations. Circulation 63:87–95.

93. Warshaw JB (1970): Cellular energy metabolism during fetal development. III. Deficient acetyl-CoA synthetase, acetylcarnitine transferase and oxidation of acetate in the fetal bovine heart. Biochim Biophys Acta 233:409–415.

94. Warshaw JB (1972): Cellular energy metabolism during fetal development. IV. Fatty acid activation, acyl transfer and fatty acid oxidation during development of the chick and rat. Dev Biol 28:537–544.

95. Watson RM, Markle DR, Young MR, Goldstein SR, McGuire DA, Peterson JI, Patterson RE (1984): Transmural pH gradient in canine myocardial ischemia. Am J Physiol 246:H232–H238.

96. Way GL, Wolfe RR, Eshaghpour E, Bender RL, Jaffe RB, Ruttenberg HD (1979): The natural history of hypertrophic cardiomyopathy in infants of diabetic mothers. J Pediatr 95:1020–1025.

97. Way GL, Wolfe RL, Pettett GP, Merenstein GB, Simmons MA, Spangler RD, Nora JJ (1975): Echocardiographic assessment of ventricular dimension and myocardial function in infants of diabetic mothers (abstr). Pediatr Res 9:273.

98. Werner JC, Whitman V, Fripp RR, Schuler HG, Morgan HE (1981): Carbohydrate metabolism in isolated, working newborn pig heart. Am J Physiol 241:E364–E371.

99. Werner JC, Whitman V, Vary TC, Fripp RR, Musselman J, Schuer HG (1983): Fatty acid and glucose utilization in isolated, working newborn pig hearts. Am J Physiol 244:E19–E23.

100. Wesselhoeft H, Fawcett JS, Johnson AL (1964): Anomalous origin of the left coronary artery from the pulmonary trunk. Its clinical spectrum, pathology and pathophysiology based on a review of 140 initial cases with 7 further cases. Circulation 38:511.

101. Wildenthal K (1973): Fetal maturation of cardiac metabolism. In Comline RE, Cross KW, Dawes GS (eds.): Fetal and Neonatal Physiology. Cambridge, Cambridge University Press, pp 181–185.

102. Williamson JR, Safer B, Rich T, Schaffer S, Kobayashi K (1975): Effects of acidosis on myocardial contractility and metabolism. Acta Med Scand 487 (Suppl 1):95–112.

103. Wright NL, Baue AE, Baum S, Blakemore WS, Zinsser HF (1970): Coronary artery steal due to an anomalous left coronary artery originating from the pulmonary artery. J Thorac Cardiovasc Surg 59:461–467.

104. Wyler F, Rohner F, Olafsson A et al (1976): Cardiomegaly in neonatal hypoglycemia. Eur J Pediatr 1121:119–124.

105. Zierler KL (1976): Free fatty acids as substrates for heart and skeletal muscle. Circ Res 38:459–463.

41 TACHYARRHYTHMIAS

Arthur Garson, Jr.

Richard T. Smith, Jr.

Jeffrey P. Moak

It has been less than 100 years since the first description of a tachyarrhythmia in a child, then referred to as "paroxysmal hurry of the heart."[2] Buckland wrote in 1892:

On one occasion when running upstairs, the patient became giddy, fell and could not rise for three to four minutes. When I saw her, the rate was well over 200/minute... and then it stopped suddenly. When it began again, citrate of iron and ammonium and spirit of chloroform was prescribed and a visit to the country recommended; nonetheless, the heart riot was unaffected. Neither digitalis nor strophanthidin seemed to have any effect. We then applied mustard to the neck and subsequently blisters appeared but without effect. I applied constant current (5–6 milliamperes) to the pneumogastric of the neck. This reduced the rate of the cardiac cycles from 210 to 202. I repeated this on the following day, but since the patient complained of the prickling and heat from the electrode, and seemed to dread the proceeding, I gave it up.

More than 25 years later, the first case of tachyarrhythmia was reported in an infant. The title was all that was necessary: "Paroxysmal Tachycardia with Ventricular Rate of 307 in a Child Four Days Old."[19] The term *paroxysmal tachycardia* persisted through the 1940s and even to the landmark article by Nadas and coworkers in 1952: "Paroxysmal Tachycardia in Infants and Children."[13] This report was the first large series describing the features of tachyarrhythmias in infancy and separated supraventricular arrhythmias (38 cases) from ventricular arrhythmias (3 cases).

Treatment of tachyarrhythmias has not changed dramatically over the years. Digitalis was tried in the first case of paroxysmal tachycardia in a child in 1892 and was called the drug of choice in the 1940s.[10] The first cases of external cardioversion in children were reported by Paul and Miller in 1962.[14] Three older children with congenital heart disease underwent successful conversion of atrial flutter with 60-cycle alternating current. Two years later, Pryor and Blount[15] successfully used synchronized direct-current cardioversion to convert a supraventricular tachyarrhythmia in a 3-month-old child.

We have built on these milestones and improved in both our diagnostic ability and therapy. Arrhythmias in the newborn are being recognized more frequently, probably because of the increased use of monitoring in the newborn nursery. The heart rates of arrhythmias in this age group are statistically much faster than those seen in older children and adults, and an entirely different set of criteria are necessary for their recognition. In addition, the QRS duration in newborns is normally so narrow that a "wide QRS"

tachycardia in a newborn would be "narrow" by adult standards.

Arrhythmias are relatively common in normal newborns. We will begin with a discussion of the range of normal, then progress through the various tachyarrhythmias (including premature beats) in terms of their identification and need for treatment, and finish with the properties of antiarrhythmic drugs used to treat newborns.

THE RANGE OF NORMAL

In beginning an analysis of neonatal arrhythmias it is important to understand the variation in normal heart rate. Southall and his associates[16] performed a study using 24-hour ECGs. It was found that over the 24-hour period, the lowest heart rate (when the rate over six consecutive beats was averaged) averaged 87 beats per minute (bpm), with a standard deviation of 12 bpm. The mean minus two standard deviations, the lower limit of normal, was 63 bpm in this study. At this low heart rate, 80 per cent of these normal infants were in sinus rhythm whereas 20 per cent had junctional rhythm with a transient rate in the 60s or 70s. The highest heart rate in 24 hours averaged 179 bpm, with a standard deviation of 19 bpm. Two standard deviations above the mean, or the upper limit of normal, was 217 bpm.

In Southall's study, 31 of the 3383 infants studied (0.9 per cent) had an arrhythmia on routine ECG taken within the first 4 days of life, which is approximately the same incidence as structural congenital heart disease. The most common neonatal arrhythmia was premature atrial contractions, followed by premature ventricular contractions, supraventricular tachycardia, and atrial flutter. In Southall's series, no patient had ventricular tachycardia. Wolff-Parkinson-White syndrome was found in two of these asymptomatic normal newborns, an incidence of 0.06 per cent, which is approximately one tenth the incidence of structural congenital heart disease.

PREMATURE ATRIAL CONTRACTIONS

Criteria

The criterion for a premature atrial contraction is a premature P wave. A premature atrial contraction may conduct

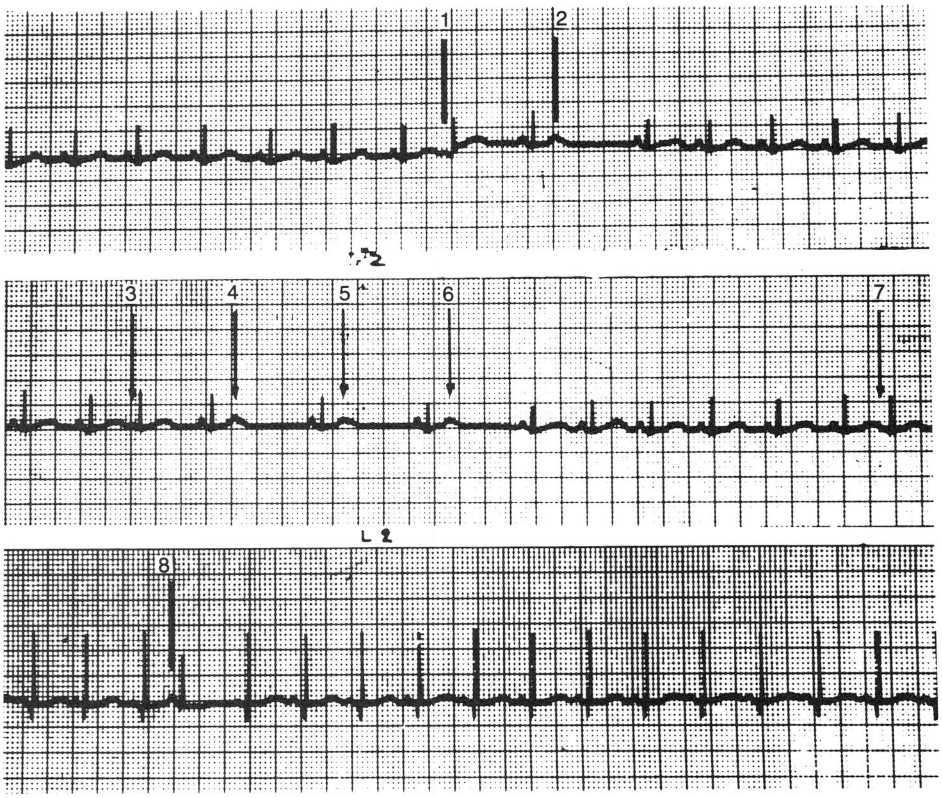

Figure 41–1. Premature atrial contractions in a newborn infant. The premature atrial contractions are numbered. Those numbered 1, 3, and 7 conduct normally. Number 8 conducts with aberration. Numbers 2, 4, 5, and 6 do not conduct. Note that the coupling interval of the blocked premature atrial contractions is shorter that those that conduct.

normally, giving a premature P wave followed by a premature normal QRS complex, or it may conduct aberrantly. Aberrant conduction may simulate a premature ventricular contraction, especially if the preceding P wave is not noticed. Finally, the P wave may not conduct at all, simulating sinus bradycardia if the premature P wave is not noted (Fig. 41–1).

Clinical Situations

Premature atrial contractions usually occur in infants with an otherwise normal heart. Occasionally, an infant with premature atrial contractions may have underlying atrial enlargement due to congenital heart disease or cardiomyopathy or may have mechanical atrial irritation from a central venous pressure catheter. Finally, toxic levels of sympathomimetic drugs, such as isoproterenol or dopamine, rarely result in premature atrial contractions, but premature ventricular contractions are more often the result.

Course and Management

Prognosis for the infant with premature atrial contractions is generally excellent. Southall and his associates[16] found that 15 of 3300 normal newborns had premature atrial contractions on a routine ECG. Of the 15 normal newborns with premature atrial contractions, 7 had a 24-hour

ECG; on this more extended tracing, 2 of the 7 had episodes of supraventricular tachycardia. Therefore, premature atrial contractions in normal newborns may be associated with short asymptomatic periods of supraventricular tachycardia. In follow-up of the 15 patients, in 13 (87 per cent) the premature atrial contractions had disappeared within 3 months and there were no episodes of symptomatic tachyarrhythmias.

In the infant with very frequent premature atrial contractions, a chest radiograph and an echocardiogram are obtained to make sure there is no coexistent congenital heart disease or cardiomyopathy. These infants should be observed for 3 to 4 days, and then a 24-hour ECG is obtained. If there are no episodes of supraventricular tachycardia or atrial flutter, we do not treat premature atrial contractions but follow the child after 1 month with a 24-hour ECG. If supraventricular tachycardia or atrial flutter is found, these arrhythmias are treated.

SUPRAVENTRICULAR TACHYCARDIA

Criteria

In the infant under 1 month of age with supraventricular tachycardia, the QRS complex is regular and narrow. In the infant with a wide QRS tachycardia (over 0.07 second), the correct diagnosis is ventricular tachycardia.

In none of our 48 patients with supraventricular tachycardia appearing at less than 1 month of age was the QRS complex wide during tachycardia.[7] Recognition of the fact that wide QRS tachycardia in newborns is ventricular, rather than supraventricular with aberration, is extremely important, because patients with ventricular tachycardia may respond to digitalis with ventricular fibrillation. In our patients with supraventricular tachycardia presenting under 1 month of age, the rate of tachycardia varied from 210 to 310 bpm or more. In neonates, sinus tachycardia is the other important etiology of narrow QRS tachycardia. In the vast majority of infants with sinus tachycardia, heart rate is below 230 bpm. Therefore, supraventricular tachycardia is the likely diagnosis in patients with a narrow QRS tachycardias with a heart rate above 230 bpm. Finally, in this age group, P waves were visible during supraventricular tachycardia in 59 per cent of the patients but only 15 per cent had a normal P wave axis (defined by positive P waves visible in both lead I and aVF). Therefore, sinus tachycardia is likely if the heart rate is less than 230 bpm and there are positive P waves in leads I and aVF, and supraventricular tachycardia is more likely if the heart rate is over 230 bpm and the P waves are either not visible or not positive in leads I and aVF (Fig. 41–2).

In fact, we have seen only three infants with sinus tachycardia with a heart rate greater than 230 bpm; the highest heart rate was 265 bpm. Also, all three of these infants with rapid sinus tachycardia were extremely ill with sepsis.

Management

The management of supraventricular tachycardia in infants is somewhat controversial since numerous methods of treatment are effective. In most medical centers, each of several treatments might be used, but one center might start with one treatment whereas another medical center might start with another treatment. Regardless of the treatment chosen, it is important to quickly stop the tachycardia in neonates with supraventricular tachycardia because it is quite difficult to assess how close to decompensation a given infant may be. Neonates who appear to be tolerating an episode of supraventricular tachycardia well may suddenly become hemodynamically unstable.

Management of the infants with supraventricular tachycardia is begun by application of a cold, wet washcloth to the infant's face to elicit the "diving reflex." This "diving reflex" causes not only vagal stimulation but also sympathetic withdrawal. The washcloth should be placed in ice water before being placed on the infant's face, and it should be left in place for 10 to 20 seconds if necessary.[17] The infant's ECG and blood pressure should be monitored

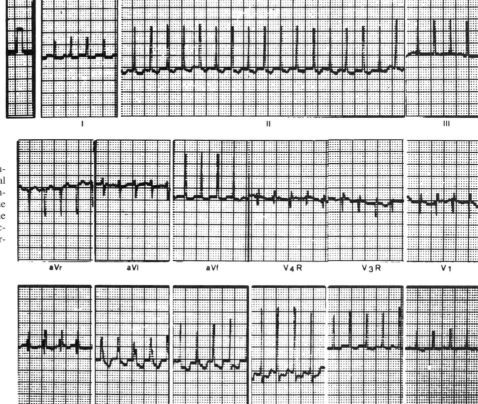

Figure 41–2. Newborn infant with supraventricular tachycardia. The atrial and ventricular rates are 230 per minute. The QRS complex is narrow. The P waves are visible as a notch in the ST segment in lead II. The mean vector of the P waves cannot be determined from this tracing.

throughout application of the cold washcloth, since asystole may rarely follow cessation of supraventricular tachycardia. In other medical centers, the infant's face is placed directly into the cold water. If facial immersion is done properly with closure of the nose and mouth, aspiration will not occur; however we have not found facial immersion to be any more effective than use of the wet washcloth.

If facial application of a cold washcloth is ineffective, overdrive pacing through the esophagus can be performed.[1] The problem with this method is that esophageal overdrive pacing requires a special stimulator with a 10-msec pulse duration. If such a stimulator is available, it is extremely simple to place a No. 4 F pacing catheter through the nose into the esophagus and overdrive pace the tachycardia. The pacing rate is set slightly faster than the tachycardia; the stimulator is turned on for 5 to 10 seconds, and on termination of pacing the tachycardia will usually stop.

In the past, edrophonium (Tensilon) has been recommended for acute treatment of supraventricular tachycardia since it is an anticholinesterase inhibitor and potentiates vagal tone. Edrophonium is effective in stopping supraventricular tachycardia approximately 50 per cent of the time; however, the drug's side effects of vomiting and bradycardia after conversion limit its usefulness. The same may be said for phenylephrine, which exerts its effect by a vagal reflex. To convert the tachycardia, sufficient phenylephrine must be given to elevate the blood pressure and then a vagal reflex slows the heart rate. We now know that acute elevations of systemic vascular resistance may cause a decrease in cardiac output; such realizations have diminished the use of phenylephrine in neonates with supraventricular tachycardia. We prefer to avoid the use of both edrophonium and phenylephrine.

Instead our next treatment choice depends on the infant's status. If there are signs of low cardiac output or respiratory distress, then the treatment of choice at our medical center and most others is direct-current electrical cardioversion. We have found no morbidity from cardioversion if it is applied correctly. Cardioversion of supraventricular tachycardia should be synchronized to the QRS complex and should be delivered in a proper dose of 2 ws/kg. In the vast majority of cases, cardioversion is effective in stopping the supraventricular tachycardia.

If the infant is not in distress, intravenous digitalis is used. In the study by Deal and colleagues,[4] intravenous digitalis was effective in converting supraventricular tachycardia in 88 per cent of infants. All of these infants had Wolff-Parkinson-White syndrome, and there were no untoward effects of digitalis. However, a single infant with Wolff-Parkinson-White syndrome has been reported to have had ventricular fibrillation after receiving digitalis for supraventricular tachycardia.[3] On balance, digitalis appears relatively safe and effective in this situation.

If digitalis is not effective, intravenous procainamide can be tried. If neither digitalis nor procainamide are effective, intravenous propranolol is used. However, propranolol may acutely reduce cardiac output and may cause severe bradycardia. Therefore, intravenous propranolol should not be used unless standby ventricular pacing is available.

Finally, there has been much discussion on the use of intravenous verapamil for supraventricular tachycardia in infants and children. One report has pointed out the dangers of verapamil in infants.[6] We have had personal experience with several infants in whom the cardiac output was severely reduced after administration of verapamil, and we prefer to avoid its use. Another dangerous side effect of verapamil in infants is apnea. The use of intravenous verapamil is not recommended in infants under 1 year of age.

The chronic management of the infant with supraventricular tachycardia depends on whether the infant has underlying Wolff-Parkinson-White syndrome. If Wolff-Parkinson-White syndrome is not present, oral therapy with digoxin is begun. If orally administered digoxin does not prevent recurrences of supraventricular tachycardia, orally administered propranolol is added. If the combination of digoxin and propranolol is not effective, the propranolol is discontinued for several days and then the combination of oral administration of digoxin and verapamil is used. Oral administration of verapamil does not appear to have the same deleterious effects as intravenous administration of the drug.

If oral administration of digoxin and verapamil proves ineffective, oral administration of propranolol and quinidine could be tried, and if this therapy is also ineffective, we would strongly consider an electrophysiology study to determine the mechanism of tachycardia.

If the infant with refractory recurrent supraventricular tachycardia does have occult Wolff-Parkinson-White syndrome, we would prefer to avoid digoxin, since there have been occasional sudden deaths in infants with Wolff-Parkinson-White syndrome treated chronically with this drug.[4] The reason for sudden death in patients with Wolff-Parkinson-White syndrome on oral therapy with digoxin is that digitalis may accelerate atrioventricular conduction over the Kent bundle, which permits early premature atrial beats to conduct to the ventricles, thus predisposing to ventricular fibrillation, and also permits rapid conduction to the ventricles during atrial flutter, thus predisposing to extremely rapid ventricular rates. We would therefore begin with propranolol and then continue with the drug sequence outlined earlier for patients without Wolff-Parkinson-White syndrome. If these drugs are not effective, electrophysiology is performed with the idea of localizing the Kent bundle for attempted surgical division.

ATRIAL FLUTTER

Criteria

The diagnosis of atrial flutter depends on the presence of flutter waves, which are regular sawtooth undulations in the baseline that are larger than P waves. Atrial flutter in infants may occur at rates between 300 and 600 bpm. The ventricular rate is usually irregular in infants with atrial flutter. Occasionally, the ventricular rate is regular with 2:1 atrioventricular conduction. The infant's atrioventricular node may occasionally conduct atrial flutter 1:1 with a ventricular rate of 400 to 500 bpm (Fig. 41–3).

Clinical Situations

Atrial flutter usually occurs in patients with an otherwise normal heart. Atrial flutter seems to be slightly more common in patients who have had intrauterine supraventricular tachycardia. Occasionally, atrial flutter is found in patients with atrial enlargement due to congenital heart disease, especially endocardial fibroelastosis, or with cardiomyopathy. It may also be found in patients with an atrial tumor.

Course and Management

The course of atrial flutter is quite variable. Moller and associates,[12] in 1969, reported 24 cases of atrial flutter in infants under 1 week of age. In 22 of the 24 infants, digoxin was used for initial treatment and 11 infants converted to sinus rhythm. In the other 11 patients, atrial flutter continued. Of these 11 infants with chronic atrial flutter, 5 died and the others continued to have atrial flutter for a median of 6 months. Digoxin was not effective in either of the 2 patients with associated atrial fibrillation. The mortality of atrial flutter was high if there was associated congenital heart disease; both patients with underlying congenital heart disease and atrial flutter died. Even if atrial fibrillation or congenital heart disease were not present, mortality was still 11 per cent, which indicates the importance of controlling continuing atrial flutter in neonates. Fortunately, methods of treatment for atrial flutter have improved; at our institution there have been no deaths in infants with atrial flutter since 1969. In one series, Dunnigan and coworkers,[5] reported 8 infants with atrial flutter; 6 presented in the first week, and the other 2 presented between 6 and 8 weeks of age. A right atrial catheter was associated with the arrhythmia in 3 of the 8 infants; the atrial flutter disappeared on withdrawal of the catheter in all three. Contrary to previous reports, the atrial flutter did not recur after initial termination in 7 of the 8 infants; 1 infant had recurrent episodes. In our experience, over 50 per cent of infants with atrial flutter have recurrent episodes with rapid ventricular rates. We would recommend chronic treatment for all infants with even a single episode of atrial flutter unless the episode is catheter induced.

Cardioversion is recommended when atrial flutter is recognized. Overdrive atrial pacing through the esophagus may be used, but it is much more difficult to overdrive pace atrial flutter than supraventricular tachycardia. Once the atrial flutter has stopped, digoxin therapy is begun unless the patient has underlying Wolff-Parkinson-White syndrome. If the digoxin proves ineffective in preventing recurrences, propranolol is added. If the combination of digoxin and propranolol proves ineffective, the combination of digoxin and quinidine can be tried. Since atrial flutter in the infant rarely continues for more than 6 months,

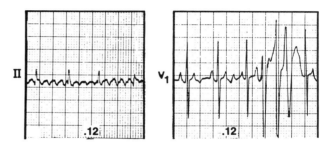

Figure 41–3. Atrial flutter in infants. In the left tracing, classic flutter waves are seen at an atrial rate of 500 per minute with 4:1 and 5:1 atrioventricular conduction. On the right, blocked premature atrial contractions follow the first two QRS complexes. Then, there are two beats of atrial flutter. The rapid wide QRS rhythm on the right results from 1:1 atrioventricular conduction of atrial flutter at a ventricular rate of 460 per minute.

therapy is stopped approximately 6 months after the last episode of atrial flutter but we continue to follow these patients quite closely.

PREMATURE VENTRICULAR CONTRACTIONS

Criteria

Premature ventricular contractions are defined by premature QRS complexes not preceded by a premature P wave. As pointed out for premature atrial contractions, it is important to examine the T wave preceding an apparently premature QRS complex quite closely to rule out the presence of a preceding premature P wave (in which case the correct diagnosis would be premature atrial contraction). In a premature ventricular contraction, the QRS complex is different from the QRS complex of sinus rhythm. However, premature ventricular contractions are not necessarily beyond the upper limits of normal in width. The most reliable criterion for diagnosis of premature ventricular contraction is occurrence of a fusion complex, which has the combined morphology of both a sinus beat and a premature ventricular contraction.

Clinical Situations

Premature ventricular contractions are usually found in newborns with otherwise normal hearts. However, premature ventricular contractions may also be found in infants with heart disease. In any patient with premature ventricular contractions, it is most important to measure the QT interval (Fig. 41–4). Prolonged QT intervals may occur in an idiopathic familial form but may also be due to hypocalcemia or asphyxia. Premature ventricular contractions may also be associated with hypoxia, hypoglycemia, myocarditis, severe ventricular hypertrophy, ventricular tumor, or ventricular catheter. Swan-Ganz catheters in the pulmonary artery are particularly prone to causing premature

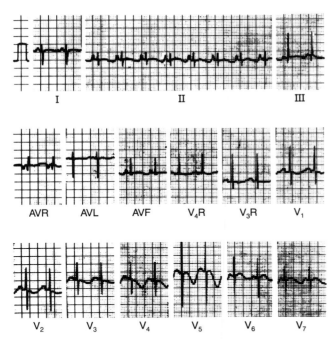

Figure 41–4. Newborn with a prolonged QT interval. QT prolongation is especially apparent in leads II and V_1 and in the midprecordial leads.

ventricular contractions, presumably as a result of the catheter loop in the right ventricle. Finally, premature ventricular contractions may be associated with drug intoxication, most commonly digitalis or sympathomimetic amines such as isoproterenol or dopamine.

Course and Management

The prognosis for the infant with premature ventricular contractions depends entirely on whether the heart is normal. In a study of 3300 normal newborns, Southall and associates found that 11 infants had premature ventricular contractions on routine ECG.[16] Of these 11 infants, 7 had a 24-hour ECG in the newborn period; 3 of the 7 had short episodes of ventricular tachycardia. None of these 11 normal infants with premature ventricular contractions was treated; in 10 of the 11, the arrhythmia completely disappeared by the age of 3 months. However, the risk of ventricular fibrillation is certainly higher when premature ventricular contractions occur in neonates with underlying cardiac problems, such as myocarditis or digitalis intoxication.

In neonates with premature ventricular contractions, we perform a chest radiograph and an echocardiogram to establish that the patient has a normal heart. We would not treat patients with a normal heart and uniform premature ventricular contractions. On the other hand, if the patient has an abnormal heart (e.g., myocarditis) we would treat frequent uniform premature ventricular contractions (defined by more than 10 uniform premature ventricular contractions per hour on a 24-hour ECG). We would treat any

patient with multiform premature ventricular contractions or couplets, whether the heart was thought to be normal or abnormal. Treatment is begun with propranolol. Therapy for premature ventricular contractions with quinidine is avoided since this drug may worsen the ventricular arrhythmia, particularly in patients with a prolonged QT interval. In patients with a prolonged QT interval, quinidine, disopyramide, procainamide, and amiodarone should all be avoided since these drugs prolong the QT interval even farther.

VENTRICULAR TACHYCARDIA

Criteria

Ventricular tachycardia is defined by occurrence of three or more consecutive premature ventricular contractions at a rate over 120 bpm. The most rapid ventricular tachycardia that we have seen is a rate of 500 bpm. In the diagnosis of ventricular tachycardia, atrioventricular dissociation is extremely helpful. Atrioventricular dissociation is defined by dissociation of the P waves and the QRS complexes. Unfortunately, atrioventricular dissociation is not always present in patients with ventricular tachycardia. The presence of fusion beats during the tachycardia is diagnostic of ventricular tachycardia, just as the presence of a fusion beat proves the presence of premature ventricular contractions. Occurrence of sinus capture beats during the tachycardia, defined as the presence of a normal QRS complex preceded by a P wave, is also diagnostic for ventricular tachycardia. Infants with ventricular tachycardia may have a relatively narrow QRS complex (as narrow as 0.06 second); however, the QRS morphology in ventricular tachycardia is always different from the QRS in sinus rhythm (Fig. 41–5). In infants, ventricular tachycardia can either be "paroxysmal" (occurring in bursts up to several times per day) or "incessant" (occurring almost all of the 24-hour period).

Clinical Situations

Neonatal ventricular tachycardia occurs in different settings, depending on whether the ventricular tachycardia is paroxysmal or incessant. Paroxysmal ventricular tachycardia occurs in situations similar to those in which premature ventricular contractions are found, except that ventricular tachycardia usually does not occur in patients with a normal heart. In their review of published literature on ventricular arrhythmias in infants under 4 months old, Stevens and coworkers found 14 cases had been reported with paroxysmal ventricular tachycardia either in the mother (meperidine intoxication, mepivicaine toxicity, heroin overdosage) or in the infant (congenital heart disease, hypercalcemia due to adrenogenital syndrome, myocarditis, long QT interval syndrome). We have seen 20 cases of incessant ventricular tachycardia in infants under 2 years of age; 3 infants presented in the neonatal period.[9] None of the 20 infants had any structural heart disease detected by

Figure 41–5. Rapid ventricular tachycardia. In *A*, note that the tachyarrhythmia, sometimes at a rate of 440 per minute, has all the characteristics of ventricular tachycardia. There is a sinus capture beat (upright QRS in the middle of the tracing), several fusion beats, atrioventricular dissociation, and a QRS complex during tachycardia completely different from that found in sinus rhythm. The ventricular tachycardia was mapped in the electrophysiology laboratory and found to originate from the left ventricular apex. The patient was taken to the operating room where a small epicardial tumor was found and excised. *B*, the postoperative tracing in sinus rhythm. The lead is the same as that in *A*. Note the single sinus capture beat in *A* has a similar morphology to the sinus beats in *B*. The patient has been in sinus rhythm for the 3 years since surgery.

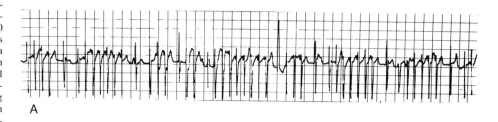

A

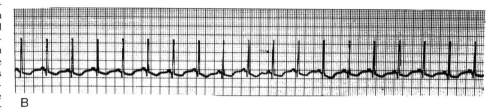

B

echocardiography or angiocardiography. Because of the incessant nature of the arrhythmia and lack of response to any medical treatment, all 20 infants were taken to the operating room; in 15 of 20 infants, a small cardiac tumor was found. Removal of the cardiac tumor cured the tachycardia in all 15 infants. In the other 5 infants, there was no visible cardiac lesion but excision of the area electrophysiologically mapped as the site of origin of the ventricular tachycardia resulted in cure of the tachycardia in each case.

Course and Management

The prognosis for the patient with ventricular tachycardia depends on whether the patient truly has a normal heart. In Southall's[16] group of normal patients, none had ventricular tachycardia on a routine ECG. Three of Southall's patients had ventricular tachycardia on a 24-hour ECG; in each case the tachycardia resolved by 3 months of age.

Of the 14 cases of paroxysmal ventricular tachycardia reported by Stevens and associates,[18] only three patients had ventricular tachycardia beyond 1 month of age. On the other hand, none of our three cases of incessant ventricular tachycardia occurring in the neonatal period resolved, and none was successfully treated with any antiarrhythmic agent, including amiodarone.[8] Surgery was undertaken in each of these three infants because the majority of such patients have died suddenly before 2 years of age.[11]

Initial management of the patient with paroxysmal ventricular tachycardia begins with stopping the tachycardia. If the patient is in sustained ventricular tachycardia (i.e., it does not stop and start) synchronized direct-current electrical cardioversion should be performed. After the initial conversion, intravenous lidocaine or procainamide can be used. If the patient has a prolonged QT interval, phenytoin

should be substituted for procainamide. Once it is established that the arrhythmia is controlled, the patient can be started on oral propranolol or phenytoin which should be continued for at least 6 months. If propranolol and phenytoin are ineffective, the patient could be tried on quinidine as long as the QT interval is not prolonged. If quinidine is also ineffective, we would recommend amiodarone.[8] Digitalis should be avoided in patients with ventricular tachycardia; we have seen three infants under the age of 6 months develop ventricular fibrillation during digitalization for an arrhythmia believed to be supraventricular tachycardia but which in reality was ventricular tachycardia.

Infants with ventricular tachycardia should be thoroughly evaluated to determine whether the heart is normal or abnormal. Important tests include a 24-hour ECG (to search for a prolonged QT interval) and an echocardiogram (to search for anatomic abnormalities).

If there is recurrent incessant ventricular tachycardia that is resistant to antiarrhythmic drugs, anatomic and electrophysiologic catheterizations are also indicated to localize the origin of the ventricular tachycardia for subsequent surgical ablation of the tachycardia.

NEONATAL ANTIARRHYTHMIC DRUGS

Digoxin should be given to newborns in a lower dose than older children. The total oral digitalizing dose in newborns for digoxin is 20 µg/kg and the intravenous dose is 80 per cent of that. Therefore, if the total intravenous digitalizing dose is 16 µg/kg (or 0.016 mg/kg), and half that dose is given initially, the initial intravenous dose is 0.008 mg/kg. Orally, the maintenance dose is 4 µg/kg every 12 hours or 0.004 mg/kg every 12 hours. Propranolol may be given intravenously in a dose of 0.025 mg/kg every 10 minutes for a total of four doses. Standby ventricular pacing should be available. Orally, propranolol may be given in a dose of 0.5 mg/kg every 6 hours. This dose may be increased to 1 mg/kg every 6 hours and even further as tolerated. The dosage of intravenous procainamide is 7 mg/kg intravenous drip over 1 hour. After this infusion, the patient may be given 3 to 9 mg/kg per dose orally every 4 hours. Intravenous quinidine is contraindicated since it causes marked hypotension; quinidine may be started orally in a dose of 4 to 12 mg/kg every 6 hours. Similarly, intravenous verapamil should not be used in infants; orally, verapamil should be given in a dose of 2 to 4 mg/kg every 8 hours. Lidocaine should be given as an intravenous bolus of 1 mg/kg, which may be repeated for a total of three doses. If a bolus of lidocaine proves effective, a lidocaine drip may be started at a dosage of 1 mg/kg/hr. Lidocaine is not available orally. Since phenytoin (Dilantin) precipitates in any kind of intravenous fluid, it is best given directly into the patient's circulation. We prefer to administer phenytoin as intravenous boluses in doses of 1 mg/kg every 5 to 10 minutes depending on the patient's clinical status. Up to 15 boluses of 1 mg/kg (total dose of 15 mg/kg) may be given over 1 to 2 hours. Bretylium is an excellent drug for recurrent ventricular fibrillation and should be given in a dose of 5 mg/kg per dose. Bretylium should not be given for ventricular tachycardia since it is much less effective for this arrhythmia. Finally, electrical energy doses of 1 to 2 ws/kg should be used for direct-current cardioversion of ventricular tachycardias. Supraventricular tachycardias can often be cardioverted with substantially less electrical energy. Energy doses of 5 to 6 ws/kg can result in severe myocardial burns, which can lead to congestive cardiomyopathy (due to reduced contractility) and death.

CONCLUSIONS

Tachyarrhythmias in newborns are extremely challenging largely because of difficulties in accurate diagnosis. However, even when the correct diagnosis is made, treatment may vary widely in different institutions. If pharmacologic therapy is to be used for neonatal arrhythmias, it is important to be fully cognizant of the differences in pharmacokinetics and dynamics the newborn exhibits in handling a given drug. Fortunately, the vast majority of tachyarrhythmias that appear in the newborn period have an extremely good prognosis. If the tachyarrhythmia can be controlled in the first month of life, the eventual outlook for neonates with tachyarrhythmias is extremely good.

References

1. Benson DW Jr, Dunnigan A, Benditt DG, Pritzker MR, Thompson TR (1983): Transesophageal study of infant supraventricular tachycardia: Electrophysiologic characteristics. Am J Cardiol 52:1002–1006.
2. Buckland FO (1892): Case of rapid heart. Trans Clin Soc Lond 25:92–96.
3. Byrum CJ, Wahl RA, Behrendt DM, Dick M (1982): Ventricular fibrillation associated with use of digitalis in a newborn infant with Wolff-Parkinson-White syndrome. J Pediatr 101:400–403.
4. Deal BJ, Keane JF, Gillette PC, Garson A (1983): Wolff-Parkinson-White and atrial tachycardia in infancy: Long-term follow-up. Pediatr Cardiol 17:111A.
5. Dunnigan A, Benson W Jr, Benditt DG (1985): Atrial flutter in infancy: Diagnosis, clinical features, and treatment. Pediatrics 75:725–729.
6. Epstein ML, Kiel EA, Victorica BE (1985): Cardiac decompensation following verapamil therapy in infants with supraventricular tachycardia. Pediatrics 75:737–740.
7. Garson A, Gillette PC, McNamara DG (1981): Supraventricular tachycardia in children: Clinical features, response to treatment and long-term follow-up in 217 patients. J Pediatr 98:875–882.
8. Garson A, Gillette PC, McVey P, Hesslein P, Porter CJ, Hittner HM, Angell LK, Kaldis LC (1984): Amiodarone treatment of clinical arrhythmias in children and young adults. J Am Coll Cardiol 4:749–755.
9. Garson A, Gillette PC, Titus JL, Hawkins EP, Kearney D, Ott C, Cooley DA, McNamara DG (1984): Surgical treatment of ventricular tachycardia in infants. N Engl J Med 310:1443–1445.
10. Hubbard JP (1941): Paroxysmal tachycardia and its treatment in young infants. Am J Dis Child 61:687–709.
11. James TN, Beeson, CW, Sherman EB (1975): De Subitaneis Mortibus XIII: Multifocal Purkinje tumors of the heart. Circulation 52:333–344.
12. Moller JH, Davachi F, Anderson RC (1969): Atrial flutter in infancy. J Pediatr 75:643–651.
13. Nadas AS, Daeschner CW, Roth A, Blumenthal SL (1952): Paroxysmal tachycardia in infants and children: Study of 44 cases. Pediatrics 9:167–178.
14. Paul MH, Miller RA (1962): External electrical termination of supraventricular arrhythmias in congenital heart disease. Circulation 25:604–609.
15. Pryor R, Blount SG (1964): Refractory supraventricular tachycardia in infancy: External countershock termination. Am J Dis Child 107:428–430.
16. Southall DP (1979): Study of cardiac rhythm in healthy newborn infants. Br Heart J 43:14–20.
17. Sperandeo V, Pieri D, Palazzolo P, Donzelli M, Spataro G (1983): Supraventricular tachycardia in infants: Use of the "diving reflex." Am J Cardiol 51(2):286–287.
18. Stevens DC, Schreiner RL, Hurwitz RA, Gresham EL (1979): Fetal and neonatal ventricular arrhythmia. Pediatrics 63:771–777.
19. Werley G (1925): Paroxysmal tachycardia with ventricular rate of three hundred and seven in child four days old. Arch Pediatr 42:825–826.

42 ATRIOVENTRICULAR BLOCK

Paul C. Gillette

Derek A. Fyfe

Bertrand A. Ross

Congenital complete atrioventricular (AV) block occurs once in every 15,000 to 20,000 live births. It is defined as complete electrical dissociation of the atria from the ventricles. The atrial rate is faster than the ventricular rate. The QRS complexes are almost always narrow and normal. The QT interval may be prolonged. If there are any short RR intervals with the same QRS, the block is said to be advanced second-degree block rather than complete. The pacemaker that controls the ventricles is usually in the bundle of His, as shown by intracardiac electrophysiologic studies. This pacemaker is under control of both the sympathetic and parasympathetic nervous systems. A few patients with congenital complete AV block have their block in the middle of the His bundle with the escape pacemaker in the distal bundle of His. The third electrophysiologic substrate is block within the bundle branch system with the escape pacemaker in one of the bundle branches. There is less and less autonomic control and a slower resting rate as the pacemaker is lower in the conduction system.

HISTORICAL PERSPECTIVE

Concern about congenital AV block appears to have begun near the beginning of the 20th century. Early reports dealt mainly with diagnosing the child early in life by providing graphic proof of AV block with no evidence of a cause found by history or physical examination. Van den Heuvel in 1908 was able for the first time to report the ECG findings in complete AV block.[34] By 1927, the first presumptive diagnosis of congenital complete AV block in utero was made by Witt on the basis of a slow in utero heart rate and an ECG at 2 days of age that showed complete AV block with a ventricular rate almost identical to the previously recorded fetal rate.[36] In 1929 Yater reported a case of congenital third-degree AV block diagnosed in utero.[38] Diagnosis was again made without graphic proof of the AV block in utero, but instead relying on the ECG after delivery to prove the diagnosis.

By 1947, over 100 cases of congenital AV block were recorded, but no in utero diagnosis had been corroborated graphically since the technology was not yet available.[33] Plant and Steven reported a case of an infant with congenital AV block who had a fetal ECG that showed a ventricular rate of 56 beats per minute (bpm).[20] The atrial rate, however, could not be clearly seen.

The first graphic proof of an antenatal diagnosis of complete AV block was not until 1968 when Teteris, Chisholm, and Ullery reported a case diagnosed just prior to delivery with the aid of fetal scalp electrodes.[32] Sokol also reported a case using the fetal ECG to diagnose congenital AV block in utero.[27] Recently, with the advent of fetal echocardiography, there have been numerous reports of the antenatal diagnosis of AV block.[3,7,14]

PATHOLOGY

Three histologic types of congenital complete AV block have been reported that seem to correlate with the three electrophysiologic mechanisms. They are absence of communication between the atrium and the AV node, interruption of the His bundle, and improper alignment of the AV node and the distal conduction system. Each type can occur with either normal hearts or in association with minor or major congenital heart defects.

Autopsy studies in maternal connective tissue disease–associated congenital AV block demonstrate that the sinus node, AV node, and proximal conduction bundle are fibrosed and often have dystrophic calcification. Frequently the AV node itself cannot be identified. Endomyocardial calcification and fibrosis are common accompaniments.[4,7]

INCIDENCE

From the Association of European Pediatric Cardiologist Collaborative (AEPC) Study it appears that congenital AV block occurs in approximately 1 in 20,000 live births and is associated with congenital heart malformations in approximately one third of cases.[18] The most common cardiac lesions occurring with congenital complete AV block are ventricular inversion syndromes and abnormalities of the AV septum such as AV canal defects.[1,18] The natural history of patients with congenital complete AV block in association with congenital heart disease is frequently lethal. There is a sevenfold increase in death by 1 year of age when compared with patients with isolated heart block. Additionally, patients with slow ventricular rates of less than 55 bpm have the highest mortality.[18]

In the AEPC study of 593 cases of congenital AV block, only 15 familial cases were noted.[18] The current view is that congenital complete AV block is acquired during gestation, which is supported by the observation that in 67 children with congenital AV block whose mothers had connective tissue disorders, 22 other siblings were also affected. Congenital AV block associated with maternal connective tissue disorders is most frequently complete, although incomplete, progressive, and even transient AV block have occurred in some infants.[7]

ETIOLOGY

Serologic Studies

The etiology and mechanism of this apparent injury to the conduction system is of intense interest due to its association with the presence or later development of connective tissue disorders in many mothers of offspring with congenital complete AV block.[16,17] Most frequently systemic lupus erythematosus has been present in mothers of children with congenital complete AV block, but Sjögren's syndrome, rheumatoid arthritis, and dermatomyositis have also been found.[7,8] Many asymptomatic mothers of children with congenital complete AV block have only serologic abnormalities associated with connective tissue diseases. It has been proposed that systemic lupus erythematosus can cause congenital complete AV block by the passage of maternal immunologic factors to the fetus. In 1981, Franco provided suggestive evidence demonstrating that antibodies to SICCA syndrome antigens (SS-A) were present in infants with neonatal lupus syndrome and that these correlated with the presence of similar antibodies in the mother.[8]

Further evidence that placental transfer of maternal anti-SICCA antibodies has been provided by Scott and associates who demonstrated that antisoluble ribonuclear protein antibodies, anti-RO (SS-A), were present in 34 of 41 mothers who had given birth to children with complete congenital AV block and also were present in seven of eight blood samples from both mothers and their infants at age under 3 months with complete congenital AV block.[21] These antibodies were not detectable in infants after 3 months of age and were not present in mothers of infants with congenital heart diseases not associated with congenital complete AV block.[21]

Postmortem Studies

Postmortem studies have demonstrated diffuse deposition of IgA and IgG within the right atrium of a 25-week fetus dying 4 weeks after the diagnosis of complete congenital AV block.[21] Sera from both the mother and the fetus were strongly positive for antinuclear antibody and also contained anti-RO (SS-A) antibodies. Microscopic pathology demonstrated dystrophic calcification of the right atrium, atrial septum, and the AV node. Singsen and coworkers reported the postmortem finding of a fetus examined at 34 weeks' gestation.[26] In this case a heart rate of 144 bpm was present at 18 weeks' gestation, but decreased to 48 bpm at 24 to 26 weeks' gestation. Postmortem immunoflorescence studies at 34 weeks failed to demonstrate deposition of IgG or IgM, or antibodies to complement components C3 or C4; inflammatory cells were likewise absent, despite the presence of fibrosis of the sinoatrial and AV nodes and positive serology for SS-A antibodies. It is possible that immunoglobulin deposition may only be demonstrable around the time of the active pathologic process causing congenital complete AV block and may not be detectable subsequently. Most recently, Taylor and colleagues demonstrated maternal IgG antibody capable of reacting with fetal cardiac tissues in sera from 21 of 41 mothers of children with congenital complete AV block.[31] Similar antibodies were also present in three of eight affected infants. Of note is the fact that no specificity for the conduction system could be demonstrated.

Possible Immune Pathogenesis

From these data it appears that most cases of congenital complete AV block are associated with maternal immunologic factors that are capable of placental transfer and that may be demonstrable in the serum of both mothers and affected infants. In some cases these immunoglobulins may be shown to be deposited on the endocardial surfaces of the heart. The coincident demonstration of destruction of the proximal conduction system implies that there is a causal relationship between this maternal antibody and the development of congenital complete AV block. However, antibodies have not been shown to be cytotoxic or truly pathogenic in this disease. It is possible that they may represent an epiphenomenon. Furthermore, there is no explanation for the unique susceptibility of the conduction system to presumed immunologic damage despite the apparent nonspecificities of the antibodies demonstrated thus far.

DIAGNOSIS OF CONGENITAL COMPLETE AV BLOCK

The intrauterine diagnosis of congenital complete AV block is most frequently suspected during pregnancy by the presence of sustained fetal heart rates of less than 100 bpm noted by the obstetrician during routine prenatal evaluation. Although brief episodes of fetal bradycardia are common during early pregnancy, sustained bradycardias are usually abnormal. In a series of echocardiograms of fetuses with sustained bradycardia, 13 of 15 had congenital complete AV block.[1] Only 2 of the 15 had sinus bradycardia. In 6 of these patients with AV block, associated cardiac malformations involving the AV septum were present.

In addition to the presence of bradycardia, the obstetrician may also note the presence of features of hydrops fetalis, indicating chronic intrauterine fetal compromise. Although most infants with congenital complete AV block do not develop intrauterine congestive heart failure, the presence of hydrops in an infant with congenital complete AV block has grave implications, especially if a cardiac malformation is present, in which case the condition is frequently fatal despite optimal medical therapy.[11,12,24,127]

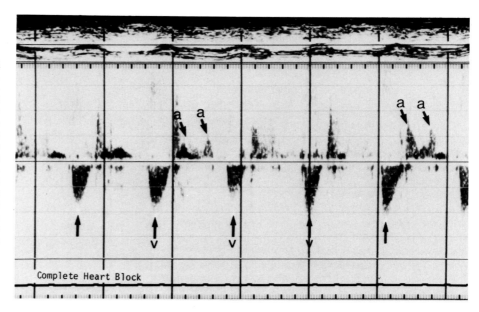

Figure 42–1. Example of AV block recorded from a patient with complete AV block. The tracing is recorded in the left ventricular outflow, capturing ejection from the ventricle below baseline and the flow into the ventricle above baseline. The ventricular contraction at about 55 beats per minute (v and arrows) is shown. The atrial rate at about 150 beats per minute can be seen (a) during ventricular diastole. a = atrial ejection; v = ventricular ejection. (Reproduced with permission of Silverman NH et al [1986]: The uses of pulsed utrasound in the human fetus. Pediatric Cardiology, Proceedings of the Second World Congress 1986. New York, Springer-Verlag, Inc, pp 44–51.)

Echocardiographic Evaluation

Since fetal electrocardiography is limited in its ability to define AV conduction characteristics due to the failure to record either satisfactory R wave amplitude or to display adequate P waves, the most accurate assessment of the presence of congenital complete AV block requires echocardiography.[2,23] Before a fetal echocardiographic examination is performed, however, it is mandatory to carry out complete fetal ultrasonographic evaluation. The goals of this examination are to define the presence of coexistent somatic or structural abnormalities in the child, to demonstrate the presence of polyhydramnios or oligohydramnios, or to discover evidence of fetal distress (see Chapter 17), such as ascites, hepatomegaly, and chest wall or scalp edema. In addition, the presence of pericardial effusion or ventricular dilatation and the measurement of systolic contractility are helpful indicators of cardiac decompensation.[12] When the heart is evaluated with fetal ultrasound, two-dimensional cardiac imaging must be performed to define the fetal cardiac connections and anatomy (see Chapter 15) because of the previously mentioned association of congenital complete AV block with serious cardiac malformations.

Defining the nature of the cardiac arrhythmia is best done using two-dimensional sector echocardiographic guidance and M-mode examination of simultaneously visualized cardiac structures (see Chapter 16). In this way the timing and relationships of atrial and ventricular wall motions may be analyzed, providing an indirect indicator of the electrical depolarizations of the cardiac chambers. This approach has been validated with concurrent use of ECGs.[37]

The onset of atrial wall movement is a useful marker for the initiation of atrial systole and approximates the P wave.[13,14,15,23,37] Ventricular wall motion or thickening may be used as an indicator of ventricular systole. Similarly, aortic valve opening may also be used as an indicator of ventricular systole.

M-mode echocardiographic recording of the anterior mitral leaflet is also helpful, since atrial contractions are indicated by a waves. By careful examination, the E point of the anterior mitral leaflet motion that indicates the beginning of ventricular diastole can also be determined.[14] The dissociation of the A and E points with more rapid a waves, defines the AV block.

Doppler Echocardiography

Pulsed Doppler echocardiography has great utility in the rapid diagnosis and definition of fetal arrhythmias.[25,28,30] Since pulsed Doppler is range gated, sample volumes from specific locations within the heart may be selected for comparison of blood flow patterns. Sampling blood flow in the inlet region of AV valves reflects ventricular inflow patterns caused by atrial contractions. These may then be compared with blood flow through the ventricular outlets or great vessels that represent ventricular systole (Fig. 42–1). Since the sample volume of the most conventional Doppler machines is relatively large compared with chamber sizes of the fetal heart, records of both blood flow into and out of the ventricle may be obtained concurrently.[25] Such recordings may allow an instantaneous comparison of blood flow patterns due to atrial and ventricular systole.

In addition, the presence of mitral or tricuspid regurgitation can be identified and quantitated (see Chapter 14). Global cardiac dysfunction may be suspected if severe regurgitation is present.[24]

TREATMENT

History of Pacing

The era of treatment for complete AV block and asystole began in the late 1920s and early 1930s. Hyman, in the 1930s, developed a practical machine to be used as an artificial pacemaker in experimental animals. However, after his first report was published, he received a great deal of public derision even though he only recorded the work in animals.[11]

As reported by Mond et al, the first pacemaker may have been developed by a fellow Australian, Mark C. Lidwell, who used it on a stillborn child who was successfully resuscitated after pacing was accomplished with this machine.[19] It is certainly clear in both accounts that pacing might have evolved much more quickly had it been more readily accepted by the medical community and public at the time.

It is difficult to be certain when devices to externally pace the heart were first used in a clinical setting for complete AV block, but certainly one of the first devices if not the first, was used by Lillehei's group and reported on by Weirich et al.[35] This device required insertion of a fine copper wire into the right ventricular myocardium; energy was supplied by an external power source. The device was used successfully in 18 postoperative patients beginning January 30, 1957.[35] Furman and Schwedel used a pacing catheter transvenously in a similar manner in July 1958.[9] Glenn and colleagues reported placing a radiofrequency stimulator and coil in a patient so that the patient could be paced without being connected to an external power source by cables![10]

The transition from external pacing source to implantable pacing devices was quickly accelerated with a rechargeable implantable unit by Senning[22] in 1959 and a permanent unit by Chardrack et al in 1960.[22] This last device opened the door to the modern era of pacing for complete AV block. The implanted mercury cell power source soon became the standard for the industry.

Prenatal Therapy

Unfortunately, our ability to treat congenital complete AV block in utero has not kept pace with our ability to diagnose it. Experience has shown us that if the fetus is in no distress no treatment is necessary and the child can be delivered vaginally without problem. The asymptomatic fetus with complete AV block can withstand labor and delivery in spite of the fact that the ability of the heart rate to increase is severely blunted.

The presence of evidence of fetal cardiac decompensation in a patient with complete AV block has led to the maternal administration of numerous cardiotonic agents to increase fetal ventricular rates. The conclusion of the AEPC collaborative study in 1972 was that none of these agents was effective.[18] These workers did recommend using digoxin, and although the benefit of this drug is unproven, no detrimental effect on heart rate was noted. Medical therapy of the moribund hydropic newborn without cardiac pacing is likewise futile. The recent attempt at in utero ventricular pacing by Strasburger[29] and colleagues of a near moribund fetus is the logical next step when early delivery and immediate placement of an artificial pacemaker are not viable options.[5]

Postnatal Therapy

When the infant with congenital complete AV block is delivered and found to have signs and symptoms of congestive heart failure, rapid treatment is required. Since the escape pacemaker is often under autonomic control, drugs such as atropine or isoproterenol may increase the ventricular rate and cardiac output.

Other standard anticongestive measures such as intubation and positive pressure ventilation with positive end-expiratory pressure should also be used. Digoxin can increase ventricular performance. It rarely decreases ventricular rate.

Indications for Pacing

Any infant with congenital complete (or second-degree) AV block and congestive heart failure should be considered for pacing. Even if medical treatment results in an initial improvement, one episode of congestive heart failure should be considered indication for pacing. Another indication for pacemaker implant in the neonate is a ventricular rate less than 55 bpm in an infant with a normal heart or less than 65 bpm in an infant with a significant structural heart disease. Attempts to break this rule in infants who appear very well clinically have resulted in death.

Temporary Pacing

Temporary pacing may be carried out by transumbilical, transfemoral, or subclavian puncture. A soft 4 or 5 F bipolar catheter may be passed across the tricuspid valve and positioned in the right ventricular apex. Balloon electrode catheters are also available. Care should be taken not to pass the catheter across the foramen ovale into the left side of the heart because of the possibility of thromboembolism. The same is true of patients with right-to-left shunts. It must also be remembered that even the softest catheters may result in tricuspid insufficiency. Prevention of tricuspid insufficiency is more important in the neonate since the right ventricular pressure is high. Tricuspid insufficiency may result in a high right atrial pressure and right-to-left shunting and cyanosis. We have seen severe cyanosis result from pacing catheter-induced tricuspid insufficiency.

Permanent Pacing

Although temporary transvenous pacing may be lifesaving, the above problems, together with the possibility of perforating the neonatal heart, necessitate consideration of primary permanent epicardial pacing. Permanent epicardial pacing may be performed via a thoracotomy or by a subxiphoid approach. It is possible to place epicardial atrial and ventricular leads by either approach. Modern dual-chamber fully automatic pacemakers may be implanted in the rectus sheath in a normal-sized newborn.

Although it has not been documented in neonates, physiologic dual-chamber pacing has been shown to increase exercise cardiac output over single chamber ventricular pacing in adults and older children. Since we have found dual-chamber pacing to be feasible in neonates, we believe that it should be used in neonates as well as older children.

Technical Considerations

In small premature infants, it may be impossible to use dual-chamber pacemakers because of the infant's size. In such cases, smaller single-chamber ventricular demand pacemakers must be used. Very small units are now available that are multiprogrammed and that have lithium batteries designed to last for 5 years. Although sensor-driven pacemakers increase the rate in response to a physiologic signal such as bodily activity, they have not been tested in neonates or young children. It is possible that the physiologic signals will be so different in neonates that sensor-driven pacemakers will not function properly. Furthermore, the rate settings of the sensor-driven pacemakers are not currently appropriate for neonates. However, when a physiologic dual-chamber pacemaker is used, the infant's sinus node will control the pacing rate. The maximum upper rate limit should be used (usually 175–180 bpm). An appropriate lower rate limit should also be set (80–100 bpm) in case the sinus node is also abnormal. The AV interval should be set appropriately for a neonate (usually 100 msec). If the neonate has been tested for retrograde conduction and found not to have have it, which is usually the case, the shortest possible atrial sensing refractory period should be set to allow the upper rate limit to function as programmed. If the sum of the AV interval and the atrial sensing refractory period is greater than the cycle length of the upper rate limit, then 2:1 block will occur at the rate identified by the sum of the AV interval and atrial refractory period rather than Wenckebach block at the upper rate limit. Great care must be taken in selecting a dual-chamber pacemaker. Some pacemakers are available that have upper rate limits of only 150 bpm and that only have 2:1 block as a response to upper rate limit. Pacemakers are also available that have very small batteries and may only last 1 year when implanted.

When the infant is very small and it is necessary to use a ventricular demand pacemaker, a rate must be selected that is a compromise between that necessary during activity and that during rest. Consideration should also be given to battery size and programmable parameters in this setting. It is not in the patient's best interest to use the smallest, least expensive pacemaker. Pediatric epicardial pacing is difficult to maintain because of high battery drain from frequent increases in threshold requiring higher output setting and because of rapid heart rates.

Multiprogrammability offers many advantages. The use of integrated circuits has put to rest the old adage of pediatric cardiologists to use the simplist pulse generator. A microchip that works initially will virtually always continue to work.

Follow-Up

Follow-up is extremely important in paced neonates. Both transtelephonic and "hands on" follow-up are necessary. Major pulse generator or lead problems will be detected by transtelephonic follow-up, whereas more minor problems such as atrial capture will only be detected by hands on follow-up. The determination of capture threshold is particularly important in epicardial pacemakers, because of frequent instances of high thresholds. These occur most frequently in the first 6 to 8 weeks after implantation. After this period, if the thresholds are low, the output of the pulse generator may be decreased to prolong battery life.

Follow-up is also critical in neonates who do not meet criteria for pacing in the first few days of life. Twenty-four-hour ambulatory monitoring may be used to ensure that severe bradycardia or ventricular ectopy do not occur. Close observation for signs of congestive heart failure is also important. The majority of deaths in patients with congenital complete AV block occur in the first year of life in infants with associated structural congenital heart disease. It is in these infants where we can make gains by aggressive use of pacemakers. It should be possible to prevent virtually all deaths in infants with normal hearts. In infants with structural heart disease, it is usually the structural cardiac abnormalities that result in death, although the complete AV block may play an important ancillary role.

References

1. Allan LD (1985): A review of fetal echocardiography. Echocardiography 2:351–375.
2. Allan LD, Anderson RH, Sullivan ID, Campbell S, Holt DW, Tynan M (1983): Evaluation of fetal arrhythmias by echocardiogram. Br Heart J 50:240–245.
3. Allan LD, Crawford DC, Anderson RH, Tynan M (1984): Evaluation and treatment of fetal arrhythmias. Clin Cardiol 7:467–473.
4. Bharati S, de la Fuente DJ, Kallen DJ, Freij M, Lev M (1975): Conduction system in systic lupus erythematosus with atrioventricular block. Am J Cardiol 35:299–305.
5. Carpenter RJ, Strasburger JF, Garson A, Smith RT, Deter RL, Engelhardt HT (1986): Fetal ventricular pacing for hydrops secondary to complete atrioventricular block. J Am Coll Cardiol 8:1434–1436.
6. Chardrack WM, Gage AA, Greatbatch W (1960): A transistorized self-contained, implantable pacemaker for the long-term correction of complete heart block. Surgery 48:643–654.
7. Esscher E, Scott JS (1979): Congenital heart block and maternal systemic lupus erythematosus. Br Med J 1:1235–1238.
8. Franco HL, Weston WL, Peebles C, Forstot L, Phanuphak P (1981): Autoantibodies directed against sicca syndrome antigens in the neonatal lupus syndrome. Am Acad Dermatol 4:67–72.
9. Furman S, Schwedel JB (1959): An intracardiac pacemaker for Stokes-Adams seizures. N Engl J Med 261:943–948.
10. Glenn WWL, Mauro A, Longo E, Lavietes PH, Mackay FJ (1959): Remote stimulation of the heart by radiofrequency transmission. N Engl J Med 261:948–951.
11. Hyman AS (1930): Resuscitation of the stopped heart by intracardiac therapy. Arch Intern Med 46:283–305.
12. Kleinman CS, Donnerstein RL, DeVore FR, Jaffe CC, Lynch DC, Berkowitz RL, Talner NS, Hobbins JC (1982): Fetal echocardiography for evaluation of in utero congestive heart failure. N Engl J Med 306:568–575.
13. Kleinman CS, Donnerstein RL, Jaffe CC, DeVore GR, Weinstein EM, Lynch DC, Talner NS, Berkowitz RL, Hobbins JC (1983): Fetal echocardiography: A tool for evaluation of in utero cardiac arrhythmias and monitoring of in utero therapy: Analysis of 71 patients. Am J Cardiol 51:237–243.
14. Kleinman CS, Hobbins JC, Jaffe CC, Lynch DC, Talner NC (1980):

Echocardiographic studies of the human fetus: Prenatal diagnosis of congenital heart disease and cardiac dysrhythmias. Pediatrics 65:1059–1066.

15. Kleinman CS, Donnerstein RL (1985): Ultrasonic assessment of cardiac function in the intact human fetus. J Am Coll Cardiol 5 (Suppl 1):845–945.

16. Litsey SE, Noonan JA, O'Connor WN, Cottrill CM, Mitchell B (1985): Maternal connective tissue disease and congenital heart block. N Engl J Med 312:98–100.

17. Madison JP, Sukhum P, Williamson DP et al (1979): Echocardiography and fetal heart sounds in the diagnosis of fetal heart block. Am Heart J 98:505–509.

18. Michaelsson M, Engle MA (1972): Congenital complete heart block: An international study of the natural history. Cardiovasc Clin 4:86–101.

19. Mond HG, Sloman JF, Edwards RH (1982): The first pacemaker. PACE 5:278–282.

20. Plant RK, Steven RA (1945): Complete AV block in a fetus. Am Heart J 30:615–618.

21. Scott JS, Maddison PJ, Taylor PV, Esscher E, Scott O, Skinner RP (1983): Connective tissue disease, antibodies to ribonucleoprotein, and congenital heart block. N Engl J Med 309:209–212.

22. Senning A (1959): Discussion of a paper by Stephenson SE et al. J Thorac Surg 38:639.

23. Shenker L (1979): Fetal cardiac arrhythmias. Obstet Gynecol Surv 34:561–572.

24. Silverman NH, Kleinman CS, Rudolph AM, Copel JA, Weinstein EM, Enderlein MA, Golbus M (1985): Fetal atrioventricular valve insufficiency associated with nonimmune hydrops: A two-dimensional echocardiographic and pulsed Doppler ultrasound study. Circulation 72:825–832.

25. Silverman NH, Ramaciotti C, Enderlein MA (1986): The uses of pulsed ultrasound in the human fetus. In Doyle EF et al (eds): Pediatric Cardiology, Proceedings of the Second World Congress 1986. New York, Springer-Verlag, pp 44–51.

26. Singsen BH, Akhter JE, Weinstein MM, Sharp GC (1985): Congenital complete heart block and SSA antibodies: Obstetric implications. Am J Obstet Gynecol 152:655–658.

27. Sokol RJ, Hutchison P, Kaouskop RW, Brown EG, Reed G, Vasquez H (1974): Congenital complete heart block diagnosed during intrauterine fetal monitoring. Am J Obstet Gynecol 120:1115–1119.

28. Steinfeld L, Rappaport HL, Rossbach HC, Martinex E (1986): Diagnosis of fetal arrhythmias using echocardiographic and Doppler techniques. J Am Coll Cardiol 8:1425–1433.

29. Strasburger J, Carpenter R, Smith RT, Deater R, Garson A (1986): Fetal transthoracic pacing for advanced hydrops fetalis secondary to complete atrioventricular block (abstr). PACE 9:295.

30. Strasburger JF, Huhta JC, Carpenter RJ, Garson A, McNamara DG (1986): Doppler echocardiography in the diagnosis and management of persistent fetal arrhythmias. J Am Coll Cardiol 7:1386–1391.

31. Taylor PV, Scott JS, Gerlis LM, Esscher E, Scott O (1986): Maternal antibodies against fetal cardiac antigens in congenital complete heart block. N Engl J Med 315:667–672.

32. Teteris NJ, Chisholm JW, Ullery JC (1968): Antenatal diagnosis of congenital heart block. Obstet Gynecol 32:851–853.

33. Turner LB (1947): Asymptomatic congenital heart block in an Army Air Force pilot. Am Heart J 34:426–431.

34. Van den Heuvel GCJ (1908): Die Ziekle van Stokes-Adams en een genal van aangeboren Hartblock. Proefschrift aan de Ryks, Universitat, Gronigen.

35. Weirich WL, Paneth M, Gott VL, Lillehei CW (1958): Control of complete heart block by use of an artificial pacemaker and a myocardial electrode. Circ Res 6:410–415.

36. Witt DB (1934): Congenital complete auriculoventricular heart block. Am J Dis Child 47:380–387.

37. Wren C, Hunter S, Campbell R (1986): The use of echocardiography in the assessment of arrhythmias. Echocardiography 3:129–141.

38. Yater WM (1929): Congenital heart block. Am J Dis Child 38:112–136.

43 TRICUSPID ATRESIA

P. Syamasundar Rao

Tricuspid atresia is a cyanotic, congenital cardiac anomaly and has been commonly defined as congenital absence or agenesis of the morphologic tricuspid valve.[53] It is the third most common cyanotic congenital heart defect and is the most common cause of cyanosis with left ventricular hypertrophy. There is considerable controversy with regard to whether most cases of tricuspid atresia are examples of univentricular heart.[2,8,55] However, the author is of the opinion that tricuspid atresia is a distinct entity and prefers to retain the term "triscupid atresia" for reasons detailed elsewhere.[55]

Although some authors[21,76] state that this malformation was first described in 1906 by Kühne or in 1824 by Holmes, a methodical and thorough review by Rashkind[74] suggests that the first documented case of tricuspid atresia was that of Kreysig in 1817;[74] although the 1812 report by the editors of London Medical Review[74] appears to fit the description of tricuspid atresia, they did not use the specific term for us to be sure of the diagnosis.

The true prevalence of tricuspid atresia is not known. Extensive review of the literature revealed an autopsy prevalence rate of 2.9 per cent and a clinical prevalence rate of 1.4 per cent among subjects with congenital heart disease.[56] The clinical prevalence of tricuspid atresia in neonates with congenital heart defects is also similar at 1.5 per cent. With the known prevalence of congenital heart defects of 0.8 per cent of live births, it is estimated that tricuspid atresia occurs in approximately 1 of 10,000 live births.[56] A slight male predominance has been suggested[76] for tricuspid atresia, but detailed analysis of sex incidence[56] did not support the claim of male predominance (p > 0.1). However, the observation about male predominance in tricuspid atresia patients with associated transposition of the great arteries[21] is borne out by our analysis;[56] the male-to-female ratio was 66:34.

In this chapter I will discuss classification; anatomic, physiologic, and clinical features; noninvasive and invasive evaluation; differential diagnosis; management; and prognosis of tricuspid atresia in the neonate.

CLASSIFICATION

Tricuspid atresia may be classified on the basis of valve morphology,[89] radiographic appearance of pulmonary vascular markings,[5] and associated cardiac defects.[25,38,42] In considering the morphology of the atretic tricuspid valve, Van Praagh classified it into muscular, membranous, valvular, Ebstein, and atrioventricular canal types.[87,89] The muscular type, constituting 89 per cent of cases[57] is char-

acterized by a dimple or a localized fibrous thickening in the floor of the right atrium at the usual site of the tricuspid valve.[38] No valvular material can be identified by either gross or microscopic examination.[38] A classification based solely on the radiographic appearance of pulmonary vascular markings was put forward by Astley,[5] who divided tricuspid atresia into two groups: Group A, decreased pulmonary vascular markings; and Group B, increased pulmonary vascular markings. Dick et al[21] added another group to Astley's classification: Group C, transition from increased to decreased pulmonary vascular markings in serial chest films. The above two classifications have some clinical value, but a classification based on associated cardiac defects appears to be more useful clinically.[53,57] A classification based on great artery interrelationship was first proposed by Kühne in 1906.[42] This classification was later expanded by Edwards and Burchell,[25] and was further refined and popularized by Keith, Rowe, and Vlad.[38,39,90] Because of some apparent inconsistencies in subgrouping and the need for inclusion of all variations in great artery anatomy, we proposed a new, unified classification,[53,57] which is listed in Table 43–1. First, the tricuspid atresia is classified into four major types based on the interrelationship of the great arteries. Each type is identified with a Roman number: Type I, normally related great arteries; type II, d-transposition of the great arteries; type III, malpositions of the great arteries other than d-transposition; and type IV, truncus arteriosus. Type III is again further divided into several subtypes (see Table 43–1) identified with an Arabic number (1 through 5). Each type and subtype are further divided into subgroups on the basis of pulmonary arteries; each subgroup is indicated by a lower case letter: subgroup a, pulmonary atresia; subgroup b, pulmonary stenosis or hypoplasia; and subgroup c, normal pulmonary arteries (no pulmonary stenosis).[53,57] Once a patient with tricuspid atresia is thus classified, the status of the interventricular septum, i.e., intact, small, or large ventricular septal defect (VSD) or multiple VSDs and the other associated malformations, should be described. If one wants to follow the terminology of congenital heart disease proposed and reemphasized by Van Praagh,[88] one could include the remaining segmental subsets, namely visceroatrial situs and ventricular loop. Each case could be described by notations [S,D,S], [S,D,D], [S,D,L] and so on as the case may be.[88,92]

PATHOLOGIC ANATOMY

The most common type of tricuspid atresia, muscular variety, is characterized by a dimple or a localized fibrous

Table 43–1. CLASSIFICATION OF TRICUSPID ATRESIA

Type I	Normally related great arteries	Each type and subtype are divided:
Type II	*d*-transposition of the great arteries	Subgroup a Pulmonary atresia
Type III	Malpositions other than *d*-transposition	Subgroup b Pulmonary stenosis or hypoplasia
	Subtype 1 *l*-transposition of great arteries	Subgroup c Normal pulmonary arteries (no pulmonary
	Subtype 2 Double outlet right ventricle	stenosis)
	Subtype 3 Double outlet left ventricle	
	Subtype 4 *d*-malposition of the great arteries	
	(anatomically corrected malposition)	
	Subtype 5 *l*-malposition of the great arteries	
	(anatomically corrected malposition)	
Type IV Persistent truncus arteriosus		

Reproduced with permission from Rao PS (1980): A unified classification for tricuspid atresia. Am Heart J 99:799–804.

thickening in the floor of the right atrium at the expected site of the tricuspid valve[38] and constitutes 89 per cent of the cases.[57] No valvular material can be identified by either gross or microscopic examination.[38] Other anatomic types, namely, membranous type (4 per cent) with the atrioventricular portion of the membranous septum forming the floor of the right atrium,[23,87,89,91] valvular type (3 per cent) with minute valve cusps that are fused,[3,13,26,36,38,40,91] Ebstein type (4 per cent) with Ebstein deformity of the tricuspid valve leaflets (and valve leaflet fusion),[3,69,89] and common atrioventricular canal type in which a leaflet of the common atrioventricular canal completely seals off the only entry into the right ventricle[65,87,92] have also been described.

The right atrium is usually enlarged and its wall thickened and hypertrophied. The interatrial communication, which is necessary for survival, is usually a stretched patent foramen ovale, sometimes an ostium secundum atrial septal defect and rarely an ostium primum atrial septal defect. Occasionally, the interatrial communication is obstructive and may form an aneurysm of the fossa ovalis, causing obstruction to the mitral flow.[29] The left atrium is enlarged and may be more so if the pulmonary blood flow is increased.

The mitral valve is morphologically a mitral valve, usually bicuspid; the mitral orifice is large and rarely incompetent. The left ventricle is clearly a morphologic left ventricle with only occasional abnormalities;[8,9,55] however, it is enlarged and hypertrophied.

The VSD may be large, small or nonexistent (intact ventricular septum), or multiple VSDs may be present. When present, the VSD may be (1) conoventricular or perimembranous VSD (located inferior to the septal band), (2) conal septal malalignment VSD (located in between the anterosuperior and posteroinferior limbs of septal band), (3) muscular VSD (located inferiorly when compared with 1 and 2), and (4) atrioventricular canal type VSD.[92] In the author's experience, muscular VSDs are most common.[52,60,70,71] Also, most of these VSDs are restrictive and act as subpulmonic stenosis in the type I patients and as subaortic stenosis in the type II patients.[52,60,62,70,71,92]

The right ventricle is small and hypoplastic; even the largest of the right ventricles that are present in patients with large VSDs and/or transposition of the great arteries are smaller than normal. Right ventricular size, by and large, is determined by anatomic type. The right ventricle may be extremely small, so that it may escape detection on gross examination of the specimen, as in type Ia cases. Usually, such diminutive right ventricles can be identified at the right upper aspect of the ventricular mass, but on occasion, they can be identified only on microscopic examination.[25,38] However, in most cases the ventricle is a true right ventricle,[8,9] consisting of (1) a sharply demarcated infundibulum with septal and parietal bands and (2) a sinus with trabeculae that communicates with the left ventricle via a VSD. The inflow region of the right ventricle, by definition, is absent, although papillary muscles may be present occasionally.[90]

The relative position of the great vessels is quite variable and has been the basis for classification of this anomaly, as has been described in the preceding section. The ascending aorta may be normal in size, or it may be larger than normal. Pulmonary outflow obstruction may be either subvalvular or valvular in patients with transposition of the great arteries; in patients with normally related great arteries, pulmonary obstruction is often at the VSD level. In a few cases, subvalvular pulmonic stenosis, narrow tract of the hypoplastic right ventricle, and, rarely, valvular pulmonary stenosis may also be responsible for pulmonary outflow tract obstruction. With pulmonary atresia, either a patent ductus arteriosus or aortopulmonary collateral vessels may be present.

A large number of additional abnormalities may be present in 30 per cent of tricuspid atresia patients.[17,22] Significant among these are persistent left superior vena cava and coarctation of the aorta; the latter is much more common in type II (transposition) patients. The possible physiologic reason for this association is discussed in the next section.

PATHOPHYSIOLOGY

Prenatal Circulation

Tricuspid atresia is not detrimental to normal fetal development. In a normally formed fetus, the highly saturated inferior vena caval blood is preferentially shunted into the left atrium via the patent foramen ovale and from there into the left ventricle and aorta. The superior vena caval blood containing desaturated blood is directed toward the tricuspid valve and right ventricle, and from there into the pulmonary arteries, ductus arteriosus, and descending aorta. Thus, in a normal fetus, the head and upper extremities are supplied with blood at higher PO_2 and the lungs, the lower part of the body, and placenta with blood at lower PO_2. In tricuspid atresia, both vena caval streams have to be shunted across the foramen ovale into the left atrium and left ventricle. Therefore, the PO_2 differential to various parts of the fetal body that is normally present does not exist. Whether or not this higher fetal lung PO_2 influences pulmonary arteriolar smooth muscle development is not known.[78] The lower than normal fetal brain and upper body PO_2 does not seem to impair development, at least as observed clinically.

In type I (normally related great arteries) fetuses with intact ventricular septum and/or pulmonary atresia (type Ia) and in type II (transposition of the great arteries) fetuses with pulmonary atresia (type IIa), the pulmonary blood flow must be derived entirely through the ductus. Since the ductus is carrying only the pulmonary blood flow, representing 8 to 10 per cent of combined ventricular output in contrast to 66 per cent in the normal fetus,[78] the ductus arteriosus is likely to be smaller than normal. Intrauterine reduction in and reversal of direction of ductus flow may render the ductus less responsive to the usual postnatal stimuli.[78]

In type I fetuses with VSD, the amount of antegrade blood flow from the left ventricle through the VSD into the right ventricle, pulmonary artery, and ductus arteriosus versus the amount of retrograde blood flow from the aorta to the ductus arteriosus varies with the size of the VSD such that the larger the VSD, the greater the amount of fetal antegrade ductal flow.

In type I fetuses with a small or no VSD, most of the left ventricular blood is ejected into the aorta, which is then carried to the entire body, including the placenta and lower part of the body. Thus, the aortic isthmus carries a larger proportion of ventricular output than normal; presumably this increase in aortic isthmus flow is the reason for the rarity of associated coarctation of the aorta in these subgroups of tricuspid atresia patients. In type II (transposition of the great arteries) patients without significant pulmonary stenosis, the VSD is usually smaller than the pulmonary valve ring,[47] and a larger proportion of blood traverses the pulmonary artery and ductus arteriosus. As a result, the isthmic flow decreases, thus accounting for the high incidence of coarctation of the aorta and aortic arch anomalies seen with these types of tricuspid atresia.[47,78]

Postnatal Circulation

An obligatory right-to-left shunt occurs at the atrial level in all types and subtypes of tricuspid atresia. Usually, this shunting is through a patent foramen ovale, but on occasion, secundum or primum atrial septal defects may be present. Thus the systemic and coronary venous blood mixes with pulmonary venous return in the left atrium. This mixed pulmonary, coronary, and systemic venous returns enter the left ventricle.

In type I (normally related great arteries) patients with a VSD, left-to right ventricular shunt occurs, thus perfusing the lungs. In the absence of a VSD, the pulmonary circulation is derived either via a patent ductus arteriosus

or through bronchopulmonary or persistent embryonic aortopulmonary collateral vessels. The presence of either a VSD or other means of blood supply to the lungs is crucial for the patient's survival. The aortic blood flow is derived directly from the left ventricle.

In type II (with d-transposition of the great arteries) patients, the pulmonary blood flow is directly derived from the left ventricle. The systemic blood flow is via the VSD and the right ventricle. In type III and type IV patients, the systemic and pulmonary blood flows are determined by the size of the VSD and other associated defects.

Other Physiologic Principles

Arterial Desaturation

Because of complete admixture of the systemic, coronary, and pulmonary venous returns in the left atrium and left ventricle, systemic arterial desaturation is always present. The oxygen saturation is proportional to the magnitude of the pulmonary blood flow.[35,78] The data from our group of patients are plotted in Figure 43–1; the pulmonary-to-systemic blood flow ratio (Qp:Qs), which represents the pulmonary

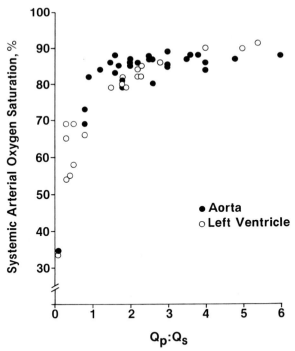

Figure 43–1. The systemic arterial saturations, left ventricular (LV) or aortic (Ao), in tricuspid atresia are plotted against the pulmonary-to-systemic blood flow ratio (Qp:Qs). Both type I and type II anatomy are included. Note curvilinear relationship between two parameters. At low Qp:Qs levels, a slight increase in Qp:Qs produces large increases in systemic O_2 saturation, and at higher Qp:Qs levels a further increase does not produce significant increase in O_2 saturation. Ideal Qp:Qs appears to be between 1.5 and 2.5, giving O_2 saturations in the low 80s. Aortic saturations are marked as solid circles and LV saturations as open circles. Qp:Qs = ratio of pulmonary blood flow to systemic blood flow. (Reproduced with permission from Rao PS [1982]: Tricuspid Atresia. Mt. Kisco, Futura Publishing Co, p 155.)

blood flow, has a curvilinear relationship with the arterial oxygen saturation. A Qp:Qs of 1.5 to 2.5 appears to result in adequate oxygen saturation.[58] Further increase in Qp:Qs does not result in better oxygen saturation but may subject the left ventricle to large volume overloading and therefore is not advisable.[58]

Pulmonary Blood Flow

The magnitude of pulmonary blood flow is the major determinant of clinical features in tricuspid atresia. An infant with markedly decreased pulmonary blood flow will present early in the neonatal period with severe cyanosis, hypoxemia, and acidosis. An infant with markedly increased pulmonary flow does not have significant cyanosis but usually presents with signs of heart failure. Although there is some overlap, patients with decreased pulmonary flow usually belong to type I (normally related great arteries), and those with increased pulmonary blood flow are usually type II (transposition of the great arteries) and occasionally type Ic.

The magnitude of pulmonary blood flow in an unoperated patient is dependent on the magnitude of obstruction to the pulmonary outflow tract and on patency of the ductus arteriosus. The pulmonary outflow obstruction is either valvular, subvalvular in type II patients; and valvular, subvalvular, or at VSD level in type I patients. In our own experience with tricuspid atresia, we have repeatedly found the obstruction to be located most commonly at the VSD level.[52,60,70,71] When the VSD is large and nonrestrictive and the pulmonary valve nonstenotic, the pulmonary flow is proportional to the pulmonary-to-systemic vascular resistance ratio. When a systemic-to-pulmonary artery shunt has been performed, the pulmonary blood flow is proportional to the size of the anastomosis.

Left Ventricular Volume Overloading

Because the entire systemic, coronary, and pulmonary venous returns are pumped by the left ventricle, the left ventricle has a greater volume overload than normal. This volume overloading is further increased if the Qp:Qs is higher either because of mild or no obstruction to pulmonary blood flow or because of surgically created shunts of large size; heart failure may result. Normal left ventricular function is critical for a successful Fontan-type procedure later in life and should be maintained within normal range. Several studies have shown that the left ventricular function tends to decrease with increasing age, Qp:Qs, and arterial desaturation.[1,33,45,48,79]

Size of the Interatrial Communication

The interatrial communication is usually a patent foramen ovale. Because of the obligatory shunting, this fetal pathway persists in the postnatal period; persistent foramen ovale patency is in part related to low left atrial pressure. However, the entire systemic venous return must pass through the patent foramen ovale, and it is therefore not surprising to find interatrial obstruction; nevertheless, very few patients with tricuspid atresia have clinically significant obstruction.[21] The right-to-left shunt occurs in late atrial diastole with augmentation during atrial systole (a wave).[61] A mean atrial pressure gradient greater than 5 mmHg is usually associated with interatrial obstruction. A markedly increased a wave in the right atrium also indicates interatrial obstruction.

Changing Hemodynamics

With growth and development, several changes may take place in patients with tricuspid atresia. Closure of the ductus arteriosus in the early neonatal period may result in severe hypoxemia. The size of the interatrial communication may diminish either in absolute terms or relative to the volume of the systemic venous return and cause systemic venous congestion; atrial septostomy may be required. The ventricular septal defect may close spontaneously,[31,52,60,70,71] causing pulmonary oligemia and hypoxemia in type I patients or subaortic obstruction in type II patients. Such VSD closures occur over a period of months and years and are not germane to our discussion of tricuspid atresia in neonates; therefore, they will not be discussed further.

CLINICAL FEATURES

Approximately one half of the patients with tricuspid atresia present with symptoms on the first day of life, and 80 per cent have symptoms by the end of the first month of life.[21,22] As previously mentioned, the magnitude of pulmonary blood flow determines the clinical features. Two modes of presentation are recognized: those with decreased pulmonary blood flow and those with increased pulmonary blood flow.

Infants with pulmonary oligemia present with symptoms of cyanosis within the first few days of life; with more severe pulmonary oligemia, clinical presentation is on the first day of life. These hypoxemic infants may have hyperpnea and acidosis if the pulmonary blood flow is markedly decreased. The majority of these infants belong to type Ib. Patients with pulmonary atresia (subgroup a) irrespective of the type will also present with early cyanosis, especially when the ductus begins to close. Hypoxic spells are not common in the neonate, although the spells can occur later in infancy. Physical examination reveals central cyanosis, tachypnea or hyperpnea, normal pulses, prominent a waves in the jugular venous pulse (if there is significant interatrial obstruction), and no hepatic enlargement. (Presystolic hepatic pulsations may be felt if there is severe interatrial obstruction.) Quiet precordium and absence of thrills are usual. The second heart sound is usually single. A holosystolic murmur suggestive of VSD may be heard at the left lower or midsternal border. No diastolic murmurs are heard. In patients with associated pulmonary atresia, no murmurs are usually heard; although in an occasional patient, a continuous murmur of patent ductus arteriosus may be heard. Signs of clinical congestive heart failure are notably absent.

Infants with pulmonary plethora usually present with signs of heart failure within the first few weeks of life, although an occasional infant may present within the first week of life.[77] Such infants are only minimally cyanotic but present with symptoms of dyspnea, fatigue, feeding difficulties, and marked perspiration. Recurrent respiratory tract infection and failure to thrive are another mode of presentation. The majority of these patients belong to type IIc, although a small number may be of type Ic. The association of coarctation of the aorta with type II patients has already been mentioned; coarctation, when present, predisposes to early cardiac failure. Examination reveals tachypnea, tachycardia, decreased femoral pulses (when associated with coarctation of the aorta but without significant-sized patent ductus arteriosus), minimal cyanosis, prominent neck vein pulsations, and hepatomegaly. Prominent a waves in jugular veins and/or presystolic hepatic pulsations may be observed with associated interatrial obstruction. The precordial impulses are increased and hyperdynamic. The second heart sound may be single or split. A holosystolic murmur of VSD is usually heard at the left lower sternal border. An apical mid-diastolic murmur may be heard. Clear-cut signs of congestive heart failure are usually present.

NONINVASIVE EVALUATION

Chest Radiograph

Chest radiographic appearance is, by and large, dependent on the total pulmonary blood flow. In patients with diminished pulmonary flow (the majority of infants will fall into this category), the heart size is either normal or minimally enlarged, whereas in those with increased pulmonary blood flow, the heart size is moderately to severely enlarged. Several patterns of cardiac configuration have been described, namely "characteristic" tricuspid atresia appearance;[85] *coeur en sabot* configuration;[94] and "egg-shaped,"[90] "ball-shaped,"[26] and square[5] heart; but in the author's experience and that of others,[90] there is no consistent pattern that would be diagnostic of tricuspid atresia. There may be concavity in the region of the pulmonary artery segment in patients with pulmonary oligemia and a small pulmonary artery. The right atrial shadow may be prominent.

Right aortic arch is present in approximately 8 per cent of patients with tricuspid atresia[90] and is less commonly observed than in tetralogy of Fallot (25 per cent) and truncus arteriosus (40 per cent). An unusual contour of the left border of the heart suggestive of *l*-transposition may be seen in association with or confused with tricuspid atresia.

The greatest use of the chest radiograph is in categorizing infants into those with decreased pulmonary vascular markings and those with increased pulmonary vascular markings (Fig. 43–2). Often the chest radiograph is all that is necessary to make a correct diagnosis once a history, physical examination, and electrocardiogram have been obtained.[17]

Electrocardiogram and Vectorcardiogram

The electrocardiogram can be virtually diagnostic of tricuspid atresia in an infant with cyanotic congenital heart

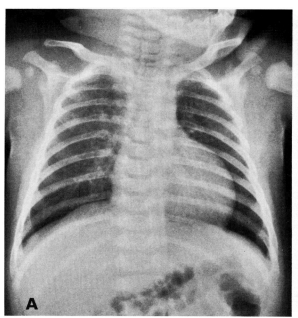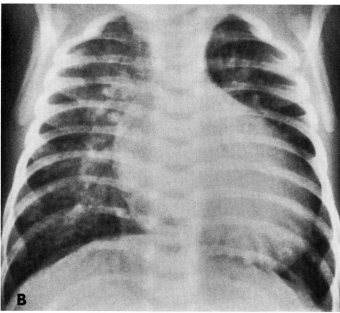

Figure 43–2. *A*, Posteroanterior view of a chest radiograph of a neonate showing normal to mildly enlarged cardiac size and decreased pulmonary vascular markings. A diagnosis of tricuspid atresia, type Ib was confirmed by cardiac catheterization. *B*, Chest radiograph of a 3-week-old infant with type IIc tricuspid atresia showing severe cardiomegaly and markedly increased pulmonary vascular markings. Note that there is nothing characteristic in these radiographs to suggest the diagnosis of tricuspid atresia, but these radiographs are useful in assessing the status of the pulmonary blood flow.

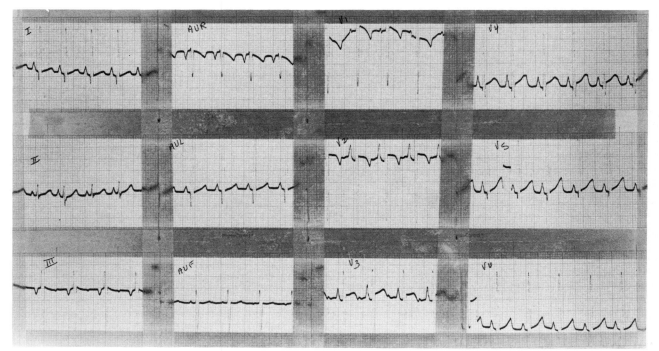

Figure 43–3. Twelve-lead electrocardiogram showing abnormal, superiorly oriented mean QRS vector in frontal plane (−45°, left axis deviation), left ventricular hypertrophy, and diminished anterior (R waves in leads V_1 and V_2) and rightward (S waves in leads V_5 and V_6) forces. Prominent P waves are also seen in several leads. This electrocardiogram is highly suggestive of tricuspid atresia.

disease. The characteristic features include right atrial hypertrophy, an abnormal, superiorly oriented major QRS vector (so-called left axis deviation) in the frontal plane, left ventricular hypertrophy, and diminished right ventricular forces (Fig. 43–3).

The right atrial hypertrophy, manifested by tall, peaked P waves exceeding 2.5 mm in amplitude, is present in three fourths of the patients with tricuspid atresia.[44] Although it has been claimed that the amplitude of the P wave in lead II is directly proportional to the interatrial pressure gradient and inversely proportional to the size of the interatrial communication, detailed analysis of these parameters does not suggest a consistent relationship.[21,50] A double peak spike and dome configuration of the P wave, referred to as "P-tricuspidale"[32] may be present. The first taller peak is contributed by the right atrial depolarization, and the second smaller peak is presumed to be due to left atrial depolarization.[44]

Abnormal, superiorly oriented major QRS vector (ASV), more popularly called left axis deviation, between 0 to −90 degrees in the frontal plane is present in the majority of the patients with tricuspid atresia. ASV is present in excess of 80 per cent of patients with type I anatomy (normally related great arteries), while only less than 50 per cent of patients with type II (transposition of great arteries) and type III (malpositions of great arteries other than *d*-transposition) anatomy show such a typical electrocardiographic pattern.[44] Normal (0 to +90 degrees) or right axis deviation is present in a minority of patients, and most of these patients belong to type II or III anatomy. It has been suggested that the ASV may be related

to destructive lesions in the left anterior bundle,[32] fibrosis of left bundle branch,[51] or abnormal distribution[7,24,34] of the conduction system (unusually long right bundle branch and origin of left bundle branch very close to the nodal-His bundle junction). More recently, data on ventricular activation from our group[43,44] suggested that this characteristic QRS pattern in tricuspid atresia is produced by interaction of several factors, the most important being the right-to-left ventricular disproportion and the asymmetrical distribution of the left ventricular mass favoring the superior wall.

Regardless of the frontal plane mean QRS vector, electrocardiographic criteria for left ventricular hypertrophy are present in the vast majority of patients. LVH may be manifested by increased (beyond the ninety fifth percentile) S waves in right chest leads and R waves in left chest leads or by adult progression of the QRS in the chest leads in the neonates and infants. ST-T wave changes suggestive of left ventricular strain are present in 50 per cent of patients.[32] Left ventricular hypertrophy is due to both left ventricular volume overload and lack of right ventricular forces. Occasionally, biventricular hypertrophy may be present; the majority of such patients have type II or III anatomy with a good-sized right ventricle. Diminished R waves in right chest leads and S waves in left chest are related to right ventricular hypoplasia.

Vectorcardiographic features closely resemble the scalar electrocardiogram. Characteristically, the QRS loop on the frontal plane is oriented superiorly with counterclockwise rotation. The horizontal plane QRS loop is also counterclockwise, and the major vector is directed to the left and

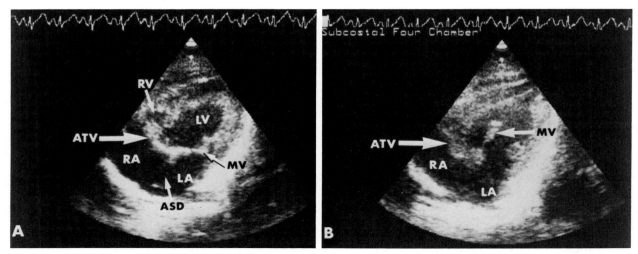

Figure 43–4. Subcostal four-chamber two-dimensional echocardiographic view of a neonate with tricuspid atresia showing an enlarged left ventricle, a small right ventricle, and a dense band of echoes at the site where the tricuspid valve echo should be. Atrial and ventricular septal defects and the mitral valve are also seen. Note the attachment of the anterior leaflet of the detectable atrioventricular valve to the left side of the interatrial septum. ASD = secundum atrial septal defect; ATV = atretic tricuspid valve; LA = left atrium; LV = left ventricle; MV = mitral valve; RA = right atrium; RV = right ventricle.

posterior. Davachi et al[18] have reported narrow QRS loops in patients with decreased pulmonary blood flow and wide QRS loops in those with increased pulmonary blood flow.

Echocardiogram

M-mode echocardiographic features include a large left atrium (usually proportional to the magnitude of pulmonary blood flow), dilated left ventricle with normal to decreased left ventricular shortening fraction, a large posterior atrioventricular valve in continuity with the posterior semilunar valve, and a small right ventricle.[17,82] The pulmonary valve may or may not be recorded. The tricuspid valve is conspicuously absent.[17] Occasionally, tricuspid valve-like echoes of low amplitude may be recorded, and this feature should not exclude the diagnosis of tricuspid atresia.[83,84] Contrast echocardiography with injection of saline or a similar substance into a peripheral vein may be of help in the diagnosis. While recording left atrium, aorta, and right ventricular outflow tract, sequential contrast echo visualization of the left atrium, aorta, and right ventricular outflow tract, in that order, is seen with type I tricuspid atresia. When both ventricles are recorded, earlier opacification of the left ventricle than the right ventricle is typically seen.

Two-dimensional echocardiography, apart from showing an enlarged right atrium, left atrium, and left ventricle and small right ventricle, will demonstrate the atretic tricuspid valve directly. In the most common muscular type, a dense band of echoes is seen at the site where the tricuspid valve should be,[6,17] and the anterior leaflet of the detectable atrioventricular valve is attached to the left side of the interatrial septum (Fig. 43–4). Apical and subcostal four-chamber views are best used to demonstrate the anatomy. Atrial and ventricular septal defects can also be demonstrated by two-dimensional echocardiography. Shunting across these

defects can be demonstrated by Doppler studies (Fig. 43–5). Semilunar valves can be identified as pulmonic or aortic by following the great vessel until the bifurcation of the pulmonary artery or the arch of the aorta is seen; such maneuvers help determine whether there is associated transposition of the great arteries. Suprasternal notch imaging is of use in demonstrating coarctation of the aorta, which is often seen in type II patients. Contrast echocardiography with two-dimensional imaging can clearly demonstrate sequential opacification of the right atrium, left atrium, left ventricle, and then the right ventricle.

CARDIAC CATHETERIZATION AND SELECTIVE CINEANGIOGRAPHY

The diagnosis of tricuspid atresia based on clinical, electrocardiographic, and echocardiographic features is relatively simple, and cardiac catheterization and selective cineangiography, rarely, if ever, are essential for arriving at the diagnosis.[58] Neonates with significant arterial desaturation should undergo cardiac catheterization and selective cineangiography even if the diagnosis of tricuspid atresia is clear-cut on the basis of clinical and noninvasive evaluation, so as to define the detailed anatomy and associated defects prior to any palliative surgical intervention. In many patients with tricuspid atresia presenting in the neonatal period, the pulmonary blood flow is ductal dependent. The ductus arteriosus may be kept patent by infusion of prostaglandin E_1 (see the section Medical Management at the Time of Initial Presentation for details) to improve hypoxemia and the attendant metabolic acidosis prior to performing cardiac catheterization. Additional precatheterization preparation of the neonates includes monitoring

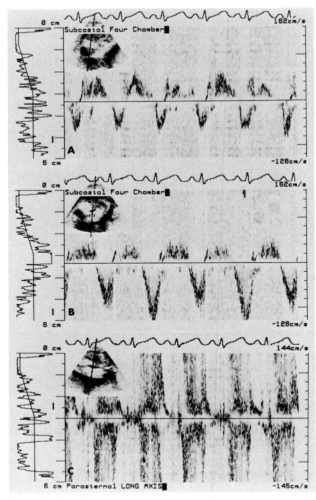

Figure 43–5. Pulsed Doppler echocardiography demonstrating left-to-right (*A*) and right-to-left (*B*) shunting across the interatrial communication in a subcostal four-chamber view in an infant with tricuspid atresia. The right-to-left shunt is as expected in tricuspid atresia, but the left-to-right shunt, although unexpected, has been explained on the basis of instantaneous pressure differences between the atria (see text and Fig. 43–6). *C* shows Doppler left-to-right shunting across the ventricular septal defect.

for and prompt restoration of a neutral thermal environment, normal acid-base status, normocalcemia, and normoglycemia.[73]

Catheter Insertion and Course

Percutaneous right femoral venous catheterization using Desilets-Hoffman modification[20] (using a sheath) of the Seldinger technique[81] is the preferred approach.

Because of an atretic tricuspid valve, the right ventricle cannot be directly catheterized from the right atrium. The catheter can easily be maneuvered into the left atrium across the patent foramen ovale. The catheter may follow a similar course in patients with pulmonary atresia (or severe stenosis) with intact ventricular septum and hypoplastic

right ventricle or severe tricuspid stenosis. Inability to enter the right ventricle from the right atrium is not necessarily diagnostic of tricuspid atresia, but in experienced hands it is highly suggestive of tricuspid atresia.

From the left atrium, the catheter can easily be manipulated into the left ventricle. With the previous conventional catheters, the left ventricle is the farthest structure that could be catheterized in tricuspid atresia. However, with the use of balloon-tipped catheters and other maneuvers using guide wires, the aorta, the right ventricle, and the pulmonary artery can be catheterized, particularly in older infants and children. But in neonates, once an adequate left ventricular angiogram is performed, we terminate the procedure because further manipulation of the catheter may precipitate spells or arrhythmias and the additional information obtained by further catheter manipulation may not be of much value.

In infants with clinical and/or pressure evidence of aortic arch obstruction, retrograde arterial catheterization (again using the percutaneous Seldinger technique) may be necessary, especially if the aortic arch anatomy is not clearly demonstrated by left ventricular angiography. When the ductus is patent, the retrograde catheter may be advanced into the pulmonary artery via the patent ductus arteriosus.

Oxygen Saturations

Systemic venous oxygen saturations are usually diminished, and the extent of decrease is related to systemic arterial desaturation and the severity of congestive heart failure.

Because of the obligatory right-to-left shunting across the patent foramen ovale, it is generally believed that the right atrial saturations are similar to vena caval saturations. However, our group found left-to-right atrial shunting, represented by an increase of 6 per cent or more in oxygen saturation from the superior vena cava to the right atrium in two or more sets of saturations, in 29 of 50 (58 per cent) catheterizations in which the data were adequate.[61] Anatomic causes, such as large ostium primum atrial septal defect and anomalous pulmonary venous return, were found in only two catheterizations. Comparison of age, pulmonary-to-systemic flow ratio (Qp:Qs), and mean atrial pressure difference between the shunt and the nonshunt group did not reveal any difference (p > 0.1).[61] However, in the shunt group the left atrial v waves were equal to or higher than the right atrial v waves, thus accounting for the left-to-right atrial shunting. Simultaneous pressure recordings (in one tricuspid atresia patient with left-to-right atrial shunting) from the left atrium and the right atrium with isosensitized miniature pressure transducers mounted 5 cm apart revealed a higher pressure in the left atrium than in the right atrium during atrial diastole (Fig. 43–6). From that study[61] it was concluded that (1) left-to-right shunt across the atrial septal defect occurs frequently in tricuspid atresia and (2) that the left-to-right shunt is a result of instantaneous pressure differences between atria and such shunts are "physiologic."

The pulmonary venous saturations are usually in the normal range. A significant decrease in left atrial saturation is expected because of obligatory right-to-left shunting across the patent foramen ovale. Falsely high or falsely low saturations may be measured in the left atrium because of streaming. The left ventricular saturations are usually well mixed and are more reliable. The saturations in the left atrium and left ventricle as well as those in the right ventricle, the pulmonary artery, and the aorta are nearly identical. Systemic arterial desaturation is always present, and the extent of desaturation is proportional to the Qp:Qs (see Fig. 43–1).[58]

The vena caval, left atrial, left ventricular, and aortic oxygen saturations are usually lower in type I patients than those in type II patients.[58] Lower saturations are presumably related to the greater preponderance of pulmonary oligemia in type I patients.

Pressures

The right atrial mean pressure is minimally elevated. In the absence of interatrial obstruction, it is dependent on the left ventricular end-diastolic and left atrial pressures. The right atrial a waves are usually prominent. A mean pressure gradient of 5 mmHg across the foramen ovale in favor of the right atrium and giant a waves in the right atrium are indicative of an obstructive foramen ovale. However when there is marked elevation of the left ventricular end-diastolic pressure and left atrial pressure, lack of a pressure gradient across the interatrial communication does not exclude interatrial obstruction.[58]

The left atrial mean pressures are usually in the normal range. Elevated mean left atrial pressure is present with a large pulmonary blood flow or with poor left ventricular function and occasionally with mitral insufficiency. The left atrial v waves are smaller than the a waves in patients with reduced pulmonary flow. In patients with increased pulmonary blood flow the v waves are taller.

The left ventricular end-diastolic pressure is usually normal and rises with increasing Qp:Qs and decreasing left ventricular function.

The right ventricular pressure is proportional to the size of the ventricular septal defect in type I patients, while it is at systemic level in type II patients. Systolic pressure gradient across the VSD may be seen if the VSD is restrictive.[52,60] Pulmonary artery pressure may be normal or increased depending on the size of the VSD in type I patients or on the presence or absence of subvalvular or valvular stenosis in type II patients. Aortic pressures are usually normal. If coarctation of the aorta is present, systolic hypertension and pressure gradient across the coarctation may be present.

Calculated Variables

Systemic and pulmonary blood flows and resistances and shunts can be calculated by the Fick principle either by measuring oxygen consumption or by assuming it from

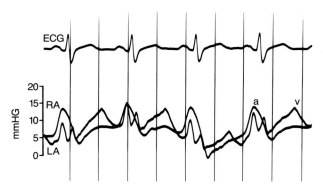

Figure 43–6. Simultaneous pressure tracings from the left atrium and right atrium in an infant with tricuspid atresia are recorded by means of high fidelity miniature pressure transducers mounted on a catheter 5 cm apart. Note higher RA pressure during atrial systole and higher LA pressure during atrial diastole; the later finding may help explain the "physiologic" left-to-right shunting at the atrial level in tricuspid atresia patients. a = a wave; ECG = electrocardiogram; LA = left atrial pressure tracing; RA = right atrial pressure tracing; V = v wave. (Reproduced with permission of Rao PS [1983]: Left to right shunting in tricuspid atresia. Br Heart J 49:345–349.)

tables or normal values.[58] The principles and methods of calculation have been detailed elsewhere[58] and will not be discussed here. Although most of the calculations can be performed, Qp:Qs is the most useful calculated value in the neonate. The Qp:Qs is diminished in type I hypoxemic infants with small or no VSD. It is markedly increased in type I patients with moderate to large VSDs and in most patients with type II anatomy.

Cineangiography

Since the original description by Campbell and Hills[12] and Cooley et al,[16] two signs, namely, "typical sequence of tricuspid atresia" and "right ventricular window," on right atrial angiography have been very helpful in the diagnosis of tricuspid atresia. Selective right atrial or superior vena caval angiography will reveal successive opacification of the left atrium and left ventricle without immediate opacification of the right ventricle (Fig. 43–7). The negative shadow, the so-called right ventricular window (Fig. 43–7) seen in earlier frames of right atrial angiography is due to failure of direct right ventricular filling, but the right ventricle is seen subsequent to left ventricular opacification. Although this area can be profiled well in the elongated right anterior oblique and the four-chamber views,[80] the posteroanterior view is most commonly used to demonstate these signs and is perhaps far superior.[90] The above described signs were initially thought to be pathognomonic of tricuspid atresia, but it is now well recognized that such an appearance can be seen in patients with pulmonary atresia or severe stenosis with intact ventricular septum and large right-to-left shunting at the atrial level, with tetralogy of Fallot with atrial septal defects (the so-called pentology of Fallot), and with total anomalous pulmonary venous drainage to the coronary sinus.[76,90]

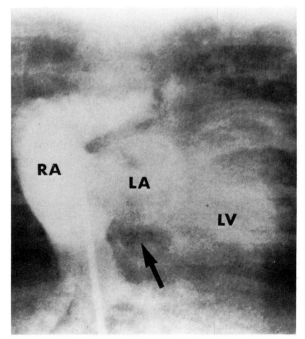

Figure 43–7. Selected frame from a posteroanterior view of a right atrial angiogram in an infant with tricuspid atresia showing successive opacification of the left atrium and left ventricle. There was no direct and immediate opacification of the right ventricle; the negative shadow, the so-called right ventricular window, is shown with an arrow. LA = left atrium; LV = left ventricle; RA = right atrium.

Although right atrial angiography is helpful in the diagnosis, selective left ventricular angiography (Fig. 43–8) should also be performed in order to delineate the anatomy and size of the right ventricle, the size and type of ventricular septal defect(s), the relationship of great arteries, and the source of the pulmonary blood flow. Frontal and lateral views of the ventriculogram are most commonly used, although the left anterior oblique view, long axial oblique view, or four-chamber view may provide information specific to a given patient.

In most neonates, selective right atrial and left ventricular angiograms are all that will be necessary. Selective antegrade or retrograde aortography to demonstrate either the pulmonary arterial anatomy or aortic coarctation may occasionally be needed.

DIFFERENTIAL DIAGNOSIS

Differential diagnostic considerations differ with the mode of presentation: (1) moderate to severely cyanotic infants with decreased pulmonary vascular markings on the chest radiograph and (2) mildly cyanotic infants with increased pulmonary vascular markings with or without signs of congestive heart failure.

Decreased Pulmonary Blood Flow

Once decreased pulmonary blood flow is recognized on the chest film, several possibilities, as listed in Table 43–2,

should be considered. Most often, they can be differentiated with the help of an electrocardiogram (Fig. 43–9),[63] and occasionally, echocardiography and/or cineangiography may be necessary for confirming the diagnosis.

1. Patients with *tetralogy of Fallot* (including VSD with pulmonary atresia) will have a frontal plane mean QRS vector between 90 and 180 degrees and right ventricular hypertrophy. M-mode and two-dimensional echocardiography will show a large right ventricle, a large aorta that overrides the interventricular septum, a large subaortic VSD, and pulmonary outflow tract obstruction. Angiographic features are characteristic for this anomaly.

2. Infants with *pulmonary atresia* (or stenosis) with intact ventricular septum and hypoplastic right ventricle are likely to have a mean frontal plane vector between 0 to 90 degrees without right ventricular hypertrophy; left ventricular hypertrophy may be present, and right ventricular forces may be decreased. Echocardiography will show a large left ventricle, a hypoplastic right ventricle, and small but demonstrable tricuspid valve leaflets. Angiocardiography will confirm the diagnosis.

3. *Tricuspid atresia* patients will not only have abnormal superiorly oriented vector (0 to −90 degrees) on the frontal plane but will also have left ventricular hypertrophy and decreased right ventricular forces.

4. The final group, those with *complex pulmonary stenosis*, includes several defects, namely, single ventricle, double outlet right ventricle, transposition of the great arteries with VSD, ventricular inversion and others, all associated with severe pulmonary stenosis or atresia. The electrocardiographic mean frontal plane vector and ventricular hypertrophy patterns vary markedly. Echocardiography and/or angiography are often necessary for accurate diagnosis.

Increased Pulmonary Blood Flow

The differential diagnostic considerations are also listed in Table 43–2. Although the characteristic electrocardiographic pattern (abnormal, superior vector or "left axis deviation") is helpful, it is not present in all cases of tricuspid atresia with transposition. Furthermore, some of the conditions listed in Table 43–2, Part B also have similar displacement mean frontal plane vector. Often, echocardiography and angiocardiography are necessary for the final diagnosis.

MANAGEMENT

Recently described physiologically "corrective" operations for tricuspid atresia[27,41] and their modifications[10,30,37] have improved the prognosis of patients with tricuspid atresia. Such physiologic correction is usually performed in patients older than 3 to 5 years.[10,14,27,30,37,41,67] As stated previously, most patients present with symptoms in the neonatal period and should be effectively palliated to enable them to reach the age at which surgical correction could be undertaken. The objective of any management plan, apart from providing symptomatic relief and increased survival

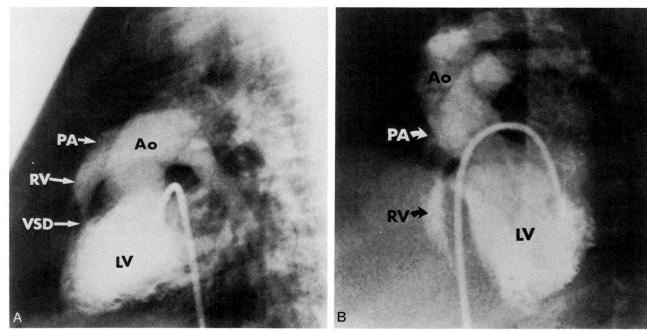

Figure 43–8. Selective left ventricular cineangiograms in an infant with tricuspid atresia in lateral (*A*) and four-chamber (*B*) views demonstrating clearly the relative position of the aorta and pulmonary artery. The ventricular septal defect is also clearly seen. Ao = ascending aorta; LV = left ventricle; PA = pulmonary artery; RV = right ventricle; VSD = ventricular septal defect.

rate, should be to preserve, protect, and restore anatomy (good-sized and undistorted pulmonary arteries) and physiology (normal pulmonary artery pressure and preserved left ventricular function) to normal such that a "corrective" procedure could later be performed. Keeping the above objective in mind, the management plan could be discussed under the following headings: (1) medical management at the time of initial presentation, (2) palliative treatment of specific physiologic abnormalities, (3) medical management following palliative surgery, (4) physiologically corrective surgery, and (5) follow-up following corrective operation. Items 3 to 5 are not germane to a chapter on tricuspid atresia in neonates and therefore will not be discussed.

Medical Management at the Time of Initial Presentation

The need for prompt identification and rapid transfer of a cyanotic/distressed neonate with suspected serious heart disease to a regional pediatric cardiology center has been stressed elsewhere.[63,72] During the process of identification, transfer to a pediatric cardiology center, initial workup, cardiac catheterization, and palliative surgery as well as following surgery, neutral thermal environment, normal acid-base status, normoglycemia, and normocalcemia should be maintained by appropriate monitoring and correction if needed. No more than 0.4 FIO_2 is necessary unless there is associated pulmonary pathology.

Table 43–2. DIFFERENTIAL DIAGNOSIS OF TRICUSPID ATRESIA IN THE NEONATE

A. Decreased pulmonary blood flow
1. Tetralogy of Fallot including pulmonary atresia with ventricular septal defect
2. Pulmonary atresia or severe stenosis with intact ventricular septum
3. Tricuspid atresia
4. Complex cardiac defects with severe pulmonary stenosis or atresia.

B. Increased pulmonary blood flow.
1. *d*-Transposition of the great arteries with large ventricular septal defect
2. Coarctation of the aorta with ventricular septal defect
3. Multiple left-to-right shunts (ventricular septal defect, common atrioventricular canal and patent ductus arteriosus)
4. Single ventricle, double outlet right ventricle, and other complex cardiac defects without pulmonic stenosis
5. Total anomalous pulmonary venous drainage without obstruction
6. Rarely, hypoplastic left-heart syndrome

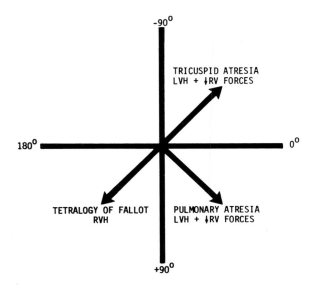

ECG-FRONTAL PLANE MEAN QRS VECTOR ("AXIS")

Figure 43–9. Use of electrocardiographic mean QRS vector (axis) in the frontal plane in the differential diagnosis of a cyanotic newborn with decreased pulmonary blood flow. Associated ventricular hypertrophy patterns and decreased right ventricular (RV) forces are also helpful (see text for details) in differential diagnosis. (Reproduced with permission from Rao PS [1984]: Management of the neonate with suspected serious heart disease. King Faisal Splst Hosp Med J 4:209–216.)

In infants with low arterial PO_2 and oxygen saturation and with ductal-dependent pulmonary blood flow, the ductus should be kept open by intravenous administration of prostaglandin E_1.[15,28,54] The ductal dilating effect of this drug results in an increase in pulmonary blood flow, thereby improving oxygenation and reversing the metabolic acidosis so that further diagnostic studies and surgical intervention can be performed with relative safety. Current recommendations are for intravenous infusion of PGE_1 at a dose of 0.05 to 0.1 µg/kg/min. We usually begin with a dose of 0.05 µg/kg/min and reduce the rate of infusion, provided the desired oxygen tension levels are maintained; minimizing the PGE_1 infusion rate has been most helpful in reducing the incidence and severity of some of the drug's bothersome side effects, namely, apnea and hyperpyrexia. The PGE_1 infusion rate may be increased if there is no increase in PO_2.

The occasional infant that presents with signs of congestive heart failure (more common in type II patients) should be treated with routine anticongestive measures.[73] Patients with associated severe coarctation of the aorta may also be helped with PGE_1 infusion; in such cases ductal dilation improves systemic perfusion.

Palliative Treatment of Specific Physiologic Abnormalities

The palliation of patients with tricuspid atresia would largely depend on the hemodynamic abnormality produced by the basic lesion and associated cardiac defects. These may be broadly grouped[67,73,90] into (1) decreased pulmonary blood flow, (2) increased pulmonary blood flow, and (3) intracardiac obstruction.

Decreased Pulmonary Blood Flow

Since the description of subclavian artery-to-ipsilateral pulmonary artery anastomosis in 1945 by Blalock and Taussig,[11] several other types of operations have been devised to improve the pulmonary blood flow. These include other types of systemic-pulmonary artery shunts, namely, the Potts anastomosis (descending aorta-to-left pulmonary artery shunt), ascending aorta-to-main pulmonary artery anastomosis, Waterston-Cooley shunt (ascending aorta-to-right pulmonary artery anastomosis), and aorta-to-pulmonary artery Gore-Tex shunt, superior vena cava-to-right pulmonary artery anastomosis (Glenn procedure), and formalin infiltration of the ductus arteriosus. Systemic-pulmonary artery shunts are most commonly used in the palliation of pulmonary oligemia. Because of the problems associated with the Potts anastomosis at the time of total surgical repair, the Waterston shunt became the procedure of choice in the neonate and small infant with pulmonary oligemia. Despite initial enthusiasm, however, a large number of complications have been reported in association with Waterston anastomosis, the most notable of which are elevated pulmonary artery pressure or resistance (and pulmonary vascular obstructive disease in some instances), left ventricular dysfunction, and marked distortion (kinking and obstruction) of the pulmonary arteries.[67,68]

The difficulty in creating successful Blalock-Taussig shunts, pointed out in earlier studies, has been used as evidence against recommending such shunts in neonates and small infants. However, if the mortality and long-term results of this shunt are compared with those reported for Potts and Waterston shunts,[67] it becomes apparent that the subclavian artery-to-pulmonary artery shunt is similar to central aortopulmonary shunts. Furthermore, recent experience with Blalock-Taussig shunts is encouraging.[67] Microsurgical techniques and modifications of the Blalock-Taussig shunt, such as subclavian arterioplasty[46] and the use of Gore-Tex grafts to extend the length of the subclavian artery[67] or for interposition between the subclavian artery and the ipsilateral pulmonary artery,[19] have made this procedure safer, with effective palliation. At present, a modified Blalock-Taussig shunt with a Gore-Tex graft interposed between the subclavian artery and the ipsilateral pulmonary artery appears to be the first choice for surgical palliation of the neonate and young infant with pulmonary oligemia (see Chapter 60).

Enlargement of the VSD and/or resection of the right ventricular outflow tract stenosis has been performed and recommended by Annecchino and his colleagues[4] as a palliative procedure to augment the pulmonary blood flow. This ingenious approach attacks the site of obstruction rather than bypassing it but is an open heart procedure, which may not be feasible or necessary in the neonatal period.[4,67]

In summary, despite the availability of many types of palliative procedures to increase pulmonary blood flow, most of them are either not effective or, if effective, may produce serious enough complications to deter a successful Fontan-Kreutzer procedure from being performed subsequently. The Blalock-Taussig anastomosis or one of its modified versions is the preferred procedure because it has the fewest long-term complications and at the same time preserves suitable anatomy for subsequent corrective procedures. Blalock-Taussig anastomosis is therefore the procedure of choice for palliation of tricuspid atresia patients with decreased pulmonary blood flow.

Increased Pulmonary Blood Flow

Infants with a modest increase in pulmonary blood flow do not have any significant symptomatology and indeed are less cyanotic than the pulmonary oligemic patients. Markedly increased pulmonary blood flow, however, can produce congestive heart failure. Only type Ic and type IIc patients, i.e., those without associated pulmonic stenosis, will fall into this category of pulmonary plethora. A majority of these patients will have type II anatomy and will usually present during early infancy.

In type I patients aggressive anticongestive measures should be promptly instituted. The natural history of the VSD has been well documented in this group;[31,47,52,60,70,71] as the VSD becomes smaller, patients with pulmonary plethora will, in due course, develop pulmonary oligemia requiring palliative surgical shunts. These patients can also develop right ventricular outflow tract obstruction with a resultant decrease in pulmonary blood flow. Therefore, it is recommended that pulmonary artery banding not be performed in type I patients. Among our 40 consecutive patients with tricuspid atresia,[59,67] only two with type I anatomy required pulmonary artery banding.[86,93] If optimal anticongestive therapy with some time delay does not produce adequate relief of symptoms,[67] pulmonary artery banding should be considered in type I patients. In those that did not have pulmonary artery banding performed, careful follow-up studies with measurement of pulmonary artery pressure and appropriate treatment are necessary to prevent pulmonary vascular obstructive disease.[50]

In type II patients, banding of the pulmonary artery should be performed once the infant is stabilized with anticongestive therapy.[21,47,67,93] If there is associated coarctation of the aorta or aortic arch interruption or hypoplasia, adequate relief of the aortic obstruction should be provided at the time of pulmonary artery banding, and the patent ductus arteriosus should be ligated, if present. The importance of PGE_1 administration in the control of congestive heart failure when aortic arch obstruction is present has already been mentioned. The role of balloon dilation angioplasty of the coarctation[66] in these complicated lesions has not yet been completely delineated.

Intracardiac Obstruction

Intracardiac obstruction can occur at two different levels, namely, patent foramen ovale and VSD.

INTERATRIAL OBSTRUCTION

Since the entire systemic venous return must egress through the patent foramen ovale, it should be of adequate

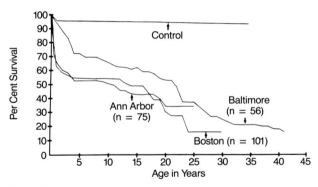

Figure 43–10. Actuarial survival curves in tricuspid atresia from three reported clinical series compiled by Dick and Rosenthal[22] showing (1) high initial mortality in the first year of life, (2) a plateau between the first year and middle of the second decade of life, and (3) a second bout of mortality from the middle of second decade onward, presumably related to impaired left ventricular function. (Reproduced with permission from Dick M, Rosenthal A [1982]: The clinical profile of tricuspid atresia. In Rao PS (ed): Tricuspid Atresia. Mt. Kisko, Futura Publishing Co, p 107.)

size. A mean atrial pressure difference of 5 mmHg or more with very prominent a waves (15 to 20 mmHg) in the right atrium is generally considered to represent obstructed interatrial septum.[67] Balloon atrial septostomy,[75] or if that is unsuccessful, blade atrial septostomy,[49,64] and rarely surgical atrial septostomy may be necessary to relieve the obstruction. Significant interatrial obstruction requiring atrial septostomy in the neonate is rare and unusual, although interatrial obstruction can be a significant problem later in infancy.[52,64]

INTERVENTRICULAR OBSTRUCTION

Spontaneous closure of the VSD causing severe pulmonary oligemia in type I patients and subaortic obstruction in type II patients can occur; such closure usually takes months to years to develop. For further discussion of this subject, the reader is referred elsewhere.[31,52,59,60,70]

PROGNOSIS

Untreated, the prognosis of liveborn infants with tricuspid atresia is poor; only 10 to 20 per cent may survive their first birthday.[21,77] Palliative surgery to normalize the pulmonary blood flow has markedly improved the survival rate. But, as one can see from survival curves from several large studies (Fig. 43–10),[22] there is still considerable early mortality. Because of recent improvement in surgical mortality for the palliative surgery, the initial mortality should decrease. Introduction of physiologic corrective surgery in the early 1970s should, to some degree, improve the second bout of mortality (Fig. 43–10) seen in children beyond 15 years of age. However, this improvement in late mortality remains to be documented. Because of the potential for improved prognosis, each neonate with tricuspid atresia should be offered aggressive medical and surgical therapy.

CONCLUSON

Tricuspid atresia is the third most common cyanotic congenital heart defect. There are significant variations in the morphology of the atretic tricuspid valve, the associated cardiac defects, and physiology, resulting in different clinical presentations. The diagnosis is relatively simple and can often be made on clinical features and simple laboratory studies (chest radiograph and electrocardiogram), which can be confirmed by echocardiography, cardiac catheterization, and selective cineangiography. Aggressive management to normalize the pulmonary blood flow and to correct physiologically important associated defects (for example coarctation of the aorta) should be undertaken at the time of presentation. Follow-up and treatment plans should strive to maintain or normalize cardiac structure and function (pulmonary artery anatomy and pressure, and left ventricular function). Finally, performing Fontan-Kreutzer type of corrective surgery prior to deterioration of the left ventricular function should markedly improve the prognosis for tricuspid atresia patients.

References

1. Alpert BS, Rao PS (1982): Left ventricular function in tricuspid atresia. In Rao PS (ed): Tricuspid Atresia. Mount Kisco, Futura Publishing Co, pp 197–200.
2. Anderson RH, Becker AE, Macartney FJ, Shinebourne EA, Wilkinson JL, Tynan MJ (1979): Special article: A question of definition. Is "Tricuspid Atresia" a univentricular heart? Pediatr Cardiol 1:51–56.
3. Anderson RH, Wilkinson JL, Gerlis LM, Smith A, Becker AE (1977): Atresia of the right atrioventricular orifice. Br Heart J 39:414–428.
4. Annecchino FP, Fontan F, Chauve A, Quaegebeur J (1980): Palliative reconstruction of the right ventricular outflow tract in tricuspid atresia: A report of five patients. Ann Thorac Surg 29:317–321.
5. Astley R, Oldham JS, Parson G (1953): Congenital tricuspid atresia. Br Heart J 15:287–297.
6. Beppu S, Nimura Y, Tamai M, Nagata S, Matsuo H, Kawashima Y Kozuka T, Sakakibara H (1978): Two dimensional echocardiography in diagnosing tricuspid atresia: Differentiation from other hypoplastic right heart syndromes and common atrioventricular canal. Br Heart J 40:1174–1183.
7. Bharati S, Lev M (1977): The conduction system in tricuspid atresia with and without regular d-transposition. Circulation 56:423–429.
8. Bharati S, Lev M (1979): The concept of tricuspid atresia complex as distinct from that of the single ventricle complex. Pediatr Cardiol 1:57–62.
9. Bharati S, McAllister HA Jr, Tatooles CJ, Miller RA, Weinberg M, Bucheleres G, Lev M (1976): Anatomic variations in underdeveloped right ventricle related to tricuspid atresia and stenosis. J Thorac Cardiovasc Surg 72:383–400.
10. Björk VO, Olin CL, Bjarke BB, Thorén CA (1979): Right atrial-right ventricular anastomosis for correction of tricuspid atresia. J Thorac Cardiovasc Surg 77:452–458.
11. Blalock A, Taussig HB (1945): The surgical treatment of malformations of the heart in which there is pulmonary stenosis or pulmonary atresia. J Am Med Assoc 128:189–202.
12. Campbell M, Hills TH (1950): Angiocardiography in cyanotic congenital heart disease. Br Heart J 12:65–95.
13. Chiche P (1952): Etude anatomique et clinique des atrésies tricuspidiennes. Arch Mal Coeur 45:980–1015.
14. Choussat A, Fontan F, Besse P, Vallot F, Chauve A, Bricaud H (1977): Selection criteria for Fontan's procedure. In Anderson RH, Shinebourne EA (eds): Paediatric Cardiology. Vol 11, Edinburgh, Churchill Livingstone, pp 559–566.
15. Coceani F, Olley P (1983): Prostaglandins and the ductus arteriosus. Pediatr Cardiol 4(Suppl 2):33–37.
16. Cooley RN, Sloan RD, Hanlon CR, Bahnson HT (1950): Angiocardiography in congenital heart disease of cyanotic type. II. Observations on tricuspid stenosis or atresia with hypoplasia of the right ventricle. Radiology 54:848–867.
17. Covitz W, Rao PS (1982): Noninvasive evaluation of patients with tricuspid atresia (roentgenography, echocardiography, and nuclear angiography). In Rao PS (ed): Tricuspid Atresia. Mount Kisco, Futura Publishing Co, pp 127–145.
18. Davachi F, Lucas RV Jr, Moller JH (1970): The electrocardiogram and vectorcardiogram in tricuspid atresia: Correlation with pathologic anatomy. Am J Cardiol 25:18–27.
19. deLeval MR, McKay R, Jones M, Stark J, Macartney FJ (1981): Modified Blalock-Taussig shunt: Use of subclavian artery orifice as flow regulator in prosthetic systemic-pulmonary artery shunts. J Thorac Cardiovasc Surg 81:112–119.
20. Desilets DT, Hoffman R (1965): A new method of percutaneous catheterization. Radiology 85:147–148.
21. Dick M, Fyler DC, Nadas AS (1975): Tricuspid atresia: Clinical course in 101 patients. Am J Cardiol 36:327–337.
22. Dick M, Rosenthal A (1982): The clinical profile of tricuspid atresia. In Rao PS (ed): Tricuspid Atresia. Mount Kisco, Futura Publishing Co, pp 83–111.
23. Dickinson DF, Wilkinson JL, Smith A, Anderson RH (1979): Atresia of the right atrioventricular orifice with atrioventricular concordance. Br Heart J 42:9–14.
24. Dickinson DF, Wilkinson JL, Smith A, Becker AE, Anderson RH (1979): Atrioventricular conduction tissues in univentricular hearts of left ventricular type with absent right atrioventricular connection ("tricuspid atresia"). Br Heart J 42:1–8.
25. Edwards JE, Burchell HB (1949): Congenital tricuspid atresia: A classification. Med Clin North Am 33:1117–1196.
26. Elster SK (1950): Congenital atresia of pulmonary and tricuspid valves. Am J Dis Child 79:692–697.
27. Fontan F, Baudet E (1971): Surgical repair of tricuspid atresia. Thorax 26:240–248.
28. Freed MD, Heymann MA, Lewis AB, Roehl SL, Kensey RC (1981): Prostaglandin E₁ in infants with ductus arteriosus-dependent congenital heart disease. Circulation 64:899–905.
29. Freedom RM, Rowe RD (1976): Aneurysm of the atrial septum in tricuspid atresia: Diagnosis during life and therapy. Am J Cardiol 38:265–267.
30. Gago O, Salles CA, Stern AM, Spooner E, Brandt RL, Morris JP (1976): A different approach for the total correction of tricuspid atresia. J Thorac Cardiovasc Surg 72:209–214.
31. Gallaher ME, Fyler DC (1967): Observations on changing hemodynamics in tricuspid atresia without associated transposition of the great vessels. Circulation 35:381–388.
32. Gamboa R, Gersony WM, Nadas AS (1966): The electrocardiogram in tricuspid atresia and pulmonary atresia wih intact ventricular septum. Circulation 34:24–37.
33. Graham TP Jr, Erath HJG Jr, Boucek RJ Jr, Boerth RC (1980): Left ventricular function in cyanotic congenital heart disease. Am J Cardiol 45:1231–1236.
34. Guller B, DuShane JW, Titus JL (1969): The atrioventricular conduction system in two cases of tricuspid atresia. Circulation 40:217–226.
35. Guller B, Kincaid OW, Ritter DG, Titus JL (1969): Angiocardiographic findings in tricuspid atresia: Correlation with hemodynamic and morphologic features. Radiology 93:531–540.
36. Henriette (1861): Rapport au sujet d'une note de M. le docteur Henriette sur un cas de cyanose generale, Liée a un vice congenitale du coeur, par M. Van Kempen. Gaz Med Paris 16:618.
37. Henry JN, Devloo RA, Ritter DG, Mair DD, Davis GD, Danielson GK (1974): Tricuspid atresia: Successful surgical "correction" in two patients using porcine xenograft valves. Mayo Clin Proc 49:803–810.
38. Keith JD, Rowe RD, Vlad P (1958): Heart Disease in Infancy and Childhood. New York, Macmillan, pp 434–470.

39. Keith JD, Rowe RD, Vlad P (1966): Heart Disease in Infancy and Childhood. 2nd ed. New York, Macmillan, pp 664–681.

40. Kelly C (1868): Malformations of the heart in a case of cyanosis. Trans Pathol Soc London 19:185.

41. Kreutzer G, Bono H, Galindez E, dePalma C, Laura JP (1971): Una operacion para la correccion de la atresia tricuspidea. Ninth Argentinean Congress of Cardiology, Buenos Aires, Argentina, Oct 31 to Nov 6, 1971.

42. Kühne M (1906): Über zwei falle kongenitaler atreside des ostium venosum dextrum. Jahrb Kinderh 63:235–249.

43. Kulangara RJ, Boineau JP, Moore HV, Rao PS (1981): Ventricular activation and genesis of QRS in tricuspid atresia (abstr). Circulation 64(Suppl IV):225.

44. Kulangara RJ, Boineau JP, Moore HV, Rao PS (1982): Electrovectorcardiographic features of tricuspid atresia. In Rao PS (ed): Tricuspid Atresia. Mount Kisco, Futura Publishing Co, pp 113–126.

45. LaCorte MA, Dick M, Scheer G, LaFarge CG, Fyler DC (1975): Left ventricular function in tricuspid atresia: Angiographic analysis in 28 patients. Circulation 52:996–1000.

46. Laks H, Castaneda AR (1975): Subclavian arterioplasty for the ipsilateral Blalock-Taussig shunt. Ann Thorac Surg 19:319–321.

47. Marcano BA, Riemenschneider TA, Ruttenburg HD, Goldberg SJ, Gyepes M (1969): Tricuspid atresia with increased pulmonary blood flow: An analysis of 13 cases. Circulation 40:399–410.

48. Nishioka K, Kamiya T, Ueda T, Hayashidera T, Mori C, Konishi Y, Tatsuta N, Jarmakani JM (1981): Left ventricular volume characteristics in children with tricuspid atresia before and after surgery. Am J Cardiol 47:1105–1110.

49. Park SC, Neches WH, Zuberbuhler JR, Lenox CC, Mathews RA, Fricker FJ, Zoltun RA (1978): Clinical use of blade atrial septostomy. Circulation 58:600–606.

50. Patel R, Fox K, Taylor JFN, Graham GR (1978): Tricuspid atresia: Clinical course in 62 cases (1967–1974). Br Heart J 40:1408–1414.

51. Puri PS, Neill CA (1966): Vectorcardiographic study in ten cases of tricuspid atresia. In Cassels DE, Ziegler RF (eds): Electrocardiography in Infants and Children: A symposium. New York, Grune and Stratton, p 269.

52. Rao PS (1977): Natural history of the ventricular septal defect in tricuspid atresia and its surgical implications. Br Heart J 39:276–288.

53. Rao PS (1980): A unified classification for tricuspid atresia. Am Heart J 99:799–804.

54. Rao PS (1981): Present status of surgery in congenital heart disease. Indian J Pediatr 48:349–361.

55. Rao PS (1982): Terminology: Tricuspid atresia or univentricular heart. In Rao PS (ed): Tricuspid Atresia. Mount Kisco, Futura Publishing Co, pp 3–6.

56. Rao PS (1982): Demographic features of tricuspid atresia. In Rao PS (ed): Tricuspid Atresia. Mount Kisco, Futura Publishing Co, pp 13–24.

57. Rao PS (1982): Classification of tricuspid atresia. In Rao PS (ed): Tricuspid Atresia. Mount Kisco, Futura Publishing Co, pp 41–47.

58. Rao PS (1982): Cardiac catheterization in tricuspid atresia. In Rao PS (ed): Tricuspid Atresia. Mount Kisco, Futura Publishing Co, pp 153–178.

59. Rao PS (1982): Natural history of ventricular septal defect in tricuspid atresia. In Rao PS (ed): Tricuspid Atresia. Mount Kisco, Futura Publishing Co, pp 201–229.

60. Rao PS (1983): Further observations on the spontaneous closure of physiologically advantageous ventricular septal defects in tricuspid atresia: Surgical implications. Ann Thorac Surg 35:121–131.

61. Rao PS (1983): Left to right shunting in tricuspid atresia. Br Heart J 49:345–349.

62. Rao PS (1983): Physiologically advantageous ventricular septal defects (letter). Pediatr Cardiol 4:59–61.

63. Rao PS (1984): Management of the neonate with suspected serious heart disease. King Faisal Splst Hosp Med J 4:209–216.

64. Rao PS (1984): Transcatheter blade atrial septostomy. Cath Cardiovasc Dgn 10:335–342.

65. Rao PS (1987): Atrioventricular canal tricuspid atresia: Echocardiographic and angiographic features. Br Heart J 58:409–412.

66. Rao PS (1986): Transcatheter treatment of pulmonary stenosis and coarctation of the aorta: Experience with percutaneous balloon dilatation. Br Heart J 56:250–258.

67. Rao PS, Covitz W, Moore HV (1982): Principles of palliative management of patients with tricuspid atresia. In Rao PS (ed): Tricuspid Atresia. Mount Kisco, Futura Publishing Co, pp 233–253.

68. Rao PS, Ellison RG (1978): The cause of kinking of the right pulmonary artery in the Waterston anastomosis: A growth phenomenon. J Thorac Cardiovasc Surg 76:126–129.

69. Rao PS, Jue KL, Isabel-Jones J, Ruttenberg HD (1973): Ebstein's malformation of the tricuspid valve with atresia: Differentiation from isolated tricuspid atresia. Am J Cardiol 32:1004–1009.

70. Rao PS, Linde LM, Liebman J, Perrin E (1974): Functional closure of physiologically advantageous venticular septal defects: Observations in three cases with tricuspid atresia. Am J Dis Child 127:36–40.

71. Rao PS, Sissman NJ (1971): Spontaneous closure of physiologically advantageous ventricular septal defects. Circulation 43:83–90.

72. Rao PS, Strong WB (1974): Early identification of neonates with heart disease. J Med Assoc Georgia 63:430–433.

73. Rao PS, Strong WB (1981): Congenital heart disease. In Conn HB (ed): Current Therapy. Philadelphia, WB Saunders, pp 185–209.

74. Rashkind WJ (1982): Tricuspid atresia: A historical review. Pediatr Cardiol 2:85–88.

75. Rashkind WJ, Waldhausen JA, Miller WW, Friedman S (1969): Palliative treament of tricuspid atresia: Combined balloon atrioseptostomy and surgical alteration of pulmonary blood flow. J Thorac Cardiovasc Surg 57:812–818.

76. Rosenthal A, Dick M II (1983): Tricuspid atresia. In Adams FH, Emmanouilides GC (eds): Moss' Heart Disease in Infants, Children, and Adolescents. 3rd ed. 1983. Baltimore, Williams & Wilkins, pp 271–283.

77. Rowe RD, Freedom RM, Mehrizi A, Bloom KR (1981): The Neonate with Congenital Heart Disease. Major Problems in Clinical Pediatrics. Vol 5. 2nd ed. Philadelphia, WB Saunders, pp 456–479.

78. Rudolph AM (1974): Congenital Disease of the Heart. Chicago, Year Book Medical Publishers, pp 429–461.

79. Sauer U, Mocellin R (1979): Left ventricular volume determination in tricuspid atresia. Herz Kardiovascular Erkankungen 4:248–255.

80. Schwartz D (1982): Angiography in tricuspid atresia. In Rao PS (ed): Tricuspid Atresia. Mount Kisco, Futura Publishing Co, pp 179–196.

81. Seldinger SI (1953): Catheter replacement of the needle in percutaneous arteriography: A new technique. Acta Radiol 39:368–376.

82. Seward JB, Tajik AJ, Hagler DJ, Ritter DG (1978): Echocardiographic spectrum of tricuspid atresia. Mayo Clin Proc 53:100–112.

83. Silverman NH, Payot M, Stanger P (1978): Simulated tricuspid valve echoes in tricuspid atresia. Am Heart J 95:761–765.

84. Takahashi O, Eshaghpour E, Kotter MN (1979): Tricuspid and pulmonic valve echoes in tricuspid and pulmonic atresia. Chest 76:437–440.

85. Taussig H (1936): The clinical and pathologic findings in congenital malformations of the heart due to defective development of the right ventricle associated with tricuspid atresia or hypoplasia. Bull Johns Hopkins Hosp 59:435–445.

86. Tingelstad JB, Lower RR, Howell TR, Eldredge WJ (1971): Pulmonary artery banding in tricuspid atresia without transposed great arteries. Am J Dis Child 121:434–437.

87. Van Praagh R (1973): Discussion after paper by Vlad P (1973): Pulmonary atresia with intact venticular septum. In Barrett-Boyes BG, Neutze JM, Harris EA (eds): Heart Disease in Infancy: Diagnosis and Surgical Treatment. London, Churchill Livingston, pp 246–247.

88. Van Praagh R (1977): Terminology of congenital heart disease: Glossary and commentary. Circulation 56:139–143.

89. Van Praagh R, Ando M, Dungan WT (1971): Anatomic types of tricuspid atresia: Clinical and developmental implications (abstr). Circulation 44(Suppl II):115.

90. Vlad P (1978): Tricuspid atresia. In Keith JD, Rowe RD, Vlad P (eds): Heart Disease in Infancy and Childhood. 3rd ed. New York, Macmillan, pp 518–541.

91. Weinberg PM (1980): Anatomy of tricuspid atresia and its relevance to current forms of surgical therapy. Ann Thorac Surg 29:306–311.

92. Weinberg PM (1982): Pathologic anatomy of tricuspid atresia. In Rao PS (ed): Tricuspid Atresia. Mount Kisco, Futura Publishing Co, pp 49–66.

93. Williams WG, Rubis L, Fowler RS, Rao MK, Trusler GA, Mustard WT (1976): Tricuspid atresia: Results of treatment in 160 children. Am J Cardiol 38:235–240.

94. Wittenborg MH, Neuhauser EBD, Sprunt WH (1951): Roentgenographic findings of congenital tricuspid atresia with hypoplasia of the right ventricle. Am J Roentgenol 66:712–727.

44 OTHER TRICUSPID VALVE ANOMALIES

P. Syamasundar Rao

In this chapter abnormalities of the morphologic tricuspid valve other than tricuspid atresia, namely, Ebstein malformation of the tricuspid valve, Ebstein anomaly of the left atrioventricular valve, tricuspid stenosis, and tricuspid insufficiency will be discussed; tricuspid atresia is discussed in Chapter 43.

EBSTEIN MALFORMATION OF THE TRICUSPID VALVE

Ebstein anomaly of the tricuspid valve is a congenital cardiac malformation in which the septal and posterior leaflets of the tricuspid valve are displaced downward into and are adherent to the inflow portion of the right ventricle. In addition, there is a redundancy or dysplasia of the tricuspid valve apparatus. In 1866, Wilhelm Ebstein[15] described the autopsy findings of the tricuspid valve and right ventricle in a 19-year-old laborer who had a history of cyanosis and dyspnea since early childhood. This tricuspid valve abnormality is now known by its eponym, Ebstein anomaly. Although several reports of autopsy cases of this anomaly appeared in the literature in the later part of 19th century and early part of 20th century, it was not until 1949 that the first report of diagnosis during life appeared in the literature.[53] Ebstein anomaly is a rare cardiac anomaly comprising 0.3 to 0.6 per cent of congenital heart defects in pediatric patients.[26,44] Both sexes are equally affected.[26,56] Although familial cases have been reported, the majority are sporadic. Exposure to lithium during prenancy has been implicated in the causation of this anomaly.[35,36,60]

Pathologic Anatomy

The two characteristic features of Ebstein anomaly are downward displacement of the tricuspid valve leaflets with adherence to the right ventricular muscle and redundancy or dysplasia of the tricuspid valve leaflets. There is a marked variability in the pathology. The septal and posterior leaflets are displaced downward, away from the true tricuspid valve annulus, and adhere to the right ventricular wall. The extent of the displacement varies from patient to patient, ranging from small (with the true and apparent or false tricuspid valve annuli close to each other) to extensive (so that the false annuli is displaced down to the level of the parietal band and crista supraventricularis). The inflow portion of the right ventricle between the true and false annuli of the tricuspid valve forms a common chamber with the right atrium and is described as the "atrialized"

portion of the right ventricle. The nonatrialized portion of the right ventricle is usually normal. The degree of adherence of the displaced tricuspid leaflets is also variable; it ranges from superficial attachment to the trabeculae carneae with minimal loss of right ventricular muscle to extensive adherence such that the right ventricular wall becomes a paper-thin, fibrous sac simulating Uhl's anomaly.[54] The anterior leaflet of the tricuspid valve is usually spared in the above-described pathologic process. The redundancy and dysplasia are seen in the free portions of the valve leaflets, and again the anterior leaflet is less affected. The free portions of the tricuspid valve leaflets are abnormally formed with nodular appearance. The effective or false orifice of the tricuspid valve may be unobstructed and is usually incompetent. It may be stenotic,[52] is rarely atretic,[40] and may have more than one opening. Sometimes the redundant tricuspid valve causes right ventricular outflow obstruction mimicking pulmonary valve stenosis or atresia.[34]

In Ebstein anomaly, right atrial enlargement is usual and massive. Interatrial communication, usually a patent foramen ovale or a secundum atrial septal defect, is present in most cases. Other associated defects, especially in the neonatal period, include pulmonary stenosis, pulmonary atresia, and ventricular septal defect. Occasionally, patent ductus arteriosus, tetralogy of Fallot, right aortic arch, coarctation of the aorta, transposition of the great arteries, and mitral prolapse may be associated with Ebstein malformation.

Pathophysiology

The pathophysiology of Ebstein malformation is as variable as the pathology. In patients with only minor degrees of abnormality, the tricuspid valve function may be normal and the malformation may not be detected until adulthood. In moderate-to-severe cases, elements of stenosis (or even atresia) and insufficiency of the tricuspid valve raise the right atrial pressure above that in the left atrium; resultant right-to-left atrial shunt across the patent foramen ovale or atrial septal defect can cause systemic arterial desaturation. With each right atrial contraction, the blood is propelled into the atrialized right ventricle. With ventricular contraction, a major portion of the blood in the right ventricle is forced back into the right atrium, only to be propelled back into the atrialized ventricle with the next atrial contraction. This "ping-pong" effect further increases right atrial pressure and consequent right-to-left atrial shunting. As a result of the right-to-left shunting, the pulmonary blood flow is decreased.

In the immediate neonatal period, pulmonary artery pressure and resistance and right atrial pressure are high; as a result, tricuspid regurgitation, right-to-left atrial shunting, and systemic arterial desaturation can be exacerbated if Ebstein anomaly is present. Thus, neonates with Ebstein anomaly can have quite severe cyanosis at birth, which spontaneously improves over several days as pulmonary vascular resistance and pressure fall. However, as the efficiency of the tricuspid valve apparatus deteriorates, cyanosis can recur during late childhood and early adolescence even in infants who become totally asymptomatic after the neonatal period.

Clinical Features

Approximately one half of the patients with Ebstein malformation have cyanosis during the neonatal period.[26,48] Among infants who become symptomatic during the neonatal period, cyanosis is the initial complaint in most, if not all neonates.[32,44] Cardiac murmurs and signs of congestive heart failure occur less often as presenting complaints. Occasionally supraventricular tachycardia may be a presenting finding.

Physical examination in an average case of Ebstein anomaly shows no distress, cyanosis, normal pulses and blood pressure, and a quiet precordial impulse without thrills. Despite increased right atrial pressure, distended neck veins and hepatomegaly are not prominent features because of the compliant right atrium and systemic veins. If there is severe tricuspid insufficiency, hyperdynamic precordium and a thrill at the lower sternal border may be felt and neck vein distention and hepatomegaly may be observed.

The first heart sound in Ebstein malformation may be normal, diminished, or loud, but it is delayed when referenced to the onset of the QRS complex on the ECG. In neonates with Ebstein anomaly, the second heart sound is usually single but may be split. Loud third and fourth heart sounds are usually heard, giving the so-called triple or quadruple rhythm, which is a characteristic feature of this anomaly. Faint or no cardiac murmurs are the usual findings. However, in the presence of severe tricuspid insufficiency, loud holosystolic murmur may be heard at the left lower sternal border. A scratchy, superficial sounding mid-diastolic murmur may be heard that is presumed to be related to absolute or relative tricuspid stenosis. These murmurs tend to change intensity with respiration, although respiratory variation is more difficult to demonstrate in the newborn because of rapid breathing.

Noninvasive Evaluation

The chest radiograph in Ebstein malformation usually shows severe cardiomegaly (Fig. 44–1A), and a substantial portion of this enlargement is due to massive right atrial enlargement. The lung fields are oligemic. Some infants may have normal to minimally enlarged heart size (Fig. 44–1B); presumably these are mild cases.

Classic ECG features of Ebstein anomaly in childhood (namely, right atrial enlargement, low QRS precordial voltages, and right bundle branch block pattern) are also present in neonates (Fig. 44–2), although right bundle branch block is not as common as in older children.

The rhythm in Ebstein malformation is usually sinus, although occasionally supraventricular tachycardia or atrial flutter may be present. Right atrial enlargement with tall peaked P waves in lead II and right chest leads is present in most of the patients. Prolonged PR interval is present in more than two thirds of the neonates.[44] Wolff-Parkinson-

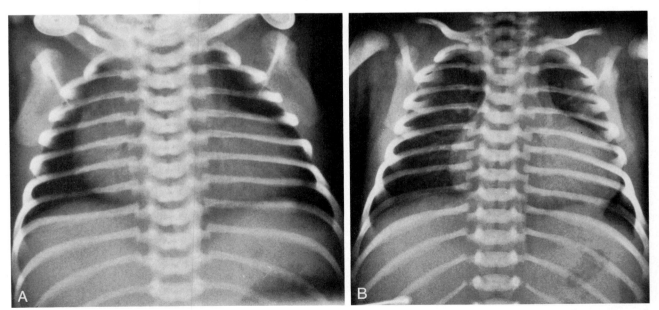

Figure 44–1. *A,* Chest radiograph of a 1-day-old infant with severe cyanosis secondary to Ebstein anomaly of the tricuspid valve diagnosed by cardiac catheterization and later by autopsy. Note markedly enlarged heart, dilated right atrium, and decreased pulmonary vascular markings. *B,* Chest radiograph of a 2-day-old infant with Ebstein anomaly diagnosed by catheterization. Note mildly enlarged heart with decreased pulmonary vascular markings. This infant improved with supportive measures.

White syndrome (short PR interval with delta wave) pattern may be present in some neonates. There is usually a right axis deviation of the QRS complex, but sometimes left axis deviation occurs.[11,28,44,48] Right bundle branch block is less common than in older children. When present, the QRS voltages in right precordial leads are low. When associated with other lesions, such as pulmonary stenosis or atresia and ventricular septal defect, right ventricular hypertrophy pattern may be present, especially in the absence of right bundle branch block.

Features from both M-mode and two-dimensional echocardiography are helpful in the diagnosis of Ebstein anomaly of the tricuspid valve. On M-mode study, the anterior leaflet of the tricuspid valve can be recorded farther to the left of the sternum than normal,[16] tricuspid valve closure is delayed (0.06 second later than mitral valve closure)[31] (Fig. 44–3), and the interventricular septal motion is abnormal.[62] The late closure of the tricuspid valve was initially thought to be due to the right bundle branch block, but in view of its presence in patients without right bundle branch block and even in patients with preexcitation syndrome,[51] delayed tricuspid valve closure is thought to be related to some other factor, possibly a mechanical factor.[31] These M-mode features, although helpful, may not be diagnostic because they can be seen in patients with other types of right ventricular volume overload.[21]

Two-dimensional echocardiographic findings are more reliable than the M-mode features and include enlarged right atrium, thick and dysplastic tricuspid valve leaflets, and displacement of the attachment of the tricuspid valve leaflets into the right ventricle[38] (Fig. 44–4). In addition, the status of the pulmonic valve and the presence and extent of right-to-left shunting across the patent foramen

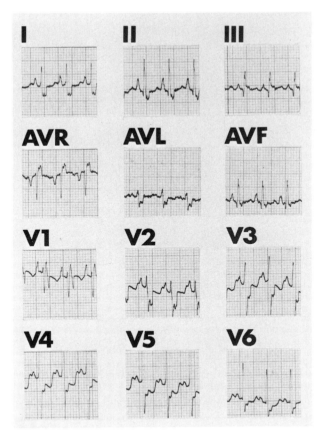

Figure 44–2. Twelve-lead electrocardiogram of a 7-day-old infant with Ebstein anomaly of the tricuspid valve. Note right atrial enlargement, right bundle branch pattern, and low QRS voltages in the right chest leads.

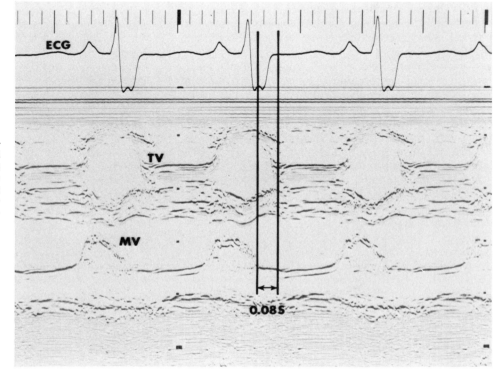

Figure 44–3. M-mode echocardiogram of an infant with Ebstein anomaly of the tricuspid valve showing delayed closure of the tricuspid valve. The tricuspid valve closure occurred 0.08 second after mitral valve closure. ECG = electrocardiogram; MV = mitral valve; TV = tricuspid valve.

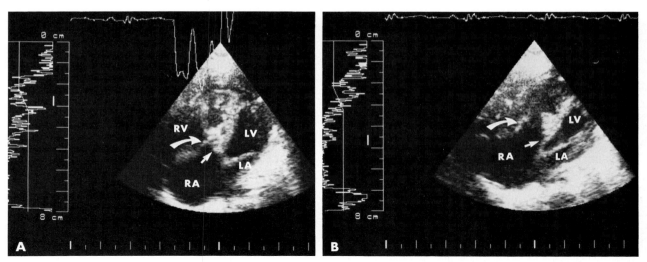

Figure 44–4. Four-chamber two-dimensional echocardiographic views of a neonate with Ebstein malformation of the tricuspid valve. Note displacement of the septal leaflet of the tricuspid valve onto the septum (small, straight arrows). Closed (A) and open (B) tricuspid valve leaflets are shown. The large curved arrow shows the anterior leaflet of the tricuspid valve. Also, note thickened, "dysplastic" valve leaflets. LA = left atrium; LV = left ventricle; MV = mitral valve; RA = right atrium; RV = right ventricle.

ovale by contrast study can also be evaluated by two-dimensional echocardiography.

Doppler evaluation may be of value in determining the degree of tricuspid insufficiency and right-to-left interatrial shunting and in the assessment of tricuspid and pulmonic flows.

Invasive Studies

Because of the incidence of dysrhythmias and deaths associated with cardiac catheterization in patients with Ebstein anomaly,[12,32,59] it has been recommended in the past that catheterization not be performed. However, because of the availability of more flexible catheters and balloon catheters, greater experience in catheterization, and better monitoring and treatment modalities, cardiac catheterization in patients with Ebstein anomaly does not currently carry any higher risk than in other anomalies. Nevertheless, the availability of noninvasive techniques, particularly two-dimensional echocardiography, makes accurate diagnosis of Ebstein anomaly easy, and catheterization may not be necessary for diagnosis, especially in neonates.

Entrance into the right ventricle may be difficult, and the catheter may coil-up in a large right atrium. These features, although suggestive, are not diagnostic of Ebstein anomaly. It is easy to advance the catheter into the left atrium (from the femoral approach) across the patent foramen ovale and from there into the left ventricle.

Systemic venous oxygen saturations are usually decreased, and the extent of decrease is related to the systemic arterial desaturation. There is usually no evidence for left-to-right shunt in the right side of the heart, unless there is associated ventricular septal defect or patent ductus arteriosus. There is usually evidence for right-to-left shunting at the atrial level with resultant systemic arterial

desaturation. Right-to-left shunting and arterial desaturation are inversely proportional to the pulmonary flow; pulmonary blood flow is in turn related to the degree of dysplasia and obstruction caused by the malformed tricuspid valve.

The mean right atrial pressure may be normal or slightly increased. The right atrial a waves are prominent but may be extremely tall if there is associated tricuspid obstruction (stenosis) and restrictive patent foramen ovale. The v waves may be prominent in the presence of tricuspid insufficiency, but more often than not they are not that well seen because of dissipation of the pressure wave in the large, compliant right atrium. The right ventricular systolic pressures are usually normal, although they may be elevated because of pulmonic stenosis, large ventricular septal defect, or elevated pulmonary artery pressure, especially in the neonate. The right ventricular end-diastolic pressure may be elevated. The pulmonary artery pressures are normal unless increased because of a large ventricular septal defect or the normal newborn elevation of pulmonary vascular resistance. The left atrial pressures are normal to low. The left ventricular and aortic pressures are normal.

The use of intracavitary ECG studies to confirm the diagnosis of Ebstein anomaly of the tricuspid valve was first suggested by Sodi-Pallares and Marsico.[50] The simultaneous recording of the intracavitary ECG and pressure at cardiac catheterization to confirm the diagnosis of Ebstein anomaly was first reported by Hernandez and associates.[23] In three patients with this malformation, these investigators showed that recording of typical right ventricular intracavitary ECG pattern with simultaneously obtained atrial-type pressure curves was diagnostic of this condition. This observation was confirmed in subsequent reports by other investigators.[19,22,58,61] As a platinum-tipped, end-hole catheter (with which the intracavitary ECG and pressure could be simultaneously recorded) is withdrawn from the right

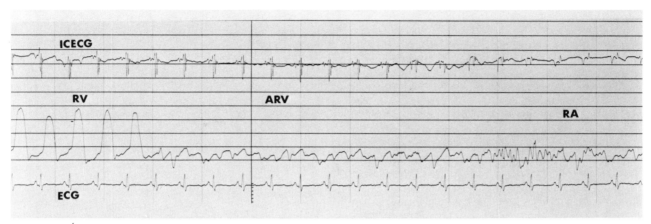

Figure 44–5. Simultaneous intracavitary electrocardiogram and pressures as the catheter is withdrawn from the right ventricular body to the right atrium. Surface electrocardiogram is shown at the bottom. Note the ventricular pressure and ventricular ECG in the body of the right ventricle, ventricular ECG and atrial pressure in the atrialized right ventricle, and atrial ECG and atrial pressure in the right atrium. This pattern is characteristic of Ebstein anomaly of the tricuspid valve. ARV = atrialized right ventricle; ECG = surface electrocardiogram; ICECG = intracavitary electrocardiogram; RA = right atrium; RV = right ventricle.

ventricle, ventricular ECG and ventricular pressure, ventricular ECG and atrial pressure ("atrialized" ventricle), and atrial ECG and atrial pressure (Fig. 44–5) are successively recorded. Although such a recording is characteristic of Ebstein anomaly, it is not always present in the neonate. It should also be pointed out that a false-negative recording may be obtained if the catheter slides along the normally attached anterior leaflet of the tricuspid valve, especially when the femoral approach is used during the catheterization.

Selective right ventricular angiography is optimal for diagnosing this anomaly and will show displaced tricuspid

valve leaflets (Fig. 44–6), size and function of the right ventricle, and the pulmonary valve and artery anatomy. Tricuspid insufficiency may also be observed. Opacification of the entire right side of the heart, either during right ventricular angiography or after right atrial angiography, reveals a tri-lobed right-sided heart consisting of right atrium, atrialized right ventricle, and the distal right ventricle. The notch separating the first two structures is formed by a true tricuspid annulus, while the notch separating the last two is formed by the origin of the displaced tricuspid valve leaflets.

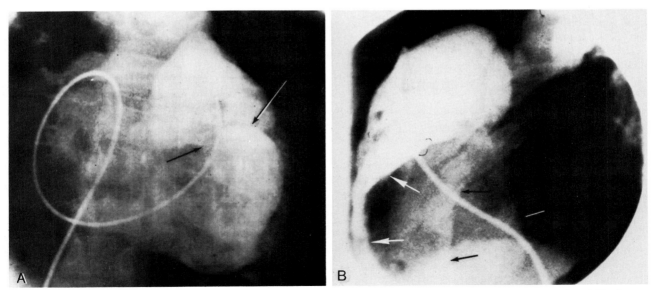

Figure 44–6. Right ventricular cineangiogram in a patient with Ebstein anomaly of the tricuspid valve; posteroanterior (A) and lateral (B) views are shown. Regurgitation through the displaced tricuspid valve leaflets (at arrows) is shown in A. In B, the black, small arrows point to the true tricuspid valve annulus, and the white, large arrows show the false annulus with displaced tricuspid valve leaflets.

Differential Diagnosis

Severe cardiomegaly and pulmonary oligemia in a cyanotic neonate are highly suggestive of Ebstein anomaly of the tricuspid valve, but they can also be seen in patients with severe or critical pulmonary stenosis with intact septum, pulmonary atresia with intact ventricular septum, and "functional pulmonary atresia."

In critical pulmonary stenosis, right ventricular hypertrophy is clearly discernible and the right atrial enlargement is proportional to the degree of right ventricular hypertrophy. In pulmonary atresia with intact ventricular septum, left ventricular hypertrophy pattern on ECG, and a single second heart sound (in contrast to split second sound in Ebstein anomaly) are helpful in the diagnosis. Two-dimensional echocardiographic studies have distinctive features in both these conditions.

Functional pulmonary atresia, because of grossly ineffective forward flow,[17,44] apart from severe Ebstein anomaly, can be caused by tricuspid valve dysplasia, severe tricuspid insufficiency, and Uhl anomaly and may simulate pulmonary atresia with intact ventricular septum. Even selective right ventricular angiography may not be able to distinguish anatomic from functional pulmonary atresia because in the latter angiographically demonstrable right ventricular forward flow may be absent secondary to massive tricuspid insufficiency. Although passage of a catheter across the pulmonic valve excludes anatomic pulmonary atresia, this is not always possible. Freedom and coworkers[17] have shown that functional pulmonary atresia can be identified by aortography. Aortic contrast injection opacifies the pulmonary artery via the ductus, and pulmonary insufficiency permits contrast regurgitation into the right ventricle, thus confirming the patency of the pulmonic valve. Prostaglandin E_1 administration to maintain ductal patency may be necessary prior to aortography. Two-dimensional echocardiography may be helpful in demonstrating the pulmonic valve and in differentiating anatomic or functional pulmonary atresia from Ebstein anomaly.

Tricuspid atresia, transposition of the great arteries, and tetralogy of Fallot rarely mimic Ebstein anomaly, and their clinical, roentgenographic, ECG, and echocardiographic features are distinctive.

Management

Cyanotic neonates with Ebstein anomaly, who are otherwise asymptomatic, do not need any treatment unless they are markedly hypoxemic. They will improve as the pulmonary vascular resistance and pressure fall.

If severe hypoxemia is present, infusion of E-type prostaglandins (prostaglandin E_1, 0.05 to 0.1 µg/kg/min) may open the ductus arteriosus, increase the pulmonary flow, and improve systemic arterial saturation. As the neonatal pulmonary vascular resistance regresses, the need for prostaglandin may be obviated. Some of these infants may become candidates for systemic artery-to-pulmonary artery anastomosis if they do not tolerate discontinuing prostaglandins.

Neonates with signs of congestive heart failure secondary to tricuspid insufficiency will be benefited by anticongestive measures (digitalis and diuretics).

Although replacement of the tricuspid valve with a prosthetic valve with the exclusion of the abnormally contracting atrialized ventricle[30,40] may be beneficial in older children and adults, such procedures in the neonatal period have not been successful and are not recommended.[33]

Prognosis

Ebstein anomaly diagnosed during infancy appears to have higher mortality than when diagnosed during childhood and adulthood.[20] Approximately 50 per cent of patients whose disease is diagnosed during the neonatal period do not survive through their first birthday.[44] Congestive heart failure, tricuspid insufficiency, very tall P waves on the ECG, complete right bundle branch block, or an arrhythmia in the newborn period are considered to be poor prognostic signs.[44]

EBSTEIN ANOMALY OF THE LEFT ATRIOVENTRICULAR VALVE WITH CONGENITAL CORRECTED TRANSPOSITION OF THE GREAT ARTERIES

Corrected transposition of the great arteries (CTGA) was originally described by von Rokitansky[57] in 1875. Although only a few cases were reported by 1950, several large series of cases[2,9,18,29,49] have since been published and have defined the pathologic, clinical, and hemodynamic features of this entity. In congenital CTGA, the atria are normal, the coarsely trabeculated morphologic right ventricle is left sided and gives rise to the anterior aorta, and the finely trabeculated morphologic left ventricle is right sided and gives rise to the posterior pulmonary artery (Fig. 44–7). Thus, there is atrioventricular and ventriculoarterial discordance. In essence, the ventricles are inverted. However, the normal hemodynamics are preserved: the systemic venous blood is directed into the morphologic left ventricle and from there into the pulmonary artery, while the pulmonary venous blood is directed into the morphologic right ventricle and from there into the aorta. In CTGA, the atrioventricular valves correspond to the ventricular chamber.[37,46,49] Therefore, the left atrioventricular valve is the morphologic tricuspid valve. Malformations of this left-sided tricuspid valve are very common and were considered an integral part of this pathologic entity by Paul and associates.[37] The occurrence of an anomaly of Ebstein type in the left-sided morphologic right atrioventricular valve is well described.[7,29,49,55] Schiebler and associates[49] examined 13 specimens of hearts with CTGA and found a deformed left atrioventricular valve in 11. In seven cases, the deformity assumed the pattern of Ebstein anomaly. Other, more commonly associated defects in CTGA

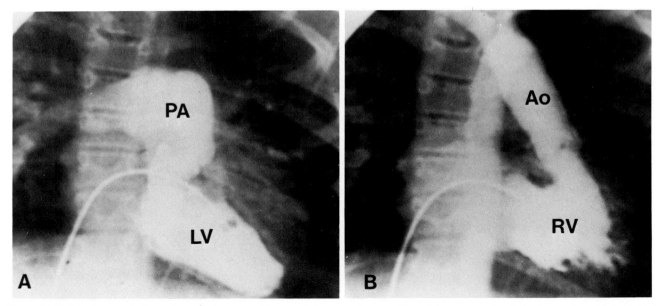

Figure 44–7. Selective ventricular angiography in a case with congenital corrected transposition of the great arteries. *A,* Angiogram from the right-sided, morphologic left ventricle shows a smooth-walled ventricular cavity, with opacification of the pulmonary artery. The pulmonary valve is inferior and rightward (also posterior on the lateral view of the cineangiogram; not shown). *B,* Cineangiographic frame from the left-sided, morphologic right ventricle. The catheter had been advanced into the ventricle via a patent foramen ovale and left-sided atrioventricular valve. Note heavily trabeculated ventricle consistent with right ventricular morphology. The aorta is opacified and is located superiorly and to the left of pulmonary valve. The aorta is also anterior in the lateral view, not shown here. The aorta descends on the left side of the spine. Ao = ascending aorta; LV = left ventricle; PA = pulmonary artery; RV = right ventricle.

are ventricular septal defect, pulmonary outflow tract obstruction, or both. Heart block is also seen with notable frequency.

Although the majority of patients with CTGA are symptomatic during the first month of life, more often than not these symptoms are related to left-to-right shunting through the ventricular septal defect or to pulmonary oligemia and right-to-left shunting because of the ventricular septal defect and pulmonic stenosis. Occasionally, the Ebstein malformation of the left atrioventricular valve with insufficiency either contributes greatly to the symptomatology or is the sole reason for the symptoms.[43] Findings on physical examination include a loud single heart sound (because of anteriorly located aortic valve) and a holosystolic murmur of left atrioventricular valve insufficiency heard best at the apex and left lower sternal border; the latter could easily be confused with the murmur of ventricular septal defect. The chest radiograph may show signs of left atrial enlargement and a peculiar contour of the left-sided heart border highly suggestive of CTGA, which is due to abnormal aortic origin and course. The ECG may show reversal of initial ventricular depolarization (no Q waves in left chest leads and Q waves in right chest leads) because of the inverted conduction system in CTGA. Left atrial enlargement may also be seen. Echocardiographic features of inability to demonstrate the continuity between left atrioventricular valve and aortic valve and the ventricular morphology suggest the CTGA diagnosis. Delayed closure of the left atrioventricular valve and visualization of the abnormal attachments of the left atrioventricular

valve may suggest Ebstein malformation of this valve. Angiography confirms the diagnosis of CTGA (see Fig. 44–7) and demonstrates left atrioventricular valve insufficiency (Fig. 44–8). Simultaneous recording of intracavity ECG and pressures is helpful in diagnosing this anomaly[43] in a manner similar to Ebstein anomaly of the normally located tricuspid valve.

Treatment essentially consists of management of heart failure. Some of these infants may require surgical repair or replacement of the atrioventricular valve later in life.

TRICUSPID VALVE STENOSIS

Congenital tricuspid valve stenosis may occur alone or in association with other defects. The isolated form is extremely rare. It is more common in females and has a familial tendency. Pathologically, there may be hypoplasia of the entire valve apparatus (though it is formed normally), formation of two cusps (mitralized) with abnormal attachments to the papillary muscles, or conversion to a sheet of valve structure attached to short chordae and small or markedly abbreviated papillary muscles.[10] Moderate-to-severe hypoplasia of the right ventricle may be noted. Clinical features, all similar to those observed in tricuspid atresia, include cyanosis (secondary to right-to-left shunting across the interatrial septum), right atrial enlargement, left axis deviation,[25] left ventricular hypertrophy, diminished or absent right ventricular forces on ECG, and diminished pulmonary vascular markings on the chest radiograph. This

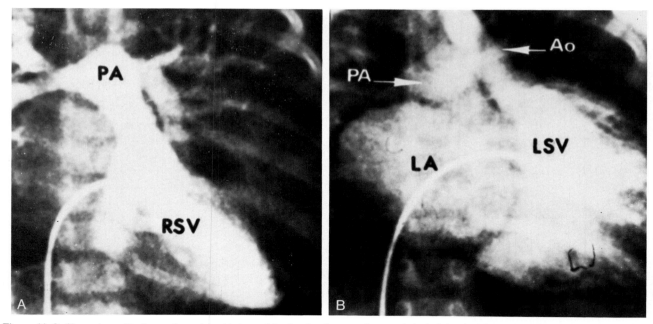

Figure 44–8. Cineangiographic frames from right-sided ventricle showing features of a morphologic left ventricle (A) and a left-sided ventricle showing features of a morphologic right ventricle (B) essentially similar to those shown in Figure 44–7B. Note opacification of the left atrium because of insufficiency of the left-sided atrioventricular valve. This infant was shown to have Ebstein malformation of this valve, proved by simultaneous recording of the pressures and intracardiac electrocardiogram.[43] Pulmonary artery is opacified through a ventricular septal defect (not shown). Ao = ascending aorta; LA = left atrium; LSV = left-sided ventricle; PA = pulmonary artery; RSV = right-sided ventricle. (Reproduced with permission of Rogers JH Jr, Rao PS [1971]: Ebstein's anomaly of the left atrioventricular valve with congenital corrected transposition of the great arteries: Diagnosis by intracavitary electrocardiography. Chest 72:253–256.)

lesion is indeed difficult to distinguish from tricuspid atresia, even with cineangiography. However, on two-dimensional echocardiography, the patency of the tricuspid valve may be demonstrable. The treatment approach is similar to that of tricuspid atresia;[39] however, some of these patients could be treated by commissurotomy or valve excision or replacement.

Most commonly, however, congenital tricuspid valve stenosis is associated with severe pulmonary valve stenosis or atresia with hypoplastic right ventricle. Other lesions in which tricuspid stenosis has been reported to coexist include double-outlet right ventricle, mitral stenosis, polyvalvular disease, single ventricle, tetralogy of Fallot, transposition of the great arteries, ventricular septal defect, and Uhl anomaly. The clinical features largely depend on the associated cardiac defects. Treatment should be directed toward the primary defect.

TRICUSPID INSUFFICIENCY

Tricuspid valve insufficiency in the neonate may be transient, may be associated with other significant cardiac abnormalities, or may occur as an isolated abnormality. The transient form of tricuspid insufficiency may be related to severe persistent pulmonary hypertension of the newborn syndrome or myocardial ischemia in the stressed neonate.[13,14,42,45] These subjects are discussed in Chapters 51 and 40, respectively.

Most frequently, tricuspid insufficiency is associated with other congenital abnormalities, namely, severe stenosis or atresia of the pulmonary valve.[4,6,24] With these lesions, the tricuspid valve may be normally formed, but regurgitation is functional, owing to extremely high pressure in the right ventricle, or the valve may be dysplastic and abnormally formed with short chordae tendineae causing tricuspid incompetence. The tricuspid insufficiency may also be seen with Ebstein malformation, Uhl anomaly, and endocardial cushion defects. Rarely, straddling (or overriding) tricuspid valve may also be incompetent.

Isolated, congenital tricuspid insufficiency is extremely rare but is well documented.[1,3–6,8,17,27,41,47] The pathologic abnormality may vary from case to case, ranging from nodular thickening of the tricuspid valve leaflets with normal chordae tendineae and papillary muscles to markedly thickened, elongated or partially absent, abnormally formed valve leaflets with thickened, shortened abnormally inserted chordae tendineae, and underdeveloped papillary muscles.[6]

Clinical Features

The clinical presentation of neonates with tricuspid valve insufficiency, whether isolated or associated with other abnormalities, is very similar[4,8,17] and, indeed, it is extremely difficult to differentiate these two groups.[4,8,17] Clinical features include cyanosis at or shortly after birth, signs of congestive heart failure, single second heart sound, precordial thrill with a holosystolic murmur at the left lower sternal border, and sometimes a soft mid-diastolic scratchy murmur at the left lower sternal border. Chest radiographs show severe cardiomegaly with pulmonary oligemia. The ECG shows right atrial enlargement, right axis deviation, and right ventricular hypertrophy. Some authors report a right bundle branch block pattern. Echocardiography combined with Doppler studies show enlarged right atrium and right ventricle with Doppler evidence for tricuspid insufficiency.

Invasive Studies

Cardiac catheterization findings include systemic arterial desaturation with evidence for right-to-left shunting at the atrial level, elevated mean right atrial pressure with prominent v waves and mild-to-moderate elevation of the right ventricular pressure. When the pulmonary artery has been catheterized, the pressures are normal to moderately elevated; however, in the most severe forms, the pulmonary artery is difficult to catheterize even with the use of guide wires and flow-directed catheters.[8,17] Selective right ventricular angiography reveals an enlarged right ventricle with free regurgitation across the tricuspid valve. In severe forms, there is no antegrade flow into the pulmonary artery, which is apparently related to the inability of the right ventricle to generate enough pressure to open the pulmonary valve. This "functional" pulmonary atresia causes considerable confusion with anatomic pulmonary atresia.[8,17] It is very important to differentiate these two conditions[8,17] because the treatment approach to these two clinically similar conditions is markedly different. Berman and coworkers[8] suggested that isolated tricuspid insufficiency (functional pulmonary atresia) is more likely if there is a large right ventricle, right ventricular systolic pressure is equal to or less than systemic pressure, arterial oxygen saturation is above 65 per cent, and a moderate-sized diverticulum-like deformity of the right ventricular outflow tract is present. They also suggested administration of 100 per cent oxygen or tolazoline immediately prior to right ventricular outflow tract angiogram to encourage pulmonary artery opacification in cases with functional pulmonary atresia. Freedom and his colleagues[17] demonstrated that aortography, in the presence of patent ductus arteriosus, is an excellent tool in differentiating these cases. Opacification of the pulmonary artery was followed by right ventricular outflow tract opacification (because of pulmonary regurgitation) in each case of functional pulmonary atresia. These investigators advocate the infusion of prostaglandins to allow better visualization of the pulmonary root via the ductus in this group of patients.[17]

Management

Treatment of isolated tricuspid insufficiency consists initially of differentiating infants with this insufficiency from those with anatomic pulmonary atresia, especially in view of poor surgical results and preferred medical man-

agement of infants with isolated tricuspid insufficiency. Prostaglandin infusion to keep the ductus open is not only helpful in arriving at diagnosis but also relieves arterial hypoxemia. Aggressive anticongestive measures with digitalis and diuretics should be instituted promptly. Supportive therapy includes the prevention of hypoglycemia and hypocalcemia, monitoring of acid-base and blood gas status, prompt and appropriate treatment of metabolic and/or respiratory acidosis, and provision of increased inspired oxygen concentration. Surgical intervention by repair or replacement of the tricuspid valve has uniformly resulted in death and should be the last resort in the desperately ill neonates whose condition does not improve with aggressive medical management.

References

1. Adams APS, Venables AW, Jenner B, Goh TH, Edis B (1978): The management of congenital tricuspid incompetence. Eur J Cardiol 8:599–606.
2. Anderson RC, Lillehei CW, Lester RG (1957): Corrected transposition of the great vessels of the heart: A review of 17 cases. Pediatrics 20:626–646.
3. Antia AU, Osunkoya BO (1969): Congenital tricuspid incompetence. Br Heart J 31:664–666.
4. Barr PA, Celermajer JM, Bowdler JD, Cartmill TB (1974): Severe congenital tricuspid incompetence in the neonate. Circulation 49:962–967.
5. Barritt DW, Urich H (1956): Congenital tricuspid incompetence. Br Heart J 18:133–136.
6. Becker AE, Becker MJ, Edwards JE (1971): Pathologic spectrum of dysplasia of the tricuspid valve: Features in common with Ebstein's malformation. Arch Pathol 91:167–178.
7. Becu LM, Swan HJC, DuShane JM, Edwards JE (1955): Ebstein malformation of the left atrioventricular valve in corrected transposition of the great vessels with ventricular septal defect. Proc Mayo Clin 30:483–490.
8. Berman W Jr, Whitman V, Stanger P, Rudolph AM (1978): Congenital ticuspid incompetence simulating pulmonary atresia with intact ventricular septum: A report of two cases. Am Heart J 96:655–661.
9. Berry WB, Roberts WC, Morrow AG, Braunwald E (1964): Corrected transposition of the aorta and pulmonary trunk: Clinical, hemodynamic and pathologic findings. Am J Med 36:35–53.
10. Bharati S, McAllister HA, Tatooles CJ, et al (1976): Anatomic variations in underdeveloped right ventricle related to tricuspid atresia and stenosis. J Thorac Cardiovasc Surg 72:383–400.
11. Bialostozky D, Medrano GA, Munoz L, Contreras R (1972): Vectorcardiographic study and anatomic observations in 21 cases of Ebstein's malformation of the tricuspid valve. Am J Cardiol 30:354–361.
12. Blacket RB, Sinclair-Smith BC, Palmer AJ, Halliday JH, Maddox JK (1952): Ebstein's disease: A report of five caes. Australas Ann Med 1:26–41.
13. Boucek RJ Jr, Graham TP Jr, Morgan JP, Atwood GT, Boerth RC (1976): Spontaneous resolution of massive congenital tricuspid insufficiency. Circulation 54:795–800.
14. Bucciarelli RL, Nelson RM, Egan EA II, Eitzman DV, Gessner IH (1977): Transient tricuspid insufficiency of the newborn: A form of myocardial dysfunction in stressed newborns. Pediatrics 59:330–337.
15. Ebstein W (1866): Uber einen sehr seltenen Fall von Insufficienz der Valvula tricuspidalis, bedingt dwich eine tangeborene hochgradige Missbildung derselben. Arch Anat Physiol Wissensch Med 238–254 (Translation appears in Am J Cardiol [1968] 22:867–873).
16. Farooki ZQ, Henry JG, Green EW (1976): Echocardiographic spectrum of Ebstein's anomaly of the tricuspid valve. Circulation 53:63–68.

17. Freedom RM, Culham G, Moes F, Olley PM, Rowe RD (1978): Differentiation of functional and structural pulmonary atresia: Role of aortography. Am J Cardiol 41:914–920.

18. Friedberg DZ, Nadas AS (1970): Clinical profile of patients with congenital corrected transposition of the great arteries: A study of 60 cases. N Engl J Med 282:1053–1059.

19. Gandhi MJ, Datey KK (1963): The value of electrophysiologic changes at the tricuspid valve in the diagnosis of Ebstein's anomaly. Am J Cardiol 12:169–174.

20. Giuliani ER, Fuster V, Brandenberg RO, Mair DD (1979): Ebstein's anomaly: The clinical features and natural history of Ebstein's anomaly of the tricuspid valve. Mayo Clin Proc 54:163–173.

21. Gussenhoven WJ, Spitaels SEC, Bom N, Becker AE (1980): Echocardiographic criteria for Ebstein's anomaly of tricuspid valve. Br Heart J 43:31–37.

22. Hansen JF, Wennevold A (1971): The diagnosis of Ebstein's disease of the heart. Acta Med Scand 189:515–520.

23. Hernandez FA, Rochkind R, Cooper HR (1958): The intracavitary electrocardiogram in the diagnosis of Ebstein's anomaly. Am J Cardiol 1:181–190.

24. Kanjuh VI, Stevenson JE, Amplatz K, Edwards JE (1964): Congenitally unguarded tricuspid orifice with coexistent pulmonary atresia. Circulation 30:911–917.

25. Keefe JF, Wolk MJ, Levine HJ (1970): Isolated tricuspid valvular stenosis. Am J Cardiol 25:252–257.

26. Keith JD, Rowe RD, Vlad P (1978): Heart disease in Infancy and Childhood. 3rd ed. New York, Macmillan, pp 1–13, 847–855.

27. Kincaid OW, Swan HJC, Ongley PA, Titus JL (1962): Congenital tricuspid insufficiency: Report of two cases. Mayo Clin Proc 37:640–650.

28. Kumar AE, Fyler DC, Miettinen OS, Nadas AS (1971): Ebstein's anomaly: Clinical profile and natural history. Am J Cardiol 28:84–95.

29. Lev M, Rowlatt UF (1961): The pathologic anatomy of mixed levocardia: A review of 13 cases of atrial or ventricular inversion with or without corrected transposition. Am J Cardiol 8:216–263.

30. Lillehei CW, Kalke BR, Carlson RG (1967): Evolution of corrective surgery for Ebstein's anomaly. Circulation 35(suppl):111–118.

31. Lundström NR (1973): Echocardiography in the diagnosis of Ebstein's anomaly of the tricuspid valve. Circulation 47:597–605.

32. Mayer FE, Nadas AS, Ongley PA (1957): Ebstein's anomaly: Presentation of ten cases. Circulation 16:1057–1069.

33. McFaul RC, Davis Z, Giuliani ER, Ritter DG, Danielson GK (1976): Ebstein's malformation: Surgical experience at the Mayo Clinic. J Thorac Cardiovasc Surg 72:910–915.

34. Newfeld EA, Cole RB, Paul MH (1967): Ebstein's malformation of the tricuspid valve in the neonate: Functional and anatomic outflow obstruction. Am J Cardiol 19:727–731.

35. Nora JJ, Nora AH, Toews AH (1974): Lithium, Ebstein's anomaly and other congenital heart defects. Lancet 2:594–595.

36. Park JM, Sridaromont S, Ledbetter EO, Terry WM (1980): Ebstein's anomaly of the tricuspid valve associated with prenatal exposure to lithium carbonate. Am J Dis Child 134:703–704.

37. Paul MH, Van Praagh S, Van Praagh R (1968): Corrected transposition of the great arteries. In Watson H (ed): Paediatric Cardiology. St. Louis, CV Mosby, p 611.

38. Ports TA, Silverman NH, Schiller NB (1978): Two-dimensional echocardiographic assessment of Ebstein's anomaly. Circulation 58:336–343.

39. Rao PS (1989): Tricuspid atresia. In Long WA (ed): Fetal and Neonatal Cardiology. Philadelphia, WB Saunders, p. 534.

40. Rao PS, Jue KL, Isabel-Jones J, Ruttenberg HD (1973): Ebstein's malformation of the tricuspid valve with atresia. Am J Cardiol 32:1004–1009.

41. Reisman M, Hipona FA, Bloor CM, Talner NS (1965): Congenital tricuspid incompetence: A cause of massive cardiomegaly and heart failure in the neonate. J Pediatr 66:869–876.

42. Riemenschneider TA, Nielsen HC, Ruttenberg HD, Jaffe RB (1976): Disturbances of the transitional circulation: Spectrum of pulmonary hypertension and myocardial dysfunction. J Pediatr 89:622–625.

43. Rogers JH Jr, Rao PS (1977): Ebstein's anomaly of the left atrioventricular valve with congenital corrected transposition of the great arteries: Diagnosis by intracavitary electrocardiography. Chest 72:253–256.

44. Rowe RD, Freedom RM, Mehrizi A, Bloom KR (1981): The neonate with congenital heart disease. In Major Problems in Clinical Pediatrics. 2nd ed. Philadelphia, WB Saunders, Vol 5, pp 101–109, 515–528.

45. Rowe RD, Hoffman T (1972): Transient myocardial ischemia of the newborn infant: A form of severe cardiorespiratory distress in full-term infants. J Pediatr 81:243–250.

46. Ruttenberg HD (1983): Corrected transposition (l-transposition) of the great arteries and splenic syndromes. In Adams FH, Emmanouilides GC (eds): Moss' Heart Disease in Infants, Children, and Adolescents. Baltimore, Williams & Wilkins, pp 333–350.

47. Sanyal SK, Bhargava SK, Saxena HM, Ghosh S (1968): Congenital insufficiency of the tricuspid valve: A rare cause of massive cardiomegaly and congestive cardiac failure in neonate. Indian Heart J 20:214–218.

48. Schiebler GL, Adams P Jr, Anderson RC, Amplatz K, Lester RG (1959): Clinical study of twenty-three cases of Ebstein's anomaly of the tricuspid valve. Circulation 19:165–187.

49. Schiebler GL, Edwards JE, Burchell HB, Dushane JW, Ongley PA, Wood EH (1961): Congenital corrected transposition of the great vessels: A study of 33 cases. Pediatrics 27(suppl):849–888.

50. Sodi-Pallares D, Marsico F (1955): The importance of electrocardiographic patterns in congenital heart disease. Am Heart J 49:202–217.

51. Tajik AJ, Gau GT, Giuliani ER, Ritter DG, Schattenberg TT (1973): Echocardiogram in Ebstein's anomaly with Wolff-Parkinson-White preexcitation syndrome, type B. Circulation 47:813–818.

52. Takayasu S, Obunai Y, Konno S (1978): Clinical classification of Ebstein's anomaly. Am Heart J 95:154–162.

53. Tourniaire A, Deyrieux F, Tartulier M (1949): Maladie d'Ebstein: Essai de diagnostic clinique. Arch Mal Coeur 42:1211.

54. Uhl HSM (1952): A previously undescribed congenital malformation of the heart: Almost total absence of the myocardium of the right ventricle. Bull Johns Hopkins Hosp 91:197–209.

55. Van Mierop LH, Alley RD, Kausel HW, Stranahan A (1961): Ebstein's malformation of the left atrioventricular valve in corrected transposition with subpulmonary stenosis and ventricular septal defect. Am J Cardiol 8:270–274.

56. Van Mierop LHS, Schiebler GL, Victoria BE (1983): Ebstein's anomaly. In Adams FH, Emmanouilides GC (eds): Moss' Heart Disease in Infants, Children, and Adolescents. Baltimore, Williams & Wilkins, pp 283–296.

57. Von Rokitansky K (1875): Die Defekte der Scheidewände des Herzens. Vienna, Wilhelm Braumüller, pp 83–85.

58. Watson H (1966): Electrode catheters and the diagnosis of Ebstein's anomaly of the tricuspid valve. Br Heart J 28:161–171.

59. Watson H (1974): Natural history of Ebstein's anomaly of the tricuspid valve in childhood and adolescence: An international cooperative study of 505 cases. Br Heart J 36:417–427.

60. Weinstein MR, Goldfield MD (1975): Cardiovascular malformations with lithium use during pregnancy. Am J Psychol 132:529–531.

61. Yim BJB, Yu PN (1958): Value of an electrode catheter in diagnosis of Ebstein's disease. Circulation 17:543–548.

62. Yuste P, Minguez I, Aza V, Señor J, Asin E, Martinez-Bordiu C (1974): Echocardiography in the diagnosis of Ebstein's anomaly. Chest 66:273–277.

45 PULMONARY VALVE ABNORMALITIES

Howard P. Gutgesell

FETAL CIRCULATION

In the fetus with mild right ventricular outflow obstruction and intact ventricular septum, the fetal circulation is not appreciably different from normal. The fetal myocardium has the capacity to respond to increased pressure work with very rapid and dramatic hyperplasia. Although right ventricular systolic pressure is increased, the right ventricular contribution to combined ventricular output is maintained.

At the other end of the spectrum of right ventricular outflow obstruction, i.e., pulmonary atresia with intact ventricular septum, the fetal circulation is markedly altered. Since the right ventricular outflow tract ends blindly, all blood returning to the heart from the inferior and superior vena cavae and the coronary sinus must cross the foramen ovale to the left atrium and left ventricle. Whereas the ascending aorta normally carries about 33 per cent of combined ventricular output,[75] in the fetus with pulmonary atresia and intact ventricular septum, the left ventricle and ascending aorta must carry the total cardiac output, about three times the normal amount.

The ductus arteriosus normally carries 35 to 60 per cent of total cardiac output from the pulmonary artery to the descending aorta.[15,75] In the fetus with pulmonary atresia, the ductus carries only the pulmonary blood flow (from the aorta toward the lungs). Since pulmonary flow represents only 8 to 10 per cent of combined ventricular output in the fetus, the ductus arteriosus might be expected to be hypoplastic in the fetus with pulmonary atresia. Unfortunately, angiographic and autopsy studies do not clearly distinguish ductal hypoplasia from postnatal constriction.

Since all venous blood returning to the heart is completely mixed in the left atrium of the fetus with pulmonary atresia and intact ventricular septum, the resultant PO_2 of blood distributed to the fetal myocardium and brain is slightly lower than normal. (In the normal fetus, the oxygenated blood from the placenta is preferentially directed from the inferior vena cava across the foramen ovale to the left atrium and hence to the coronary arteries and ascending aorta.) Likewise, the lungs receive blood with slightly higher PO_2 than normal via the ductus arteriosus.

In the fetus with pulmonary stenosis and ventricular septal defect (tetralogy of Fallot), flows across the tricuspid valve and foramen ovale are normal, but a variable portion of right ventricular output is directed across the ventricular septal defect and into the ascending aorta. Thus, the size of the ascending aorta is directly related to the severity of the pulmonary stenosis, and the size of pulmonary arteries is inversely related to the severity of the stenosis.

The peak systolic pressures in the right ventricle, left ventricle, and aorta are the same in tetralogy of Fallot. The presence of pulmonary stenosis will produce a lower systolic pressure in the pulmonary arterial tree. Thus, blood flows from the aorta into the pulmonary arteries via the ductus, as opposed to the normal fetal flow pattern from the pulmonary artery to the descending aorta.

The angle between the ductus arteriosus and the thoracic aorta may be altered in tetralogy of Fallot, especially if there is actual pulmonary atresia. Normally, there is an obtuse inferior angle between the descending aorta and the ductus, but in neonates with severe forms of tetralogy of Fallot, this angle is quite acute, with the ductus often appearing to descend from the inferior surface of the transverse arch. It has been suggested that this change in orientation is due to the abnormal ductal flow pattern in utero.[75] The lack of this abnormal orientation in most infants with pulmonary atresia and intact ventricular septum has led to speculation that this condition may develop at a later stage of embryonic development than pulmonary atresia with ventricular septal defect.[77]

TRANSITIONAL CIRCULATION

In neonates with pulmonary stenosis and intact ventricular septum, circulatory changes after birth depend on the severity of the pulmonary stenosis. If the stenosis is mild or moderate, right ventricular output, and hence pulmonary blood flow, is normal. The closure of the ductus arteriosus is of little consequence and as the lungs expand and pulmonary blood flow and pulmonary venous return increase, rising left atrial pressure closes the foramen ovale.

In more severe forms of pulmonary stenosis and certainly in pulmonary atresia, intracardiac right-to-left shunting continues at the atrial level as a result of elevated right ventricular end-diastolic pressure and hence elevated right atrial pressure. Systemic arterial saturation is determined by the amount of pulmonary blood flow, which, in cases of pulmonary atresia, is directly related to the size of the ductus arteriosus. If the ductus closes, extreme hypoxemia and ultimately acidemia result.

In neonates with tetralogy of Fallot, the removal of the low resistance placenta at the time of birth reduces right-to-left ventricular shunt and may actually increase pulmonary blood flow compared with prenatal levels. However, the postnatal elevation in systemic resistance caused by loss of the placenta is to a large degree offset by closure of the ductus arteriosus. The resultant systemic arterial PO_2 is directly related to the amount of pulmonary blood flow, which in turn is determined by the severity of the pulmonary stenosis, the systemic arterial pressure, and the degree of ductal patency.

PULMONARY VALVE STENOSIS

Historical Aspects

Morgagni is given credit for first describing pulmonary stenosis in 1761, and Fallot for distinguishing this condition from tetralogy in 1888 (cited by Emmanouilides and Baylen[24]). Precise hemodynamic and anatomic diagnosis in the neonate was not possible until the development of cardiac cathetherization techniques in the 1930s and 1940s. In 1948 Brock[8] and Sellors[78] independently described closed surgical methods for opening a stenosed pulmonary valve; open heart techniques followed the development of cardiopulmonary bypass in the 1950s.

Incidence

Pulmonary stenosis is a relatively common congenital defect, although many mild cases are not detected in the neonatal period. Pulmonary stenosis was the fourth most common lesion seen in the cardiac clinic of the Hospital for Sick Children from 1950 to 1973, accounting for 9.9 per cent of patients.[44] It was the second most common cardiac lesion in a prospective study by Mitchell et al of 56,109 births[60] and occurred with a frequency of 1 per 1516 births. Isolated pulmonary stenosis accounted for 5 per cent of all cardiac catheterizations of infants under 6 months of age at Texas Children's Hospital in Houston between 1968 and 1978[33] and for 3 per cent of all infants enrolled in the New England Infant Cardiac Program between 1968 and 1975.[30]

Pathology

Right ventricular outflow obstruction may occur at the level of the pulmonary valve, in the subvalvular or infundibular portion of the right ventricle, or in the pulmonary arteries themselves. The most frequent lesion is isolated pulmonary valvular stenosis, in which the valve orifice is reduced by fusion of the three cusps.[22] A less common form of pulmonary stenosis, termed "pulmonary valvular dysplasia," has also been described[41,46,53] and accounts for 10 to 15 per cent of cases of pulmonary stenosis. In the latter lesion, the leaflets are not fused, but thickened and immobile, formed of disorganized myxomatous tissue. Dysplastic pulmonary valves may be present in multiple family members and represent the type of pulmonary stenosis in the majority of patients with Noonan syndrome.[63]

In isolated pulmonary valve stenosis, the main pulmonary artery and its branches are usually normal at birth. Poststenotic dilation takes weeks or months to develop.

Pulmonary arterial hypoplasia is relatively uncommon in pulmonary stenosis with intact ventricular septum except in cases associated with diffuse cardiovascular disease, such as seen in Williams syndrome[4] or congenital rubella.[89]

Right ventricular cavity size may be normal, enlarged, or clearly diminutive. Hypoplasia of the right ventricle is present in a substantial proportion of neonates with *critical* pulmonary stenosis.[27,57] The ventricular walls are hypertrophied, especially in the infundibular region, producing an appearance of subvalvular stenosis. The right ventricular endocardium is frequently thickened, and the right atrium is dilated and hypertrophied. The foramen ovale is usually patent, and occasionally a secundum defect of the atrial septum is present.

Histologic evidence of more widespread cardiac disease has been reported in some patients with pulmonary stenosis. Harinck et al[37] found *left* ventricular hypertrophy and fibrosis in 18 patients with isolated pulmonary valve stenosis. Becu et al[3] found myocardial dysplasia and abnormal aortic and coronary artery histology in a series of patients with dysplastic pulmonary valves.

Hemodynamics

Right ventricular pressure is elevated, frequently to suprasystemic levels. Cyanosis is present in severe forms and is due to right-to-left shunting through the foramen ovale. Pulmonary artery pressure is low, although the pulmonary artery is rarely entered at cardiac catheterization and attempts to do so are inadvisable.

Clinical Features

The presenting manifestation of pulmonary stenosis in the neonate is either a murmur (mild to moderately severe cases) or cyanosis (severe cases). The murmur of pulmonary stenosis is typically a crescendo-decrescendo murmur at the upper left sternal border. In the neonate, this murmur may be obscured by a continuous murmur from a patent ductus arteriosus. An ejection click is audible in approximately one half of cases; its absence suggests either very severe stenosis or a dysplastic pulmonary valve. The second heart sound is usually single.

In the neonate with pulmonary stenosis, the ECG may be normal[57] or demonstrate right ventricular hypertrophy (Fig. 45–1). Enlarged P waves indicative of right atrial enlargement are common. In severe cases associated with right ventricular hypoplasia, there is often left ventricular hypertrophy with decreased right ventricular forces.

The chest radiograph reveals a normal or slightly enlarged heart. Cardiomegaly is most conspicuous in patients with severe tricuspid insufficiency and an enlarged right atrium. The pulmonary vascular markings are normal or decreased.

The anatomic features of pulmonary stenosis can be demonstrated by echocardiography. Thickening of the pulmonary valve leaflets can be seen on M-mode echocardiography,[35] but is more easily detected by two-dimensional

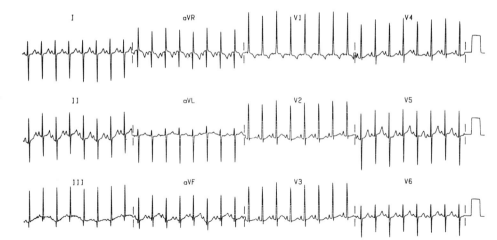

Figure 45–1. Electrocardiogram from 2-week old infant with moderately severe pulmonary stenosis. Note evidence of right ventricular hypertrophy as manifested by the tall R waves and lack of S waves in V_1 and prominent S waves in V_6.

echocardiography (Fig. 45–2). Although absolute volume determination is difficult to gauge by two-dimensional echocardiography, it is generally possible to classify the right ventricular cavity as diminutive, normal, or enlarged. Likewise, tricuspid annulus diameter can be determined and compared with normal values for body size.[34,45]

Doppler echocardiography is useful to estimate the pressure gradient across the pulmonary valve[36,39,52] and to distinguish severe pulmonary stenosis from pulmonary atresia.

Right ventricular angiocardiography is the definitive method for illustrating right ventricular size and function in pulmonary stenosis. It also distinguishes the usual form of valvular stenosis (Fig. 45–3) from obstruction due to a dysplastic valve or peripheral pulmonary arterial stenosis or hypoplasia.

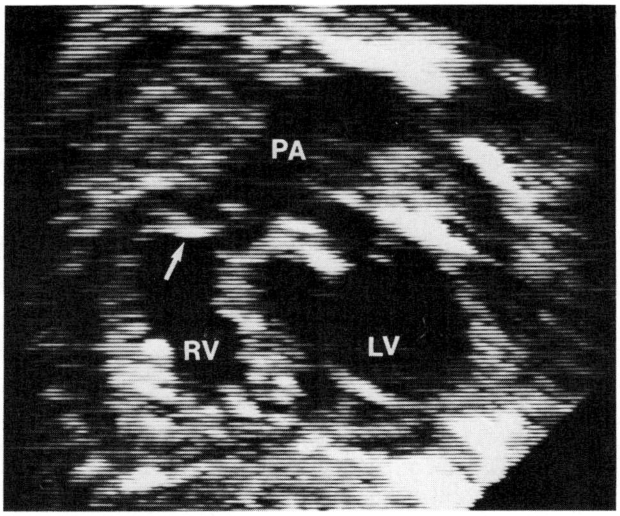

Treatment

Neonates with mild to moderate pulmonary stenosis may require no treatment, at least in the first few months of life. Close observation is warranted, however, because serial hemodynamic studies demonstrate that the severity of the obstruction is often progressive.[13]

In infants with marked cyanosis, systemic oxygenation may be improved by a prostaglandin infusion (PGE_1, 0.05 to 0.1 µg/kg/min) to maintain patency of the ductus arteriosus. Until recently, subsequent therapy was primarily surgical and consisted of either a pulmonary valvotomy or

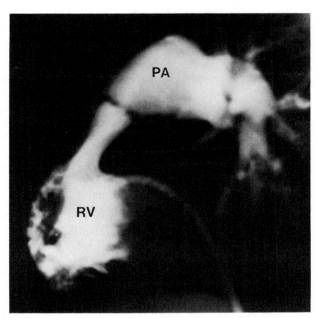

Figure 45–3. Lateral projection of right ventricular angiocardiogram in a neonate with pulmonary valve stenosis. The right ventricular cavity is of normal size. The pulmonary valve leaflets are thick and form a "dome" in systole. Note the jet of contrast material through the small orifice and the poststenotic dilation of the main pulmonary artery. PA = pulmonary artery; RV = right ventricle.

Figure 45–2. Two-dimensional echocardiogram obtained from the subxyphoid region in a neonate with severe pulmonary valve stenosis. The pulmonary valve leaflets (arrow) are thickened and were observed to "dome" with systole. LV = left ventricle; PA = pulmonary artery; RV = right ventricle.

a valvotomy plus a systemic-to-pulmonary artery anastomosis (the latter procedure generally reserved for cases with right ventricular hypoplasia or persistent hypoxemia after a valvotomy). Recently, percutaneous transluminal balloon angioplasty has been used in the treatment of pulmonary valve stenosis,[42,43,48] and this technique has been used to treat a small number of neonates and young infants.[83,87]

Prognosis

The prognosis for neonates with pulmonary stenosis and intact ventricular septum is related to the severity of valvular obstruction, the size of the right ventricle, and the competence of the tricuspid valve. Patients with mild or moderate stenosis remain asymptomatic and may require no therapy, or at most elective pulmonary valvotomy or balloon valvuloplasty, both of which can be accomplished with low morbidity or mortality. Accurate survival rates for neonates with critical pulmonary stenosis are difficult to obtain, since many studies include these patients together with reports of pulmonary atresia and intact ventricular septum, a lesion with a poor prognosis. Although the prognosis is thought to be better if the valve is severely stenotic rather than atretic,[27,57] infants with a hypoplastic right ventricle often require a shunt as well as valvotomy, have continued cyanosis, and ultimately require a second operation for closure of the shunt and the atrial septal defect or foramen ovale.

PULMONARY ATRESIA WITH INTACT VENTRICULAR SEPTUM

Historical Aspects

Peacock[68] credits Hunter with the first anatomic description of pulmonary atresia with intact ventricular septum in 1783. As with the other lesions described in this chapter, consistent clinical diagnosis was not possible until the development of cardiac catheterization and angiocardiographic techniques in the 1930s and 1940s, with application to neonates in the 1950s.

Pathology

The atretic pulmonary valve consists of a thick membrane, often with visible raphes. The infundibulum is usually hypoplastic, and about 20 per cent of cases have infundibular as well as valvular atresia.[61]

Right ventricular size is variable but is usually smaller than normal.[88,92] Several classification systems have been proposed based on either right ventricular volume[14] or the presence or absence of the three anatomic portions of the normal right ventricle (inlet, trabecular, and outlet).[9,31] The right ventricular cavity was markedly hypoplastic in 50 per cent of cases examined by Van Praagh et al,[88] moderately hypoplastic in 26 per cent, and normal in only 10 per cent.

The tricuspid valve ring is usually proportional to the right ventricular cavity size, but the leaflets are often hypoplastic with thick, short chordae resulting in tricuspid stenosis.[28,88,92]

Pulmonary artery size is likewise variable, although often not as small as might be anticipated considering that the pulmonary valve is completely obstructed. Van Praagh et al[88] analyzed 52 cases and found the main pulmonary artery absent in two. Clearly diminutive pulmonary arteries (0 to 3 mm in diameter) were found with the following frequency: main pulmonary artery, 9.6 per cent; right pulmonary artery, 6.4 per cent; left pulmonary artery, 17.8 per cent.

Unusual coronary artery–myocardial sinusoidal communications are present in many patients with pulmonary atresia and intact ventricular septum.[50,81] These channels serve as a means of egress of blood from the hypertensive right ventricle. Angiographic studies often demonstrate flow from the right ventricular cavity into the sinusoids and thus into the coronary arteries in systole and coronary-to-right ventricular flow in diastole.

Incidence

Pulmonary atresia with intact ventricular septum is a very uncommon malformation. Estimates of occurrence in live births range from 1 per 8016[60] to 1 per 144,000,[30] and it accounts for only 3 to 4 per cent of cases of congenital heart disease diagnosed in the first year of life.[30,33]

Hemodynamics

Since the right ventricular outflow tract ends blindly, all systemic venous return to the right atrium ultimately must cross the atrial septum to the left atrium. There is mixing of systemic and pulmonary venous blood in the left atrium and left ventricle, with systemic arterial desaturation. Systemic saturation depends on the amount of pulmonary blood flow, which is determined by the size of the ductus arteriosus. Systemic arterial saturation may range from 20 to 88 per cent,[19,57,80] but is usually below 60 per cent.

Right ventricular peak systolic pressure is elevated and is often greater than left ventricular pressure.[19,57,80] A right ventricular systolic pressure of 120 to 130 mmHg is not uncommon. Right atrial pressure is elevated, especially the a wave, and exceeds left atrial pressure.

Clinical Features

Cyanosis is the most prominent finding on physical examination. The first and second heart sounds are single. The presence of cardiac murmurs is variable. If the ductus arteriosus is still patent, there may be a systolic ejection murmur or continuous murmur at the upper left sternal border. A harsh, holosystolic murmur at the mid- and lower left sternal border may be heard in patients with tricuspid insufficiency. If the atrial septal defect is restrictive, hepatic enlargement is often present.

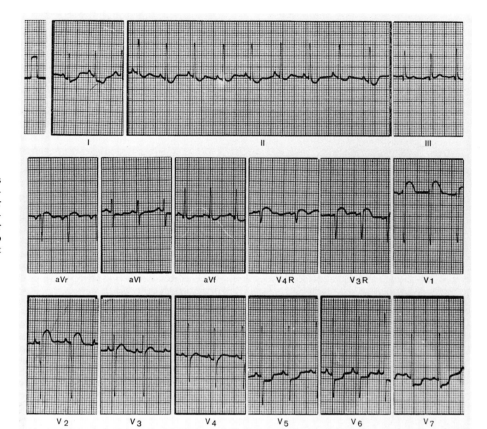

Figure 45–4. This electrocardiogram is from a 1-week-old infant with pulmonary atresia and an intact ventricular septum. There is left ventricular hypertrophy with a paucity of right ventricular forces. Note the small R waves and deep S waves in V_1. These findings suggest right ventricular hypoplasia.

Arterial blood gas values reveal marked hypoxemia, which ultimately leads to metabolic acidosis. The chest radiograph is not diagnostic and may be normal or show cardiomegaly, especially if the right atrium is dilated. Pulmonary vascular markings reflect the size of the shunt through the ductus arteriosus.

The electrocardiogram in infants with pulmonary atresia and intact ventricular septum is largely influenced by the size of the right ventricle. If the right ventricle is extremely small, the electrocardiogram typically shows an axis of 30 to 90 degrees and left ventricular hypertrophy (Fig. 45–4).[14,19,80] In patients with larger right ventricles, the electrocardiogram may be normal or may even show right ventricular hypertrophy. Prominent P waves are present in patients with marked right atrial enlargement.

The anatomic features of this condition are clearly demonstrated by two-dimensional echocardiography (Fig. 45–5). The right ventricular cavity is typically small and thick walled.[2,85] The tricuspid valve is smaller than normal, but the leaflets move, distinguishing this condition from tricuspid atresia. The pulmonary valve image is variable. At times, only an immobile mass of echoes is seen separating the right ventricular cavity from the main pulmonary artery. In other patients, a thin, mobile but imperforate valve is seen protruding toward the pulmonary artery in systole and collapsing into the right ventricle in diastole. Doppler echocardiography is valuable in analyzing the flow pattern

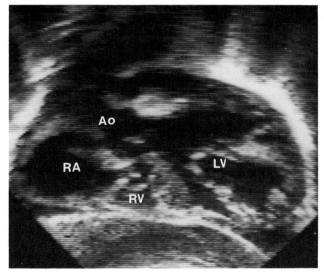

Figure 45–5. Two-dimensional echocardiogram obtained from the subxyphoid region in a neonate with pulmonary atresia and an intact ventricular septum. The right ventricle is spherical and extremely hypoplastic. The left ventricle is enlarged and connected normally to the aortic root. Ao = ascending aorta; LV = left ventricle; RA = right atrium; RV = right ventricle.

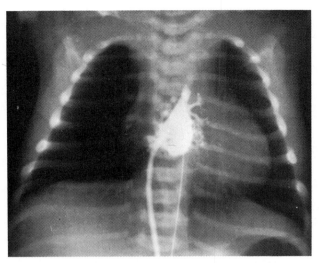

Figure 45–6. Right ventricular angiocardiogram in a neonate with pulmonary atresia and an intact ventricular septum. The right ventricular cavity is extremely hypoplastic and ends blindly.

in the main pulmonary artery and thereby distinguishing pulmonary atresia from severe pulmonary valve stenosis. Additional anatomic features that may be demonstrated by two-dimensional echocardiography are the size of the interatrial communication and the size of the ductus arteriosus.

Right ventricular angiocardiography is useful to confirm the diagnosis and to determine the size of the right ventricle,[67] the degree of tricuspid insufficiency, and the presence of myocardial sinusoids (Fig. 45–6). Freedom et al[29] have described a double catheter technique with simultaneous injection in the right ventricle and the thoracic aorta to allow for the precise characterization of the site of atresia. Since all pulmonary blood flow is via the ductus arteriosus, the thoracic aortogram will establish the size of the pulmonary arteries.

Treatment

Initial treatment is aimed at relieving hypoxemia by infusion of type E prostaglandins to increase flow through the ductus arteriosus. Subsequent therapy is surgical and consists of pulmonary valvotomy, creation of systemic-to-pulmonary shunt, or both.[7,17,18,51,59,86] To a large degree the choice of surgical procedure will be dictated by the size of the right ventricular cavity and the tricuspid annulus; if these structures are extremely hypoplastic, a systemic-to-pulmonary shunt will be necessary, whether or not pulmonary valvotomy can be performed. When right ventricular size approaches normal, pulmonary valvotomy alone is most likely to suffice. If the right ventricular cavity and tricuspid annulus are extremely hypoplastic, balloon atrial septostomy should be performed at the time of cardiac catheterization to ensure adequate interatrial communication.

Prognosis

The outlook for infants with pulmonary atresia and intact ventricular septum is poor despite the variety of surgical procedures utilized in their management. One year survival rates were 36 and 23 per cent, respectively, in prospective series from the Texas Children's Hospital in Houston[33] and the New England Regional Cardiac Program.[30] Although several studies have demonstrated that the right ventricular cavity may grow if continuity to the pulmonary artery is established,[32,55] such growth is by no means universal. Patients with right ventricular hypoplasia who survive infancy may be candidates for a right ventricular bypass procedure (Fontan operation) if their pulmonary arteries are of adequate size.

ABSENT PULMONARY VALVE SYNDROME

Historical Aspects

Chevers is credited with the first published description in 1847 of absent pulmonary valve with annular stenosis and aneurysmal dilation of the pulmonary arteries.[12] Individual cases were described by Royer and Wilson in 1908[74] and by Kurtz et al in 1927.[47] However, it was not until the 1950s and 1960s that this constellation of pulmonary and cardiac anomalies was widely recognized.

Incidence

Absent pulmonary valve syndrome is a rare anomaly. It has been noted in 3 to 6 per cent of autopsied cases of tetralogy of Fallot.[30,62] Emmanouilides and Baylen[23] found only 12 reported cases with intact ventricular septum in the literature.

Pathology

Although the lesion is often called tetralogy of Fallot with absent pulmonary valve, the external appearance of the heart and great vessels is unlike tetralogy of Fallot. The heart is enlarged and the pulmonary trunk and its branches are markedly dilated, often reaching aneurysmal proportions. The pulmonary valve leaflets are not actually absent but are present as rudimentary nodules of gelatinous tissue.[58] The pulmonary annulus is restrictive, and the infundibulum is hypoplastic. A large, subaortic ventricular septal defect is usually present. The ductus arteriosus is usually not patent and "agenesis" of the ductus has been associated with the lesion.[25]

The massively enlarged pulmonary arteries compress the main stem bronchi, often producing emphysema of the affected lung.[5] In addition, Rabinovitch et al[72] have demonstrated that in some cases there is an abnormal pulmonary arterial branching pattern, with peripheral vessels entwining and compressing small intrapulmonary bronchi.

Hemodynamics

The combination of rudimentary pulmonary valve cusps with a narrow annulus produces pulmonary stenosis and insufficiency. Right ventricular pressure is equal to left ventricular pressure. In the neonate, the predominant shunt is often right to left, but bidirectional and ultimately left-to-right shunting occur as pulmonary resistance falls after birth, especially if the respiratory insufficiency is not severe.[49] Hiraishi et al[38] have suggested that the volume and compliance of the central pulmonary arteries are directly related to the degree of respiratory insufficiency and right ventricular dysfunction.

Clinical Features

The two hallmark features of this syndrome in early infancy are respiratory insufficiency and a to-and-fro murmur along the left sternal border.[6,16,49,58] Many of the infants are cyanotic. The compression of the bronchi produces tachypnea, intercostal retractions, wheezes, and rhonchi. The first and second heart sounds are single. A harsh systolic ejection murmur and a low pitched diastolic murmur are separated by a pause (during which the second heart sound is audible) and can be easily distinguished from the continuous murmur of patent ductus arteriosus.

The chest radiograph reveals cardiomegaly. The dilation of the pulmonary arteries is often apparent, as is hyperexpansion of one or more pulmonary segments (Fig. 45–7).[16,26,69,71] The electrocardiogram reveals right ventricular hypertrophy, occasionally with right atrial enlargement.

The anatomic and physiologic features of this syndrome are well demonstrated by echocardiography.[11,20,84] M-mode and two-dimensional echocardiography demonstrate marked enlargement of the right ventricle, often with paradoxical septal motion.[11] The two-dimensional echocardiogram is useful to visualize the enlarged pulmonary arteries (Fig. 45–8) and the ventricular septal defect.

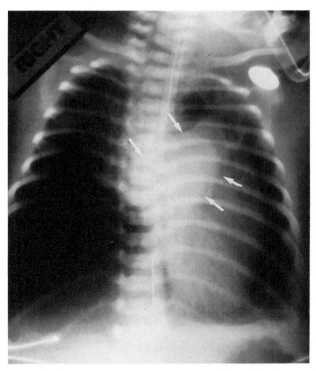

Figure 45–7. Chest radiograph from a newborn infant with absent pulmonary valve syndrome and respiratory insufficiency. Both lungs are hyperinflated and the mediastinum and heart are displaced toward the left. The pulmonary arteries are markedly enlarged (arrows).

Doppler echocardiography confirms the presence of pulmonary stenosis and insufficiency and clearly demonstrates the to-and-fro flow pattern in the main pulmonary artery.[11]

Right ventricular angiocardiography demonstrates the narrow pulmonary annulus and the dilated pulmonary arteries.[16] The infundibulum is frequently long and narrow

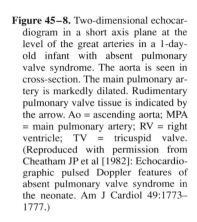

Figure 45–8. Two-dimensional echocardiogram in a short axis plane at the level of the great arteries in a 1-day-old infant with absent pulmonary valve syndrome. The aorta is seen in cross-section. The main pulmonary artery is markedly dilated. Rudimentary pulmonary valve tissue is indicated by the arrow. Ao = ascending aorta; MPA = main pulmonary artery; RV = right ventricle; TV = tricuspid valve. (Reproduced with permission from Cheatham JP et al [1982]: Echocardiographic pulsed Doppler features of absent pulmonary valve syndrome in the neonate. Am J Cardiol 49:1773–1777.)

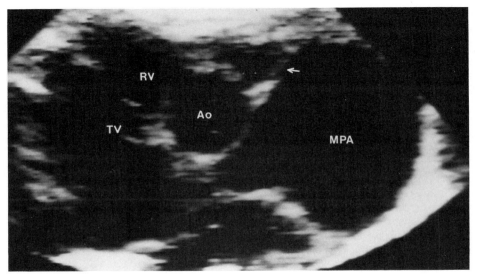

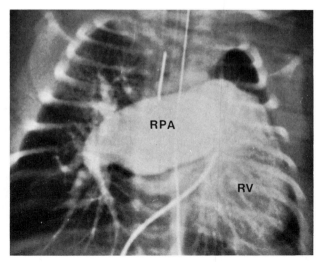

Figure 45–9. Pulmonary arteriogram in a neonate with respiratory distress secondary to absent pulmonary valve syndrome. Note the huge right pulmonary artery and the reflux of contrast material back into the right ventricle. RPA = right pulmonary artery; RV = right ventricle.

and oriented toward the pulmonary artery segment with the greatest dilation.[49] Pulmonary angiography is useful to demonstrate the pulmonary arterial dilation (Fig. 45–9) and the degree of pulmonary regurgitation.

Treatment and Prognosis

The prognosis is largely determined by the degree of respiratory insufficiency in early infancy. Infants with the severe form of the syndrome frequently die from respiratory distress and hypoxemia. Bronchial compression by the enlarged pulmonary arteries often produces a "ball-valve" effect, in which air can enter the lungs but cannot exit, thereby creating progressive hyperinflation. Intubation and assisted ventilation are frequently unsuccessful in achieving adequate oxygenation, although positive end-expiratory pressure may help prevent expiratory collapse of the airways. Unlike the other lesions discussed in this chapter, prostaglandin infusion is unlikely to be beneficial in absent pulmonary valve syndrome.

A variety of surgical procedures have been employed to palliate or correct this condition. These include aneurysmorrhaphy,[66] aneurysmectomy with suspension of the pulmonary artery,[6] pulmonary artery banding,[65] and transection of the dilated pulmonary arterial segment with anastomosis to the superior vena cava or main pulmonary artery.[54,90] Because of the high mortality rates associated with these procedures in early infancy, it has been recommended that surgery be deferred until later in childhood.[49,70] Successful results in a small group of recently reported infants[1,21,73] have led some to advocate surgery in symptomatic patients, even in the first year of life.

The prognosis is much better for infants with lesser degrees of respiratory involvement. Intracardiac repair of the lesion with or without replacement of the pulmonary valve has been performed in older children with good results.[10,40,56,70,82,91]

References

1. Agarwal KC, Ali Khan MA, Karpawich PP, Amato JJ (1985): Successful surgical repair of absent pulmonary valve syndrome in infancy. Am Heart J 109:174–177.
2. Andrade JL, Serino W, deLeval M, Somerville J (1984): Two-dimensional echocardiographic evaluation of tricuspid hypoplasia in pulmonary atresia. Am J Cardiol 53:387–388.
3. Becu L, Somerville J, Gallo A (1976): "Isolated" pulmonary valve stenosis as part of more widespread cardiovascular disease. Br Heart J 38:472–482.
4. Beuren AJ, Schulze C, Eberle P, Harmjanz D, Apitz J (1964): The syndrome of supravalvular aortic stenosis, peripheral pulmonary stenosis, mental retardation and similar facial appearance. Am J Cardiol 13:471–483.
5. Borg SA, Young LW, Roghair GC (1975): Congenital avalvular pulmonary artery and infantile lobar emphysema. A diagnostic correlation. Am J Roentgenol Radium Ther Nucl Med 125:412–421.
6. Bove EL, Snaher RM, Alley RM, McKneally M (1972): Tetralogy of Fallot with absent pulmonary valve and aneurysm of the pulmonary artery: Report of two cases presenting as obstructive lung disease. J Pediatr 81:339–343.
7. Bowman FO Jr, Malm JR, Hayes J, Gersony WM, Ellis K (1971): Pulmonary atresia with intact ventricular septum. J Thorac Cardiovasc Surg 61:85–95.
8. Brock RC (1948): Pulmonary valvulotomy for the relief of congenital pulmonary stenosis: Report of 3 cases. Br Med J 1:1121–1126.
9. Bull C, de Leval MR, Mercanti C, Macartney FJ, Anderson RH (1982): Pulmonary atresia and intact ventricular septum: A revised classification. Circulation 66:266–272.
10. Calder AL, Brandt PW, Barratt-Bowes BG, Neutze JM (1980): Variant of tetralogy of Fallot with absent pulmonary valve leaflets and origin of one pulmonary artery from the ascending aorta. Am J Cardiol 46:106–116.
11. Cheatham JP, Latson LA, Gutgesell HP (1982): Echocardiographic pulsed Doppler features of absent pulmonary valve syndrome in the neonate. Am J Cardiol 49:1773–1777.
12. Chevers N (1847): Recherches sur les maladies de l'artere pulmonaire. Arch Gen Med 15:488–508.
13. Danilowicz D, Hoffman JI, Rudolph AM (1975): Serial studies of pulmonary stenosis in infancy and childhood. Br Heart J 37:808–818.
14. Davignon AL, Greenwold WE, DuShane JW, Edwards JE (1961): Congenital pulmonary atresia with intact ventricular septum. Clinicopathologic correlation of two anatomic types. Am Heart J 62:591–602.
15. Dawes GS, Mott JC, Widdicomb JG (1954): The foaetal circulation in the lamb. J Physiol 126:563–587.
16. Dee PM, Hubbell MM Jr, Rheuban KR, Tompkins DG, Carpenter MA (1981): Congenital absence of the pulmonary valve. Cardiovasc Intervent Radiol 4:158–166.
17. de Leval M, Bull C, Stark JG, Anderson RH, Path FRC, Taylor JFN, Macartney F (1982): Pulmonary atresia and intact ventricular septum: Surgical management based on a revised classification. Circulation 66:272–280.
18. de Leval M, Bull C, Hopkins R, Rees P, Deanfield J, Taylor JFN, Gersony W, Stark J, Macartney FJ (1985): Decision making in the definitive repair of the heart with a small right ventricle. Circulation 72(Suppl II):52–60.
19. Dhanavaravibul S, Nora JJ, McNamara DG (1970): Pulmonary valvular atresia with intact ventricular septum: Problems in diagnosis and results of treatment. J Pediatr 77:1010–1016.
20. DiSegni E, Einzig S, Bass JL, Edwards JE (1983): Congenital absence of pulmonary valve associated with tetralogy of Fallot: Diagnosis by 2-dimensional echocardiography. Am J Cardiol 51:1798–1800.

21. Dunnigan A, Oldham HN, Benson DW (1981): Absent pulmonary valve syndrome in infancy: Surgery reconsidered. Am J Cardiol 48:117–122.

22. Edwards JE (1968): Congenital malformations of the heart and great vessels. In Gould SE (ed): Pathology of the Heart. 3rd ed. Springfield, Charles C Thomas, p 320.

23. Emmanouilides GC, Baylen BG (1983): Congenital absence of the pulmonary valve. In Adams FH, Emmanouilides GC (eds): Moss' Heart Disease in Infants, Children, and Adolescents. Baltimore, Williams & Wilkins, p 228.

24. Emmanouilides GC, Baylen BG (1983): Pulmonary stenosis. In Adams FH, Emmanouilides GC (eds): Moss' Heart Disease in Infants, Children, and Adolescents. Baltimore, Williams & Wilkins, p 234.

25. Emmanouilides GC, Thanopoulos B, Siassi B, Fishbein M (1976): "Agenesis" of ductus arteriosis associated with syndrome of tetralogy of Fallot and absent pulmonary valve. Am J Cardiol 37:403–409.

26. Fischer DR, Neches WH, Beerman LB, Fricker FJ, Siewers RD, Lenox CC, Park SC (1984): Tetralogy of Fallot with absent pulmonic valve: Analysis of 17 patients. Am J Cardiol 53:1433–1437.

27. Freed MD, Rosenthal A, Bernhard WF, Litwin SB, Nadas AS (1973): Critical pulmonary stenosis with diminutive right ventricle in neonates. Circulation 48:875–881.

28. Freedom RM, Dische MR, Rowe RD (1978): The tricuspid valve in pulmonary atresia and intact ventricular septum: A morphological study of 60 cases. Arch Pathol Lab Med 102:28–31.

29. Freedom RM, White RI Jr, Ho CS, Gingell RL, Hawker RE, Rowe RD (1974): Evaluation of patients with pulmonary atresia and intact ventricular septum by double catheter technique. Am J Cardiol 33:892–895.

30. Fyler DC, Buckley LP, Hellenbrand WE, Cohn HE, Kirklin JW, Nadas AS, Cartier JM, Breibart MH (1980): Report of the New England Regional Cardiac Program. Pediatrics 65(Suppl):375–461.

31. Goor DA, Lillehei CW (1975): Congenital Malformations of the Heart. New York, Grune & Stratton, p 11.

32. Graham TP Jr, Bender HW, Atwood GF, Page DL, Sell CGR (1974): Increase in right ventricular volume following valvulotomy for pulmonary atresia or stenosis with intact ventricular septum. Circulation 49(Suppl I):69–79.

33. Gutgesell HP, Garson A Jr, Hesslein P, Park I, McNamara DG (1982): Prognosis for the neonate and infant with congenital heart disease (abstr). Pediatr Cardiol 2:168.

34. Gutgesell HP, Bricker JT, Colvin EV, Latson LA, Hawkins EP (1984): Atrioventricular valve annular diameter: Two-dimensional echocardiographic-autopsy correlation. Am J Cardiol 53:1652–1655.

35. Gutgesell HP, Paquet M (1978): Atlas of pediatric echocardiography. Hagerstown, Harper and Row, pp 128–132.

36. Hagler DJ, Tajik AJ, Seward JB, Ritter DG (1986): Noninvasive assessment of pulmonary valve stenosis, aortic valve stenosis and coarctation of the aorta in critically ill neonates. Am J Cardiol 57:369–372.

37. Harinck E, Becker AE, Gittenberger-De Groot AC, Oppenheimer-Dekker A, Versprille A (1977): The left ventricle in congenital isolated pulmonary valve stenosis: A morphological study. Br Heart J 39:429–435.

38. Hiraishi S, Bargeron LM, Isabel-Jones JB, Emmanouilides GC, Friedman WF, Jarmakani JM (1983): Ventricular and pulmonary artery volumes in patients with absent pulmonary valves: Factors affecting the natural course. Circulation 67:183–190.

39. Houston AB, Sheldon CD, Simpson IA, Doig WB, Coleman EN (1985): The severity of pulmonary valve or artery obstruction in children estimated by Doppler ultrasound. Eur Heart J 6:786–790.

40. Ilbawi MN, Idriss FS, Muster AJ, Wessel HU, Paul MH, DeLeon SY (1981): Tetralogy of Fallot with absent pulmonary valve: Should valve insertion be part of the intracardiac repair? J Thorac Cardiovasc Surg 81:906–915.

41. Jeffrey RF, Moller JH, Amplatz K (1972): The dysplastic pulmonary valve: A new roentgenographic entity. Am J Roentgenol 114:322–339.

42. Kan JS, White RI Jr, Mitchell SE, Anderson JH, Gardner TJ (1984): Percutaneous transluminal balloon valvuloplasty for pulmonary valve stenosis. Circulation 69:554–560.

43. Kan JS, White RI Jr, Mitchell SE, Gardner TJ (1982): Percutaneous balloon valvuloplasty: A new method for treating congenital pulmonary valve stenosis. N Engl J Med 307:540–542.

44. Keith JD (1978): Prevalence, incidence, and epidemiology. In Keith JD, Rowe RD, Vlad P (eds): Heart Disease in Infancy and Childhood. 3rd ed. New York, Macmillan, p 5.

45. King DH, Smith EO, Huhta JC, Gutgesell HP (1985): Mitral and tricuspid valve anular diameter in normal children determined by two-dimensional echocardiography. Am J Cardiol 55:787–789.

46. Koretzky E, Moller JH, Korns ME, Schwartz CJ, Edwards JE (1969): Congenital pulmonary stenosis resulting from dysplasia of valve. Circulation 40:43–53.

47. Kurtz CM, Sprague HD, White PD (1927): Congenital heart disease: Interventricular septal defects with associated anomalies in a series of three cases examined postmortem, and a living patient fifty-eight years old with cyanosis and clubbing of the fingers. Am Heart J 3:77–90.

48. Lababidi Z, Wu J-R (1983): Percutaneous balloon pulmonary valvuloplasty. Am J Cardiol 52:560–562.

49. Lakier JB, Stanger P, Heymann MA, Hoffman JIE, Rudolph AM (1974): Tetralogy of Fallot with absent pulmonary valve: Natural history and hemodynamic considerations. Circulation 50:167–175.

50. Lauer RM, Fink HP, Petry EL, Dunn MI, Diehl AM (1964): Angiographic demonstration of intramyocardial sinusoids in pulmonary valve atresia with intact ventricular septum and hypoplastic right ventricle. N Engl J Med 271:68–72.

51. Lewis AB, Wells W, Lindesmith GG (1983): Evaluation and surgical treatment of pulmonary atresia and intact ventricular septum in infancy. Circulation 67:1318–1323.

52. Lima CO, Shan DJ, Valdes-Cruz LM, Goldberg SJ, Barron JU, Allen HD, Grenadier E (1983): Non-invasive prediction of transvalvular pressure gradient in patients with pulmonary stenosis by quantitative two-dimensional echocardiographic Doppler studies. Circulation 67:866–871.

53. Linde LM, Turner SW, Sparkes RS (1973): Pulmonary valvular dysplasia: A cardiofacial syndrome. Br Heart J 35:301–304.

54. Litwin SB, Rosenthal A, Fellows K (1973): Surgical management of young infants with tetralogy of Fallot, absence of pulmonary valve and respiratory distress. J Thorac Cardiovasc Surg 65:552–558.

55. Luckstead EF, Mattioli L, Crosby IK, Reed WA, Diehl AM (1972): Two-stage palliative surgical approach for pulmonary atresia with intact ventricular septum (Type I). Am J Cardiol 29:490–496.

56. McCaughan BC, Danielson GK, Driscoll DJ, McGoon DC (1985): Tetralogy of Fallot with absent pulmonary valve—Early and late results of surgical treatment. J Thorac Cardiovasc Surg 89:280–287.

57. Miller GAH, Restifo M, Shinebourne EA, Paneth M, Joseph MC, Lennox SC, Kerr IH (1973): Pulmonary atresia with intact ventricular septum and critical pulmonary stenosis presenting in first month of life: Investigation and surgical results. Br Heart J 35:9–16.

58. Miller RA, Lev M, Paul MH (1962): Congenital absence of the pulmonary valve. The clinical syndrome of tetralogy of Fallot with pulmonary regurgitation. Circulation 26:266–278.

59. Milliken JC, Laks H, Hellenbrand W, George B, Chin A, Williams RG (1985): Early and late results in the treatment of patients with pulmonary atresia and intact ventricular septum. Circulation 72(Suppl II):61–69.

60. Mitchell SC, Korones SB, Berendes HW (1971): Congenital heart disease in 56,109 births: Incidence and natural history. Circulation 43:323–332.

61. Morgan BC, Stacy GS, Dillard DH (1965): Pulmonary and infundibular and valvular atresia with intact ventricular septum. Am J Cardiol 16:746–749.

62. Nagao GI, Daoud GI, McAdams AJ, Schwartz DC, Kaplan S (1967): Cardiovascular anomalies associated with tetralogy of Fallot. Am J Cardiol 20:206–215.

63. Noonan JA (1968): Hypertelorism with Turner phenotype. Am J Dis Child 116:373–380.

64. Nudel DB, Berman MA, Talner NS (1976): Effects of acutely increasing systemic vascular resistance on oxygen tension in tetralogy of Fallot. Pediatrics 58:248–251.

65. Opie JC, Sandor GG, Ashmore PG, Patterson MW (1983): Successful palliation by pulmonary artery banding in absent pulmonary valve syndrome with aneurysmal pulmonary arteries. J Thorac Cardiovasc Surg 85:125–128.

66. Osman MQ, Meng CCL, Girdany BR (1969): Congenital absence of the pulmonary valve: Report of eight cases with review of the literature. Am J Roentgenol Radium Ther Nucl Med 106:58–69.

67. Patel RG, Freedom RM, Moes CAF, Bloom KR, Olley PM, Williams WG, Trusler GA, Rowe RD (1980): Right ventricular volume determinations in 18 patients with pulmonary atresia and intact ventricular septum: Analysis of factors influencing right ventricular growth. Circulation 61:428–440.

68. Peacock TB (1858): On Malformations, & C., of the Human Heart. London, J. Churchill, p 51.

69. Pernot C, Hoeffel JC, Henry M, Worms AM, Stehlin H, Louis JP, (1972): Radiological patterns of congenital absence of the pulmonary valve in infants. Radiology 102:619–622.

70. Pinsky WW, Nihill MR, Mullins CE, Harrison G, McNamara DG (1978): The absent pulmonary valve syndrome. Circulation 57:159–162.

71. Portman MA, Riggs TW, Port RB, Young LW (1984): Radiological case of the month. Tetralogy of Fallot with absent pulmonary valve. Am J Dis Child 138:697–698.

72. Rabinovitch M, Grady S, David I, Van Praag R, Sauer U, Buhlmeyuer K, Castaneda AR, Reid L (1982): Compression of intrapulmonary bronchi by abnormally branching pulmonary arteries associated with absent pulmonary valves. Am J Cardiol 50:804–813.

73. Rao PS, Lawrie GM (1983): Absent pulmonary valve syndrome. Surgical correction with pulmonary arterioplasty. Br Heart J 50:586–589.

74. Royer BF, Wilson JD (1908): Incomplete heterotaxy with unusual heart malformations: Case report. Arch Pediatr 25:881–896.

75. Rudolph AM (1974): Congenital Diseases of the Heart. Chicago, Year Book Medical Publishers, p 364.

76. Ibid, p 405.

77. Santos MA, Moll JN, Drumond C, Araujo WB, Romao N, Reis NB (1980): Development of the ductus arteriosus in right ventricular outflow tract obstruction. Circulation 62:818–822.

78. Sellors TH (1948): Surgery of pulmonic stenosis. Lancet 1:988–989.

79. Shah PM, Kidd L (1967): Circulatory effects of propranolol in children with Fallot's tetralogy. Am J Cardiol 19:653–657.

80. Shams A, Fowler RS, Trusler GA, Keith JD, Mustard WT (1971): Pulmonary atresia with intact ventricular septum: Report of 50 cases. Pediatrics 47:370–377.

81. Sissman NJ, Abrams HL (1965): Bidirectional shunting in a coronary artery–right ventricular fistula associated with pulmonary atresia and intact ventricular septum. Circulation 32:582–588.

82. Stafford EG, Mair DD, McGoon DC, Danielson GK (1973): Tetralogy of Fallot with absent pulmonary valve. Surgical considerations and results. Circulation 48(Suppl III):24–30.

83. Sullivan ID, Robinson PF, Macartney FJ, Taylor JFN, Rees PG, Bull C, Deanfield JE (1985): Percutaneous balloon valvuloplasty for pulmonary valve stenosis in infants and children. Br Heart J 54:435–441.

84. Tenorio AM, Ortiz J, Villela A, Atik E, Ebaid M, del Nero E Jr, Pileggi F (1984): Cross-sectional echocardiographic features of "absent" pulmonary valve. Report of two cases. Int J Cardiol 5:155–161.

85. Trowitzsch E, Colan SD, Sanders SP (1985): Two-dimensional echocardiographic evaluation of right ventricular size and function in newborns with severe right ventricular outflow tract obstruction. J Am Coll Cardiol 6:388–393.

86. Mustard WT (1976): Surgical treatment of pulmonary atresia with intact ventricular septum. Br Heart J 38:957–960.

87. Tynan M, Jones O, Joseph MC, Deverall PB, Yates AK (1984): Relief of pulmonary valve stenosis in first week of life by percutaneous balloon valvuloplasty (Letter). Lancet 1:273.

88. Van Praagh R, Ando M, Van Praagh S, Senno A, Hougen TJ, Novak G, Hastreiter AR (1976): Pulmonary atresia: Anatomic considerations. In Kidd BSL, Rowe RD (eds): The Child with Congenital Heart Disease After Surgery. Mt. Kisco, Futura Publishing Company, pp 105–112.

89. Venables AW (1965): The syndrome of pulmonary stenosis complicating maternal rubella. Br Heart J 27:49–55.

90. Waldhausen JA, Friedman S, Nicodemus H, Miller WW, Rashkind W, Johnson J (1969): Absence of the pulmonary valve in patients with tetralogy of Fallot: Surgical management. J Thorac Cardiovasc Surg 57:669–674.

91. Weldon CS, Rowe RD, Gott VL (1968): Clinical experience with the use of aortic valve homografts for reconstruction of the pulmonary artery, pulmonary valve, and outflow portion of the right ventricle. Circulation 37(Suppl II):51–61.

92. Zuberbuhler JR, Anderson RH (1979): Morphological variations in pulmonary atresia with intact ventricular septum. Br Heart J 41:281–288.

46 CONOTRUNCAL ABNORMALITIES

Thomas P. Graham, Jr.
Howard P. Gutgesell

Conotruncal abnormalities comprise transposition of the great arteries (TGA), tetralogy of Fallot, including pulmonary atresia with ventricular septal defect, and truncus arteriosus. In these lesions severe abnormalities of cardiac development occur early in development with conotruncal septation completed by approximately 34 days' gestation. The probable vulnerable period for teratogenic influences on cardiovascular development for these malformations is between 18 and 29 days' gestation.[37] These lesions do not normally cause abnormalities of fetal cardiovascular function. Diagnosis usually is apparent early after birth because of cyanosis or abnormal cardiac physical findings.

TRANSPOSITION OF THE GREAT ARTERIES

Historical Perspective

The earliest recorded anatomic descriptions of transposition of the great arteries were by Steno (1672), Morgagni (1761), and Baillie (1797).[26] The clinical and radiologic descriptions of TGA by Fanconi[12] and later by Taussig[50] resulted in premorbid diagnosis of this condition long before angiography was available. The landmark publication by Rashkind and Miller[42] in 1966 was the first successful nonsurgical palliation of this condition and ushered in the era of pediatric interventional catheterization. For a review of the surgical history of TGA, the reader is referred to Chapter 66.

Incidence

Transposition is the malformation in which the aorta arises from the right ventricle and the pulmonary artery arises from the left ventricle with parallel pulmonary and systemic circuits. There are normal atrioventricular connections and abnormal ventriculoarterial connections. Patients with TGA include approximately 10 per cent of all infants born with critical congenital heart disease, or 2 in 10,000 live births, and represent the second most common diagnostic group in the first year of life.[15]

The authors would like to thank Joy Phillips and Marge Hampton for their tireless efforts in manuscript preparation and Dolores Garrison and Judy Burger for help in preparing the echocardiographic illustrations.

The most common group comprises those neonates with simple transposition in which ventricular septal defect and significant pulmonary stenosis are absent. Complex transposition includes those with significant ventricular septal defect(s) with or without significant pulmonary stenosis and represents only approximately 25 per cent of the total patients with TGA.[15]

Pathology

In simple transposition, intracardiac anatomy is normal and at birth the left and right ventricles are similar in size to those of patients without cardiovascular disease.[18,22] Ventricular septal defects can occur in all areas of the ventricular septum but are most common in the perimembranous or outlet region, the midportion of the muscular septum, the apical muscular septum, and the muscular septum at the junction with the right ventricular freewall anteriorly.[2]

Pulmonary stenosis is usually subvalvular.[2] As left ventricular pressure falls postnatally there is commonly a small, dynamic gradient from the left ventricle to the pulmonary artery because of the upper part of the septum bulging over into the left ventricular outflow tract. This abnormality usually is of no hemodynamic consequence. A fixed subvalvular tunnel-type of narrowing of the left ventricular outflow tract can lead to severe restriction of pulmonary flow but is rarely significant in the neonate. Finally, valvular pulmonary stenosis, anomalous mitral valve insertion, and tissue tags in the left ventricular outflow tract are all rare causes of outflow obstruction.[2]

Ventricular pump function of both ventricles usually is normal when determined shortly after birth.[18,22] With time there is evidence suggesting progressive decrease in right ventricular function, possibly as a consequence of myocardial hypoxia with subsequent myocardial damage.[18] Abnormalities of left ventricular function are seldom noted in the infant with transposition. Usually this ventricle is subjected to a low afterload with pulmonary resistance significantly less than systemic resistance, and thus delineation of left ventricular dysfunction is more difficult.

Clinical Features

Patients with TGA and intact ventricular septum generally present shortly after birth with intense cyanosis. The majority of patients are male, birthweight is normal to slightly increased, and there is no history of preceding

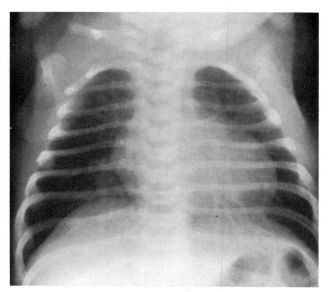

Figure 46–1. Posteroanterior chest film of a newborn infant with simple transposition of the great arteries. There is a narrow mediastinum, mild cardiomegaly, and normal pulmonary vascular markings.

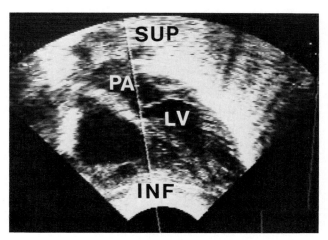

Figure 46–2. Echocardiogram obtained from subcostal view with "anatomic" presentation from an infant with transposition of the great arteries . Left ventricle gives rise to main pulmonary artery, which is identified by its branching into right and left pulmonary arteries. INF = inferior; LV = left ventricle; PA = pulmonary artery; SUP = superior.

maternal or fetal distress. Rarely patients with a large atrial septal defect and open ductus will appear normal to mildly cyanotic. Ductal constriction in all patients results in a marked increase in cyanosis. In patients with small atrial defects, severe clinical deterioration can occur.

The physical examination in the infant with TGA and intact septum usually reveals an intensely cyanotic infant. Cyanosis increases with crying and is poorly responsive to increases in FIO_2. Cardiac examination can be normal with the exception of a right ventricular parasternal lift. The second heart sound may be single or closely split. Murmurs are uncommon in infants with intact septum, but a soft pulmonary ejection murmur or a soft ductus murmur is occasionally present.

Arterial blood gas analysis in the infant with TGA and intact septum usually shows a PO_2 in room air ranging from 20 to 35 mmHg, with a normal to slightly decreased PCO_2 and generally a normal pH. With an increase in FIO_2, the PO_2 generally rises minimally. There is one caution in interpreting PO_2 determinations. Infants with transposition occasionally will show normal to increased PO_2 in umbilical artery samples due to shunting of oxygenated pulmonary artery blood to the aorta. The diagnosis of transposition can easily be made in this situation if simultaneous right radial artery PO_2 and umbilical artery PO_2 reveal a higher PO_2 in the descending aorta.

The chest radiograph in the infant with TGA and intact septum can be normal, or it can show a narrow mediastinum due to the anteroposterior relationship of the aorta and pulmonary artery. The heart size is usually normal to slightly increased, and pulmonary vascularity is normal (Fig. 46–1). The ECG in the infant with TGA and intact septum is normal or suggestive of right ventricular hypertrophy.

These findings will be modified for patients with TGA and a large ventricular septal defect. Such patients gen-

erally show mild cyanosis and may or may not have a murmur of a ventricular septal defect in the first 1 or 2 days after birth. With falling pulmonary resistance over the first week of life, the ventricular septal defect murmur will become audible. These patients are more likely to present with signs of congestive heart failure at age 2 to 4 weeks with physical findings of an active precordium, cardiac enlargement, typical murmur of ventricular septal defect, and an apical diastolic rumble of increased pulmonary blood flow.

Initial radiographs early after birth in patients with TGA and ventricular septal defect generally show mild cardiac enlargement. Increased pulmonary blood flow becomes apparent only after the fall in pulmonary resistance over the first several weeks of life. The ECG usually shows biventricular hypertrophy and biatrial enlargement.

Patients with TGA and ventricular septal defect plus significant pulmonary stenosis will present like those with tetralogy of Fallot; symptoms and the degree of cyanosis will be related to the degree of pulmonary stenosis. The murmur of pulmonary stenosis usually will be present at birth, a characteristic that should distinguish this group.

Echocardiography/Doppler Findings

The hallmark of current diagnostic techniques is echocardiography/Doppler evaluation for all cyanotic congenital cardiac abnormalities.[45] The diagnosis of TGA is usually evident by finding a great artery arising from the left ventricle that bifurcates into the right and left pulmonary arteries (Fig. 46–2). A second useful echocardiographic image from the same subcostal location will show the aorta arising from the anatomic right ventricle (Fig. 46–3). The presence of outflow obstruction as well as the presence or absence of significant ventricular septal defects can usually be readily determined from echocardiography/Doppler studies. The finding of diastolic flow in the pulmonary artery indicates an

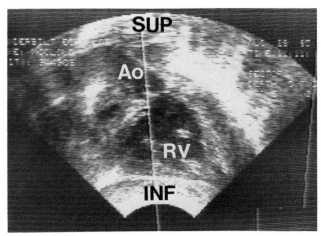

Figure 46–3. Echocardiogram from an infant with transposition of the great arteries from a similar transducer location as that in Figure 46–2, with the aorta shown arising from the anatomic right ventricle. Ao = aorta; INF = inferior; RV = right ventricle; SUP = superior.

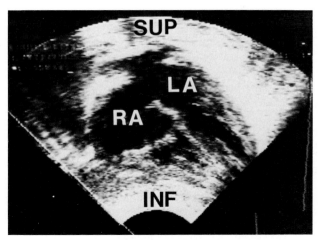

Figure 46–4. Echocardiogram from an infant with transposition of the great arteries from views similar to those in Figures 46–2 and 46–3, showing large atrial septal defect following septostomy. INF = inferior; LA = left atrium; RA = right atrium; SUP = superior.

associated patent ductus with aortic to pulmonary shunting.

In patients with TGA and ventricular septal defects, questions regarding straddling or overriding of atrioventricular valves should be clearly ascertained. The distinction between transposition plus large ventricular septal defect versus double-outlet right ventricle of the Taussig-Bing variety frequently can be determined by echocardiography, although this distinction is not always clear. Finally, coarctation is associated with TGA and ventricular septal defect, as well as Taussig-Bing abnormality; careful echocardiographic and Doppler studies should be conducted to exclude coarctation when TGA and ventricular septal defect coexist.

Management

Intravenous administration of prostaglandin E_1 (PGE_1) is indicated early in the course of the cyanotic infant with transposition. Dilatation of the ductus is associated with marked improvement in PO_2 and allows further therapy to be instituted with the infant in an improved physiologic condition. Infusion rates of 0.05 μg/kg/min are used initially, and an improvement in PO_2 usually occurs within 10 to 20 minutes. A doubling of this infusion rate can be used in infants who are markedly cyanotic or acidotic. High infusion rates are associated with an increased incidence of central nervous system effects, including jitteriness and apnea. These infants should be monitored closely for these problems. Additional side effects of PGE_1 include fever, vasodilatation, and peripheral edema. If PGE_1 is needed for longer than a few hours, the initial infusion that produces effective ductal dilatation can usually be decreased by a factor of one fourth to one half with continued ductal patency and a decrease in the associated side effects.

Most infants with TGA and an intact atrial septum require cardiac catheterization. Cardiac catheterization can

clarify the diagnosis if there are unclear features after echocardiographic and Doppler study but is mainly indicated to perform a balloon atrial septostomy to enlarge the atrial defect. A number of centers have reported effective atrial septostomy without cardiac catheterization using only echocardiographic guidance.[1,39] Echocardiographic-guided balloon septostomy can be performed in the nursery as long as appropriate facilities are available for monitoring and maintaining sterile technique. Septostomy can be performed through the umbilical vein if the ductus venosus is open, but usually percutaneous femoral vein puncture is required. Echocardiography is quite useful to assess atrial septal defect size following septostomy (Fig. 46–4).

Angiography is useful for those patients with TGA in whom further characterization of ventricular septal defect size and location or left ventricular outflow obstruction is required. Angiography is particularly useful in evaluating associated coarctation, the echocardiographic and Doppler diagnosis of which can be difficult during PGE_1 infusion.

Patients with TGA and intact ventricular septum will usually show an acceptable systemic PO_2 in the range of 30 to 35 mmHg with systemic oxygen saturation above 75 per cent when balloon septostomy is successful and the atrial defect has been enlarged effectively. There are occasional patients, however, who show continued significant cyanosis despite balloon atrial septostomy. The reasons for persistent cyanosis after septostomy include inadequate atrial defect size, abnormal compliance of the ventricular chambers such that adequate bidirectional shunting at the atrial level does not take place, inadequate pulmonary blood flow due to elevated pulmonary vascular resistance, and/or left ventricular outflow tract obstruction. Frequently improvement in systemic oxygen can be obtained with an increase in inspired FIO_2, continued therapy with PGE_1, or passage of time. The effect of the increase in FIO_2 is generally to lower pulmonary resistance and increase pulmonary blood flow. PGE_1 can also lower pulmonary resistance but also maintains ductal patency. Frequently oxygen and/or PGE$_1$ can be weaned as pulmonary resistance slowly falls, and the infant will maintain a reasonable PO$_2$ for discharge. A systemic PO$_2$ above 30 mmHg with saturation above 75 per cent generally results in normal newborn growth and development without acidosis. When the PO$_2$ remains in the low 20s, it is usually necessary to proceed with further therapy. If the atrial defect appears small after septostomy, surgical creation of a large atrial defect via the Blalock-Hanlon operation usually will produce an improved PO$_2$. Other options include neonatal intra-atrial baffle repair, which carries with it a probable slight increase in overall risk versus repair at 3 to 6 months of age. Finally, arterial switch can be performed (see Chapter 66); a number of centers have reported good results with this therapy.[7,40] If arterial repair is to be performed, consideration must be given to ensuring that the left ventricular volume and muscle mass are adequate to maintain systemic blood flow and pressure following operation. With repairs done in the first week of life and the echocardiogram on short axis showing a round left ventricular cavity, there is usually no problem in this regard. When operation is performed later, measurement of left ventricular pressure prior to proceeding with arterial repair is advisable. This procedure is rapidly becoming the treatment of choice in most centers.

Patients with TGA and a large ventricular septal defect generally do not require neonatal surgery but present with symptoms of congestive heart failure in the first few weeks to months of life. Their initial congestive failure frequently can be controlled with the use of cardiac glycosides and diuretics. Patients with TGA do have an accelerated pulmonary vascular response such that pulmonary vascular disease occurs at a much earlier time than in patients with similar left-to-right shunts without transposition.[17] Surgery generally is required in the first 3 months of life. Options include pulmonary artery banding for the infant in severe failure or with multiple ventricular defects. Use of the arterial switch repair is probably the treatment of choice for most patients in this situation. This operation is associated with a higher mortality than with simple TGA, probably because of the time required for both the arterial switch and closure of the ventricular septal defect. Arterial switch does, however, appear to be the most useful operative approach for TGA with ventricular septal defect at the present time.[40]

Patients with TGA, ventricular septal defect, and left ventricular outflow tract obstruction are candidates for Blalock-Taussig shunts when cyanosis is severe. These shunts frequently are required in the first 6 to 18 months of life. In most patients with TGA and ventricular septal defect, the defect remains sizeable; these patients are therefore candidates for Rastelli operation, in which left ventricular output is tunneled through the ventricular septal defect to aorta and a conduit or homograft is placed to connect the right ventricle to pulmonary artery. The Rastelli operation is usually reserved for patients with TGA who are approximately 3 years of age or older and who have had earlier palliative shunts. There is evidence to suggest that progressive myocardial dysfunction occurs in patients with TGA, ventricular septal defect, and left

ventricular outflow obstruction, and thus earlier repair would seem a reasonable future direction.[21]

There is continued evolution in the surgical treatment of simple transposition. Currently considerable enthusiasm for an early arterial switch prevails at a few centers in hopes of preventing the long-term problems that have been found with atrial repair of transposition (including right ventricular dysfunction, baffle obstruction, and atrial rhythm disorders). Short-term follow-up appears to be excellent in most of these arterial switch patients, but problems with right ventricular to pulmonary artery obstruction and higher surgical mortality when beginning this operative approach have dampened enthusiasm in many centers. Further follow-up data in regard to the questions of supravalvular aortic stenosis, growth of coronary anastomoses, possible development of aortic regurgitation, and right ventricular to pulmonary artery stenosis are needed in patients who have undergone arterial repair. Current follow-up of patients with the Senning atrial repair indicate improved systemic ventricular function over that found in patients who have undergone repair 5 to 10 years earlier and the virtual elimination of baffle obstruction.[19] Thus the operative approach to TGA varies in different centers, and comparisons of long-term follow-up of patients with recent atrial versus arterial repair will be required to determine the best operative approach for these infants.

TETRALOGY OF FALLOT

In tetralogy of Fallot there is a large ventricular septal defect, severe right ventricular outflow tract obstruction, and significant right-to-left shunting. Included in this definition is pulmonary atresia with ventricular septal defect.

Historical Perspective

Nicholas Stensen is credited with providing the first anatomic description of tetralogy of Fallot in 1671.[53] Fallot's series of articles in 1888[11] described the four characteristic features of the lesion and distinguished it from other causes of cyanosis. However, the diagnosis of tetralogy during life was not made with any consistency until the 1930s and 1940s. In 1945, Blalock and Taussig[4] reported success with an operation in which a subclavian artery was anastomosed to a pulmonary artery to relieve cyanosis in patients with tetralogy of Fallot. Open-heart procedures for intracardiac repair of tetralogy were first applied by Lillehei and colleagues in 1955.[33] Each of the surgical procedures was initially performed in older children and gradually adapted to younger infants.

Incidence

Tetralogy of Fallot is estimated to occur approximately two times per 10,000 live births.[15,36] It is among the three most common cardiac lesions necessitating cardiac catheterization or surgery in the first year of life[15,23] and accounts for about 10 per cent of patients seen in large pediatric cardiology clinics.[30]

Pathology

Of the four elements of Fallot's "tetralogy," the most variable is the degree of pulmonary stenosis. The subvalvular portion of the right ventricle, the infundibulum, is so invariably hypoplastic that some have considered this abnormality the true hallmark of the malformation.[52] The pulmonary valve itself is commonly bicuspid and stenotic, and the pulmonary annulus is frequently hypoplastic. Pulmonary artery anatomy is variable, ranging from near normal to extremely hypoplastic. The left and right pulmonary arteries may be stenotic at their origins or discontinuous, and either may be isolated from the main pulmonary artery and perfused from a patent ductus arteriosus or collateral vessel.

The ventricular septal defect in tetralogy of Fallot is located in the perimembranous portion of the ventricular septum and is bordered superiorly by the aortic annulus.[44] The defect is typically large and nonrestrictive. Rarely, it may be occluded by portions of the tricuspid valve. The conduction system passes posterior and inferior to the defect.[31] In 4 to 7 per cent of cases, there are additional muscular ventricular septal defects.[13]

The aortic root overrides or straddles the ventricular septum to a variable degree, a finding that is well demonstrated by echocardiography and angiocardiography. In general, there is an inverse relationship between the size of the main pulmonary artery and that of the aortic root. Thus, in patients with extremely hypoplastic pulmonary arteries, the aorta tends to be very large and half or more of its diameter appears to be "committed" to the right ventricle.

The final element of the tetralogy is right ventricular hypertrophy, which is simply the result of the systemic pressure in the right ventricle.

The most extreme form of tetralogy of Fallot is the lesion called pulmonary atresia with ventricular septal defect, sometimes referred to as pseudotruncus arteriosus. In this lesion, the right venticular outflow tract ends blindly with atresia of the pulmonary valve and in some cases the entire main pulmonary artery. The anatomy of the distal pulmonary arteries is quite variable, and pulmonary blood flow is provided by collateral vessels arising from the descending aorta and occasionally from the subclavian or innominate arteries.[27,29,32,41,51]

Additional associated anatomic findings in tetralogy include right aortic arch in 20 to 25 per cent of cases, origin of the anterior descending coronary artery from the right coronary artery,[9,28,35] and secundum atrial septal defect.

Hemodynamics

The presence of the large ventricular septal defect and pulmonary stenosis produces virtually identical pressures in the left and right ventricles. Shunting across the ventricular septal defect is typically bidirectional. If there is only mild right ventricular outflow obstruction, the predominant shunt will be left to right and systemic arterial saturation may be normal. With more severe degrees of right ventricular outflow obstruction, there is a greater degree of right-to-left shunting through the ventricular septal defect and thus increasing systemic arterial desaturation. In the neonate, the foramen ovale is patent and there may be additional intracardiac right-to-left shunting at atrial level.

The degree of right ventricular outflow obstruction in many patients is relatively fixed and determined by the degree of pulmonary valvular stenosis and pulmonary arterial hypoplasia; thus, on a moment-to-moment basis the systemic arterial saturation is largely determined by systemic vascular resistance. The degree of hypoxenia will increase if systemic arterial pressure and resistance fall as a result of hypovolemia, fever, exercise, or drugs that produce peripheral vasodilation.[46] Conversely, systemic arterial saturation is increased by conditions that increase systemic pressure and thus decrease the amount of intracardiac right-to-left shunting. For this reason, the knee-chest position and systemic vasoconstrictors such as methoxamine and phenylephrine are used to treat hypercyanotic spells.

Conversely, some infants have a variable degree of infundibular pulmonary stenosis that can increase with increases in heart rate and sympathetic stimulation. These patients can often be improved with beta blockade during a hypercyanotic spell. In addition, chronic therapy can abolish spells in selected patients.

Clinical Features

In patients with severe pulmonary stenosis, cyanosis is present immediately after birth. In patients with less severe pulmonary stenosis, cyanosis may not be apparent until later in the first year of life. Likewise, the cyanosis may be variable and present only during times of exertion such as feeding or crying.

Patients with tetralogy of Fallot who have forward flow out the right ventricle to the pulmonary artery have systolic murmurs that are present at birth. The murmur is due to the pulmonary stenosis since flow across the ventricular septal defect does not reach the velocity necessary for audible turbulence. There is an inverse relationship between intensity of the systolic murmur and degree of pulmonary blood flow and therefore intensity of cyanosis. Precordial examination reveals a right ventricular parasternal lift and a single second sound. Patients with pulmonary atresia may have no murmur, a typical patent ductus murmur at the upper left sternal border, or continuous murmurs throughout both lung fields consistent with major pulmonary collateral arteries. These patients may have an aortic ejection click.

Patients with pulmonary atresia usually will have a PO_2 similar to that found in patients with TGA. With a widely patent ductus, a PO_2 in the 50s is common and cyanosis is absent. These patients can show rapid and severe deterioration with ductal constriction.

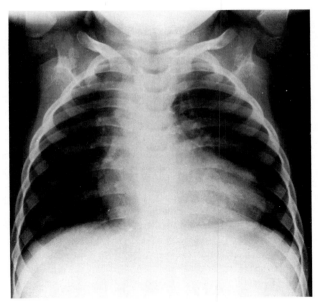

Figure 46–5. Posteroanterior chest film of a newborn infant with pulmonary atresia and large ventricular septal defect. There is a narrow mediastinum, concave main pulmonary artery segment, right aortic arch, and dark lung fields with decreased pulmonary vascular markings.

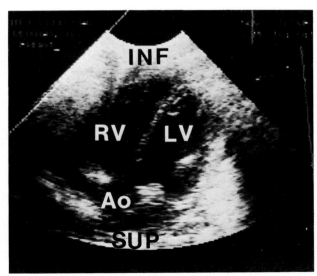

Figure 46–6. Echocardiogram from an apical four-chamber view showing a large ventricular septal defect with overriding aorta in an infant with tetralogy of Fallot. Ao = aorta; INF = inferior; LV = left ventricle; RV = right ventricle; SUP = superior.

A chest radiograph in this situation frequently shows a similar cardiac configuration to that found in TGA with a narrow mediastinum and concave main pulmonary artery segment (Fig. 46–5). Pulmonary blood flow is usually decreased except in those patients with prominent major pulmonary collateral arteries or widely patent ductus. A right aortic arch is formed in about 25 per cent of patients. Occasionally neonates with tetralogy have a virtually normal chest radiograph. The ECG usually shows right ventricular dominance and may show right atrial enlargement. If right ventricular hypertrophy is not present, an alternative diagnosis should be considered.

Echocardiography/Doppler Findings

Echocardiography/Doppler evaluation will demonstrate a large subaortic ventricular septal defect and a large aorta that overrides the ventricular septum (Fig. 46–6). The defect is usually well seen on precordial long axis, subcostal, and apical four-chamber views. Demonstration of right ventricular outflow tract hypoplasia, a thickened pulmonary valve, and hypoplastic pulmonary arterial tree confirm the diagnosis and exclude truncus arteriosus, which also has an overriding root. Precordial and suprasternal views can be used to demonstrate continuity or lack of continuity between the main pulmonary artery and the major branches, the diameter of the main pulmonary artery, right and left pulmonary arteries, the presence of a ductus arteriosus, and the anatomy of the aortic arch and its branch vessels.[24] Doppler echocardiography can be used to provide additional confirmation of antegrade pulmonary flow and/or continuous or diastolic pulmonary flow, indicating that a patent ductus or major pulmonary collateral arteries are present. Doppler studies are useful in order to determine whether there is antegrade flow from the right ventricle to the pulmonary artery or whether there is only continuous or diastolic flow, indicating that the patient is either ductal dependent or has major pulmonary collateral arteries.

Management

Prostaglandin E_1 is indicated in all patients with severe cyanosis who are ductal dependent or questionably ductal dependent. Patients who are minimally cyanotic and whose clinical findings and echocardiographic data indicate antegrade flow from the right ventricle to the pulmonary artery and no patent ductus usually do not require cardiac catheterization as neonates. Patients whose pulmonary blood flow appears ductal dependent or questionably ductal dependent usually will require catheterization to delineate the sites of origin of the pulmonary flow. Right ventricular angiography in the "sitting-up" view can delineate the extent and severity of infundibular stenosis, valvular stenosis, annular size, pulmonary artery size, and the presence or absence of branch stenosis (Fig. 46–7). Aortic root angiography will delineate the ductus, and descending aortic injection can detect whether major pulmonary collateral arteries are present. In addition, the pulmonary artery anatomy should be delineated with aortic injections in patients with pulmonary atresia. Particular data should be obtained in regard to the size of the main pulmonary artery and branches, continuity between main and major branches, the question of branch stenosis, and major pulmonary collateral arteries. When collateral arteries are present they will require careful delineation in regard to the bronchopulmonary segments that are supplied by both the true pulmonary artery and collateral arteries. Such studies

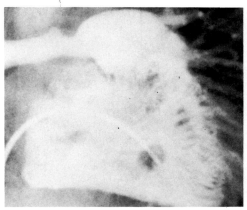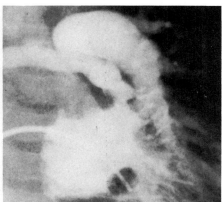

Figure 46–7. Right ventricular diastolic (A) and systolic (B) angiograms in the sitting-up view showing severe infundibular pulmonary stenosis, mildly thickened pulmonary valve, large left pulmonary artery, relatively small right pulmonary artery, and aortic opacification.

A   B

involving selective injection of collaterals and/or pulmonary venous wedge angiography are usually reserved for the older infant with stable pulmonary flow.

In patients who have limited pulmonary blood flow or who are ductal dependent, systemic pulmonary shunting (see Chapter 60) or primary repair (see Chapter 64) is required. The Blalock-Taussig anastomosis is the shunt of choice with modification using a 5-mm Gore-Tex tube or the standard shunt giving equally good palliation in most centers. The classic Blalock-Taussig shunt is performed on the side opposite the aortic arch in order to use the innominate artery and to avoid kinking of the subclavian artery as it is brought down into the mediastinum. Patients with aberrant origin of the subclavian artery from the descending aorta usually cannot have this vessel used for shunting, and thus an approach using a Gore-Tex interposition graft is required.

Patients who have ductal origin of the left pulmonary artery with either severe stenosis or atresia of the left pulmonary–main pulmonary artery junction must be delineated early in infancy in order to put a shunt into the left pulmonary artery and save this vessel for future reparative operation.

Operative repair of tetralogy of Fallot is most commonly done in patients who are over 12 to 18 months of age.[6,25] Occasionally patients who reach 6 to 9 months of age have good pulmonary artery anatomy (main pulmonary artery greater than or equal to one third the size of the ascending aorta) can be candidates for primary repair at this time. Primary repair in younger patients has been performed, but mortality appears to be slightly higher.[25] More recent results with neonatal primary repair of symptomatic infants with favorable anatomy appear to be encouraging (see Chapter 64).

Patients with hypoplastic pulmonary arteries are difficult to treat because the arteries themselves are abnormal and may not dilate with shunts. In such patients the right and left pulmonary arteries prior to branching are usually only 1 to 2 mm in diameter. Attempts to enlarge these arteries with the use of preliminary shunts or by establishment of continuity between the right ventricle and main pulmonary artery without ventricular septal defect closure have met with mixed success.[14] These procedures are suc-

cessful in some patients in achieving adequate pulmonary arteries for later reparative operation. Generally, surgery in the first year of life is required to achieve optimal growth of these pulmonary arteries.

In older patients careful delineation of the collateral arteries in regard to their distribution is extraordinarily important. In situations in which the main pulmonary artery does not distribute to all lobes, attempts at unifocalization of pulmonary blood flow have been attempted. In this procedure collarteral arteries are anastomosed to the main pulmonary artery or to other collateral arteries, the aortic connection is ligated, and a Blalock-Taussig or modified Blalock-Taussig shunt is performed to provide blood supply to an entire lung. In complex cases, this procedure usually has to be performed on both right and left lungs at separate operations.

Long-term results for these patients depend on the size of their pulmonary arteries and the ability to perform effective repair with resultant postoperative right ventricular pressure that is half systemic or less. Of particular importance in the neonate is palliation without distortion of the pulmonary arteries for future repair. Patients with pulmonary regurgitation and elevated pulmonary artery pressure either due to distorted pulmonary arteries, peripheral pulmonary stenosis, or pulmonary vascular disease do poorly and frequently require a homograft or another type of valved conduit from right ventricle to pulmonary artery. Pulmonary regurgitation in the absence of elevated pulmonary artery pressure is tolerated well with excellent long-term results.

TRUNCUS ARTERIOSUS

Historical Perspective

The first clinical and pathologic descriptions of truncus arteriosus are attributed to Buchanan (1864),[5] who described a 6½-month-old child. Collett and Edwards[8] described the pathologic features of 80 cases in 1949 and provided the first classification system. Rastelli and associates[43] demonstrated the feasibility of using a homograft and the modern era of treatment for this complex

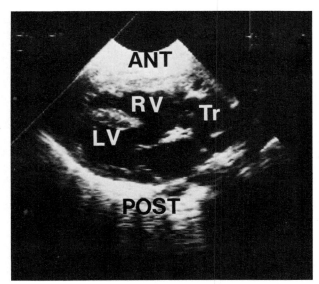

Figure 46-8. Long axis parasternal view from an infant with truncus arteriosus showing a large ventricular septal defect, overriding the truncal root and the pulmonary artery origin from the truncus. ANT = anterior; LV = left ventricle; POST = posterior; RV = right ventricle; Tr = truncus.

malformation was ushered in by McGoon and associates[34] in 1968, with their report of successful repair.

Incidence

Truncus arteriosus is a relatively rare malformation that accounts for approximately 1.5 per cent of critical congenital heart disease occurring in infancy.[15] The overall occurrence is 3 in 100,000 live births, and females slightly outnumber males (58:42).[15] Extracardiac anomalies are relatively common, and the DiGeorge syndrome should be considered in any infant with this defect.

Pathology

Truncus arteriosus is a large truncal root overriding a large outlet ventricular septal defect with the pulmonary arteries arising from the ascending aorta. Associated anomalies in this situation include right aortic arch and occasionally patent ductus. In addition, mild abnormalities of the truncal valve are relatively common but significant truncal regurgitation occurs in a relatively small number and truncal stenosis is very rare. The pulmonary artery origins are usually unobstructed and can be either the so-called truncus type I in which there is a main pulmonary artery segment that then branches into right and left pulmonary arteries or the combined types II or III in which the pulmonary arteries arise separately or as a single orifice from the truncal root without a significant length of main pulmonary artery. The surgical distinction between these groups is minimal.

Patients with truncus arteriosus usually have unobstructed pulmonary blood flow and show signs of pro-

gressive congestive heart failure with the postnatal fall in pulmonary vascular resistance. Congestive heart failure occurs somewhat earlier than in patients with isolated ventricular septal defect, and clinical signs of significant congestive failure can occur in the first 1 or 2 weeks of life. Low aortic diastolic pressures are common and result in a wide pulse pressure and decreased coronary perfusion pressure. It has been postulated that the combination of high myocardial oxygen demand and relatively decreased supply makes these patients susceptible to subendocardial ischemia. Subendocardial ischemia may account for the frequent clinical deterioration of these patients early in infancy after severe congestive heart failure develops.

Clinical Features

Physical examination in the patient with truncus arteriosus shows increased pulse pressure with bounding pulses, increased precordial activity, and mild to insignificant cyanosis. A constant ejection click is frequently present. A prominent diastolic rumble of increased pulmonary blood flow is common, and there may be a systolic murmur that can go into diastole at the upper left sternal border. A diastolic decrescendo murmur of truncal insufficiency may be present but is difficult to characterize as separate from the loud apical diastolic rumble.

Arterial blood gas determinations in the patient with truncus arteriosus show mild desaturation and usually improve very little if any with hyperoxia.

The chest radiograph in the patient with truncus arteriosus shows a relatively narrow mediastinum with cardiomegaly and increased pulmonary blood flow. A right aortic arch is found in about 25 per cent of patients, as is the case with tetralogy of Fallot. The ECG usually shows biventricular hypertrophy and biatrial enlargement. ST segment depression and negative T waves over the lateral precordium can be present and are suggestive of subendocardial ischemia.

Echocardiography/Doppler studies are extremely helpful in the diagnosis of truncus arteriosus. The long axis view usually shows the large outlet ventricular defect with overriding large truncal root (Fig. 46-8). With careful attention to the aortic root, the aortic arch position and pulmonary artery origin are frequently ascertained. Clinically, truncus arteriosus and aorticopulmonary window are similar. In aorticopulmonary window, however, there is no ventricular septal defect and a pulmonary valve can be found. Doppler studies are helpful in determining whether truncal regurgitation is present.

Catheterization usually is indicated in truncus arteriosus to determine the size and branching pattern of the main pulmonary artery if present. Of particular importance is an aortogram (Fig. 46-9) to rule out truncal insufficiency and also any major stenoses in pulmonary arteries, which are rare. Patients with hemitruncus, in which only one pulmonary artery arises from the aorta, can be readily differentiated angiographically since they have a pulmonary valve and right ventricular origin of one of the pulmonary arteries.

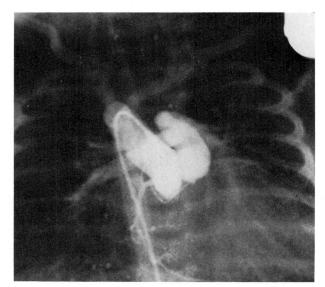

Figure 46–9. Truncal root angiogram in an infant with truncus arteriosus in posteroanterior orientation showing the pulmonary artery arising from the sinus of Valsalva, no truncal regurgitation, and the right aortic arch.

Management of truncus arteriosus consists of vigorous treatment for congestive failure with cardiac glycosides and diuretics. In general, these patients are poorly responsive to medical therapy and severe congestive failure along with inadequate growth and nutrition persist despite medical treatment. Early surgical repair is the treatment of choice. A homograft is placed between the right ventricle and pulmonary artery, and the ventricular septal defect is closed; the left ventricle alone remains in continuity with aorta. Patients with significant truncal regurgitation have an increased operative risk. In the absence of truncal regurgitation, mortality ranges from 10 to 20 per cent.[3,10,47–49]

Those patients who survive the initial operative repair generally require reoperation within 3 to 5 years for either progressive conduit stenosis or simply because they have outgrown their initial graft. The use of homografts as conduits may delay the need for a second operation.

Patients with truncus arteriosus who undergo repair of the defect in infancy have usually shown reasonably good right and left ventricular function when assessed several years after surgery.[38] However, patients who are palliated initially and have a conduit or homograft operation later frequently show myocardial dysfunction.[38] These data support the earlier observation that chronic cyanosis and volume or pressure overloading can cause ventricular dysfunction,[16,20] and give further impetus for early operative repair.

CONCLUSIONS

Conotruncal abnormalities constitute the majority of infants who present with symptomatic cyanotic congenital heart disease during the first year of life. Early diagnosis and appropriate management can result in normal growth and development for most of these children. Significant problems still remain in determining optimal management strategies and appropriate timing of surgical intervention. These issues represent a continued challenge to the cardiologists and surgeons caring for these infants.

References

1. Allan LD, Leanage R, Wainwright R, Joseph MC, Tynan M (1982): Balloon atrial septostomy under two-dimensional echocardiographic control. Br Heart J 47:41–43.
2. Anderson RH, Becker AE, Lucchese FA, Meier MA, Rigby ML, Sato B (1983): Morphology of Congenital Heart Disease. Tunbridge Wells, Castle House, pp 84–100.
3. Applebaum A, Bargeron LM, Pacifico AD, Kirklin JW (1976): Surgical treatment of truncus arteriosus, with emphasis on infants and small children. J Thorac Cardiovasc Surg 71:436–442.
4. Blalock A, Taussig HB (1945): The surgical treatment of malformations of the heart in which there is pulmonary stenosis or pulmonary atresia. JAMA 128:189–202.
5. Buchanan A (1864): Malformation of the heart: Undivided truncus arteriosus: Heart otherwise double. Trans Path Soc Lond 15:89.
6. Castañeda AR, Freed MD, Williams RG (1977): Repair of tetralogy of Fallot in infancy: Early and late results. J Thorac Cardiovasc Surg 74:372–380.
7. Castañeda AR, Norwood WI, Jonas RA, Colan SD, Sanders SP, Lang P (1984): Transposition of the great arteries and intact ventricular septum: Anatomical repair in the neonate. Ann Thorac Surg 38:438–443.
8. Collett RW, Edwards JE (1949): Persistent truncus arteriosus: A classification according to anatomic types. Surg Clin North Am 29:1245–1270.
9. Dabizzi RP, Giuseppe C, Aiazzi L, Castelli C, Baldrighi G, Parenzan L, Baldrighi V (1980): Distribution and anomalies of coronary arteries in tetralogy of Fallot. Circulation 61:95–102.
10. Ebert PA, Robinson SJ, Stanger P, Engle MA (1976): Pulmonary artery conduits in infants younger than six months of age. J Thorac Cardiovasc Surg 72:351–356.
11. Fallot A (1888): Contribution of l'anatomie pathologique de la maladie (bleue cyanose cardiaque). Marseille Med Med 25:77, 138, 297, 341, 403.
12. Fanconi G (1932): Die transposition der grossen Gefässe (das charakteristsche Röntgenbild). Arch Kinderheilkd 95:202.
13. Fellows KE, Smith J, Keane JF (1981): Preoperative angiography in infants with tetrad of Fallot: Review of 36 cases. Am J Cardiol 47:1279–1285.
14. Freedom RM, Pangiglione G, Williams WG, Trusler GA, Rowe RD (1983): Palliative right ventricular outflow tract construction of patients with pulmonary atresia, ventricular septal defect, and hypoplastic pulmonary arteries. J Thorac Cardiovasc Surg 86:24–36.
15. Fyler DC, Buckley LP, Hellenbrand WE, Cohn HE, Kirklin JW, Nadas AS, Cartier JM, Breibart MH (1980): Report of the New England Regional Cardiac Program. Pediatrics 65(suppl):375–461.
16. Graham TP (1982): Ventricular performance in adults after operation for congenital heart disease. Am J Cardiol 50:612–620.
17. Graham TP (1982): Hemodynamic residua and sequelae following intra-atrial repair of transposition of the great arteries: A review. Pediatr Cardiol 2:203–213.
18. Graham TP, Atwood GF, Boucek RJ, Boerth RC, Nelson JH (1975): Right heart volume characteristics in transposition of the great arteries. Circulation 51:881–889.
19. Graham TP, Burger J, Bender HW, Hammon JW, Boucek RJ, Appleton S (1985): Improved right ventricular function after intra-atrial repair of transposition of the great arteries. Circulation 72(suppl II):45–51.
20. Graham TP, Erath HG, Boucek RJ, Boerth RC (1980): Left ventricular function in cyanotic congenital heart disease. Am J Cardiol 45:1231–1236.
21. Graham TP, Franklin RCG, Wyse RKH, Gooch V, Deanfield JE (1987): Left ventricular wall stress and contractile function in transposition of the great arteries following Rastelli operation. J Thorac Cardiovasc Surg 93:775–784.

22. Graham TP, Jarmakani JM, Canent RV, Jewett PH (1971): Quantification of left heart volume and systolic output in transposition of the great arteries. Circulation 51:889–909.

23. Gutgesell HP, Garson A Jr, Hesslein P, Park I, McNamara DG (1982): Prognosis for the neonate and infant with congenital heart disease (abstr). Pediatr Cardiol 2:168.

24. Gutgesell HP, Huhta JC, Cohen MH, Latson LA (1984): Two-dimensional echocardiographic assessment of pulmonary artery and aortic arch anatomy in cyanotic infants. J Am Coll Cardiol 4:1242–1246.

25. Hammon JW, Henry CL, Merrill WH, Graham TP, Bender HW (1985): Tetralogy of Fallot: Selective surgical management can minimize operative mortality. Ann Thorac Surg 40:280–284.

26. Harris JS, Farber S (1939): Transposition of the great arteries with special reference to the phylogenetic theory of Spitzer. Arch Pathol 28:427–502.

27. Haworth SB, Macartney FJ (1980): Growth and development of pulmonary circulation in pulmonary atresia with ventricular septal defect and major aortopulmonary collateral arteries. Br Heart J 44:14–24.

28. Hurwitz RA, Smith W, King H, Girod DA, Caldwell RL (1980): Tetralogy of Fallot with abnormal coronary artery: 1967 to 1977. J Thorac Cardiovasc Surg 80:129–134.

29. Jefferson K, Rees S, Somerville J (1972): Systemic arterial supply to the lungs in pulmonary atresia and its relation to pulmonary artery development. Br Heart J 34:418–427.

30. Keith JD (1978): In Keith JD, Rowe RD, Vlad P (eds): Heart Disease in Infancy and Childhood. 34th ed. New York, Macmillan, p 5.

31. Lev M (1959): The architecture of the conduction system in congenital heart disease: II. Tetralogy of Fallot. Arch Pathol 67:527–587.

32. Liao P-K, Edwards WD, Julsrud PR, Puga FJ, Danielson GK, Feldt RH (1985): Pulmonary blood supply in patients with pulmonary atresia and ventricular septal defect. J Am Coll Cardiol 6:1343–1350.

33. Lillehei CW, Cohen M, Warden HE, Read RC, Aust JB, DeWall RA, Varco RL (1955): Direct vision intracardiac surgical correction of the tetralogy of Fallot, pentalogy of Fallot, and pulmonary atresia defects. Ann Surg 142:418–445.

34. McGoon DC, Rastelli GC, Ongley PA (1968): An operation for the correction of truncus arteriosus. JAMA 205:69–73.

35. Meyer J, Chiariello L, Hallman GL, Cooley DA (1975): Coronary artery anomalies in patients with tetralogy of Fallot. J Thorac Cardiovasc Surg 69:373–376.

36. Mitchell SC, Korones SB, Berendes HW (1971): Congenital heart disease in 56,109 births: Incidence and natural history. Circulation 43:323–332.

37. Nora JJ (1983): Etiologic aspects of heart diseases. In Adams FH, Emmanouilides GC (eds): Heart Disease in Infants, Children, and Adolescents. 3rd ed. Baltimore, Williams & Wilkins, pp 2–10.

38. Palik I, Graham TP, Burger J (1986): Ventricular pump performance in patients with obstructed right ventricular-pulmonary artery conduits. Am Heart J 112:1271–1278.

39. Perry LW, Ruckman RN, Galioto FM, Shapiro SR, Potter BM, Scott LP (1982): Echocardiographically assisted balloon atrial septostomy. Pediatrics 70:403–408.

40. Quaegebeur JM, Rohmer J, Ottenkamp J, Buis T, Kirklin JW, Blockstone EH, Brown AG (1986): The arterial switch: An eight year experience. J Thorac Cardiovasc Surg 92:361–384.

41. Rabinovitch M, Herrera-deLeon V, Casteneda AR, Reid L (1981): Growth and development of the pulmonary vascular bed in patients with tetralogy of Fallot with or without pulmonary atresia. Circulation 64:1234–1249.

42. Rashkind WJ, Miller WM (1966): Creation of an atrial septal defect without thoracotomy: A palliative approach to complete transposition of the great arteries. JAMA 196:991–992.

43. Rastelli GC, Titus JL, McGoon DC (1967): Homograft of ascending aorta and aortic valve as a right ventricular outflow: An experimental approach to repair of truncus arteriosus. Arch Surg 95:698–707.

44. Rosenquist GC, Sweeney LJ, Stemple DR, Christianson SD, Rowe RD (1973): Ventricular septal defect in tetralogy of Fallot. Am J Cardiol 31:749–754.

45. Sanders SP (1984): Echocardiography and related techniques in the diagnosis of congenital heart defects: III. Conotruncus and great arteries. Echocardiography 1:443–493.

46. Shah PM, Kidd L (1967): Circulatory effects of propranolol in children with Fallot's tetralogy. Am J Cardiol 19:653–657.

47. Spicer RL, Behrendt D, Crowley DC, Dick M, Rocchini AP, Uzark K, Rosenthal A, Sloan H (1984): Repair of truncus arteriosus in neonates with the use of a valveless conduit. Circulation 70(suppl I):26–29.

48. Stark J, Gandhi D, deLeval M, Macartney F, Taylor JFN (1978): Surgical treatment of truncus arteriosus in the first year of life. Br Heart J 40:1280–1287.

49. Sullivan H, Sulayman R, Repogle R, Arcilla RA (1976): Surgical correction of truncus arteriosus in infancy. Am J Cardiol 38:113–117.

50. Taussig HB (1949): Complete transposition of the aorta and a levoposition of the pulmonary artery: Clinical physiological and pathological findings. Am Heart J 37:551–559.

51. Thiene G, Frescura C, V Bortolotti U, Del Maschio A, Valente M (1981): The systemic pulmonary circulation in pulmonary atresia with ventricular septal defect: Concept of reciprocal development of the fourth and six aortic arches. Am Heart J 101:339–344.

52. Van Praagh R, Van Praagh S, Nebesar RA, Muster AJ, Sinha SN, Paul MH (1970): Tetralogy of Fallot: Underdevelopment of the pulmonary infundibulum and its sequelae. Am J Cardiol 26:25–33.

53. Willius FA (1948): Cardiac Clinics CXXIV: An unusually early description of the so-called tetralogy of Fallot. Proc Staff Mayo Clin 23:316–320.

47 NEONATAL CARDIAC INFECTIONS

William Jackson
William Pinsky

HISTORICAL PERSPECTIVE

Pathologists have recognized vegetations within the neonatal heart since at least the late nineteenth century. In 1885, Ayrolles described impressive cardiac vegetations at autopsy in a 10-day-old child whose mother had developed sepsis-like findings just prior to delivery.[2] The first report of bacterial cardiac vegetations in a newborn was in 1894 by Bidone, who identified a probable streptococcus.[5]

The first well-described pathologic findings in neonatal myocarditis were probably described in a 1926 report of a 13-day-old infant with a fairly prolonged course of bronchitis.[42] Most cases of neonatal myocarditis reported in the first half of the nineteenth century were idiopathic. The coxsackieviruses were not described until 1947. With the advent of modern virology, the number of cases of idiopathic myocarditis has decreased rapidly.

ENDOCARDITIS

Epidemiology

Neonatal endocarditis has long been considered exceedingly rare, but sound data on its incidence are lacking. Almost all instances of neonatal endocarditis reported between 1852 and 1953 were individual case reports. Macaulay's 1954 summary of the literature on endocarditis included 109 cases in infants less than 2 years of age; nine (8 per cent) of these were neonatal patients.[25] In the largest pediatric autopsy study of endocarditis, 1535 patients less than 2 years of age underwent autopsy between 1930 and 1972; the incidence of endocarditis was 0.2 per cent (12/1535).[19] No case of neonatal endocarditis was identified.[19] From these observations it seems clear that neonatal endocarditis was indeed rare in the preantibiotic and early antibiotic eras.

The success of increasingly intensive neonatal care over the past 20 years has resulted in more cases of neonatal endocarditis and, again, more individual case reports. A review of these cases suggests that neonates with indwelling intravascular catheters are predisposed to endocarditis, especially when gastrointestinal surgery is also required. Premature infants and term infants with congenital heart diseases also appear frequently in these case reports of neonatal endocarditis.

Etiology

The newborn infant has increased susceptibility to infection for several reasons. Although the uterus and placenta are impervious to many pathogens, a large number of pathogens can gain access to the fetus through the placenta or membranes or can infect the fetus during vaginal delivery. Protective maternal antibodies are passively received by the fetus, but other components of the fetal and neonatal immune system are well documented to be defective. Neonatal antibody synthesis does not seem effective when compared with that of older infants and children. Complement activity and T-lymphocyte function are decreased in neonates. Phagocytic migration and microbicidal activity are diminished. Despite these immune defects, endocarditis remains very rare in newborns without additional risk factors such as indwelling intravascular catheters, gastrointestinal surgery, or congenital heart disease.

Low-Risk Infants

Beta-hemolytic streptococcus appears to be the most frequent cause of neonatal endocarditis in low-risk neonates, and streptococcal maternal sepsis is usually present. Large vegetations within the neonatal heart have been documented in three of these cases.[27,40] Vegetations are more frequently located on the mitral valve or its chordae tendineae cordis than on the tricuspid valve; involvement of the pulmonic and aortic valves has not been reported. In neonatal endocarditis due to *Staphylococcus aureus*, another focus of infection is often evident clinically that obscures cardiac involvement, and endocarditis is not recognized until autopsy.[6,11] Common foci of staphylococcal infection-obscuring endocarditis include skin and umbilical infections. One case of neonatal endocarditis secondary to *Escherichia coli* infection has been reported; a large mitral vegetation was present.[27]

High-Risk Infants

The incidence of neonatal endocarditis is highest in patients with indwelling intravascular catheters. Endothelial injury from venous catheter contact with the superior vena cava, inferior vena cava, right atrial surface (most commonly the atrial septum in the region of the fossa ovalis), left atrial surface, or the atrial surface of the tricuspid valve may predispose to endocarditis.[27,37,41] In animal models of endocarditis a catheter is left in place for varying periods before bacteria are injected into the blood, either peripherally or through the catheter. The endothelial damage produced by the catheter has been shown to allow more rapid endothelial adherence of bacteria.[4,9,33,39] Staphylococci have been shown to stimulate the production of tissue

571

thromboplastin after endothelial adherence. Tissue thromboplastin activates coagulation by the extrinsic pathway, which causes deposition of fibrin at the site of endothelial injury and subsequent vegetation accretion. Unfortunately, the mechanism by which bacteria stimulate tissue thromboplastin production has not been demonstrated. The release of lipoteichoic acid or cytotoxin may mediate this effect.

Even in the absence of bacteria, in animals catheters can cause sterile vegetations that mimic similar sterile vegetations found in infants. Such sterile vegetations are usually termed non-bacterial thrombotic endocarditis (NBTE); less is known of the cellular processes that produce NBTE than of those that cause bacterial infections. A number of investigators have suggested that NBTE lesions are more common than currently appreciated.[30,37] Lesions of NBTE can be found incidentally in the right heart at autopsy; usually in such cases numerous small fibrinous pulmonary emboli can also be found if the lungs are carefully studied. NBTE lesions have also been found in the aorta near the ductus arteriosus (presumably secondary to high umbilical arterial catheters), but distal embolization is poorly documented. Such sterile vegetations at whatever location offer a nidus of infection for bacteria or fungi. *S. epidermidis* and *S. aureus* are the most common pathogens in neonates who develop endocarditis during the use of vigorous supportive measures, including indwelling catheters. The duration of catheter placement prior to infection has been as short as 5 days in one reported case of neonatal endocarditis.[37] The most common fungal pathogen in neonatal endocarditis is *Candida albicans*. Case reports of *Candida* endocarditis suggest that indwelling catheters and parenteral hyperalimentation are significant risk factors.[7,13,16,20]

Clinical Findings

Early signs and symptoms of neonatal endocarditis are indistinguishable from those of neonatal sepsis. The sudden appearance of temperature imbalance with even brief periods of hyper- or hypothermia may be the earliest indication. Tachypnea, relative tachycardia, apnea (especially the reappearance of apneic episodes), vomiting, diarrhea, lethargy, and disinterest in feeding may occur as initial manifestations. Petechiae, major embolic events, jaundice, seizures, and hepatosplenomegaly are usually seen as later findings. Few physical findings suggestive of endocarditis in older infants and children are reported in neonates with endocarditis. Isolated splenomegaly, splinter hemorrhages, conjunctival hemorrhages, a new or changing murmur, Osler nodes, Janeway lesions, and Roth spots are apparently rare in neonatal endocarditis. In most reported cases with vegetations at subsequent autopsy, recognition of any abnormal signs or symptoms has preceded death by only 48 to 72 hours. This rapidly progressive course following the onset of recognizable signs has made neonatal bacterial endocarditis an autopsy diagnosis in the majority of reported cases. The most important clinical finding is the history of indwelling catheters or previous surgical manipulation during the infant's clinical course.

Laboratory Findings

Laboratory findings of importance are positive blood cultures, especially of *S. epidermidis* in the presence of a catheter, thrombocytopenia, anemia, and hematuria. Echocardiographic confirmation of a significant vegetation is the single most helpful diagnostic study (Fig. 47–1). The lesions must usually be greater than 2 mm for the echo-

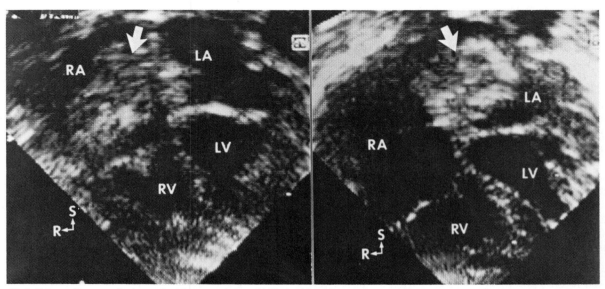

Figure 47–1. Echocardiogram of a 1-month-old preterm infant (1100 g) with a history of an umbilical venous catheter for 3 weeks. The mass, which migrated through the foramen ovale, is shown within the right atrium initially and later within the left atrium. Multiple blood cultures were positive for *Staphylococcus epidermidis*. LA = left atrium; LV = left ventricle; R = right; RA = right atrium; RV = right ventricle; S = superior.

cardiogram to be specific. The increasing use of color flow Doppler echocardiography should offer better specificity for small vegetations associated with minor valvular regurgitation.

Differential Diagnosis

Neonatal endocarditis presents as a nonspecific systemic illness and therefore has a wide differential diagnosis. Sepsis from any etiology may precede endocarditis and cause a fulminant course in neonates. Thrombocytopenia and intravascular coagulation as a result of sepsis or other etiologies may simulate the course of neonatal endocarditis. Neonatal hematuria is most often associated with renal deformities or noncardiac infection. Echocardiography may confuse rare intracardiac tumors with endocarditis, although only the very rare small tumor limited to valvular surfaces should resemble valvular vegetations.

Clinical Course

Most reports of neonatal endocarditis have described a rapidly fatal course despite appropriate intervention for presumed sepsis. The patients routinely had blood and urine cultures and less frequently cerebral spinal fluid cultures. These were done when the initial signs of sepsis were noted. Variations in the clinical course of these reported cases then became more evident. McGuinness, Schieken, and Maguire[27] described a preterm infant who presented with apnea and bradycardia requiring reintubation at 4 weeks of age. *S. epidermidis* grew from the initial (drawn through a central venous line) and subsequent blood cultures despite therapy with methicillin sodium. By 7 weeks of age, a murmur had developed along with massive hepatosplenomegaly. An echocardiogram confirmed a mass in the right atrium attached to the tricuspid valve. Even after well-monitored antibiotic therapy with cephalothin, blood cultures remained positive for the same appropriately sensitive *S. epidermidis* until the patient's death at 11 weeks of age. A second pathogen, *Serratia* sp., grew from late skin and post-mortem blood cultures. This case constitutes the longest well-documented survival after recognition of neonatal endocarditis and is the exception that proves the rule of brief fulminant courses in neonatal endocarditis. Most of the events described in this case occurred over a brief 2- to 4-day period after onset of the illness.

Outcome

The prognosis of neonatal endocarditis during the antibiotic era has remained as grave as that reported in the preantibiotic era. Optimal use of antibiotics with careful monitoring of bacterial sensitivities, concentrations of antibiotic in the blood, and Schlichter levels does not seem to alter outcome. Blood cultures often remain positive despite optimal antibiotic therapy, leading to discussion of surgical removal of the intracardiac vegetations.[27] However,

intracardiac surgery for endocarditis remains impractical in these infants, who are usually small and premature. Very careful echocardiographic monitoring of infants requiring indwelling catheters could result in earlier detection of endocarditis; one infant whose endocarditis was recognized early survived.[3]

MYOCARDITIS

Epidemiology

Neonatal viral myocarditis can occur alone or as a component of a more generalized illness with accompanying encephalitis and hepatitis. In cases of generalized viral illness myocarditis is often severe. Group B coxsackieviruses are most commonly implicated in neonatal myocarditis. Other viruses documented to cause neonatal myocarditis include ECHO virus,[10] rubella virus,[1] and herpes.[14,43]

Group B Coxsackievirus

Group B coxsackieviruses have been identified in numerous epidemics over the past 30 years within newborn nurseries.[18,21,22,28] In this setting, the spread of the virus is by feces as well as by airborne contamination. The prevalence of maternal coxsackievirus infections during late gestation follows trends in the general population; peak periods of enteroviral illnesses occur during the summer months. Maternal illnesses with coxsackieviruses may manifest as minimal upper respiratory tract infections or more pronounced gastroenteritis, meningoencephalitis, hepatitis, pneumonia, and carditis. No data are available to suggest that maternal coxsackievirus infections in early and midgestation cause damage to the fetal heart. Late-gestation maternal coxsackievirus infections can cause late fetal and early neonatal infections.[22] The neonatal manifestations of coxsackievirus infection vary widely. At least 50 per cent of these neonatal infections are entirely asymptomatic and undetectable despite meticulous observation. In one of the larger nursery outbreaks, only 5 per cent of the infected newborns exhibited cardiac manifestations.[8] Group B coxsackievirus serotypes 1 through 6 have been associated with myocarditis in infants and children; types 3 and 4 are associated with more severe cases.[21,22] Serotypes have not always been identified in reported nursery epidemics of group B coxsackievirus, but these are assumed to follow the prevalence of serotypes in the remainder of the population.

Rubella Virus

The rubella virus has been shown to persist in the fetus for prolonged periods after initial infection in the first 4 months of gestation.[1] While the teratogenic effects of rubella virus are well known, studies done prior to rubella immunization programs showed a 21 per cent incidence of myocarditis at birth. Of those neonates with rubella myocarditis, 70 per cent had active disease, and 40 per cent subsequently died.

Etiology

Gross Pathology

Pathologic findings in the hearts of neonates with viral myocarditis are similar to those in similarly afflicted older infants and children. On gross examination, the heart is variably pale with occasional mottling. The external myocardial conformation is frequently described as flabby. All four chambers are usually enlarged, and either decreased ventricular wall thickness or myocardial hypertrophy is described. Cardiac weight is increased in the majority of cases diagnosed prior to death. In occasional cases cut sections show marked edema. Such pathologic findings are not specific to a particular etiologic agent. Studies from a broader age range including young infants have suggested at least one consistent finding indicative of group B coxsackievirus infections: hemorrhagic petechiae over large areas of the epicardium with corresponding thinly blood-tinged pericardial fluid.[17]

Another common finding in neonates, infants, and children with myocarditis is endocardial thickening and whitening. Several investigators have examined the possible relationship between endocardial fibroelastosis and myocarditis[15,17] and concluded that congestive cardiomyopathy found in patients with endocardial fibroelastosis could be a consequence of acute viral myocarditis. Because of recent diagnostic and therapeutic advances in fetal cardiology, the study by Hutchins and Vie published in 1972[17] may have new implications for understanding fetal and neonatal myocarditis. They examined more than 60 hearts from children diagnosed with either endocardial fibroelastosis or myocarditis. Using fairly strict criteria, the cases were re-examined, and it was shown that 64 per cent of the patients had clear features of both diseases, 28 per cent had findings only of endocardial fibroelastosis, and 8 per cent had findings only of myocarditis. These three groups had different durations of illness. When the duration of illness prior to death was longer than 4 months, the group with endocardial fibroelastosis predominated. When the duration of illness prior to death was 2 weeks to 4 months, the group with both diseases (the largest group) predominated. When duration of illness prior to death was less than 2 weeks, the group with only myocarditis predominated. This study confirmed several earlier studies linking viral myocardial involvement to endocardial fibroelastosis.[12,15] One of these earlier studies isolated group B coxsackievirus type 3 from the myocardium of 13 of 27 infants with endocardial fibroelastosis.[12]

Microscopic Pathology

Microscopic findings in viral myocarditis include interstitial collections of lymphocytes, eosinophils, and occasionally plasma cells. These collections are usually diffuse throughout the myocardium but may be focal. Unfortunately, useful microscopic markers of viral myocarditis, such as inclusion bodies, viral particles, or mononuclear cells with obvious viral involvement, are very rare.[35] However, a consistent predominance of mononuclear cells around very small vessels within the myocardium has been described in patients with group B coxsackievirus myocarditis (Fig. 47–2). Although a similar pattern has been observed in other forms of myocarditis, these other agents have not been described in neonates. As a result, perivascular mononuclear infiltrates in neonatal myocarditis are highly suggestive of group B coxsackievirus infection.

Pathophysiology

The pathophysiology of myocarditis begins with direct or indirect myocardial cell damage and concomitant interstitial inflammation. The reduced myocardial contractility resulting from this diffuse process leads to chamber enlargement over a highly variable period of time. In the presence of decreased contractility, the usual Starling mechanism (which normally increases the force of contraction and improves ejection fraction and cardiac output in response to increases in filling volume) is impaired. In fulminant myocarditis cardiac output can be increased only by increases in heart rate, and arterial pressure can be maintained only by sympathetic peripheral vasoconstriction. Such compensation is effective only for brief periods in the neonate. As ventricular dilation progresses, elevations in filling pressures are substantial; eventually, both pulmonary venous and systemic venous hypertension result. In myocarditis pulmonary edema is more common in older infants and children than in neonates, in whom clinical manifestations of classic right heart failure are more common. Neonatal patients with viral myocarditis are also more likely to develop concomitant hepatitis or meningoencephalitis.

Clinical Findings

Neonatal myocarditis, like myocarditis in older infants and children, has a wide range of severity. However, severe myocarditis with a fulminant, rapidly progressive course leading to early death is encountered more often in neonates. Such fulminant myocarditis is caused more frequently by group B coxsackieviruses than by herpes virus or rubella virus. Clinical presentation of myocarditis in the neonatal period is too often manifested by rapid circulatory collapse. In less rapidly progressive cases, the patient may initially appear quiet and listless. Fever, an unusual finding in the newborn nursery, may develop and is usually accompanied by tachycardia. Gradual pallor is noted, with eventual cooling of the skin. Tachypnea is evident with gradually increasing work of respiration and eventual grunting respirations. Heart sounds are frequently distant with indistinct splitting of the second heart sound. A gallop cadence is frequently present; once severe myocardial dysfunction develops, a loud S_3 is usually noted (as often occurs in older infants and children with severe myocarditis).

Differential Diagnosis

Myocarditis presenting during the newborn period may be difficult to recognize in its early stages. The effects of

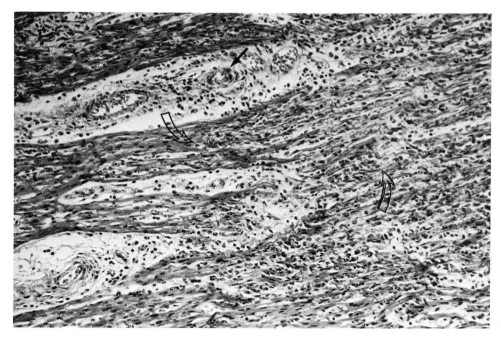

Figure 47–2. Light microphotograph of myocardium in a neonate with fatal myocarditis due to group B coxsackievirus. Note perivascular lymphocytic infiltrates (solid arrow) and patchy areas of myocyte necrosis replacing normal cellular architecture (open arrows) (hematoxylin-eosin stain, original magnification × 100).

perinatal asphyxia with variable pulmonary hypertension may frequently cause myocardial enlargement and congestive failure in the newborn (see Chapter 40). A complete, detailed gestational history and review of delivery room records may confirm fetal distress even in the absence of low Apgar scores.

Physical Examination

In the early stages of myocarditis, physical examination may not differentiate birth asphyxia from myocarditis. Distant heart sounds, especially with a pronounced third heart sound, may be more common in myocarditis. A long, harsh systolic ejection murmur clearly localized to the lower left and right sternal borders and to the hepatic area is consistent with tricuspid regurgitation secondary to birth asphyxia. This murmur must be localized carefully to differentiate it from mitral regurgitation, also an unusual finding in newborn infants with myocarditis.

Laboratory Studies

Arterial blood gas sampling may reveal hypercarbia or metabolic acidosis as the cause of myocardial dysfunction, although metabolic acidosis is also frequently found in patients with myocarditis. Low serum glucose and calcium values are frequent after birth asphyxia and can by themselves cause cardiac enlargement and congestive heart failure. A chest radiograph may demonstrate meconium aspiration and may also document unexpected findings of interstitial lung disease, such as hyaline membrane disease or pneumonia.

The echocardiogram, especially with color flow Doppler studies, may differentiate between asphyxia and myocarditis by several important findings.

In myocarditis, profoundly decreased contractility and diffuse chamber enlargement may be found on the echocardiogram at a time when clinical findings are minimal or mild. A small pericardial effusion may be present, suggesting cardiac inflammation. The usual indices of left ventricular function may be normal or only slightly depressed after birth asphyxia; echocardiograms in asphyxia frequently show enlargement of the right rather than the left ventricle and atrium. Tricuspid regurgitation suggests birth asphyxia and is often evident on color flow Doppler studies even when inaudible clinically.

Shock

Myocarditis presenting as shock in the newborn can be even more difficult to recognize. Sepsis and the hypoplastic left-heart syndrome are the most common causes of shock in the newborn infant. Sepsis with circulatory collapse and myocarditis present with similar physical findings: Infants are usually unresponsive or lethargic; have pale, gray, or mottled skin and weak or thready pulses; have hypothermia or, rarely, fever; and have hypotension with narrow pulse pressure and tachycardia. Physical findings more likely present with myocarditis than sepsis include hepatic and splenic congestion and quiet, muffled heart sounds. Findings more indicative of sepsis include obvious sources of infection (such as omphalitis or scalded skin, findings suggestive of staphylococcal infection), and a maternal history consistent with prenatal intrauterine bacterial infection. A maternal upper respiratory infection in the weeks preceding delivery may correlate with a subsequent diagnosis of myocarditis.

Clinical Course

Neonatal myocarditis has a fulminant and deadly course compared with the usual course of myocarditis in older infants and children. Given the rapid natural history of neonatal myocarditis, early treatment is essential if outcome is to be optimized. Supplemental oxygen and, if needed, prompt intubation and assisted ventilation should be instituted at once while other diagnostic or therapeutic measures are being organized. Inotropic support should also be administered early. Digoxin has significant risks because the injured myocardium is prone to arrhythmias and cannot maintain renal output. However, if low total digitalizing doses of digoxin (0.02 to 0.03 μg/kg) are given cautiously over a longer time period than usual, digoxin can be quite helpful and safe. The oral route should be used unless shock is present. Intravenous dopamine or dobutamine may be used acutely with less risk to improve contractility. The tachycardia and consequent reduction in myocardial perfusion associated with isoproterenol make this drug less attractive. Diuretics should be used when congestive heart failure develops, but careful monitoring is mandatory to prevent rapid reduction of the intravascular volume and subsequent shock. Central venous pressures as high as 12 to 15 mmHg may be necessary for filling the compromised ventricular myocardium and maintaining cardiac output. Strict, frequent monitoring of urine output, tissue perfusion, heart rate, and central venous pressure is necessary. Volume infusions of albumin, whole blood, fresh frozen plasma, or crystalloids should be utilized to achieve the optimum ventricular filling pressure. Afterload reducing agents may become necessary to improve perfusion. Nitroprusside acutely and hydralazine chronically have traditionally been used in the most severely affected infants, but captopril is presumably a better agent than hydralazine, since it is a venodilator as well as an arterial dilator. Arrhythmias noted in infants and children have been reported less frequently in neonates. Complete heart block may require temporary pacing. The appearance of supraventricular tachycardia may necessitate digoxin for adequate control.

Treatment

Current treatment for neonatal myocarditis is symptomatic rather than specific, but a number of experimental studies support the current therapy recommended for myocarditis. The rationale for maintaining blood oxygen levels within a normal range came from studies by Pearce,[32] which showed that hypoxia increased the severity of myocarditis. Adequate oxygenation is desirable, but hyperoxia may increase viral replication in mouse myocardium and double the mortality rate.[31] The fulminant course of neonatal myocarditis has not been adequately explained, although lack of interferon and serum gamma globulins in neonates could potentiate rapid viral replication. Norris and Loo[29] infected mice with Group B coxsackievirus type 3 and found that an interferon inducer had a protective effect when given 12 to 36 hours before the virus was introduced. Limitation of enteroviral infections was subsequently shown to be more

effective when type-specific antibodies were used with macrophages.[34]

The use of steroids has been debated for many years. The studies of Kilbourne, Wilson, and Perrion[23] suggested that corticosteroids given during the acute phase of myocarditis increased viral replication and myocardial necrosis. Cortisone impairment of interferon function has been demonstrated in coxsackievirus–infected mice,[36] which suggests that steroids could be harmful in coxsackievirus–induced human myocarditis. Immunosuppressive agents have been used to treat myocarditis in animals and humans; improvements in cardiac function and decreases in myocardial infiltrates were thought to occur.[18,26] However, controlled clinical trials have not been conducted in neonates or infants.

Outcome

The lowest mortality rate in a large series of neonatal myocarditis with good documentation of the disease was 75 per cent.[21,22] Most of the deaths occurred within 5 to 7 days of recognition of the illness. The late natural history of survivors remains unknown. Early and vigorous supportive measures could improve outcome, which currently is dismal, but new insights into the pathogenesis of the disease and new therapies are needed. It is possible that extracorporeal membrane oxygenator therapy or even cardiac transplantation could have a therapeutic role in the future.

References

1. Ainger, LE, Lawyer NG, Fitch CW (1966): Neonatal rubella myocarditis. Br Heart J 28:691–692.
2. Ayrolles P (1885): Endocardite congenitale generalisee: Obliteration de l'orifice mitral: cloissonnement de l'orifice tricuspide. Rev Mens Mal Enf (Paris) 3:222.
3. Barton CW, Crowley DC, Uzark K, Dick M (1984): A neonatal survivor of group B β-hemolytic streptococcal endocarditis. Am J Perinatol 3:214–215.
4. Bayer AS, Lam K (1985): Efficacy of vancomycin plus rifampin in experimental aortic valve endocarditis due to methicillin-resistant *Staphylococcus aureus*: In vitro–in vivo correlations. J Infect Dis 151:157–165.
5. Bidone E (1894): Erisipela materna: Endocardite streptococcica fetale. Teratologia 1:182.
6. Blieden LO, Morehead RR, Burke B, Kaplan EL (1972): Bacterial endocarditis in the neonate. Am J Dis Child 124:747–749.
7. Boeckman CR, Krill CE Jr (1970): Bacterial and fungal infections complicating parenteral alimentation in infants and children. J Pediatr Surg 5:117–126.
8. Brightman VJ, Scott TF, Westphal M, et al (1966): An outbreak of Coxsackie B-5 virus infection in a newborn nursery. J Pediatr 69:179–192.
9. Drake TA, Scheld WM, Sande MA (1985): Effects of sub-bactericidal concentrations of antibiotics in experimental models of endocarditis. J Antimicrob Chemother 15(Suppl A):293–296.
10. Drew JH (1973): ECHO 11 virus outbreak in a nursery associated with myocarditis. Aust Paediatr J 9:90–95.
11. Edwards K, Ingall D, Czapek E, Davis AT (1977): Bacterial endocarditis in 4 young infants: Is this complication on the increase? Clin Pediatr 16:607–609.
12. Frühling L, Korn R, Lavillaurex J, Surjus A (1962): Chronic fibroelastotic myoendocarditis of the newborn and the infant (fibroelastosis). Ann Anat Pathol 7:227–303.

13. Groff DB (1969): Complications of intravaneous hyperalimentation in newborns and infants. J Pediatr Surg 4:460–464.

14. Harris LC, Nghiem QX (1972): Cardiomyopathies in infants and children. Prog Cardiovasc Dis 15:255–261.

15. Hastreiter AR, Miller, RA (1964): Management of primary endomyocardial disease. The myocarditis–endocardial fibroelastosis syndrome. Pediatr Clin North Am 11:401–430.

16. Heird WC, Driscoll JM, Schullinger JN, Grebin B, Winters RW (1972): Intravenous alimentation in pediatric patients. J Pediatr 80:351–372.

17. Hutchins GH, Vie SA (1972): The progression of interstitial myocarditis to idiopathic endocardial fibroelastosis. Am J Pathol 66:483–496.

18. Javett SN, Heymann S, Mundell B, Pepler WJ, Lurie HI, Gear J, Measroch V, Kirsch Z (1956): Myocarditis in the newborn infant: A study of an outbreak associated with Coxsackie group B virus infection in a maternity home in Johannesburg. J Pediatr 48:1–22.

19. Johnson DH, Rosenthal A, Nadas AS, (1975): Bacterial endocarditis in children under 2 years of age. Am J Dis Child 129:581–588.

20. Joshi VV, Wang N-S (1973): Repeated pulmonary embolism in an infant with subacute *Candida* endocarditis of the right side of the heart. Am J Dis Child 125:257–259.

21. Kibrick S, Benirschke K (1956): Acute aseptic myocarditis and meningoencephalitis in the newborn child infected with coxsackie virus group B, type 3. N Engl J Med 255:883–889.

22. Kibrick S, Benirschke K (1958): Severe generalized disease (encephalohepatomyocarditis) occurring in the newborn period and due to infection with Coxsackie virus, group B. Pediatrics 22:857–875.

23. Kilbourne ED, Wilson CB, Perrior D (1956): The induction of gross myocardial lesions via Coxsackie (pleurodymic) virus and cortisone. J Clin Invest 35:362–370.

24. Lerner AM, Wilson FM (1973): Virus myocardiopathy. Prog Med Virol 15:63–91.

25. Macaulay D (1954): Acute endocarditis in infancy and early childhood. Am J Dis Child 88:715–731.

26. Mason JW, Billingham ME, Ricci DR (1980): Treatment of acute inflammatory myocarditis assisted by endomyocardial biopsy. Am J Card 45:1037–1044.

27. McGuinness GA, Schieken RM, Maguire GF (1980): Endocarditis in the newborn. Am J Dis Child 134:577–580.

28. Montgomery J, Gear J, Prinsloo FR, Kahn M, Kirsch ZG (1955): Myocarditis of the newborn. S Afr Med J 29:608–612.

29. Norris D, Loh PC (1973): Coxsackie virus myocarditis: Prophylaxis and therapy with an interferon stimulator. Proc Soc Exp Biol Med 142:133–136.

30. Oelberg DG, Fisher DJ, Gross D, Denson SE, Adcock EW (1983): Endocarditis in high-risk neonates. Pediatrics 71:392–397.

31. Orsi EV, Mancini R, Barriso J (1970): Hyperbaric enhancement of Coxsackie infection in mice. Aerosp Med 41:1169–1172.

32. Pearce JM (1960): Heart disease and filtrable viruses. Circulation 21:448–455.

33. Pulliam L, Dall L, Inokuchi S, Wilson W, Hadley WK, Mills J (1985): Effects of exopolysaccharide production by viridans streptococci on penicillin therapy of experimental endocarditis. J Infect Dis 151:153–156.

34. Rager-Zisman B, Allison AC (1973): The role of antibody and host cells in resistance of mice against infection by Coxsackie B-3 virus. J Gen Virol 19:329–338.

35. Rosenberg HS, McNamara DG (1964): Acute myocarditis in infancy and childhood. Prog Cardiovasc Dis 7:179–197.

36. Rytel MW (1969): Interferon response during Coxsackie B-3 infection in mice. I. The effect of cortisone. J Infect Dis 120:379–382.

37. Symchych PS, Krauss AN, Winchester P (1977): Endocarditis following intracardiac placement of umbilical venous catheters in neonates. J Pediatr 90:287–289.

38. Tilles JG, Elson SH, Shaka JA, Abelmann WH, Lerner AM, Finland M (1964): Effect of exercise on Coxsackie A-9 myocarditis in adult mice. Proc Soc Exp Biol Med 117:777–782.

39. Tsao MMP, Katz D (1984): Central venous catheter-induced endocarditis: Human correlate of the animal experimental model of endocarditis. Rev Infect Dis 6:783–790.

40. Weinberg AG, Laird WP (1978). Group B streptococcal endocarditis detected by echocardiography. J Pediatr 92:335–336.

41. Wheeler JG, Weesner KM (1984): *Staphylococcus aureus* and pericarditis in an infant with a central venous catheter. Clin Pediatr 23:46–47.

42. White PD (1926): Incidence of endocarditis in earliest childhood. Am J Dis Child 32:536–549.

43. Wright HT Jr, Miller A (1965): Fatal infection in a newborn infant due to Herpes simplex virus: Report of a case diagnosed before death. J Pediatr 67:130–133.

48 CHROMOSOMAL ABNORMALITIES

Jacqueline A. Noonan

It is estimated that 6 to 10 per cent of newborns with a congenital cardiac malformation have some chromosomal abnormality.[88] Among 965 children with congenital heart disease undergoing postmortem examination, Ary[4] noted a chromosomal abnormality in 9.6 per cent. Greenwood and colleagues[42] reported 6 per cent of 1566 symptomatic infants with a cardiac abnormality to have a chromosomal disorder, and Kramer and associates[57] reported 5.5 per cent of 1016 infants and children with chromosomal abnormalities. Without a chromosome study, some infants with a chromosomal abnormality will not be recognized. Many infants with chromosomal abnormalities die shortly after birth before cardiac disease is evident. Thus it is likely that reported clinical studies underestimate the true incidence of chromosomal abnormalities among liveborn infants with a congenital cardiac malformation. Cardiac defects are among the most common malformations occurring in chromosomal syndromes. A large number of structural chromosomal abnormalities have already been described, and additional new abnormalities continue to be reported.

Chromosomal imbalance usually results from meiotic nondisjunction. Full trisomy, producing an extra chromosome, occurs when a full extra chromosome is accidentally incorporated into a gamete prior to fertilization. A karyotype with 47 chromosomes results, such as Down syndrome or trisomy 21. Meiotic nondisjunction can also result in loss of a full chromosome. Most full monosomies are nonviable. Forty-five XO Turner syndrome, in which there is loss of one X chromosome, may result in a viable newborn, although the great majority of XO fetuses are spontaneously aborted. The most common structural chromosomal aberration is translocation. During meiosis, breakage and then reunion between parental chromosomes may occur. If the translocation is balanced with no loss or excess of chromatin material, the phenotype is normal. Unbalanced translocation with extra chromosome material will result in a partial trisomy, whereas deletion will cause a partial monosomy. Most infants born with a chromosomal abnormality have parents with normal chromosomes. A parent, however, with a balanced translocation will have a normal phenotype but may produce offspring with full or partial trisomy or partial monosomy.

Any newborn with a cardiac malformation and associated extracardiac anomalies should be suspect for a chromosomal abnormality. Clinical features particularly common in chromosomal syndromes include low birthweight, especially if small for gestational age, dysmorphic facial features such as abnormal ears, obvious central nervous system malformation, abnormalities of the hands or feet, redundant nuchal skin, or severe hypotonia. A partial deletion of chromosome 5 (5p monosomy) called cri-du-chat syndrome may be suspected in a newborn because of a characteristic shrill cry resembling that of a kitten. Many chromosomal syndromes are not readily apparent in the newborn, and certainly the phenotypes may not be so specific that diagnosis is apparent by physical examination alone. Chromosomal analysis, therefore, is often needed to evaluate fully the infant with a multiple malformation syndrome.

DOWN SYNDROME (TRISOMY 21)

Down syndrome, or trisomy 21, is the most common chromosome disorder, with an incidence of 1:700 live births. The phenotype is so specific that it is usually readily recognized even in the newborn.

Historical Perspective

Langdon Down,[28] in 1866, described a condition characterized by mental retardation and characteristic facies that he named mongolian idiocy. His use of the term *mongolian* was based on his perception that such patients might represent a retrogression to the Mongolian race. Such a theory was consistent with contemporary scientific thought, which was highly influenced by Darwin's work on evolution. Down's ethnic theory received little support, but the term *mongol* or *mongolian* came into general use even though such patients do not really resemble Mongolian people. In 1876, Fraser and Mitchell,[36] apparently unaware of Down's earlier report, reported on 62 similar cases they called Kalmuck idiocy, named for a Mongolian people. In their papers, an autopsy description of the brain was reported and attention was drawn to the association of brachycephaly and increased maternal age in such patients. Many clinical reports followed, and in 1894, Garrod[39] described the association of congenital heart disease with mongolism.

For the next 30 years there were many papers reporting the genetic aspects and theories as to the etiology of this syndrome. As early as 1932, Waardenburg[114] suspected that a chromosomal aberration caused by nondisjunction might be implicated as a cause of mongolism. In 1956, Tjio and Levan[108] confirmed that the normal human diploid chromosome number was 46. Studies of karyotyping began, and in 1959 Lejeune and associates[64] reported 47 chromosomes to be present in Down syndrome patients. This finding was immediately confirmed by many other workers. In 1960, Polani and coworkers[90] reported a translocation chromosomal abnormality in a Down syndrome child born to a young mother and Penrose and colleagues[86] demonstrated in two siblings with Down syndrome that

578

there was familial transmission of translocation in three generations. Mosaicism in Down syndrome was reported in 1961 by Clarke and associates.[23] Hanhart and coworkers,[46] in 1961, reported the first demonstration of secondary nondisjunction in humans by studying the chromosomes of both a mother and a child with trisomy 21.

Once amniocentesis became available and it was feasible to culture cells in the fetus, the prenatal diagnosis of Down syndrome became commonplace. Because the risk of trisomy is associated with increasing maternal age, prenatal screening for Down syndrome is recommended for mothers over 35 years of age and for those mothers at any age who have had a previously affected child.

Epidemiology

In 94 per cent of the cases of Down syndrome, there is full trisomy 21. Some form of translocation accounts for 4 to 5 per cent, and mosaicism accounts for 1 to 2 per cent. At birth the incidence of Down syndrome is close to 1:700 and occurs worldwide. It is estimated, however, that over one half of the embryos with trisomy 21 terminate in spontaneous abortion.[49]

For the great majority of patients with Down syndrome, the cause of chromosomal nondisjunction is unknown. The risk of trisomy 21 is, however, strongly related to maternal age.[48] At age 15 to 29 years, the risk is 1:1500; at 30 to 34 years, 1:800; at 35 to 39 years, 1:270; at 40 to 45 years, 1:100; and over 45 years, 1:50. The reason for the increasing risk with age is unknown, but it is postulated that natural aging of the nucleus of the ovum may somehow predispose to nondisjunction. The role of environmental toxins and hormonal influences on meiosis related to aging is still unknown. It is known, however, that a variety of environmental toxins such as radiation or viral infections can predispose to aneuploidy.

For a small number of patients with Down syndrome, a strong genetic influence is present. A mother with trisomy 21 has a 50 per cent risk of having a child with trisomy 21. In the 5 per cent of infants with translocation-type Down syndrome,[93] there is a 70 to 75 per cent chance that the translocation occurred de novo and that both parents will have normal chromosomes. However, among the translocation patients, a maternal-balanced translocation will be found in 25 per cent, whereas in 2 per cent a paternal translocation will be identified. Known balanced translocation carrier mothers have been found to have only 10 per cent of offspring to be affected rather than the expected one third. This surprisingly low incidence of affected offspring may well be attributed to the high fetal loss in early pregnancy of an abnormal conceptus. The mosaic form of Down syndrome occurs in 1 to 2 per cent and usually results from nondisjunction de novo. However, a mother with mosaicism of the 46/47 type may give birth to a full trisomy 21 infant.

It is important to emphasize that repetitive Down syndrome in young mothers is usually regular, full trisomy 21 and not due to translocation. Although the overall risk of recurrent Down syndrome in a young mother with normal chromosomes is only slightly above control risk at 1 per cent,[31] there are families with multiple cases of Down syndrome. The hypothesis that there may be a genetic predisposition to nondisjunction could explain multiple cases of Down syndrome in some families. One of the mothers with normal chromosomes I studied gave birth to an infant with 45,XO Turner syndrome and later an infant with trisomy 21.

In liveborn infants with Down syndrome, about 40 per cent have a congenital cardiac defect.[26,98] In the great majority, a ventricular septal defect is present, which is often associated with a complete atrioventricular septal defect. The distribution of cardiac defects in several series is shown in Table 48–1. Atrioventricular septal defects

Table 48–1. PER CENT DISTRIBUTION OF CONGENITAL CARDIAC DEFECTS AMONG 3104 LIVEBORN INFANTS COMPARED WITH 612 DOWN SYNDROME PATIENTS

Lesion	Liveborn Infants With Cardiac Defects	Down Syndrome Infants			
	Hoffman and Christianson[47]	*Tandon and Edwards*[107]*	*Greenwood and Nadas*[42]†	*Greenwood and Nadas*[42]	*Park, et al*[84]
Ventricular septal defect	30.3	29	17.1	28.7	31.9
Patent ductus arteriosus	8.6	1.8 (45.4)‡	6.7 (19.7)	6.9 (6.1)	4.4 (16)
Atrial septal defect	6.7	1.8 (47.3)	1.3 (5.2)	2.6	9.5
Atrioventricular septal defect	3.2	60	56.5	45.7	43
Pulmonary stenosis	7.4	(5.5)	(3.9)	< 1	< 1
Aortic stenosis	5.2	(5.5)			< 1
Coarctation of aorta	5.7	(14.5)	(3.9)	(< 1)	(< 1)
Tetralogy of Fallot	5.1	5.4	7.9	8.3	6.4
Transposition of great arteries	4.7				< 1
Other	23.2		10.5	4.8	4.8

*Autopsy series
†Infants under 1 year of age
‡( ), associated defect

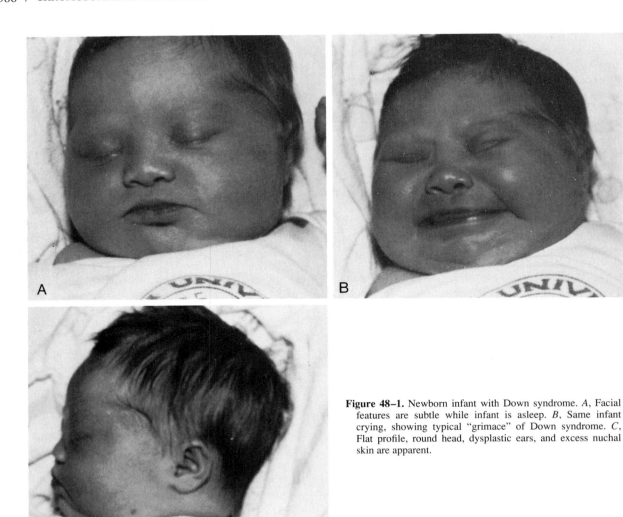

Figure 48–1. Newborn infant with Down syndrome. *A*, Facial features are subtle while infant is asleep. *B*, Same infant crying, showing typical "grimace" of Down syndrome. *C*, Flat profile, round head, dysplastic ears, and excess nuchal skin are apparent.

were found in 3.2 per cent of unselected patients with cardiac defects, whereas among Down syndrome patients, the incidence was 43 to 60 per cent. Isolated pulmonary stenosis, aortic stenosis, and coarctation of the aorta are uncommon in Down syndrome, and transposition of the great arteries is quite rare. Only two cases of transposition were noted among the 612 total Down syndrome patients listed in Table 48–1. Down syndrome patients with atrioventricular septal defect or ventricular septal defect have a high incidence of associated lesions, especially patent ductus arteriosus and secundum atrial septal defects. Tandon and Edwards[107] in their autopsy series noted one or both as additional lesions in nearly one half of their cases. A right-sided aortic arch and anomalous right subclavian artery are more common in patients with Down syndrome than controls. Between 10 and 15 per cent of patients with Down syndrome have decreased pulmonary blood flow due either to tetralogy of Fallot or atrioventricular septal defect with right ventricular outflow obstruction. The explanation for the high incidence of atrioventricular septal defects in patients with Down syndrome is unknown.

Rosenquist and associates[97] made an important observation in their study of 14 heart specimens from patients with Down syndrome who did not have any structural heart disease; the percentage of the ventricular septal area occupied by the membranous ventricular septum was over four times larger than the average percentage measured in control normal hearts. These investigators speculated that if somehow Down syndrome results in an abnormality of cellular growth so that malalignment or underdevelopment of the muscle at the base of the cardiac ventricles occurs, a spectrum of anomalies including atrioventricular septal defect could result. White and colleagues,[119] in 1984, showed that fibroblasts from lung and cardiac tissue of trisomy 21 fetuses have increased adhesiveness compared with normal controls, and they speculated that the increased adhesiveness in cardiac cells could predispose to atrioventricular and other septal defects characteristic of Down syndrome. Kurnit and colleagues[59] have further suggested that the genetic defect present in Down syndrome could result in the wide variety of atrioventricular septal defects depending partly on chance. They developed a computer program demonstrating support for this hypothesis. Cooney and Thurlbeck[25] reported pulmonary hypoplasia in six of seven Down syndrome patients studied by morphometry. The number of alveoli in relation to the acini was diminished, as were the total number of alveoli and alveolar surface area; individual alveoli and alveolar ducti were enlarged.[25] Wright and coworkers[119] have speculated that the increased adhesiveness found in cells from lung tissue might be responsible for these pulmonary findings.

Clinical Findings

It is usually possible to diagnose Down syndrome at birth because of the characteristic physical findings. In the newborn, some of the most characteristic findings include marked muscular hypotonia, absent or decreased Moro reflex, weak cry, and generalized decreased motor activity compared with that of the normal newborn.[45] The typical facial features include a flat facial profile, flat nasal bridge, a round shape to the head, upward slanting of the palpebral fissures, small and often dysplastic ears, and excess skin on the back of the neck (Fig. 48–1). Short midphalanx of the fifth finger, a simian crease (Fig. 48–2), and wide spacing between the great and second toe are also often present. As a group, children with Down syndrome tend to be slightly below average for birthweight and 20 per cent are born prematurely. Moessinger and associates[72] noted that infants with Down syndrome have significantly shorter umbilical cords than normal infants. Patients with Down syndrome had a mean umbilical cord length of 45.1 cm compared with 57.6 cm for matched standards. These investigators suggested that decreased fetal motor activity might be implicated as a cause of the decreased umbilical cord length.

The labia majora have a typical appearance in female newborns with Down syndrome. Iancu[52] has described a "labial index." The labia majora are measured in the vertical axis and the horizontal axis. The ratio between the vertical axis and the horizontal axis is designated as the labial index. The mean index for normal control group was 2.33, whereas among 11 female newborns with Down syndrome, the labial index ranged from 1.31 to 1.79. Iancu suggested that this objective sign might be useful in the newborn, especially in doubtful cases.[52] Another objective measurement discriminating between normal children and infants with Down syndrome is the "iliac index,"[78] which is significantly lower in Down syndrome children.

The reported incidence of congenital heart disease in Down syndrome is variable, ranging from over 60 per cent in autopsy series to 25 per cent in Hoffman and associates' report.[47] No study has been reported using echocardiography in an unselected group of newborns with Down syndrome to more accurately evaluate the true incidence of cardiac anomalies in this syndrome. It is likely that the true incidence is close to 50 per cent and therefore every newborn with Down syndrome should be evaluated for the possible presence of a cardiac malformation.

A newborn with Down syndrome frequently has acrocyanosis of the hands and feet. Generalized cyanosis also

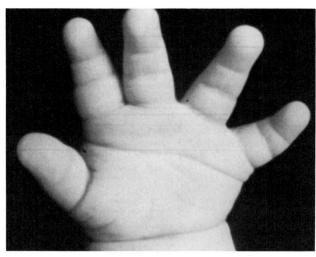

Figure 48–2. Hand of Down syndrome patient showing simian crease.

occurs. Polycythemia and hypoventilation may cause cyanosis in the absence of an underlying cardiac defect. It is not at all uncommon for an infant with a large ventricular septal defect or complete atrioventricular septal defect to have no audible murmur in the immediate newborn period. A prominent murmur in the newborn with Down syndrome should suggest associated right ventricular outflow obstruction, which might be due to tetralogy of Fallot or an atrioventricular septal defect with associated pulmonary stenosis. An occasional newborn with Down syndrome will present in congestive heart failure because of severe atrioventricular valve insufficiency, but this presentation is quite unusual in spite of the high incidence of atrioventricular septal defects. In contrast, severe atrioventricular valve insufficiency is a relatively common cause of fetal cardiac failure with hydrops. Ultrasound studies performed on fetuses with suspected intrauterine cardiac failure have thus far identified a disproportionately high number of infants with atrioventricular septal defects and valvular insufficiency.[1,54] It is likely that most fetuses with severe atrioventricular valve insufficiency die in utero.

The physical findings in the typical newborn with a large atrioventricular septal defect will be quite subtle. The second heart sound is generally accentuated, and there may be slightly increased precordial activity. Physical examination, therefore, is not sufficient to evaluate the infant for the presence of congenital heart defect. An ECG showing left anterior hemiblock or other abnormalities may provide a clue, but clearly an echocardiogram is very helpful in diagnosing a significant cardiac malformation. Cardiac failure generally does not occur before the first or second month of life, but a few patients with an atrioventricular septal defect and an associated coarctation of the aorta who developed cardiac failure in the first week of life have been seen. By 1 to 2 months of age a heart murmur not previously heard may become audible, but many infants with a large atrioventricular septal defect and severe pulmonary artery hypertension never develop a prominent murmur. A number of children with Down syndrome have not been recognized as having congenital heart disease until pulmonary vascular obstructive disease was far advanced. Since the majority of defects present in infants with Down syndrome are potentially treatable by surgical repair, it is important to recognize the presence of the cardiac defect before pulmonary vascular disease progresses.

In Down syndrome there is an increased incidence of several serious congenital malformations in addition to congenital heart disease. Duodenal atresia or stenosis, tracheoesophageal fistula with or without esophageal atresia, imperforate anus, malrotation, and Hirschsprung's disease all occur more often in children with Down syndrome than in the general newborn population. Meckel diverticulum is also a common additional anomaly. Umbilical hernias occur in about 12 per cent, and diastasis recti is also common. Hypospadias, which occurs in 0.3 per cent of liveborn males, occurred in 6.5 per cent of Down syndrome infants in a report by Lang and coworkers.[60] Cleft lip and palate occur in 1 to 2 per cent. Rare reduction malformations of upper/lower extremities have also been reported.[10]

Nonimmune hydrops fetalis occurs in about 1 in 3748 births. A variety of causes have been identified, but many remain labeled as idiopathic. In 61 cases of nonimmune hydrops fetalis,[51] there were two patients with Down syndrome, and in another report,[87] one of eight patients had Down syndrome. In addition, Fujimoto and associates[37] reported nonimmune fetal hydrops in six Down syndrome infants. Among these six patients, three had congenital cardiac malformation, which included tetralogy of Fallot in two and a patent ductus in one. None of these cardiac defects would be expected in itself to have caused heart failure in utero; thus the cause of nonimmune fetal hydrops and its relationship to Down syndrome remain obscure.

The incidence of acute leukemia in children with Down syndrome is reported to be 30 times higher than that in the general population. Congenital acute leukemia and a congenital leukemoid reaction have been reported in newborns with Down syndrome.[58,113,117] The tendency for some Down syndrome patients to have polycythemia has been attributed to congenital marrow dysfunction. So-called transient congenital leukemia, which is characterized by a marked leukemoid reaction and sometimes skin infiltrates, often undergoes spontaneous remission. Long-lasting cure may result, but a number of children have been reported to develop leukemia 1 to 2 years later.[20] A transient leukemoid reaction occurring in some Down syndrome newborns may mimic acute myeloblastic leukemia. Down syndrome patients who develop acute leukemia, like the general pediatric population, more commonly develop acute lymphoblastic leukemia.

With the advent of newborn screening for congenital hypothyroidism, Fort and coworkers[35] confirmed either persistent or transient congenital hypothyroidism in 11 of 1130 newborns with Down syndrome studied in New York. The incidence of persistent primary congenital hypothyroidism in Down syndrome was 1:141, which was 28 times more frequent than in the general population; the incidence of transient congenital hypothyroidism was 1:377. The cause of congenital hypothyroidism in infants with Down syndrome remains unknown. In none of these pa-

tients was athyreosis found. Older children and adults with Down syndrome have an increased incidence of autoimmune diseases affecting the thyroid gland. In none of the newborns, however, was it possible to detect any thyroid antibodies.

Differential Diagnosis

Congenital hypothyroidism, like Down syndrome, is characterized by sluggish motor activity, flat nasal bridges, and frequently an umbilical hernia. Careful physical examination, however, should allow differentiation. Several other chromosomal abnormalities may have some of the findings present in Down syndrome such as 9P– and 20P. Females with XXXXX syndrome and males with XXXXY syndrome show some superficial facial resemblance to Down syndrome. A Prader-Willi infant in the newborn period has poor motor activity and occasionally has prominent eyes, which are confusing findings. Newborns with Zellweger syndrome, an autosomal recessive condition due to cytochrome oxidase enzyme deficiency, have some similar features. However, the presence of an enlarged liver and spleen, limb contractures, as well as the high forehead in Zellweger syndrome should help in differentiation. Zellweger syndrome is generally fatal by 6 months of age.

Medical Management

Early accurate diagnosis of Down syndrome in the newborn is essential for appropriate management. The likelihood of a serious associated congenital malformation requires careful evaluation. Karyotyping is very helpful in confirming the diagnosis and identifying the exact chromosomal abnormality present. When the diagnosis of Down syndrome is made in a newborn, both parents should be informed by a physician with knowledge and understanding of the condition. A positive physician attitude is both appropriate and needed to support the parents.

The majority of infants born with Down syndrome will survive, and most will be raised at home by their family. Parent education through reading material and parent support groups is important. For a wholesome family situation, it is essential that the parents accept that the infant has Down syndrome and also that they accept the infant. The natural flow of affection between parent and child is usual and is helped if the physicians also accept and feel positive toward the infant.

Because of the high incidence of serious congenital heart disease, consultation by a pediatric cardiologist is appropriate. An infant with congenital heart disease and Down syndrome should be treated as any other child with a similar defect. Since complete atrioventricular septal defect and a large ventricular septal defect have a high incidence of severe pulmonary artery hypertension, there is a high risk for the development of pulmonary hypertensive vascular disease.[17,118] Close observation and early cardiac catheterization, if warranted, are often required to plan for the most appropriate time for surgical treatment. Among normal children with ventricular septal defects, small to moderate defects predominate. There is a tendency for many ventricular septal defects to decrease in size and for some defects to undergo spontaneous closure. In my experience, small or moderate ventricular septal defects are the exception rather than the rule in Down syndrome children; as a result, the tendency in normal children for improvement or spontaneous closure of the ventricular septal defect is unlikely in an infant with Down syndrome.

Severe failure to thrive and congestive cardiac failure frequently develop after the first 1 to 2 months of age. Appropriate medical treatment with digoxin and diuretics will often bring some improvement. If there is a large atrioventricular septal defect and severe pulmonary artery hypertension, medical management will usually be of limited value and surgical treatment (see Chapter 65) should be considered before pulmonary vascular disease develops.[77]

The natural history of a complete atrioventricular septal defect treated medically is poor. Death from congestive heart failure or an intercurrent respiratory infection occurred in over 60 per cent of symptomatic infants with an atrioventricular septal defect reported by Greenwood and Nadas.[42] In their same report, over 60 per cent of their patients treated by pulmonary artery banding also died. The mortality from surgical treatment of atrioventricular septal defect in infancy by pulmonary artery banding has been high, with an average reported mortality of 32 per cent in several collected series. More recent studies have shown that with improved postoperative care of infants, pulmonary artery banding can be carried out with a mortality rate closer to 5 per cent.[102] Pulmonary artery banding, however, is a palliative procedure and requires further surgery. Prior to 1975, the risk of complete repair of the atrioventricular septal defect in infancy was prohibitively high. Since that time there has been significant improvement in the surgical results.[8,21] For infants with an atrioventricular septal defect who have favorable anatomy and no pulmonary vascular disease, there is over an 80 per cent chance of survival with good long-term results.[19] Mitral valve dysfunction is one of the major causes of operative mortality from total repair of an atrioventricular septal defect in infancy. The presence of a solitary left ventricular papillary muscle appears to carry a high risk. Chin and coworkers[18] found by echocardiography that 3 of 31 infants with complete atrioventricular septal defect had a single left ventricular papillary muscle. Twenty-five infants had two left ventricular papillary muscles, and 3 infants had three papillary muscles. Among the 25 infants with two papillary muscles, there was only one operative and one late death. Five of the 6 infants with either one or three left ventricular papillary muscles underwent surgical repair, and 4 died in the early postoperative period. Other unfavorable anatomic findings include hypoplasia of either ventricle and significant outflow obstruction. Chapter 65 reviews surgical repair of atrioventricular septal defect in detail.

Repair of a ventricular septal defect in infants with Down syndrome, if carried out prior to the development of pulmonary vascular disease, should be possible with a low operative mortality of under 5 per cent. Cyanotic congenital heart disease in Down syndrome is usually due to te-

tralogy of Fallot or an atrioventricular septal defect with pulmonary stenosis. Surgical repair of tetralogy of Fallot in Down syndrome patients should be similar to that in normal children. Surgical repair of atrioventricular septal defect with severe pulmonary stenosis carries a high mortality so that in infancy a "shunt" operation may be more appropriate if severe cyanosis develops.

Many infants with Down syndrome and congenital heart disease die of pneumonia or other infections. Prompt treatment of respiratory infections is, therefore, essential. Respiratory syncytial virus infections are of particular concern in infants with congenital heart disease and Down syndrome. In the past, several of my patients have died of this complication, but more recently I have had several critically ill infants survive with vigorous medical management and the use of ribavirin.

Prognosis

The prognosis for an infant with Down syndrome continues to improve. The presence of congenital heart disease clearly affects the prognosis.[5] Greenwood and Nadas[42] reported a 53.9 per cent mortality rate among 76 infants with Down syndrome who had symptomatic congenital heart disease and were enrolled in the New England Regional Infant Cardiac Program. Park and colleagues,[84] on the other hand, reported 82 newborns with Down syndrome and congenital heart disease followed for 1 year or more and noted a 13 per cent mortality rate. Their series included 19 patients undergoing cardiac surgery in the first year of life with 15 survivors. My experience regarding the mortality of infants with Down syndrome and congenital heart disease is similar to that reported by Park. I am aggressive in my treatment of infants with atrioventricular septal defect and large ventricular septal defect, and most of the mortality in infancy is now related to the surgical repair of a high-risk atrioventricular septal defect. The prognosis, of course, in a patient with Down syndrome is influenced by the presence of other congenital malformations, such as duodenal atresia, Hirschsprung's disease, or tracheoesophageal fistula. Fortunately, all of these conditions are amenable to surgical treatment. Without aggressive surgical treatment of atrioventricular septal defect in early infancy, the likelihood of pulmonary vascular obstructive disease is high. Infants and children with Down syndrome who develop progressive pulmonary vascular disease usually survive childhood but become symptomatic in the second to fourth decades. I am currently following a sizeable number of Down syndrome patients 18 to 30 years of age with polycythemia, cyanosis, and typical Eisenmenger physiology. Death occasionally comes suddenly, but often there is a slow, progressive downhill course. In contrast, my Down syndrome patients with atrioventricular septal defect who survived early surgical repair are now asymptomatic and doing well at 10 to 15 years of age and are likely to continue to do well.[7]

Although children with Down syndrome have an increased risk of developing leukemia and an increased incidence of scoliosis, prognosis is relatively good at least up

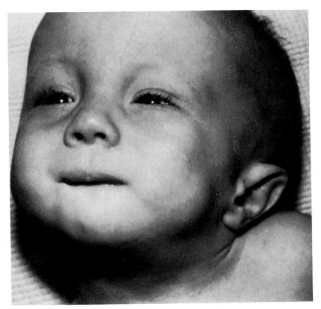

Figure 48–3. Facies of infant with trisomy 18 showing small facial features, short palpebral fissures, low set malformed ears, and micrognathia.

to the fifth to sixth decades. Premature aging, including an increased risk of Alzheimer's disease, has been reported in the older Down syndrome patient.[27]

TRISOMY 18 (EDWARDS SYNDROME)

Trisomy 18 is the second most common trisomy, occurring in 1 in 7000 live births. Some cardiac malformation is present in virtually 100 per cent of patients.

Historical Perspective

In 1960, Edwards and coworkers[29] were the first to describe an extra 18th chromosome in infants with a distinctive pattern of multiple malformations; later that same year Smith and associates[105] reported the same syndrome. Many additional cases have been reported, and the clinical picture is now well documented. Milunsky and colleagues[71] reported one case of trisomy 18 at 31 weeks from among 100 amniocenteses, and Hsu and coworkers[50] reported prenatal cytogenic diagnosis in a 20-week pregnancy and noted the recognizable phenotype of trisomy 18 in the fetus.

Epidemiology

In the majority of cases, trisomy for all of chromosome 18 is present. Translocation cases may occur as the result of

chromosome breakage; in such patients the parents' chromosomes should be studied to exclude a balanced translocation carrier. Mosaicism may also occur and is usually associated with longer survival and more variation in phenotype. In addition to full trisomy 18, partial trisomy 18 may occur. If the long arm is trisomic, the clinical picture is quite similar to full trisomy 18. Less severe malformations and prolonged survival may occur if the partial trisomy occurs on the short arm of the chromosome. The incidence of trisomy 18 is 1 in 7000 live births, but as in other trisomies, a much higher number are spontaneously aborted. There is a 3:1 female predominance. Eighty per cent of the cases are nondisjunction, 10 per cent translocation, and 10 per cent mosaic. As in Down syndrome, there is an increasing risk of nondisjunction type trisomy 18 with increasing maternal age. The risk of recurrence in younger mothers with normal chromosomes is less than 1 per cent.

Clinical Findings

The newborn with trisomy 18 usually has a low birthweight with a mean reported of 2340 g. Polyhydramnios, small placenta, and a single umbilical artery are often present. One third are born prematurely, and one third are postmature.[104] The infant is feeble and often requires resuscitation following delivery. The head is dolichocephalic with small facial features, including a narrow nasal bridge, short palpebral fissures, low-set malformed ears, narrow palate, and micrognathia (Fig. 48–3). Characteristic hand findings include a clenched hand with overlapping of the index finger over the third finger and of the fifth finger over the fourth finger (Fig. 48–4). The distal crease of the fifth finger is often absent, and nails of the fifth finger and toes are often hypoplastic. The sternum is short, and nipples are small. There is limited hip abduction. Excessive lanugo hair, rocker-bottom feet, and a calcaneovalgus deformity are relatively frequent.[53] Cryptorchidism occurs in about one half of the males, and in one half of the females the clitoris and labia minora are hypoplastic. Cleft lip or palate may occur less frequently. Renal anomalies are relatively frequent. Cataracts, choanal atresia, microphthalmia, imperforate anus, radial aplasia, and biliary atresia occur in less than 10 per cent.

Infants with trisomy 18 are very feeble and have limited capacity for survival. During the neonatal period apneic episodes are frequent and a poor suck is common. Even with maximal care and tube feedings, failure to thrive is the rule.

Congenital cardiac anomalies have been present in almost every trisomy 18 case studied at postmortem. A large ventricular septal defect is most common, and associated lesions are frequent. Coarctation of the aorta has been reported in 20 to 40 per cent of cases, usually in association with a ventricular septal defect. Both bicuspid aortic valves and bicuspid pulmonary valves are frequently associated findings. Polyvalvular disease involving all four valves was present in all the cases reported by Matsuoka and colleagues.[69] The dysplastic process in the valves consisted of vacuoles and lacunar degeneration in the spongiosa and distinct lack of elastic tissue in the proximalis and the spongiosa. In a patient reported by Anderson and associates,[3] a congenital papillary tumor of the dysplastic tricuspid valve caused right ventricular outflow obstruction. High origin of the right coronary artery, aberrant right subclavian artery, and bilateral superior venae cavae have also been noted frequently. Evidence for early development of pulmonary vascular disease was reported by Butler and associates,[12] who noted intimal changes in the small pulmonary vessels of two infants dying at 60 and 66 days of life. Both had large ventricular septal defects. No intimal changes were noted in 11 other infants who were stillborn to 49 days of age. The few patients I have studied by cardiac catheterization have had severe pulmonary artery hypertension, and one infant at 4 months of age had a severely elevated pulmonary vascular resistance.

Differential Diagnosis

Sometimes clinical features of trisomy 18 and trisomy 13 may overlap, particularly if the infant has a cleft palate. Trisomy 18 may also resemble the VATER syndrome or a CHARGE association. A number of infants appear to have a phenocopy of trisomy 18 but have normal chromosomes; etiology is unknown in such cases.

Medical Management

The diagnosis of trisomy 18 is usually suspected at birth but should be confirmed by chromosomal analysis. Both parents should be told the diagnosis and the prognosis. Although most infants do not survive infancy, many do stabilize enough to be discharged from the nursery. The parents of infants with trisomy 18 require much emotional support and counseling. The infant's inability to suck may require tube feedings for nutrition or even a feeding gastrostomy. A monitor may be helpful if apneic episodes occur. Although all of these children are severely retarded, some progress in development does occur. With love and stimulation, the survivors do learn to smile and respond to the family.

Severe congenital heart disease or other associated anomalies clearly affect the prognosis of trisomy 18. For those infants with congenital heart disease surviving past 1 to 2 months of age, cardiac failure may become a significant problem. Although I have treated such infants with digitalis and diuretics and have performed cardiac catheterization in a few, none of my patients with trisomy 18 has undergone open heart surgery, but one improved after ligation of a large patent ductus arteriosus. Depending on the patient's status and the relative risk-benefit ratio from surgery, it is possible that surgical repair will occasionally be warranted for a rare patient. In general, the very poor prognosis of trisomy 18 discourages aggressive medical management. The infant with trisomy 18 should be kept comfortable and the condition allowed to run its usual natural course.

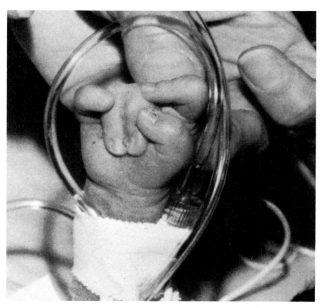

Figure 48–4. Characteristic hand findings in infant with trisomy 18.

Prognosis

Reports regarding the prognosis for infants with trisomy 18 vary, although all agree the prognosis is poor and survival beyond 1 year of age is unlikely. In an attempt to better evaluate the prognosis, Carter and coworkers[15] studied 48 cases of trisomy 18. Five were identified by amniocentesis and not further considered. Of the remaining 43 infants with trisomy 18 recognized postnatally, there were 4 with mosaicism. The 39 infants with full trisomy 18 born by spontaneous delivery included 16 males and 23 females. Twenty per cent of the male fetuses but none of the females were stillborn. The median life expectancy for liveborn infants with trisomy 18 was 5 days, with a range of 1 hour to 18 months. The mean age at death was 48 days. In nine patients without a serious cardiac defect or other serious congenital anomalies, the median life expectancy was 40 days, ranging from 4 hours to 18 months. Three of the 4 patients with mosaic-type trisomy 18 died at 2 hours, 1 week, and 7 weeks; the remaining patient was alive at 9 years of age but severely retarded. In this study, less than 4 per cent of infants with trisomy 18 survived to the first birthday.[15]

In general, patients with partial trisomy 18, as well as mosaic trisomies, have a somewhat longer life expectancy, although all have mental retardation and a poor prognosis.

TRISOMY 13 (PATAU SYNDROME)

Trisomy 13 is a syndrome of multiple congenital anomalies with an incidence of about 1 in 7000 births. Cardiac malformations are present in over 80 per cent.

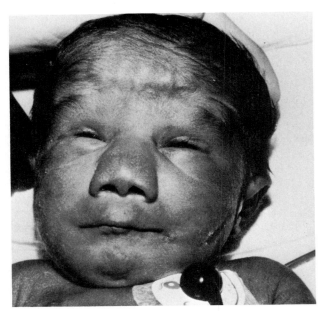

Figure 48–5. Infant with trisomy 13 showing microphthalmia, absent philtrum, and abnormal nose.

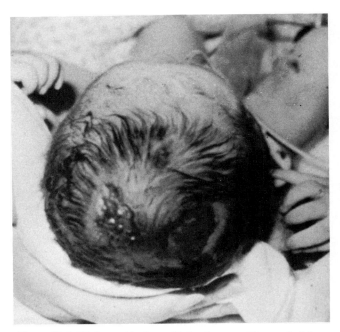

Figure 48–6. Newborn with trisomy 13 showing several large scalp defects.

Historical Perspective

The phenotype was apparently first described by Bartholin in 1657,[115] but the trisomic etiology was first reported in 1960 by Patau and coworkers.[85] Since that time hundreds of cases have been reported.

Epidemiology

The nondisjunction form of trisomy 13, which accounts for 80 per cent of the cases, is associated with increased maternal age. Partial trisomy 13 for the proximal segment (13pter → q14) has a nonspecific phenotype with severe mental retardation and a good likelihood of long-term survival. Partial trisomy for the distal segment (13q14 → qter) has a characteristic phenotype with severe mental retardation, and about one fourth of these patients die in early postnatal life.[104]

Clinical Findings

The newborn with trisomy 13 has an average birthweight of 2500 g. Facial cleft, microphthalmia, polydactyly, low-set ears, and rocker-bottom feet are obvious on external examination (Fig. 48–5). A holoprosencephalic defect of the central nervous system is present with incomplete development of the forebrain and of the olfactory and optic nerves. Moderate microcephaly with a sloping forehead and wide sagittal sutures and fontanelles are usual. Frequent findings are localized scalp defects (Fig. 48–6); colobomas, cataracts, and anophthalmia; capillary hemangiomas, especially on the forehead; and loose skin in the posterior neck. Internal abnormalities include du-

plication or polycystic kidneys; cardiac malformations are present in about 80 per cent. Other anomalies reported include omphalocele, diaphragmatic hernia, incomplete rotation of the colon, and Meckel's diverticulum. Hand deformities similar to those of trisomy 18 may be seen. Simian creases are more common than in either trisomy 21 or 18. Frequently, abnormalities in rib number and structure are present.

Minor motor seizures with a hypsarrhythmic pattern on the electroencephalogram and frequent apnea are common manifestations of the central nervous system anomalies. Severe mental retardation, deafness, often blindness, and severe failure to thrive are found. Other interesting features include an abnormal elevation of fetal hemoglobin F and an increased frequency of nuclear projections in polymorphonuclear cells.[104]

Patients with trisomy 13 and mosaicism have a less severe and more variable phenotype that does not resemble full trisomy 13. Partial trisomy for the proximal segment of chromosome 13 is characterized by a large nose, short upper lip, receding mandible, fifth finger clinodactyly, and usually severe mental retardation. Partial trisomy for the distal segment of chromosome 13 is a more characteristic phenotype that is also associated with severe mental deficiency. These latter infants have a prominent frontal capillary hemangioma, short nose with an upturned tip, elongated philtrum, bushy eyebrows, long incurved lashes, and a prominent helix.

Cardiac malformations in trisomy 13 are variable, but ventricular septal defect is most common. Similar to trisomy 18, bicuspid aortic valves and bicuspid pulmonary valves are relatively frequent, as is coarctation of the aorta. Polyvalvular dysplasia has been reported,[9] similar to that characteristic of trisomy 18.[69] Although cardiac failure may occur secondary to congenital heart disease, the central nervous system malfunction predominates. Because of the poor prognosis, plastic and orthopedic surgical procedures should be postponed until there is some indication of how well the patient will do.

Differential Diagnosis

Nonchromosomal disorders with holoprosencephaly must be considered in the differential diagnosis of trisomy 13, as must other chromosomal malformations such as short-arm 18 deletion syndrome, 4p–, partial 10qs, triploidy s, 13q–, and 18p–. Meckel-Gruber syndrome may also need to be considered as well as the CHARGE association. Karyotyping is important for a definitive diagnosis of trisomy 13 and for identification of those infants with translocation so that appropriate genetic counseling can be given.

Medical Management

Although the diagnosis of trisomy 13 can be suspected by physical examination, karyotyping is appropriate to confirm the diagnosis and to aid in genetic counseling. Similar to trisomy 18, parental support and counseling are needed. Infants with trisomy 13 require much nursing care during their usually short lives. Severe mental retardation, deafness, and blindness are the rule. Elective surgical procedures should be delayed until the child's prognosis can be better assessed.

In my limited experience, pulmonary artery hypertension is frequent in infants with trisomy 13 and a large ventricular septal defect. One of my patients had evidence of severe pulmonary vascular obstructive disease by 4 months of age. Apnea and aspiration (related to the brain defect) are usually the causes of death, but renal and cardiac failure may contribute. Cardiac evaluation can usually be accomplished by echocardiography; for rare patients, cardiac catheterization and angiocardiography may be appropriate. In some instances even surgical repair of a cardiac defect may be recommended if the procedure is expected to improve the quality of life at a reasonable surgical risk.

Prognosis

The prognosis of trisomy 13 is very poor, with a mean life expectancy of 130 days; survival is rare beyond 1 year of age. Mental and growth retardation are severe. There is no survival difference between sexes. About one half of the patients die in the first month after birth. Survival to 19 years in a patient with full trisomy 13 has been reported.[96]

XO SYNDROME (TURNER SYNDROME)

XO or sex chromatin–negative females are often referred to as having Turner syndrome and may present

with a distinctive phenotype. The majority of XO fetuses, however, are nonviable.

Historical Perspective

Probably the first description of a patient with pterygium colli, which we now call Turner syndrome, was by Funke[38] in 1902. Ullrich,[111] in 1930, reported several patients with lymphedema who likely had Turner syndrome. Turner,[109] in 1938, described a more expanded syndrome stressing short stature, webbed neck, cubitus valgus, and sexual infantilism. The eponym Turner syndrome has been used by many since then. In 1943, Flavell[33] noted a male with features resembling those reported by Turner and coined the term *male Turner syndrome*. In 1947, Lisser and associates[68] published 25 cases similar to those reported by Turner and suggested that a chromosomal defect was a likely etiology. Polani and colleagues,[91] in 1954, demonstrated a negative nuclear sex chromatin pattern characteristic of the male to be present in these phenotypic female subjects. In 1959, Ford[34] showed that patients with Turner syndrome had a missing X chromosome with a 45,XO karyotype. Ferrier and coworkers,[32] in 1961, described a patient with Turner phenotype who was chromatin positive and had mosaicism. In 1965, Carr[13] demonstrated that 5.5 per cent of a series of abortuses had a 45,XO karyotype. Singh and Carr,[103] in 1966, described the fetal manifestation of 45,XO karyotype as widespread edema associated with lymphangiectasis and a nuchal cystic hygroma (Fig. 48–7). They also noted internal abnormalities such as coarctation of the aorta and a variety of renal anomalies. Interestingly, up to the third month of gestation, ovarian development in XO fetuses appears normal but afterward evidence of ovarian dysgenesis becomes more apparent. Later on in fetal life, the primordial follicle formation decreases or ceases and connective tissue

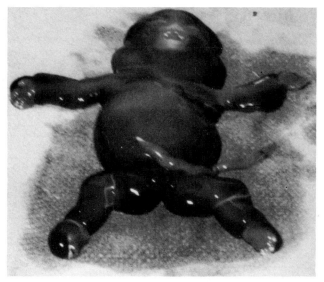

Figure 48–7. XO fetus with cystic hygroma and widespread edema.

of the gonad increases. Bove[11] has speculated that developmental arrest at the stage of primordial follicle formation and subsequent regression of germinal structures is the most likely morphologic basis for ovarian dysgenesis characteristic of the XO karyotype.

In 1963, Noonan and Ehmke[79] reported nine children with pulmonary stenosis who had similar characteristic facies, short stature, and other skeletal anomalies with some superficial resemblance to the phenotype of Turner syndrome. There were six males and three females, and these patients had no chromosomal abnormalities. In 1965, Opitz[81] proposed the name Noonan syndrome as an eponym for these patients. Chromosome studies clearly differentiate Noonan syndrome from Turner syndrome. Palmer and Richardson, in 1976, reported the chromosome findings in 110 females with Turner syndrome. An XO karyotype was present in 64, whereas 21 had an isochromosome X and the remaining 25 had a variety of mosaic patterns. Only 12 of the 110 were suspected in the newborn period because of lymphedema or loose nuchal skin folds, and all had an 45,XO karyotype.

Epidemiology

Complete absence of the X chromosome or 45,XO monosomy is usually lethal. It is estimated that 99.9 per cent of such XO fetuses do not survive beyond 28 weeks' gestation.[116] An XO karyotype is found in about 1 in 15 cases of spontaneous abortion, whereas the reported incidence in live births varies between 1 in 5000 and 1 in 20,000. Only one half of liveborn infants with Turner syndrome have full or partial monosomy of the X chromosome; the remainder have mosaicism or an isochromosome for the long arm of the X chromosome.[82] Monosomy X is unrelated to increasing maternal age, as is true of trisomic conception. In fact, Warburton[116] has demonstrated that among spontaneous abortions, monosomy X is associated with a young maternal age. Because mean maternal age is not increased, it is suspected that maternal meiotic nondisjunction is not an important cause of monosomy X, but the true cause remains unknown. Postfertilization events, such as anaphase lag in early mitosis or loss of a damaged sex chromosome, have been proposed as an explanation for the high frequency of mosaicism found in live births. Infants with mosaicism or only partial deletion of an X chromosome are usually viable, and rarely are they found among abortuses. Cases of Turner syndrome are generally sporadic, with a low risk of recurrence.

Among 45,XO fetuses, cystic hygroma of the neck is the most consistent feature.[99] The prenatal use of ultrasonography has allowed detection of cystic hygroma in utero and a better opportunity to study the karyotype. Of 15 consecutive cases of nuchal hygroma detected prenatally, 11 (73 per cent) had a karyotype consistent with Turner syndrome.[16] Poland and colleagues[89] reported 22 fetuses with cystic hygroma and female external genitalia among 813 embryos studied. They noted edema of the limbs in 15 cases and generalized edema in 9 cases. Twenty of the 22 fetuses had associated anomalies. Sex chromatin was negative in 5; karyotyping was successful in only 2, and both were XO. Four cases had coarctation of the aorta. The cause of fetal cystic hygroma is believed to be failure of the jugular lymphatic sac to connect with the jugular vein, which occurs at approximately 40 days' gestation.

Clinical Findings

The most striking feature of the typical newborn with XO karyotype is a webbed neck, which is often accompanied by some residual fluid in the posterior neck area,[106] as well as pedal and hand edema (Fig. 48–8). Short stature is often evident even at birth, and the chest

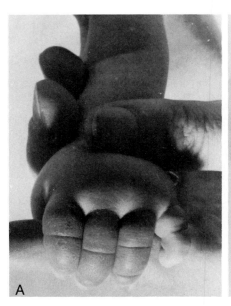
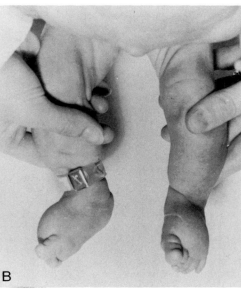

Figure 48–8. Newborn infant with XO Turner syndrome showing lymphedema. *A*, Hand. *B*, Feet.

appears broad with widely spaced nipples. The maxilla is narrow, and the mandible is relatively small. The ears are often prominent, and often there is a prominent crease below the orbits.[41] The posterior hairline appears low, and there is often lax skin at the posterior neck area (Fig. 48–9). The mean birthweight is 2900 g. Skeletal abnormalities include a cubitus valgus deformity and a short fourth metacarpal or metatarsal. Nails are described as narrow and hyperconvex and may be quite deep set. Pigmented nevi are often excessive in number but generally are not present in the newborn period and become more apparent with increasing age. Common internal anomalies include renal malformations, most commonly a horseshoe kidney or a double or cleft renal pelvis. Minor renal abnormalities may also occur. Cardiac defects occur in at least 20 per cent.[44,65]

Many patients with XO-XX mosaicisms or infants with only partial deletion of the X chromosome may appear quite normal at birth or have only very subtle findings. Redundant nuchal skin and lymphedema in the newborn should alert the clinician to the possibility of Turner syndrome. If the condition is not recognized in the neonatal period, features that later will suggest the possibility of Turner syndrome include short stature and failure to develop secondary sex characteristics as adolescence approaches.[61] Although sexual infantilism with streak ovaries is a characteristic finding in Turner syndrome, there is considerable variation. A number of patients with mosaicism do develop secondary sex characteristics, and a rare patient may be fertile.[55,75]

There is little information regarding the true incidence of congenital heart defects in Turner syndrome since there are no large series of cases diagnosed from birth. Coarctation of the aorta has long been recognized as a frequently associated malformation in patients with Turner syndrome. The incidence of coarctation of the aorta in patients appears to be higher in those with XO Turner syndrome than in those with XO-XX mosaicism or only partial deletion of the X chromosome.[40] Miller and colleagues[70] reported a high incidence of biscuspid aortic valve in older patients with Turner syndrome, as well as idiopathic dilatation of the aortic root and mitral valve prolapse. In that series of 80 patients with Turner syndrome, 13 had coarctation of the aorta.[70] Thirty-five patients with Turner syndrome who had no history or clinical evidence of congenital heart disease were studied by echocardiography. An M-mode study was obtained in all, and 29 of the 35 had two-dimensional echocardiography as well. Twelve of the 35 patients (34 per cent) were shown to have a biscuspid aortic valve. Two patients had mitral valve prolapse, and two had a dilated aortic root. Allen and associates[2] reported 28 patients with Turner syndrome ranging in age from 11 to 26 years. Twenty-four of the 28 had chromosome studies revealing a 45,XO karyotype in 14 and a mosaic or isochromosome X in 10. Two of their 28 (7 per cent) had coarctation of the aorta, 5 of 28 (18 per cent) had a bicuspid aortic valve, and 8 of 28 (29 per cent) had an aortic root diameter that was greater than 90 per cent of the control group of similar body surface area. The pathologic association of cystic medial necrosis with aortic dissection in patients

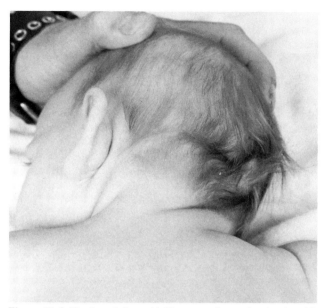

Figure 48–9. Newborn infant with Turner syndrome showing lax skin at posterior neck and low hairline.

with Turner syndrome was first noted by Kostich and Opitz[56] and has subsequently been confirmed by several authors. Although there is an increased risk of aortic dissection in those Turner syndrome patients who also have coarctation of the aorta or a bicuspid aortic valve, Allen[2] did note several patients who had only an isolated dilatation of the aortic root. The majority of patients reported with aortic dissection with Turner syndrome have been adults,[66] but there has been one report[67] of a fatal rupture in a 4-year-old child with Turner syndrome.

No large series of newborns with Turner syndrome has been reported. Gordon and O'Neal,[41] however, reported 10 infants with the Turner infantile phenotype. Three of their patients had serous effusions, 9 had edema of the feet, and 7 had a loose neck fold. Two patients died at 3 days and 4 days of age, but in neither was significant congenital heart disease reported. Follow-up of the cardiac findings in the other 8 infants was not given. Eller and associates,[30] in 1971, described the prognosis in newborns with X chromosomal abnormalities. Routine screening of the chromatin constitution of 21,214 consecutive newborns identified 32 infants with gross X chromosomal abnormalities. They noted 3 patients with XO karyotype who had the typical features of Turner syndrome as neonates. All 3 had prominent dorsal pedal edema at birth. One of the 3 died by 13 days of age with coarctation of the aorta. The other 2 survived, but follow-up of their cardiac status was not given. They also noted 6 patients with 45,XO/46,XX karyotype. None of these had classic features of Turner syndrome, and all had a normal phenotype as neonates. Greenwood and colleagues[43] reported that there were 5 infants with XO Turner syndrome among 1566 infants in the New England Regional Infant Cardiac Program. Heart lesions in these 5 infants included one case each of severe coarctation of the aorta, aortic atresia and hypoplastic left-heart syndrome, levocardia and asplenia, transposition with an intact ventricular septum, and truncus arteriosus. Ary[4] noted 5 patients with gonadal dysgenesis among 652 autopies. It is of great interest to note that of 12 cases of premature closure of the foramen ovale reported by Ary, there were seven males and five females and four of the five females had gonadal dysgenesis. Three of the four infants with Turner syndrome with premature closure of the foramen ovale had hypoplastic left-heart syndrome, whereas the fourth had a double-outlet right ventricle with a hypoplastic left ventricle. The fifth patient with gonadal dysgenesis had coarctation of the aorta.

My own experience would suggest that severe congenital heart disease may cause death in the newborn with Turner syndrome. I have seen five infants with Turner syndrome who died in early infancy. Three had aortic atresia and hypoplastic left-heart syndrome, another had severe aortic stenosis with endocardial fibroelastosis, and the fifth had a patent ductus arteriosus and stenosis of the left coronary artery. Natowicz and Kelley[76] reported an association of Turner syndrome with hypoplastic left-heart syndrome. Among 91 autopsy cases of hypoplastic left-heart syndrome, there were three examples of Turner syndrome, including two fetuses and one liveborn. The association of hypoplastic left-heart syndrome and Turner syndrome was first noted by Conen and Glass[24] in 1963.

Some early studies reported pulmonary stenosis among the cardiac defects seen in Turner syndrome, but these studies probably included some patients with Noonan syndrome.[94,100] To my knowledge there has not been any patient with documented XO Turner syndrome who has had pulmonary stenosis,[80] which is a lesion commonly seen in Noonan syndrome. Left-sided lesions, such as bicuspid aortic valve, aortic stenosis, aortic atresia, and dilatation of the aortic root, are strongly associated with Turner syndrome.[112] It is of interest that all of these lesions have an increased incidence in males.

Partial anomalous pulmonary venous drainage with an intact atrial septum is an uncommon lesion and is more frequently found in males than females. There are six patients reported in the literature with Turner syndrome who had partial anomalous pulmonary venous drainage.[40,62,92,110] In none of them was an atrial septal defect confirmed. My experience would suggest that partial anomalous pulmonary venous drainage may be quite common in patients with XO Turner syndrome. In five patients with Turner syndrome studied by cardiac catheterization, I found partial anomalous pulmonary venous drainage in three. Two of these patients also had a coarctation of the aorta. Two underwent surgical correction of the partial anomalous pulmonary venous drainage, and the atrial septum was intact in both. The third patient had a single left upper pulmonary vein into the innominate vein that was not believed to be of sufficient functional significance to require repair. In two of the patients, an atrial septal defect was suspected because of clinical findings, whereas in the third the partial anomalous pulmonary venous drainage was only diagnosed because a pulmonary artery angiogram had been done to visualize the left side of the heart since a catheter could not be passed across the coarctation. An additional patient with aortic atresia and premature closure of the foramen ovale at postmortem had partial anomalous pulmonary venous drainage of both upper pulmonary veins.

Clark,[22] in 1984, speculated that there was an association between neck web and congenital heart disease in patients with Turner syndrome. He noted that the incidence of congenital heart disease was significantly different between those patients with the neck web and those without. Congenital heart disease occurred in 30 per cent of those with a webbed neck compared with 9 per cent with a normal neck. Twenty-five per cent of patients with neck webbing had coarctation of the aorta whereas only 3 per cent with a normal neck had coarctation. Clark believed the association between webbed neck and congenital heart disease suggested a pathogenic relationship. He proposed that increased lymphatic pressure associated with jugular lymphatic sac obstruction was the mechanism for neck webbing and suggested that thoracic duct distention might compress the ascending aorta and alter intracardiac blood flow. Small changes in left-sided heart blood flow might result in a bicuspid aortic valve, whereas very severe reductions in left-sided heart blood flow could lead to aortic atresia. Dilated lymphatics could also increase lymphatic pressure in the splanchnic space separating the developing lung bud and left atrium. It is certainly very tempting to speculate that some alteration in intracardiac blood flow in utero could be responsible for the spectrum of cardiac defects found in Turner syndrome, namely the tendency for premature closure of the foramen ovale, partial anomalous pulmonary venous drainage with an intact atrial septum, as well as the left-sided obstructive lesions ranging from bicuspid aortic valve to aortic valve atresia. Thus the cardiac defects found in Turner syndrome could be secondary to fetal thoracic pressure alterations caused by the lymphatic abnormalities.

Differential Diagnosis

With the increasing use of fetal ultrasound, fetal cystic hygroma is being recognized more commonly. Turner syndrome should certainly be suspected in cases of fetal cystic hygroma and probably accounts for the majority of those cases in which a definitive diagnosis is made. A report by Carr and colleagues[14] recommended that karyotyping be carried out in all cases of fetal cystic hygroma since a number of other conditions can be associated with cystic hygroma. Other chromosomal anomalies associated with cystic hygroma include trisomy 21, 18, 13, 13q–, 18q–, partial 11q trisomy, and trisomy 22. Fetal cystic hygroma may also occur with normal chromosomes; in such cases Noonan syndrome should be considered in the differential diagnosis. There are five reports that describe fetal cystic hygroma occurring in multiple sibships of a family, suggesting that this condition may occur as an autosomal recessive syndrome.[14]

Noonan syndrome should also be considered in a newborn with lymphedema or a webbed neck. Multiple pterygium syndrome has webbing not only of the neck but also of the axilla, elbows, and knees and should not lead to confusion. A karyotype should be obtained in infants with unexplained lymphedema, particularly if there is redundant skin at the nape of the neck.[101]

Medical Management

A neonate with a persistent cystic hygroma of the neck with accompanying lymphedema is very likely to have XO Turner syndrome. The majority of infants with Turner syndrome, however, will have more subtle features. The diagnosis may well be missed in the newborn period. Coarctation of the aorta and aortic atresia are both lesions found more commonly in males than females. Any female neonate with these lesions should be evaluated for the possibility of Turner syndrome. In my experience, four of five Turner syndrome newborns dying of a severe cardiac malformation had a typical phenotype with a webbed neck and lymphedema but the fifth had a normal phenotype. Routine karyotyping at postmortem examination revealed a mosaic form of Turner syndrome in that patient. Hypoplastic left-heart syndrome has been reported in at least one other mosaic form of Turner syndrome.[63] Although a buccal smear demonstrating a negative nuclear sex chromatin pattern might be helpful as a screening test for Turner syndrome, it is important to remember that Turner syndrome may be present with a positive nuclear sex chromatin pattern if the patient has mosaicism. Even if the buccal smear is negative, karyotyping should be carried out to rule out the rare XO-XY mosaicism known as mixed gonadal dysgenesis. Such patients often have genitalia that are ambiguous; in some there are somatic signs of Turner syndrome with female-appearing external genitalia. Gonadal tumors, especially gonadal blastomas, are reported to have increased frequency in patients with mixed gonadal dysgenesis.[73,74] Chromosomal analysis should be carried out on all patients suspected of Turner syndrome; should a mixed gonadal dysgenesis be found, surgical removal of the gonads should be carried out at some point because of the increased incidence of gonadal neoplasia.

Lymphedema present at birth gradually subsides without therapy. The redundant nuchal skin also improves, but a short webbed neck may persist. Because of the tendency for keloid formation in these patients, plastic surgery on the webbed neck should be avoided. In order to evaluate the aortic root and aortic valve, an echocardiogram should be performed in patients with Turner syndrome even if they have no clinical evidence of congenital heart disease. A newborn with Turner syndrome should be suspect for serious congenital heart disease. An ultrasound examination of the abdomen should be helpful in defining a renal abnormality.

In the absence of significant cardiac or renal disease, the patient with Turner syndrome requires little in the way of medical management throughout childhood. Primary amenorrhea and failure of secondary sex characteristics to develop in adolescence are usual. However, some patients with mosaicism do develop secondary sex development, menses, and even fertility. Hormonal treatment with estrogens will promote breast development and other secondary sex characteristics as well as the initiation of menses. Replacement therapy with estrogens should be deferred until 13 to 15 years of age to avoid early closure of the epiphyses, since short stature is the rule.

Prognosis

The prognosis for the XO fetus is very poor; over 99 per cent are spontaneously aborted. Probably the majority of Turner syndrome infants born alive have some degree of mosaicism. Those infants with a full-blown clinical picture of Turner syndrome at birth are more likely to have the XO karyotype without definite evidence of mosaicism. My experience and the reports from the literature suggest that a significant number of these infants will develop symptoms of cardiac failure in early infancy. Serious congenital cardiac defects are probably more common than previously suspected.

Coarctation of the aorta, if present, should be corrected. Beyond the newborn period, the operative mortality for coarctation is usually very low. Ravelo and associates[95] reported 8 patients with Turner syndrome among 353 patients undergoing surgical repair of coarctation of the aorta. Three of the 8 had severe perioperative hemorrhage from the aortic wall, resulting in one death and one paraplegia. In 2 others the aorta wall appeared so thin that a patch angioplasty was carried out instead of resection with end-to-end anastomosis. These authors caution that surgical treatment of coarctation of the aorta in patients with Turner syndrome should be carried out with great care and caution. Van der Hauwaert and coworkers[112] reported one of their three patients with Turner syndrome undergoing surgical repair of coarctation died 1 week later from acute necrotizing arteritis of the superior mesenteric artery. In none of the three fatal cases reported was there evidence of cystic medial necrosis. Why the aorta is so friable is not clear, but the increased incidence of aortic root dilatation with risk of dissection should be kept in mind. For those patients without clinical evidence of congenital heart disease, echocardiography may reveal an unsuspected bicuspid aortic valve or dilatation of the aorta. Such patients will require periodic reevaluation.

There is surprisingly little in the literature regarding the life expectancy of patients with Turner syndrome. The stature is almost always below the third percentile,[83] and an adult height of more than 58 inches is rare. As mentioned previously, dissecting aortic aneurysm is a rare complication that has been reported in a number of adults with Turner syndrome. Patients with Turner syndrome have an increased incidence of lymphocytic thyroiditis, systemic hypertension, intestinal telangiectasia, and diabetes, as well as hearing and cognitive problems.[6]

References

1. Allan LD, Crawford DC, Anderson RH, Tynan MJ (1984): Echocardiographic and anatomical correlations in fetal congenital heart disease. Br Heart J 52:542–548.

2. Allen DB, Hendricks MD, Levy JM (1986): Aortic dilation in Turner syndrome. J Pediatr 109:302–305.

3. Anderson KR, Fiddler GI, Lie JT (1977): Congenital papillary tumor of the tricuspid valve. Mayo Clin Proc 52:665–669.

4. Ary JB (1984): Cardiovascular Pathology in Infants and Children. Philadelphia, WB Saunders, pp 34, 73–74.

5. Baird PA, Sadovnick AD (1987): Life expectancy in Down syndrome. J Pediatr 110:849–854.

6. Bender B, Puck M, Salbenblatt J, Robinson A (1984): Cognitive development of unselected girls with complete and partial X monosomy. Pediatrics 73:175–182.

7. Berger TJ, Blackstone EH, Kirklin JW, Bargeron LM, Hazelrig JB, Turner ME (1979): Survival and probability of cure without and with operation in complete atrioventricular canal. Ann Thorac Surg 27:104–111.

8. Berger TJ, Kirklin JW, Blackstone EH, Pacifico AD, Kouchoukos NT (1978): Primary repair of complete atrioventricular canal in patients less than 2 years old. Am J Cardiol 41:906–913.

9. Bharati S, Lev M (1973): Congenital polyvalvular disease. Circulation 47:575–586.

10. Bofinger MK, Dignan PSJ, Schmidt RE, Warkany J (1973): Reduction malformations and chromosome anomalies. Am J Dis Child 125:135–143.

11. Bove KE (1970): Gonadal dysgenesis in a newborn with XO karyotype. Am J Dis Child 120:363–366.

12. Butler LJ, Snodgrass GJAI, France NE, Sinclair L, Russell A (1965): E (16–18) trisomy syndrome: Analysis of 13 cases. Arch Dis Child 40:600–611.

13. Carr DH (1965): Chromosome studies in spontaneous abortions. Obstet Gynecol 26:308–326.

14. Carr RF, Ochs RH, Ritter DA, Kenney JD, Fridey JL, Ming PL (1986): Fetal cystic hygroma and Turner syndrome. Am J Dis Child 140:580–583.

15. Carter PE, Pearn JH, Bell J, Martin N, Anderson NG (1985): Survival in trisomy 18. Clin Genet 27:59–61.

16. Chervenak FA, Isaacson G, Blakemore KJ, Breg WR, Hobbins JC, Berkowitz RL, Tortora M, Mayden K, Mahoney MJ (1983): Fetal cystic hygroma: Cause and natural history. N Engl J Med 309:822–825.

17. Chi TLC, Krovetz LJ (1975): The pulmonary vascular bed in children with Down syndrome. J Pediatr 86:533–538.

18. Chin AJ, Bierman FZ, Sanders SP, Williams RG, Norwood WI, Castaneda AR (1983): Subxyphoid 2-dimensional echocardiographic identification of left ventricular papillary muscle anomalies in complete common atrioventricular canal. Am J Cardiol 51:1695–1699.

19. Chin AJ, Keane JF, Norwood WI, Castaneda AR (1982): Repair of complete common atrioventricular canal in infancy. J Thorac Cardiovasc Surg 84:437–445.

20. Chu JY, Weldon BC (1982): Acute leukemia in a patient with Down syndrome and transient congenital leukemia. Am J Dis Child 136:367.

21. Clapp SK, Perry BL, Farooki ZQ, Jackson WL, Karpawich PP, Hakimi M, Arciniegas E, Green EW (1987): Surgical and medical results of complete atrioventricular canal: A ten year review. Am J Cardiol 59:454–458.

22. Clark EB (1984): Neck web and congenital heart defects: A pathogenic association in 45 X-O Turner syndrome? Teratology 29:355–361.

23. Clarke CM, Edwards JH, Smallpiece V (1961): 21 trisomy/normal mosaicism in an intelligent child with some mongoloid characters. Lancet 1:1028–1030.

24. Conen PE, Glass IH (1963): 45/XO Turner syndrome in the newborn: Report of 2 cases. J Clin Endocrinol 23:1–10.

25. Cooney TP, Thurlbeck WM (1982): Pulmonary hypoplasia in Down syndrome. N Engl J Med 307:1170–1173.

26. Cullum L, Liebman J (1969): The association of congenital heart disease with Down syndrome (mongolism). Am J Cardiol 24:354–357.

27. Cutler NR, Heston LL, Davies P, Haxby JV, Schapiro MB (1985): Alzheimer's disease and Down syndrome. Ann Intern Med 103:566–578.

28. Down JL (1866): Observation on an ethnic classification of idiots. Clin Lect Rep Lond Hosp 3:259–262.

29. Edwards JH, Harden DG, Cameron AH, Crosse VM, Wolff OH (1960): A new trisomic syndrome. Lancet 1:787–790.

30. Eller E, Frankenburg W, Puck M, Robinson A (1971): Prognosis in newborn infants with X-chromosomal abnormalities. Pediatrics 47:681–688.

31. Eunpu DL, McDonald DM, Zackai EH (1986): Trisomy 21: Rate in second-degree relatives. Am J Med Genet 25:361–363.

32. Ferrier P, Shepard TH, Gartler S, Burt B (1961): Chromatin positive gonadal dysgenesis and mosaicism. Lancet 1:1170–1171.

33. Flavell G (1943): Webbing of the neck with Turner syndrome in the male. Br J Surg 31:150–153.

34. Ford CE, Jones KW, Polani PE, de Almeida JC, Briggs JH (1959): A sex chromosome anomaly in a case of gonadal dysgenesis (Turner syndrome). Lancet 1:711–713.

35. Fort P, Lifshitz F, Bellisario R, Davis J, Lanes R, Pugliese M, Richman R, Post EM, David R (1984): Abnormalities of thyroid function in infants with Down syndrome. J Pediatr 104:545–549.

36. Fraser J, Mitchell A (1876): Kalmuck idiocy: Report of case with autopsy with notes on 62 cases by A. Mitchell. J Ment Sci 22:169–179.

37. Fujimoto A, Broom DL, Shinno NW, Wilson MG (1983): Nonimmune fetal hydrops and Down syndrome. Am J Med Genet 14:533–537.

38. Funke O (1902): Pterygium colli. Dtsch Z Chir 63:162–167.

39. Garrod AE (1894): On the association of cardiac malformations with other congenital defects. St Barth Hosp Rep 30:53.

40. Goldberg MB, Scully AL, Solomon IL, Steinbach HL (1968): Gonadal dysgenesis in phenotypic female subjects. Am J Med 45:529–543.

41. Gordon RR, O'Neill EM (1969): Turner infantile phenotype. Br Med J 1:483–485.

42. Greenwood RD, Nadas AS (1976): The clinical course of cardiac disease in Down's syndrome. Pediatrics 58:893–897.

43. Greenwood RD, Rosenthal A, Parisi L, Fyler DC, Nadas AS (1975): Extracardiac abnormalities in infants with congenital heart disease. Pediatrics 55:485–492.

44. Haddad HM, Wilkins L (1959): Congenital anomalies associated with gonadal aplasia. Pediatrics 23:885–902.

45. Hall B (1966): Mongolism in newborn infants. Clin Pediatr 5:4–12.

46. Hanhart E, Delhanty JDA, Penrose LS (1961): Trisomy in mother and child. Lancet 1:403.

47. Hoffman JIE, Christianson R (1978): Congenital heart disease in a cohort of 19,502 births with long-term follow-up. Am J Cardiol 42:641–647.

48. Hook EB (1981): Down syndrome frequency in human populations and factors pertinent to variations in rate. In de La Cruz FF, Gerald PS (eds): Trisomy 21 (Down Syndrome) Research Perspectives. Baltimore, University Park Press, pp 3–67.

49. Hook EB (1978): Spontaneous deaths of fetuses with chromosomal abnormalities diagnosed prenatally. N Engl J Med 299:1036–1038.

50. Hsu LYF, Strauss L, Dubin E, Hirschhorn K (1973): Prenatal diagnosis of trisomy 18. Am J Dis Child 125:290–292.

51. Hutchison AA, Drew JH, Yu VYH, Williams ML, Fortune DW, Beischer NA (1982): Nonimmunologic hydrops fetalis: A review of 61 cases. Obstet Gynecol 59:347–352.

52. Iancu T (1975): The "labial index" in Down syndrome. Clin Genet 8:81–84.

53. James AE, Belcourt CL, Atkins L, Janower ML (1969): Trisomy 18. Radiology 92:37–43.

54. Kleinman CS, Donnerstein RL, DeVare GR, Jaffe CC, Lynch DC, Berkowitz RL, Talner NS, Hobbins JC (1982): Fetal echocardiography for evaluation of in utero congestive heart failure: A technique for study of non-immune fetal hydrops. N Engl J Med 306:568–575.

55. Kohn G, Yarkoni S, Cohen MM (1980): Two conceptions in a 45,X woman. Am J Med Genet 5:339–343.

56. Kostich ND, Opitz JM (1965): Ullrich-Turner syndrome associated with cystic medial necrosis of the aorta and great vessels. Am J Med 39:943–950.

57. Kramer HH, Majewski F, Trampisch HJ, Rammos S, Bourgeois M (1987): Malformation patterns in children with congenital heart disease. Am J Dis Child 141:789–795.

58. Krivitt W, Good RA (1956): The simultaneous occurrence of leukemia and mongolism. Am J Dis Child 94:289–293.

59. Kurnit DM, Layton WM, Matthysse S (1986): Genetics and chance: Inheritance of congenital heart defects. Pediatr Res 20:338A.

60. Lang DJ, Van Dyke DC, Heide F, Lowe PL (1987): Hypospadias and urethral abnormalities in Down syndrome. Clin Pediatr 26:40–42.

61. Leao JC, Voorhess ML, Schlegel RJ, Gardner LI (1966): XX/XO mosaicism in nine preadolescent girls: Short stature as presenting complaint. Pediatrics 38:972–980.

62. Lebecque P, Bosi G, Lentermans J, Stijns M, Germanes J, Chalant CH, Vliers A (1984): Myxomatous degeneration of the mitral valve in a child with Turner syndrome and partial anomalous pulmonary venous return. Eur J Pediatr 141:228–230.

63. Lee JC, Perrin J, Blomberg D (1973): Mosaic Turner syndrome in a newborn (letter). JAMA 226:9.

64. Lejeune J, Gautier M, Turpin R (1959): Études des chromosomes somatiques de neuf enfants mongoliens. C R Acad Sci 248:1721–1722.

65. Lemli L, Smith DW (1963): The XO syndrome: A study of the differential phenotype in 25 patients. J Pediatr 63:577–588.

66. Lin AE, Lippe BM, Geffner ME, Gomes A, Lois JF, Barton CW, Rosenthal A, Friedman WF (1986): Aortic dilation, dissection, and rupture in patients with Turner syndrome. J Pediatr 109:820–826.

67. Lippe BM, Kogus MD (1972): Aortic rupture in gonadal dysgenesis (letter). J Pediatr 80:895–896.

68. Lisser H, Curtis LE, Escamilla RF, Goldberg MB (1947): The syndrome of congenitally aplastic ovaries with sexual infantilism, high urinary gonadotropins, short stature, and other congenital anomalies: Tabular presentation of twenty-five previously unpublished cases. J Clin Endocrinol 7:665–687.

69. Matsuoka R, Misugi K, Goto A, Gilbert EF, Ando M (1983): Congenital heart anomalies in the trisomy 18 syndrome, with reference to congenital polyvalvular disease. Am J Med Genet 14:657–668.

70. Miller MJ, Geffner ME, Lippe BM, Itami RM, Kaplan SA, DiSessa TG, Isabel-Jones JB, Friedman WF (1983): Echocardiography reveals a high incidence of bicuspid aortic valve in Turner syndrome. J Pediatr 102:47–50.

71. Milunsky A, Atkin L, Littlefield J (1972): Lessons from one hundred amniocenteses for prenatal genetic studies. Pediatr Res 6:356A.

72. Moessinger AC, Mills JL, Harley EE, Ramakrishnan R, Berendes HW, Blanc WA (1986): Umbilical cord length in Down syndrome. Am J Dis Child 140:1276–1277.

73. Moshang T Jr, Vallet HL, Cintron C, Bongiovanni AM, Eberlein WR (1972): Gonadal function in mosaic XO/XY or XX/XY Turner syndrome. J Pediatr 80:460–464.

74. Muller J, Skakkebaek NE, Ritzen M, Ploen L, Petersen KE (1985): Carcinoma in situ of the testis in children with 45,X/46,XY gonadal dysgenesis. J Pediatr 106:431–436.

75. Nakashima I, Robinson A (1971): Fertility in a 45,X female. Pediatrics 47:770–772.

76. Natowicz M, Kelley RI (1987): Association of Turner syndrome with hypoplastic left-heart syndrome. Am J Dis Child 141:218–220.

77. Newfeld EA, Sher M, Paul MH, Nikaidoh H (1977): Pulmonary vascular disease in complete atrioventricular canal defect. Am J Cardiol 39:721–726.

78. Nicolis FB, Sacchetta G (1963): A nomogram for the x-ray evaluation of some morphological anomalies of the pelvis in the diagnosis of mongolism. Pediatrics 1074–1076.

79. Noonan JA, Ehmke DA (1963): Associated non-cardiac malformations in children with congenital heart disease (abstr). J Pediatr 63:469.

80. Nora JJ, Torres FG, Sinha AK, McNamara DG (1970): Characteristic cardiovascular anomalies of XO Turner syndrome, XX and XY phenotype and XO/XX Turner mosaic. Am J Cardiol 25:639–641.

81. Opitz JM, Summitt RL, Sarto GE (1965): Noonan syndrome in girls: A genocopy of the Ullrich-Turner syndrome (abstr). J Pediatr 67:968.

82. Palmer CG, Reichmann A (1976): Chromosomal and clinical findings in 110 females with Turner's syndrome. Hum Genet 35:35–49.

83. Park E, Bailey JD, Cowell CA (1983): Growth and maturation of patients with Turner syndrome. Pediatr Res 17:1–7.

84. Park SC, Mathews RA, Zuberbuhler JR, Rowe RD, Neches WH, Lenox CC (1977): Down syndrome with congenital heart malformation. Am J Dis Child 131:29–33.

85. Patau K, Smith DW, Therman E, Inhorn SL, Wagnes HP (1960): Multiple congenital anomaly caused by an extra chromosome. Lancet 1:790–793.

86. Penrose LS, Ellis JR, Delhanty JDA (1960): Chromosomal translocation in mongolism and in normal relatives. Lancet 2:409–410.

87. Perlin BM, Pomerance JJ, Schifrin BS (1981): Nonimmunologic hydrops fetalis. Obstet Gynecol 57:584–588.

88. Pierpont MEM, Goolin RJ, Moller JH (1987): Chromosomal abnormalities. In Pierpont MEM, Moller JH (eds): Genetics of Cardiovascular Disease. Norwell, Martinus Nijhoff, pp 69–94.

89. Poland BJ, Dill F, Paradice B (1980): A Turner-like phenotype in the aborted fetus. Teratology 21:361–365.

90. Polani PE, Briggs JH, Ford CE, Clarke CM, Berg JM (1960): A mongol girl with 46 chromosomes. Lancet 1:721–724.

91. Polani PE, Hunter WF, Lennox B (1954): Chromosomal sex in Turner syndrome with coarctation of the aorta. Lancet 2:120–121.

92. Price WH, Willey RF (1980): Partial anomalous pulmonary venous return in two patients with Turner syndrome. J Med Genet 17:133–134.

93. Pulliam LH, Huether CA (1986): Translocation Down syndrome in Ohio 1970–1981: Epidemiologic and cytogenetic factors and mutation rate estimates. Am J Hum Genet 39:361–370.

94. Ranier-Pope CR, Cunningham RD, Nadas AS, Crigler JF (1964): Cardiovascular malformations in Turner syndrome. Pediatrics 33:919–925.

95. Ravelo HR, Stephenson LW, Friedman S, Chatten J, Rashkind WJ, Vidas M, Edmunds LH Jr (1980): Coarctation resection in children with Turner's syndrome. J Thorac Cardiovasc Surg 80:427–430.

96. Redheendran R, Neu RL, Bannerman RM (1981): Long survival in trisomy-13 syndrome: 21 cases including prolonged survival in two patients 11 and 19 years old. Am J Med Genet 8:167–172.

97. Rosenquist GC, Sweeney LJ, Amsel J, McAllister HA (1974): Enlargement of the membranous ventricular septum: An internal stigma of Down syndrome. J Pediatr 85:490–493.

98. Rowe RD, Uchida IA (1961): Cardiac malformations in mongolism: Prospective study of 184 mongoloid children. Am J Med 31:726–735.

99. Rushton DI, Faed MJW, Richards SEM, Bain AD (1969): The fetal manifestations of the 45XO karyotype. J Obstet Gynaecol Br Commonw 76:266–272.

100. Seggers DC, Polani PE (1972): Congenital heart disease in male and female subjects with somatic features of Turner syndrome and normal sex chromosome: Ullrich's and related syndromes. Br Heart J 34:41–46.

101. Shapiro LR, Hsu LYF, Hirschhorn K (1970): Extra posterior cervical skin: A possible sign of chromosomal aberration in infancy. J Pediatr 77:690–691.

102. Silverman N, Levitsky S, Fisher E, DuBrow I, Hastreiter A, Scagliotti D (1983): Efficacy of pulmonary artery banding in infants with complete atrioventricular canal. Circulation 68(suppl II):48–53.

103. Singh RP, Carr DH (1966): The anatomy and histology of XO human embryos and fetuses. Anat Rec 155:369–383.

104. Smith DW (1982): Recognizable Patterns of Human Malformation. 3rd ed. Philadelphia, WB Saunders, pp 10–23, 72–75.

105. Smith DW, Patau K, Therman E, Inhorn SL (1960): A new autosomal trisomy syndrome. J Pediatr 57:338–345.

106. Sunderland WA (1970): Fluid-filled pterygium colli (XO Turner syndrome). Am J Dis Child 119:352–353.

107. Tandon R, Edwards JE (1973): Cardiac malformations associated with Down syndrome. Circulation 47:1349–1355.

108. Tjio JH, Levan A (1956): The chromosome number of man. Hereditas 42:1–6.

109. Turner HH (1938): A syndrome of infantilism, congenital webbed neck, and cubitus valgus. Endocrinology 23:566–574.

110. Uhrenholdt A, Wilton B, Djernes B, Efsen F (1975): Partial anomalous pulmonary venous drainage in a patient with Turner syndrome. Dan Med Bull 22:37–39.

111. Ullrich O (1930): Uber typische Kombinationsbilder multiper Abantungen. Z Kinderheilkd 49:271–276.

112. Van der Hauwaert LG, Fryns JP, Dumoulin M, Logghe N (1978): Cardiovascular malformations in Turner and Noonan syndrome. Br Heart J 40:500–509.

113. Vesterhus P, Moe PJ (1974): Bone marrow dysfunction in a newborn twin with Down syndrome. Clin Pediatr 13:347–349.

114. Waardenburg PJ (1932): Das menschlicke Auge und seine Erbaulagen. The Hague, Martinus Nijhoff.

115. Warburg M, Mikkelsen M (1963): A case of 13–15 trisomy or Bartholin-Patau's syndrome. Acta Ophthalmol 41:321–334.

116. Warburton D (1980): Monosomy X: A chromosomal anomaly associated with young maternal age. Lancet 1(8161):167–169.

117. Wegelius R, Vaananer I, Koskela SL (1967): Down's syndrome and transient leukemia-like disease in a newborn. Acta Paediat 56:301–306.

118. Wilson SK, Hutchins GM, Neill CA (1979): Hypertensive pulmonary vascular disease in Down syndrome. J Pediatr 95:722–726.

119. Wright TC, Orkin RW, Destrempes M, Kurnit DM (1984): Increased adhesiveness of Down syndrome fetal fibroblasts in vitro. Proc Natl Acad Sci USA 81:2426–2430.

49 TERATOGENIC AGENTS

Herbert S. Harned, Jr.

Genetic factors and chromosomal aberrations are well known to cause congenital malformations, but several important human teratogens have also been identified. Even with the future discovery of additional agents currently thought to be safe, it is unlikely that more than 10 per cent of congenital malformations will be shown to be due to specific exogenous teratogens. A greater number of malformations probably occur as a result of a combination of genetic and environmental factors, including teratogens, but the biochemical mechanisms involved in these interrelationships are only beginning to be perceived.

The thalidomide tragedy emphasized dramatically the extraordinarily deleterious effects that a prescribed drug might have on the developing fetus.[50,54] Although other agents previously had been shown to be teratogenic,[39,71,74,80] the serious nature of the defects produced and the delay in incrimination of thalidomide highlighted the need for more effective research in teratology. Improved monitoring of agents that might cause embryopathies has resulted, and there has been impetus to avoid all potentially harmful agents during human gestation.

Although the latter is a legitimate goal, it cannot be achieved at this time, because certain prescribed drugs, with known but infrequent teratogenic effects, are needed to treat serious disorders occurring in pregnant women, including seizures, depression, malignancy, and potentially thrombotic states. Unfortunately, widespread prescribed and nonprescribed drug use occurs among women, especially during the early stages of gestation before pregnancy is known. Many of these agents are potential teratogens. Finally, accidental environmental exposures to teratogens also cause congenital defects.

Considerable overlap exists in the clinical features of various teratogenic syndromes, probably indicating similar cellular derangements. In many cases, specific teratogens can be suspected strongly from the clinical findings and questions can be directed toward maternal use of those agents. Furthermore, accurate anatomic diagnosis of the cardiac lesion may help to identify the offending teratogen. A partial listing of the agents to be discussed is presented in Table 49–1.

The cardiologist usually becomes involved with patients suspected of having a teratogen-induced malformation when he is called on to evaluate a cardiac murmur in an unusual-appearing child. On the other hand, sometimes the murmur will be the primary finding and the syndromic features may only be appreciated after close observation.

As communications between obstetricians and pediatricians have improved, information about exposure of the mother to possible teratogens may be available to the cardiologist. A history of prescribed drugs is easier to obtain than a history of drug abuse or exposure to environmental toxins. In evaluating cardiac murmurs, questions should be asked about the use of all the drugs indicated by asterisks in Table 49–1, since each one appears to be associated with cardiac malformations. In addition, even broader questioning might reveal previously unknown associations, as well as contributing to the general care of the infant and anticipating problems with future pregnancies.

Despite similar exposures to known teratogens, not all fetuses, even twins, develop embryopathies. The genetic predisposition to develop embryopathies including cardiac malformations, in response to teratogens, has not been well delineated but is under active investigation. None of the known human teratogens, including thalidomide, invariably produces fetal disorders. The dose of the offending agent is important, as evidenced by an increased incidence of fetal cardiac malformations with increased maternal ingestion of alcohol or trimethadione. Up to 30 per cent of infants so exposed may develop cardiac defects, a percentage similar to that found with severe rubella infection or poorly controlled maternal diabetes.[74]

REQUIRED THERAPEUTIC DRUGS

Anticonvulsants

One in 200 women require anticonvulsant therapy. When possible, anticonvulsant drugs should be discontinued during the period of fetal organogenesis. Even phenobarbital has not been ruled out as a teratogen in high doses,[89] but this drug appears to carry much less teratogenic risk than several other anticonvulsant agents. Anticonvulsant-induced teratogenic syndromes are all serious and are all associated with congenital cardiac defects.

Hydantoin

The fetal hydantoin syndrome is especially important, since it is a widely studied, easily identifiable condition that nicely illustrates the interplay of environmental and genetic factors in drug-induced embryopathies. The association between anticonvulsant medication of the mother and appearance of congenital anomalies in the fetus was suggested first by Meadow in 1968.[59,60] Subsequently, many others have confirmed this association.

The estimated risk for an exposed infant to develop classic fetal hydantoin syndrome is 7 to 10 per cent, but the incidence of developing partial hydantoin syndromic features is as high as 40 per cent.[33–35, 62,100]

Table 49–1. TERATOGENIC AGENTS

Categories	References
Required Therapeutic Drugs	
Anticonvulsants	
Hydantoin*	7, 8, 9, 23, 33, 34, 35, 62, 81, 91, 100, 101
Valproic acid*	6, 41, 44, 68
Trimethadione*	27, 91, 103
Primidone*	47, 64, 82, 84
Phenobarbital	79, 80
Antidepressives	
Lithium*	52, 75, 96
Anticoagulants	
Warfarin*	91
Antineoplastics	
Aminopterin	91
Others	
Drugs of Abuse	
Alcohol*	11, 15, 42, 43, 45, 48, 49, 53, 57, 87, 91, 97
Tobacco–nicotine	2, 10, 21, 22, 58, 66, 67, 95
Amphetamines*	76, 77, 94
Diazepam (Valium)	18, 28, 86
Cocaine	5, 14
Other street drugs	25, 26, 30, 51, 65
Marginally Necessary Drugs	
Propranolol*	29
Estrogens and progestagens	4, 37, 38, 72, 73, 102
Bendectin	17, 83, 90, 93
Antihistaminics	
Salicylates	78, 85
Ferrous sulfate	55, 70
Environmental Agents and Conditions	
Hyperthermia*	13, 16, 19, 20, 24, 32, 56, 61, 91, 92
Methyl mercury	3, 36, 46
Lead	69
Hexachlorophene (pHisoHex)	31
Povidone-iodine (Betadine)	12, 99
Polybrominated biphenyls (PBBs)	88
Polychlorinated biphenyls (PCBs)	1
Dioxin	98
Ionizing radiation	63

*Associated with cardiac malformations.

Characteristic features of fetal hydantoin syndrome are hypoplasia of the nails and distal phalanges. These findings were once believed to be quite specific or "sentinel" characteristics, but they have also been observed in several other teratogenic syndromes. The classic fetal hydantoin syndrome includes hypertelorism, prominent metopic suture, broad nasal bridge, cleft lip and palate, syndactyly, polydactyly, club foot, and congenital hip disease, as well as hypoplasia of the nails and distal phalanges. Ambiguous genitalia, anal ectopia, renal disorders, diaphragmatic and umbilical hernias, pyloric stenosis, and duodenal atresia have also been reported.[91]

Cardiac malformations are common in fetal hydantoin syndrome. Ventricular and atrial septal defects, coarctation of the aorta, and patent ductus arteriosus are most frequent. More complex conditions, such as tetralogy of Fallot, transpositions, and hypoplastic left-heart syndrome, may also be present.

The argument as to whether the embryopathy results from hydantoin therapy or from the disorder resulting in maternal seizures has been settled. A higher incidence of this disorder has been demonstrated in progeny of treated epileptic women than in epileptic women not treated with hydantoin.[101] Animal model studies comparing "quaking" and "nonquaking" mice of the same strain revealed that the incidence of deformed offspring was dose related.[35]

Various biochemical studies have attempted to identify the toxic products responsible for fetal hydantoin syndrome. Wells and Harbison[101] showed that hydantoin may be activated in vitro to a toxic arene by the cytochrome P-450 transport system. However, the arene mechanism has been questioned by Finnell and DiLiberti,[23] who showed that ethotoin, which is not metabolized via an arene oxide intermediate, produced a similar syndrome in three siblings. An additional proposed mechanism is that the inhibition of cell growth by hydantoin may be related to inhibition of ornithine decarboxylase and lowered levels of putrescine.[7]

An important report of discordant expression of fetal hydantoin syndrome in heteropaternal dizygotic twins appeared recently.[81] Twin A was a girl with black pigmentation; twin B was a white girl. By 4 years of age, twin A was progressing reasonably well, with an intellectual performance in the low normal range; she had normal finger and toe development. Twin B had an estimated IQ of 66, facial features highly suggestive of fetal hydantoin syndrome, small fingernails, and hypoplastic fifth toes. Genotypic analysis indicated near certainty that the twins were fathered by different persons. These twins were studied further by Buehler,[8,9] who used an artificial substrate to quantitate the specific activity of epoxide hydralase, which detoxifies arene oxide. Epoxide hydralase activity was less in twin B than in twin A, despite the similar exposures to hydantoin. Other affected infants have shown lower epoxide hydralase levels when compared with their unaffected nontwin siblings. These studies demonstrate that a specific, genetically determined enzymatic defect in a fetus may potentiate the teratogenic effects resulting from maternal drug ingestion.

Valproic Acid

Valproic acid is another antiepileptic drug that at times must be administered during pregnancy. Reports have indicated that this drug produces an embryopathy distinct from that seen with hydantoin, primidone, and trimethadione.[6,41,44,68] Valproic acid–affected infants have a different facial appearance, which includes a high forehead, brachycephaly, flat nasal bridge, small nose, shallow or bits, long upper lip, thin vermilion border, macrostomia, and low-set, rotated ears. The fingers are long and overlapping, as are the toes, and the nails are hyperconvex. Mild hypospadias may be present. In a group of 14 infants reported by Jager-Roman and colleagues,[41] whose mothers received valproic acid only, two had congenital heart disease. One had a patent ductus that supposedly closed after 6 months, and one had a nondefined congenital cardiac malformation. The infants who were more severely affected generally were the products of mothers who had received higher doses of valproic acid and who had higher serum levels during pregnancy. Jager-Roman and colleagues advise amniocentesis, ultrasonography, maternal serum valproic acid monitoring during pregnancy to minimize the dose, and careful obstetric care. Good obstetric care is important because the incidence of fetal distress during labor appears to be increased and Apgar scores are often low.

Trimethadione

German and coworkers[27] and Zackai[103] have described the embryopathy associated with trimethadione and paramethadione. Since the incidence of fetal anomalies is 50 to 60 per cent, elective abortion should be considered when women taking these drugs become pregnant. Septal defects, tetralogy of Fallot, transpositions, and hypoplastic chamber defects have been reported.

The general features of the trimethadione syndrome are variable, but hypoplasia of the midface and unusual upward slanting of the eyebrows, strabismus, and maldeveloped rectangular or cupped and overlapping helices have been noted frequently. Other features include a short, upturned nose, low nasal bridge, prominent forehead, cleft lip and palate, micrognathia, ambiguous genitalia, and simian creases. Growth is affected, even prenatally, and mental retardation is common.[91]

Primidone

Primidone appears to have teratogenic properties quite similar to those of hydantoin.[64,82,84] In one report of four siblings,[47] all of whom developed a similar embryopathy, two were treated with primidone and hydantoin and two with primidone alone. The latter two infants exhibited telecanthus, short and antiverted nares, and long upper lips. One of these children had a venticular septal defect, confirmed by echocardiography. Neither of the two infants whose mothers were treated with primidone alone was mentally retarded.

Phenobarbital

A specific embryopathy from maternal phenobarbital use has not been confirmed, but phenobarbital may potentiate the effects of other agents given concurrently. Also, phenobarbital is a strong teratogenic agent in rodents.[79]

Antidepressive Medication

Lithium

The presence of a specific congenital condition can provide a clue to a particular teratogenic agent, as illustrated by the occurrence of a rare congenital cardiac malformation, Ebstein anomaly, in an abnormally high percentage of infants of mothers receiving lithium salts for treatment of psychiatric conditions.[75] Nora screened 733 cases with malformations in which detailed histories of maternal drug ingestion were available. Both mothers in this series who received lithium had infants with Ebstein anomaly of the tricuspid valve. Nora also uncovered six instances of congenital cardiac conditions among the offspring of 118 pregnancies of women receiving lithium. Other lesions of the tricuspid valve, including insufficiency and atresia, have also been found associated with maternal lithium ingestion.[75] At the North Carolina Memorial Hospital a case of Ebstein anomaly associated with maternal lithium use was diagnosed readily by two-dimensional echocardiography.[52] Cardiovascular defects have been produced in fetal mice, along with palatal defects.[96]

Like other major congenital cardiac conditions, Ebstein anomaly, if severe, can be identified by fetal ultrasonography by observing the characteristic displacement of the medial leaflet of the tricuspid valve toward the apex of the right ventricle.

Anticoagulant Medication

Warfarin

Although warfarin has not been observed to cause cardiac lesions in the fetus, it remains important for the cardiologist since warfarin may be essential for anticoagulation of women of child-bearing age who have prosthetic valves. This drug causes abortion in one sixth of pregnancies and a noncardiac embryopathy in another one sixth. Warfarin's fetal embryopathy apparently develops as early as the sixth or ninth week of gestation. Nasal hypoplasia often is accompanied by a deep groove betwen the nasal tip and the alae nasae, stippling of epiphyses, and fetal growth retardation. Warfarin-affected infants may also show some hypoplasia of the nails. Central nervous system disorders, including microcephaly, optic atrophy, seizures, and mental retardation, have been described. Microhemorrhages may account for some of the delayed neurologic defects, but many of the defects described have developed before the major blood factors have been formed.[91]

Heparin, with a molecular weight of 1000 daltons, cannot pass through the placental membrane but is not an ideally adequate substitute for warfarin because it may cause maternal hemorrhage. Heparin is recommended for treatment of thromboembolism in pregnant women because it lacks teratogenic effects.

Antineoplastic Medications

Aminopterin

When aminopterin was used to induce abortions, the fetuses were observed to have a variety of defects. Methotrexate, which is used more widely now than aminopterin as an antineoplastic medication, also has been observed to be teratogenic. The cardiac manifestations that have been observed with aminopterin exposure, including dextroposition, have not been as prominent as other defects, including prenatal growth deficiency, microcephaly with hypoplasia of the bones of the skull, upsweeping of the frontal scalp hair, broad bridging of the nose, prominent eyes, micrognathia, shortness of the forearms, syndactyly, and hypotonia. The number of aminopterin embryopathies has been limited because the underlying condition being treated is usually serious enough to preclude pregnancy.[91]

Other antineoplastic agents that are possibly teratogenic are busulfan (Myleran), chlorambucil (Leukeran), nitrogen mustard, vincristine (Encovin), and procarbazine (Metulane).

DRUGS OF ABUSE

Alcohol

The fetal alcohol syndrome is relatively common, occurring as a full embryopathy in 0.2 per cent of infants in Seattle,[91] and often the heart is affected.

The risk of harm to the fetus from maternal alcohol ingestion was appreciated in ancient times, but fetal alcohol syndrome was only defined clearly very recently by Jones and Smith.[42,43] The Bible has a clear-cut reference to the potential danger of maternal alcohol ingestion. In Judges 13, Manoah's wife is described as being barren. In verse 3 of the King James version, it is stated, "And the angel of the Lord appeared unto the woman, and said unto her, Behold now thou art barren, and bearest not: but thou shall conceive, and bear a son." Verse 4 states "Now therefore beware, I pray thee, and drink not wine nor strong drink, and eat not any unclean thing." Verse 24 states, "And the woman bore a son, and called his name Samson," who turned out to be especially robust. Also, Carthaginian laws prohibited couples from drinking on their wedding nights to keep them from developing bad habits.[43]

The full fetal alcohol syndrome involves growth deficit, mental retardation, and facial abnormalities, which appear to be linked to the amount of alcohol consumed. Perhaps more important are the implications of alcohol causing less obvious findings. Ulleland[97] reinforced Lemoine's[48,49] earlier description of presumed bad effects from maternal alcohol ingestion by describing underweight conditions in infants who also were irritable and hyperactive.

The general features of fetal alcohol syndrome must be known to all those professionals caring for neonates.[91] Many of these features overlap with those described for other drug-induced embryopathies, but several signs are specific enough to suggest alcohol as the embryopathic agent.

Facial features include short palpebral fissures, a short, up-turned nose, hypoplastic philtrum, hypoplastic mandible, thin upper vermilion, retrognathia in infancy, and micrognathia developing later. Neurologic conditions include mild-to-moderate mental retardation, microcephaly, poor coordination, hypotonia, irritability, and hyperactivity. Growth deficiency may be severe but can be found as a mild condition in pregnancies associated with mild drinking (approximately two drinks per day).

The differential diagnosis may not be difficult, but seriously involved infants may resemble those with the deLange syndrome. The Noonan and Williams syndromes may resemble the fetal alcohol syndrome to a degree.

Although the full-blown syndrome is observed primarily in mothers who have averaged four or more drinks daily during the pregnancy, the growth retardation with relatively low alcohol consumption and the possible effects of binge drinking during the active states of organogenesis are of great concern. Some physicians might even challenge the consumption of one daily glass of wine as inadvisable.[15]

Fetal alcohol syndrome can be accompanied by a variety of cardiac lesions. Sandor[87] described 31 patients, 15 of whom had isolated ventricular septal defects and 5 of whom had ventricular septal defects complicated by subpulmonic and subaortic stenoses, aortic regurgitation, coarctation of the aorta, or secundum atrial septal defect. Three isolated secundum atrial septal defects were also noted along with two cases of peripheral pulmonic stenosis.

On the other hand, Loser and Majewski[53] found 10 instances of isolated secundum atrial septal defects and only 2 of ventricular septal defects among 16 fetal alcohol syndrome cases studied by cardiac catheterization.

The biochemical mechanisms causing fetal alcohol syndrome have not been clarified. Some investigators have attributed alcohol's toxicity to its acetaldehyde breakdown product,[57] but ethanol itself may be the toxic product.

There are other interesting aspects of the fetal alcohol syndrome. Nutritional deficiency may potentiate the fetal alcohol syndrome. Keppen and coworkers[45] have shown that zinc deficiency acts as a co-teratogen in animals. There also is a surprisingly high incidence of tumors appearing later in children with fetal alcohol syndrome, especially neural crest tumors and lymphomas. Cavdar[11] raised the possibility that low zinc levels might decrease cellular immunity in the infant of an alcoholic. In Turkey, where zinc deficiency is common, there is a high incidence of MC-type of Hodgkin disease. Alcohol appears to be oncogenic in the adult, but the tumors of the mouth, esophagus, and larynx observed in adult alcoholics are not the same as those observed in the fetal alcohol syndrome.

In summary, alcohol is the most common teratogen in present use and may be the most common drug causing congenital heart disease. The fetal effects of maternal use of other agents in combination with alcohol and the genetic factors that may potentiate alcohol's harmful effects on the fetus remain to be defined.

Tobacco and Nicotine

Cleft lip and palate[21] and cardiac defects[22] have been reported to be associated with maternal smoking but these observations have not been confirmed. However, infants with other congenital defects whose mothers smoked appear to have an increased mortality over those whose mothers did not smoke.[66]

Maternal smoking results in formation of placentas that are small. Peripheral ischemic changes have been observed in these placentas,[67] as well as changes in the villar morphology.[2] The birthweights of infants born to smoking mothers are low, and neonatal mortality is increased.[67] Nicotine alone can have important effects, since nicotine chewing gum results in placental passage of nicotine and interference with fetal breathing.[58] Smoking is a risk factor in sudden infant death syndrome[10] and, when associated with alcoholism in mothers, results in increased neonatal mortality.[95]

Amphetamines

Nora has proposed a relationship between maternal amphetamine use and fetal congenital cardiac conditions, especially septal defects, patent ductus arteriosus, and transpositions, which have been observed in retrospective studies only.[77] Unlike medications such as anticonvulsant drugs that have to be continued during pregnancy, amphetamines are not essential prescribed drugs, but they are used widely on the street. The proof of human teratogenicity of amphetamines has not been established, but animal studies have shown teratogenicity to a degree that warrants further investigation.[76,94] Since there may be a predilection for cardiac conditions, the cardiologist should consider possible maternal amphetamine abuse when evaluating neonates with congenital heart disease.

Diazepam

One report has associated diazepam (Valium) use with fetal cleft lip and palate.[86] Whether this association is true or not, use of diazepam during labor causes decreased Apgar scors and other signs of neonatal depression.[18] Diazepam preferentially crosses the placenta and produces very high serum levels in the fetus that persist for up to a week after delivery.[28]

There are no known reports of cardiac teratogenicity in humans, but widespread use of diazepam warrants concern about additional, as yet unrecognized, deleterious fetal effects.

Cocaine

Cocaine is used so widely as a street drug that concern must be raised about its possible teratogenicity. Although no cardiac conditions have been documented, there is no question that cocaine can cause abruptio placentae after intravenous injection, presumably from its norepinephrine effects. The vasoconstrictive, tachycardic, and hypertensive responses that provide some of cocaine's "kick" also result in decreased placental blood flow, placental vasoconstriction, and increased uterine contractility.[5,14]

There is much controversy about the effects on infants resulting from maternal cocaine abuse, especially as related to interactive behavior and emotional states. The possibility of a higher incidence of sudden infant death syndrome in infants whose mothers abused cocaine needs more scientific evaluation of prenatal and postnatal influences. Animal studies of possible teratogenicity have also been inconclusive, despite a report of "prune belly" in cocaine-treated mice.[14] Obviously, much more information bearing on cocaine's effects during pregnancy will be forthcoming as cocaine abuse continues.

Other Street Drugs

Heroin-addicted mothers may produce infants who have withdrawal symptoms and disturbances in behavior. Also, a higher infant mortality has been documented.[25,26,65] Maternal phencyclidine (angel dust) use has been associated with a case with an unusual facial appearance, behavioral abnormalities, and spasticity.[30] Marijuana is teratogenic in animals, resulting in embryonic death, congenital anomalies, and retardation. However, marijuana and LSD appear to be surprisingly nonteratogenic in humans.[51]

MARGINALLY NECESSARY DRUGS

Propranolol

Maternal use of propranolol does not appear to produce congenital cardiac malformations, but it does have deleterious effects on the fetal heart. Propranolol can cause fetal sinus bradycardia and may delay fetal growth and produce neonatal hypoglycemia.[29] Therapeutic use of beta blockers for hypertension and arrhythmias in women of child-bearing age needs to be restricted to avoid these consequences.

Estrogens and Progestagens

The wide use of estrogens and progestagens as contraceptives has raised concerns about their possible role in fetal malformations. Several retrospective studies have shown increased incidences of ventricular septal defects, tetralogies, and transpositions.[73] One collaborative study[37] apparently revealed a risk for congenital heart disease 2.3 times higher when these hormonal contraceptives were used than when these drugs had not been taken. The spectrum of cardiac anomalies observed in this study was quite similar to that observed overall in the human population.

It has been difficult to establish statistical validity of the teratogenicity of estrogens and progestagens since the incidence of malformations must be very low. However, the pattern of lesions found in the VACTERL association has been related to an unusually high incidence of hormonal contraceptive use.[72] The evidence at the present time appears to be insufficient to alter contraceptive recommendations.

The roles of progestin therapy in virilizing female offspring[38] and of diethylstilbestrol (DES) in causing late-appearing carcinomas in female offspring and urinary tract anomalies in males[4,102] have been well delineated.

Bendectin

Bendectin was a widely used drug that was taken off the market because of litigations relating to its possible teratogenicity. One study[83] appeared to show a weak association of maternal Bendectin use and congenital cardiac conditions. Bendectin contained three constituents initially: doxylamine (an antihistaminic), dicyclomine (an antispasmodic), and pyridoxine (an antinausea agent). Later dicyclomine was removed from the compound.[39]

Other extensive studies did not reveal significant teratogenicity of Bendectin.[17,90,93] Its unavailability means that there is no effective antinausea agent for treating pernicious vomiting of pregnancy in this country.

Antihistamines

Antihistamines have not been convincingly shown to be teratogenic in humans, although they are teratogenic in animals. Their use in late pregnancy has been associated with neonatal respiratory depression.

Salicylates

Concern about salicylates' teratogenicity is derived from their very widespread use (they are present in over 200 over-the-counter formulations) and their demonstrated teratogenicity in animals. Cardiac anomalies have been produced in animals, but somewhat surprisingly no such teratogenicity has been shown in humans. By inhibiting platelet formation, aspirin can promote bleeding during the immediate perinatal period that can jeopardize the neonate.

The effects of maternal ingestion of aspirin and other prostaglandin inhibitor drugs on closure of the fetal ductus have been of concern.[85] Aspirin-induced ductal closure in utero has been proposed as a possible mechanism for some cases of persistent pulmonary hypertension of the newborn syndrome.[78]

Ferrous Sulfate

Conflicting results have been reported in studies of the teratogenicity of ferrous iron in humans.[55,70] Since there is some concern, ferrous iron should be avoided during the period of active organogenesis.

ENVIRONMENTAL CONDITIONS

Heat

There is strong evidence that maternal hyperthermia, either from fever or from exposure to high ambient temperatures, can produce fetal anomalies. In animals, maternal fever appears to slow and alter neural cell growth so that neural tube defects, microcephaly, microphthalmia, and hypotonia may develop.[13,16,19,20,24,32,56,61,91,92] Studies by Smith[91] of pregnant women who were febrile during the period of fetal organogenesis from influenza, pyelonephritis, or streptococcal pharyngitis also have suggested that neural disorders and facial maldevelopment might be related to hyperthermia. Interestingly, for three offspring with neurologic defects and mental retardation, a history was obtained of maternal use of sauna facilities and hot tubs during fetal organogenesis. These observations are of concern since an earlier report by McDonald[56] indicated women working in hot laundries had a higher incidence of children with congenital anomalies, including congenital heart anomalies. The neurologic syndromes of fetal animals and humans have been strikingly similar.

Methyl Mercury

Severe teratogenic effects of methyl mercury entering the food chain have been demonstrated on three occasions.[3,36,46] Severe muscular signs and mental deficiency have been observed, but the heart has not been conspicuously involved.

MISCELLANEOUS AGENTS

Lead has been shown to produce increased stillbirths, abortions, and prematurity during pregnancies of exposed mothers. There does not appear to be a syndromic pattern, but an overall increase in malformations has been shown.[69] In particular, learning disabilities have been observed in animal offspring of exposed mothers.

Hexachlorophene (pHisoHex) exposure of a group of Swedish nurses during pregnancy resulted in a 15 per cent incidence of congenital anomalies in their children.[31] Hexachlorophene has been superseded by other sterilizing solutions.

Povidine-iodine (Betadine) is of concern since it is used for treatment of vaginal infections. Absorption of povidine-iodine after such usage can cause great increases in maternal serum iodine levels, which are as high as those observed in neonates who were washed in this solution and developed hypothyroidism.[12,99]

Other agents deserving attention, but which have not been shown to be associated with cardiac defects, include polybrominated biphenyls (PBBs),[88] polychlorinated biphenyls (PCBs),[1] and dioxin. PBBs and PCBs may be incriminated as adversely affecting fetal neural development. Dioxin bears watching because it is teratogenic in small quantities in animals.[98]

The use of ultrasonography has not been shown to adversely affect the fetus (see Chapter 14) and has proven to be an excellent substitute for iodizing radiation. The risks from the latter, which include producing fetal malformation, abortion, abnormalities in fetal chromosomes, and growth and mental retardation, are so well documented that x-rays should be avoided entirely during the period of fetal organogensis.[63] Microwaves have been shown to have possible teratogenic effects in animals and need to be studied in humans.[40]

CONCLUSIONS

The teratogens described are dangerous predominantly during the period of fetal organogenesis. As determined from thalidomide studies, the most vulnerable period for fetal cardiac conditions starts on the 18th day of gestation and ends earlier for conotruncal disorders (29th day) than for atrioventricular septal defects (33rd day), ventricular septal defects (39th day), and secundum atrial septal defects (50th day).[74] Coarctation of the aorta and ductal patency may result from later deleterious factors, and ductal closure is influenced significantly by postnatal events, especially in the premature infant. The periods of vulnerability may be broader for other teratogen-induced disorders, particularly those of the central nervous system.

In the search for "sentinel" lesions, the observation that lithium may be associated with Ebstein anomaly remains the most specific.[75] As more data are accumulated, it is expected that other particular cardiac lesions will be related to specific teratogens, since specific patterns of cardiac lesions have been observed already in infants infected with rubella virus (peripheral pulmonic stenoses, patent ductus, septal defects), in infants of diabetic mothers (transpositions and cardiomyopathies), and in infants whose mothers have connective tissue disorders (congenital heart blocks).

Perinatologists and geneticists have made very important contributions in defining some of the syndromes described. The powers of clinical observation, which were valued so highly in the past, have obviously not been lost, as was illustrated by the truly remarkable ability of some observers to define new and important syndromes. It is

hoped that new investigators will continue to discover new syndromes, refine the descriptions of those already noted, and visualize new methods of avoiding the devastating effects of these teratogenic agents.

References

1. Allen JR, Barsotti DA, et al (1979): Reproductive effects of halogenated aromatic hydrocarbons on nonhuman primates. Ann NY Science 320:419–425.
2. Asmussen I (1980): Ultrastructure of the villi and fetal capillaries in placentas from smoking and nonsmoking mothers. Br J Obstet Gynaecol 87:239–245.
3. Bakir F, Damluji SF, et al (1973): Methylmercury poisoning in Iraq. Science 181:230–241.
4. Bibbo M, Gill WG, et al (1977): Follow-up study of male and female offspring of DES-exposed mothers. Obstet Gynecol 49:1–7.
5. Bingol N, Fuchs M, et al (1985): Teratogenicity of cocaine in humans. Am J Hum Genet 37(suppl):A45.
6. Browne TR (1980): Valproic acid. N Engl J Med 302:661–666.
7. Buehler BA (1980): Polyamine, Dilantin, teratogenesis and neoplasia. Presented at the conference on malformations and morphogenesis, San Diego, September 4–6.
8. Buehler BA (1983): Epoxide hydralase activity and fetal hydantoin syndrome. Proc Greenwood Genetic Center 3:109.
9. Buehler BA (1985): Epoxide hydralase and the fetal hydantoin syndrome. Am J Hum Genet 37(suppl):A7.
10. Butler NR, Goldstein H, Ross EM (1972): Cigarette smoking in pregnancy: Its influence on birth weight and perinatal mortality. Br Med J 2:127–130.
11. Cavdar AO (1984): Fetal alcohol syndrome, malignancies and zinc deficiency (letter). J Pediatr 105:335.
12. Chabrolle JP, Rossier A (1978): Goitre and hypothyroidism in the newborn after cutaneous absorption of iodine. Arch Dis Child 53:495–498.
13. Chance PF, Smith DW (1978): Hyperthermia and meningomyelocele and encephaly (letter to the editor). Lancet 1:769.
14. Chasnoff IJ, Burns WJ, et al (1985): Cocaine use in pregnancy. N Engl J Med 13:666–669.
15. Clarren SK, Smith DW (1978): The fetal alcohol syndrome. N Engl J Med 298:1063–1067.
16. Clarren SK, Smith DW, Harvey MA, et al (1979): Hyperthermia—a prospective evaluation of a possible teratogenic agent in man. J Pediatr 95:81–83.
17. Cordero JF, Oakley GP, et al (1981): Is Bendectin a teratogen? JAMA 245:2307–2310.
18. Cree JE, Meyer J, Hailey DM (1973): Diazepam in labour: Its metabolism and effect on the clinical condition and thermogenesis of the newborn. Br Med J 4:251–255.
19. Edwards MJ (1967): Congenital defects in guinea pigs following induced hyperthermia during gestation. Arch Pathol 84:42–48.
20. Edwards MJ (1969): Congenital defects in guinea pigs: Prenatal retardation of brain growth of guinea pigs following hyperthermia during gestation. Teratology 2:329–336.
21. Ericson A, Kallen B, Westerholm P (1979): Cigarette smoking as an etiologic factor in cleft lip and palate. Am J Obstet Gynecol 135:348–351.
22. Fedrick J, Alberman ED, Goldstein H (1971): Possible teratogenic effect of cigarette smoking. Nature 231:529–530.
23. Finnell RH, DiLiberti JH (1983): Hydantoin-induced teratogenesis: Are arene oxide intermediates really responsible? Helv Paediatr Acta 38:171–177.
24. Fisher NL, Smith DW (1980): Hyperthermia as a possible cause for occipital encephalocele. Clin Res 28:116A.
25. Fraser AC (1976): Drug addiction in pregnancy. Lancet 1:896–899.
26. Fricker HS, Segal S (1978): Narcotic addiction, pregnancy and the newborn. Am J Dis Child 132:360–366.
27. German J, Kowal A, Ehlers KH (1970): Trimethadione and human teratogenesis. Teratology 3:349–361.
28. Gillberg C (1977): "Floppy infant syndrome" and maternal diazepam (letter to the editor). Lancet 2:244.

29. Gladstone GR, Hardof A, Gersony WM (1975): Propranolol administration during pregnancy: Effects on fetus. J Pediatr 86:962–964.

30. Golden NL, Sokol RJ, Rubin IL (1980): Angel dust: Possible effects on the fetus. Pediatrics 68:18–20.

31. Halling H (1979): Suspected link between exposure to hexachlorophene and malformed infants. Ann NY Acad Sci 320:426–435.

32. Halperin LR, Wilroy RS (1978): Maternal hyperthermia and neural tube defects (letter to the editor). Lancet 2:212.

33. Hanson JW, Smith DW (1975): The fetal hydantoin syndrome. J Pediatr 87:285–290.

34. Hanson JW, Myrianthopoulos NC, et al (1976): Risks to the offspring of women treated with hydantoin anticonvulsants, with emphasis on the fetal hydantoin syndrome. J Pediatr 89:662–668.

35. Hanson JW, Buehler BA (1982): Fetal hydantoin syndrome: Current status. J Pediatr 101:816–818.

36. Harada Y (1968): Congenital Minimata disease: Study group of Minimata disease. Kumamoto, Japan, Kumamoto University, pp 93–117.

37. Heinonen OP, Slone D, et al (1977): Cardiovascular birth defects and antenatal exposure to female sex hormones. N Engl J Med 296:67–70.

38. Herbst AL (ed) (1978): Intrauterine exposure to diethylstilbestrol in the human. Proceedings of Symposium on DES by the American College of Obstetricians and Gynecologists.

39. Hill LM, Kleinberg F (1984): Effects of drugs and chemicals on fetus and the newborn. Mayo Clin Proc 59:707–716; 59:755–765.

40. Inouye M, Galvin MJ, et al (1983): Effects of 2.45 MHz microwave radiation on the development of the rat brain. Teratology 28:413–419.

41. Jager-Roman E, Diechi A, et al (1986): Fetal growth, major malformations and minor anomalies in infants born to women receiving valproic acid. J Pediatr 108:997–1004.

42. Jones KL, Smith DW (1973): Recognition of the fetal alcohol syndrome in early infancy. Lancet 2:999–1001.

43. Jones KL, Smith DW, et al (1973): Pattern of malformation in offspring of chronic alcoholic mothers. Lancet 1:1267–1271.

44. Kaneko S, Otani K, et al (1983): Transplacental passage and half-life of sodium valproate in infants born to epileptic mothers. Br J Clin Pharmacol 15:503–506.

45. Keppen LD, Pysher T, Rennert OM (1985): Zinc deficiency acts as a co-teratogen with alcohol in fetal alcohol syndrome. Pediatr Res 19:944–947.

46. Koos BJ, Longo LD (1976): Mercury toxicity in the pregnant woman, fetus, and newborn infant. Am J Obstet Gynecol 126:390–409.

47. Kraus CM, Holmes LM, et al (1984): Four siblings with similar malformations after exposure to phenytoin and primidone. J Pediatr 105:750–755.

48. Lemoine P, Harousseau H, et al (1967): Les infants de parents alcooliques: Anomalies observées, à propos de 127 cas (abstr). Arch Fr Pediatr 25:830–831.

49. Lemoine P, Harousseau H, et al (1968): Les infants de parents alcooliques. Ouest Med 21:476.

50. Lenz W, Knapp K (1962): Thalidomide embryopathy. Arch Environ Health 5:100–105.

51. Long SY (1981): Does LSD induce chromosomal damage and malformations? A review of the literature. Teratology 6:75–90.

52. Long WA, Willis PW IV (1984): Maternal lithium and neonatal Ebstein's anomaly: Evaluation with cross-sectional echocardiography. Am J Perinatol 1:182–184.

53. Loser H, Majewski M (1977): Type and frequency of cardiac defects in embryofetal alcohol syndrome: Report of 16 cases. Br Heart J 39:1374–1379.

54. McBride WG (1961): Thalidomide and congenital anomalies (letter to the editor). Lancet 2:1358.

55. McBride WG (1963): The teratogenic action of drugs. Med J Aust 2:689–693.

56. McDonald AD (1958): Maternal health and congenital defect: A prospective investigation. N Engl J Med 258:767–773.

57. Majewski F (1981): Alcohol embryopathy: Some facts and speculations about pathogenesis. Neurobehav Toxicol Teratol 3:129–144.

58. Manning FA, Feyerabend C (1976): Cigarette smoking and fetal breathing movements. Br J Obstet Gynecol 83:262–270.

59. Meadow SR (1968): Anticonvulsant drugs and congenital anomalies (letter). Lancet 2:1296.

60. Meadow SR (1970): Congenital anomalies and anticonvulsant drugs. Proc R Soc Med 63:48–49.

61. Miller P, Smith DW, Shepard T (1978): Maternal hyperthermia as a possible cause of encephalopathy. Lancet 1:519–520.

62. Monson RR, Rosenberg L, Hartz SC, et al (1973): Diphenylhydantoin and selected congenital malformations. N Engl J Med 289:1049–1052.

63. Mossman KL, Hill LT (1982): Radiation risks in pregnancy. Obstet Gynecol 60:237–242.

64. Myhre SA, Williams R (1981): Teratogenic effects associated with maternal primidone therapy. J Pediatr 99:160–162.

65. Naeye RL, Blanc W, et al (1973): Fetal complications of maternal heroin addiction: Abnormal growth, infections and episodes of stress. J Pediatr 83:1055–1061.

66. Naeye RL (1978): Relationship of cigarette smoking to congenital anomalies and perinatal death: A prospective study. Am J Pathol 90:289–293.

67. Naeye RL (1980): Abruptio placentae and placenta previa: Frequency, perinatal mortality, and cigarette smoking. Obstet Gynecol 55:701–704.

68. Nau H, Rating D, et al (1981): Valproic acid and its metabolites: Placental transfer, neonatal pharmacokinetics, transfer via mother's milk and clinical status in neonates of epileptic mothers. J Pharmacol Exp Ther 219:768–777.

69. Needleman HL, Rabinowitz M, et al (1984): The relationship between prenatal exposure to lead and congenital anomalies. JAMA 251:2956–2959.

70. Nelson MM, Forfar JO (1971): Associations between drugs administered during pregnancy and congenital abnormalities of the fetus. Br Med J 1:523–527.

71. Nora JJ, Fraser FC (1981): Medical Genetics: Principles and Practice. Philadelphia, Lea & Febiger, pp 357–378.

72. Nora JJ, Nora AH (1975): A syndrome of multiple congenital anomalies associated with teratogenic exposure. Arch Environ Health 30:17–20.

73. Nora JJ, Nora AH (1976): Congenital abnormalities and first trimester exposure to progestagen/estrogen (letter). Lancet 1:313.

74. Nora JJ, Nora AH (1978): Genetics and Counseling in Cardiovascular Disease. Springfield, Charles C Thomas, pp 134–148.

75. Nora JJ, Nora AH, Toews WH (1974): Lithium, Ebstein's anomaly and other congenital heart defects (letter). Lancet 2:594–595.

76. Nora JJ, Vargo TA (1969): Congenital malformations in four animal species following maternal exposure to dextroamphetamine (abstr). South Med J 62:1550.

77. Nora JJ, Vargo TA, Nora AH, Love KE, McNamara OG (1970): Dexamphetamine: A possible environmental trigger in cardiovascular malformations (letter). Lancet 1:1290–1291.

78. Perkin RM, Levin DL, Clark R (1980): Serum salicylate levels and right to left ductus shunts in newborn infants with persistent pulmonary hypertension. J Pediatr 96:721–726.

79. Persaud TVN (1968): The foetal toxicity of barbiturates. Wisen Z Univ Rostock 18:571–575.

80. Persaud TVN (1985): Causes of developmental defects. In Basic Concepts of Teratology. New York, Alan R. Liss, pp 69–102.

81. Phelan MC, Pellock JM, Nance WE (1982): Discordant expression of fetal hydantoin syndrome in heteropaternal dizygotic twins. N Engl J Med 307:99–101.

82. Rating D, Nau H, et al (1982): Teratogenic and pharmacokinetic studies of primidone during pregnancy and in the offspring of epileptic women. Acta Paediatr Scand 71:301–311.

83. Rothman KJ, Fyler DC, et al (1979): Exogenous hormones and other drug exposures of children with congenital heart disease. Am J Epidemiol 109:433–439.

84. Rudd NL, Freedom RM (1979): A possible primidone embryopathy. J Pediatr 94:835–837.

85. Rudolph AM (1981): Effects of aspirin and acetaminophen in pregnancy and in the newborn. Arch Intern Med 141:358–363.

86. Safra MJ, Oakley GP Jr (1975): Association of cleft lip with or without cleft palate and prenatal exposure to diazepam. Lancet 2:478–480.

87. Sandor GGS, Smith DW, MacLeod PM (1981): Cardiac malformations in the fetal alcohol syndrome. J Pediatr 98:771–773.

88. Seagull EAW (1983): Developmental abilities of children exposed to polybrominated biphenyls (PBB). Am J Public Health 73:281–285.

89. Seip M (1976): Growth retardation, dysmorphic facies and minor malformations following massive exposure to pentabarbitone in utero. Acta Paediatr Scand 65:617–621.

90. Shapiro S, Henionen OP, et al (1977): Antenatal exposure to doxylamine succinate and dicyclomine hydrochloride (Bendectin) in relation to congenital malformations, perinatal mortality rate, birth weight and intelligent quotient score. Am J Obstet Gynecol 128:480–485.

91. Smith DW (1982): Recognizable Patterns of Human Malformation. Genetic, Embryologic and Clinical Aspects. 3rd ed. Philadelphia, WB Saunders.

92. Smith DW, Clarren SK, Harvey MA (1978): Hyperthermia as a possible teratogenic agent. J Pediatr 92:878–883.

93. Smithells RW, Sheppard S (1978): Teratogenicity testing in humans: A method of demonstrating safety of Bendectin. Teratology 17:31–35.

94. Snyder SH, Meyerhoff JL (1973): How amphetamine acts in minimal brain dysfunction. Ann NY Acad Sci 205:310–320.

95. Sokol RJ, Miller SI, Reed G (1980): Alcohol abuse during pregnancy: An epidemiologic study. Alcoholism 4:135–145.

96. Szabo KT (1970): Teratogenic effects of lithium carbonate in the foetal mouse. Nature 225:73–75.

97. Ulleland CN (1972): The offspring of alcoholic mothers. Ann NY Acad Sci 197:167–169.

98. Van Miller JP, Marlar RJ, Allen JR (1976): Tissue distribution and excretion of tritiated tetrachlorodibenzo-p-dioxin in nonhuman primates and rats. Food Cosmet Toxicol 14:31–34.

99. Vorherr H, Vorherr UF, et al (1980): Vaginal absorption of povidine-iodine. JAMA 244:2628–2629.

100. Watson JD, Spellacy WN (1971): Neonatal effects of maternal treatment with the anticonvulsant drug diphenylhydantoin. Obstet Gynecol 37:881–885.

101. Wells JW, Harbison RD (1980): Significance of the phenytoin reactive arene oxide intermediate, its oxepin tautomer, and clinical factors modifying their roles in phenytoin-induced teratology. In Hassell TM, Johnston MC, Dudley KH (eds): Phenytoin-induced Teratology and Gingival Pathology. New York, Raven Press, pp 83–108.

102. Wilson JG, Brent RL (1981): Are female sex hormones teratogenic? Am J Obstet Gynecol 141:567–580.

103. Zackai EH, Mellman WJ, et al (1975): The fetal trimethadione syndrome. J Pediatr 87:280–284.

50 SYNDROMES

Jacqueline A. Noonan

With the exception of cleft lip and myelomeningocele, all of the major anomalies recognizable at birth have an increased incidence of associated congenital heart disease.[73] The reported incidence of associated extracardiac anomalies in infants with congenital heart disease is variable, with autopsy series reporting a range from 24 to 45 per cent[55,81,114] depending on what is defined as a significant malformation. Among 1566 infants with symptomatic congenital heart disease, Greenwood and coworkers[36] reported 25.2 per cent to have one or more significant extracardiac anomalies. Importantly, in 60 per cent of such infants, more than one extracardiac anomaly was present. Extracardiac anomalies occur nearly twice as frequently among low birthweight infants compared with those weighing over 2500 g. Multiple extracardiac anomalies are especially common in the low birthweight group.

When a pattern of malformations presumably having the same etiology is recognized, the term *syndrome* may be applied. Among infants with congenital heart disease and associated extracardiac anomalies, Greenwood and coworkers found one third to have a well-defined syndrome. Syndromes may result from chromosomal abnormalities, mutant gene disorders, or environmental teratogens, but in many cases the etiology is not yet defined.

Multiple extracardiac anomalies may also reflect a malformation sequence in which a single problem in morphogenesis leads to a single localized abnormal formation of tissue, which in turn initiates a chain of subsequent defects. One example is the DiGeorge sequence in which the primary defect is in the fourth branchial arch and derivations of the third and fourth pharyngeal pouches. This defect subsequently leads to defects of development in the thymus, parathyroids, and great vessels. The term *association* is applied to nonrandom association of a number of specific defects occurring in a person in whom the etiology is unknown. The VATER and CHARGE associations are two good examples. The concept of the developmental field complex elaborated by Opitz and coworkers[82] may explain the multiple anomalies present in these associations. The postulate of developmental field complex implies that a particular part of the embryo reacts as a temporally and spatially coordinated unit to localized forces of organization and differentiation. Disruption of a developmental field complex can be caused by a variety of agents and will result in multiple usually contiguous but also distally located anomalies that may vary in nature and number.

It is important to recognize if there is a pattern of multiple malformations in an infant with congenital heart disease. Recognition of a specific syndrome will be helpful in suggesting the most likely cardiac lesion, will help to predict prognosis, and will be vital in genetic counseling.[73]

In this chapter some of the more common nonchromosomal, nonteratogenic syndromes and associations are considered. Those most likely to be recognized in the newborn will be stressed.

NONCHROMOSOMAL SYNDROMES WITH CHARACTERISTIC FACIES

Noonan Syndrome

Noonan syndrome is estimated to have an incidence between 1 in 1000 and 1 in 2500 live births.[66] About 50 per cent of these newborns have a cardiac defect. Noonan syndrome is the most common (1 to 1.4 per cent) nonchromosomal syndrome in patients with congenital heart disease.

Historical Perspective

Kobylinski,[52] in 1883, reported the first case of a patient who would now fit the diagnosis of Noonan syndrome. The patient's most striking finding was webbed neck or pterygium colli. Funke,[27] in 1902, probably reported the first description of another syndrome with pterygium colli, which is now called Turner syndrome. Ullrich,[105] in 1930, and Turner,[104] in 1938, reported the phenotypic findings of patients with Turner syndrome, with Turner noting the sexual infantilism that was not apparent to Ullrich, whose patients were young children. In 1943, Flavell[21] noted a male with features resembling those reported by Turner and coined the term *male Turner syndrome*. In 1959, Ford and associates[22] defined the XO sex chromosomal abnormality in many of the females with features of Turner syndrome, and it is this sex chromosomal abnormality that is now labeled as Turner syndrome. The term *male Turner syndrome* was applied to a variety of patients, many with some form of testicular insufficiency without the facial features described by Ullrich. In 1963, Ehmke and I[72,77] reported nine children with pulmonary stenosis who shared similar characteristic facies, short stature, and other skeletal anomalies. There were six males and three females. No chromosomal abnormalities were present. In order to distinguish this group of patients from those with a sex chromosomal abnormality of Turner syndrome, Opitz and colleagues,[83] in 1965, proposed the name Noonan syndrome for this condition. Other eponyms that have been used include Ullrich, Bonnevie-Ullrich, Ullrich-Turner, as well as XX Turner phenotype or XY Turner phenotype.[79] Since the mid 1970s, the eponym Noonan syndrome[66] has been generally accepted as the appropriate designation.

Epidemiology

The cause of Noonan syndrome is not yet completely understood. The family data reported are most consistent with an autosomal dominant inheritance of a highly variable trait. Only fairly severely affected newborns are usually identified as having Noonan syndrome, whereas those with mild manifestations are likely to be considered normal. Once a newborn is identified as having Noonan syndrome, frequently other family members, particularly one parent, will be recognized as sharing some of the characteristics of the infant and then identified as having a mild form of Noonan syndrome. Allanson and associates[3] reported a study of 109 patients with Noonan syndrome in which photographs of persons from the same family and the same person at different ages were studied independently by several dysmorphologists. Patients were divided by consensus into groups of "look-alikes." Instead of "look-alikes" occurring within the same family, it became apparent that one of the major dividing characteristics between groups was age. Their study showed that persons with Noonan syndrome have a characteristic but dynamic phenotype that changes predictably with age. These authors believe that careful examination of parents and siblings of Noonan syndrome patients, taking into account the age-specific phenotype, will uncover affected persons previously regarded as normal (Fig. 50–1).

Since Noonan syndrome is so frequent, genetic heterogeneity must be considered. Mendez and Opitz[66] suggest some cases occurring only in siblings with sometimes consanguineous parents could represent an autosomal recessive trait. Several autosomal dominant genes could be responsible for other cases. It is of particular interest that neurofibromatosis, a known autosomal dominant disorder, has been reported in association with Noonan syndrome.[84] Many cases of Noonan syndrome appear to be sporadic. Since there is no specific diagnostic test or specific marker at the present time, the diagnosis is purely clinical. It is hoped that with more definitive studies of specific genes the underlying defect in Noonan syndrome will be identified.

Clinical Findings

The characteristic facies include hypertelorism, prominent eyes, ptosis, epicanthus, antimongoloid slant of palpebral fissures, posteriorly rotated fleshy ears that appear low set, and malar flattening. The neck is short and may be webbed. Curly hair is common. Other findings include short stature, low posterior hairline, and a chest deformity such as pectus excavatum and/or carinatum. Undescended testes are frequent in male patients. Mental retardation, which is frequently mild, is a common feature. Other less common findings include renal anomalies, large head,

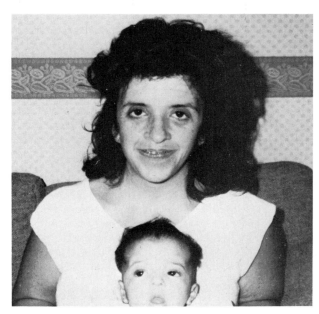

Figure 50–1. Mother and infant, both with Noonan syndrome, showing changes in phenotype with age.

hepatosplenomegaly, scoliosis, skin manifestations, and lymphatic abnormalities resulting in limb lymphedema, chylous thorax, and intestinal lymphangiectasis.

Congenital heart disease occurs in about 50 per cent of patients. Valvular pulmonary stenosis, frequently with a dysplastic pulmonary valve, is the most common lesion. An atrial septal defect and mild peripheral pulmonary artery stenoses, with or without associated valvular pulmonary stenosis, are also common. Virtually every kind of congenital heart disease has been reported. Hypertrophic cardiomyopathy, both obstructive and nonobstructive, has been described. In addition to the pulmonary valve, both the mitral valve and the tricuspid valve may be dysplastic and both tricuspid and mitral valve prolapse may occur. In these patients with a dysplastic valve, the physical findings of pulmonary stenosis may be atypical. The systolic murmur tends to transmit widely, and an ejection click is frequently not present. Often the chest deformity obscures the expected dilatation of the main pulmonary artery seen on a chest radiograph. The ECG frequently shows left anterior hemiblock, and a deep S wave may be present in all precordial leads. Although the ECG findings may reflect an associated left ventricular myopathy, patients with both mild and severe pulmonary stenosis may have these atypical findings in the absence of left ventricular disease. An echocardiogram and Doppler study should be very helpful in evaluating the degree of pulmonary valve obstruction and the presence of left ventricular disease.

Without a positive family history, it is unlikely mild Noonan syndrome would be recognized in the newborn. Noonan syndrome is not easy to recognize at birth but should be considered in newborns with edema and/or redundant nuchal skin. Typically, the infants are of normal or high normal birthweight. Some of this weight may be

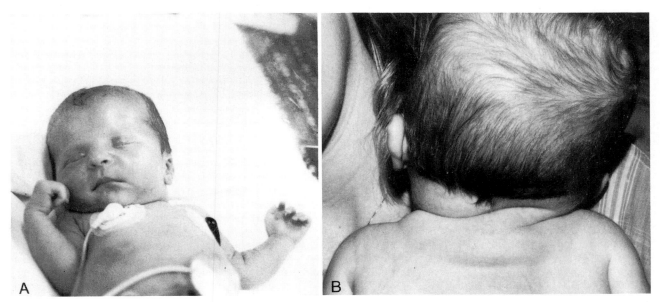

Figure 50–2. *A*, Newborn with Noonan syndrome. *B*, Redundant nuchal skin.

due to edema so that rapid weight reduction occurs soon after birth with subsequent slow weight gain; a diagnosis of failure to thrive is common. The forehead is often broad and sloping, and there is apparent hypertelorism and a downward slant of the palpebral fissures. The ears appear fleshy and posteriorly rotated. The neck is short and frequently shows redundant nuchal skin (Fig. 50–2). It is not uncommon for newborns with Noonan syndrome to develop cyanosis, lethargy, and hypotonia resulting in a workup for suspected sepsis or hypoglycemia. Some of these infants have severe failure to thrive and undergo extensive testing with negative results. Fortunately, both the failure to thrive and muscular hypotonia improve with time. Seldom can the cardiac diagnosis be implicated as the cause of the symptoms, although congenital heart disease can be expected in at least 50 per cent. The classic ECG with left anterior hemiblock may be present at birth and, when present, should make one suspicious that Noonan syndrome is indeed present. Critical pulmonary valvular obstruction in the newborn appears to be rare in Noonan syndrome, but a dysplastic pulmonary valve may lead to a rapid progression of valvular obstruction in an infant with Noonan syndrome. Since almost every kind of congenital heart disease has been reported in patients with Noonan syndrome, a complete cardiac evaluation is indicated to exclude a cardiac cause of cyanosis or other symptoms in neonates with suspected Noonan syndrome. Cardiomyopathy has been noted soon after birth in several infants with Noonan syndrome. Hirsch and colleagues[38] reported two infants with obstructive cardiomyopathy, one dying at 6 months and another at 22 months. I have also seen several infants who have developed progressive obstructive cardiomyopathy during infancy. A dysplastic mitral valve may result in significant mitral insufficiency.

Beyond the newborn period up to about 2 years of age, the more typical features of Noonan syndrome appear (Fig.

50–3). The head appears relatively large with turricephaly and a relatively flat malar eminence. The eyes may be quite prominent and round with hypertelorism. The nasal bridge is flat and the nasal tip bulbous. The philtrum is deep. The ears remain posteriorly rotated. The neck is short, but the redundant skin is no longer present. The chest deformity becomes more prominent. There is often failure to thrive, and mild muscular hypotonia is frequent. By 12 to 18 months the upper body appears stocky and square whereas the limbs become relatively longer and thinner. There is occasional hepatosplenomegaly. In infancy, the hair is often relatively sparse and wispy but often becomes quite curly and woolly as childhood approaches.

With the increasing use of ultrasonography, two newborns who had edema on prenatal ultrasonography[6] have been recognized after birth as having Noonan syndrome, suggesting that prenatal ultrasonography may be helpful in detection of a fetus known to be at risk for Noonan syndrome. Unfortunately, both the infants who presented with nonimmune hydrops fetalis and Noonan syndrome died 10 days and 5 weeks, respectively, after birth because of severe hypoproteinemia and renal failure.

Differential Diagnosis

A careful pregnancy and family history should be taken in all patients with suspected Noonan syndrome to avoid confusion with other entities, such as the fetal alcohol syndrome and fetal hydantoin syndrome, both of which share some of the physical findings. The differential diagnosis also includes Aarskog syndrome, which is characterized by short stature, peculiar facies, saddle deformity of the scrotum, and abnormalities of the hands and feet. Congenital heart disease is not common in Aarskog syndrome, and from the published pedigree an X-linked recessive mode of inheritance has been proposed. Leopard

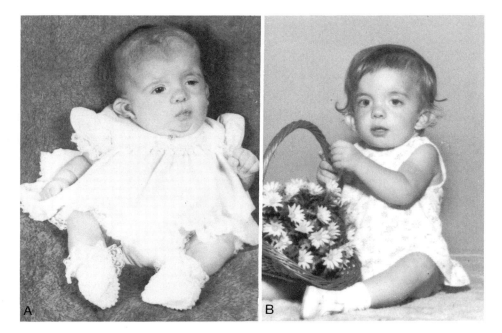

Figure 50–3. *A*, Patient with Noonan syndrome at 2½ months. *B*, Same patient at 10 months.

or multiple lentigines syndrome shares so many features in common with Noonan syndrome that it is considered by many to be a variant of Noonan syndrome.

Medical Management

The possibility of Noonan syndrome in any newborn infant with the clinical features described should be considered. Chromosomal studies should be normal. Recognition of the natural history of some infants with Noonan syndrome should discourage the use of repeated studies to evaluate the cause of failure to thrive. Echocardiography is helpful in evaluating and following the cardiac problem. Should symptoms related to the cardiac disease develop, surgical repair will usually be of more value than medical management. Balloon angioplasty may be tried, but it is less likely to be successful in these patients with pulmonary stenosis because the valve is frequently dysplastic and an associated atrial septal defect is not uncommon.

Patients with Noonan syndrome have an increased incidence of inguinal hernias and undescended testes so that surgical repair may be needed at some time during childhood. The limb lymphedema requires no specific treatment and usually disappears during childhood. The possibility of a malabsorption syndrome secondary to intestinal lymphangiectasis should be considered if a protein-losing enteropathy is present.

Pulmonary lymphangiectasis is a rare finding but has been reported to result in spontaneous chylothorax in infancy and has led to chylothorax as a complication of cardiac surgery (Fig. 50–4). Partial deficiency of factor XI was reported by Kitchens and Alexander[51] in some non-Jewish patients with Noonan syndrome, suggesting that preoperative evaluation of this blood factor should be considered. Malignant hyperthermia has been reported in several patients with Noonan syndrome so that this pos-

sibility should be considered prior to any surgical procedure.

Although mild mental retardation is a relatively frequent finding in Noonan syndrome, evaluation of hearing should be carried out to be sure that deafness is not a contributing factor to a delay in speech and poor school performance.

Prognosis

In many patients Noonan syndrome is so mild that it is never recognized and apparently has an excellent prognosis. The more severe forms of Noonan syndrome, in general, also have a good prognosis. The cardiac lesions can usually be treated with a low risk by surgery if warranted. The presence of a dysplastic pulmonary valve may require a pulmonary valvectomy, and sometimes an annular patch is needed to relieve the obstruction.

The prognosis for those infants who develop obstructive cardiomyopathy would appear poor, but fortunately such patients are quite uncommon. In general, hypertrophic cardiomyopathy carries a guarded prognosis, but the natural history of this problem in patients with Noonan syndrome is still not defined. I have placed several patients on verapamil who appeared to have progressive obstructive cardiomyopathy. With this therapy the cardiac findings have appeared to stabilize. Hypotonia and failure to thrive, common in infancy, improve with time, and the great majority of patients with Noonan syndrome, unless significantly retarded, are able to lead a normal life.

Williams Syndrome

Williams syndrome[116] is an eponym used to describe patients with elfin facies who frequently have supravalvular

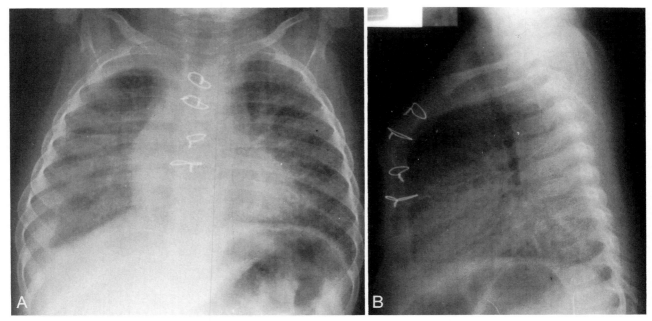

Figure 50–4. *A,* Chest radiograph showing dilated lymphatics and right pleural effusion in postoperative patient with Noonan syndrome (PA view). *B,* Same patient in lateral view.

aortic stenosis and peripheral pulmonary artery stenoses. Although some patients with Williams syndrome have had documented hypercalcemia, it is an uncommon feature. Abnormal teeth, hoarse voice, mild-to-moderate growth retardation, and moderate mental retardation are additional features. The etiology remains unknown, and most cases are sporadic.

Historical Perspective

Fanconi and coworkers,[20] in 1952, described a severe form of infantile hypercalcemia that was characterized by elfin facies, severe failure to thrive, vomiting, irritability, muscular hypotonia, generalized osteosclerosis, and renal impairment. A relationship to vitamin D intake was suspected because at that time in England 1000 units of vitamin D was being added to each quart of milk and vitamin D was also added to many other food products.[60] About 100 cases of infantile hypercalcemia (with a serum calcium level 12 mg/dl or greater) were diagnosed in England during 1953 and 1954. When the vitamin D content of milk was reduced to 400 units per quart, the number of new cases virtually ceased.[85] Although heart murmurs were reported in such patients, little attention was paid to the cardiovascular system.

In 1961, supravalvular aortic stenosis was first described by Perou[88] in a mentally retarded 8-year-old boy. In that same year, Wooley and associates[117] described the first cases of familial supravalvular aortic stenosis and Williams described four unrelated children with similar facies described as elfin who were mentally retarded and had supravalvular aortic stenosis. In 1963, Black and Bonham-Carter[8] recognized that the patients described by Williams shared similar facies with the earlier patients reported with se-

vere hypercalcemia. In 1964, Garcia and colleagues[30] were the first to observe an infant with idiopathic hypercalcemia who had supravalvular aortic stenosis, peripheral pulmonary artery stenoses, mental retardation, and elfin facies. This patient had elevated vitamin D activity. The theory evolved that abnormalities seen in such patients began during pregnancy and were in some way related to vitamin D metabolism. Friedman and Roberts[26] gave large amounts of vitamin D to pregnant rabbits and were able to produce supravalvular aortic stenoses in the offspring.

However, as more cases of Williams syndrome were described, the association with hypercalcemia became quite uncommon. It is now well documented that Williams elfin facies syndrome can occur without any symptoms of hypercalcemia, and even when looked for hypercalcemia is an unusual feature. Excessive intake of vitamin D by the mother is seldom documented. Supravalvular aortic stenosis, often with peripheral pulmonary artery stenosis, is a frequent associated cardiac defect, but a variety of other cardiac defects have been described and some patients have no evidence of cardiac disease. In addition to the ascending aorta and pulmonary arteries, virtually every systemic artery can be involved and isolated renal artery stenoses may occur.

Epidemiology

Although the early reports suggested a relationship to vitamin D metabolism, the etiology of Williams syndrome remains obscure.[64] It is still possible that there is an underlying metabolic defect present that under appropriate circumstances may result in hypercalcemia, but clearly this syndrome can occur without any evidence of hypercalcemia. Of considerable interest is the fact that supravalvular aortic stenosis may occur as a syndromic

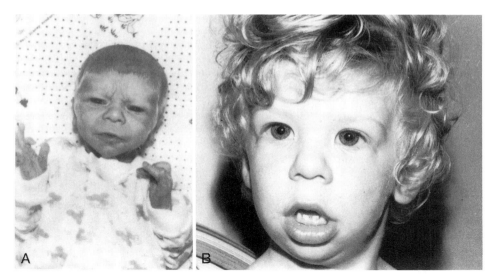

Figure 50–5. *A,* Patient with Williams syndrome as a newborn. *B,* Same patient at 2½ years of age.

form (Williams syndrome)[7] or as an autosomal dominant familial form[96] with normal facies and mentality, or it may be sporadic. In all three forms there is generalized arterial fibromuscular dysplasia. Microscopic examination shows disorganization of the medial elements with a fibrotic intima sometimes containing lacunae. On electron microscopy,[80] the ultrastructure shows irregular elastic fibers with abundant whirling collagen, hypertrophied smooth muscle cells, and scant ground substance. It is possible that the hemodynamics during fetal life predispose to the localized area of stenosis in the supravalvular region, but the cause of the mural dysplasia remains unknown.

Clinical Findings

Mild-to-moderate prenatal growth deficiency is present. Jones and Smith[43] reported an average birthweight of 2900 g (10th percentile) in their report of 16 patients and an average length of 47 cm (3rd percentile). Postnatal growth deficiency persists with a linear growth rate about 75 per cent of normal. Although the typical elfin facies may become more prominent during the first few years of life, abnormal facies may be present at birth. There is median eyebrow flare, short palpebral fissures, ocular hypotelorism, depressed nasal bridge, epicanthal folds, periorbital fullness, strabismus, stellate pattern in the iris, anteverted nares, long philtrum, prominent lips, and malar hypoplasia. Additional findings include mild microcephaly, hoarse voice, abnormal dentition, mental retardation, hypoplastic nails, and fifth finger clinodactyly. A heart murmur is commonly heard, with supravalvular aortic stenosis and peripheral pulmonary stenoses the most frequently reported cardiovascular lesions. However, a wide variety of cardiac malformations have been described.

Failure to thrive in early infancy may be a feature; in such patients the possibility of hypercalcemia should be considered, but it is unlikely to be present. Although the newborn with Williams syndrome may appear "dysmorphic," typical facies often become much more apparent

with time. Figure 50–5 shows a newborn with Williams syndrome and his more typical appearance at 2 years of age. Later in childhood the irritability seen in the infant is replaced by a friendly outgoing nature often described as a "cocktail personality."

Differential Diagnosis

Fetal alcohol syndrome, Noonan syndrome, fetal hydantoin syndrome, and a variety of chromosomal deletions may have some overlapping features.

Medical Management

There have been no reports of infants with Williams syndrome who were symptomatic from either supravalvular aortic stenosis or peripheral pulmonary artery stenoses in the newborn period. Periodic follow-up examinations are indicated since rapidly progressive obstruction can occur. One of my patients by age 19 months had a 175-mm pressure gradient at cardiac catheterization across the supravalvular aortic stenosis. Another infant with failure to thrive developed severe left ventricular hypertrophy and at 4 months of age was noted to have severe systemic hypertension. Subsequent studies documented a renal artery stenosis on the left. There was improvement with surgical treatment, but on follow-up recurrent hypertension was noted. A repeat study indicated renal artery stenoses had developed in the right renal artery. Both of these children support the hypothesis that the underlying malformation appears to be a generalized arterial fibromuscular dysplasia, which may develop, regress, or remain static on follow-up.

Surgical treatment of the supravalvular aortic stenosis is generally successful. Fortunately, most cases of pulmonary artery stenosis are relatively mild. Except for localized areas of constriction at the site of major branching of the pulmonary arteries, surgical treatment is of limited value. Balloon angioplasty may play a role in treatment of localized areas of pulmonary artery constrictions, but the results so far have been somewhat disappointing. In those patients with severe multiple peripheral pulmonary artery stenoses, neither surgery nor balloon angioplasty is likely to be successful. Renal artery stenosis may be managed by angioplasty or a surgical procedure. Improvement is likely, although it is possible that the renal artery obstructions may recur or that obstruction may develop at additional sites.

Prognosis

Long-term prognosis for patients who have undergone successful treatment of supravalvular aortic stenosis must remain somewhat guarded. Since almost any systemic artery may be involved, central nervous system complications such as strokes may occur with increasing time. Premature coronary artery disease has been reported. A review of the literature would suggest that there is an increased incidence of sudden unexpected death among patients with supravalvular aortic stenosis and peripheral pulmonary stenosis. Postmortem studies in such patients often show unsuspected coronary artery lesions with evidence of significant myocardial ischemia. These children also appear to have an increased risk of sudden death at cardiac catheterization.[75] Nonspecific renal failure requiring dialysis and renal transplantation has been reported in some patients with Williams syndrome in the teenage and young adult years.

Asymmetrical Crying Facies

The association of asymmetrical crying facies with congenital heart disease was reported by Cayler in 1967.[11,12] This minor congenital anomaly is due to congenital hypoplasia of the depressor anguli oris muscle.

Historical Perspective

Cayler[11] was the first to draw attention to the association of asymmetrical crying facies with congenital heart disease in 1967. Nelson and Eng,[70] in 1972, pointed out the important differences between congenital hypoplasia of the depressor anguli oris muscle and true seventh nerve palsy. In 1972, Pape and Pickering[87] reviewed 44 children with asymmetrical crying facies being followed at a large children's hospital. They noted only 10 of the 44 were otherwise normal or had only a minor associated congenital anomaly. Twenty-seven of the 44 had a known major associated anomaly, and 22 had congenital heart disease. Their study indicated that when asymmetrical crying facies is associated with congenital heart disease, multiple system involvement should be suspected. In 1976, Alexiou and associates[2] conducted a prospective study of 6487 newborns and found an incidence of asymmetrical crying facies of 6.7 per 1000 births. Additional anomalies were noted in 20 newborns. Congenital heart disease was present in 3 of 44, for an incidence of 6.8 per cent compared with a 0.45 per cent incidence in the remaining infants without asymmetrical facies. Their findings suggest that asymmetrical crying facies should be considered a sign at least comparable in value to the finding of a single um-

bilical artery. If present, it is prudent to look for associated anomalies. Asymmetrical crying facies has been found in both the VATER association and the CHARGE association. The velocardiofacial syndrome described by Shprintzen and associates in 1973[97] and the conotruncal anomaly face described by Kinouchi and coworkers in 1976[48] are probably similar syndromes, and asymmetrical crying facies has been noted in both entities in a few of these reported cases.

Epidemiology

Cayler,[11] in his first report, suggested there was an epidemic of asymmetrical crying facies; however, he was unable to establish any specific predisposing factor. Since asymmetrical crying facies is present in a variety of syndromes and associations, the patients represent a heterogeneous mix with diverse predisposing factors. Some cases may be attributed to genetic factors, others to teratogens, but in the majority no specific cause has been found.

Clinical Findings

Clinical findings associated with congenital hypoplasia of the depressor anguli oris muscle include the following. One corner of the mouth does not move downward or outward symmetrically with the other corner. This asymmetry is most evident with crying. Forehead wrinkling, eye closure, nasolabial fold depth, and tearing are all symmetrical and mentalis function is normal. There is usually palpable thinning of the lateral portion of the lower lip on the affected side. Junction times and nerve excitability studies, if carried out, are normal. This condition occurs equally in both males and females. Low birthweight is common in those newborns with associated congenital defects. Asymmetry may occur on either the right or the left side. If an associated unpaired anomaly is present, it is likely to occur on the same side as the facial weakness.

Differential Diagnosis

Conditions to be considered in the differential diagnosis include a central facial palsy. When central facial palsy occurs in the neonate, it is often associated with birth anoxia. In this condition there is flattening of the nasolabial fold, apparent drooping of the affected side of the face at rest, and widening of the palpable fissure; electrical testing is normal. Peripheral seventh nerve palsy must also be considered. This condition is often associated with birth trauma, particularly forceps delivery. In these patients there are abnormalities of eye closure, forehead wrinkling, and nasolabial fold depth. Electrical testing will be abnormal. Peripheral seventh nerve palsy may also be part of first branchial arch malformation, and such infants will have other congenital anomalies.

Medical Management

Recognition of asymmetrical crying facies in a newborn should alert one to the possibility of an associated malformation. If congenital heart disease is recognized in such an infant, an additional anomaly should be suspected. A careful look at the chest radiograph for an associated vertebral or other skeletal anomaly is warranted. If a skeletal anomaly is detected, congenital anomalies of the gastrointestinal or genitourinary system should be suspected. Since there is an association of asymmetrical crying facies with the CHARGE association, careful evaluation of the affected newborn, including searching for a coloboma of the eye, choanal atresia, ear anomalies, or cleft palate, should be undertaken.

Almost every kind of congenital heart disease has been reported with asymmetrical crying facies. In those infants with multiple anomalies, conotruncal cardiac defects, especially tetralogy of Fallot and right aortic arch, are common. One of the patients reported by Pape and Pickering[87] had a truncus arteriosus and absent thymus and probably had DiGeorge syndrome.

Prognosis

Prognosis will depend primarily on the associated defects. Fortunately, the facial palsy improves with time. It is probable that other muscle groups are able to compensate for the hypoplastic muscle. Usually there is no cosmetic problem later on in life. Asymmetry during crying may remain quite prominent throughout infancy.

Alagille Syndrome (Arteriohepatic Dysplasia)

The association of intrahepatic biliary hypoplasia with characteristic facies and pulmonary artery stenoses was described by Alagille. It is an uncommon but now well-recognized syndrome that is frequently familial.

Historical Perspective

Alagille and associates first described this syndrome in the French literature in 1970. Watson and Miller,[111] in 1973, unaware of Alagille's report, reported arteriohepatic dysplasia as a familial disease with neonatal liver disease, characteristic facies, and pulmonary artery stenosis in the English literature. In 1975, Alagille[1] then reported 15 cases in the English literature, all with intrahepatic biliary hypoplasia and characteristic facies. Twelve of the 15 patients had a murmur compatible with pulmonary artery stenosis, and 8 of the 15 had a vertebral anomaly. Three patients had a positive family history. In 1976, Greenwood and coworkers[35] reported 14 patients with intrahepatic biliary dysgenesis, all of whom had peripheral pulmonary artery stenoses, either alone (8 patients) or associated with an additional cardiac malformation (6 patients). Unlike Alagille and Watson, they did not note unusual facial features. Among their 14 cases were two siblings. Riely and associates,[92] in 1978, reported a father and son with the syndrome compatible with an autosomal dominant form of inheritance.

In 1979, Riely and associates[91] reported the interesting association of characteristic eye findings in five patients with the syndrome. All had bilateral posterior embryotoxon, and four had pigmentary changes in the retina. These researchers suggested that the embryotoxon might serve as a specific marker for Alagille syndrome much as a Kayser-Fleischer ring serves as a marker for hepatolenticular degeneration (Wilson disease). In 1982, Dahms and colleagues[16] presented a longitudinal study of six patients with serial liver biopsies that added to better understanding of the pathogenesis of the liver findings.

In 1983, Sokol and associates[100] suggested that the characteristic facies present in Alagille syndrome might be related to congenital intrahepatic cholestasis rather than being specific for Alagille syndrome. Of their 15 patients with congenital intrahepatic cholestatic liver disease, 7 had a diagnosis of Alagille syndrome. Photographs of all patients were reviewed by a group of pediatric hepatologists to see if patients diagnosed as having Alagille syndrome would be identified as having characteristic facies by the reviewers. Of five subjects identified as having characteristic facies by more than 75 per cent of the hepatologists, only two actually had Alagille syndrome, with three having other forms of cholestasis. Fewer than one half of the examiners identified the remaining five patients with Alagille syndrome as having characteristic facies. In 1984, Shulman and coworkers[98] described a three-generation family with five family members with striking differences in the degree of severity of the clinical finding, demonstrating marked intrafamilial variability.

Epidemiology

From the cases reported so far, an autosomal dominant form is well documented. In some families recessive inheritance has been suggested, and in a few sibships a consanguineous mating was reported. Greenwood and coworkers suggested that intrahepatic biliary dysgenesis frequently resulted from intrauterine infection because there were signs of inflammation on liver biopsies obtained in some of their patients. As the natural history of this syndrome has evolved, it is apparent that biopsy of the liver in early infancy will often show portal inflammation as well as cholestasis and bile ductular proliferation suggesting an inflammatory process. The inflammation in the liver and peripheral pulmonary artery stenosis are similar to the findings in rubella syndrome. Search for an infectious agent or any specific teratogen so far, however, has been unrewarding. Biopsies taken later on in life show no signs of inflammation. The striking finding is paucity or absence of intralobular bile ducts.

There is clear evidence in the literature that Alagille syndrome may be inherited as an autosomal dominant disorder and, like other dominant conditions, there may be considerable variation within a family.

In 1981, my colleagues and I[53] reported a case of extrahepatic biliary atresia in an infant who had the characteristic facies and a cardiac lesion associated with Alagille syndrome, suggesting that the liver involvement may not always be intrahepatic. In reviewing Alagille's report, it was interesting to note that in two separate families a proband with typical Alagille syndrome had a sibling with extrahepatic biliary atresia and possibly had other features of Alagille syndrome.

Although the generally benign nature of this liver condition has been stressed, a family reported by Shulman and coworkers[98] included one patient who developed cirrhosis and portal hypertension and died before 5 years of age. The 31-year-old mother, on the other hand, had characteristic facies, mild peripheral pulmonary stenosis, and normal findings on liver function tests. At the present time Alagille syndrome should be considered a complex syndrome with multisystemic involvement. Although sporadic cases have been reported, many cases demonstrate autosomal dominant inheritance. It is apparent that careful study of additional families will be necessary before the spectrum of this syndrome will be completely understood.

Clinical Findings

A typical infant born with Alagille syndrome is small for gestational age, usually weighing under 6 pounds. There is equal sex distribution. Early jaundice with hepatomegaly occurs. The urine may be dark or normal in color, and the stools may be clay colored or pigmented. Early-onset conjugated hyperbilirubinemia is evident. Typical facies may not be recognizable in the newborn, although a wizened postmature-appearing infant of low birthweight should arouse suspicion. Characteristic facies include a prominent forehead, deep-set eyes with mild hypertelorism, straight nose, malar flattening, and a pointed chin.

Careful eye examination should be carried out. Schwalbe's line (a posterior embryotoxon) and pigmentary retinopathy are common findings. Sometimes the posterior embryotoxon is obvious on gross examination, but in most cases examination with a slit lamp is required. The retina should be examined for hyperpigmentation. Other eye findings have included esotropia, ectopic pupils, and infantile myopia. Eye findings have been reported as early as 7 months of age. Unfortunately, detailed reports of eye examinations have been few.

A variety of skeletal abnormalities have been reported, with the most characteristic being vertebral anomalies, especially butterfly vertebrae. Clinodactyly and, in general, short proximal phalanges have also been frequent features.

Peripheral pulmonary artery stenosis is the characteristic cardiac lesion, so that a widely transmitted ejection systolic murmur is usually heard. The murmur of peripheral pulmonary stenosis is also a frequently "normal" murmur present transiently in full-term and premature infants in early infancy. A variety of associated cardiac defects occur, with ventricular septal defect, atrial septal defect, and patent ductus arteriosus among the more commonly reported. Severe tetralogy of Fallot, including pulmonary valve atresia and ventricular septal defect, has also been reported and may result in early death from severe hypoxia. Physical findings on cardiac examination will, of course, depend on what cardiac lesions are present.

A careful family history should be obtained and both parents examined for subtle findings. In general, patients with Alagille syndrome improve and may appear quite normal as adults. Careful examination of parents and siblings, including eye examinations, may be required to rule out a mild variant of the syndrome.

Differential Diagnosis

Congenital heart disease associated with neonatal cholestasis is rare. Greenwood and colleagues[35] reported 1566 newborns with symptomatic heart disease seen in the New England Regional Infant Cardiac Program between 1968 and 1972, and only two of these had biliary atresia. One of these infants had the "cat eye" syndrome, and the other had heterotaxy syndrome and complex congenital heart disease. Zukin and associates[119] reviewed the literature in 1981 regarding extrahepatic biliary atresia associated with cyanotic congenital heart disease and found only five reported cases. They added two additional cases and noted that four of the seven patients had some degree of heterotaxy and no evidence of Alagille syndrome. Thus, cyanotic heart disease and neonatal cholestasis should suggest some form of heterotaxy, and the likelihood of extrahepatic biliary atresia, rubella syndrome, trisomy 18, "cat eye" syndrome, and Zellweger syndrome should also be ruled out.

As mentioned previously, it may be difficult by liver biopsy to differentiate Alagille syndrome from other forms of neonatal liver disease. Early in infancy the microscopic findings may suggest neonatal hepatitis. Microscopic findings might also suggest the possibility of extrahepatic biliary atresia. It is important to remember that at least in one patient, extrahepatic biliary atresia has been present along with typical features of Alagille syndrome.

Medical Management

In an infant with conjugated hyperbilirubinemia and an associated heart murmur, the possibility of Alagille syndrome could be considered. Careful eye examination and a search for a skeletal anomaly should be carried out. Since the liver disease generally follows a benign and improving course, unnecessary invasive studies should be avoided. Pruritus may become a significant symptom, and treatment with diet or cholestyramine should be instituted. Xanthomas may develop after 6 months of age. Serum triglyceride and cholesterol levels may be only mildly elevated in the newborn period but rapidly rise, with cholesterol reaching levels of 700 to 3000 mg/dl. Triglyceride levels frequently rise to between 1000 and 5000 mg/dl. The alkaline phosphatase concentration is also increased, and the serum transaminase value is usually moderately elevated. Tests for hepatitis-associated antigens and evidence of intrauterine infection are negative. Triglyceride and cholesterol levels should be monitored and treated with appropriate diet and drug therapy.

Fortunately, the peripheral pulmonary stenosis is generally mild or moderate and usually nonprogressive. An occasional patient, however, may have severe peripheral pulmonary stenosis with progressive cardiac impairment. Echocardiography should be helpful in determining whether additional associated cardiac lesions are present. In general, the associated lesions are amenable to surgical treatment.

Prognosis

Unlike most other forms of congenital intrahepatic cholestatis, Alagille syndrome carries a fairly good prognosis. The benign nature of this condition has been noted in many reports. There are, however, a number of reports describing patients who died in infancy. One of these was an infant who had stenosis of the right coronary ostium at autopsy and died in congestive heart failure at 18 months. Another report describes a 9-month old who died of progressive renal failure. As mentioned earlier, one patient died under 5 years of age of cirrhosis with portal hypertension. In Alagille's report, two of his patients died at 6 months and 3 months of age of septicemia. Mueller and coworkers[69] described a 23 per cent mortality rate under age 5 years in their review of 62 patients with Alagille syndrome, emphasizing that there may be significant morbidity and mortality for this condition. Beyond early childhood a benign course has been the rule.

UPPER LIMB DEFECTS

Defects of the upper limb are frequently associated with congenital heart disease. The limb buds and shaft of the radius form at the same time as the atrial and ventricular septa are developing at 4 to 6 weeks of fetal development. Chromosomal, genetic, and teratogenic syndromes must be considered. Two genetic syndromes, Ellis-van Creveld, an autosomal recessive condition, and Holt-Oram, an autosomal dominant condition, are discussed.

Ellis-van Creveld Syndrome

Ellis-van Creveld syndrome is a rare condition characterized by polydactyly, ectodermal dysplasia, and chondrodystrophy with symmetrical shortening of the extremities.

Historical Perspective

In 1940, Ellis and van Creveld[19] reported a syndrome they called chondroectodermal dysplasia. In 1959, Walls and coworkers[110] reviewed 28 cases and suggested that there was an autosomal recessive mode of inheritance and that congenital heart disease was present in about one half of the cases. Six of the 28 patients, all with significant congenital heart disease, died in infancy. Relatively few additional cases were added until 1964 when McKusick and colleagues[65] reported 52 cases from an inbred Amish population. Their study clearly defined the inheritance as autosomal recessive. Mahoney and Hobbins,[61] in 1977, reported the first prenatal diagnosis of this syndrome using fetoscopy and ultrasonography.

Epidemiology

Ellis van-Creveld syndrome is a rare autosomal recessive condition with the majority of cases appearing in consanguineous matings. It has been reported in a variety of countries, although the largest number of cases has occurred in an inbred Amish population.

Clinical Findings

The most easily recognized feature at birth is polydactyly of the fingers, with the extra digit almost always being located on the ulnar aspect of the hand (Fig. 50–6). Polydactyly may also occur in the lower extremities. The extremities are short, especially in the distal portions. The thorax is often relatively hypoplastic. In the infant the upper lip is attached by numerous heavy frenula to the mucosa of the alveolar process, eliminating the mucobuccal space or sulcus in the anterior part of the mouth (Fig. 50–7). This finding is an important feature of the Ellis-van Creveld syndrome in early infancy. Another common oral feature is a notched mandibular alveolar process. Often there are

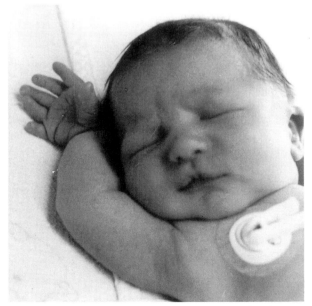

Figure 50–6. Infant with Ellis-van Creveld syndrome showing six fingers.

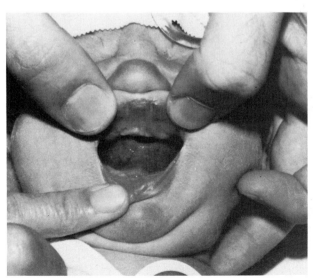

Figure 50–7. Infant with Ellis-van Creveld syndrome showing characteristic frenula.

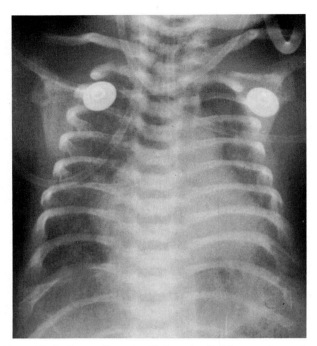

Figure 50-8. Chest radiograph of infant who died from respiratory insufficiency.

natal teeth. The heavy frenula of the upper lip seen in the newborn change as the maxilla increases in height. They become narrower and recede so that the mucobuccal fold becomes visible but numerous frenula remain present on the anterior part of the maxilla. The teeth are often peg shaped, and some are missing. Fingernails are dystrophic. The hair is often sparse and fine. There is no involvement of the sweat glands.

Fifty to 60 per cent of patients have a congenital malformation of the heart.[33] A single atrium with a cleft mitral valve has been the most common cardiac defect in my experience. Ventricular septal defects, atrioventricular septal defects, anomalous pulmonary venous drainage, as well as other defects, have been reported. The combination of a small thorax and congenital heart disease may cause severe respiratory problems in the newborn, and death from respiratory insufficiency may occur (Fig. 50-8).

Radiographs will show disproportionate shortening of the tibia and fibula in comparison to the femur. In the upper extremities, the capitate and hamate bones are fused. Bones of the distal extremities are very short and thickened. The proximal end of the ulna and distal end of the radius are greatly enlarged. Bony changes in the tibia result in a genu valgum deformity that increases as the child grows and becomes ambulatory. Although mental retardation has been reported, the great majority of patients have normal intelligence.

Differential Diagnosis

Other forms of achondroplasia must be considered, but the presence of polydactyly and the major shortening of

the distal rather than the proximal portion of the extremities is helpful in the differential diagnosis. Jeune thoracic dystrophy occasionally includes polydactyly. These patients have a small thorax and hypoplastic lungs. Death may occur in early infancy from respiratory insufficiency similar to that in the Ellis-van Creveld syndrome. Lack of ectodermal dysplasia in Jeune thoracic dystrophy helps distinguish these two conditions, both of which are inherited as autosomal recessive disorders.

Medical Management

Since Ellis-van Creveld syndrome is an autosomal recessive condition, accurate diagnosis is essential to provide genetic counseling to the family. The most serious problem anticipated in the newborn period is that of respiratory insufficiency because of the small thorax. The high incidence of congenital heart disease should alert the clinician to search for evidence of a cardiac lesion. The cardiac defects present in these patients usually result in increased pulmonary blood flow. Fortunately, should the heart disease become symptomatic, the lesions are generally amenable to surgical treatment. Orthopedic consultation should be sought. The surgical procedure involved in treating the polydactyly in these patients is much more complicated than the simple removal of an extra finger. Additional surgical procedures on the lower extremities to correct the genu valgum deformity may also be required. Dental consultation will also be necessary to provide the best cosmetic result for the child.

It is important early in life to inform the parents that the child will be short. Adult stature in the range of 43 to 60 inches has been reported. Every effort should be made to anticipate and prevent emotional disability that may result from short stature. Every attempt should be made to allow these patients to lead a productive life since they are mentally normal. This disorder is a rare autosomal condition, and patients can be expected to bear unaffected children in the future.

Prognosis

The prognosis depends on the severity of the cardiac lesion present and the degree of thoracic hypoplasia. In those patients with severe hypoplasia of the chest, death in early infancy is the rule. Surgical repair of the single atrium with cleft mitral valve or any other cardiac lesion usually results in an excellent result so that a good long-term prognosis from a cardiac point of view can be anticipated. Dental and skeletal deformities frequently require ongoing care and treatment. Unfortunately, these patients will be quite short as adults, and ongoing counseling and support should be provided to prevent emotional disability.

Holt-Oram Syndrome

The association of upper extremity skeletal defects with congenital heart disease transmitted as an autosomal dominant is known as the Holt-Oram syndrome.

Historical Perspective

In 1960, Holt and Oram[40] reported a family in which upper extremity malformations were associated with a secundum atrial septal defect. Subsequent reports confirmed an autosomal dominant transmission of this syndrome but demonstrated a variety of skeletal and cardiac defects. In 1965, Lewis and associates[59] and Holmes[39] reported additional families with more severe upper extremity abnormalities, including absent radii, and noted that ventricular septal defect as well as atrial septal defect could occur. Kaufman and colleagues,[46] in 1974, stressed the variable expression of the Holt-Oram syndrome both between families and within families.

Epidemiology

An autosomal dominant form of inheritance is well documented. Like other autosomal dominant conditions, there may be a great variation in expression of the gene.

Clinical Findings

Marked gradations of defects in the upper limb and shoulder girdle may occur from thumb hypoplasia to phocomelia. The thumb is frequently triphalangeal or fingerlike but may be hypoplastic or absent. The radius may be hypoplastic or absent, and defects of the ulna, humerus, clavicle, scapula, and sternum may occur. Absence of the pectoralis major muscle is occasionally noted as well as pectus excavatum, scoliosis, or vertebral anomalies (Fig. 50–9).

Smith and associates[99] reported detailed clinical findings of 39 patients with the syndrome and emphasized the asymmetry of skeletal involvement. Although skeletal involvement is usually bilateral, it was more severe on the left side in 69 per cent. These investigators confirmed the finding of other observers that congenital heart disease is a frequent feature, and only 5 of the 39 patients were believed to have normal hearts. A variety of rhythm disturbances including first-degree atrioventricular block or nodal rhythm was almost a uniform finding among those patients with congenital heart disease. An atrial septal defect alone or associated with a ventricular septal defect was the most common cardiac lesion, but a wide variety was found. They noted in their families that there were no members with congenital heart disease without skeletal anomalies. However, within a family there might be a family member with skeletal defects and a normal cardiovascular system. An important observation noted by Smith and associates and mentioned by Holt and Oram was the finding of hypoplastic peripheral blood vessels at cardiac catheterization in a 22-year-old woman and a 7-week-old infant. Of interest is that 7 of their 27 patients developed complications following cardiac catheterizations that could be attributed to hypoplastic vessels. Both males and females appear to be affected equally, although in some families females appear to have more severe skeletal deformities. In several families the high number of affected offspring suggested that abnormal segregation may occur in the Holt-Oram syndrome.

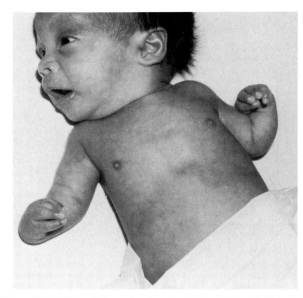

Figure 50–9. Bilateral absent thumb and radius in infant with Holt-Oram syndrome.

Differential Diagnosis

Absent radii, usually bilateral, may occur as part of an autosomal recessive condition called Fanconi syndrome. Such patients are small and develop pancytopenia that is usually fatal by late childhood. Associated congenital heart disease is reported but not frequent. Another autosomal recessive condition with absent radii is accompanied by thrombocytopenia and only occasionally by congenital heart disease. Thalidomide embryopathy may have severe upper limb deformities and congenital heart disease. Perhaps the most important condition to be distinguished is that of the VATER association in which absent radius may occur but is usually unilateral.

Medical Management

The most important part of management is establishing whether the patient has Holt-Oram syndrome, since this is an autosomal dominant disorder with a 50 per cent chance of recurrence. Careful examination of parents and other family members for even subtle abnormalities in the upper extremities should be performed. The newborn with a hypoplastic thumb should be a suspect for associated congenital heart disease.

Clinical findings of an atrial septal defect may not be present in the newborn period, but an echocardiogram may help establish that diagnosis. An ECG should be obtained since conduction defects and rhythm disorders are common. If there is no family history to support the diagnosis of Holt-Oram syndrome, the possibility of VATER association should be considered. Anomalies of the genitourinary or gastrointestinal tract are frequent in the VATER association. Fortunately, the heart defects present in the Holt-Oram syndrome are usually amenable to cardiac surgery, although an occasional patient will have complex cardiac defects.

Prognosis

Generally the prognosis is good since the heart defects are amenable to surgical repair. Long-term prognosis, however, must be somewhat guarded because of the tendency for arrhythmias, such as sick sinus syndrome or atrial flutter, to occur on follow-up. I have already seen one patient who required a pacemaker in her early 20s because of sick sinus syndrome following repair of a large atrial septal defect in childhood and another patient who has persistent atrial flutter following repair of an atrial septal defect in childhood. Genetic counseling indicating that there is a 50 per cent chance of recurrence in offspring should be provided to the patient.

IVEMARK SYNDROME (CARDIOSPLENIC OR HETEROTAXY SYNDROME)

Ivemark syndrome implies some degree of heterotaxy usually associated with asplenia or polysplenia. There is a tendency for the symmetrical development of normally asymmetrical organs or pairs of organs. The term *bilateral right sidedness* is associated with asplenia whereas *bilateral left sidedness* is related to polysplenia.

Historical Perspective

Asplenia with cyanotic congenital heart disease was first described by Martin in 1826.[63] In 1952, Polhemus and Schafer[89] reported additional cases and reviewed the literature. Willi and Gasser[114] made the first premortem diagnosis of asplenia based on findings in the peripheral blood smear. Ivemark,[42] in 1955, reviewed 55 cases and added 14 of his own in a monograph on asplenia that included some discussion of polysplenia. In 1962, Van Mierop and Wiglesworth[108] noted the *bilateral right sidedness* in asplenia, whereas Moller and coworkers,[68] in 1967, described *bilateral left sidedness* in polysplenia. In 1975, Rose and colleagues[93] reviewed 60 cases and compared the clinical features of asplenia with polysplenia, noting among their cases three families, each with two affected siblings.

Epidemiology

Although the cardiac defects in asplenia vary significantly compared with those found in polysplenia, there is much overlap.[106] Both have some degree of heterotaxy. It is likely that they share a common etiology related to failure to achieve normal visceral asymmetry. Normally, the viscera and the heart undergo dextrorotation. Complete situs inversus is infrequent, occurring in approximately 0.01 per cent of the population. With complete situs inversus, normal cardiac development is usual but there is a significantly increased incidence of congenital heart disease compared with situs solitus. In 1938, Cockayne[14] noted that developmental anomalies are more likely to occur with sinistral rather than dextral rotation of the viscera and that if that rotation is incomplete, developmental anom-

alies are likely to be more severe. Torgersen[103] pointed out that "situs inversus is no simple alternative to normal situs. It is the most complicated among anomalies concerning not only the situs but all details of structures." Cockayne postulated that situs inversus was due to a single recessive autosomal gene. He further suggested that incomplete forms of situs inversus were probably similarly inherited. Although most cases of Ivemark syndrome are sporadic, many familial cases have been reported, including families with multiple cases of asplenia or polysplenia as well as families with an example of each.

Considerable insight into autosomal recessive inheritance of situs inversus has been provided by Layton's interesting work in an inbred strain of mice who have a mutant gene given the symbol IU. This mutant gene is inherited as an autosomal recessive. Early studies in the mouse were confusing since only 50 per cent of IU/IU mice had situs inversus. Layton,[57] in 1976, hypothesized that the developmental control mechanism that normally determines situs solitus was missing in these mice so that the visceral situs was determined by chance. The IU/IU mouse embryo would by chance develop either situs inversus or situs solitus. This hypothesis would explain the 50 per cent rather than 100 per cent incidence of situs inversus noted in the homozygous mouse. In the mouse model, heterotaxy was frequent and occurred with both situs solitus and inversus, suggesting heterotaxy could be attributed to loss of developmental control. Layton[58] also noted that complex congenital heart disease occurred in over 20 per cent of the affected mice similar in type to that present in the human with heterotaxy. Study of the cardiac loop in the mouse embryo showed, as Layton had hypothesized, one half with a *d* cardiac loop and one half with an *l* loop. Thus the cardiac malformation like the heterotaxy could be attributed to loss of the developmental process that determines asymmetry. For a complete total situs inversus to occur, the visceral and cardiac loop need to be concordant by chance. It is not surprising that with loss of developmental control there is failure of normal asymmetry to occur. With bilateral left-sidedness as seen in the polysplenia syndrome, the cardiac lesions tend to be less severe than in those patients with bilateral right sidedness characteristic of the asplenia syndrome.

Autosomal recessive inheritance of some cases of heterotaxy in humans is well documented.[41] Gatrod and colleagues[32] noted a relationship between consanguinity and complex congenital anomalies with situs ambiguus. There was a 10-fold increase in the incidence of Ivemark syndrome in Asian Muslems, who have a very high rate of consanguinity when compared with English patients.

Although teratogens such as trypan blue and x-irradiation have produced conotruncal malformations and reversed loops in experimental animals, these teratogens usually produce severe malformations of the central nervous system and other organs as well as the heart. In general, heterotaxy is not a striking feature. In humans rarely has a teratogen been implicated in this syndrome, but such a pathogenesis is, of course, possible.

It is interesting to note that in thoracopagus conjoined twins there is a high incidence of heterotaxy and cardiac

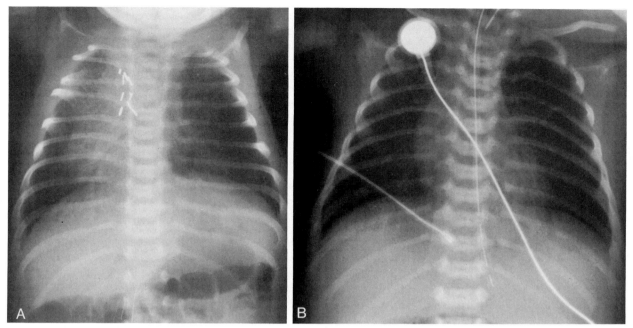

Figure 50–10. *A*, Chest radiograph of an infant with asplenia showing a symmetrical liver (dextrocardia). *B*, Chest radiograph of an infant with asplenia showing a symmetrical liver (levocardia).

lesions similar to that present in the Ivemark syndrome.[75] Mirror-image monozygous twins have also been reported with one twin having situs solitus and the other complete situs inversus. It is difficult to explain the latter finding on a genetic basis. The possibility of a mechanical factor related to the twinning process could be implicated. At the present time it is not clear how much human heart development is governed by genetic factors and how much by mechanical ones, but it is likely that heterotaxy may be the result of either or both factors.

Clinical Findings

ASPLENIA

It is important to consider the asplenia syndrome in every newborn with cyanotic congenital heart disease. There is a male predominance, with about two thirds of the cases reported in boys. About one third have dextrocardia. A symmetrical liver is evident (Fig. 50–10). The liver edge may be palpable across the entire upper abdomen. A normal birthweight is usual, and the mother's pregnancy history is usually unremarkable.

The cardiac findings will, of course, depend on the defects present. Decreased pulmonary blood flow with severe cyanosis is the rule. The great majority of patients have transposition or malposition of the great arteries and either pulmonary stenosis or atresia. Total anomalous pulmonary venous drainage and a common atrioventricular valve are present in over 70 per cent. There is usually a common atrium, and almost one half will have a single ventricle. Bilateral superior vena cavae are frequent.

In about one half the cases, the stomach is located on the right side. Partial malrotation of the jejunum and ileum is frequent. The liver is bilateral and symmetrical. Isomerism of the lungs with bilateral tri-lobed lungs is expected. The spleen is absent. The presence of Howell-Jolly and Heinz bodies in the peripheral red cells is strong evidence for the asplenia syndrome. A splenic scan may be useful but may not be appropriate in a sick newborn.

The chest radiograph should be evaluated carefully. Sometimes bilateral eparterial bronchi can be identified. The position of the cardiac apex, stomach bubble, and liver shadow should be noted.[23] Elliott and coworkers[18] have pointed out that if the inferior vena cava and aorta are located on the same side of the spine, which may be either to the right or left, asplenia is very likely. The pulmonary vascularity is generally decreased.

The ECG does not provide helpful specific findings.

POLYSPLENIA

In the polysplenia syndrome, there appears to be no sex predominance, although an increased number of females has been noted by some authors. Unlike the infants with asplenia, these infants are usually acyanotic and have increased pulmonary blood flow. Only one third have significant pulmonary outflow obstruction. Like patients with asplenia, bilateral superior venae cavae and a common atrioventricular valve are frequent findings. Transposition of the great vessels, however, is uncommon. Partial rather than total anomalous pulmonary venous drainage is a common finding. The most characteristic malformation is absence of the hepatic portion of the inferior vena cava with an azygous vein connection.

Abdominal heterotaxy is frequent. The stomach is usually on the right side, and there is partial malrotation of the small bowel similar to that in asplenia. There are bilateral hyparterial bronchi and bilateral bi-lobed lungs. The liver is often symmetrical and bilateral. Absence of the gallbladder and extrahepatic biliary atresia occur occasionally.

Careful attention to the chest radiograph will demonstrate some degree of heterotaxy, alerting the clinician to the possibility of this syndrome. Multiple spleens may be identified by splenic scintigraphy.[25] Absence of the inferior vena cava shadow on the chest radiograph, as well as a prominent azygous vein, is a helpful sign suggesting the polysplenia syndrome.

The ECG frequently has a superiorly oriented P wave axis with negative P waves in leads II, III, and AVF. There also is an increased incidence of congenital complete heart block in patients with polysplenia syndrome. Garcia and colleagues[29] have pointed out that in any infant presenting with complete heart block, complex congenital heart disease, and a superiorly oriented P wave axis, the diagnosis of left isomerism is likely.

Differential Diagnosis

When a chest radiograph demonstrates the heart shadow to be on the right side, a number of possibilities other than the Ivemark syndrome must be considered. There may be complete mirror-image dextrocardia with situs inversus, which, of course, may occur in the absence of any cardiac anomaly. There may be dextroposition of the heart because of an abnormality of the lung. Dextroversion can occur with the heart rotated to the right in the absence of any heterotaxy. Since the heterotaxy syndrome varies significantly in its manifestations and severity, it may be difficult to rule out a mild form of the syndrome, particularly in the absence of complex congenital heart disease.

Medical Management

A high index of suspicion is essential if heterotaxy is to be recognized in the cyanotic newborn. A very cyanotic newborn with asplenia is likely to have a ductal dependent form of cyanotic congenital heart disease. Although a prostaglandin infusion to maintain patency of the ductus arteriosus may be lifesaving, it may also unmask the presence of obstructed total anomalous pulmonary venous drainage.[24] Delisle and associates[17] reported 23 cases of heterotaxy with total anomalous pulmonary venous drainage; pulmonary veins were obstructed in 11 and nonobstructed in 12. Fourteen of their patients had asplenia, and 9 had polysplenia; obstructed pulmonary veins occurred in both groups. In 7 patients pulmonary venous drainage was to the subdiaphragmatic area and all veins were obstructed. Of 10 patients with pulmonary veins entering the supracardiac area, obstruction was present in 4. Only the 6 patients with pulmonary veins that entered the heart directly had no evidence of obstruction. It is very important to identify pulmonary venous connections by cardiac catheterization or echocardiography prior to any palliative surgical procedure. In all their obstructed cases, Delisle and associates

found that there was a horizontal vein present that would be suitable for anastomosis to the dorsal wall of the left atrium.

Because of the very complex heart disease present in the cyanotic infant with asplenia syndrome, there was a tendency in the past to be quite conservative in recommending palliative surgical treatment. There appears to be more optimism for survival today. A number of children with asplenia have had long-term survival following palliative surgery, and a number of such children have undergone a successful Fontan procedure with a satisfactory result.

Infants with asplenia have an increased susceptibility to bacterial infections. Pneumococcal vaccine and continuous prophylactic antibiotics are recommended and should be continued indefinitely. Waldman and his associates[109] noted that in the young infant there was a greatly increased risk of either *Klebsiella* or *Escherichia coli* infection, whereas pneumococcus and *Haemophilus influenzae* were common in infants 6 months of age or older. These authors recommended that, instead of penicillin, amoxicillin, 25 mg/kg/day in two divided doses, be prescribed once the diagnosis of asplenia syndrome is made.

It is important to examine the peripheral blood for presence of Howell-Jolly bodies, which are highly suggestive of absence of the spleen in a cyanotic newborn.

Patients with polysplenia syndrome tend to have increased pulmonary blood flow so that congestive cardiac failure rather than severe cyanosis is a more likely problem. The usual medical treatment of congestive cardiac failure is indicated. The high incidence of complete atrioventricular septal defect (sometimes associated with left ventricular outflow obstruction and often with double-outlet right ventricle) may make corrective cardiac surgery in early infancy of such high risk that palliative pulmonary artery banding may be indicated initially. There is a wide range of cardiac lesions with the polysplenia syndrome. Absence of the inferior vena cava with an azygous vein connection is highly characteristic of polysplenia. This venous anomaly may complicate cardiac catheterization, but with flow-directed catheters absent inferior vena cava is less of a problem than in the past. It is helpful, however, to make the diagnosis of absent inferior vena cava prior to cardiac catheterization.

In both asplenia and polysplenia, partial malrotation of the small intestines is common[67] and may lead to intestinal obstruction. Jaundice in an infant with evidence of congenital heart disease should prompt a search for heterotaxy because of the increased incidence of extrahepatic biliary atresia in this syndrome.[13]

Prognosis

There is a high mortality in infants with complex congenital heart disease and asplenia. In the series of Rose and associates, by 1 year of age death had occurred in 79 per cent of the infants with asplenia and 61 per cent of those with polysplenia.[95] Among the symptomatic infants reported by Fyler and coworkers,[28] 70 per cent of the infants with asplenia or polysplenia were dead by age 1 year. The prognosis today for the infants with severe cyanotic heart disease has improved. The availability of prostaglandin E_1 permits stabilization of the critically ill cyanotic newborn so that cardiac catheterization and palliative surgery can be carried out with the infant in a stable condition. The prognosis of infants with asplenia can be improved with prophylactic antibiotics and prompt treatment of any infections. As mentioned previously, the combination of obstructive pulmonary veins and severe pulmonary stenosis or atresia may be lethal unless the obstructed pulmonary veins are recognized and treated at the time of shunt placement. Since many of these children have single ventricle or a double-outlet right ventricle with common atrioventricular valve, complete surgical repair is frequently unsuccessful. Sridaromont and colleagues[101] reported the extremely poor surgical results for patients with double-outlet right ventricle and common atrioventricular valve, particularly when associated with heterotaxy. Ando and associates,[4] however, did report a single patient who had successful repair of double-outlet right ventricle with transposition of the great arteries, total anomalous pulmonary venous drainage, pulmonary stenosis, a sinus venosus type atrial septal defect, an atrioventricular septal defect, patent ductus arteriosus, bilateral superior vena cavae, and an inferior vena cava entering the left atrium. Although an occasional patient with such complex heart disease may undergo complete correction of the defects, it is more likely that the Fontan procedure later in life will be more successful in those newborns with severe pulmonary stenosis or atresia.

Cardiac lesions in the polysplenia syndrome vary so much in their severity that the prognosis is dependent on the specific cardiac defects. It is likely that this syndrome is not recognized in many instances, since patients may have only mild cardiac defects and minimal evidence of heterotaxy. In most series there is a much higher reported incidence of asplenia than polysplenia, which may partly be explained by the high mortality rate in the former. A postmortem examination may reveal a previously unsuspected absence of the spleen. If the cardiac lesion is mild, the diagnosis of polysplenia may not be considered and unless specifically searched for will not be evident clinically.

CHARGE ASSOCIATION

The mnemonic CHARGE (*coloboma, heart disease, atresia choanae, retarded growth and development, genital hypoplasia,* and *ear anomalies and/or deafness*) was proposed by Pagon and coworkers[86] to describe the interesting association of choanal atresia and/or ocular coloboma with a number of other nonrandomly associated multiple congenital anomalies.

Historical Perspective

Congenital choanal atresia was first reported by Roederer in 1755. This anomaly occurs with the frequency of about 1 in 8000 live births. Buckfield and associates,[10] in 1971, reported congenital choanal atresia associated with anomalies of the foregut and noted a wide range of associated abnormalities including colobomas and congenital heart disease. In 1979, Hall[37] first reported that choanal atresia was nonrandomly associated with multiple congenital anomalies in patients who had normal chromosomes. His 17 patients demonstrated a regularly recurring pattern of associated features, which included mental retardation, postnatal growth deficiency, hypogonadism in males, small ears, cardiac defects, and ocular coloboma. In the same year, Hittner and colleagues reported 10 patients with ocular coloboma who also had heart disease, abnormalities of the external ear with hearing loss, and mental retardation. These patients were remarkably similar to the ones reported by Hall. In 1981, Pagon and coworkers[86] proposed the mnemonic CHARGE association to emphasize that both coloboma and choanal atresia are associated with each other and with a number of other abnormalities in a nonrandom fashion. They proposed the term *association* rather than *syndrome,* suspecting that there was a heterogeneous etiology. In 1985, Kaplan[44] reviewed the charts of all the inpatients with choanal atresia seen at Boston Children's Hospital over a 15-year period. Forty-one patients were identified. Fifty-nine per cent of these patients had at least one additional anomaly. If the choanal atresia were bilateral, 75 per cent had at least one other abnormality. Although Kaplan only noted three patients (7 per cent) to have all of the features associated with the CHARGE association, the remaining patients with associated abnormalities had a high incidence of postnatal growth retardation, sensorineural hearing deficit, congenital heart disease, and coloboma.

Epidemiology

Thus far, most cases of CHARGE association are sporadic and the etiology is unknown. Most of the anomalies present in the CHARGE association may be attributed to altered morphogenesis between days 35 and 45 of gestation. The cause of this arrested growth is probably heterogeneous. Familial cases compatible with an autosomal dominance have been reported, and there are also reports of affected siblings with normal parents, suggesting that autosomal recessive inheritance may also be present in some cases. For normal parents of a child with CHARGE association, the risk for a subsequent affected child appears to be low but not negligible.

It has been suggested that the CHARGE association involves a number of tissues derived from the cephalic neural crest and that the association of choanal atresia with craniofacial anomalies may be due to faulty development of the neural crest. Maldevelopment of the neural crest may help explain the association between anomalies of the craniofacial region and the cardiovascular system. Kirby and colleagues[49] have reported that the mesenchyme of the aorticopulmonary septum is derived from cells of the occipital neural crest. The association of craniofacial and conotruncal anomalies in the DiGeorge syndrome,[107] fetal alcohol syndrome, and holoprosencephaly support this observation. The velocraniofacial syndrome and asymmetrical crying facies both have some overlap with the CHARGE association. There are a number of patients who fit well into the CHARGE association who also have DiGeorge syndrome. In addition, Kallmann syndrome (hypogonadotropism and hypogonadism) has been reported with choanal atresia. The concept of a developmental field defect proposed by Opitz and associates[82] may explain the diversity as well as the nonrandom association of these defects, which may share a common locus within the developing embryo. Disruption of a developmental field complex could be caused by a variety of agents, including genetic, environmental, or a combination of both.

Clinical Findings

An infant with CHARGE association may present with respiratory distress and cyanosis in the delivery room. Such signs are the expected presentation for an infant with bilateral choanal atresia. Since newborns are nasal breathers, bilateral obstruction of the nares will result in cyanosis and severe respiratory distress. Affected newborn infants may be quite blue when quiet but turn pink when stimulated to cry and breathe through the mouth. The inability to pass a catheter through the nares in the delivery room may establish the diagnosis, and prompt establishment of an oral airway may be lifesaving. An occasional infant with the CHARGE association may also have esophageal atresia with a tracheoesophageal fistula. Respiratory distress shortly after birth or after the first feeding should alert the clinician to this possibility. In the presence of bilateral choanal atresia, associated esophageal atresia may be overlooked unless this known association is considered.

Choanal atresia is present in about 60 per cent of the patients with the CHARGE association. In the absence of choanal atresia, the clinician should consider the possibility of CHARGE association in a newborn with an abnormal external ear, unilateral facial palsy, coloboma of the iris, or hypoplastic male genitalia (Fig. 50–11). Colobomas are reported in about 80 per cent of these infants but may involve only the retina or optic nerve so that a careful eye examination is warranted if the infant has any findings suggestive of the CHARGE association. A small number of patients have cleft palate and micrognathia, and microcephaly is relatively common.

Although retarded growth and development are almost constant findings in patients with the CHARGE association, it is not uncommon for these infants to have normal length and weight at delivery. Retardation of growth is primarily postnatal, but some low birthweight infants have been reported. The presence of choanal atresia and/or coloboma in a small-for-dates infant should alert the clinician to the possibility of a chromosomal abnormality. The CHARGE association is a diagnosis of exclusion; therefore, chromosomal abnormalities that may have some of the features present in the CHARGE association must be ruled out in the newborn.

Congenital heart disease occurs in about 80 per cent of patients with the CHARGE association. A variety of cardiac lesions have been reported.[118] Patent ductus arteriosus alone or with an associated ventricular septal defect is most common. Complex congenital heart diseases such as atrioven-

tricular septal defect, double-outlet right ventricle, pulmonary atresia with hypoplastic right ventricle, and tetralogy of Fallot have also been reported. It is important for the clinician to remember that there is a high incidence of associated congenital heart disease with bilateral choanal atresia. Cardiac evaluation including echocardiography should be part of the neonatal assessment of such infants.

Differential Diagnosis

A number of chromosomal syndromes share phenotypic features with the CHARGE association. Trisomy 13, trisomy 18, 8q− trisomy, 4p− syndrome, and cat eye syndrome should be ruled out. Several monogenetic syndromes, especially Treacher Collins and Crouzon, may have choanal atresia and offer some confusion. Both the DiGeorge and Kallmann syndromes may share several features of the CHARGE association, and in some patients there is an overlap between the CHARGE and VATER associations.

Medical Management

The newborn presenting with respiratory distress and cyanosis requires prompt and accurate evaluation. In addition to considering diaphragmatic hernia, tracheoesophageal fistula, primary lung disease, and cyanotic heart disease, bilateral choanal atresia must also be considered. It is essential that bilateral nasal obstruction be recognized promptly so that an oral airway can be established as soon as possible. Until definitive surgery to relieve the choanal atresia can be performed, an oral airway must be ensured. The treatment of choanal atresia is surgical.[9] The obstruction may be membranous or bony and may be approached either intranasally or transpalatally. In general, a transnasal procedure is preferred in infants because of the lower morbidity. Postoperative results are usually good but postsurgical stenosis may occur requiring postoperative follow-up rhinoscopy. If the clinical diagnosis of CHARGE association is considered, chromosome studies should be carried out to rule out a specific chromosome abnormality. Detailed family history and pregnancy history are essential. Because of the high incidence of associated malformations,[54] any infant with choanal atresia should have thorough evaluation for the possibility of congenital heart disease. Fundoscopic examination in a search for coloboma will often uncover optic nerve coloboma not noted on external inspection. Careful measurement of the head circumference is indicated, and further evaluation of the central nervous system may be warranted since there is a high incidence of mental retardation and central nervous system malformations. The male with CHARGE association often has a microphallus and cryptorchidism so that both genitourinary and endocrine abnormalities should be considered. An occasional infant will have a cleft palate without a facial cleft, so that this sometimes partially hidden anomaly should be ruled out.

Delayed growth and development are the rule in children with CHARGE association. Mild to profound mental retardation is likely. Infants with bilateral choanal atresia are at risk for postpartum asphyxia. It is important, there-

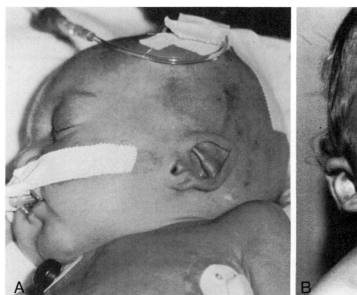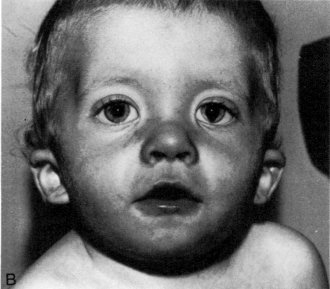

Figure 50–11. *A*, A patient with CHARGE association. Note abnormal ear and airway in place because of choanal atresia. *B*, A patient with CHARGE association. Note coloboma of iris as well as abnormal ears.

fore, to prevent any hypoxia that may contribute to mental retardation. There is also a high incidence of deafness, which may be both conductive and sensorineural. Prompt treatment of otitis media and careful hearing evaluation should be carried out in infancy so that these children will have the best chance to reach their full potential. The most important part of medical management in these children is early identification of the many anomalies found in the CHARGE association. A true multidisciplinary approach, as emphasized by Goldson and coworkers,[34] is necessary for these children to achieve their full potential.

Prognosis

In the reported cases of CHARGE association, there is a fairly high mortality rate that is usually attributed to severe associated malformations such as complex congenital heart disease or associated tracheoesophageal fistula. In the review of Greenwood and colleagues,[36] 11 of 63 children with choanal atresia had congenital heart disease. Seven of the 11 died in infancy, whereas none of those with isolated choanal atresia died. Certainly the association of congenital heart disease and bilateral choanal atresia is a bad combination. Nevertheless, most of the cardiac lesions found in these children represent treatable conditions, and early recognition and treatment of congenital heart defects should improve the prognosis.

There are only a few patients who have had a long-term follow-up. Although male hypogonadism has been stressed as a part of the syndrome, Goldson and associates[34] reported a female patient with delayed puberty who was found at age 17 years by laparoscopy to have ovarian atrophy. Growth retardation, one of the cardinal features of the CHARGE association, may reflect varying degrees of hypo-

pituitarism. A patient reported by August and coworkers[5] showed evidence of growth hormone and gonadotropin deficiencies as well as features compatible with the CHARGE association. Careful endocrine workup would, therefore, seem appropriate in the evaluation of growth failure in these patients.

VATER OR VACTERL ASSOCIATION

Quan and Smith,[90] in 1973, coined the acronym VATER association to describe the nonrandom occurrence of *v*ertebral defects, *a*nal atresia, *t*racheoesophageal fistula with *e*sophageal atresia, *r*enal defects, and *r*adial limb dysplasia. Since that time the acronym has been expanded to VACTERL to include *c*ardiovascular anomalies and *l*imb defects. The diagnosis of VACTERL association requires three or more of these defects and absence of chromosomal abnormalities or other known syndromes.

Historical Perspective

In 1963, Ehmke and I[73,77] noted in a study of associated noncardiac malformations in children with congenital heart disease that 13 of 14 children with congenital heart disease and a vertebral anomaly had multiple other anomalies including 5 patients with four body systems involved. In 1965, Kirkpatrick and coworkers[50] reported 5 patients with tracheoesophageal fistula and esophageal atresia with imperforate anus and additional renal, cardiac, or skeletal malformations. These 5 patients were among 67 patients with esophageal atresia encountered over an 8-year period. In 1968, Say and Gerald[95] proposed the association of imperforate anus, tracheoesophageal fistula, vertebral anomalies, and polydactyly as a new syndrome. Nelson and Forbar,[71] in 1969, noted vertebral anomalies to occur as a single malformation only 15 per cent of the time, whereas in 85 per cent they were part of a multiple anomaly malformation. In 1973, Quan and Smith[90] noted a broader association of these defects and coined the term VATER association. Kaufman,[45] in 1973, and Nora and Nora,[78] in 1975, expanded the acronym to VACTERL, stressing the association of cardiac and limb defects in addition to the vetebral, anal atresia, tracheoesophageal fistula, and renal anomalies.

Epidemiology

In 1983, Khoury and colleagues[47] using population-based data from the Metropolitan Atlanta Congenital Defects Program, noted an incidence of VACTERL association of 1.6 per 10,000 live births. They investigated the interrelation of the six defects that are part of VACTERL association, and they analyzed 76 cases in patients with three or more defects recognized as part of the association. Five of these patients had known chromosomal abnormalities, and 2 were known to have single gene disorders, whereas 19 others appeared to fit into a clinically recognized phenotype or syndrome of unknown etiology, such as Potter syndrome, sirenomelia, or Goldenhar syndrome. The remaining 50 cases were believed to represent the VACTERL association. The authors noted no relation to maternal age or birth order. Fifty-four per cent of newborns weighed 2500 g or less, and one third were born at 37 weeks of gestation or less. There was an increased incidence of the disorder in white males. Twelve per cent of their cases were stillbirths.

Kaufman and coworkers[45] and Nora and Nora[78] had each suggested a causal relation between maternal intake of progesterone/estrogen medication and the VACTERL association. Czeizel and Ludanyi[15] in another population-based study found no correlation between VACTERL association and exogenous female sex hormones. Their findings were similar to those of Khoury and colleagues[47] in that there was a male predominance and a 12 per cent incidence of stillbirths, and 57.6 per cent of their patients weighed 2500 g or less. They noted no specific familial occurrence in 143 first-degree relatives of their indexed cases.

Most authors postulate that the common denominator is defective mesodermal development during embryogenesis. Russell and coworkers[94] have proposed the term *axial mesodermal dysplasia spectrum* to explain the spectrum of overlapping defects. It is suspected that a variety of causative agents could result in this spectrum of defects. Gardner and associates[31] have postulated that anomalies of the heart, gastrointestinal tract, kidneys, and limbs could all be caused by overdistention of the neural tube during embryogenesis. Experimental production of neural tube swelling by a variety of agents such as hypoxia and dimethyl sulfoxide has created a variety of different defects. The same pathogenesis could be proposed for the VACTERL association as has been proposed for the CHARGE association, namely a developmental field complex. Disruption of a developmental field complex could be caused by a variety of agents and could result in multiple anomalies, none of which would always have to be present. Until further data are available from both animal and human studies, the pathogenesis and etiology of this interesting association will remain speculative.

Clinical Findings

The six major defects of the VACTERL association are vertebral anomalies, anal/rectal atresia, cardiovascular anomalies, tracheoesophageal fistula, renal anomalies, and limb defects. The clinical picture will vary considerably depending on what combination of defects is present. Tracheoesophageal fistula, anal/rectal atresia, or a severe limb deformity will be readily recognized in the newborn period. If any of these anomalies is present and particularly if associated with any other component of the VACTERL association, the clinician should be alerted to search for additional hidden renal or vertebral anomalies and to consider the possibility of congenital heart disease. Although the occurrence of even two of the mentioned six major defects is unlikely to be due to chance alone, for most reports three or more of the defects have been required for the diagnosis of VACTERL association.

The typical newborn with this condition will be of low birthweight and more likely be a white male. Several authors have stressed the high incidence of a single umbilical artery.[102,112] Careful examination of the newborn may reveal dysmorphic features that might suggest a known chromosomal or genetic syndrome. Careful pregnancy, maternal, and family histories are essential to rule out a known cause for these malformations. Careful examination of any stillborns for this condition should be carried out, since 12 per cent of the patients with VACTERL association were stillbirths in two population-based studies.

Vertebral anomalies often result in scoliosis but may not be apparent on gross examination of the newborn. Vertebral anomalies are varied, but hemivertebrae, butterfly vertebrae, and sacral agenesis are the most frequent findings. Anal and rectal anomalies include anal atresia with or without rectovaginal, rectourethral, or rectovesical fistulae. Esophageal fistula is usually associated with esophageal atresia, but either esophageal atresia alone or tracheoesophageal fistula alone may occur. Infants with forearm anomalies may have either unilateral or bilateral involvement. Absence or hypoplasia of the thumb is very common, although an extra thumb may occur. Radial agenesis or hypoplasia may occur in association with the thumb anomaly.

Renal malformations tend to be unilateral, ranging from renal agenesis to horseshoe kidney; duplicated collecting systems and obstructive lesions may also occur.

In most clinical reports congenital heart disease has been present in 50 to 80 per cent of the cases. Ventricular septal defects are most common, either alone or in association with additional anomalies such as tetralogy of Fallot, atrial septal defect, or patent ductus arteriosus. However, a wide variety of cardiac defects have been reported, including transposition of the great vessels, dextrocardia, and coarctation of the aorta.

Other defects that occur more often than expected by chance include lower limb defects, rib anomalies, cleft lip and/or palate, omphalocele, neural tube defects, and diaphragmatic hernia. Weaver and associates[112] reported 5 of their 46 patients to have choanal atresia and 2 of these had defects that would overlap both the CHARGE and VACTERL association.

Although there is a high early mortality rate because of the serious multiple malformations present, patients who do survive beyond infancy eventually show some catchup in growth and exhibit normal brain function.

Differential Diagnosis

A number of known syndromes may share many of the defects present in the VACTERL association. Chromosome disorders to be considered include trisomy 13, trisomy 18, 5p deletion, and 13q– deletion. Chromosome studies should be carried out to rule out any known chromosome disorder. Single gene disorders that may be confusing include Meckel syndrome and Zellweger syndrome. It is important not to diagnose Holt-Oram syndrome in a patient with a cardiac defect and radial dysplasia who has other features of the VACTERL association. The Holt-Oram syndrome is an autosomal dominant disorder. The VACTERL association thus far is of unknown etiology and carries a low risk of recurrence in a subsequent pregnancy. A number of recognized phenotypes or syndromes of unknown cause such as Potter syndrome and Goldenhar syndrome may have overlapping features with the VACTERL association. There is considerable overlap between the caudal regression syndrome usually associated with maternal diabetes and the VACTERL association. Therefore, it is important to rule out maternal diabetes before labeling such a patient as having the VACTERL association.

Medical Management

The most important part of medical management is to suspect this association and to look for the life-threatening defects that may be present. Any newborn with an upper limb abnormality (especially a hypoplastic thumb) should be suspect for having an associated serious abnormality such as anal atresia, tracheoesophageal atresia, or a defect of the heart or kidney. The mortality rate in all series of patients with either anal atresia or esophageal atresia who have multiple defects is very high. An ultrasound examination of the abdomen looking for kidney anomalies and an echocardiogram to diagnose a congenital heart defect are important in medical management of these sometimes seriously ill newborns.

Fortunately, most of the defects present in patients with the VACTERL association are amenable to surgical correction. The low birthweight and multiple anomalies, however, often pose a substantial medical challenge. Long-term hospitalization and multiple operative procedures must be ex-

pected. Fortunately, involvement of the central nervous system is uncommon. The majority of patients surviving infancy have exhibited normal brain function. Aggressive medical management in the newborn period, therefore, seems warranted.

Prognosis

The prognosis for infants with the VACTERL association in general is poor. Twelve per cent apparently are stillborn, and in the report by Khoury and coworkers[47] 48 per cent died in the first year of life. Czeizel and Ludanyi[15] reported only 7 of 43 liveborns to survive the first year. This high infant mortality reflects the serious malformations present in such infants and the need for early recognition of those abnormalities that require early surgical treatment. In 46 patients reported by Weaver and associates,[112] 14 died, with seven deaths occurring within 2 weeks of birth and the rest occurring between 6 and 26 months of age.

Following successful surgery the prognosis for tracheoesophageal fistula and anal atresia in patients without associated defects is generally very good. The cardiac defects found in the VACTERL association for the most part can undergo surgical correction with an expected good result. Renal anomalies may prove difficult to manage if there is bilateral involvement such as bilateral renal agenesis or hypoplasia. Fortunately for the most part, renal agenesis has been unilateral. Many of the renal anomalies are amenable to surgical correction. If renal failure develops, peritoneal dialysis until renal transplantation can be effected would improve the long term prognosis. Lawhon and coworkers[56] reviewed the orthopedic aspects of the VACTERL association and pointed out that orthopedic anomalies may be overlooked until the more life-threatening problems have been treated. Some of the orthopedic problems may become more apparent and progressive with time. Careful orthopedic evaluation and follow-up are essential.

As mentioned earlier, low birthweight is common in these patients as is postnatal growth deficiency. Weber and colleagues,[113] who studied 30 patients with the VACTERL association, noted that the average weight gain in those who survived to 3 years of age and beyond was below the 5th percentile. Mapstone and associates[62] outlined the growth of 31 patients with the VACTERL association. In 14 of their patients in whom height and weight were greater than the 5th percentile during the majority of the first 3 years of life, growth tended to remain below the 50th percentile. However, beyond 3 years of age these patients tended to move closer to the mean. In contrast, 17 patients with growth below the 5th percentile for the first 3 years of life tended to show continued growth deficiency and little evidence of catchup growth after 3 years of age. The authors noted that severe cardiac disease was found in approximately one half of the patients with the growth deficiency and that it was the only defect found in the VACTERL association that was significantly correlated with growth deficiency. Additional long-term studies are needed in these patients before the prognosis can be accurately predicted.

References

1. Alagille D, Odievre M, Gautier M, Dommergues JP (1975): Hepatic ductular hypoplasia associated with characteristic facies, vertebral malformations, retarded physical, mental, and sexual development, and cardiac murmur. J Pediatr 86:63–71.

2. Alexiou D, Maniolidis C, Papaevangellow G (1976): Frequency of other malformations in congenital hypoplasia of depressor anguli oris muscle syndrome. Arch Dis Child 51:891–893.

3. Allanson JE, Hall JG, Hughes HE, Preus M, Witt RD (1985): Noonan syndrome: The changing phenotype. Am J Med Genet 21:507–514.

4. Ando F, Shirotoni H, Kawai J, Kangaki Y, Setsuie N, Yamguchi K, O'Kamato F, Yokoyama T, Makino S, Tateishi K, Nashi K (1976): Successful total repair of complicated cardiac anomalies with asplenia syndrome. J Thorac Cardiovasc Surg 72:33–38.

5. August GP, Rosenbaum KN, Friendly D, Hung W (1983): Hypopituitarism and the CHARGE association. J Pediatr 103:424–425.

6. Bawle EV, Black V (1986): Non-immune hydrops fetalis in Noonan's syndrome. Am J Dis Child 140:758–760.

7. Beuren AJ, Schulze C, Eberle P, Harmjanz D, Opitz J (1964): The syndrome of supravalvular aortic stenosis, peripheral pulmonary stenosis, mental retardation and similar facial appearance. Am J Cardiol 13:471–483.

8. Black JA, Bonham-Carter RE (1963): Association between aortic stenosis and facies of severe infantile hypercalcemia. Lancet 2:745–749.

9. Blasberg B, Stool S, Oka S (1975): Choanal atresia: A cryptic congenital anomaly. Cleft Palate J 12:409–416.

10. Buckfield PM, Holdaway MD, Horowitz S, Kean MR (1971): Bilateral congenital choanal atresia associated with anomalies of the foregut. Aust Paediat J 7:37–44.

11. Cayler GC (1967): An epidemic of congenital facial paresis and heart disease. Pediatrics 40:666–668.

12. Cayler GC (1969): Cardiofacial syndrome: Congenital heart disease and facial weakness, a hitherto unrecognized association. Arch Dis Child 44:69–75.

13. Chandra RS (1974): Biliary atresia and other structural anomalies in the congenital polysplenia syndrome. J Pediatr 85:649–655.

14. Cockayne EA (1938): The genetics of transposition of the viscera. Q J Med 7:479–493.

15. Czeizel A, Ludanyi I (1985): An aetiological study of the VACTERL association. Eur J Pediatr 144:331–337.

16. Dahms BB, Petrelli M, Henoch MS, Halpin TC, Morrison S, Park MC, Tavell AS (1982): Arteriohepatic dysplasia in infancy and childhood: A longitudinal study of six patients. Hepatology 2:350–358.

17. Delisle G, Ando M, Calder AL, Zuberbuhler JR, Rochenmacher S, Alday LE, Mangini O, Van Praagh S, Van Praagh R (1976): Total anomalous pulmonary venous connection: Report of ninety-three autopsied cases with emphasis on diagnostic and surgical considerations. Am Heart J 91:99–122.

18. Elliott LP, Cramer GG, Amplatz K (1966): The anomalous relationship of the inferior vena cava and abdominal aorta as a specific angiocardiographic sign in asplenia. Radiology 87:859–863.

19. Ellis RWB, Van Creveld S (1940): A syndrome characterized by ectodermal dysplasia, polydactyly, chondrodysplasia and congenital morbus cordis: Report of three cases. Arch Dis Child 15:65–84.

20. Fanconi G, Giaodet P, Schlesinger B, Butler H, Black JS (1952): Chronische hypercalcamia kombiniert mit osteosklerose, hyperazotemie, minderwuschs und kongenital missbildungen. Helv Paediatr Acta 7:314–334.

21. Flavell G (1943): Webbing of the neck with Turner's syndrome in the male. Br J Surg 31:150–153.

22. Ford CE, Jones KW, Polani PE, de Almeida JC DE, Briggs JH (1950): A sex chromosome anomaly in a case of gonadal dysgenesis (Turner's syndrome). Lancet 1:711–713.

23. Freedom RM, Fellows KE (1973): Radiographic visceral patterns in the asplenia syndrome. Radiology 106:387–391.

24. Freedom RM, Olley PM, Coceani F, Rowe RD (1978): The prostaglandin challenge: Test to unmask obstructed total anomalous pulmonary venous connections in asplenia syndrome. Br Heart J 40:91–94.

25. Freedom RM, Treves S (1973): Splenic scintigraphy and radionuclide venography in the heterotaxy syndrome. Radiology 107:381–386.

26. Friedman WF, Roberts WC (1966): Vitamin D and the supravalvular aortic stenosis syndrome: The transplacental effects of vitamin D on the aorta of the rabbit. Circulation 34:77–86.

27. Funke O (1902): Pterygium colli. Dtsch Z Chir 63:162–167.

28. Fyler DC, Buckley LP, Hellenbrand WE, Cohn HE, Kirklin JW, Nadas AS, Cartier JM, Breibart MH (1980): Report of the New England Regional Infant Cardiac Program. Pediatrics 65(suppl):377–461.

29. Garcia OL, Mehta AV, Pickoff AS, Tamer DF, Ferrer PL, Wolff GS, Gelband H (1981): Left isomerism and complete atrioventricular block: A report of six cases. Am J Cardiol 48:1103–1107.

30. Garcia RE, Friedman WF, Kaback MM, Rowe RD (1964): Idiopathic hypercalcemia and supravalvular aortic stenosis. N Engl J Med 271:117–120.

31. Gardner WJ, Breuer AC (1980): Anomalies of heart, spleen, kidneys, gut, and limbs may result from an overdistended neural tube: A hypothesis. Pediatrics 65:508–514.

32. Gatrod AR, Read AP, Watson GH (1984): Consanguinity and complex cardiac anomalies with situs ambiguous. Arch Dis Child 59:242–245.

33. Giknis FL (1963): Single atrium and the Ellis-van Creveld syndrome. J Pediat 62:558–564.

34. Goldson E, Smith AC, Stewart JM (1986): The CHARGE association: How well can they do? Am J Dis Child 140:918–921.

35. Greenwood RD, Rosenthal A, Crocker AC, Nadas AS (1976): Syndrome of intrahepatic biliary dysgenesis and cardiovascular malformations. Pediatrics 58:243–247.

36. Greenwood RD, Rosenthal A, Parisi L (1975): Extracardiac anomalies in children with congenital heart disease. Pediatrics 55:485–492.

37. Hall BD (1979): Choanal atresia and associated multiple anomalies. J Pediatr 95:395–398.

38. Hirsch HD, Gelband H, Garcia O, Gottlieb S, Tamer DM (1975): Rapidly progressive obstructive cardiomyopathy in infants with Noonan's syndrome: Report of two cases. Circulation 52:1161–1165.

39. Holmes LB (1965): Congenital heart disease and upper extremity deformities: A report of two families. N Engl J Med 272:437–444.

40. Holt M, Oram S (1960): Familial heart disease with skeletal malformations. Br Heart J 22:236–242.

41. Hurwitz RC, Caskey CT (1982): Ivemark syndrome in siblings. Clin Genet 22:7–11.

42. Ivemark BI (1955): Implications of agenesis of the spleen on the pathogenesis of conotruncus anomalies in childhood. An analysis of the heart malformations in the splenic agenesis syndrome, with fourteen new cases. Acta Paediatr 44(suppl):1–110.

43. Jones KL, Smith DW (1975): The Williams elfin facies syndrome: A new perspective. J Pediatr 86:718–723.

44. Kaplan LC (1985): Choanal atresia and its associated anomalies. Further support for the CHARGE association. Int J Pediatr Otorhinolaryngol 8:237–242.

45. Kaufman RL (1973): Birth defects and oral contraceptive. Lancet 1:1396.

46. Kaufman RL, Rimoin DC, McAlister WH, Hartmann AF (1974): Variable expression of the Holt-Oram syndrome. Am J Dis Child 127:21–25.

47. Khoury MJ, Cordero JF, Greenberg F, James LM, Erickson JD (1983): A population study of the VACTERL association: Evidence for its etiologic heterogeneity. Pediatrics 71:815–820.

48. Kinouchi A, Mori K, Ando M, et al (1976): Facial appearance of patients with conotruncal anomalies. Pediatr Jpn 17:84.

49. Kirby ML, Gale TF, Stewart DE (1983): Neural crest cells contribute to normal aorticopulmonary septation. Science 220:1059–1061.

50. Kirkpatrick JA, Wagner ML, Pilling GP (1965): A complex of anomalies associated with tracheoesophageal fistula and esophageal atresia. AJR 95:208–211.

51. Kitchens CS, Alexander JA (1983): Partial deficiency of coagulation factor XI as a newly recognized feature of Noonan syndrome. J Pediatr 102:224–227.

52. Kobylinski O (1883): Ueber eine flughautahnlicke Ausbreitung Am Halse. Arch Anthropol 14:342–348.

53. Kocoshis SA, Cottrill CM, O'Connor WN, Haugh R, Johnson GL, Noonan JA (1981): Congenital heart disease, butterfly vertebrae and extrahepatic biliary atresia: A variant of arteriohepatic dysplasia? J Pediatr 99:436–439.

54. Koletzko B, Majewski F (1984): Congenital anomalies in patients with choanal atresia. Eur J Pediatr 142:271–275.

55. Landtman B (1971): Clinical and morphological studies in congenital heart disease: A review of 777 cases. Acta Paediatr Scand 213(suppl):1–27.

56. Lawhon SM, MacEwen GD, Bunnell WP (1986): Orthopedic aspects of the VATER association. J Bone Joint Surg 68:424–429.

57. Layton WM Jr (1976): Random determination of a developmental process: Reversal of normal visceral asymmetry in the mouse. J Hered 67:336–338.

58. Layton WM Jr (1978): Heart malformations in mice homozygous for a gene causing situs inversus. Birth Defects 14:277–293.

59. Lewis KB, Bruce RA, Baum D, Motulsky AG (1965): The upper limb cardiovascular syndrome. JAMA 193:98–104.

60. Lightwood R, Sheldon W, Harris C, Stapleton T (1956): Hypercalcemia in infants with vitamin D. Br Med J 2:149.

61. Mahoney MJ, Hobbins JC (1977): Prenatal diagnosis of chondroectodermal dysplasia (Ellis-van Creveld syndrome): with fetoscopy and ultrasound. N Engl J Med 297:258–260.

62. Mapstone CL, Weaver DD, Yu P (1986): Analysis of growth in the VATER association. Am J Dis Child 140:386–390.

63. Martin G (1826): Observation d'une deviation organique de l'estomac, d'une anomalie dans la situation, dans la configuration du coeur et des vaisseaux quie en partent ou qui s'y rendent. Bull Soc Anat de Paves 1:40.

64. Martin NDT, Snodgrass GJAI, Cohen RD (1984): Idiopathic infantile hypercalcemia: A continuing enigma. Arch Dis Child 59:605–613.

65. McKusick VA, Egeland JA, Eldridge R, Hostetler JA (1964): Dwarfism in the Amish. Bull Johns Hopkins Hosp 115:306–336.

66. Mendez HMM, Opitz JM (1985): Noonan syndrome: A review. Am J Med Genet 21:493–506.

67. Moller JH, Amplatz K, Wolfson J (1971): Malrotation of the bowel in patients with congenital heart disease associated with splenic anomalies. Radiology 99:393–398.

68. Moller JH, Nakib N, Anderson RC, Edwards JE (1967): Congenital cardiac disease associated with polysplenia: A developmental complex of bilateral "left-sidedness." Circulation 36:789–799.

69. Mueller RF, Pagon RA, Haas JE, Stephan MJ (1981): Arteriohepatic dysplasia: A potentially lethal disorder of intrahepatic cholestasis and/or congenital heart disease. Am J Hum Genet 33:87A.

70. Nelson KB, Eng GD (1972): Congenital hypoplasia of the depressor anguli oris muscle: Differentiation from congenital facial palsy. J Pediatr 81:16–20.

71. Nelson MM, Forbar JO (1969): Congenital abnormalities at birth and their association in the same patient. Dev Med Child Neural 11:3–16.

72. Noonan JA (1968): Hypertelorism with Turner phenotype. Am J Dis Child 116:373–380.

73. Noonan JA (1978): Association of congenital heart disease with syndromes or other defects. Pediatr Clin North Am 25:797–816.

74. Noonan JA (1980): Syndromes associated with cardiac defects. Cardiovasc Clin 11:97–116.

75. Noonan JA (1978): Twins, conjoined twins and cardiac defects. Am J Dis Child 132:17–18.

76. Noonan JA, Cottrill CM, O'Connor WN (1982): Supravalvular aortic stenosis: A developmental complex with an increased risk of death at cardiac catheterization (abstr). Pediatr Cardiol 3:342–343.

77. Noonan JA, Ehmke DA (1963): Associated non-cardiac malformations in children with congenital heart disease (abstr). J Pediatr 63:469.

78. Nora AH, Nora JJ (1975): A syndrome of multiple congenital anomalies associated with teratogenic exposure. Arch Environ Health 30:17–21.

79. Nora JJ, Sinka AK (1970): Direct male-to-male transmission of the XY Turner phenotype. Lancet 1:250–251.

80. O'Connor WN, Davis JB Jr, Geissler R, Cottrill CM, Noonan JA, Todd EP (1985): Supravalvular aortic stenosis, clinical and pathologic observations in six patients. Arch Pathol 109:179–185.

81. Okada R, Johnson D, Lev M (1968): Extracardiac malformations associated with congenital heart disease. Arch Pathol 85:649–657.

82. Opitz JM, Herrmann J, Pettersen JC, Bersu ET, Colacino SC (1979): Terminological, diagnostic, nosological, and anatomical developmental aspects of developmental defects in man. Adv Hum Genet 9:71–164.

83. Opitz JM, Summitt RL, Sarto GE (1965): Noonan's syndrome in girls: A genocopy of the Ullrich-Turner syndrome (abstr). J Pediatr 67:968.

84. Opitz JM, Weaver DD (1985): Editorial comment: The neurofibromatosis Noonan syndrome. Am J Med Genet 21:477–490.

85. Oppe TE (1964): Infantile hypercalcemia, nutritional rickets, and infantile scurvy in Great Britain. Br Med J 1:1659–1661.

86. Pagon RA, Graham JM, Zonana J, Yong SL (1981): Coloboma, congenital heart disease, and choanal atresia with multiple anomalies: CHARGE association. J Pediatr 99:223–227.

87. Pape KE, Pickering D (1972): Asymmetric crying facies: An index of other congenital anomalies. J Pediatr 81:21–30.

88. Perou ML (1961): Congenital supravalvular aortic stenosis. Arch Pathol 71:453–466.

89. Polhemus DW, Schafer WB (1952): Congenital absence of the spleen: Syndrome with atrioventriculosis and situs inversus. Pediatrics 9:696–708.

90. Quan L, Smith DW (1973): The VATER association. J Pediatr 82:104–107.

91. Riely CA, Cotlier E, Jensen PS, Klatskin G (1979): Arteriohepatic dysplasia: A benign syndrome of intrahepatic cholestasis and multiple organ involvement. Ann Intern Med 91:520–527.

92. Riely CA, La Brecque DR, Ghent C, Horwich A, Klatskin G (1978): A father and son with cholestasis and peripheral pulmonic stenosis. J Pediatr 92:406–411.

93. Rose V, Iziukawa T, Moes CA (1975): Syndromes of asplenia and polysplenia. A review of cardiac and non-cardiac malformations in sixty cases with special references to diagnosis and prognosis. Br Heart J 37:840–852.

94. Russell LJ, Weaver DD, Bull MJ (1981): The axial mesodermal dysplasia spectrum. Pediatrics 67:176–182.

95. Say B, Gerald PS (1968): A new polydactyly, imperforate anus, vertebral anomalies syndrome. Lancet 2:688.

96. Schmidt RE, Gilbert EF, Amend TC, Chamberlain CR, Lucas RV (1969): Generalized arterial fibromuscular dysplasia and myocardial infarction in familial supravalvular aortic stenosis syndrome. J Pediatr 74:576–584.

97. Shprintzen RJ, Goldberg RB, Lewin ML (1978): A new syndrome involving cleft palate, cardiac anomalies, typical facies, and learning disabilities: Velo-cardiofacial syndrome. Cleft Palate J 15:56–62.

98. Shulman SA, Hyams JS, Gunta R, Greenstein RM, Cassidy SB (1984): Arteriohepatic dysplasia (Alagille syndrome): Extreme variability among affected family members. Am J Med Genet 19:325–332.

99. Smith AT, Sack GH, Taylor GJ (1979): Holt-Oram syndrome. J Pediatr 95:538–543.

100. Sokol RJ, Heubi JE, Balisteri WF (1983): Intrahepatic "cholestasis facies": Is it specific for Alagille syndrome? J Pediatr 103:205–208.

101. Sridaromont S, Feldt RH, Ritter DG, David GD, McGoon DC, Edwards JE (1975): Double-outlet right ventricle associated with persistent common atrioventricular canal. Circulation 52:933–942.

102. Temtamy SA, Miller JD (1974): Extending the scope of the VATER association: Definition of the VATER syndrome. J Pediatr 85:345–349.

103. Torgersen J (1949): Genetic factors in visceral asymmetry and in the development and pathologic changes of lungs, heart, and abdominal organs. Arch Pathol 47:566–593.

104. Turner HH (1938): A syndrome of infantilism, congenital webbed neck, and cubitus valgus. Endocrinology 23:566–574.

105. Ullrich O (1930): Uber typische Kombinationsbilder multiper Abantungen. Z Kinderheilkd 49:271–276.

106. Van Mierop LHS, Gessner IH, Schiebler GL (1972): Asplenia and polysplenia syndromes. Birth Defects VIII:36–44.

107. Van Mierop LHS, Kutsche LM (1986): Cardiovascular anomalies in DiGeorge syndrome and importance of neural crest as a possible pathogenetic factor. Am J Cardiol 58:133–137.

108. Van Mierop LHS, Wiglesworth FW (1962): Isomerism of the cardiac atria in the asplenia syndrome. Lab Invest 11:1303–1315.

109. Waldman JD, Rosenthal A, Smith AL, Shurin S, Nadas AS (1977): Sepsis and congenital asplenia. J Pediatr 90:555–559.

110. Walls WL, Altman DH, Winslow OP (1959): Chondroectodermal dysplasia (Ellis-van Creveld syndrome). Am J Dis Child 98:242–248.

111. Watson GH, Miller V (1973): Arteriohepatic dysplasia. Arch Dis Child 48:459–466.

112. Weaver DD, Mapstone CL, Yu P (1986): The VATER association: Analysis of forty-six patients. Am J Dis Child 140:225–229.

113. Weber TR, Smith W, Goosfeld JL (1980): Surgical experience in infants with the VATER association. J Pediatr Surg 15:849–854.

114. Wiland OK (1956): Extracardiac anomalies in association with congenital heart disease. Lab Invest 5:380–388.

115. Willi H, Gasser C (1955): The clinical diagnosis of the triad splenic agenesis, defects of the heart and vessels, and situs inversus. Etudes Neonatales 4:25–63.

116. Williams JCP, Barratt-Boyes BG, Lowe JB (1961): Supravalvular aortic stenosis. Circulation 24:1311–1318.

117. Wooley CF, Hosier DM, Booth RW, Molnar W, Sirak HD, Ryan JM (1961): Supravalvular aortic stenosis. Am J Med 31:717–725.

118. Zagnoeo M, Milner S, Levin SE (1981): Choanal atresia and congenital heart disease. South Med J 21:815–817.

119. Zukin DD, Liberthson RR, Lake AM (1981): Extrahepatic biliary atresia associated with cyanotic congenital heart disease. Clin Pediatr 20:64–66.

51

PERSISTENT PULMONARY HYPERTENSION OF THE NEWBORN SYNDROME (PPHNS)

Walker A. Long

Moreover, I would not willingly lay an aspersion of falsehood upon any that is desirous of the truth, nor blemish any man by accusing him of an error; but I follow the truth only, and have bestowed both my pains and charges to that purpose, that I might bring forth something which might be both acceptable to good men, agreeable to learned men, and profitable to literature.

William Harvey, 1628

Patterns of circulation similar to those of fetal life frequently persist or recur in neonates because the anatomic pathways and physiologic mechanisms responsible for the fetal circulation remain intact in the newborn. A great variety of disorders can cause neonatal persistence or reemergence of fetal circulatory patterns. The purposes of this chapter are to establish the fact that persistence of fetal circulatory patterns is truly a syndrome rather than a disease, to define that syndrome, to establish a uniform terminology, to clarify diagnostic criteria, and to review the syndrome's many causes. Application of consistent terminology and diagnostic criteria will improve recognition of the syndrome and will eventually lead to better understanding of its many pathogenetic mechanisms and treatments.

HISTORICAL PERSPECTIVE

The fetal circulation has been recognized for 350 years. In 1628 William Harvey published *Exercitatio Anatomica De Motu Cordis et Sanguinis in Animalibus* describing his discovery of the circulation of blood.[132] In that same book Harvey also brilliantly deduced the pathways of the fetal circulation and described postnatal persistence of circulation through those pathways.

...in the unripe births of mankind, and likewise in others...the heart by its motion brings forth the blood from the *vena cava* openly and by very patent wayes, by the drawing of both its ventricles. For the right receiving blood from the ear, thrusts it forth through the *vena arteriosa*, and its branch called *canalis arteriosus*, into the great arterie. Likewise, the left at the time by the mediation of the motion of the ear, receives blood through that oval hole from the *vena cava*, and by its tention and constriction thrusts it through the root of the Aorta into the great artery likewise. So in Embryons whilst the lungs are idle, and have no action or motion (as if there were none at all) Nature makes use of both ventricles of the heart, as of one for transmission of blood. And so the condition of Embryons that have lungs and make no use of them, is like to the condition of creatures which have none at all.[132]

Despite Harvey's description in *De Motu Cordis*, the most famous book in all of medicine, of the fact that "unripe births

of mankind" and "likewise others" can exhibit postnatal circulatory patterns similar to those of fetal life, his observations have been overlooked until today. The syndrome Harvey described as occurring in "unripe births of mankind" and "likewise others" was independently rediscovered in recent times by several investigators. In 1950 at the first World Congress of Cardiology in Paris, Novelo et al presented a paper describing postnatal persistence of fetal circulatory patterns.[227] In that same year Keith and Forsythe[160] mentioned a newborn with coarctation in whom "a patent ductus was delivering blood into the aorta," and Everett and Johnson[85a] observed right-to-left ductal shunts up to 15 days of age in puppies. In 1952 Lind and Wegelius[189] injected contrast material via the umbilical vein and demonstrated that in asphyxiated infants "the foramen ovale has either failed to close or reopened." In that same paper[189] Lind and Wegelius also observed two cases in which "the ductus arteriosus was found to be open with a direction of the foetal flow from the pulmonary artery to the aorta." In 1953 Burchell et al[39] showed that hypoxia exacerbated right-to-left ductal shunting in older children with patent ductus arteriosus and pulmonary hypertension. In 1954 Lind and Wegelius[189a] reported venous angiocardiographic findings in 12 normal newborn infants. Right-to-left atrial shunt was demonstrated in three of six infants after upper extremity venous injections and six of six infants after lower extremity venous injections; as a result, Lind and Wegelius noted[189a] "Since blood mainly from the inferior vena cava is shunted into the left atrium in fetal life, it is advisable to inject contrast media from below to demonstrate atrial patency in the newborn infant. It is of interest to note that in several instances it was possible to demonstrate atrial patency in newborn infants only when contrast was injected from below."

In that same study[189a] Lind and Wegelius also performed venous angiocardiography during the first week of life in 30 infants with persistent or recurrent cyanosis. Right-to-left atrial shunts were noted in all; in three cases, "a reversed flow, from the pulmonary artery to the aorta, was observed in the ductus arteriosus." Lind and Wegelius observed that "In cases in which the pulmonary circulation

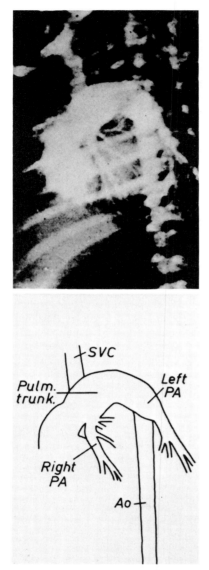

Figure 51–1. Third published (1964) angiocardiographic demonstration of PPHNS. Note that the right ventricle perfuses not only the lungs but also the lower body via right-to-left ductal shunt. Ao = descending aorta; left PA = left pulmonary artery; pulm. trunk = main pulmonary artery; right PA = right pulmonary artery; SVC = superior vena cava. (From Lind J, Stern L, Wegelius CE [1964]. Human Fetal and Neonatal Circulation. Courtesy of Charles C Thomas Publishers, Springfield, p 49.)

does not function properly at birth, the hemodynamic equilibrium becomes disturbed. The blood fails to pass through the lungs because of increased resistance, and is shunted to the aorta descendens through the ductus arteriosus, which remains open or reopens." Lind and Wegelius's 1954 report[189a] included what appears to be the first published angiographic demonstration of neonatal right-to-left ductal shunt.

Also in 1954, Eldridge, Hultgren, and Wigmore[81a] observed lower extremity cyanosis in newborn infants and postulated that "this cyanosis of the lower extremities occasionally seen in the newborn might be due to a flow of blood in the fetal direction through an open ductus."

Stimulated by this observation, Eldridge, Hultgren, and Wigmore measured simultaneous arterial saturations in room air in the hands and feet at various times after birth and documented lower saturations in the lower extremities through 3 days of age. In a subsequent study[82] published the following year, they placed normal newborn infants in 12 per cent oxygen, observed greater falls in arterial saturations in the lower extremities than in the upper extremities, and concluded that hypoxia caused right-to-left ductal shunting in normal newborns. Also in 1955 Berglund[22] angiographically demonstrated right-to-left atrial shunt in an infant with respiratory distress and Berglund, Korlberg, and Lind[23] reported similar findings in additional infants with respiratory distress. Yet again in 1955 Prec and Cassels[240] demonstrated peculiar diphasic dye dilution curves in 7 of 24 normal newborns studied within 26 hours of birth. These peculiar diphasic curves were characterized by a small initial curve, followed by a much larger second curve after a time interval appropriate for recirculation, and were interpreted as suggesting that only part of the dye reached the sampling site (the ear) on the first pass. They suggested that right-to-left ductal shunt accounted for this phenomenon.[240]

In 1957 James and Rowe[153] reported the effects of hypoxia on pulmonary artery pressure in normal newborns and suggested that "venous blood was almost certainly shunting from the pulmonary artery into the aorta during the hypoxic period." In that same paper, they also noted right-to-left atrial shunts and concluded that:

If the neonatal circulatory adjustments involving the lungs and the ductus have taken place, the response to hypoxia will be the same as in the older infants and adults. However, if this readjustment is incomplete, a short period of anoxia may produce a dramatic change in the circulatory dynamics, so that venous blood may by-pass the lungs at both the foramen ovale and ductus arteriosus level, producing a precipitous fall in arterial saturation.[153]

Also in 1957 Adams and Lind[1a] reported cardiac catheterization findings in eight normal newborns and noted right-to-left shunts and systemic pulmonary artery pressures in some infants. In that same year Mitchell[210a] reported that anatomic closure of the ductus arteriosus takes place at 7 days of age; included in her paper were the case history of an infant with trisomy 21 and complete atrioventricular septal defect who exhibited persistent cyanosis and a frame from his right ventriculogram, which demonstrated right-to-left ductal shunt. Mitchell's angiocardiogram was probably the second published angiographic demonstration of right-to-left ductal shunting in the newborn.

In 1959 Rowe described ill newborns with right-to-left ductal and atrial shunting, noted associations with various types of cardiac and pulmonary disease, and termed such persistence of fetal circulatory patterns a "transitional circulation."[249] In 1961 Rudolph et al[260] documented right-to-left atrial shunting and occasionally right-to-left ductal shunting in infants with respiratory distress syndrome. Also in 1961 James, Burnard, and Rowe[152] observed that asphyxia caused transitory left-to-right atrial shunting as well. In 1964, 10 years after publishing what was probably the first angiographic demonstration of right-to-left ductal shunting in a newborn infant, Lind, Stern, and Wegelius[188] published another angiographic demonstration of right-to-

Table 51–1. NAMES FOR PERSISTENT POSTNATAL RIGHT-TO-LEFT DUCTAL SHUNTING, RIGHT-TO-LEFT ATRIAL SHUNTING, OR BOTH

Name	Acronym	Reference	Year
La persistance du canal arterial avec hypertension pulmonaire	—	227	1950
Transitional circulation	—	249	1959
Reversed ductus syndrome	—	188	1964
Hypoperfusion syndrome	—	56	1965
Neonatal pulmonary ischemia	—	49	1967
Pulmonary hypoperfusion syndrome	—	168	1969
Persistent fetal circulation	PFC	108	1969
Persistent pulmonary vascular obstruction	—	279	1971
Progressive pulmonary hypertension	—	41	1972
Primary pulmonary hypertension in infants	—	305	1973
Persistent transitional circulation	—	33	1974
Syndrome of persistent pulmonary vascular obstruction of the newborn	—	16	1974
Persistence of the fetal cardiopulmonary pathway	—	179	1975
Persistence of the fetal circulation	—	19	1976
Persistent fetal cardiopulmonary circulation	—	35	1976
Persistent transitional circulation syndrome	—	226	1976
Primary pulmonary hypertension of the newborn	—	200	1976
Persistent pulmonary hypertension of the newborn	PPHN	180	1976
Persistent fetal circulation syndrome	—	95	1977
Persistence of fetal circulation syndrome	—	247	1977
Pulmonary vasoreactive hypoxemia	—	281	1981
Persistence of the fetal circulation syndrome	—	105	1982
Persistent pulmonary hypertension syndrome of the newborn	—	245	1982
Persistent pulmonary hypertension syndrome	—	285a	1985
Persistent neonatal pulmonary hypertension	—	317	1986
Persistent pulmonary hypertension of the newborn syndrome	PPHNS	this chapter	1989

left ductal shunting in a newborn (Fig. 51–1), termed such shunting the "reversed ductus syndrome," and noted that "anything which will either raise the pulmonary artery pressure or lower the systemic arterial pressure can reverse the flow in the ductus and revert it to the foetal situation." Lind and his colleagues subsequently published detailed descriptions of postnatal right-to-left ductal and atrial shunting.[304,318] Also in 1964, Rowe and colleagues[253] showed that 10 per cent oxygen reopened the ductus, increased left-to-right shunt, and caused systemic pulmonary artery pressures in newborn piglets, but right-to-left ductal shunting was not detected. Stahlman[290] reported in 1964 that large right-to-left atrial shunts occurred in one half of infants with moderate respiratory distress syndrome, that small right-to-left atrial shunts occurred in another one third of infants with moderate respiratory distress syndrome, and that one fifth of infants with moderate respiratory distress syndrome had right-to-left ductal shunts. In 9 of 10 infants with severe respiratory distress syndrome, Stahlman observed extrapulmonary right-to-left shunting.[290] Both right-to-left atrial and ductal shunts were present in half the infants with severe respiratory distress syndrome, which Stahlman said implied "persistent levels of pulmonary artery pressure exceeding aortic."[290] Stahlman also noted extrapulmonary right-to-left shunts in all infants with meconium aspiration (including some instances of right-to-left ductal shunting) and termed this syndrome "acute cor pulmonale associated with meconium aspiration pneumonia."[290] The following year Stahlman et al[290a] noted that "Situations, therefore, which either increase pulmo-

nary resistance or lower systemic resistance, or both, will promote resumption of the fetal direction of shunting through both the foramen ovale and ductus arteriosus."

In 1969 Gersony, Duc, and Sinclair[108] described two newborns with pulmonary hypertension and right-to-left ductal shunting and coined the term "persistent fetal circulation"; subsequently, the acronym PFC gained wide usage to describe this syndrome. After their description, the syndrome of persistent fetal circulatory patterns became widely recognized, and a large number of clinical and experimental observations have followed, including reports from journals all over the world,[242,310] and recent descriptions of the syndrome in horses.[55,70]

Thus, a great many different individuals independently recognized PPHNS. Although Gersony, Duc, and Sinclair certainly published the paper that brought PPHNS to general attention, Sir William Harvey should be credited with discovering the syndrome; and Novelo and his colleagues, Lind and his colleagues, Eldridge and his colleagues, and Rowe and his colleagues deserve much credit for independently rediscovering the syndrome in modern times.

TERMINOLOGY

Postnatal persistence of right-to-left ductal shunting, right-to-left atrial shunting, or both has been given many different names (Table 51–1). The most popular name for this syndrome has been persistent fetal circulation, or PFC, probably because persistent fetal circulation was the term used by the authors who brought the syndrome to general attention[108] and because persistent fetal circulation is self-explanatory, easy to say, and yields a concise and memorable acronym (PFC). However, strictly speaking, the term persistent fetal circulation is not accurate because the placenta is not part of the postnatal circulation in neonates who exhibit persistent right-to-left ductal shunting, right-to-left atrial shunting, or both. Others have suggested that "persistent pulmonary hypertension of the newborn" would be a more accurate designation,[71,180,307] but strictly speaking this latter term is also inaccurate—many infants who do not have pulmonary hypertension exhibit similar physiology. Recently Gersony suggested that persistent pulmonary hypertension of the newborn would be the appropriate term for cases of persistent fetal circulatory patterns due to identifiable predisposing factors and that the term persistent fetal circulation should be reserved for idiopathic cases.[106]

In this chapter and throughout this book a new terminology will be employed. Postnatal persistence of right-to-left ductal shunting, right-to-left atrial shunting, or both will be termed "persistent pulmonary hypertension of the newborn syndrome," or PPHNS. Idiopathic cases will not be termed persistent fetal circulation but instead "idiopathic PPHNS." This terminology has been adopted because postnatal persistence of right-to-left ductal shunting or right-to-left atrial shunting or both is not a disease but a common physiologic response to a wide variety of disorders, many of which are not even accompanied by pulmonary hypertension. As long as indirect diagnostic criteria are used in place of pulmonary arterial pressure measurements, newborns who may or may not actually have elevated pulmonary arterial pressures but who do have other reasons for right-to-left atrial or ductal shunting will be incorrectly categorized as having persistent pulmonary hypertension if the term persistent pulmonary hypertension of the newborn is used. Newborns exhibiting circulatory patterns similar to those of fetal life should not be presumed to have persistent pulmonary hypertension. For these reasons, persistent right-to-left ductal shunting or right-to-left atrial shunting or both can be most accurately described as persistent pulmonary hypertension of the newborn syndrome, or PPHNS.

DEFINITION

PPHNS is characterized by postnatal persistence of right-to-left ductal shunting or right-to-left atrial shunting or both. These extrapulmonary right-to-left shunts result in cyanosis, which often proves refractory to supplemental oxygen. Pulmonary arterial pressures in infants with PPHNS can be elevated,[108] normal,[246] or reduced. In most cases of PPHNS, pulmonary arterial pressures are elevated and are in fact responsible for the extrapulmonary right-to-left shunts. However, in an important minority of PPHNS cases, identical physiology is present, as determined by noninvasive means, and the extrapulmonary right-to-left shunts are unrelated to the status of the pulmonary circulation. Pulmonary arterial pressures in such cases can be elevated, normal, or even low.

DIAGNOSTIC CRITERIA

In the two idiopathic PPHNS cases described by Gersony, Duc, and Sinclair,[108] pulmonary hypertension was proved by pulmonary pressure measurements at cardiac catheterization. Angiographic demonstration of right-to-left ductal shunting has also been thought to be diagnostic of pulmonary hypertension, but of course this concept is inaccurate. The combination of systemic hypotension, normal neonatal pulmonary arterial pressures, and a patent ductus arteriosus can result in right-to-left ductal shunting that is angiographically indistinguishable from that due to pulmonary hypertension.[246] Since cardiac catheterization in newborns with PPHNS is largely reserved for research protocols,[103,307] noninvasive evidence of right-to-left ductal or atrial shunting (such as positive right radial–umbilical arterial oxygen gradients, or right-to-left atrial passage of contrast on echocardiography) has come to be accepted as evidence of the presence of pulmonary hypertension. However, much of the confusion in the literature on PPHNS can be attributed to the fact that there has been little agreement on what diagnostic criteria must be met to make the diagnosis of PPHNS. On the other hand, early diagnosis of PPHNS appears to be important; in Hageman et al's study of 62 infants with PPHNS,[124] 80 per cent of infants diagnosed prior to 6 hours of age survived (35 of 44), whereas only 50 per cent of those diagnosed after 6 hours of age survived (9 of 18). However, the conclusion that early diagnosis accounted for this difference has been questioned.[272]

Cardiac Catheterization

The most conclusive diagnostic test in PPHNS is cardiac catheterization. Documentation of systemic or suprasystemic pressures in the pulmonary artery is unassailable evidence of PPHNS. Of course, normal pulmonary arterial pressures vary with postnatal age.[85,252] Angiographic demonstration of right-to-left ductal shunting is also diagnostic of PPHNS, but of course not diagnostic of pulmonary hypertension because right-to-left shunting through the ductus arteriosus can occur with normal newborn pulmonary artery pressures if systemic hypotension is severe.[246] Detailed angiographic studies demonstrate that most ductal shunts are bidirectional, though flow in one direction usually predominates.[289] Right-to-left ductal shunting can be diagnosed angiographically by left heart injections (Fig. 51–2) as well as right heart injections (see Fig 51–1). However, the hazards and expense of cardiac catheterization restrict its use in PPHNS to either investigational protocols[103,307] or to exclusion of congenital heart disease when noninvasive methods fail.[106] The diagnostic criteria for PPHNS outlined in the following sections are either less sensitive or less specific than cardiac catheterization but

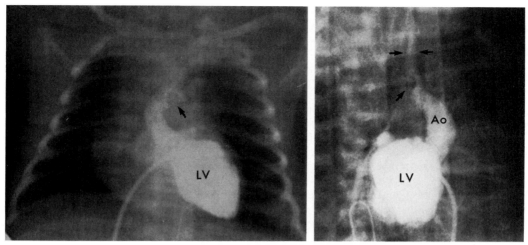

Figure 51–2. Left ventriculogram. First published (1984) angiocardiographic demonstration of a "negative jet" in PPHNS from unopacified pulmonary arterial blood retrogradely perfusing the aortic arch. In such infants positive arterial PO_2 gradients between the right radial artery and umbilical artery are often absent. In this infant pulmonary hypertension was secondary to left ventricular failure caused by congenital endocardial fibroelastosis. The single arrow in the left panel and the lower arrow in the right panel point out the "negative jet;" the upper arrows in the right panel point out the right carotid artery. Note left ventricular dilation at end-systole. LV = left ventricle. (Reproduced with permission from Long, WA [1984]. Structural cardiovascular abnormalities presenting as persistent pulmonary hypertension of the newborn. Clin Perinatol 11:601–626.)

nevertheless very useful as long as the limitations of each approach are recognized.

Physical Examination

Differential Cyanosis

The presence of obvious differential cyanosis can be considered pathognomonic for PPHNS. Typical findings are present when the right arm and head remain pink, while the left arm and lower body are cyanotic. Changes in pulmonary vascular resistance, systemic vascular resistance, left heart function, or right heart function can cause migration of the cyanosis. For example, additional deterioration in left heart function or further elevation in pulmonary vascular resistance can be inferred from spreading of cyanosis to include the head and right arm. Conversely, improvement in left heart function or diminution of pulmonary vascular resistance can be inferred from disappearance of cyanosis from the left arm and eventually the lower body. Unfortunately, despite the very high specificity of differential cyanosis for PPHNS, this finding is relatively rare and thus lacks sensitivity.

Loud Pulmonic Valve Closure

When pulmonary hypertension is present, closure of the pulmonary valve is more forceful than normal; as a result, the second component of the second heart sound (P_2) is accentuated. Clinical detection of a loud P_2 has been considered sufficient for diagnosis of PPHNS in at least two studies,[144,184] and the utility of the loudness of P_2 in both diagnosis and management of PPHNS was recently re-emphasized.[136] Loud pulmonic closure is most reliably detected when splitting of the second sound is heard over the cardiac apex; normally, only aortic closure is heard over the apex. However, reliable detection of any splitting of the second heart sound in tachycardic, mechanically ventilated neonates, much less recognition of a loud P_2 in such infants (not to speak of changes in the intensity of a loud P_2), is beyond the skill of most neonatologists. Pediatric cardiologists are trained to appreciate such subtleties, but usually it is the neonatologist rather than the pediatric cardiologist who is at the bedside taking care of the patient. Observers untrained in cardiac physical diagnosis are likely to attribute any loud sound in the pulmonic area to pulmonary hypertension, when in reality the loud sound in the pulmonary area (depending upon whether or not both components of the second sound are present) could reflect anything from a normal heart to aortic atresia, to pulmonary atresia, to transposition of the great vessels, to truncus arteriosus. In addition, some infants with PPHNS have such severe pulmonary hypertension that the right ventricle is unable to open the pulmonary valve at all.[282] Further, in other infants with PPHNS, pulmonary hypertension may or may not be present, but the pulmonary valve does not open because of right ventricular dysfunction, tricuspid valve incompetence, or pulmonary atresia. Thus, quantification of the intensity of pulmonary valve closure lacks both sensitivity and specificity as a diagnostic test for PPHNS.

Oximetry

Positive PO₂ Gradients

Another excellent diagnostic criterion for PPHNS is occurrence of a positive PO_2 gradient between the right radial artery and the descending aorta.[94,192,307] In a study of 110 infants with respiratory difficulties, only five exhibited a greater than 20 mmHg difference in upper and lower extremity PO_2,[268] so such gradients are relatively rare. Positive PO_2 gradients greater than 10 to 15 mmHg between the right radial artery and the descending aorta are usually considered indicative of PPHNS.[27,94,148,192] However, simultaneous sampling of oxygen tensions in the right arm and descending aorta does not assess right-to-left atrial shunts, nor does it identify pulmonary hypertension when the arterial duct is closed. Further, simultaneous right radial and descending aorta PO_2 determinations cannot be used to diagnosis PPHNS when the right ventricle is perfusing (via the arterial duct) both the right arm and the descending aorta.[192] In addition, if high thoracic umbilical arterial catheters are used, false-positive right radial–umbilical arterial positive PO_2 gradients can occur if the tip of the catheter crosses the arterial duct into the pulmonary artery;[5] such a possibility can be excluded by comparing right radial, umbilical arterial, and posterior tibial PO_2. Thus, a positive PO_2 gradient between the right radial artery and the descending aorta, like differential cyanosis, is virtually 100 per cent specific for PPHNS (unless a high umbilical catheter is used), but this finding is not highly sensitive.

Positive transcutaneous PO_2 gradients between the right upper chest and lower body are also diagnostic of PPHNS,[30,37,61,135,329,335] but caution is warranted in interpreting results if tolazoline is being administered.[228a] Oxygen saturations of capillary blood are useful in diagnosing congenital heart disease.[147] However, fetal hemoglobin is fully saturated at low PO_2 levels; as a result, transcutaneous arterial saturation gradients between the upper and lower body are more useful in following than diagnosing PPHNS.

Negative PO_2 Gradients

In other infants with severe pulmonary hypertension, including those with transposition of the great vessels, Taussig-Bing double outlet right ventricle, and supracardiac obstructed total anomalous pulmonary venous drainage, oxygen saturation values in the pulmonary artery exceed those of the ascending aorta. In such cases right-to-left ductal shunting is indicated by negative rather than positive PO_2 gradients between the right arm and descending aorta, i.e., umbilical arterial PO_2 is higher than right radial PO_2. The occurrence of such negative PO_2 gradients[15] is rare, but nevertheless diagnostic for PPHNS,[191,333] and more importantly, diagnostic for major structural congenital heart disease.

Hyperoxia Test

In the past, documenting a rise in arterial PO_2 above 100 mmHg during inhalation of 100 per cent oxygen was thought to exclude cyanotic congenital heart disease,[174,175,302] and to suggest that PPHNS was not present.[27,96] In a series of 386 infants under 1 year of age, Jones et al[157] found that in 8 of 109 infants with cyanotic congenital heart disease, hyperoxia caused arterial PO_2 in excess of 100 mmHg, and in two infants with cyanotic congenital heart disease, hyperoxia raised arterial PO_2 in excess of 150 mmHg. Jones et al[157] also noted that all infants with acyanotic congenital heart disease (many types of which can cause PPHNS [see Tables 51–2 to 51–7]) had arterial PO_2 in excess of

150 mmHg in hyperoxia but that only 7 of 23 infants with lung disease had arterial PO_2 in excess of 150 mmHg in hyperoxia. A recent reappraisal suggested that the hyperoxia test still had value.[333] Nevertheless, the level of hyperoxia-induced arterial PO_2 asserted to exclude the presence of congenital heart disease has steadily risen in recent years; exceptions to every PO_2 level claimed to exclude congenital heart disease have become apparent. We have observed arterial PO_2 levels in excess of 350 mmHg on 100 per cent oxygen in infants with the hypoplastic left-heart syndrome and PPHNS. Even infants with transposition of the great vessels[15] and infradiaphragmatic total anomalous pulmonary venous drainage[194] may have descending aorta PO_2 values greater than 200 mmHg, and some infants with both idiopathic and secondary PPHNS have dramatic increases in arterial PO_2 with oxygen alone. A recent review concluded that a less than 20 mmHg change in arterial PO_2 on 100 per cent oxygen can indicate either congenital heart disease or severe PPHNS;[307] similar refractory hypoxemia can be seen in severe lung disease as well. In fact, the predictive value of changes in arterial PO_2 on 100 per cent oxygen in separation of heart disease and lung disease, or in identification of PPHNS among such infants, is poor.[192,333] Yabek[333] has pointed out the physiology behind large increases in arterial PO_2 during hyperoxia in some newborns with cyanotic congenital heart disease. On the other hand, measurement of umbilical venous PO_2 during inhalation of 100 per cent oxygen can be quite useful in determining which infants with PPHNS have infradiaphragmatic total anomalous pulmonary venous drainage.[84,192,194,283]

Hyperoxia-CPAP Test

Shannon et al introduced a modification of the hyperoxia test in an attempt to improve its sensitivity and specificity.[275] Applying 10 cm H_2O constant positive airway pressure (CPAP) via facemask appeared to provide greater separation of cardiac and lung disease in neonates.[275] However, Yabek has recently noted that large increases in arterial PO_2 during the hyperoxia-CPAP test cannot exclude cyanotic congenital heart disease.[333] At the time of Shannon et al's publication (1976), the fact that PPHNS occurs among both infants with lung disease and infants with heart disease was not recognized. However, in an accompanying editorial[307a] published in 1976, Tooley and Stanger observed that CPAP could markedly increase arterial PO_2 in infants with the hypoplastic left-heart syndrome, one of the structural cardiac disorders now known to cause PPHNS.[192,249] Subsequently, Rao et al[243] have found that the hyperoxia-CPAP test cannot differentiate idiopathic PPHNS from congenital heart disease;[243] such differentiation is of course impossible when PPHNS is secondary to congenital heart disease.

Hyperoxia-Hyperventilation Test

More recently, dramatic increases in arterial PO_2 with hyperventilation have been asserted to be the best diagnostic criterion for PPHNS.[74,96,124,307] In this test, the infant is hyperventilated at fast rates and whatever pressures are necessary to achieve a PCO_2 in the low 20s and a pH higher than 7.55. Arterial PO_2 increases of 50^{307} to 100^{124} mmHg have been considered diagnostic of PPHNS. One publication has asserted that the magnitude of PO_2 response to the hyperoxia-hyperventilation test is predictive of the type of PPHNS; those infants who respond with an increase in PO_2 from less than 100 mmHg to greater than 200 mmHg have idiopathic PPHNS, and those who respond with an increase to between 150 and 200 mmHg have secondary PPHNS.[123]

Despite the common misconception that hyperventilation should provide no additional increase in arterial PO_2 over 100 per cent oxygen in infants with congenital heart disease, increases in arterial PO_2 above 200 mmHg during hyperventilation have been reported in infants with PPHNS secondary to transposition of the great vessels[15] and PPHNS secondary to obstructed total anomalous pulmonary venous drainage.[98,192,194] Further, in some infants with refractory PPHNS, neither hyperventilation, or anything else for that matter, will elevate arterial PO_2 above 100 mmHg. In other infants without PPHNS but with significant lung or cardiac disease, hyperventilation will dramatically increase arterial PO_2.[192] Thus, the hyperoxia-hyperventilation test is not sufficiently accurate to be blindly relied upon in diagnosis of PPHNS. Further, intubating and hyperventilating infants in an attempt to diagnose PPHNS when clinical circumstances do not call for such aggressive measures is inappropriate. Noninvasive diagnostic approaches to PPHNS are far preferable.

Refractory Hypoxemia

Persistent hypoxemia despite aggressive medical management has also been used as a diagnostic criterion for PPHNS.[313] However, this criterion is unreliable because infants without PPHNS but with refractory lung disease or cyanotic congenital heart disease often exhibit persistent hypoxemia.

Electrocardiogram

Presence of an abnormal electrocardiogram (ECG) has been said to differentiate congenital heart disease from PPHNS.[190] However, infants with idiopathic PPHNS can exhibit electrocardiographic abnormalities.[94,136] Further, the ECG can be normal in infants with PPHNS secondary to congenital[195,306] or acquired[29,251] heart disease. As discussed earlier, at least five groups of congenital heart diseases can present as PPHNS,[192] and in most such cases the ECG is abnormal. Thus, an abnormal ECG cannot separate PPHNS from congenital heart disease because congenital heart disease is one of the most important causes of PPHNS. Further, an abnormal ECG occurs in idiopathic PPHNS, and a normal ECG occurs in infants with PPHNS secondary to cardiac disease.

On the other hand, there are electrocardiographic abnormalities that can be quite useful in identifying infants with PPHNS in whom congenital heart disease is present. Electrocardiographic evidence of left axis deviation or left ventricular hypertrophy in infants with PPHNS appears to be pathognomonic (100 per cent specific) for underlying congenital heart disease, although only 30 per cent sensitive.[221]

Rebreathing Techniques

Rebreathing studies have been reported to differentiate congenital heart disease from PPHNS.[99] However, as considered previously, at least five groups of congenital heart diseases can present as PPHNS,[192] and it is unlikely that rebreathing techniques could distinguish which infants with PPHNS have underlying congenital heart disease and which do not.

Echocardiography

M-Mode Echocardiography: Systolic Time Intervals

Several M-mode echocardiogaphic findings, including mid-systolic partial closure of the pulmonary valve ("notching"), delayed opening of the pulmonary valve, and lack of atrial opening of the pulmonary valve in early systole, are indicative of pulmonary hypertension when present, particularly in the adult. Some suggest that systolic time intervals are the most reliable M-mode indicators of pulmonary hypertension in newborn infants.[156,247,313] In a prospective study of 115 normal neonates and 51 neonates requiring FiO_2 greater than 0.25, all 10 infants diagnosed as having PPHNS but none of the others had prolonged systolic ejection times of both ventricles (RPEP/RVET > 0.50; LPEP/LVET > 0.38).[313] However, neither delayed right ventricular emptying alone or delayed left ventricular emptying alone predicted PPHNS. Further, despite suggestions to the contrary in a previous study,[247] systolic time intervals did not predict clinical course or clinical outcome.[313]

In addition, one of the two criteria for diagnosis of PPHNS in the latter study[313] was suspect. The criterion of severe right-to-left atrial shunting demonstrated by peripheral venous injection of contrast material from the right arm or hand was acceptable (see the following), but the criterion of increasing hypoxemia despite FiO_2 equaling 1.0, respiratory paralysis, and full mechanical ventilatory support (i.e., refractory hypoxemia) permitted diagnosis of infants with refractory lung disease (or even congenital heart disease) as having PPHNS.

In view of the latter criterion, it is perhaps not surprising that none of the 10 infants diagnosed as having PPHNS in that study[313] had positive right radial–umbilical arterial PO_2 gradients—a "harder" diagnostic criterion. Although some believe that prolongation of systolic time intervals in both ventricles is probably a valid M-mode diagnostic criterion for PPHNS, the relationship between systolic time intervals and pulmonary artery pressure is probably too variable (see Chapter 25) to be relied upon for diagnosis of PPHNS, and better diagnostic methods are available (see below).

Contrast M-Mode Echocardiography

M-mode detection of right-to-left atrial shunting with contrast injections, even when combined with careful analysis of the time sequence in which the various chambers opacify, lacks predictive value in diagnosis of PPHNS.[207]

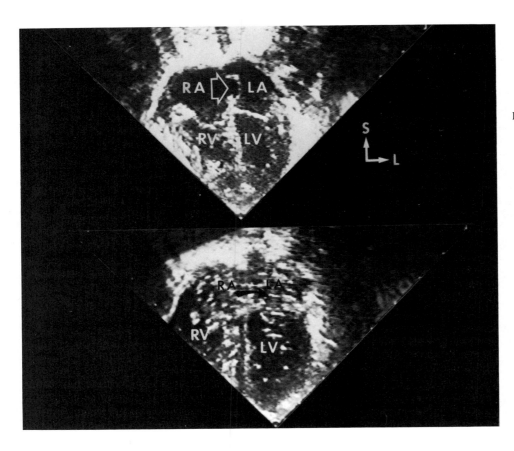

Figure 51–3. Two-dimensional contrast echocardiographic demonstration of right-to-left atrial shunt in an infant with PPHNS. In the *upper panel*, an apical four-chamber view taken immediately prior to contrast injection into a right arm vein, the white arrow points out right-to-left bulging of the atrial septum. In the *lower panel*, an apical four-chamber view taken immediately after contrast injection into a right arm vein, the black arrow indicates passage of contrast across the foramen ovale into the left atrium. Note that left atrial opacification equals right atrial opacification. L = left; LA = left atrium; LV = left ventricle; RA = right atrium; RV = right ventricle; S = superior.

In the great majority of adults with patent foramen ovale, at least some opacification of the left heart is noted on M-mode echocardiography after venous injection of contrast material.[120,162] Nearly all newborns ill with lung disease have right-to-left atrial shunts as seen on contrast M-mode echocardiography.[263,264,313] Further, in one series, 3 of 10[313] and in another series 10 of 10[263] normal newborns exhibited right-to-left atrial passage of contrast material on M-mode echocardiography. Streaming of inferior vena caval blood across the foramen ovale is detectable by angiography[189] and by indicator dilution dye technique[240] for several hours after birth; as a result, lower extremity injections of contrast medium are particularly likely to opacify the left heart,[192,263] as originally observed by Lind and Wegelius.[189a] Thus, contrast M-mode detection of right-to-left atrial shunts cannot be considered diagnostic for PPHNS. However, Valdez-Cruz et al[239] and others[192] have suggested that contrast M-mode echocardiography can be diagnostic of PPHNS when left heart opacification after upper extremity venous injection of saline exceeds right heart opacification, an assertion that is probably true.

Contrast Cross-Sectional Echocardiography

Contrast cross-sectional echocardiography is more useful than contrast M-mode echocardiography in the diagnosis of PPHNS,[192] because contrast cross-sectional echocardiography appears to be less sensitive in detecting right-to-left atrial contrast passage with a patent foramen ovale.[120]

(Other investigators have reported that contrast cross-sectional echocardiography is more sensitive than contrast M-mode echocardiography in detection of atrial septal defects.[97]) In any case some right-to-left atrial passage of contrast is apparent with cross-sectional echocardiography in nearly all sick newborns, particularly after lower extremity injection of saline. Employing a qualitative approach to contrast cross-sectional echocardiographic studies in which left heart opacification after saline injection via an upper extremity vein has to equal (Fig. 51–3) or exceed (see Fig. 51–11B) right heart opacification appears to be a valid criterion for diagnosis of PPHNS. Cross-sectional contrast techniques have been used to detect left-to-right ductal shunts,[83,107,126,128] but are not commonly used to detect right-to-left ductal shunts.

Cross-Sectional Echocardiography: Atrial Septal Position

Determination of the position of the atrial septum with cross-sectional echocardiography accurately indicates whether right and left atrial pressures are approximately equal or whether one atrial pressure is significantly higher than the other (Fig. 51–4). When the atrial septum is bulging right-to-left (Figs. 51–4 and 51–5), it can safely be assumed that right atrial pressure exceeds left atrial pressure and that significant right-to-left atrial shunt (i.e., PPHNS) is present.[192] Infants with poor right ventricular function are diagnosed as having PPHNS by this criterion, whether

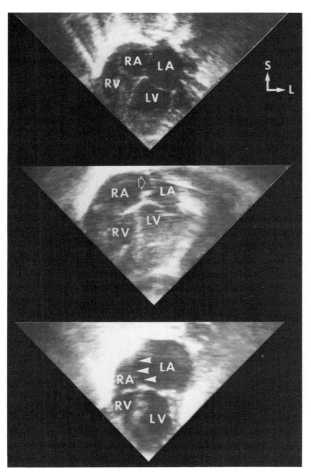

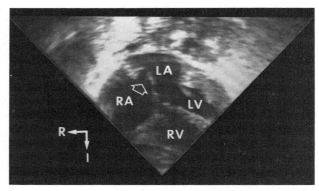

Figure 51–5. Two-dimensional subxiphoid four-chamber echocardiographic demonstration of right-to-left bulging of the atrial septum (at the arrow) in an infant with PPHNS secondary to infradiaphragmatic total anomalous pulmonary venous drainage. Such right-to-left bulging of the atrial septum is diagnostic of PPHNS when it is persistent throughout the cardiac cycle. I = inferior; LA = left atrium; LV = left ventricle; R = right; RA = right atrium; RV = right ventricle.

Figure 51–4. Two-dimensional apical four-chamber echocardiographic demonstration of three different atrial septal positions. In the *top panel*, the atrial septum is in the midline, indicating approximately equal right and left atrial pressures and equal bidirectional atrial shunting. This pattern is seen in infants without PPHNS, or in PPHNS infants with only right-to-left ductal shunting. In the *middle panel*, the atrial septum is bulging right to left (hollow arrow), indicating that right atrial pressure is higher than left atrial pressure and that predominantly right-to-left atrial shunting is present. This pattern is diagnostic of PPHNS and is typical of PPHNS associated with right ventricular dysfunction, lung diseases, or infradiaphramatic total anomalous pulmonary venous drainage. In the *lower panel*, the atrial septum is bulging left to right (solid arrow heads), indicating that left atrial pressure is higher than right atrial pressure and that predominantly left-to-right atrial shunting is present. This pattern is virtually diagnostic of congenital heart disease (whether or not PPHNS is present) and is typical of PPHNS (as documented by right-to-left ductal shunting) associated with left ventricular dysfunction, coarctation, or interrupted arch. Thus, even when PPHNS is already proved by documentation of right-to-left ductal shunt, determining atrial septal position still provides important information. L = left; LA = left atrium; LV = left ventricle; RA = right atrium; RV = right ventricle; S = superior.

or not elevation of pulmonary vascular resistance is responsible for right ventricular dysfunction, because the position of the atrial septum is a function not only of the afterloads of the two ventricles but also of ventricular filling capacities.[169]

Left-to-right bulging of the atrial septum (see Fig. 51–4) is a very important sign in infants with respiratory distress

whether or not simultaneous right radial and umbilical arterial PO$_2$ indicates PPHNS because the atrial septum bulges left-to-right when left ventricular dysfunction is present, whether it is congenital or acquired. When left-to-right bulging of the atrial septum and positive PO$_2$ gradients between the right radial artery and umbilical artery coexist, some form of heart disease is responsible for PPHNS.[192]

Doppler and Color Flow Doppler

Echocardiography Doppler techniques can accurately determine the direction and velocity of blood flow in both the fetus (see Chapter 14) and newborn (see Chapter 25) and is finding increasing use.[67,198] Doppler techniques are particularly valuable in assessing both the direction and magnitude of ductal shunt,[49a] but are also valuable in assessing atrial shunts.[330] When the arterial duct is well visualized by two-dimensional echocardiography (Fig. 51–6), placement of a pulse Doppler probe within the duct permits remarkably accurate assessment of both right-to-left and left-to-right shunts.[49a] Similar sampling at the foramen ovale is routine. As a result, demonstrations of right-to-left atrial and ductal shunts with Doppler and color flow Doppler echocardiography are increasingly useful in the diagnosis of PPHNS. Doppler is also useful in noninvasive estimation of pulmonary artery pressures[163] (see Chapter 25) and is more accurate than M-mode estimates derived from systolic time intervals.[298]

EPIDEMIOLOGY

The incidence of PPHNS is not well characterized, but there is little doubt that the syndrome is fairly rare. Goetzman and Riemenschneider have estimated that PPHNS occurs in 1 per 1500 live births,[113] which would mean that approximately 2300 cases occur in the United States each year. In concert with this estimate, Brown and Pickering

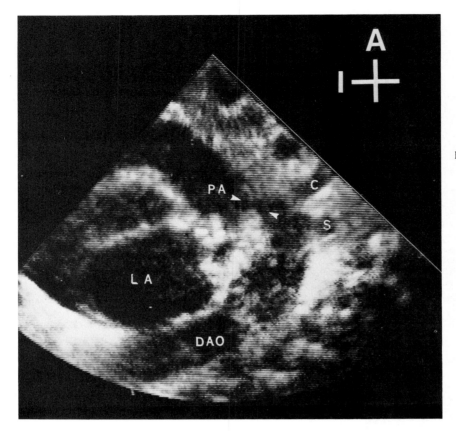

Figure 51–6. High parasternal two-dimensional echocardiographic demonstration of the arterial duct. When the arterial duct can be so visualized, determining the direction of flow in the duct is straightforward with pulse Doppler ultrasound (see Chapters 25 and 30). If right-to-left ductal shunt predominates, the diagnosis of PPHNS can be made with confidence. A = anterior; C = carotid artery; DAO = descending aorta; I = inferior; LA = left atrium; PA = pulmonary artery; S = subclavian artery.

noted a PPHNS incidence of 1 per 1454 live births.[33] In contrast, Philips et al[57,236] have estimated that 6000 idiopathic cases occur in the United States each year and that several times that number of secondary cases occur each year.

The incidence of PPHNS among admissions to neonatal intensive care units is much higher. Wille et al[329] noted 7 cases among 345 admissions, for an incidence of 2 per cent; Heritage and Cunningham[138] noted 71 cases among 1257 admissions, for an incidence of 5.6 per cent; Horgan et al[144] noted 48 cases among 535 full-term admissions, for an incidence of 9 per cent.

Although data from many publications have demonstrated that PPHNS occurs more commonly in males, this fact has escaped comment until recently.[144,241a] Geographical differences may also exist, probably as a result of differences in altitude; the incidence of PPHNS in Denver appears to be high (Kurt Stenmark, personal communication). The great majority of PPHNS cases have identifiable predisposing factors; idiopathic PPHNS accounts for only approximately 1 in 5 cases. In any case, most neonates who develop PPHNS are term infants who experienced either acute or chronic intrauterine asphyxia. PPHNS remains an important cause of neonatal death in term infants.[79]

NATURAL HISTORY

In most cases PPHNS runs a relatively short course culminating in either death or complete recovery. However, prolonged courses have been described.[41,42] Neurologic outcome in survivors appears to be good even in hyperventilated infants,[12,24,32,34,271] but chronic lung disease is an increasing problem[18,96,129] and both cerebral infarction[167] and sensorineural hearing loss[224] have been reported. Even an association with later sudden infant death syndrome has been suggested.[314] Prognosis depends on the underlying cause and is probably better in idiopathic cases. Treatment, which is fully covered in Chapter 55, is best directed at gently correcting hypothermia, hypoxia and acidosis; treating any underlying diseases; and waiting for the infant to improve spontanously. As a general rule, less therapy is better therapy; time is a much better treatment than any currently approved therapy. Making the diagnosis of PPHNS does not dictate use of hyperoxia or aggressive mechanical ventilation; both are toxic and should be instituted only when absolutely necessary. Instead, infants with PPHNS should be managed as gently and noninvasively as possible. My own bias is that surfactant deficiency[125,150,334] and pulmonary vasospasm play critical roles in most cases of PPHNS and that prostacyclin[159,194c] and surfactant replacement therapy[195a] will eventually replace hyperoxia, tolazoline,[2–4,26, 52,72,73,111,112,134,146,165,170,214,261,295–297,310,319,320] hyperventilation,[87,197,215,287] nitroprusside,[20] dopamine,[69,110,134] other drugs,[172,199,312,324] paralysis,[137,265] and extracorporeal membrane oxygenator (ECMO) therapy[8,14] in treatment of PPHNS. Indeed, some centers do manage PPHNS infants successfully without aggressive intervention.[332] Certainly, the reductions in functional residual capacity and pulmonary compliance observed in infants with PPHNS[278] should

Table 51–2. PULMONARY DISORDERS ASSOCIATED WITH PPHNS

Pulmonary Disease	Right-to-Left Ductal Shunt	Right-to-Left Atrial Shunt	Reference
Meconium aspiration	+	+	71, 77, 95, 118, 122, 141, 177 222
Amniotic fluid aspiration	+	+	95
Blood aspiration	+	+	95, 124, 125
Hyaline membrane disease	+	+	49, 114, 168, 184, 203, 208, 212, 241, 248, 260, 290, 290a, 291, 295, 299a, 299b
Transient tachypnea	+	+	35
Diaphragmatic hernia	+	+	50, 53, 64, 81, 92, 100, 103, 185, 213, 214, 276, 299, 302, 327
Pulmonary infection	+	+	212
Pulmonary hypoplasia	+	+	178, 223, 303
Tracheoesophageal fistula	+	+	100
Misalignment of pulmonary vessels	+	+	317
Microthrombi	+	+	144, 184, 216
Peripheral pulmonary vascular occlusion	+	+	204
Thromboemboli	+	+	11, 216
Congenital alveolar dysplasia	+	+	205, 206
Congenital alveolar capillary dysplasia	+	+	155, 166
Phrenic nerve agenesis	+	+	117
Phlebectasia	+	+	230
Diaphragmatic amyoplasia	+	+	117
Surfactant deficiency	+	+	125, 150, 334
Chest tubes	+	+	53
Pulmonary hemorrhage	+	+	213
Cystic adenomatoid malformation	+	+	234

respond to surfactant and to an effective pulmonary vasodilator. (Despite contrary observations in lambs,[44] pulmonary hypertension appears to reduce pulmonary compliance in human infants [see Chapter 7]). Continuous monitoring of mixed venous saturation would appear to be an excellent way to follow critically ill or deteriorating infants.[161]

ETIOLOGY

PPHNS, like most syndromes, has many different causes (see Table 51–2 to Table 51–8), but the majority of cases are associated with lung disease of one kind or another. Common pathogenetic factors in many of the disorders known to cause PPHNS include acidosis and hypoxia, both of which are powerful neonatal pulmonary vasoconstrictors (see Chapter 7). On the other hand, several types of PPHNS may not be accompanied by pulmonary hypertension.

Idiopathic PPHNS

Approximately one fifth of infants with PPHNS have no known predisposing factors.[68,71] Nevertheless, there can be little doubt that a cause is present in every case of PPHNS, and future investigative efforts are likely to make the unexplained PPHNS group smaller and smaller. In the interim, accurately identifying which cases are truly idiopathic and which cases are secondary to known disorders

is critical, for many secondary forms of PPHNS are completely reversible if the underlying disorder is accurately identified and treated.

Pulmonary Disorders

PPHNS is most commonly observed in association with lung diseases. Although a wide variety of pulmonary diseases can cause PPHNS (Table 51–2), the single most common association with PPHNS is meconium aspiration.[71,118,122,141,177,195] Whether meconium has substances in it that are pulmonary vasoconstrictors is unknown, but even without such substances the combination of intrauterine compromise (signified by intrauterine passage of meconium) and postnatal hypoxia and acidosis is sufficient to account for postnatal pulmonary vasoconstriction in infants with meconium aspiration. PPHNS is also commonly observed in association with diaphragmatic hernia,[53,64,81,100,103,213,226,299,302,327] and hyaline membrane disease,[49,114,184,203,208,241,248,260] and can accompany transient tachypnea of the newborn.[35]

Pulmonary thromboembolism[11,216] is an important but usually neglected pulmonary cause of PPHNS, which should be reversible with thrombolytic therapy if the diagnosis is recognized. The role of microthrombosis in other forms of PPHNS remains largely unexplored, but it is possible that the putative success of ECMO therapy in refractory PPHNS is really due to systemic anticoagulation. The apparent benefit of prostacyclin in some infants with PPHNS[159] could

Table 51–3. CARDIAC DISORDERS ASSOCIATED WITH PPHNS: GROUP 1: OBSTRUCTIONS TO PULMONARY VENOUS DRAINAGE

Lesion	Right-to-Left Ductal Shunt	Right-to-Left Atrial Shunt	Reference
OTAPVD*	+	+	98, 192, 194, 249
Cor triatriatum	+	+	171, 249
Congenital pulmonary venous stenosis	+	+	62
Mitral stenosis	+	–	192, 249

*OTAPVD = obstructed total anomalous pulmonary venous drainage.

be due to prostacyclin's inhibition of platelet aggregation, rather than its pulmonary vasodilating effects.[194c]

Cardiac Disorders

A wide variety of cardiac disorders has been reported to cause PPHNS (see Tables 51–3 to 51–7). The various reported cardiac causes of PPHNS have been grouped into five major types based on the physiology of the lesion.[192] However, the lists of cardiac causes of PPHNS found in Tables 51–3 through 51–7 should not be considered complete because any cardiac lesion that exhibits similar physiology can cause PPHNS.

Group 1: Obstructions to Pulmonary Venous Drainage

Lesions that result in pulmonary venous obstruction cause pulmonary hypertension and are often accompanied by right-to-left ductal shunting if the arterial duct is patent. Whether right-to-left ductal shunting is detectable by oximetry in infants with pulmonary venous obstruction depends on a number of factors considered earlier. Whether pulmonary venous obstruction is accompanied by right-to-left atrial shunting or left-to-right atrial shunting depends on the site of obstruction.

When pulmonary venous obstruction is proximal to the left atrium (as in obstructed total anomalous pulmonary venous drainage), right atrial pressures are elevated, and the right atrium decompresses right-to-left across the atrial septum into the left atrium. When pulmonary venous obstruction is at the mitral valve, as in supravalvular mitral ring and congenital mitral stenosis, left atrial pressures are elevated instead, and left-to-right atrial shunting rather than right-to-left atrial shunting is present.

PPHNS has been reported in association with several types of pulmonary venous obstruction (Table 51–3). One of the most difficult cardiac causes of PPHNS to exclude is obstructed total anomalous pulmonary venous drainage. A number of diagnostic pitfalls have been reported.[98,192,194] For example, despite common misconceptions to the contrary, infants with obstructed total anomalous pulmonary venous drainage below the diaphragm can (and often do) exhibit positive right radial–umbilical arterial PO_2 gradients, arterial PO_2 levels in excess of 200 mmHg, dramatic arterial PO_2 responses to hyperventilation, and spontaneous improvement with successful temporary weaning from mechanical ventilation.[98,192,194] In addition, even pulmo-

nary angiography can fail to demonstrate the anomalous pulmonary venous drainage.[194]

In infradiaphragmatic total anomalous pulmonary venous drainage, as in most lesions accompanied by pulmonary venous obstruction, aortic oxygen saturations are higher than pulmonary artery oxygen saturations.[99a,194] As a result, right-to-left ductal shunts are detectable by positive arterial PO_2 gradients between the right arm and descending aorta.[98,192,194] Despite assertions to the contrary,[86] positive arterial PO_2 gradients between the right arm and descending aorta are common because streaming of oxygenated inferior vena caval blood across the foramen ovale into the left atrium causes higher saturations in the aorta than in the pulmonary artery, and pulmonary venous obstruction causes pulmonary hypertension and right-to-left ductal shunt.[194] In contrast, in infants with supracardiac obstructed total anomalous pulmonary venous drainage, oxygenated blood from the lungs streams from the superior vena cava into the right ventricle and pulmonary artery; as a result, pulmonary artery oxygen saturations exceed aortic saturations, and positive right radial–umbilical arterial PO_2 gradients do not occur. Further, in obstructed supracardiac total anomalous pulmonary venous drainage, changes in pulmonary venous oxygen content are not usually reflected in the systemic arterial blood, and refractory systemic arterial hypoxemia is the rule. However, infants with supracardiac total anomalous pulmonary venous drainage can exhibit negative rather than positive arterial PO_2 gradients between the right arm and umbilical artery if the arterial duct is patent.

The diagnosis of PPHNS can be made readily in infants with any form of obstructed total anomalous pulmonary venous drainage by echocardiographic examination of the position of the atrial septum; marked right-to-left bulging is present (see Fig. 51–5) because the entire left heart output must cross the atrial septum right to left. This flow pattern is nicely demonstrated by color Flow Doppler.[315] Echocardiographic diagnosis of obstructed total anomalous pulmonary venous drainage in infants with PPHNS is usually straightforward (see Chapter 34), but echocardiographic exclusion of that possibility can be difficult. In infants with infradiaphragmatic total anomalous pulmonary venous drainage, the anomalous common pulmonary venous trunk can often be readily visualized within the abdomen by two-dimensional echocardiography (Fig. 51–7), and the identity of that structure can be proved by contrast echocardiography (Fig. 51–8). However, on occasion pulmonary blood flow in infradiaphragmatic total anom-

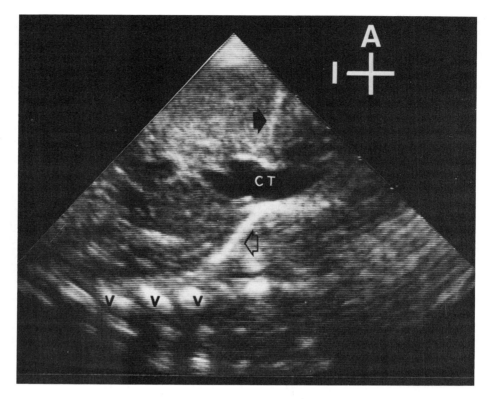

Figure 51–7. Two-dimensional echocardiographic view showing diagnosis of infradiaphragmatic total anomalous pulmonary venous drainage in an infant with PPHNS. The anomalous common pulmonary venous trunk is demonstrated traversing the diaphragm; the black solid and hollow arrows indicate the anterior and posterior aspects of the diaphragm respectively. A = anterior; CT = anomalous common pulmonary venous trunk; I = inferior; V = vertebrae.

alous pulmonary venous drainage is greatly reduced, or even absent,[62] which makes echocardiographic visualization of the anomalous pulmonary venous connection exceedingly difficult. Further, technical problems such as hyperinflation from hyperventilation can interfere with accurate echocardiographic visualization of the pulmonary veins. When echocardiography cannot delineate the drainage of the pulmonary veins, bedside umbilical venous catheterization can make and sometimes exclude the diagnosis of infradiaphragmatic total anomalous pulmonary venous drainage.[194,283,311] Radionuclide angiography (see Chapter 26) can also be used to diagnose infradiaphragmatic total anomalous pulmonary venous drainage.[194b] When other diagnostic methods fail and when obstructed total anomalous pulmonary venous drainage cannot be excluded in infants with PPHNS and a congested chest radiograph, cardiac catheterization must be performed. However, the limitations of cardiac catheterization in both the diagnosis and exclusion of obstructed total anomalous pulmonary venous drainage should be recognized.[192] If pulmonary venous drainage cannot be visualized angiographically, even cardiac catheterization cannot exclude obstructed total anomalous pulmonary venous drainage.[192]

Less common forms of pulmonary venous obstruction that also cause PPHNS include congenital pulmonary venous stenosis[62] and cor triatriatum (Fig. 51–9).

Group 2: Congenital Cardiomyopathies

Congenital as well as acquired cardiomyopathies can present as PPHNS (Table 51–4). Important differences in

the physiology and therefore the diagnosis of cardiomyopathy-induced PPHNS can occur, depending on whether left heart or right heart dysfunction predominates. Infants with cardiomyopathies in whom left ventricular dysfunction predominates are likely to have elevated left atrial pressures, left-to-right bulging of the atrial septum (see Fig. 51–4), minimal right-to-left atrial shunting, and pulmonary hypertension. If the arterial duct is patent in infants with left ventricular dysfunction, the diagnosis of PPHNS can often be made from differential cyanosis or a positive PO_2 gradient between the right arm and descending aorta.[192,193] However, when left ventricular function is exceedingly poor, the right ventricle may perfuse virtually the entire systemic circuit via the ductus arteriosus and prevent any pre- and postductal differences in oxygen tension.[192]

In contrast, when right ventricular dysfunction predominates, whether due to elevated pulmonary vascular resistance or not, right atrial pressures exceed left atrial pressures, the atrial septum bulges right-to-left (see Fig. 51–4), and massive right-to-left atrial shunting occurs (see Figs. 51–3 and 51–11B). Pulmonary hypertension and right-to-left ductal shunting may or may not accompany the ensuing hypoxemia. Simultaneous right radial and descending aorta PO_2 values can be equal if right-to-left ductal shunting is masked by massive right-to-left atrial shunting, which equalizes oxygen tensions in the two great vessels.

When both ventricles are impaired, whether right-to-left ductal shunting is present or right-to-left atrial shunting is present depends on which ventricle is most impaired. If

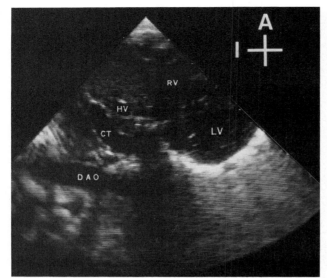

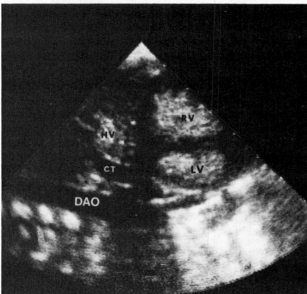

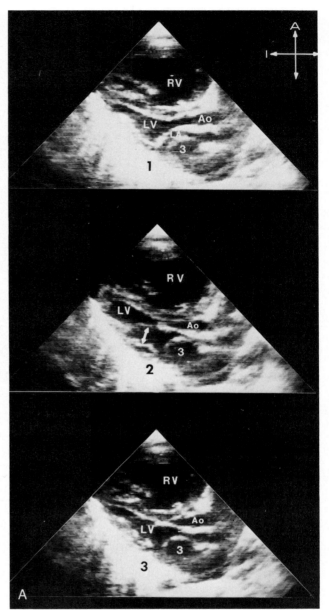

Figure 51–8. Two-dimensional contrast-enhanced echocardiographic view showing diagnosis of infradiaphragmatic total anomalous pulmonary venous drainage in an infant with PPHNS. In the *upper panel*, an epigastric view taken immediately prior to contrast injection into a right foot vein, the anomalous common pulmonary venous trunk was visualized below the diaphragm. In the *lower panel*, an epigastric view taken immediately after contrast injection into a right foot vein, the hepatic vein, right ventricle, and left ventricle opacified, but the anomalous common pulmonary venous trunk did not. In subsequent frames, the descending aorta also opacified, but the anomalous common pulmonary venous trunk never did. Such a contrast pattern is pathognomonic of infradiaphragmatic total anomalous pulmonary venous drainage, for the pulmonary capillary bed filters out contrast. A = anterior; CT = anomalous common pulmonary venous trunk; DAO = descending aorta; HV = hepatic vein; I = inferior; LV = left ventricle; RV = right ventricle.

Figure 51–9. Cor triatriatum, another cause of pulmonary venous obstruction and PPHNS, is illustrated. *A,* The *top frame* (frame 1) is a systolic frame, which demonstrates right ventricular dilation (secondary to pulmonary hypertension) and the membrane dividing the left atrium. The *middle frame* (frame 2) is an early diastolic frame; the anterior and posterior mitral leaflets are indicated by the double arrowhead. The *bottom frame* (frame 3) demonstrates a late diastolic frame; the mitral leaflets are now fully open, and the membrane within the left atrium remains unchanged.

the left ventricle is predominantly affected, as in congenital endocardial fibroelastosis, pulmonary hypertension will occur, and right-to-left ductal shunting (manifest by positive right radial–umbilical arterial PO$_2$ gradients) can be observed.[192,193] If the right ventricle is predominantly affected, as in congenital Pompe disease[192] or in prenatal myocarditis,[193] right-to-left atrial shunting is likely to predominate.

In any case the most common cause of cardiomyopathy-induced PPHNS is asphyxia. Asphyxia can affect either ventricle,[40,43,90] and thus can cause either right-to-left ductal shunts or right-to-left atrial shunts.[36,246] In 1972 Rowe and

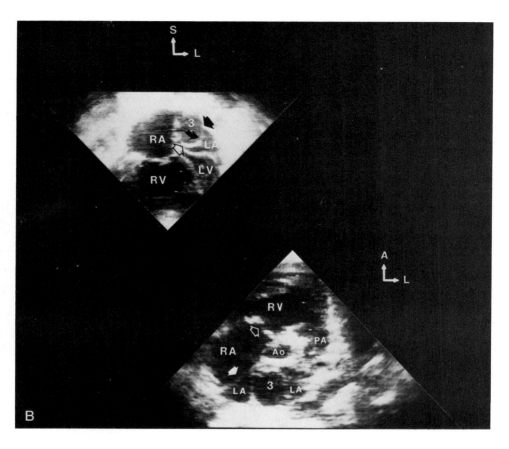

Figure 51–9 *Continued. B,* The *top frame* is an apical four-chamber view demonstrating right ventricular dilation, and the membrane dividing the left atrium and obstructing pulmonary venous return. The curved arrow demonstrates the tiny fenestration in the membrane permitting egress of pulmonary venous blood. The other two arrows indicate the lateral margins of the membrane. The *bottom frame* is a parasternal short axis view demonstrating the "third atrium" within the left atrium. The solid arrow indicates the atrial septum; the hollow arrow indicates the tricuspid valve. A = anterior; Ao = ascending aorta; I = inferior; L = left; LA = left atrium; LV = left ventricle; PA = pulmonary artery; RA = right atrium; RV = right ventricle; 3 = third atrium (cor triatriatum); S = superior.

Hoffman[251] reported three PPHNS infants with cardiomegaly and marked impairment of left ventricular function. All improved dramatically with oxygen, diuretics, and digoxin. Hypoxic pulmonary vasoconstriction was postulated to be responsible for cardiac dysfunction. Since that time, there has been increasing recognition that myocardial dysfunction itself, whether left ventricular or right ventricular or both, can cause extrapulmonary right-to-left shunting and cyanosis. In 1976, Riemenschneider et al[246] described a group of 10 neonates with PPHNS characterized by severe heart failure and systemic hypotension. Perinatal hypoxemia was suspected to have caused the cardiac dysfunction, which responded to inotropic measures. Similarly, in 1980 Fiddler et al[88] described four PPHNS infants with congestive heart failure, each of whom improved dramatically after diuretic and inotropic therapy. In all of these cases of PPHNS secondary to myocardial dysfunction, the cardiac problem appeared to be acquired from perinatal asphyxia. In 1976 Boucek et al[29] described four infants with transitory congenital tricuspid insufficiency that appeared to be due to an intrauterine insult occurring during late gestation. However, Apgar scores were not provided, and one of the four infants required resuscitation; further, one of the four infants had pulmonary hypertension at cardiac catheterization. Nevertheless, the report of Boucek et al[29] does suggest that occult episodes of intrauterine asphyxia during gestation can result in postnatal tricuspid insufficiency and PPHNS unaccompanied by signs of acute perinatal asphyxia.

The pathogenesis of asphyxia-induced cardiomyopathies may involve coronary artery thrombosis or embolism,[63] and such possibilities should be considered in every case of cardiomyopathy-induced PPHNS. In a recent example, left coronary artery embolism caused myocardial infarction, left

Table 51–4. CARDIAC DISORDERS ASSOCIATED WITH PPHNS: GROUP 2: CONGENITAL CARDIOMYOPATHIES

Type	Right-to-Left Ductal Shunt	Right-to-Left Atrial Shunt	Reference
Endocardial fibroelastosis	+	−	190, 192, 193, 234, 249
Asphyxia	+	+	88, 225, 246, 250, 251
Myocarditis	−	+	193
Pompe disease	−	+	192
Infarction	+	+	122, 273, 292
Endocardial thrombosis	+	+	216
Congenital tricuspid insufficiency	−	+	29

Table 51–5. CARDIAC DISORDERS ASSOCIATED WITH PPHNS: GROUP 3: OBSTRUCTIONS TO LEFT VENTRICULAR OUTFLOW

Lesion	Right-to-Left Ductal Shunt	Right-to-Left Atrial Shunt	Reference
Aortic atresia	+	−	249
Critical aortic stenosis	+	−	192, 249
Interrupted aortic arch	+	−	61, 148, 306
Coarctation	+	−	37, 61, 182, 192, 249, 300

ventricular failure, systemic hypotension, pulmonary hypertension, and right-to-left ductal shunt.[122]

Group 3: Obstructions to Left Ventricular Outflow

Left ventricular pressure loads are obvious causes of left ventricular failure and pulmonary hypertension. PPHNS has been reported in association with critical aortic stenosis,[192] interrupted aortic arch,[61,148,306] and coarctation (Table 51–5).[37,61,182,190,192] Usually, echocardiographic diagnosis of these lesions is straightforward; Doppler techniques can be particularly helpful. Nevertheless, on occasion, cardiac catheterization may be required to exclude one of these lesions in infants with PPHNS. For example, in some infants with critical aortic stenosis, two-dimensional echocardiography may only show a poorly functioning left ventricle without other characteristic findings such as a small aortic annulus and poststenotic dilation of the ascending aorta (Fig. 51–10), and cardiac output may be so low that no pressure gradient is detectable across the aortic valve by Doppler techniques. Similarly, echocardiographic visualization of the transverse arch to exclude interrupted arch or coarctation can be difficult in hyperventilated infants (lung can herniate over the mediastinum). Cardiac catheterization must be performed in infants with PPHNS secondary to unexplained left ventricular dysfunction because surgically treatable lesions may be responsible.

Group 4: Obligatory Left-to-Right Shunts

The concept of obligatory left-to-right shunt was put forward by Rudolph in 1970.[255] In most shunt lesions, elevations in pulmonary vascular resistance limit the shunt and reduce pulmonary blood flow. For example, in ventricular and atrial septal defects, increases in pulmonary vascular resistance limit flow across the defects into the right heart and protect the pulmonary vascular bed by reducing continued excess pulmonary blood flow. In certain shunt lesions, the magnitude of the left-to-right shunt is the same regardless of pulmonary vascular resistance; such shunts are "obligatory." When obligatory shunts are present, early and severe pulmonary vascular disease is the rule. Hemitruncus, a disorder in which one pulmonary artery arises from the right ventricle and the other arises from the aorta, is such a lesion; the normally connected lung receives twice normal pulmonary blood flow (the entire cardiac output) regardless of pulmonary artery pressure. Obligatory shunts that have been noted to cause

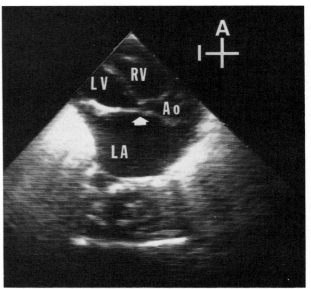

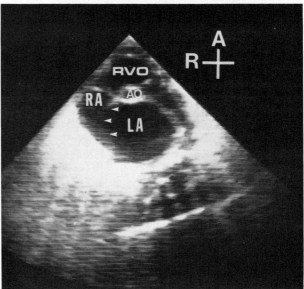

Figure 51–10. Two-dimensional echocardiographic view confirming diagnosis of critical aortic stenosis in an infant with PPHNS. The *top panel* is a parasternal long axis view demonstrating left atrial dilation, a small aortic annulus (at the arrow), and poststenotic dilation of the ascending aorta. The *bottom panel* is a parasternal short axis view demonstrating left atrial dilation, left-to-right bulging of the atrial septum (at the arrowheads), and a small aortic annulus. A = anterior; Ao = ascending aorta; I = inferior; LA = left atrium; LV = left ventricle; R = right; RA = right atrium; RV = right ventricle; RVO = right ventricular outflow tract.

Table 51–6. CARDIAC DISORDERS ASSOCIATED WITH PPHNS:
GROUP 4: OBLIGATORY LEFT-TO-RIGHT SHUNTS

Lesion	Right-to-Left Ductal Shunt	Right-to-Left Atrial Shunt	Reference
Cerebral arteriovenous malformation	+	+	59, 142, 192, 231
Hepatic arteriovenous malformation	+	–	13
Complete atrioventricular septal defect	+	–	61, 192, 210a

PPHNS include cerebral arteriovenous malformations, hepatic arteriovenous malformations, and complete atrioventricular septal defects with left ventricular–right atrial shunts (Table 51–6). Both right-to-left atrial and right-to-left ductal shunts are usually present in obligatory shunt-associated PPHNS.

The most common obligatory left-to-right shunt responsible for PPHNS is cerebral arteriovenous malformation. The clinical features of cerebral arteriovenous malformation and the diagnostic value of echocardiography and cranial ultrasonography are well characterized,[80,143,155a,219,266,267, 280,284,293,323] as is the association of cerebral arteriovenous malformation with PPHNS.[59,142,155a,192,195,231,266] In the largest series from a single institution, all 12 infants with cerebral arteriovenous malformation exhibited suprasystemic pulmonary arterial pressures, and 4 of 12 exhibited right-to-left ductal shunting.[155a] The diagnosis of cerebral arteriovenous malformation can be easy if high output congestive heart failure is obvious and if bounding arterial and cervical pulsations are present. However, more often than not cardiac failure is so pronounced that cardiac output is diminished rather than increased, and cardiomegaly and congestive heart failure are the only obvious findings. Cranial bruits, although they should be sought in every neonate with either heart failure or PPHNS, are often absent,[155a] and bounding pulses are the exception rather than the rule.[155a] Helpful diagnostic signs include dilation of the descending aorta on the chest radiograph[267] or on echocardiography,[195,267] dilation of the ascending aorta and superior vena cava on echocardiography,[280,284] evidence of myocardial ischemia on electrocardiogram,[155a] and aneurysmal right-to-left bulging of the atrial septum on echocardiography.[266] As considered earlier, the latter sign is of course in itself diagnostic of PPHNS.[192] However, the key diagnostic test, which should be performed in every neonate with unexplained congestive heart failure or PPHNS,

is cranial ultrasonography.[219] Visualization of a lucency in the brain by cranial ultrasonography, which by Doppler or contrast injection[284] contains blood flow or can be seen to pulsate,[195] is diagnostic of cerebral arteriovenous malformation. The lucency is the dilated great vein of Galen, which receives the blood coursing through the arteriovenous malformation.

The day has passed when cerebral arteriovenous malformation should be recognized only during the levophase of a pulmonary angiogram done to investigate unexplained congestive heart failure or PPHNS; cranial ultrasonography permits accurate noninvasive diagnosis of cerebral malformation and should be used frequently. Cardiac catheterization is particularly hazardous in infants with cerebral arteriovenous malformation and should be avoided.[195,293] Instead, the small volumes of contrast material these infants can tolerate are best used during cerebral angiography (after the diagnosis is made noninvasively); cerebral angiography is necessary to determine the location of the arteriovenous malformation and plan therapy. Successful outcomes have been reported.[293]

Group 5: Miscellaneous Cardiac Disorders

A wide variety of miscellaneous cardiac disorders can cause PPHNS (Table 51–7). Most of these disorders are readily recognized with two-dimensional echocardiography. However, on occasion some of these lesions present substantial difficulties in either diagnosis or management. For example, differentiating functional pulmonary atresia[282] from anatomic pulmonary atresia can be quite difficult unless pulmonary insufficiency can be detected. Further, when the pulmonary valve fails to open in neonates with Ebstein's anomaly, determining whether tricuspid incompetence, pulmonary hypertension, or pulmonary atresia is responsible (Fig. 51–11) can be a conundrum.

Table 51–7. CARDIAC DISORDERS ASSOCIATED WITH PPHNS:
GROUP 5: MISCELLANEOUS CARDIAC DISORDERS

Lesion	Right-to-Left Ductal Shunt	Right-to-Left Atrial Shunt	Reference
Ebstein anomaly	–	+	29, 192, 249
Tricuspid atresia	–	+	249
Pulmonary stenosis	–	+	249
Pulmonary atresia	–	+	249
Pulmonary vascular anomalies	+	+	116
Transposition of the great vessels	+	+	15, 65, 132a
Total anomalous pulmonary venous drainage (unobstructed)	–	+	249

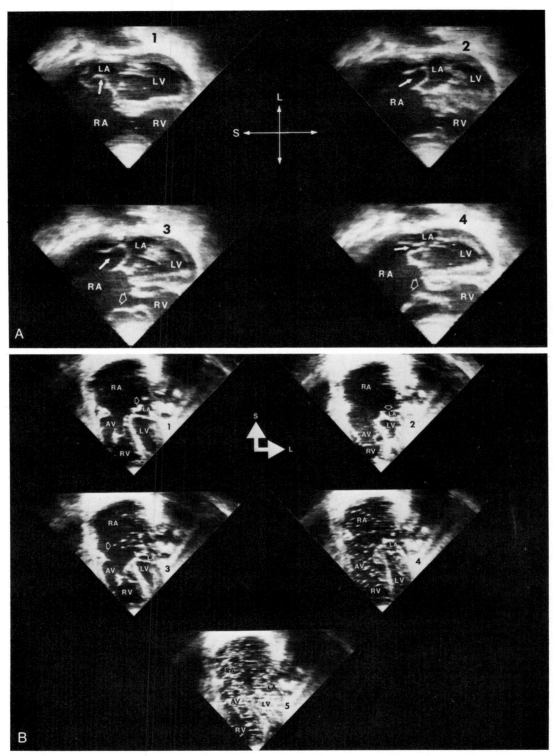

Figure 51–11. Two-dimensional echocardiographic demonstration of exaggerated atrial septal motion in an infant with Ebstein anomaly, pulmonary atresia, and PPHNS. *A*, Subxiphoid four-chamber views. The solid arrow indicates the septum secundum portion of the atrial septum; the hollow arrow indicates the tricuspid orifice. Note that the marked tricuspid regurgitation associated with ventricular systole (frame 4) drives the septum secundum all the way over to the mitral valve. *B*, Apical four-chamber contrast echocardiogram. In frames 1 and 2, note the markedly dilated right atrium, the displaced tricuspid valve, the atrialized portion of the right ventricle, and the small left atrium and left ventricle. The hollow arrows point out the foramen ovale. In frame 3, the hollow arrow points out particles of contrast entering the right atrium. In frame 5, note that left ventricular opacification exceeds right ventricular opacification.

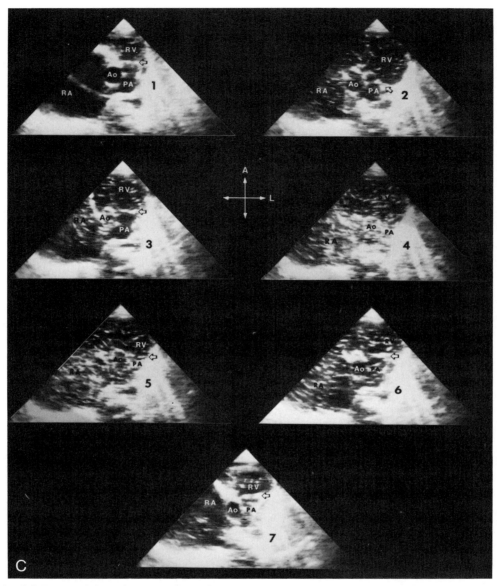

Figure 51–11 *Continued. C*, Parasternal short axis contrast echocardiogram. Frame 1 was taken immediately prior to contrast injection into a right arm vein; the arrow indicates the pulmonary valve. Note that the main pulmonary artery is of normal caliber. Frames 2 to 7 are in chronologic sequence after contrast injection into a right arm vein. Note in frame 2 that contrast has entered the right atrium and right ventricle, in frame 3 that contrast has entered the ascending aorta without entering the pulmonary artery, in frames 4 to 6 that both the ascending aorta and the pulmonary artery are opacified, and in frame 7 that contrast has cleared from the ascending aorta and remains in the pulmonary artery. This sequence indicates that there is no antegrade flow across the pulmonary valve and that the pulmonary artery fills retrogradely via left-to-right ductal shunt. When the pulmonary valve does not open, whether failure of blood to cross the pulmonary valve is due to functional pulmonary atresia (secondary to severe elevation in pulmonary vascular resistance or severe right ventricular dysfunction) or to anatomic pulmonary atresia cannot be determined echocardiographically, unless pulmonary insufficiency can be documented. In this instance the main pulmonary artery was of good size, which incorrectly suggested that the pulmonary atresia was functional rather than anatomic. A = anterior; Ao = ascending aorta; AV = atrialized portion of the right ventricle; L = left; LA = left atrium; LV = left ventricle; PA = pulmonary artery; RA = right atrium; RV = right ventricle; S = superior.

Other Etiologic Factors

PPHNS has been associated with a great many other disorders (Table 51–8). In the great majority of these associations, pulmonary hypertension is indeed responsible for PPHNS, and one or more of the three pathogenetic mechanisms for neonatal pulmonary hypertension described in Chapter 52 is responsible. Several of the more common or more interesting of these associations are considered further below.

Infectious Disorders

Group B streptococcal infections have been recognized to simulate respiratory distress syndrome for some time;[149,326] more recently, group B streptococcal infections have been

Table 51–8. OTHER DISORDERS ASSOCIATED WITH PPHNS

Category	Right-to-Left Ductal Shunt	Right-to-Left Atrial Shunt	Reference
Idiopathic	+	+	108, 279
Genitourinary			
Potter syndrome	+	+	178, 234
Infectious			
Group B streptococcus	+	+	149, 274
Listeria monocytogenes	+	+	209
Escherichia coli	+	+	280a
Haemophilus influenzae	+	+	280a
Metabolic			
Hypocalcemia	+	+	66, 125, 309
Hypoglycemia	+	+	6, 21, 104
Serum acidosis	+	+	27, 241a, 262, 269
Hypoxia	+	+	114, 143
Hyperlipidemia	+	+	232
Hematologic			
Polycythemia	+	+	93, 121, 228, 257, 304
Thrombocytopenia	+	+	95, 127, 144, 184, 216, 270
Thrombotic endocarditis	+	+	216
Acute hemorrhage	+	+	124
Gastrointestinal			
Omphalocele	+	+	202
Gut perforation	+	+	202
Gastroschisis	+	+	154
Gestational			
Chronic asphyxia	+	+	133, 285
Postmaturity	+	+	71, 94, 95
Prematurity	+	+	7, 321
Premature ductal closure	+	+	25, 139, 140
Maternal hypoxia	+	+	115, 118, 201, 218, 220
Fetopelvic disproportion	+	+	125
Fetomaternal transfusion	+	+	124, 217
Maternal fever	+	+	244
Maternal anemia	+	+	244
Breech presentation	+	+	244
Fetal distress	+	+	244
Vaginal bleeding	+	+	244
Maternal pulmonary disease	+	+	244
Chronic active hepatitis	+	+	75
Maternal hypotension	+	+	31, 109
Bone marrow transplantation	+	+	140a
Maternal Eisenmenger syndrome	+	+	218
Obstetric			
Late cord clamping	+	+	9, 187
Elective cesarean	+	+	138, 248
Drug-induced			
Aspirin	+	+	139, 183, 258
Indomethacin	+	+	58, 119, 130, 200, 254
Salicylates	+	+	140, 234
Naproxen	−	+	329
Hydantoin	−	+	308
Intralipid	+	+	176, 302
Amitriptyline	+	+	305
Lithium	+	+	89
Terbutaline	−	+	193
Prostaglandins			
Thromboxane B_2	+	+	127
$PGF_{1\alpha}$	+	+	127
Leukotrienes	+	+	294
Other			
Familial	+	+	186, 202, 277
Postoperative	+	+	100, 301
Systemic hypertension	+	−	151, 181, 210
Shock	+	+	191a
Pulmonary artery distention	−	−	17

reported in association with PPHNS.[274] The pathogenesis of this latter association is being explored,[145,325] and release of the systemic and pulmonary vasoconstrictor thromboxane appears to be responsible. PPHNS has also been observed in association with infection by *Listeria monocytogenes*[209] by *Escherichia coli*,[280a] and by *Haemophilus influenzae*[280a]; whether a similar pathogenesis is present is unknown.

Gestational Factors

The common thread among the various gestational factors associated with PPHNS (Table 51–8) appears to be either acute or chronic fetal compromise. Since the nineteenth century, asphyxia has been known to cause pulmonary hypertension. Documentation of the fact that the fetus lives in a hypoxic environment and adapts by increasing its oxygen-carrying capacity has also been extant for a substantial period.[78] In the 40 years since von Euler and Liljestrand's original observation that alveolar hypoxia without asphyxia causes pulmonary hypertension in adult cats,[316] hypoxic pulmonary vasoconstriction has been documented in fetal,[45,46,54,60,109,196,256] newborn,[153,196,229,253,256] and adult[91] animals. Similarly, acidosis is a potent pulmonary vasoconstrictor at all stages of development.[28,60,91,197,229,262] Thus, it is not surprising that PPHNS is associated with conditions that either reduce maternal oxygenation,[115,118,201,218,220,244] blood pressure,[31,109,244] or oxygen-carrying capacity;[244] interfere with placental perfusion;[94] or are associated with fetal asphyxia.[124,125,133,217,244] Most animal experiments suggest that the association of maternal hypoxia with PPHNS is best explained on the basis of fetal and neonatal polycythemia,[101,102,220] but structural changes in the pulmonary vascular bed have been observed in some experiments.[115] Recent experimental observations suggest that chronic fetal asphyxia can cause structural changes in the pulmonary vascular bed.[285]

Obstetric Factors

Late clamping of the umbilical cord permits larger placental transfusion of the newborn and increases the hematocrit. Infants whose umbilical cords are clamped late have higher pulmonary artery pressures,[9] because increases in hematocrit increase pulmonary vascular resistance more than systemic vascular resistance.[93] Polycythemia is well known to be associated with PPHNS.[93,104,106,121,178,228,304]

Elective cesarean section is also associated with PPHNS.[138] Some investigators have suggested that an altered prostaglandin milieu accounts for this association,[127] and prostaglandins are known to have important effects on the neonatal pulmonary circulation.[47,48,158,235–238,286]

Drugs

Both clinical and experimental data indicate that maternal ingestion of cyclooxygenase inhibitors such as aspirin,[139,179a,183,258] indomethacin,[58,119,130,200,254] salicylates,[140,234] and naproxen[328] can predispose to PPHNS by causing closure of the fetal arterial duct. Ductal closure in utero causes excessive pulmonary blood flow in the fetus,[259] and congestive heart failure postnatally if the fetus survives.[10] The risk to the fetus with a given cyclooxygenase inhibitor depends upon several factors, including the gestational age of the fetus, the rate of placental passage of the drug, the reversibility of cyclooxygenase inhibition, and the duration of maternal ingestion. For example, Dudley and Hardie[76] have argued that the risks of inhibiting premature labor with indomethacin are not large because indomethacin causes reversible cyclooxygenase inhibition, does not cross the placenta until late gestation,[164] and has not been associated with PPHNS in infants weighing less than 2200 g at birth. The latter observation is consistent with the facts that ductal patency is dependent on circulating prostaglandin E levels and that lower prostaglandin E levels are sufficient to maintain ductal patency in younger fetuses[51] (see Chapter 6). Such reasoning does suggest that inhibition of premature labor with cyclooxygenase inhibitors does not carry undue risk, but these arguments do not apply to term and near-term gestations or to medically unsupervised maternal ingestions of cyclooxygenase inhibitors (i.e., aspirin or ibuprofen) at any stage of gestation. The fetal risks of maternal cyclooxygenase ingestion are real and substantial, and word about these hazards must be disseminated to the general public. In the study of Csaba et al, 5 of 10 infants whose mothers received indomethacin between 35 and 41 weeks' gestation developed PPHNS, and two infants died.[58]

SUMMARY

PPHNS is not an uncommon syndrome because the anatomic pathways and physiologic mechanisms responsible for the fetal circulation remain intact in the newborn and can be reactivated by a great variety of disorders. Unless the pulmonary vascular bed is irreversibly damaged or inadequate in cross sectional area (see Chapter 52), PPHNS is usually a self-limited disorder, and supportive treatment and time are the best therapies. Prognosis is dependent on the underlying etiology. The diagnosis of PPHNS is best made by differential oximetry, two-dimensional echocardiography, contrast echocardiography, or Doppler echocardiographic techniques. PPHNS is most commonly caused by lung diseases, but cardiovascular disorders also cause PPHNS. Each infant with PPHNS should be carefully evaluated for the presence of cardiovascular disease, and in all patients the evaluation should include history, physical examination (including four extremity blood pressures and cranial auscultation), chest radiography (pulmonary venous congestion, pleural effusions,[194a] cardiomegaly, and dilation of the descending aorta[267] strongly suggest underlying cardiovascular disease), electrocardiography (left axis deviation and left ventricular hypertrophy are pathognomonic of underlying congenital heart disease; myocardial ischemia is strongly suggestive of an acquired or congenital cardiovascular disorder), and two-dimensional echocardiography. Right-to-left bulging of the atrial septum is diagnostic of PPHNS; left-to-right bulging of the atrial septum in infants with PPHNS is diagnostic of underlying cardiovascular disease. Cranial ultrasonography should be performed in infants in whom PPHNS remains unexplained after the above diagnostic measures, and umbilical venous catheterization should be conducted in infants with pulmonary venous congestion. Cardiac catheterization is indicated in infants with PPHNS in whom left ventricular dysfunction cannot be explained by noninvasive tests, and in infants in whom the connections of the pulmonary veins cannot be proved beyond doubt echocardiographically. Use of consistent terminology and a consistent, aggressive approach to noninvasive identification of underlying diseases will improve both recognition of PPHNS' many causes and understanding of its many pathogenetic mechanisms. Until more is learned about PPHNS and its treatment, attempts to "cure" the infant with aggressive but unproven therapeutic measures should be avoided; beyond gentle correction of hypothermia, hypoxia, and acidosis, treatment should be dictated only by the infant's symptoms, for the physician's first obligation is to do no harm.

References

1. Adams FH, Latta H, El-Salawy A, Nozakim (1969): The expanded lung of the term fetus. J Pediatr 75:59–66.
1a. Adams, FH, Lind J (1957): Physiologic studies on the cardiovascular status of newborn infants (with special reference to the ductus arteriosus). Pediatr 19:431–437.
2. Adams JM, Hyde WH, Procianoy RS, Rudolph AJ (1980): Hypochloremic metabolic alkalosis following tolazoline-induced gastric hypersecretion. Pediatr 65:298–300.
3. Ahlquist RP, Huggins RA, Woodbury RA (1947): The pharmacology of benzyl-imidazoline (priscol). J Pharmacol Exper Ther 9:271–288.
4. Akesode FA, Sandor GGS, MacNab AJ, Patterson MWH, Ebelt VJ, Tipple M, Pendray MR, Long E (1981): Respiratory and cardiac effects of tolazoline in persistent foetal circulation (abstract). Clin Res 29:138A.
5. Alpan G, Glick B, Peleg O, Springer C, Eyal F (1985): False diagnosis of persistent fetal circulation caused by misplacement of umbilical artery catheter. South Med J 78:1002–1004.
6. Amatayakul O, Cumming GR, Haworth JC (1970): Association of hypoglycemia with cardiac enlargement and heart failure in newborn infants. Arch Dis Child 45:717–720.
7. Amato M, deRoche B, von Muralt G (1986): Persistent pulmonary hypertension in preterm-infants. Pädiatrie Pädologie 21:25–30.
8. Andrews AF, Roloff DW, Bartlett RH (1984): Use of extracorporeal membrane oxygenators in persistent pulmonary hypertension of the newborn. Clin Perinatol 11:729–735.
9. Arcilla RA, Oh W, Lind J (1966): Pulmonary arterial pressure of newborn infants born with early and late clamping of the cord. Acta Pediatr Scand 55:305–315.
10. Arcilla RA, Thilenius DG, Ranniger K (1969): Congestive heart failure from suspected ductal closure in utero. J Pediatr 75:74–78.
11. Arnold J, O'Brodovich H, Whyte R, Coates G (1985): Pulmonary thromboemboli after neonatal asphyxia. J Pediatr 106:806–809.
12. Ballard RA, Leonard CH (1984): Developmental follow-up of infants with persistent pulmonary hypertension of the newborn. Clin Perinatol 11:737–744.
13. Bamford MF, DeBono D, Pickering D, Keeling JW (1980): An arteriovenous malformation of the liver giving rise to persistent transitional (fetal) circulation (letter). Arch Dis Child 55:244–245.
14. Bartlett RH, Roloff DW, Cornell RG, Andrews AF, Dillon PW, Zwischenberger JB (1985): Extra corporeal circulation in neonatal respiratory failure: A prospective randomized study. Pediatr 76:479–487.
15. Batton DG, Maisels MJ, Fripp RR, Heald JI (1982): Arterial hyperoxia in a newborn infant with transposition of the great vessels. J Pediatr 100:300–302.
16. Bauer CR, Tsipuras D, Fletcher BD (1974): Syndrome of persistent pulmonary vascular obstruction of the newborn: Roentgen findings. Am J Roentgenol Radium Ther Nucl Med 120:285–290.
17. Baylen BG, Emmanouilides GC, Juratsch CE, Yoshida Y, French WJ, Criley JM (1980): Main pulmonary artery distention: A potential mechanism for acute pulmonary hypertension in the human newborn infant. J Pediatr 96:540–544.
18. Beck R (1985): Chronic lung disease following hypocapneic alkalosis for persistent pulmonary hypertension (letter): J Pediatr 106:527–528.
19. Behrman RE (1976): Persistence of the fetal circulation. J Pediatr 89:636–637.
20. Benitz WE, Malachowski N, Cohen RS, Stevenson DK, Ariagno RL, Sunshine P (1985): Use of sodium nitroprusside in neonates: Efficacy and safety. J Pediatr 106:102–110.
21. Benzing G III, Schubert W, Hug G, Kaplan S (1969): Simultaneous hypoglycemia and acute congestive heart failure. Circulation 40:209–216.
22. Berglund G (1955): Studies of circulation in the neonatal period. Acta Pediatr 103:138–139.
23. Berglund G, Korlberg P, Lind J (1955): Studies of the respiration and circulation during the neonatal period. Acta Pediatr 44:136–137.
24. Bernbaum JC, Russell P, Sheridan PH, Gewitz MH, Fox WW, Peckham GJ (1984): Long-term follow-up of newborns with persistent pulmonary hypertension. Crit Care Med 12:579–583.
25. Berry TE, Muster AJ, Paul MH (1983): Transient neonatal tricuspid regurgitation: Possible relation to premature closure of the ductus arteriosus. J Am Coll Cardiol 2:1178–1182.
26. Bloss RS, Turmen T, Beardmore HE, Aranda JV (1980): Tolazoline therapy for persistent pulmonary hypertension after congenital diaphragmatic hernia repair. J Pediatr 97:984–988.
27. Bolam DL (1983): Persistent fetal circulation: Current concepts. Nebr Med J 68:60–61.
28. Bolam DL, Ruchman RN (1979): Acid base balance in persistent fetal circulation. Pediatr Res 13:490.
29. Boucek RJ Jr, Graham TP Jr, Morgan JP, Atwood GF, Boerth RC (1976): Spontaneous resolution of massive congenital tricuspid insufficiency. Circulation 54:795–800.
30. Boyle RJ, Oh W (1978): Transcutaneous PO_2 monitoring in infants with persistent fetal circulation who are receiving tolazoline therapy. Pediatr 62:605–607.
31. Bressack MA, Bland RD (1981): Intravenous infusion of tolazoline reduces pulmonary vascular resistance and net fluid filtration in the lungs of awake, hypoxic newborn lambs. Am Rev Respir Dis 123:217–221.
32. Brett C, Dekle M, Leonard CH, Clark C, Sniderman S, Roth R, Ballard R, Clyman R (1981): Developmental follow-up of hyperventilated neonates: Preliminary observations. Pediatr 68:588–591.
33. Brown R, Pickering D (1974): Persistent transitional circulation. Arch Dis Child 49:883–885.
34. Bruce DA (1984): Effects of hyperventilation on cerebral blood flow and metabolism. Clin Perinatol 11:673–680.
35. Bucciarelli RL, Egon EA, Gessner IH, Eitzman DV (1976): Persistence of fetal cardiopulmonary circulation: One manifestation of transient tachypnea of the newborn. Pediatr 58:192–197.
36. Bucciarelli R, Nelson RM, Egan EA II, Eitzman DV, Gessner IH (1977): Transient tricuspid insufficiency of the newborn: A form of myocardial dysfunction in stressed newborns. Pediatr 59:330–337.
37. Bucher HU, Arbenz U, Bucher A (1979): TcPO2 in pediatric cardiology: Application during balloon septostomy, tolazoline administration, and in children with right-to-left shunt. Birth Defects 15:355–363.
38. Buhlmeyer K, Schober JG, Lorenz HP, Muller KD, Vogel M, (1986): Early diagnosis and medical treatment of the persistent ductus arteriosus in infants. Cardiovasc Intervent Radiol 9:273–278.
39. Burchell HB, Swan HJC, Wood EH (1953): Demonstration of differential effects on pulmonary and systemic arterial pressure by variation in oxygen content of inspired air in patients with patent ductus arteriosus and pulmonary hypertension. Circulation 8:681–694.
40. Burnard ED, James LS (1961): Failure of the heart after cardiac asphyxia at birth. Pediatr 28:545–565.
41. Burnell RH, Joseph MC, Lee MH (1972): Progressive pulmonary hypertension in newborn infants: Report of two cases with no identifiable respiratory or cardiac disease. Am J Dis Child 123:167–170.

42. But WW, Bowman ED, Muton LJ (1984): Survival after prolonged persistent pulmonary hypertension. Aust Paediatr J 20:123–125.

43. Cabal LA, Devaskar U, Siassi B, Hodgman JE, Emmanouilides G (1980): Cardiogenic shock associated with perinatal asphyxia in preterm infants. J Pediatr 96:705–710.

44. Caeton AJ, Goetzman BW, Bennett SH, Millstein JM (1987): Effect of pulmonary hypertension on lung compliance in newborn lambs. Pediatr Pulm 3:324–327.

45. Cassin S (1964): The vascular resistance of the foetal and newly ventilated lung of the lamb. J Physiol 171:61–79.

46. Cassin S, Dawes GS, Ross BB (1964): Pulmonary blood flow and vascular resistance in immature foetal lambs. J Physiol 171:80–89.

47. Cassin S, Tod M, Philips J, Frisinger J, Jordan J, Gibbs C (1981): Effects of prostaglandin D_2 on perinatal circulation. Am J Physiol 240:H 755–760.

48. Cassin S, Winikor I, Tod M, Philips J, Frisinger J, Jordan J, Gibbs C (1981): Effects of prostacyclin on the fetal pulmonary circulation. Pediatr Pharmacol 1:197–207.

49. Chu J, Clements JA, Cotton EK, Klaus MH, Sweet AY, Tooley WH (1967): Neonatal pulmonary ischemia. Part 1: Clinical and physiological studies. Pediatrics 40:709–782.

49a. Cloez FL, Isaaz K, Pernot C (1986): Pulsed Doppler flow characteristics of ductus arteriosus in infants with associated congenital anomalies of the heart and great vessels. Am J Cardiol 57:845–851.

50. Cloutier R, Fournier L, Lavesseur L (1983): Reversion to fetal circulation in congenital diaphragmatic hernia: A preventable postoperative complication. J Pediat Surg 18:551–554.

51. Clyman RI, Mauray F, Rudolph AM, Heymann MA (1980): Age-dependent sensitivity of the lamb ductus arteriosus to indomethacin and prostaglandins. J Pediatr 96:94–98.

52. Cohen RS, Stevenson DK, Malachowski N, Ariagno RL, Johnson JD, Sunshine P (1980): Late morbidity among survivors of respiratory failure treated with tolazoline. J Pediatr 97:644–647.

53. Collins DL, Pomerance JJ, Travis KW, Turner SW, Pappelbaum SJ (1977): A new approach to congenital posterolateral diaphragmatic hernia. J Pediat Surg 12:149–156.

54. Cook CD, Drinker PA, Jacobson HN, Levison H, Strang LB (1963): Control of pulmonary blood flow in the foetal and newly-born lamb. J Physiol 169:10–29.

55. Cottrill CM, O'Connor WN, Cudd T, Rantanen NW (1987): Persistence of foetal circulatory pathways in a newborn foal. Equine Vet J 19:252–255.

56. Cotton EK (1965): The use of priscoline in the treatment of the hypoperfusion syndrome. Pediatr 36:149.

57. Crouse DT, Philips JB III (1987): Persistent pulmonary hypertension of the newborn. Perinatol Neonatol Sept/Oct:10–20.

58. Csaba IF, Sulyok E, Ertl T (1978): Relationship of maternal treatment with indomethacin to persistence of fetal circulation syndrome. J Pediatr 92:484.

59. Cumming GR (1980): Circulation in neonates with intracranial arteriovenous fistula and cardiac failure. Am J Cardiol 45:1019–1024.

60. Dawes GS, Mott JC (1962): The vascular tone of the foetal lung. J Physiol 164:465–477.

61. De Geeter B, Messer J, Benoit M, Willard D (1979): Right-to-left ductal shunt and transcutaneous PO_2. Birth Defects 15:387–392.

62. Delisle G, Ando M, Calder AL, Zubenbuhler JR, Rochenmacher S, Alday LE, Mangini O, Van Praagh S, Van Praagh R (1976): Total anomalous pulmonary venous connection: Report of 93 autopsied cases with emphasis on diagnostic and surgical considerations. Am Heart J 91:99–122.

63. Desa DJ (1979): Coronary arterial lesions and myocardial necrosis in stillbirths and infants. Arch Dis Child 54:918–930.

64. Dibbins AW, Wiener ES (1974): Mortality from neonatal diaphragmatic hernia. J Pediatr Surg 9:653–662.

65. Dick M II, Heidelberger K, Crowley D, Rosenthal A, Hees P (1981): Quantitative morphometric analysis of the pulmonary arteries in two patients with D–transposition of the great arteries and persistence of the fetal circulation. Pediatr Res 15:1397–1401.

66. Dickstein PJ, Trindad O, Goldberg RN, Bancalari E (1984): The effect of calcium antagonists on hypoxic pulmonary hypertension in the piglet. Pediatr Res 18:1252–1265.

67. Drayton MR, Skidmore R (1987): Doppler ultrasound in the neonate. Ultrasound Med Biol 12:761–772.

68. Drummond WH (1984): Persistent pulmonary hypertension of the

69. Drummond WH (1984): Use of cardiotonic therapy in the management of infants with PPHN. Clin Perinatol 11:715–728.

70. Drummond WH (1987): Neonatal pulmonary hypertension. Equine Vet J 19:169–171.

71. Drummond WH, Peckham GJ, Fox WW (1977): The clinical profile of the newborn with persistent pulmonary hypertension: Observations in 19 affected neonates. Clin Pediatr 16:335–341.

72. Drummond WH, Gregory GA, Heymann MA, Phibbs RA (1981): The independent effects of hyperventilation, tolazoline, and dopamine on infants with persistent pulmonary hypertension. J Pediatr 98:603–611.

73. Drummond WH, Williams BJ (1983): Effect of continuous tolazoline infusion on cardiopulmonary response to dopamine in unanesthetized newborn lambs. J Pediatr 103:278–284.

74. Duara S, Gewitz MH, Fox WW (1984): Use of mechanical ventilation for clinical management of persistent pulmonary hypertension of the newborn. Clin Perinatol 11:641–652.

75. Dubois RS, Slovia TL, Tolla V, Pensler L (1982): Chronic active hepatitis and pregnancy: A report of two cases in adolescence. Am J Gastroenterol 77:649–651.

76. Dudley DK, Hardie MJ (1985): Fetal and neonatal effects of indomethacin used as a tocolytic agent. Am J Obstet Gynecol 151:181–184.

77. Easa D, Herrman K, Holt D (1981): Management of persistent fetal circulation in a neonate. Hawaii Med J 40:355–356.

78. Eastman NJ (1930): Foetal blood studies. I. The oxygen relationships of umbilical cord blood at birth. Bull Johns Hopkins Hosp 47:221–230.

79. Eden RD, Seifert LS, Winegar A, Spellacy WN (1987): Perinatal morbidity and mortality in a regional perinatal network. J Reprod Med 32:583–586.

80. Eide J, Follis M (1978): Malformations of the great vein of Galen with neonatal heart failure. Acta Paediatr Scand 67:529–532.

81. Ein SH, Barker G, Olley P, Shandling B, Simpson JS, Stephens CA, Filler RM (1985): The pharmacologic treatment of newborn diaphragmatic hernia—a 2-year evaluation. J Pediatr Surg 15:384–394.

81a. Eldridge FL, Hultgren HN, Wigmore ME (1945): The physiologic closure of the ductus arteriosus in newborn infants: A preliminary report. Science 119:731–732

82. Eldridge FL, Hultgren HN, Wigmore ME (1955): The physiologic closure of the ductus arteriosus in the newborn infant. J Clin Invest 34:987–996.

83. Elzenga NJ, Spritzer R (1984): Countercurrent arterial contrast echocardiography in the assessment of left-to-right ductal shunting in preterm infants. Arch Dis Child 59:533–536.

84. Emmanouilides GC, Baylen BG (1979): Neonatal cardiopulmonary distress without congenital heart disease. Curr Probl Pediatr 9:1–39.

85. Emmanouilides GC, Moss AJ, Duffie ER Jr, Adams FH (1964): Pulmonary arterial pressure changes in human newborn infants from birth to 3 days of age. J Pediatr 65:327–333.

85a. Evertl NB, Johnson RT (1950): A study of the time of closure of the ductus arteriosus using radiophosphorus (abstract). Anat rec 106:194.

86. Fakhraee SH, Mathew OP, Yong E, Gutierrez FR, Marshall RE (1980): Obstructed total anomalous pulmonary venous return confused with persistent pulmonary hypertension of the newborn. Clin Pediatr 19:644–645.

87. Ferrara TB, Johnson DE, Thompson TR (1983): Hypocapneic alkalosis for treatment of persistent pulmonary hypertension (PPH) in infants with severe pulmonary pathology (abstr). Pediatr Res 17:312A.

88. Fiddler GI, Chatrath R, Williams GJ, Walker OR, Scott O (1980): Dopamine infusion for the treatment of myocardial dysfunction associated with a persistent transitional circulation. Arch Dis Child 55:194–198.

89. Filtenborg JA (1982): Persistent pulmonary hypertension after lithium intoxication in the newborn. Eur J Pediatr 138:321–323.

90. Finley JP, Howman-Giles RB, Gilday DL, Bloom KR, Rowe RD (1979): Transient myocardial ischemia of the newborn infant demonstrated by thallium myocardial imaging. J Pediatr 94:263–270.

neonate (persistent fetal circulation syndrome). Adv Pediatric 30:61–91.

91. Fishman A (1976): Hypoxia on the pulmonary circulation: How and where it acts. Circ Res 38:221–231.

92. Fong LV, Pemberton PJ (1985): Congenital diaphragmatic hernia and the management of persistent foetal circulation. Anaesth Inten Care 13:375–379.

93. Fouron J-C, Hebert F (1973): The circulatory effects of hematocrit variations in normovolemic newborn lambs. J Pediatr 82:995–1003.

94. Fox WW (1982): Arterial blood gas evaluation and mechanical ventilation in the management of persistent pulmonary hypertension of the neonate. In Peckham GJ, Heymann MA (eds): Cardiovascular Sequelae of Asphyxia in the Newborn. Report of Eighty-third Ross Conference on Pediatric Research, Ross Laboratories, Columbus, Ohio, pp 102–110.

95. Fox WW, Gewitz MW, Dinwiddie R, Drummond WH, Peckham GJ (1977): Pulmonary hypertension in perinatal aspiration syndromes. Pediatrics 59:205–211.

96. Fox WW, Duara S (1983): Persistent pulmonary hypertension in the neonate: Diagnosis and management. J Pediatr 103:505–514.

97. Fraker TD, Harris PJ, Bahar VS, Kisslo JA (1979): Detection and exclusion of intracardiac shunts by two dimensional echocardiography and peripheral venous injection. Circulation 59:379–395.

98. Fyfe D, Moodie DS, Gill CC (1982): Persistent pulmonary hypertension complicating diagnosis and treatment of total anomalous pulmonary venous return in the neonate. Clev Clin Q 49:173–180.

99. Galioto FM Jr, Brudno DS, Rivera O, Howard RP (1984): Use of the rebreathing method in the differential diagnosis of congenital heart disease and persistent fetal circulation. Am J Cardiol 54:1305–1309.

99a. Gathman GE, Nadas AS (1970): Total anomalous pulmonary venous drainage: Clinical observations in 75 patients. Circulation 42:143–154.

100. Gaulin P, Rubin SZ (1983): Persistent fetal circulation in neonates post-operatively: The value of manual ventilation. Can J Surg 26:250–251.

101. Geggel RL, Aronovitz MJ, Reid LM (1986): Effects of chronic in utero hypoxemia on rat neonatal pulmonary arterial structure. J Pediatr 108:756–759.

102. Geggel RL, Reid LM (1984): The structural basis of PPHN. Clin Perinatol 11:525–549.

103. German JC, Bartlett RH, Gazzaniga AB, Huxtable RF, Amlie R, Sperling DR (1979): Pulmonary artery pressure monitoring in persistent fetal circulation (PFC). J Pediatr Surg 12:913–919.

104. Gersony WM (1973): Persistence of the fetal circulation: A commentary. J Pediatr 82:1103–1106.

105. Gersony WM (1982): Persistence of the fetal circulation syndrome: Definition of the problem. In Peckham GS, Heyman MA (eds): Cardiovascular Sequelae of Asphyxia in the Newborn. Report of the Eighty-third Ross Conference on Pediatric Research, Ross Laboratories, Columbus, Ohio, pp 70–75.

106. Gersony WM (1984): Neonatal pulmonary hypertension: pathophysiology, classification, and etiology. Clin Perinatol 11:517–524.

107. Gersony WM (1986): Patent ductus arteriosus in the neonate. Pediatr Clin North Am 93:545–560.

108. Gersony WM, Duc GV, Sinclair JC (1969): "PFC" syndrome (persistence of the fetal circulation) (abstract). Circulation 40S:III:87.

109. Gersony WM, Morishima HO, Daniel SS, Kahl S, Cohen H, Brown W, James LS (1976): The hemodynamic effects of intrauterine hypoxia: An experimental model in newborn lambs. J Pediatr 89:631–635.

110. Godoy G, Lyrene R, Cassady G, Dew A, Philips J (1985): Hemodynamic effects of dopamine (abstract). Pediatr Res 19:171A.

111. Goetzman BW, Milstein JM (1979): Pulmonary vasodilator action of tolazoline. Pediatr Res 13:942–944.

112. Goetzman BW, Milstein JM (1980): Pulmonary vascular histamine receptors in newborn and young lambs. J Appl Physiol: Respirat Environ Exercise Physiol 49:380–385.

113. Goetzman BW, Riemenschneider TA (1980): Persistence of the fetal circulation. Pediatr 2:37–40.

114. Goetzman BW, Sunshine P, Johnson JD, Wennberg RP, Hackel A, Merten DF, Bartoletti AL, Silverman NH (1976): Neonatal hypoxia and pulmonary vasospasm: Response to tolazoline. J Pediatr 89:617–621.

115. Goldberg SJ, Levy RA, Siassi B, Betten J (1971): The effect of maternal hypoxia and hyperoxia upon the neonatal pulmonary vasculature. Pediatr 48:528–533.

116. Goldstein JD, Rabinovitch M, Van Praagh R, Reid L (1979): Unusual vascular anomalies causing persistent pulmonary hypertension in a newborn. Am J Cardiol 43:962–968.

117. Goldstein JD, Reid LM (1980): Pulmonary hypoplasia resulting from phrenic nerve agenesis and diaphragmatic amyoplasia. J Pediatr 98:282–287.

118. Gooding CA, Gregory GA (1971): Roentgenographic analysis of meconium aspiration of the newborn. Radiology 100:131–135.

119. Grella P, Zanor P (1978): Premature labor and indomethacin. Prostaglandins 16:1007–1017.

120. Gronik J (1982): Contrast echocardiography in patent foramen ovale. In Melton RS, Roelandt CJ (eds): Contrast Echocardiography. Developments in Cardiovascular Medicine 15. The Hague, Martinus Nijhoff Publishers, pp 137–152.

121. Gross GP, Hathoway WE, McGaughey HR (1973): Hyperviscosity in the neonate. J Pediatr 82:1004–1012.

122. Guller B, Bozic C (1972): Right to left shunting through a patent ductus arteriosus in a newborn with myocardial infarction. Cardiology 57:348–357.

123. Hageman JR, Adams MA, Gardner TH (1982): The use of hyperventilation in persistent pulmonary hypertension of the newborn (abstr). Clin Res 30:798A.

124. Hageman JR, Adams MA, Gardner TH (1984): Persistent pulmonary hypertension of the newborn: Trends in incidence, diagnosis, and management. Am J Dis Child 138:592–595.

125. Hallman M, Kankaanpaa K (1980): Evidence of surfactant deficiency in persistence of the fetal circulation. Eur J Pediatr 134:129–134.

126. Hammerman C, Strates E, Berger S, Zala W, Aldousany A (1986): Prostaglandins and echocardiography in the assessment of patent ductus arteriosus. Crit Care Med 14:462–465.

127. Hammerman C, Lass N, Strates E, Komar K, Bui KC (1987): Prostanoids in neonates with persistent pulmonary hypertension. J Pediatr 110:470–472.

128. Hammerman C, Strates E, Valaitis S (1986): The silent ductus: Its precursors and its aftermath. Pediatr Cardiol 7:121–127.

129. Hansen TN, Gest AL (1984): Oxygen toxicity and other ventilatory complications of treatment of infants with persistent pulmonary hypertension. Clin Perinatol 11:653–672.

130. Harker LC, Kirkpatrick SE, Friedman WF, Bloor CM (1981): Effects of indomethacin on fetal rat lungs: A possible cause of persistent fetal circulation (PFC). Pediatr Res 15:147–151.

131. Harned HS Jr (1983): Cardiovascular problems of the newborn and their etiologies. Prog Clin Biol Res 140:167–183.

132. Harvey WA (1628): Exercitatio Anatomica de Motu Cordis et Sanguinis in Animalibus. The Classics of Medicine Library, Birmingham, Alabama, 1978. The Keynes English Translation of 1928.

132a. Hawker RE, Freedam RM, Rowe RD, Krovetz LJ (1974): Persistence of the fetal circulation in transposition of the great arteries. Johns Hopkins Med J 134:107–117.

133. Haworth SC, Reid L (1976): Persistent fetal circulation: Newly recognized structural features. J Pediatr 88:614–620.

134. Hegyi T, Hiatt IM (1980): Tolazoline and dopamine therapy in neonatal hypoxia and pulmonary vasospasm. Acta Paediatr Scand 69:101–103.

135. Heinonen K, Hakulinen A (1986): Transcutaneous PO_2 recording using two sensors in a neonate with preductal coarctation of aorta. Crit Care Med 14:298–299.

136. Henry GW (1984): Noninvasive assessment of cardiac function and pulmonary hypertension in persistent pulmonary hypertension of the newborn. Clin Perinatol 11:627–640.

137. Henry GW, Stevens DC, Schreiner RL, Grosfeld JL, Ballantine TVN (1979): Respiratory paralysis to improve oxygenation and mortality in large newborn infants with respiratory distress. J Pediatr Surg 14:761–767.

138. Heritage OK, Cunningham MD (1985): Association of elective repeat cesarean delivery and persistent pulmonary hypertension of the newborn. Am J Obstet Gynecol 152:627–629.

139. Heymann MA (1986): Non-narcotic analgesics. Use in pregnancy and fetal and perinatal effects. Drugs 32:164–176.

140. Heymann MA, Rudolph AM (1976): Effects of acetyl salicylic

acid on the ductus arteriosus and circulation in fetal lambs. Circ Res 38:418–422.

140a. Hinterburger-Fischer M, Hinterburger W, Hayek Romsemayer A, Hocker P, Wagner K, Sewann H, Lechner K (1987): Pregnancy and delivery after bone marrow transplantation (BMT) for severe aplastic anemia (SAA). Blut 54:313–315.

141. Hoffman RR, Campbell RE, Decker JP (1974): Fetal aspiration syndrome. Clinical roentgenologic and pathologic features. Am J Roent Rad Ther Nucl Med 122:90–96.

142. Holden AM, Fyler DC, Shillito J, Nadas AS (1972): Congestive heart failure from intracranial arteriovenous fistula in infancy. Pediatr 49:30–39.

143. Hope R, Izzakawa T (1973): Congestive cardiac failure and intracranial arteriovenous communications in infants and children. Aust NZ J Med 3:599–605.

144. Horgan MJ, Carrasco NJM, Risemberg H (1985): The relationship of thrombocytopenia to the onset of persistent pulmonary hypertension of the newborn in the meconium aspiration syndrome. NY State J Med 85:245–247.

145. Huddleston KW, Lyrene RK, Dew A, Gray BM, Philips JB III (1986): The influence of prostaglandin D$_2$ on hemodynamic effects of group B streptococcus in neonatal lambs. Dev Pharmacol Ther 9:260–265.

146. Hughes MJ, O'Brien LJ (1977): Liberation of endogenous compounds by tolazoline. Agents Actions 7:225–230.

147. Hultgren HN, Hackett AJ (1950): Determination of the oxygen content of capillary blood in congenital heart disease. Pediatr 6:93–97.

148. Immagoulou A, Anderson RC, Miller JH (1972): Interruption of the aortic arch: Clinical features in twenty patients. Chest 61:276–282.

149. Jacob J, Edwards D, Gluck L (1980): Early–onset sepsis and pneumonia observed as respiratory distress syndrome. Am J Dis Child 134:766–768.

150. James DK, Chiswick JL, Havier A, Williams M, Hallworth J (1985): Nonspecificity of surfactant deficiency in neonatal respiratory disorders. Br Med J 105:1635–1637.

151. James LS (1959): Discussion of Dawes GS. Patterns of the transitional circulation. In Oliver TK (ed): Adaptation to Extrauterine Life. Report of Thirty-first Ross Conference on Pediatric Research, Ross Laboratories, Columbus, Ohio, pp 28–29.

152. James LS, Burnard ED, Rowe RD (1961): Abnormal shunting through the foramen ovale after birth. Am J Dis Child 102:550.

153. James LS, Rowe RD (1957): The pattern of response of pulmonary and systemic arterial pressures in newborn and older infants to short periods of hypoxia. J Pediatr 51:5–11.

154. Janik JS, Adamkin DH, Nagaraj HS, Groff DB (1982): Pulmonary hypertension after primary closure of a gastroschisis. South Med J 75:77–78.

155. Janny CG, Askin FB, Kuhn C III (1981): Congenital alveolar capillary dysplasia—an unusual cause of respiratory distress in the newborn. Am J Clin Pathol 76:722–727.

155a. Jedeikin R, Rowe RD, Freedam RM, Olley PM, Gillan JE (1983): Cerebral arteriovenous malformation in neonates: The role of myocardial ischemia. Pediatr Cardiol 4:29–35.

156. Johnson GL, Cunningham MD, Desai NS, Cottrill CM, Noonan JA (1980): Echocardiography in hyoxemic neonatal pulmonary disease. J Pediatr 96:716–720.

157. Jones RWA, Baumer JH, Joseph MC, Shinebourne EA (1976): Arterial oxygen tension and response to oxygen breathing in differential diagnosis of congenital heart disease in infancy. Arch Dis Child 51:667–673.

158. Kaapa P (1987): Platelet thromboxane B$_2$ production in neonatal pulmonary hypertension. Arch Dis Child 62:195–196.

159. Kaapa P, Koivisto M, Ylikorkala O, Kouvalainen K (1985): Prostacyclin in treatment of neonatal pulmonary hypertension. J Pediatr 107:951–953.

160. Keith JD, Forsyth C (1950): Aortography in infants. Circulation 2:977–914.

161. Kelly MA, Vincent DD, Finer NN, Etches PC (1983): Continuous monitoring of mixed venous oxygen in neonatal pulmonary hypertension. Crit Care Med 11:820–822.

162. Kisslo J (1982): Echo contrast in the detection of atrial septal defects. In Meltzer RS, Roelandt CJ (eds): Contrast Echocardiog-

raphy. Developments in Cardiovascular Medicine 15. The Hague, Martinus Nijhoff Publishers, pp 115–125.

163. Kitabatake A, Inoue M, Asao M, Masuyama T, Tanouchi J, Morita T, Mishima M, Uematsu M, Shimazu T, Hori M, Abe H (1983): Noninvasive evaluation of pulmonary hypertension by a pulsed Doppler technique. Circulation 68:302–309.

164. Klein KL, Scott WJ, Clark KE, Wilson JG (1981): Indomethacin-placental transfer, cytotoxicity, and teratology in the rat. Obstet Gynecol 141:448–452.

165. Korones SB, Eyal FG (1975): Successful treatment of "persistent fetal circulation" with tolazoline. Pediatr Res 9:367.

166. Khorsand J, Tennant R, Gillies C, Phillipps AF (1985): Congenital alveolar capillary dysplasia: A developmental vascular anomaly causing persistent pulmonary hypertension of the newborn. Pediatr Pathol 3:299–306.

167. Klesh KW, Murphy TF, Scher MS, Buchanan DE, Maxwell EP, Guthrie RD (1987): Cerebral infarction in persistent pulmonary hypertension of the newborn. Am J Dis Child 141:852–857.

168. Krahl VE (1969): Evidence of pulmonary arteriolar constriction and arteriovenous shunting in pulmonary hypoperfusion syndrome (respiratory distress syndrome of the newborn). Summary. Bibl Anat 10:220.

169. Kupferschmid C, Lang D (1983): The value of the foramen ovale in interatrial right-to-left shunt: Echocardiographic cineangiocardiographic and hemodynamic observations. Am J Cardiol 51:1489–1494.

170. Laloum D, Bonte JB, Kabilinsky G, Venezia R (1979): Hypoxemie refractaire chez le nouveau né: Traitement par la tolazoline. Arch Fr Pediatr 36:981–991.

171. Lang D, Wagonvoort CA, Kupferschmid C, Kleihauer E (1985): Cor triatriatum masked by primary pulmonary hypertension. Pediatr Cardiol 6:161–164.

172. Larsson LE, Ekstrom-Jodal B, Hjalmarson O (1982): The effect of chlorpromazine in severe hypoxia in newborn infants. Acta Paediatr Scand 71:399–402.

173. Leatham A (1958): Auscultation of the heart. Lancet 275(2):757–765.

174. Lees MH (1970): Cyanosis of the newborn. Recognition and clinical management. J Pediatr 77:484–498.

175. Lees MH, Sunderland CO (1981): Diseases of the cardiovascular system. In Behrman RE (ed): Neonatal Perinatal Medicine: Diseases of the Fetus and Infant. Philadelphia. JB Lippincott, p 572.

176. Levene MI, Wigglesworth JS, Desai R (1980): Pulmonary fat accumulation after intralipid infusion in the preterm infant. Lancet 2:815–818.

177. Levin DL (1978): Morphologic analysis of the pulmonary vascular bed in congenital left-sided diaphragmatic hernia. J Pediatr 92:805–809.

178. Levin DL (1979): Primary pulmonary hypoplasia (editorial). J Pediatr 95:550–551.

179. Levin DL, Cates L, Newfeld EA, Muster AJ, Paul MH (1975): Persistence of the fetal cardiopulmonary pathway: Survival of an infant after a prolonged course. Pediatr 56:58–64.

179a. Levin DL, Fixler DE, Morriss FC, Tyson J (1978): Morphological analysis of the pulmonary vascular bed in infants exposed in utero to prostaglandin synthetase inhibitors. J Pediatr 92:478–483.

180. Levin DL, Heymann MA, Kitterman JA, Gregory CA, Phibbs RH, Rudolph A (1976): Persistent pulmonary hypertension of the newborn infant. J Pediatr 89:626–630.

181. Levin DL, Hyman AI, Heymann MA, Rudolph AM (1978): Fetal hypertension and development of increased pulmonary vascular smooth muscle: A possible mechanism for persistent pulmonary hypertension of the newborn infant. J Pediatr 92:265–269.

182. Levin DL, Mills LJ, Parkey M (1979): Morphologic development of the pulmonary vascular bed in experimental coarctation of the aorta. Circulation 60:349–354.

183. Levin DL, Mills LJ, Weinberg AG (1979): Hemodynamic, pulmonary vascular, and myocardial abnormalities secondary to pharmacologic constriction of the fetal ductus arteriosus: A possible mechanism for persistent pulmonary hypertension and transient tricuspid insufficiency in the newborn infant. Circulation 60:360–364.

184. Levin DL, Weinberg AG, Perkin RM (1983): Pulmonary microthrombi syndrome in newborn infants with unresponsive persistent pulmonary hypertension. J Pediatr 102:299–303.

185. Levy RJ, Rosenthal A, Freed MD, Smith CD, Eraklis A, Nadas AS (1977): Persistent pulmonary hypertension in a newborn with congenital diaphragmatic hernia: Successful management with tolazoline. Pediatr 60:740–742.

186. Lin AE, Milley JR, Jaffe R, Medina J (1985): Familial persistent pulmonary hypertension (letter): J Pediatr 106:692–693.

187. Lind J (1977): Eleventh Edgar Mannheimer Lecture. Human fetal and neonatal circulation. Some structural and functional aspects. Eur J Cardiol 5:265–281.

188. Lind J, Stern L, Wegelius CE (1964): Human Fetal and Neonatal Circulation. Springfield, Charles C Thomas Publishers, p 49.

189. Lind J, Wegelius C (1952): Changes in the circulation at birth. Acta Pediatr 42:495–496.

189a. Ling J, Wegelius C (1954): Human fetal circulation: Changes in the cardiovascular system at birth and disturbance of postnatal closure of the foramen ovale and ductus arteriosus. Quant Biol 19:109–125.

190. Linday LA, Ehlers KH, O'Loughlin JE, LaGamma EF, Engle MA (1983): Noninvasive diagnosis of persistent fetal circulation versus congenital cardiovascular defects. Am J Cardiol 52:847–851.

191. Lister G (1985): Persistent pulmonary hypertension of the newborn. In Nelson NM (ed): Current Therapy in Neonatal-Perinatal Medicine 1985–1986. Toronto, BC Decker, pp 278–285.

191a. Lock JE, Fuhrman BP, Epstein ML, Rowe RD, Lucas RV Jr (1980): Pulmonary hypertension following neonatal shock. Ped Cardiol 1:109–115.

192. Long WA (1984): Structural cardiovascular abnormalities presenting as persistent pulmonary hypertension of the newborn. Clin Perinatol 11:601–626.

193. Long WA, Denfield S, Buck S, Covert R (in press): Congenital cardiomyopathies causing persistent pulmonary hypertension of the newborn syndrome. Clin Res.

194. Long WA, Lawson EE, Harned HS Jr, Henry GW (1984): Infradiaphragmatic total anomalous pulmonary venous drainage: New diagnostic, physiologic, and surgical considerations. Am J Perinatol 1:227–235.

194a. Long WA, Lawson EE, Harned HS Jr, Kraybill EN (1984): Pleural effusion in the first days of life: A prospective study. Am J Perinatol 1:190–194.

194b. Long WA, Lawson EE, Perry JR, Harned HS Jr, Henry GW (1985): Radionuclide diagnosis of infradiaphragmatic total anomalous pulmonary venous drainage. Pediatr Cardiol 6:69–76.

194c. Long WA, Rubin LJ (1987): Prostacyclin and PGE$_1$ and treatment of pulmonary hypertension. Am Rev Resp Dis 136:773–776.

195. Long WA, Schall SA, Henry GW (1984): Cerebral arteriovenous malformation presenting as persistent fetal circulation: Diagnosis by cross-sectional echocardiography. Am J Perinatol 1:236–241.

195a. Long WA, Sanders RL (1988): New treatment methods in neonatal respiratory distress syndrome: Replacement of surface active material. In Guthrie RB (ed): Neonatal Intensive Care. Clin Critical Care Med 13:21–56.

196. Lyrene RK, Philips JB (1984): Control of pulmonary vascular resistance in the fetus and newborn. Clin Perinatol 11:551–564.

197. Lyrene RK, Welch KA, Godoy G, Philips JA (1985): Alkalosis attentuates hypoxic pulmonary vasoconstriction in neonatal lambs. Pediatr Res 19:1268–1271.

198. Mahoney LT, Coryell KG, Lauer RM (1985): The newborn transitional circulation: A two-dimensional Doppler echocardiographic study. J Am Coll Cardiol 6:623–629.

199. Mammel MC, Einzig S, Kulik TJ, Thompson TR, Lock JE (1983): Pulmonary vascular effects of amrinone in conscious lambs. Pediatr Res 17:720–724.

200. Manchester D, Margolis HS, Sheldon RE (1976): Possible association between maternal indomethacin therapy and primary pulmonary hypertension of the newborn. Am J Obstet Gynecol 126:467–469.

201. Markestad T, Finne PH (1980): Effect of tolazoline in pulmonary hemorrhage in the newborn. Case report. Acta Paediatr Scand 69:425–426.

202. Martin TC, Bower RJ, Bell MJ (1982): Postoperative fetal circulation: POFC. J Pediatr Surg 17:558–562.

203. McIntosh N, Walters RO (1979): Effect of tolazoline in severe hyaline membrane disease. Arch Dis Child 54:105–110.

204. McKenzie S, Haworth SG (1981): Occlusion of peripheral pulmonary vascular bed in a baby with idiopathic persistent fetal circulation. Br Heart J 46:675–678.

205. McMahan HE (1948): Congenital alveolar dysplasia. Am J Pathol 24:919–930.

206. McMahon HE (1948): Congenital alveolar dysplasia. A developmental anomaly involving pulmonary alveoli. Pediatr 2:43–55.

207. Meijboum EJ, Cewitz MM, Wood DC, Fox WW (1982): Contrast echocardiography in persistent fetal circulation. In Meltzer RS, Roelandt CJ (eds): Contrast Echocardiography. Developments in Cardiovascular Medicine 15. The Hague, Martinus Nijhoff Publishers, pp 203–213.

208. Merten DF, Goetzman BW (1977): Persistence of the fetal circulation: A commentary. Am J Roentgenol 128:1067–1068.

209. Merten DF, Goetzman BW, Wennberg RP (1977): Persistent fetal circulation: An evolving clinical and radiographic concept of pulmonary hypertension of the newborn. Pediatr Radiol 6:74–80.

210. Milstein JM, Goetzman BW, Riemenschneider TA, Wennberg RP (1979): Increased systemic vascular resistance in neonates with pulmonary hypertension. Am J Cardiol 44:1159–1162.

210a. Mitchell SC (1957): The ductus arteriosus in the neonatal period. J Pediatr 51:12–17.

211. Mokrohisky ST, Levine RL, Blumhagen JD, Wesenberg RL, Simmons MA (1978): Low positioning of umbilical artery catheters increases associated complications in newborn infants. N Engl J Med 299:561–564.

212. Monin P, Dubrac C, Vert P, Morselli PL (1987): Treatment of persistent fetal circulation syndrome of the newborn. Comparison of different doses of tolazoline. Eur J Clin Pharm 31:569–573.

213. Moodie DS, Kleinberg P, Telander RL, Kaye MP, Feldt RH (1978): Tolazoline as adjuvant therapy for ill neonates with pulmonary hypoperfusion (letter). Chest 74:604–605.

214. Moodie DS, Telander RL, Kleinberg F, Feld RH (1978): Use of tolazoline in newborn infants with diaphragmatic hernia and severe cardiopulmonary disease. A preliminary report. J Thorac Cardiovasc Surg 75:725–729.

215. Morin FC, Vafai J, Finkelstein JN (1983): Hyperventilation decreases pulmonary vascular pressures in the newborn lamb (abstr). Pediatr Res 17:328A.

216. Morrow WR, Haas JE, Benjamin DR (1982): Nonbacterial endocardial thrombosis in neonates: Relationship to persistent fetal circulation. J Pediatr 100:117–122.

217. Moya FR, Perez A, Reece EA (1987): Severe fetomaternal hemorrhage. A report of four cases. J Reprod Med 32:243–246.

218. Mukhtar AL, Halliday HL (1982): Eisenmenger syndrome in pregnancy: A possible cause of neonatal polycythemia and persistent fetal circulation. Obstet Gynecol 60:651–652.

219. Mullaart RA, Daniels O, Hopman JCW, Krijgsman JB, Kollee LA, Rolteveel JJ, Stoelinga GB, Slouff IL, Thijssen HO (1982): Ultrasound detection of congenital arteriovenous aneurysm of the great cerebral vein of Galen. Eur J Pediatr 139:195–198.

220. Murphy JD, Aronovitz MJ, Reid LM (1986): Effects of chronic in utero hypoxia on the pulmonary vasculature of the newborn guinea pig. Pediatr Res 20:292–295.

221. Murphy JD, Meyer RA, Kaplan S (1985): Noninvasive evaluation of newborns with suspected congenital heart disease. Am J Dis Child 139:580–594.

222. Murphy JD, Vawter GF, Reid LM (1984): Pulmonary vascular disease in fatal meconium aspiration. J Pediatr 104:758–762.

223. Naeye RL, Schochat SJ, Whitman V, Maisels MJ (1976): Unsuspected pulmonary vascular abnormalities associated with diaphragmatic hernia. Pediatr 58:902–906.

224. Naulty CM, Weiss IP, Herer GR (1984): Sensorineural hearing loss in survivors of persistent fetal circulation (PFC) (abstr). Clin Res 32:918A.

225. Nelson RM, Bucciarelli RL, Eitzmann DV, Egan EA II, Gessner IH (1978): Serum creatinine phosphokinase MB fraction in newborns with transient tricuspid insufficiency. N Engl J Med 298:146–149.

226. Nielson HC, Riemenschneider TA, Jaffe RB (1976): Persistent transitional circulation. Roentgenographic findings in thirteen infants. Radiology 120:649–652.

227. Novelo S, Limon Lason R, Bouchard F (1950): Un nouveau syndrome avec cyanose congenitale: la persistence du canal arterial avec hypertension pulmonaire. Paris, ler Congres Mondial de Cardiolegie, 1950.

228. O'Connor JF, Shapiro JH, Ingall D (1968): Erythrocythemia as a

cause of respiratory distress syndrome in the newborn: Radiologic findings. Radiology 90:333–335.

228a. Peabody JL, Gregory GA, Willis MM, Tooley WH (1978): Transcutaneous oxygen tension in sick infants. Am Rev Resp Dis 118:83–87.

229. Peckham GJ, Fox WW (1978): Physiologic factors affecting pulmonary artery pressure in infants with persistent pulmonary hypertension. J Pediatr 93:1005–1010.

230. Pelet B, Godard C, Payot M, Pescia G (1982): Congenital neutropenia associated with phlebectasias and persistent fetal circulation. Helv Paediatr Acta 37:475–481.

231. Pellegrino PA, Milanesi O, Saia OS, Carollo C (1987): Congestive heart failure secondary to cerebral arterio–venous fistula. Child Nerv Syst 3:141–144.

232. Pereira GR, Fox WW, Stanley CA, Baker L, Schwartz JC (1980): Decreased oxygenation and hyperlipemia during intravenous fat infusions in premature infants. Pediatr 66:26–30.

233. Perkin RM, Anas NG (1984): Pulmonary hypertension in pediatric patients. J Pediatr 105:511–522.

234. Perkin RM, Levin DL, Clark R (1980): Serum salicylate levels and right-to-left ductus shunts in newborn infants with persistent pulmonary hypertension. J Pediatr 96:721–726.

235. Philips JB III, Lyrene RK, McDevitt M, Perlis W, Satterwhite C, Cassady G (1983): Prostaglandin D₂ inhibits hypoxic pulmonary vasoconstriction in neonatal lambs. J Appl Physiol: Respirat Environ Exercise Physiol 54:1585–1589.

236. Philips JB III, Lyrene RK (1983): Persistent pulmonary hypertension and prostaglandin D₂. In Brewer GJ (ed): Orphan Drugs and Orphan Diseases: Clinical Realities and Public Policy. New York, Alan R Liss, Inc, pp 21–32.

237. Philips JB III, Lyrene RK (1984): Prostaglandins, related compounds, and the perinatal pulmonary circulation. Clin Perinatol 11:565–579.

238. Philips JB III (1984): Prostaglandins and related compounds in the perinatal pulmonary circulation. Pediatr Pharmacol 4:129–142.

239. Pieroni DR, Valdes-Cruz LM (1982): Atrial right-to-left shunts in infants with respiratory and cardiac distress but without congenital heart disease. Pediatr Cardiol 2:1–5.

240. Prec KJ, Cassels DE (1955): Dye dilution curves and cardiac output in newborn infants. Circulation 51:781–798.

241. Purohit DM, Pai S, Levkoff AH (1978): Effect of tolazoline on persistent hypoxemia in neonatal respiratory distress. Crit Care Med 6:14–18.

241a. Radford DJ (1979): Persistent fetal circulation: Two cases with myocardial dysfunction and severe acidosis. Med J Aust 1:27–29.

242. Rao DB, Rao SS, Karan S (1979): Persistent foetal circulation syndrome. Indian Pediatr 16:363–365.

243. Rao PS, Marino BL, Robertson AF III (1978): Usefulness of continuous positive airway pressure in differential diagnosis of cardiac from pulmonary cyanosis in newborn infants. Arch Dis Child 53:456–460.

244. Reece EA, Moya F, Yazigi R, Holford T, Duncan C, Ehrenkranz RA (1987): Persistent pulmonary hypertension: Assessment of perinatal risk factors. Obstet Gynecol 70:696–700.

245. Reid L (1982): The development of the pulmonary circulation. In Peckham GJ, Heymann MA (eds): Cardiovascular Sequelae of Asphyxia in the Newborn. Report of Eighty-third Ross Conference on Pediatric Research, Ross Laboratories, Columbia, Ohio, p 7.

246. Riemenschneider TA, Nielsen HC, Ruttenberg HD, Jaffe RB (1976): Disturbances of the transitional circulation: Spectrum of pulmonary hypertension and myocardial dysfunction. J Pediatr 89:622–625.

247. Riggs T, Hirschfeld S, Fanaroff A, Liebman J, Fletcher B, Meyer R, Bormuth C (1977): Persistence of fetal circulation syndrome: An echocardiographic study. J Pediatr 91:626–631.

248. Roberton NRC, Hallidie-Smith KA, Davis JA (1967): Severe respiratory distress syndrome mimicking cyanotic heart disease in term babies. Lancet 2:1108–1110.

249. Rowe RD (1959): Clinical observation of transitional circulations. In Oliver TK (ed): Adaptation to Extrauterine Life. Report of Thirty-first Ross Conference on Pediatric Research, Ross Laboratories, Columbus, Ohio, pp 33–39.

250. Rowe RD (1977): Abnormal pulmonary vasoconstriction in the newborn. Pediatrics 59:318–321.

251. Rowe RD, Hoffman T (1972): Transient myocardial ischemia of the newborn infant: A form of severe cardiorespiratory distress in full-term infants. J Pediatr 81:243–250.

252. Rowe RD, James LS (1957): The normal pulmonary arterial pressure during the first year of life. J Pediatr 51:1–4.

253. Rowe RD, Sinclair JD, Kerr AR, Gage PW (1964): Ductal flow and mitral regurgitation during changes in oxygenation in newborn swine. J Appl Physiol 19:1159–1163.

254. Rubatelli FF, Chiazzi ML, Zanardon V, Cantarutti F (1979): Effect on neonate of maternal treatment with indomethacin. J Pediatr 4:161.

255. Rudolph AM (1970): Changes in the circulation after birth: Their importance in congenital heart disease. Circulation 41:343–359.

256. Rudolph AM (1979): Fetal and neonatal pulmonary circulation. Ann Rev Physiol 41:383–395.

257. Rudolph AM (1980): High pulmonary vascular resistance after birth. I Pathophysiologic considerations and etiologic classification. Clin Pediatr 19:585–590.

258. Rudolph AM (1981): The effects of nonsteroidal antiinflammatory compounds on fetal circulation and pulmonary function. Obstet Gynecol 58:635–675.

259. Rudolph AM (1981): Effects of aspirin and acetaminophen in pregnancy and in the newborn. Arch Intern Med 141:358–363.

260. Rudolph AM, Drorbaugh JE, Auld PAM, Rudolph AJ, Nadas AS, Smith CA, Hubbell JP (1961): Studies on the circulation in the neonatal period. The circulation in respiratory distress syndrome. Pediatrics 27:551–556.

261. Rudolph AM, Paul MH, Sommer LS, Nadas AS (1958): Effects of tolazoline hydrochloride (priscoline) on circulatory dynamics of patients with pulmonary hypertension. Am Heart J 55:424–432.

262. Rudolph AM, Yuan S (1966): Responses of the pulmonary vasculature to hypoxia and H⁺ ion concentration changes. J Clin Invest 45:399–411.

263. Sahn DJ, Allen HD, George W, Mason M, Goldberg SJ (1977): The utility of contrast echocardiographic techniques in the care of critically ill infants with cardiac and pulmonary disease. Circulation 56:959–968.

264. Sahn DJ, Friedman WF (1973): Difficulties in distinguishing cardiac from pulmonary disease in the newborn. Pediatr Clin North Am 20:293–301.

265. Sankaran K, Ninan A, Bingham W (1985): Persistent fetal circulation in neonates. In Sandor GS, McNab AJ, Rastogi RB (eds): Persistent Fetal Circulation: Etiology, Clinical Aspects, and Therapy. Mt. Kisco, Futura Media Services pp 198–199.

266. Sapire DW, Casta D (1982): Aneurysmal bulging of the interatrial septum in a newborn infant with arteriovenous fistula and congestive heart failure. Chest 82:649–651.

267. Sapire DW, Casta D, Donner HM (1979): Dilatation of the descending aorta: A radiologic and echocardiographic diagnostic sign in arteriovenous malformation in neonates and young infants. Am J Cardiol 44:493–499.

268. Schlueter MA, Tooley WH (1974): Right-to-left shunt through the ductus arteriosus in newborn infants (abstract). Pediatr Res 8:354.

269. Schreiber MD, Heymann MA, Soifer SJ (1986): Increased arterial pH, not decreased PaCO₂, attenuates hypoxia-induced pulmonary vasoconstriction in newborn lambs. Pediatr Res 20:113–117.

270. Segall ML, Goetzman BW, Schick JB (1980): Thrombocytopenia and pulmonary hypertension in the perinatal aspiration syndromes. J Pediatr 96:927–930.

271. Sell EJ, Gaines JA, Gluckman C, Williams E (1985): Persistent fetal circulation: Neurodevelopmental outcome. Am J Dis Child 139:25–28.

272. Sepkowitz S (1985): Mortality of persistent pulmonary hypertension of the newborn (letter). Am J Dis Child 139:115–116.

273. Setzer E, Ermocilla R, Tomkin I, John E, Sansa M, Cassady G (1980): Papillary muscle necrosis in a neonatal autopsy population: Incidence and associated clinical manifestations. J Pediatr 96:289–294.

274. Shankaran S, Farooki ZQ, Desai R (1982): B–hemolytic streptococcal infection appearing as persistent fetal circulation. Am J Dis Child 136:725–727.

275. Shannon DC, Lusser M, Goldblatt A (1972): The cyanotic infant—heart disease or lung disease? N Engl J Med 287:951–953.

276. Shochat SJ, Naeye RL, Ford WDA, Whitman V, Maisels MJ

(1979): Congenital diaphragmatic hernia: New concept in management. Ann Surg 190:332–341.

277. Shohet I, Reichman B, Schibi G, Brish M (1984): Familial persistent pulmonary hypertension. Arch Dis Child 59:783–785.

278. Shutack JG, Moomjian AS, Wagner HR, Peckham GJ, Fox WW (1979): Severe obstructive airway disease associated with pulmonary artery hypertension in the neonate (abstract). Pediatr Res 13:541.

279. Siassi B, Goldberg SJ, Emmanouilides GC, Higashina SM, Lewis E (1971): Persistent pulmonary vascular obstruction in newborn infants. J Pediatr 78:610–615.

280. Sivakoff M, Nouri S (1982): Diagnosis of vein of Galen arteriovenous malformation by two-dimensional ultrasound and pulsed Doppler method. Pediatrics 69:84–86.

280a. Skidmore MB, Shennan AT, Hoslans EM (1985): Tolazoline in the treatment of persistent fetal circulation. In Sandor GS, McNab AJ, Rastogi RB (eds): Persistent Fetal Circulation: Etiology, Clinical Aspects, and Therapy. Mt. Kisco, Futura Media Services pp 189–193.

281. Slack MR, Desai NS, Cunningham MD (1981): Tolazoline: Limited efficacy in pulmonary vaso-reactive hypoxemia (abstract). Pediatr Res 15:681.

282. Smallhorn JF, Isukawa T, Benson L, Freedam RM (1984): Non-invasive recognition of functional pulmonary atresia by echocardiography. Am J Cardiol 54:925–926.

283. Sneed RC (1972): Total anomalous pulmonary venous return: Diagnosis by umbilical vessel catheterization. South Med J 65:1145–1146.

284. Snider AR, Soifer SJ, Silverman NH (1981): Detection of intracranial arteriovenous fistula by two-dimensional ultrasonography. Circulation 63:1179–1185.

285. Soifer SJ, Kaslow D, Roman C, Heymann MA (1987): Umbilical cord compression produces pulmonary hypertension in newborn lambs: A model to study the pathophysiology of persistent pulmonary hypertension in the newborn. J Dev Physiol 9:239–252.

285a. Soifer SJ, Clyman RI, Heymann MA (1985): Prostaglandin D$_2$ does not lower pulmonary arterial pressure or improve oxygenation in infants with persistent pulmonary hypertension syndrome (PPHN) (abstract). Pediatr Res 19:365A.

286. Soifer SJ, Morin FC III, Heymann MA (1982): Prostaglandin D$_2$ reverses induced pulmonary hypertension in the newborn lamb. J Pediatr 100:458–463.

287. Sosulski R, Fox WW (1985): Transition phase during hyperventilation therapy for persistent pulmonary hypertension of the neonate. Crit Care Med 13:715–719.

288. Southall DP, Shinebourne EA (1980): Persistent fetal circulation and sudden infant death syndrome (letter). Lancet 2:1083.

289. Spach MS, Serwer GS, Anderson PAW, Canent RV Jr, Levin AR (1980): Pulsatile aortopulmonary pressure-flow dynamics of patent ductus arteriosus in patients with various hemodynamic states. Circulation 61:110–123.

290. Stahlman M (1964): Treatment of cardiovascular diseases of the newborn. Pediatr Clin North Am 11:363–400.

290a. Stahlman M, Shepard FM, Young WC, Gray J, Blankenship W (1965): Assessment of cardiovascular status of infants with hyaline membrane disease. In Cassels D (ed): The Heart and Circulation in the Newborn and Infant. New York, Grune & Stratton, pp 121–129.

291. Stahlman M, Blankenship WJ, Shepard KM, Gray J, Young WC, Malan AF (1972): Circulatory studies in clinical hyaline membrane disease. Biol Neonate 20:300–320.

292. St. John Sutton MG, Meyer RA (1983): Left ventricular function in persistent pulmonary hypertension of the newborn. Computer analysis of the echocardiogram. Br Heart J 50:540–549.

293. Stanbridge R deL, Westaby S, Smallhorn J (1983): Intracranial arteriovenous malformation with aneurysm of the vein of Galen as cause of heart failure in infancy: Echocardiographic diagnosis and results of treatment. Br Heart J 49:157–162.

294. Stenmark KR, James SL, Voelkel NF, Toews WH, Reeves JT, Murphy RC (1983): Leukotriene C$_4$ and D$_4$ in neonates with hypoxemia and pulmonary hypertension. N Engl J Med 309:77–80.

295. Stern L, Beaudry PH (1965): Use of priscoline in hypoperfusion (hyaline membrane) syndrome (letter). Pediatrics 36:662–663.

296. Stevens DC, Schreiner RL, Bull MJ, Bryson CQ, Lemons JA, Gresham EL, Grosfeld JL, Weber TR (1980): An analysis of tolazoline therapy in the critically-ill neonate. J Pediatr Surg 15:964–970.

297. Stevenson DK, Kasting DS, Darnall RA, Ariagno RL, Johnson JD, Malachowski N, Beets CL, Sunshine P (1979): Refractory hypoxemia associated with neonatal pulmonary disease: The use and limitations of tolazoline. J Pediatr 95:595–599.

298. Stevenson JG, Kawabori I, Guntheroth WG (1979): Noninvasive detection of pulmonary hypertension in patent ductus arteriosus by pulsed Doppler echocardiography. Circulation 60:355–359.

299. Stolar CJ, Dillon PW, Altman RP (1985): Management of the infant with congenital diaphragmatic hernia (CDH) and persistent pulmonary hypertension (PPHN). Jpn J Surg 15:438–442.

299a. Strang LB (1966): The pulmonary circulation in the respiratory distress syndrome. Pediatr Clin North Am 13:693–701.

299b. Strang LB, MacLeigh MH (1961): Ventilatory failure and right to left shunts in newborn infants with respiratory distress. Pediatrics 28:17–27.

300. Strauss A, Modanlou HD, Gyepes M, Wittner R (1982): Congenital heart disease and respiratory distress syndrome. Am J Dis Child 136:934–936.

301. Stringel G, Peterson R, Teixeira O (1985): Idiopathic post-operative pulmonary hypertension in the newborn. Can J Cardiol 1:181–184.

302. Sumner E, Frank JD (1981): Tolazoline in the treatment of congenital diaphragmatic hernias. Arch Dis Child 56:350–353.

303. Swischuk LE, Richardson CJ, Nichols MM, Ingman MJ (1979): Primary pulmonary hypoplasia in the neonate. J Pediatr 95:573–577.

304. Tahti E, Tisala R, Lind J (1964): Roentgenologic observations on the lung vascularity in early and late clamped babies. Ann Paediatr Fenn 14:94.

305. Teisberg P, Hognestad J (1973): Primary pulmonary hypertension in infancy. Acta Paediatr Scand 62:69–72.

306. Tibbits PA, Oetgen WJ, Potter BM, Chandra RS, Avery GB, Perry LW, Scott LP (1981): Interruption of aortic arch masquerading as persistent fetal circulation with definitive diagnosis by two-dimensional echocardiography. Am Heart J 102:936–938.

307. Tiefenbrunn LJ, Riemenschneider TA (1986): Persistent pulmonary hypertension of the newborn. Am Heart J 111:564–572.

307a. Tooley WH, Stanger P (1972): The blue baby—circulation, ventilation, or both? (editorial) N Engl J Med 287:329–294.

308. Truog WE, Fousner JH, Baker DL (1980): Association of hemorrhagic disease and the syndrome of persistent fetal circulation with the fetal hydantoin syndrome. J Pediatr 96:112–114.

309. Tsang R, Chen I, Hayes W, Atkinson W, Atherton H, Edwards N (1974): Neonatal hypocalcemia in infants with birth asphyxia. J Pediatr 84:428–433.

310. Tudehope DI (1979): Persistent pulmonary hypertension of the newborn. Med J Austr 1:13–15.

311. Tynan M, Behrendt D, Urquhart W, Graham GR (1974): Portal vein catheterization and selective angiography in diagnosis of total anomalous venous connexion. Br Heart J 36:1155–1159.

312. Vacanti JP, Crone RK (1983): Chronic anesthesia reduces pulmonary artery pressure in newborns with persistent fetal circulation (abstract). Pediatr Res 17:339A.

313. Valdes-Cruz LM, Dudell GG, Ferrara A (1981): Utility of M–mode echocardiography for early identification of infants with persistent pulmonary hypertension of the newborn. Pediatr 68:515–525.

314. Vesselinova-Jenkins CK (1980): Model of persistent fetal circulation and sudden infant death syndrome (SIDS): Lancet 2:831–834.

315. Vitarelli A, Scapato A, Sanguigna V, Cominiti MC (1986): Evaluation of total anomalous pulmonary venous drainage with cross-sectional colour-flow Doppler echocardiography. Eur Heart J 7:190–195.

316. Von Euler US, Liljestrand G (1946): Observations on the pulmonary arterial blood pressure in the cat. Acta Physiol Scand 12:301–320.

317. Wagenvoort CA (1986): Misalignment of lung vessels: A syndrome causing persistent neonatal pulmonary hypertension. Hum Pathol 17:727–730.

318. Walsh SZ, Lind J (1970): The dynamics of the fetal heart and circulation and its alteration at birth. In Stave U (ed): Physiology of the Perinatal Period: Functional and Biochemical Development in Mammals. Norwalk, Appleton-Century-Crofts, pp 141–208.

319. Ward RM (1984): Pharmacology of tolazoline. Clin Perinatol 11:703–713.

320. Ward RM, Daniel CH, Kending JW, Wood MA (1986): Oliguria and tolazoline pharmacokinetics in the newborn. Pediatrics 77:307–315.
321. Watchko JR (1985): Persistent pulmonary hypertension in a very low birthweight preterm infant. Clin Pediatr 24:592–595.
322. Watchko J, Bifano EM, Bergstrom WH (1984): Effect of hyperventilation on total calcium, ionized calcium, and serum phosphorus in neonates. Crit Care Med 12:1055–1056.
323. Watson DG, Smith HH, Brann AW Jr (1976): Arteriovenous malformation of the vein of Galen: Treatment in a neonate. Am J Dis Child 130:520–525.
324. Welch K, Lyrene R, Dew A, Philips J (1983): Age-related vascular effects of prostaglandin D_2 (PGD_2) (abstract). Clin Res 31:917A.
325. Welch KA, Godoy G, Dew A, Gray BM, Lyrene RK, Philips JB III (1984): Pulmonary hypertension following bolus infusions of pneumococci, other gram+ bacteria, and zymosan (abstract). Circulation 70:425.
326. Weller MH, Kutzenstein AA (1976): Radiologic findings in Group B streptococcccal sepsis. Radiology 118:385–387.
327. Wiener ES (1982): Congenital posterolateral diaphragmatic hernia: New dimensions in management. Surgery 92:670–681.
328. Wilkinson AR, Aynsley-Green A, Mitchell MD (1979): Persistent pulmonary hypertension and abnormal prostaglandin E levels in preterm infants after maternal treatment with naproxen. Arch Dis Child 54:942–945.
329. Wille L, Ulmer HE, Obladen M (1981): Persistence of fetal circulation in the newborn. J Perinatal Med 9:106–109.
330. Wilson HD, Thomas TP, Gallen WJ (1983): Differentiating persistent fetal circulation (PFC) from obstructed total anomalous pulmonary venous return (OTAPVR) by Doppler-echo analysis of foramen ovale (FO) flow pattern (abstr). Pediatr Res 17:125A.
331. Wood P (1958): The Eisenmenger syndrome: Or pulmonary hypertension with reversed central shunt. Br Med J 2:755–762.
332. Wung JT, James LS, Kilchevsky EM, James E (1985): Management of infants with severe respiratory failure and persistence of the fetal circulation, without hyperventilation. Pediatrics 76:488–494.
333. Yabek SM (1984): Neonatal cyanosis: Reappraisal of response to 100 per cent oxygen breathing. Am J Dis Child 138:880–884.
334. Yeh TF, Lilien LD (1981): Altered lung mechanics in neonates with persistent fetal circulation syndrome. Crit Care Med 9:83–84.
335. Yip WC, Ho TF, Tay JS, Wong HB (1985): Transcutaneous estimation of oxygen tension in unusual clinical situations. Ann Acad Med Singapore 14:422–426.

52 VASCULAR PATHOLOGY OF PPHNS

Marlene Rabinovitch

HISTORICAL PERSPECTIVE

Although different terminology was previously used, persistent pulmonary hypertension of the newborn syndrome (PPHNS) was recognized with increasing frequency following the report by Gersony and coworkers in 1969.[15] In 1971, Siassi and associates[54] reported hypertrophy of the medial muscular coat of the pulmonary arteries in one of three infants who died of PPHNS. In quantitative studies by Haworth and Reid[20] and by Murphy and colleagues,[36,37] the pulmonary vascular pathology of PPHNS was more consistently identified. In this chapter the varied nature of the pulmonary vascular changes associated with different disorders that have in common the physiology of PPHNS is described. There are essentially three different types of pulmonary vascular abnormalities in PPHNS: (1) those that accompany underdevelopment of the lung, (2) those that are associated with in utero maldevelopment of pulmonary vessels, and (3) those that represent maladaptation of the pulmonary arteries to postnatal life (Fig. 52–1). Recent studies have provided new insights into the mechanisms responsible for these structural changes in PPHNS, and future directions of investigation should ultimately lead to more successful therapeutic approaches.

PULMONARY VASCULAR PATHOLOGY

Underdevelopment of the Pulmonary Vascular Bed

Clinical Studies

Congenital diaphragmatic hernia is an example of a condition associated with underdevelopment of the pulmonary vascular bed[4,5,13,28] (Fig. 52–2). Peripheral pulmonary arteries in congenital diaphragmatic hernia are reduced in proportion to the diminished lung volume and the decrease in total alveolar number. Both reduced vascular cross-sectional area as well as severe hypoxia and hypercarbia (which result from the decreased surface area for gas exchange) cause increased resistance to pulmonary blood flow and account for the pulmonary hypertension and right-to-left shunting at birth. Moreover, in addition to being few in number, pulmonary arteries in congenital diaphragmatic hernia are small and have increased muscularity. There is abnormal "extension" of muscle into vessels accompanying intra-acinar airways, even to the level of alveolar ducts and walls. Although the severity of the increased muscularization may determine whether there is a "honeymoon period" following surgical correction of the diaphragmatic hernia,[13] the degree of hypoplasia of the pulmonary vascular bed probably determines whether pulmonary hypertension will either reverse after surgery and the institution of vasodilator therapy[5] or be irreversible.

In studies from the University of Toronto by Bohn and colleagues,[4,5] survival following repair of congenital diaphragmatic hernia was predictable based on the preoperative or postoperative product of PCO_2 respiratory rate and mean airway pressure (Fig. 52–3). A trial of high frequency oscillatory ventilation was effective in decreasing PCO_2, but PO_2 was only transiently improved. Postmortem analysis of the lung in seven consecutive infants revealed severe lung hypoplasia. The ratio of alveoli to arteries was normal, but the number of alveoli was reduced to less than one third normal.[25] The absolute number of pulmonary arteries was therefore severely decreased. Medial hypertrophy and extension of muscle into normally nonmuscular arteries were mild compared with findings in infants with idiopathic PPHNS but were similar to those seen in infants with left-sided obstructive congenital heart lesions in which there is potential for reversal (Fig. 52–4). Studies of extracorporeal membrane oxygenator use after repair of congenital diaphragmatic hernia would suggest that some infants with severe hypoplasia of the lung may still survive, probably because absence of barotrauma for a few days in the early postoperative period may allow postnatal proliferation of alveoli. Results with the extracorporeal membrane oxygenator in infants with PPHNS are encouraging[3] but must be interpreted with some caution since the criteria used for selection may not consistently exclude infants who might have survived with more conventional therapy.

Other causes of PPHNS with both lung and vascular hypoplasia and increased pulmonary vascular muscularity include renal agenesis or dysplasia,[24] rhesus isoimmunization,[7] prematurity,[48] asphyxiating thoracic dystrophy, absence of the phrenic nerve,[17] and, at least experimentally, amniocentesis.[23]

Experimental Studies

Clearly, the factors that govern prenatal and postnatal alveolar development must be elucidated before effective methods of inducing alveolar growth can be proposed.

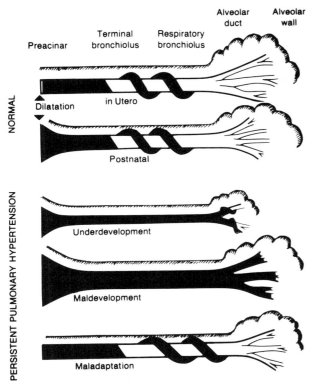

Figure 52–1. Schema showing normal (top) and abnormal (bottom) pulmonary arterial transition from fetal to neonatal circulation. When the lung is underdeveloped, the vascular bed is hypoplastic and abnormally muscular; when it is maldeveloped, the arteries are abnormally muscular; and when it is maladapted, it has not dilated appropriately at birth. (Reproduced with permission from Rabinovitch M [1985]: Morphology of the developing pulmonary bed: Pharmacologic implications. Pediatr Pharmacol 5:31–48.)

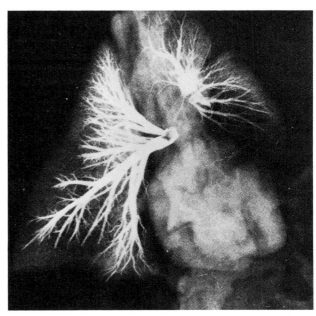

Figure 52–2. Postmortem pulmonary arteriograms in an infant with congenital diaphragmatic hernia; right lung is small, the left lung much smaller; arteries in both lungs are reduced in size and number. (Reproduced with permission of Kitigawa M et al [1971]: Lung hypoplasia in congenital diaphragmatic hernia: A quantitative study of airway artery and alveolar development. Br J Surg 51:342–345.)

have resulted from release of a protease during the early inflammatory reaction.

Maladaptation of the Pulmonary Vascular Bed

Clinical Studies

In maladaptation, postnatal dilatation of small muscular (< 250 μm) pulmonary arteries and recruitment of

Experimental studies in puppies[11] reveal that pneumonectomy increases the rate of alveolar growth in the remaining lung initially, but the final number of alveoli is normal. In studies in which congenital diaphragmatic hernia was created in fetal lambs, alveolar growth after repair is increased, but follow-up studies will be necessary to show whether a normal number of alveoli is ultimately achieved.[26] In studies in infant rats, Wilson and coworkers[64] observed that even relatively short periods of postnatal hyperoxic exposure result in a severe impairment in alveolar development that persists into adult life (Fig. 52–5). Hyperoxia decreases the ratio of arteries to alveoli during exposure, but the ratio becomes normal during recovery in room air. Nevertheless, the number of pulmonary arteries remains low after hyperoxia because of the reduction in absolute alveolar number. Moreover, the pulmonary arteries that remain after hyperoxia show increased muscularization. Studies by Collins and coworkers[8,9] suggest that connective tissue synthesis in the fetal rat lung is impaired in conditions that result in lung hypoplasia, such as smoking and amniocentesis. In studies by Todd (Todorovich-Hunter) and associates,[60] the arrest in lung development in newborn rats (Fig. 52–6) caused by the toxin monocrotaline may

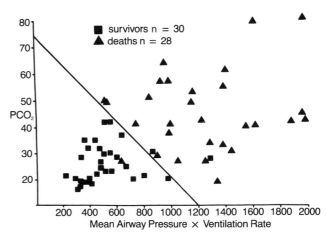

Figure 52–3. Graph comparing ventilatory parameters (PCO_2) and mean airway pressure times respiratory rate in survivors (■) and nonsurvivors (▲) with congenital diaphragmatic hernia.

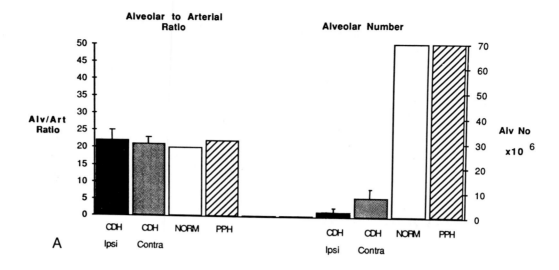

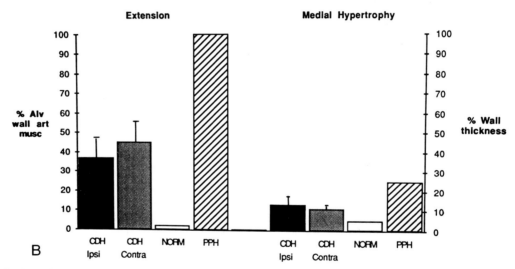

Figure 52–4. *A*, Graph depicting alveolar arterial ratio and total alveolar number in ipsilateral (ipsi) and contralateral (contra) lung from post-mortem analysis of the lung in nonsurvivors with congenital diaphragmatic hernia[14] compared with published normal values[26] and those in patients with idiopathic persistent pulmonary hypertension of the newborn syndrome.[21] Ratios are normal in patients with congenital diaphragmatic hernia (both lungs), but total alveolar number is greatly reduced. *B*, Extension of muscle as represented by alveolar wall arteries fully muscularized and medial wall thickness depicted by percentage wall thickness in arteries 100 to 300 μm in patients with congenital diaphragmatic hernia[14] compared with normals published (Haworth SG, Hislop AA: Pulmonary vascular development: normal values of peripheral vascular structure. Am J Cardiol 52:578–583, 1983) and compared with values in patients with idiopathic persistent pulmonary hypertension of the newborn syndrome.[21] Values in patients with congenital diaphragmatic hernia are abnormally elevated but not as severely as those in patients with idiopathic persistent pulmonary hypertension of the newborn syndrome. CDH = congenital diaphragmatic hernia; NORM = normal infants; PPH = idiopathic persistent pulmonary hypertension of the newborn syndrome.

peripheral pulmonary vessels may not occur because of perinatal stresses, such as hemorrhage, hypoglycemia, polycythemia, aspiration, hypoxia, or left ventricular dysfunction.[32,39,47,49] Since, at least initially, postnatal persistence of vasoconstriction rather than structural changes is responsible for the pulmonary hypertension, treatment of the underlying cause and administration of effective pulmonary vasodilators should be beneficial. However, some cases of maladaptation may reflect inadequacy of the cellular mechanisms that govern the normal fall in pulmonary vascular resistance.

Experimental Studies

When Cassin and colleagues[6] showed that prostaglandin D_2 was a pulmonary vasodilator in fetal lambs but a pulmonary vasoconstrictor in 1-week old lambs, the concept was proposed that changes in the response of the pulmonary vascular bed to certain prostaglandins at the time of birth could account for the normal fall in pulmonary vascular resistance. However, the search for a prostaglandin that is a pulmonary vasoconstrictor in utero and a pulmonary vasodilator after birth has not been fruitful.

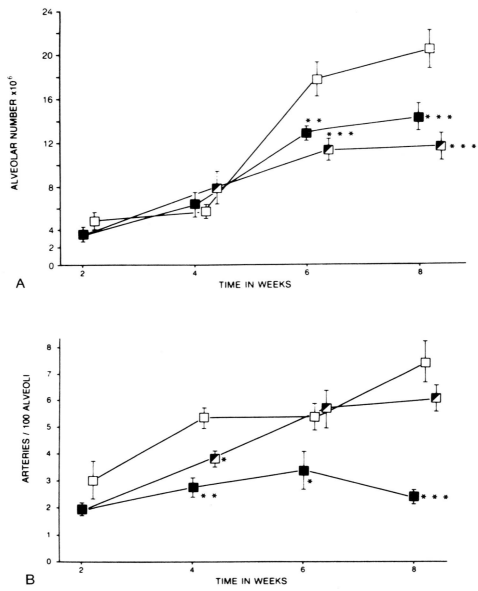

Figure 52–5. *A*, Graph depicting total alveolar number in rats continually exposed to hyperoxia (FIO$_2$ 0.8 × 8 weeks) (■) and in rats exposed for 2 weeks and then allowed to recover for the remaining 6 weeks (◪). Compared with normal alveolar development (□), there is a decrease in total alveolar number even in rats exposed to hyperoxia for a relatively short period. *B*, The number of arteries relative to the number of alveoli is reduced in rats continually exposed to hyperoxia (■), but in rats only exposed for 2 weeks (◪) the reduction is less and catches up to control (□) after removal from hyperoxia. However, since total alveolar number remains low, absolute arterial number is also low. (Reproduced with permission of Wilson WL et al [1985]: Hyperoxia-induced pulmonary vascular and lung abnormalities in young rats and potential for recovery. Pediatr Res 19:1059–1067.)

Stenmark and associates[58] reported high leukotriene levels in the lavage fluid of infants with PPHNS and suggested that these powerful vasoconstrictors may cause this condition. However, there is increasing evidence that leukotrienes may function as vasoconstrictors via release of thromboxane.[59]

The role of the vasoactive substances produced by neuroepithelial bodies (i.e., serotonin and bombesin) in maintaining fetal pulmonary vascular resistance has not

been clarified.[10] The neuroepithelial bodies are present in highest concentration in fetal airways and decrease postnatally (Fig. 52–7). Studies have shown that factors as yet incompletely characterized are produced by endothelial cells and affect smooth muscle contraction and dilatation[12,61]; as a result, a whole new avenue of investigation has opened. It is intriguing to speculate that endothelial injury or dysfunction produced by an insult at birth may alter the balance in favor of the vasoconstrictor agents.

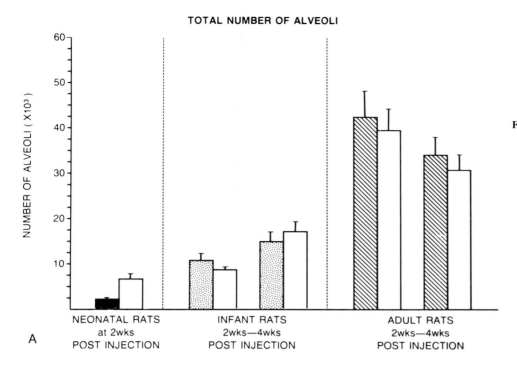

TOTAL NUMBER OF ALVEOLI

Figure 52–6. *A*, Graph of the effects of the toxin monocrotaline given to rats at 3 (neonate) (■), 8 (infant) (□), and 48 days (adult) (▨) and studied 2 to 4 weeks later. Values are compared with those in age-matched controls (□). Neonatal rats have a severe reduction in total alveolar number and do not survive for more than 2 weeks following injection.

Maldevelopment of the Pulmonary Vascular Bed

Clinical Studies

Maldevelopment of the pulmonary vascular bed can result from "arrest in development" in utero,[16] from congenital cardiac defects,[21,22] or from an unexplained intrauterine disorder that affects the pulmonary arteries[36] or veins.[62] Goldstein and colleagues[16] described an infant who presented with PPHNS and died on the first day of life. At postmortem examination, the lung vasculature was analyzed (Fig. 52–8) and there appeared to have been an "arrest in development" of the pulmonary vascular bed around the fifth week of gestation. Primitive pulmonary arteries were observed supplying the upper poles of the lung, and systemic (primitive dorsal intersegmental) arteries supplied the lower poles. Histologic examination of the lung showed airways unaccompanied by arteries.

Congenital cardiac defects that produce pulmonary venous hypertension include certain types of total anomalous pulmonary venous drainage,[22] coarctation of the aorta, aortic stenosis, mitral stenosis of varying severity, and the hypoplastic left-heart syndrome[21] and will result in structural changes in the pulmonary arteries and veins that develop in utero and are present at birth (Fig. 52–9). These pulmonary vascular changes vary in severity depending on the degree of left-sided obstruction[21] and consist of abnormal muscularization of both large and small pulmonary veins, which is a particularly prominent feature in infants with obstructed total anomalous pulmonary venous drainage.[22] On the arterial side, there is increased extension of muscle into normally nonmuscular peripheral pulmonary

arteries, and medial hypertrophy of muscular pulmonary arteries. The latter finding may reflect failure of the medial muscular coat to regress postnatally. The number of peripheral pulmonary arteries in infants with pulmonary venous hypertension is normal or even increased.

The excessive muscularity of the pulmonary vascular bed (in such infants) is potentially reversible if repair of the congenital heart lesion relieves the source of the pulmonary hypertension. However, excessive muscularity may progress if the defect is incompletely corrected and the elevation in pulmonary artery pressure persists, as has been observed in infants with total anomalous pulmonary venous drainage.[63] Excessive muscularity of pulmonary arteries and veins undoubtedly contributes to the episodes of severe pulmonary hypertension observed in the postoperative period following repair of this lesion that cause increased morbidity and mortality.[27,43] This problem of excessive muscularity of the pulmonary vascular bed is magnified when the degree of left-sided obstruction is severe and the margin for operative success is small; the Norwood procedure for correction of hypoplastic left-heart syndrome is an example.[38] Increased muscularity of the pulmonary vascular bed would decrease the compliance of the pulmonary circulation and also impair the ability of the newborn pulmonary circulation to accept volume loads or to respond to pharmacologic agents given to support the myocardium.

A third group of neonates manifest PPHNS with maldevelopment of the pulmonary arteries or veins,[62] but the cause is unexplained. Maternal ingestion of prostaglandin synthetase inhibitors such as aspirin or indomethacin has been suggested,[29,33] but this association is proably true for only a few susceptible neonates. Infants with "idiopathic"

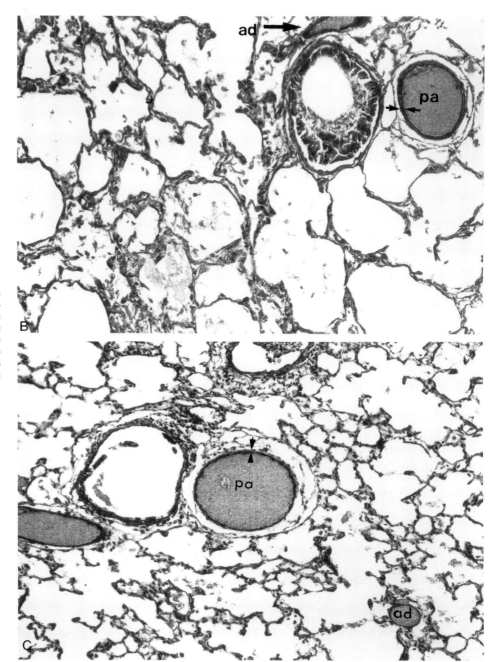

Figure 52–6 *Continued. B* and *C,* Photomicrographs comparing alveoli in neonatal rats 2 days after monocrotaline injection, *B,* and in controls, *C.* Note the marked decrease in alveoli in the former. pa = preacinar artery; ad = alveolar duct artery; small arrows denote wall thickness (Magnification × 250, elastin Van Gieson stain).

PPHNS may prove refractory to vasodilator therapy and die within the first few days of life. At postmortem examination of the lung, there is normal growth of the pulmonary vascular bed and normal dilatation of the pulmonary arteries but striking muscularization of small and peripheral pulmonary arteries.[36,37] The muscle cells are surrounded by dark-staining elastic laminae, suggesting that they had been formed in utero (Fig. 52–10). Moreover, there is a dense connective tissue sheath around the small arteries that may also contribute to decreased pulmonary arterial compliance. These structural abnormalities are also evident as early as the first day of life in infants who present with meconium aspiration and PPHNS at birth. As has been speculated, overproduction of a vasoactive substance in utero might cause vasoconstriction resulting in both structural changes in the pulmonary vascular bed and increased gastric motility leading to early passage of meconium.[36]

The structural changes seen on light microscopy in idiopathic and fatal PPHNS are not necessarily more severe in degree than those observed in neonates with congenital heart defects causing PPHNS in whom pulmonary artery pressure and resistance fall after surgical repair or palliation. There are several possible explanations for this apparent discrepancy. In infants with PPHNS of unknown etiology,

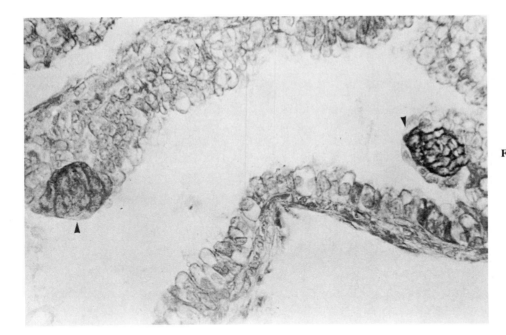

Figure 52–7. Note neuroepithelial bodies as dark staining region (immunoreactive for serotonin) in airway of a newborn infant. (Kindly supplied by E. Cutz).

the mechanism that causes vasoconstriction in utero and that induces the structural abnormalities persists, whereas in infants with PPHNS secondary to congenital heart disease the altered anatomy resulting in left-sided obstruction causes pulmonary vasoconstriction. So, after surgical repair, pulmonary artery pressure falls and the process reverses functionally and structurally. Alternatively, there may be other more subtle structural differences in idiopathic versus cardiac PPHNS that may explain their dif-

ferent clinical courses. McKenzie and Haworth[34] reported an infant with idiopathic PPHNS in whom "swollen" endothelial cells were observed to be partially or completely occluding the most peripheral precapillary pulmonary arteries. My colleagues and I made the same observation recently in lung tissue from an infant who had had mild PPHNS as a neonate but who presented at 7 months of age with severe cyanosis associated with right-to-left shunting through a large patent ductus arteriosus and died shortly

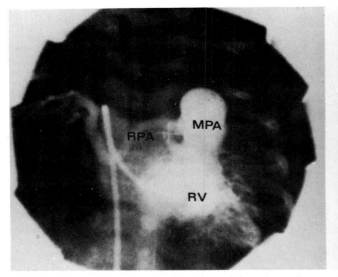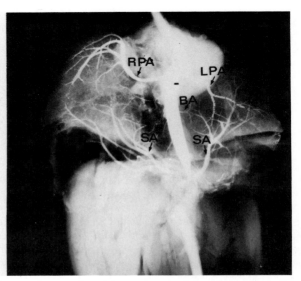

Figure 52–8. Postmortem arteriograms of a newborn infant with persistent pulmonary hypertension of the newborn syndrome show primitive hypoplastic pulmonary arteries supplying upper poles of the lungs and persistent dorsal intersegmentals to lower poles. (Reproduced with permission of Goldstein JD et al [1980]: Unusual vascular anomalies causing persistent pulmonary hypertension in a newborn. Am J Cardiol 43:962–968.) BA = bronchial artery; LPA = left pulmonary artery; MPA = main pulmonary artery; RPA = right pulmonary artery; RV = right ventricle; SA = systemic artery.

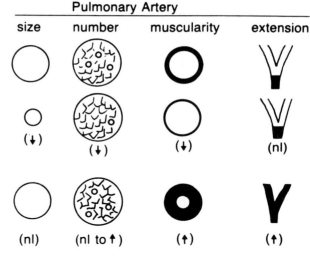

Figure 52–9. Schema showing abnormal in utero pulmonary arterial development associated with congenital heart defects. Decreased pulmonary flow is associated with hypoplasia of the peripheral pulmonary arteries and increased pulmonary venous pressure, with excessive muscularity.

thereafter. At postmortem examination, ultrastructural study of the pulmonary arteries showed enlarged endothelial cells virtually occluding the lumen of small precapillary vessels. These small precapillary pulmonary arteries were surrounded by prominent pericytes, which lacked the full characteristics of mature smooth muscle (Fig. 52–11).

Abnormal endothelial cells may contribute to pulmonary hypertension not only by occluding small pulmonary vessels but also by metabolic derangements that prevent the normal response to postnatal stimuli that initiate vasodilatation. For example, the ability of endothelial cells to handle or produce vasoactive substances may be impaired[41,45,53] and a disproportionate increase in pulmonary vasoconstrictors may result. Alternatively, endothelial cells may be unable to produce endothelium-derived (smooth muscle) relaxing factor[12] or effectively resist in situ thrombosis. Levin and associates[31] observed platelet fibrin microthrombi in the small pulmonary arteries of some infants with PPHNS, suggesting either abnormal platelet-endothelial interaction[40,46] or a perinatal coagulopathy.[2]

Another possibility is that the hypertrophied and newly differentiated fetal smooth muscle cells in infants with "idiopathic" PPHNS are functionally different from those in infants with cardiac PPHNS. Such differences could include decreased production of endogenous vasodilators (e.g., prostaglandins),[55] altered synthesis or distribution of connective tissue proteins (collagen, elastin, glycosaminoglycans), quantitative or qualitative abnormality in contractile filaments (actin, myosin), or impaired calcium metabolism.

Experimental Studies

Experimental models of PPHNS with maldevelopment have been produced in fetal rats[19] but not in guinea pigs[12] and lambs[30] by feeding prostaglandin synthetase inhibitors, either aspirin or indomethacin, to the pregnant female. The fetal lungs had both medial hypertrophy of normally muscularized pulmonary arteries and extension of muscle into

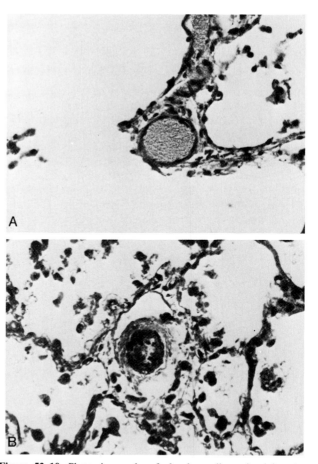

Figure 52–10. Photomicrographs of alveolar wall arteries injected at postmortem examination with a barium-gelatin suspension. *A*, A normal nonmuscular artery from a 3-day-old infant who had a normal heart and lungs. *B*, An abnormally muscularized artery from an infant with persistent pulmonary hypertension of the newborn syndrome. (Magnification: × 250, elastin Van Gieson stain). (Reproduced with permission of Murphy JD et al [1981]: The structural basis of persistent pulmonary hypertension of the newborn infant. J Pediatr 98:962–967.)

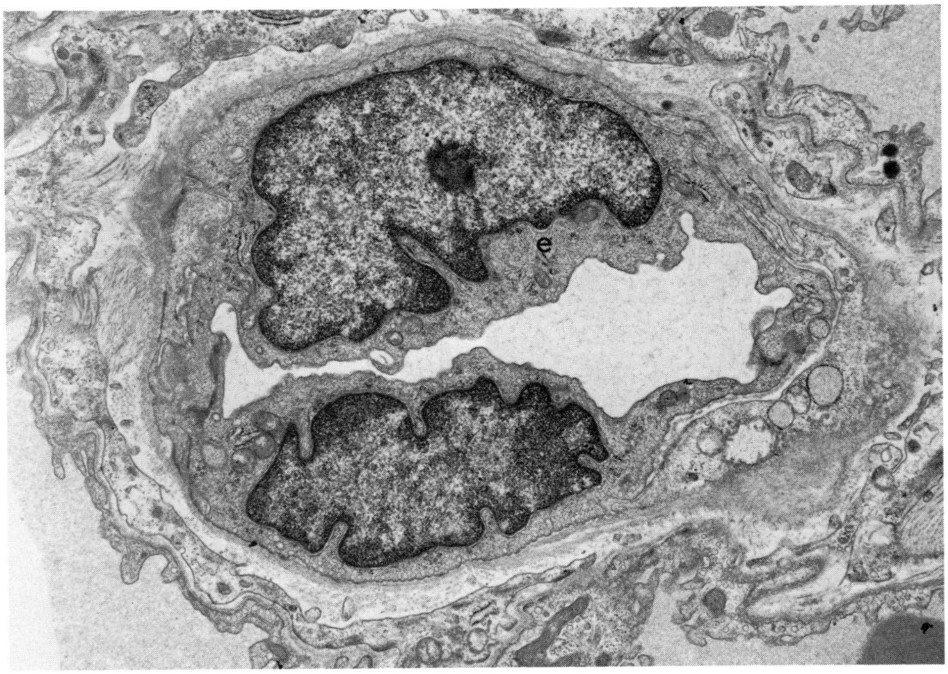

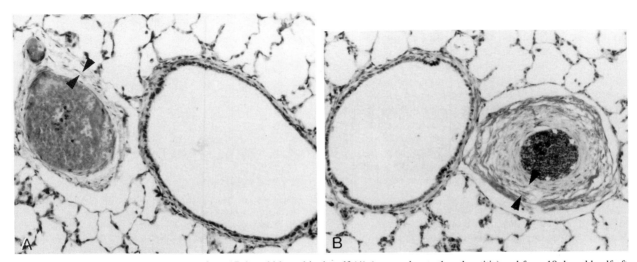

Figure 52–11. Electron photomicrograph of small precapillary artery with bulging endothelial cells (e) in a 7-month-old child with severe pulmonary hypertension and right-to-left shunting who had persistent pulmonary hypertension of the newborn syndrome as a neonate.

normally nonmuscular distal peripheral arteries. Similar morphologic changes were also produced in lambs[56] (but not in guinea pigs[35] or rats[14]) by keeping the pregnant female in hypoxia. Exposing piglets to 3 days of hypoxia starting from birth results in failure of normal postnatal regression of the fetal pulmonary vascular musculature. The "pseudohypertrophied" smooth muscle cells do not lay down any collagen or elastin.[1] When piglets are exposed to 3 days of hypoxia after birth, starting at 3 days of age (i.e., after the pulmonary arteries are dilated), the pulmonary artery

smooth muscle hypertrophy is associated with increased elastin and collagen.[1,18] These observations suggest that fetal smooth muscle cell hypertrophy may be structurally and functionally different.

In newborn calves exposed to high-altitude hypoxia, one of the most striking features observed is a tremendous increase in adventitial collagen in the pulmonary vascular bed. The effects of increased adventitial collagen on pulmonary vascular compliance reactivity are being addressed in current studies by Stenmark and coworkers[57] (Fig. 52–12).

Figure 52–12. Medium-sized pulmonary artery from 17-day-old low altitude calf (A) (arrows denote the adventitia) and from 18-day-old calf after 14 days at high altitude (B) (note large increase in adventitia [arrow heads] as well as media) (Magnification: × 100). (Kindly supplied by K. Stenmark.)

POSTNATAL EFFECTS IN THE INFANT WITH PPHNS

Judging from experimental data, it would appear that the normal newborn may be particularly susceptible to postnatal pulmonary vascular abnormalities resulting from hypoxia,[42] hyperoxia,[64] and toxins[60]; such increased susceptibility would compound the prenatal vascular changes associated with PPHNS. The abnormally muscular pulmonary vascular bed is likely to be hyperreactive to hypoxia and less responsive to the normal mechanisms causing the decrease in pulmonary vascular resistance. The barotrauma produced by ventilator therapy and hyperoxia required to manage such infants would only exacerbate the prenatal pulmonary vascular abnormalities and cause further loss of alveoli and arteries.

FUTURE DIRECTIONS

Clearly, a breakthrough in the management of infants with PPHNS will come from understanding developmental changes in pulmonary vascular cell biology and in identifying the determinants of alveolar growth. Newly described techniques of culturing endothelial and smooth muscle cells from the macropulmonary and micropulmonary circulations,[50,52] and from the ductus arteriosus[44] should be helpful in directing further investigation. My colleagues and I have shown differences in baseline and hyperoxia-stimulated prostaglandin metabolism in fetal ductal and pulmonary artery endothelial and smooth muscle cell types.[41] Methods of inducing hypertrophy of fetal pulmonary vascular smooth muscle cells in vitro[45] will be worth pursuing to identify how their biochemical function (production of prostaglandins, connective tissue proteins) and contractile behavior may be altered. Such studies could also be applied to fetal pulmonary smooth muscle cells isolated from animal models in which pulmonary vascular hypertrophy has been produced by maternal indomethacin therapy or by pulmonary venous obstruction.

References

1. Allen K, Haworth SG (1986): Impaired adaptation of intrapulmonary arteries to intrauterine life in newborn pigs exposed to hypoxia: An ultrastructural study (abstr). Fed Proc 45:879.
2. Andrew M, Bhogal M, Karpatkin M (1981): Factors XI and XII and pre-kallikrein in sick and healthy premature infants. N Engl J Med 304:1130–1133.
3. Bartlett RM, Roloff DW, Cornell RG, et al (1985): Extracorporeal circulation in neonatal respiratory failure: A prospective randomized study. Pediatrics 76:479–487.
4. Bohn D, James I, Filler RM, Ein SM, Wessen DE, Shandling B, Stephens C, Barker GA (1984): The relationship between $PaCO_2$ and ventilation parameters in predicting survival in congenital diaphragmatic hernia. J Pediatr Surg 19:166–671.
5. Bohn D, Tamura M, Perrin D, Rabinovitch M (1985): Ventilatory predictions of pulmonary hypoplasia in congenital diaphragmatic hernia confirmed by morphologic assessment. J Pediatr 111:423–431.
6. Cassin S, Tod M, Philips J, Frisinger J, Jordan J, Giggs C (1981): Effects of prostaglandin D_2 on perinatal circulation. Am J Physiol 240:H755–H760.
7. Chamberlain D, Hislop A, Hey E, Reid LM (1977): Pulmonary hypoplasia in babies with severe rhesus isoimmunization: A quantitative study. J Pathol 122:43–52.
8. Collins MH, Moessinger AC, Kleinerman J, Bassi J, Rosso P, Collins AM, James S, Blanc WA (1985): Fetal lung hypoplasia associated with maternal smoking: A morphometric analysis. Pediatr Res 19:408–412.
9. Collins MH, Moessinger A, Kleinerman J, James LS, Blanc W (1986): Morphometry of hypoplastic fetal guinea pig lungs following amniotic fluid leak. Pediatr Res 20:955–960.
10. Cutz E, Gillan JE, Track NS (1984): Pulmonary endocrine cells in the developing human lung and during neonatal adaptation. In Becker KL, Gazdar AF (eds): Endocrine Lung in Health and Disease. Philadelphia, WB Saunders, pp 210–231.
11. Davies P, McBride J, Murray GF, Wilcox BR, Shallal JA, Reid L (1982): Structural changes in the canine lung and pulmonary arteries after pneumonectomy. J Appl Physiol 53:859–864.
11a. DeMello DE, Murphy JD, Aronovitz M, Davies P, Reid LM (1987): Effects of indomethacin in utero on the pulmonary vasculature of the newborn guinea pig. Pediatr Res 22:693–697.
12. Furchgott RF (1983): Role of endothelium in responses of vascular smooth muscle. Circ Res 53:557–573.
13. Geggel RL, Murphy JD, Langleben D, Crone RK, Vacanti JP, Reid LM (1985): Congenital diaphragmatic hernia: Arterial structural changes and persistent pulmonary hypertension after repair. J Pediatr 107:457–464.
14. Geggel RL, Aronovitz M, Reid L (1986): Effects of chronic in utero hypoxemia on the rat neonatal pulmonary arterial structure (abstr). Pediatr Res 20:368A.
15. Gersony WM, Duc GV, Sinclair JC (1969): "PFC" syndrome (persistence of the fetal circulation) (abstract). Circulation 405: III:87.
16. Goldstein JD, Rabinovitch M, Van Praagh R, Reid LM (1980): Unusual vascular anomalies causing persistent pulmonary hypertension in a newborn. Am J Cardiol 43:962–968.
17. Goldstein JD, Reid LM (1980): Pulmonary hypoplasia resulting from phrenic nerve agenesis and diaphragmatic amyoplasia. J Pediatr 97:282–287.
18. Hall SM, Haworth SG (1986): Normal adaptation of pulmonary arterial intima to extrauterine life in the pig: Ultrastructural study. J Pathol 149:55–66.
19. Harker L, Kirkpatrick SE, Friedman WG, Blood CM (1980): Effects of indomethacin on fetal pulmonary circulation. Lab Invest 42:121.
20. Haworth SG, Reid LM (1976): Persistent fetal circulation: Newly recognized structural features. J Pediatr 88:614–620.
21. Haworth SG, Reid LM (1977): Quantitative structural study of the pulmonary circulation in the newborn with aortic atresia, stenosis or coarctation. Thorax 32:121–128.
22. Haworth SG, Reid LM (1977): Structural study of the pulmonary circulation in total anomalous pulmonary venous return in early infancy. Br Heart J 39:80–92.
23. Hislop A, Fairweather DVI, Blackwell RJ, Howard S (1984): The effects of amniocentesis and drainage of amniotic fluid on lung development in Macaca fascicularis. Br J Obstet Gynaecol 91:835–842.
24. Hislop A, Hey E, Reid LM (1979): The lungs in congenital bilateral renal agenesis and dysplasia. Arch Dis Child 54:32–38.
25. Hislop A, Wigglesworth JS, Desai R (1986): Alveolar development in the human fetus and infant. Early Hum Dev 13:1–11.
26. Hu L-M, Davies P, Adzick NS, Harrison M, Reid LM (1986): Morphometric growth of the residual ovine lung after left pneumonectomy in utero: A morphometric study particularly of the pulmonary arteries (abstr). Am Rev Respir Dis 133:187.
27. Jones ODH, Shore DF, Rigby ML, Leijala M, Scallan J, Shineborne EA, Lincoln JCR (1981): The use of tolazoline hydrochloride as a pulmonary vasodilator in potentially fatal episodes of pulmonary vasoconstriction after cardiac surgery in children. Circulation 64(suppl 11):134–139.
28. Kitigawa M, Hislop A, Boyden EA, Reid LM (1971): Lung hypoplasia in congenital diaphragmatic hernia: A quantitative study of airway artery and alveolar development. Br J Surg 58:341–346.
29. Levin DL, Fixler DE, Morris FC, Tyson J (1978): Morphologic analysis of the pulmonary vascular bed in infants exposed in utero to prostaglandin synthetase inhibitors. J Pediatr 83:964–972.

30. Levin DL, Mills LJ, Weinberg AG (1979): Hemodynamic, pulmonary vascular and myocardial abnormalities secondary to pharmacologic constriction of the fetal ductus arteriosus. Circulation 60:360–364.

31. Levin DL, Weinberg AG, Perkin RM (1983): Pulmonary microthrombi syndrome in newborn infants with unresponsive persistent pulmonary hypertension. J Pediatr 102:299–303.

32. Lock JE, Fuhrman BP, Epstein ML, Rowe RD, Lucas RV (1979): Pulmonary hypertension following neonatal shock. Pediatr Cardiol 1:109–115.

33. Manchester D, Margolis HS, Sheldon RE (1976): Possible association between maternal indomethacin therapy and primary pulmonary hypertension of the newborn. Am J Obstet Gynecol 126:467–469.

34. McKenzie S, Haworth SG (1981): Occlusion of peripheral pulmonary vascular bed in a baby with idiopathic persistent fetal circulation. Br Heart J 45:675–678.

35. Murphy JD, Aronovitz MJ, Reid LM (1986): Effects of chronic in utero hypoxia on the pulmonary vasculature of the newborn guinea pig. Pediatr Res 20:292–295.

36. Murphy JD, Rabinovitch M, Goldstein JD, Reid LM (1981): The structural basis of persistent pulmonary hypertension of the newborn infant. J Pediatr 98:962–967.

37. Murphy JD, Vawter G, Reid LM (1984): Pulmonary vascular disease in fatal meconium aspiration. J Pediatr 104:758–762.

38. Norwood WI, Kirklin JK, Sanders SP (1980): Hypoplastic left-heart syndrome: Experience with palliative surgery. Am J Cardiol 45:87–91.

39. Peckham GJ, Fox WW (1978): Physiologic factors affecting pulmonary artery pressure in infants with persistent pulmonary hypertension. J Pediatr 93:1005–1010.

40. Rabinovitch M, Andrew M, Thom H, Williams WG, Trusler GA, Rowe RD, Olley PM, Wilson GJ (1983): Abnormal pulmonary vascular endothelial metabolism of factor VIII in patients with pulmonary hypertension (abstr). Circulation 68:111–136.

41. Rabinovitch M, Boudreau N, Coceani F, Vella G, Olley P (1987): Prostaglandin synthesis by fetal ductus arteriosus pulmonary artery and aorta endothelial and smooth muscle cells (abstr). Pediatr Res 21:387A.

42. Rabinovitch M, Gamble WJ, Miettinen OS, Reid L (1981): Age and sex influence on pulmonary hypertension of chronic hypoxia and on recovery. Am J Physiol 240:H62–H82.

43. Rabinovitch M, Keane JF, Norwood WI, Castaneda AR, Reid L (1984): Vascular structure in lung tissue obtained at biopsy correlated with pulmonary hemodynamic findings after repair of congenital heart defects. Circulation 69:655–667.

44. Rabinovitch M, Beharry S, Bothwell T, Jackowski G (1988): Qualitative and quantitative differences in protein synthesis comparing fetal lamb ductus arteriosus endothelium and smooth muscle with cells from adjacent vascular sites. Dev Biol (in press).

45. Rabinovitch M, Bothwell T, Mullen M, Hayakawa BN (1988): High-pressure pulsation of central and microvessel pulmonary artery endothelial cells. Am J Physiol 254:C338–C343.

46. Rabinovitch M, Bothwell T, Hayakawa BN, Trusler GA, Williams WG, Rowe RD, Olley PM, Cutz E (1986): Pulmonary vascular endothelial abnormalities in patients with congenital heart defects: A correlation of light with scanning and transmission electronmicroscopy. Lab Invest 55:632–653.

47. Riemenschneider TA, Neilson HC, Ruttenberg HD, Jaffe RB (1976): Disturbances of the transitional circulation: Spectrum of pulmonary hypertension and myocardial dysfunction. J Pediatr 89:622–625.

48. Rendas A, Brown ER, Avery ME, Reid LM (1980): Prematurity, hypoplasia of the pulmonary vascular bed and hypotension: Fatal outcome in a ten-month old infant. Am Rev Respir Dis 121:873–880.

49. Rowe RD, Hoffman T (1972): Transient myocardial ischemia of the newborn infant: A form of severe cardiorespiratory distress in full-term infants. J Pediatr 81:243–250.

50. Ryan US, Clements E, Habliston D, Ryan JW (1978): Isolation and culture of pulmonary artery endothelial cells. Tissue Cell 10:535–554.

51. Ryan US, Ryan JW (1977): Correlations between the fine structure of the alveolar-capillary unit and its metabolic activities. In L'Enfant C (ed): Lung Biology in Health and Disease. New York, Marcel Dekker, vol 4.

52. Ryan US, White LA, Lopez M, Ryan JW (1982): Use of microcarriers to isolate and culture pulmonary microvascular endothelium. Tissue Cell 14:597–606.

53. Said SI (1982): Metabolic functions of the pulmonary circulation. Circ Res 50:325–333.

54. Siassi B, Goldberg SJ, Emmanouilides GC, Higashimo SM, Lewis E (1971): Persistent pulmonary vascular obstruction in newborn infants. J Pediatr 78:610–613.

55. Smith WL (1986): Prostaglandin biosynthesis and its compartmentation in vascular smooth muscle and endothelial cells. Ann Rev Physiol 48:287–362.

56. Soifer SJ, Kaslow D, Heymann MA (1983): Prolonged intrauterine hypoxia produces pulmonary hypertension in the newborn lamb. Pediatr Res 17:254–258.

57. Stenmark KR, Fasules J, Tucker A, Voelkel NF, Reeves JT (1987): Severe pulmonary hypertension and adventitial changes in newborn calves at 4300 M J Appl Physiol 62:821–830.

58. Stenmark KR, James SL, Voelkel NF, Toews WH, Reeves JT, Murphy RC (1983): Leukotriene C4 and D4 in neonates with hypoxemia and pulmonary hypertension. N Engl J Med 309:77–80.

59. Tod ML, Cassin S (1985): Thromboxane synthetase inhibition and perinatal pulmonary response to arachidonic acid. J Appl Physiol 58:710–716.

60. Todd L, Mullen M, Olley PM, Rabinovitch M (1983): Pulmonary toxicity of monocrotaline differs at critical periods of lung development. Pediatr Res 19:731–737.

61. Vanhoutte PM, Rubanyi GM, Miller VM, Hurston DS (1986): Modulation of vascular smooth muscle contraction by the endothelium. Ann Rev Physiol 48:307–320.

62. Wagenvoort CA, Losekoot G, Mulder E (1971): Pulmonary veno-occlusive disease of presumably intrauterine origin. Thorax 26:429–434.

63. Whight CM, Barratt-Boyes BG, Calder AL, Neutze JM, Brandt PWT (1978): Total anomalous pulmonary venous connection: Long-term results following repair in infancy. J Thorac Cadiovasc Surg 75:52–63.

64. Wilson WL, Mullen M, Olley PM, Rabinovitch M (1985): Hyperoxia-induced pulmonary vascular and lung abnormalities in young rats and potential for recovery. Pediatr Res 19:1059–1067.

SECTION 4
THERAPEUTIC MODALITIES

53 NEONATAL CARDIOVASCULAR PHARMACOLOGY

Adam Schneeweiss

Cardiovascular drug therapy has markedly progressed in the last two decades. New drugs and even new classes of drugs have been developed. Most of this progress appears applicable to neonatal therapy. Nonetheless, the introduction of these new achievements to neonatal cardiovascular therapy has been slow because demonstrated pharmacologic profiles in adults cannot safely be extrapolated to neonates who may require much larger or smaller doses or in fact have unexpected or even entirely opposite responses. The purpose of this chapter is to review the major cardiovascular drugs used in neonates, including those newer agents that show particular promise or hazard.

POSITIVE INOTROPIC AGENTS

Positive inotropic agents are used in patients with congestive heart failure or in those in shock to improve hemodynamics by enhancement of myocardial contractility. The concept of enhancing myocardial contractility in patients with hemodynamic deterioration is reasonable, but it has several drawbacks: (1) the failing heart is already stimulated by sympathetic activation, and further stimulation often does not enhance contractility; (2) if a considerable portion of the myocardium is damaged, stimulation of the remaining may increase the damage; (3) an increase in contractility not associated with a decrease in other determinants of oxygen consumption increases the myocardial oxygen demand and may cause myocardial ischemia; and (4) most positive inotropic agents available for clinical use have an arrhythmogenic potential. Despite all these disadvantages, under some conditions no alternative exists to the administration of positive inotropic agents.

The positive inotropic agents available for clinical use are (1) digitalis glycosides; (2) sympathomimetic amines, including isoproterenol, dopamine, and dobutamine; (3) bipyridine derivatives such as amrinone and milrinone; and (4) glucagon. The first two groups are used in neonates and are discussed in this chapter.

Several problems may complicate the use of positive inotropic agents in neonates: (1) some neonates, such as those with primary endomyocardial diseases, may require continuous treatment for long periods, which raises the question of tolerance to positive inotropics; (2) the immature heart of low birthweight neonates may respond to these agents differently from the more mature myocardium of the term infant; and (3) many neonates with congestive heart failure have congenital cardiac anomalies with mechanical disturbances. Most studies of positive agents were performed in adults without such disturbances. It is not clear how applicable data obtained in such adult studies are to neonates with congenital heart diseases.

Digitalis

Digitalis glycosides are the most widely used positive inotropic agents and the only such agents used for long-term treatment of congestive heart failure in neonates and infants. The digitalis glycoside most widely used in neonates is digoxin.

Several problems are unique to the use of digitalis glycosides in the neonate population: (1) the resting level of myocardial function in the neonate is higher than in the adult,[10] and it is not clear whether digitalis glycosides can further enhance contractility; (2) the pharmacokinetic profile of digoxin in premature neonates differs from that in older children and in adults; (3) high levels of endogenous digitalis-like substances commonly complicate interpretation of digoxin levels in neonates; and (4) under certain conditions, digitalis glycosides are the drug of choice in infancy but not at older ages. For example, in adults with

Wolff-Parkinson-White syndrome and reentrant arrhythmias, digitalis glycosides are contraindicated, whereas in neonates and small infants with this disease, they are the drug of choice.

Mechanism of Action

The positive inotropic effect of digitalis glycosides is exerted by inhibition of the membrane sodium-potassium adenosine triphosphatase, which supplies energy for maintenance of cation balance across the cell membrane. This process causes an increase in intracellular concentration of sodium and, as a result, of calcium as well.[60]

Hemodynamic Effects

The primary hemodynamic effect of digitalis glycosides is the positive inotropic effect. The increase in cardiac output resulting from the positive inotropic effect may have various secondary effects. For example an increase in cardiac output from enhanced contractility can result in sympathetic withdrawal and a decrease in peripheral vascular resistance. This process is, at least partially, opposed by a direct peripheral vasoconstricting effect of the drug. It is still controversial whether digitalis glycosides can enhance the contractility of the normal heart as well as that of the failing heart.

Almost all studies show acute hemodynamic improvement in patients with congestive heart failure after short-term administration of digitalis. The effect of long-term digitalis therapy is controversial. Some withdrawal studies performed in adults revealed hemodynamic deterioration after discontinuation of digoxin,[2] whereas others failed to show such effect.[39] Withdrawal studies have not been reported in children.

Effect of Age on Inotropic Response

Age is an important determinant of the response to digitalis glycosides and has significant implications for the use of digitalis in the pediatric age group. In most mammalian species, the sensitivity to the inotropic and toxic effects of digitalis glycosides in the neonatal period is different from that in young adulthood.[59] These differences have been attributed to variations in the effects of these agents at the cellular level,[9] as well as to maturational changes in the volume of distribution.[62] The differences are not attributable to different plasma concentrations because these concentrations are similar in animal neonates and in adults treated with digoxin.[12] The metabolism of digoxin and its protein binding do not vary with age, and the difference in effect cannot be thus explained.[11]

Because of the reduced effect of these drugs in newborn infants, these patients are treated routinely with higher doses of digoxin per kilogram of body weight than adults. These higher doses are controversial because they raise problems of tolerance.

Endocardial Fibroelastosis and Neonatal Dilated Cardiomyopathy

My colleagues and I have reviewed a series of 49 infants and children with the dilated form of primary endocardial fibroelastosis, or neonatal dilated cardiomyopathy. We have found that continued teatment with digitalis for several years may change the natural course of primary endocardial fibroelastosis. Six episodes of abrupt discontinuance of digitalis occurred in five children. In five of these episodes, congestive heart failure was worsened, or if it had disappeared during treatment, it developed again on discontinuance of digitalis.

To evaluate the late consequences in clinically "cured" patients, we studied by serial cardiac catheterization eight patients with the dilated form of primary endocardial fibroelastosis in whom congestive heart failure disappeared with treatment.[99] In six of the patients, repeated cardiac catheterization showed left ventricular dilation with poor contraction (mean ejection fraction 0.32). Left ventricular end-diastolic pressure was elevated up to 28 mmHg. Only two of these patients, with regression of the abnormal electrocardiographic findings, had no abnormal findings at repeated catheterization. These findings indicate that treatment with digitalis can cause clinical improvement in patients with the dilated form of primary endocardial fibroelastosis. The "cure" is incomplete, however. The abnormal findings may explain some of the cases of sudden death or late clinical deterioration in patients with "cured" primary endocardial fibroelastosis. The electrocardiogram is of little value in assessing these processes. Echocardiography may be useful for follow-up of the children throughout the period of treatment, however.

Left-to-Right Shunt and Congestive Heart Failure

In neonates, symptoms of heart failure may result from circulatory congestion due to anatomic defects, usually complicated ventricular septal defect or patent ductus arteriosus. Stimulation of myocardial contractility may improve the hemodynamic condition, although the myocardium is basically normal. The distinction between congestive heart failure and circulatory congestion is rarely made by pediatric cardiologists, and the usual treatment of infants and children with both conditions includes digitalis glycosides.

Several studies have demonstrated that not all infants with circulatory congestion show hemodynamic improvement after inotropic stimulation.[12,13,87] However, some infants do show hemodynamic improvement, and others show clinical improvement even in the absence of hemodynamic improvement. Thus, the mechanism by which digitalis glycosides may improve the status of infants with circulatory congestion is not settled. For example, it is possible that digitalis glycosides turn down metabolic rate. Selection of infants for treatment with digoxin may be improved if the distinction between heart failure and circulatory congestion is made.[128] Large controlled clinical trials are required to confirm the role of digitalis in patients with left-to-right shunts.

Electrophysiologic Effects

The electrophysiologic effects of digoxin have not been studied in human neonates. Karpawich and colleagues studied these effects in beagle puppies.[58] At doses of 0.04 mg/kg/day, the drug decreased the sinus rate from 176 ± 9

to 136 ± 15 beats/min and prolonged the corrected sinus node recovery time from 69 ± 4 to 198 ± 66 msec. Lower doses of digoxin did not alter the sinus node recovery time. The high dose of digoxin (0.04 mg/kg/day) prolonged the sinoatrial conduction time from 53 ± 5 to 110 ± 36 msec. Lower doses had only minimal effects on sinoatrial conduction. These findings in puppies are similar to those observed in children and adults.

Digoxin prolonged the P-R interval from 82 ± 4 to 134 ± 21 msec. In five of six puppies who received 0.04 mg/kg digoxin, second degree atrioventricular block was observed. Puppies treated with digoxin developed Wenckebach periodicity at slower pacing rates than before digoxin. The functional refractory period of the atrioventricular conduction system was increased in these puppies. The administration of atropine partially prevented the effect of digoxin.

Arrhythmias

The main use of digitalis glycosides in neonates is to terminate, control and prevent atrial tachyarrhythmias. Garson and associates reported the largest pediatric series of supraventricular tachycardia treated with digoxin.[37] Short-term treatment with digoxin was effective in 57 of 84 children (68 per cent), electrical cardioversion was effective in 60 per cent of the children, and vagal maneuvers were effective in 63 per cent. After initial treatment, 113 of 191 patients (72 per cent) received long-term treatment. Digoxin, at a dose of 0.01 mg/kg/day, was the most common drug used in the first month of treatment, either alone or in combination with propranolol or quinidine. In 116 patients, tachycardia recurred at least once. Digoxin reduced the rate of recurrences in these patients. The investigators recommend treatment for at least a year in all children with supraventricular tachycardia, regardless of spontaneous termination of the first episode.[37]

Digoxin may be used to reduce the abnormal junctional rate or to induce a second degree atrioventricular block in neonates with atrioventricular junctional tachycardia. Dick and associates recently suggested, however, that digitalis is of little value for the prophylaxis of supraventricular tachycardia in infants.[21]

Sustained supraventricular tachycardia occurring in fetuses in utero is an established cause of fetal congestive heart failure and of nonimmune hydrops fetalis. The first attempt to terminate this arrhythmia with administration of digoxin failed; the first attempt to terminate it by maternal treatment with the combination of digoxin and propranolol also failed. Several cases of sucessful termination of supraventricular tachycardia in the fetus by maternal digoxin therapy have been reported since 1980, however. In these patients, digoxin was used either alone or in combination with drugs known to terminate supraventricular tachycardia at older ages, such as verapamil and propranolol.[17,61,73] Digoxin can be used safely during pregnancy because fetuses are resistant to the arrhythmogenic effect of digitalis glycosides.[9,17] Maternal administration of digoxin is an effective and safe treatment for fetal supraventricular tachycardia.

Rowland and coworkers reviewed the experience of three institutions in the management of atrial flutter in eight infants under 2 years of age.[96] A 2-day course of digoxin was given to each infant. In the five infants with congenital atrial flutter, this course resulted in uncomplicated resolution of the arrhythmia, although one of these infants continued to suffer episodes of paroxysmal supraventricular tachycardia for 6 years. The longest period of therapy until conversion of the arrhythmia was 14 days. Digoxin was less effective in three infants with paroxysmal atrial flutter.

Clinical Pharmacology

Digoxin is the most widely used digitalis glycoside because of its favorable pharmacokinetic profile. Coadministration with food may change the rate of absorption but not its magnitude.[127] Hernandez and associates reported that in a group of 20 infants with congenital heart disease, digoxin could be detected in the plasma within 5 to 10 minutes of oral administration, and peak plasma concentrations were evident within 60 to 180 minutes.[43] Digoxin can also be given intravenously, for rapid effect.

In adults, therapeutic serum concentrations of digoxin range from 1 to 2 ng/ml.[126] In a group of 12 infants on long-term digoxin therapy, the serum digoxin concentration was 1.48 ± 0.77 ng/ml.[61] Pinsky and colleagues reported that in premature neonates, the serum digoxin concentration after a digitalizing dose of 30 μg/kg ranged from 1.4 to 7.5 ng/ml.[90] After a digitalizing dose of 20 μg/kg, the serum concentration ranged from 1.2 to 3.0 ng/ml (mean + SD 1.73 ± 0.15 ng/ml). Lang and Von Bernuth reported that the serum digoxin concentration ranged from 1.2 to 3.5 ng/ml in mature newborns and from 1.5 to 4.5 ng/ml in premature newborns.[67]

Tissue concentrations of digoxin have been reported in a few infants and children.[43,66] These concentrations are affected by age. Hastreiter and Van der Horst studied the concentration of digoxin in tissues and the content of the drug in various organs in 36 infants and children evaluated postmortem.[46] In adults and neonates, postmortem digoxin blood values were 8 and 15 ng/ml, respectively, and concentrations for ventricular myocardium were 250 and 450 ng/ml, respectively. Premature infants receiving long-term digoxin treatment had a larger fraction of digoxin in most tissues than older infants and children.[46] Pinsky and associates noted higher serum concentrations of digoxin in premature infants than in full-term infants.[90] In another study of tissue concentrations of digoxin obtained during surgical procedures, neonates had higher concentrations in the right and left ventricular myocardium than older children.[66] Reported digoxin concentrations in the liver and gastrointestinal tract were also higher in neonates than in older children.[46] These findings are probably attributable to the impaired ability of premature infants to excrete digoxin; digoxin is eliminated primarily by renal excretion of the unchanged drug. Pinsky and associates reported that the elmiination half-life of digoxin in seven premature infants ranged from 56 to 88 hours.[90] Lang and Von Bernuth found the elimination half-life of digoxin to range from 17 to 52 hours in mature newborns and from 38 to 88 hours in premature newborns.[67] However, the recent discovery of endogenous digitalis-like substances in the serum of normal neonates raises questions about many of these observations. Until a reliable assay is available to differentiate endogenous from exogenous material, the appropriate digoxin dosing schedule for the immediate newborn period must be said to remain unknown.

Treatment During Pregnancy

Digoxin readily crosses the placenta and reaches high concentrations in the fetal myocardium. The fetus may be exposed to digoxin on two occasions: (1) during treatment of heart disease in the mother, and (2) during administration of digoxin to the mother to treat a heart disease, such as supraventricular tachycardia, in the fetus. Fetal digoxin concentrations are usually high.[79]

Digitalis Toxicity

The incidence of digitalis toxicity was reported to be 8 to 20 per cent among hospitalized adults.[46] The incidence of toxicity is higher in infants, children, and elderly patients than in young and middle-aged adults. Several investigators have emphasized the lack of digitalis toxicity in premature infants,[90] whereas others have stated that the risk of digitalis toxicity in children is highest in premature infants.[67] The controversy may be explained by the finding of high serum digoxin concentrations in premature infants without toxicity. In my experience, digitalis-induced cardiac toxicity is uncommon in premature infants, despite serum concentrations higher than those found in children and adults. In a comparative study of neonatal and adult dogs, neonatal dogs developed toxicity at a higher serum concentration of digoxin than did adult dogs, in contrast to the finding of no difference in the inotropic effect of equal levels of digoxin serum concentrations in the two groups of dogs.[122] In neonates and in infants under 3 months of age, poor renal clearance of digoxin may result in high plasma levels of the drug, which may overcome the natural myocardial resistance in these age groups.

The cardiac effects of digitalis toxicity include arrhythmias and conduction disturbances. Almost all known arrhythmias and conduction disturbances have been observed in association with digitalis toxicity, with the most frequently observed being ventricular premature beats, junctional tachycardia, atrial tachycardia with block, and various degrees of atrioventricular block. The predominant extracardiac manifestations of digitalis toxicity in all age groups are related to the central nervous system and gastrointestinal system. In almost all children with digoxin toxicity the digoxin plasma concentration exceeds 2.0 ng/ml.[8]

Neonates and small infants require high levels of digoxin to develop signs of toxicity, however. They rarely develop toxic manifestations at plasma concentrations lower than 3.5 ng/ml and often have levels of 20 ng/ml or more.[47] Treatment of digitalis toxicity includes discontinuation of the drug, gastric lavage, activated charcoal, antigen-binding fragments of digoxin-specific antibodies, and correction of electrolyte disturbances (particularly hypokalemia). Arrhythmias are treated with agents such as phenytoin and lidocaine, which do not interact with digoxin and do not enhance the digoxin-induced conduction disturbances.

Drug Interactions

Coadministration of digoxin and quinidine results in elevation of plasma levels of digoxin; coadministration of verapamil and digoxin prolongs the elimination and elevates the plasma concentration of digoxin; coadministration of amiodarone and digoxin may elevate the plasma concentration of digoxin.[65]

Indomethacin is used for closure of the patent ductus arteriosus.[42,45,50] Indomethacin impairs renal function in the majority of preterm infants. Because 90 per cent of a dose of digoxin is excreted by the kidneys, indomethacin may impair the elimination of digoxin. Schimmel and coworkers reported a neonate who developed severe digitalis toxicity associated with indomethacin-induced renal insufficiency during concomitant administration of digoxin and indomethacin.[100] Koren and associates studied 11 preterm infants treated with digoxin and indomethacin. Administration of indomethacin caused a mean elevation of 50 per cent in digoxin serum concentration, which paralleled a mean reduction of 50 per cent in urine output. When indomethacin and digoxin are administered together to preterm infants, the dose of digoxin should be reduced by 50 per cent, and digoxin serum levels and urinary output should be determined.[64]

Dopamine

Dopamine is an endogenous precursor of norepinephrine. In children, this agent has been successfully used to treat cardiogenic and septic shock,[23,68] as well as low cardiac output following surgical treatment of congenital heart disease and hemodynamic disturbances of neonatal asphyxia.[22] Dopamine is preferred to isoproterenol because it has fewer tachycardiac and arrhythmogenic effects. At low concentrations, dopamine has a selective dilatory effect in the renal arterial bed.[77] At high concentrations, this effect is overcome by the generalized vasoconstricting action of the drug. Dopamine also has a positive inotropic effect. The positive inotropic effect results from both release of norepinephrine and direct stimulation by dopamine of cardiac β-adrenoreceptors.[71] This process is accompanied by various degrees of acceleration of heart rate, but the heart rate increase is usually less than that produced by isoproterenol. In a group of 14 severely asphyxiated neonates, dopamine produced no significant change in heart rate.[22]

The usual hemodynamic profile of the drug includes (1) an increase in cardiac output[95] and stroke volume; (2) a varying increase in heart rate; (3) a significant increase in systolic systemic arterial pressure, with only a slight increase, if any, in diastolic pressure; (4) a decrease in the pulmonary capillary wedge pressure because of the increase in cardiac output; or (5) no change or even an increase in pulmonary capillary wedge pressure because of systemic arterial and venous constriction. The hemodynamic effects of dopamine may be attenuated during continued therapy.

Dopamine is especially suitable for treatment of low cardiac output associated with hypotension. Roge and associates[94] reported that low doses of dopamine in mature newborn lambs increased cardiac output and decreased systemic vascular resistance without altering heart rate. Some authorities suggest that dopamine may be contraindicated in the presence of elevated pulmonary vascular resistance, but others use it.

Dobutamine

Dobutamine is a synthetic sympathomimetic amine with a potent positive inotropic effect. Dobutamine is used mainly to treat cardiogenic and septic shock. In adults, the hemodynamic changes produced include increases in myocardial contractility, cardiac output, stroke volume, ejection fraction, and systemic arterial pressure and decreases in systemic and pulmonary capillary wedge pressure, with minimal to moderate acceleration of heart rate.[74,118] Continuous infusion for more than 3 days may result in the development of hemodynamic tolerance in infants and children. The effect on pulmonary capillary wedge pressure is controversial and may differ from that observed in adults. In 12 children, dobutamine in doses of 7.75 µg/kg/min increased the cardiac index from 3.5 to 4.7 liter/min/m^2, systemic artrial pressure from 109/61 to 151/74 mmHg, mean arterial pressure from 80 to 104 mmHg, and stroke index from 38 to 49 ml/beat/m^2.[24] Cardiac index and left ventricular stroke work index were increased, and systemic ateriolar resistance index was decreased. Dobutamine is a useful drug in the management of children in shock, especially in those older than 12 months in cardiac failure not complicated by severe hypotension.[89] Dobutamine appears to be at least as effective as dopamine in increasing cardiac output, and may be tried in children in shock or congestive heart failure in whom dopamine has failed. Combined treatment with dobutamine and dopamine may be superior to treatment with high doses of either agent alone. The combination of dobutamine with intravenously administered nitrates, such as nitroglycerin and isosorbide dinitrate, may produce hemodynamic improvement in patients with congestive heart failure who are not responsive to either dobutamine or nitrate alone, but experience in neonates is limited.

Isoproterenol

Isoproterenol is a potent β-adrenoreceptor agonist that until recently was the sympathomimetic amine of choice in infants and children. Isoproterenol exerts positive chronotropic and inotropic and peripheral vasodilatory effects. Cardiac output is increased because of increases in heart rate and contractility. Driscoll and colleagues[25] found that isoproterenol produced a much greater increase in heart rate than dobutamine to achieve a similar elevation in cardiac output.

Short-term administration of isoproterenol produces at least a transient decrease in pulmonary arterial pressure and pulmonary vascular resistance in patients with primary pulmonary hypertension.[104] Side effects include tachycardia, cardiac arrhythmias, aggravation of ischemia, palpitations, headache, myocardial necrosis, and hypotension.

CALCIUM ANTAGONISTS

Calcium antagonists inhibit the slow inward calcium current and decrease the availability of intracellular calcium; as a result, negative inotropic effects are seen. Calcium antagonists are used to treat systemic hypertension, ischemic heart disease, cardiomyopathy, arrhythmias, pulmonary hypertension, and other diseases in older children and adults. Verapamil is the only calcium antagonist commonly used in infants and neonates, and it is given for arrhythmias.

Verapamil

Verapamil is usually the first-used agent of the calcium antagonists. Although the experience in neonates has been limited, verapamil has been used in many children with arrhythmias and hypertrophic cardiomyopathy and in a few young hypertensive patients with good results.

Electrophysiologic Effects

Verapamil mainly affects the slow-response action potential in the sinoatrial and atrioventricular nodes. In children, verapamil usually causes slight slowing of heart rate at rest or at any given level of submaximal exercise but not at maximal exercise.[35,125] The most important electrophysiologic effect of verapamil is prolongation of conduction time in the atrioventricular node. This effect has also been observed in children.[98,102,112] Verapamil may accelerate, inhibit, or not alter antegrade accessory pathway conduction.[44] However, in neonates and young infants, intravenous verapamil may cause cardiovascular collapse or apnea. There is an emerging consensus that intravenous verapamil is contraindicated in infants under 1 year of age (see Chapter 41). Nevertheless, in combination with oral digoxin, oral verapamil remains a relatively safe and useful supplemental agent for suppression of recurrent supraventricular tachycardia in neonates and young infants unresponsive to oral digoxin alone and to the combination of oral digoxin and oral quinidine. Further, intravenous and oral maternal verapamil may be safe and effective therapy for supression of fetal supraventricular tachycardias unresponsive to digoxin alone (see Chapter 16).

Hypertrophic Cardiomyopathy

The hemodynamic improvement produced by verapamil in patients with hypertrophic obstructive cardiomyopathy includes decreases in left ventricular systolic outflow gradient and end-diastolic pressure and better diastolic filling of the heart. The abnormal relationships between the early and late filling phases in patients with hypertrophic cardiomyopathy are redirected toward normal with verapamil. Heart rate and cardiac index are only minimally altered. Spicer and coworkers studied the short-term hemodynamic effects of verapamil in nine children and adolescents with hypertrophic cardiomyopathy.[112] At rest, verapamil increased the mean cardiac output from 3.3 ± 0.9 to 3.7 ± 0.9 liter/min/m^2 and decreased left ventricular end-diastolic pressure from 19.3 ± 8.1 to 14.5 ± 6.9 mmHg. In six patients with left ventricular outflow systolic pressure gradient, verapamil decreased the gradient from 17.5 ± 7.2 to 5.2 ± 4.5 mmHg. At maximal exercise, cardiac output increased from 6.5 ± 1.3 to 7.8 ± 1.8 liter/min/m^2, left ventricular end-diastolic pressure decreased from 29.1 ± 10.1 to 19.3 ± 10.4 mmHg, and left ventricular systolic outflow tract gradient decreased from 31.2 ± 10.5 to 1.75 ± 1.7 mmHg.[112] In summary, verapamil produces a marked hemodynamic and symptomatic improvement in pediatric patients with hypertrophic cardiomyopathy.

Clinical Pharmacology

Verapamil is rapidly and almost completely absorbed from the gastrointestinal tract after oral administration. The systemic bioavailability of the drug is low.

Effect on Arrhythmias

Verapamil is especially useful in patients with supraventricular arrhythmias. Verapamil terminates up to 90 per cent of cases of reentrant supraventricular tachycardia in adults and children.[6,92,98]

Shahar and colleagues of the Sheba Medical Center summarized the treatment of paroxysmal supraventricular tachycardia in infants and children with verapamil.[101] They studied 14 infants and children, nine of them under 2 years of age, with 53 episodes of paroxysmal supraventricular tachycardia. Stable sinus rhythm was obtained in 40 of 53 episodes (92.4 per cent) immediately or within 60 seconds of intravenous administration of verapamil. The drug was equally effective in infants and children. It terminated all 26 episodes in patients with structural anomalies and 17 of 18 episodes in patients with Wolff-Parkinson-White syndrome. Three of the four patients in whom verapamil failed to terminate the arrhythmia were under 6 weeks of age, and the fourth patient was 5 months of age. Two patients treated with propranolol prior to administration of verapamil had sinus bradycardia or atrioventricular block after receiving verapamil.[101] Several investigators have observed that in some infants under 6 months of age supraventricular tachycardia is especially resistant to conversion by verapamil, even at high doses.[93,101]

Several investigations have suggested that verapamil is the drug of choice for treatment of supraventricular tachycardia in infancy and childhood. Sapire and associates reported that verapamil failed to terminate the arrhythmia in a child with atrial flutter.[97] An important advantage of verapamil is that electrocardioversion may be safely performed even several minutes after intravenous administration of the drug.[110] Verapamil is eliminated by hepatic metabolism. The metabolites and 4 per cent of the dose in the unchanged form are excreted in the urine.

Hesslein and colleagues studied the effect of age on pharmacokinetic parameters of verapamil in pediatric patients.[49] Several age-dependent kinetic parameters were found. Younger children had faster drug uptake, lower relative bioavailability, smaller volume of distribution, and slower elimination half-life than older children. Younger children also had a diurnal variation in drug kinetics. No age-dependent difference in distribution, half-life, or elimination rate was found.

Side Effects

Cardiovascular effects include congestive heart failure, hypotension, and AV conduction disturbances. Constipation is the most common complication of treatment with verapamil. Because of a number of experiences with cardiovascular collapse after intravenous verapamil in young infants, most experts in the United States consider intravenous administration of the drug to be contraindicated in children under 1 year of age. Epstein et al[29] reported three infants with supraventricular tachycardia who demonstrated hemodynamic decompensation after intravenous verapamil. All three patients were stabilized and their tachycardia was controlled with digoxin. In the chapter on tachyarrhythmias in the newborn (see Chapter 41), Garson and coworkers reported on their experience with several infants in whom the cardiac output was severely reduced after administration of verapamil. This reduction might have resulted from increased sensitivity of neonatal myocardium to calcium antagonists.

Dosage and Administration

In neonates intravenous verapamil should not be used. Oral verapamil should be given in a dose of 2 to 4 mg/kg every 8 hours.

VASODILATORS

Vasodilators are agents that dilate blood vessels. The vasodilators may be divided into several large groups, according to their mechanism of action: (1) direct-acting vasodilators, (2) α-adrenoreceptor blocking agents, (3) angiotensin-converting enzyme inhibitors, and (4) calcium antagonists.

Hydralazine

Hydralazine is a direct-acting relaxant of vascular smooth muscle that affects mainly the arterial vascular bed. Several hypertensive children have been treated with hydralazine in combination with other antihypertensive agents. Perhaps the most important indication for hydralazine in older children is the presence of a large ventricular septal defect with left-to-right shunt. In neonates hydralazine is used to treat systemic hypertension (see Chapter 39). The mechanism of hydralazine's direct vasodilation is unknown. This effect reduces peripheral vascular resistance and arterial pressure. The systemic vasodilation causes sympathetic activation, which results in acceleration of heart rate and enhancement of myocardial contractility. Hydralazine is effective in patients with congestive heart failure. The typical hemodynamic response of these patients to intravenous administration of hydralazine is a decrease in systemic vascular resistance and, often, also of pulmonary artery pressure and an increase in cardiac output and stroke work index by 10 to 50 per cent.

Several investigators have reported that hemodynamic improvement produced by hydralazine was sustained throughout several months of treatment.[75,121] Packer and colleagues reported, however, that tolerance to the hemodynamic effects of hydralazine developed in 11 patients with chronic congestive heart failure.[86] Patients with higher systemic vascular resistance respond better to hydralazine. After the neonatal period, this fact is especially important in children with ventricular septal defect, large left-to-right shunt, and congestive heart failure, in whom hydralazine can produce sudden hemodynamic improvement. The drug may be deleterious in patients with normal systemic resistance. Therefore, in children with left-to-right shunt and congestive heart failure, it is preferable to perform hemodynamic studies before initiation of treatment with hydralazine. It is unclear whether hydralazine's beneficial hemodynamic effects are sustained during prolonged treatment.[4,84] In four children with intracardiac shunts, pulmonary hypertension, and elevated pulmonary vascular resistance, hydralazine did not alter cardiac output and pulmonary and systemic vascular resistance.[78] It would appear that hydralazine should not be used at all, or only with great caution, in patients with pulmonary vascular disease secondary to congenital cardiac lesions.

Systemic Hypertension

Hydralazine lowers blood pressure by reducing elevated peripheral vascular resistance. Reported experience with hydralazine in neonates with hypertension is limited. Plumer and colleagues studied the effects of various forms of treatment, including hydralazine, in 10 infants with systemic hypertension complicating umbilical arterial catheterization or renal artery stenosis.[91] The response to antihypertensive medication was generally poor.

Administration

Hydralazine may be administered intravenously or orally. The systemic bioavailability of hydralazine is only 10 to 40 per cent because the drug undergoes extensive first-pass hepatic metabolism. Hydralazine is widely distributed in the body and is bound by 85 per cent to serum proteins. It is eliminated by hepatic metabolism and excretion in the urine of the metabolites. Hydralazine produces side effects common to most vasodilators as well as some specific side effects such as systemic lupus erythematosus and thrombocytopenia. Doses of 0.2 to 0.3 mg/kg, injected over about a minute, have been used for short-term drug testing in infants and children. No recommended dosage for oral administration in infants and children has been established.

Nitroprusside

Nitroprusside is a potent direct-acting vasodilator that affects the arterial and venous vascular beds similarly. Its mechanism of action at the cellular level is unknown.

The hemodynamic effects of nitroprusside result from the balanced vasodilatory action: systemic vascular resistance is reduced by up to 50 per cent, left ventricular filling pressure is reduced by up to 40 per cent, and heart rate is not much altered, or it may be either slightly increased by reflex sympathetic activation or slightly reduced by general hemodynamic improvement. Nitroprusside increases cardiac output by up to 60 per cent in patients with congestive heart failure. The hemodynamic improvement induced by nitroprusside in adults with congestive heart failure has also been observed in children. For example, Beekman and coworkers evaluated the effect of a continuous infusion of nitroprusside at 20 µg/kg/min in seven children, aged 0.2 to 14.5 years with severe left ventricular dysfunction or mitral regurgitation.[5] The drug increased cardiac index by an average of 33 per cent and increased stroke index by 29 per cent; pulmonary arterial wedge pressure decreased by 28 per cent. A significant decrease of systemic vascular resistance was also observed. This early improvement was evident as symptomatic improvement in congestive heart failure when nitroprusside was replaced by oral vasodilators.[5]

Intravenous administration of nitroprusside has become conventional therapy for immediate control of severe hypertension and hypertensive emergencies in infants and older children and has been used in refractory cases of neonatal systemic hypertension. Nitroprusside has also been studied in young infants with left-to-right shunts.

Beekman and colleagues administered nitroprusside to five children with ventricular septal defect at a mean age of 2.8 months.[4] The drug increased the pulmonary-to-systemic flow ratio from 2.2 ± 0.2 to 3.4 ± 0.2, as a consequence of a marked decrease in systemic blood flow. Pulmonary flow did not change much. Right atrial pressure, mean pulmonary capillary wedge pressure, mean aortic pressure, and mean pulmonary arterial pressure decreased. However, until further studies have been conducted, use of nitroprusside in such patients cannot be recommended.

Effect After Cardiac Surgical Procedures

After neonatal cardiac surgical procedures, severe peripheral vasoconstriction can complicate myocardial dysfunction and often prevent hemodynamic recovery. Nitroprusside, by its vasodilatory effect, may reduce afterload in such patients and increase cardiac output. Appelbaum and coworkers reported that nitroprusside has a favorable effect on cardiac output in infants with elevated arterial pressure early after intracardiac operations.[1]

Prolonged infusion of high doses of nitroprusside may cause toxicity because of the accumulation of thiocyanate and cyanide, and levels should be monitored. Nitroprusside is given only intravenously. The infusion rate in children is 0.25 to 65 μg/kg/min. Nitroglycerin may be used for the same indication.[56]

Minoxidil

Minoxidil is a direct-acting potent orally available vasodilator. It lowers elevated peripheral resistance and controls hypertension. Minoxidil has been shown to be useful in patients with severe childhood hypertension refractory to other antihypertensive agents.[107] Sometimes refractory neonatal systemic hypertension can be controlled with minoxidil. Minoxidil has adverse effects of two types: (1) nonspecific effects resulting from vasodilation and (2) effects specific to minoxidil, such as pericardial damage and hypertrichosis. No neonatal dosages have been recommended.

Captopril

Captopril is a synthetic, reversible inhibitor of angiotensin-converting enzyme. It is a potent vasodilator, affecting both arteries and veins, and is used mainly for the treatment of congestive heart failure and hypertension in older children and adults. Captopril can be useful in neonates to control refractory systemic hypertension.

Effects in Hypertension

In adults, captopril has been shown to lower elevated blood pressure at rest and during exercise in the supine and standing positions. Both systolic and diastolic blood pressures are reduced. Captopril lowers elevated peripheral vascular resistance without significant alterations in heart rate and cardiac output.[30,32]

In several studies of hypertensive patients, a triphasic response to captopril was observed: (1) a favorable initial response, (2) a partial transient attenuation of the initial response during the first week of therapy, and (3) late restoration of the effect by higher doses.[15,16] The most probable mechanism of the antihypertensive effect of captopril is inhibition of the renin-angiotensin system. However, in 10 hypertensive children, no correlation was found between the pretreatment level of plasma renin activity and the magnitude of the blood pressure reduction by captopril.[108] Another mechanism of the antihypertensive effect of captopril is accumulation of bradykinin.

The first case of treatment of malignant hypertension with captopril was reported by Oberfield and coworkers in 1979.[85] They reported a 10-year-old child with hypertension that was resistant to several drugs. Captopril lowered blood pressure from 160/130 to 96/64 mmHg. Friedman and colleagues reported six children with severe hypertension resistant to several antihypertensive agents who responded favorably to captopril.[34] Sinaiko and associates studied the efficacy and safety of captopril in 10 young hypertensive patients aged 3.5 to 20 years.[108] In five of the patients, adequate control was achieved when captopril was combined with hydrochlorothiazide, whereas the other four patients required a combination of captopril and other antihypertensive drugs.

The successful use of captopril for treatment of hypertension in newborn infants without coarctation of the aorta was first reported in 1982 by Bifano and coworkers in three cases.[14]

Congestive Heart Failure

Administration of captopril to adult patients with congestive heart failure causes either no change or a decrease in heart rate; decreases in arterial pressure, systemic vascular resistance, left ventricular end-diastolic pressure, left ventricular volumes, and right atrial pressure; an increase in cardiac output; and either an increase or no change in stroke work index. The findings in infants and children have been less satisfactory than in adults. My colleagues and I and Liebau and colleagues[69] have found that patients with complex congenital heart diseases such as single ventricle and tetralogy of Fallot developed severe hypotension after administration of captopril.

Infants with severe coarctation of the aorta often have combined cardiovascular disease in the first days or week of life. They often have high plasma renin activity. My colleagues and I have recently studied two such infants, resistant to various drugs, who responded favorably to captopril.

Clinical Pharmacology

Captopril is given orally, and food may interfere with its absorption. In a study of children, the antihypertensive effect of captopril was evident within 15 minutes of oral administration and reached a peak within 1.5 hours.[108] Captopril may be transferred by breast milk. It is rapidly excreted by the kidneys. Treatment with captopril may be associated with serious side effects, including bradycardia, hypotension, hematopoietic depression, renal damage, hyperkalemia, and dysgeusia. Oral doses of 0.1 to 0.4 mg/kg, given one to four times daily, can be used in infants.

β-ADRENORECEPTOR BLOCKING AGENTS

Effect of Vasodilators on Myocardial Hypertrophy

Vasodilators can reduce myocardial hypertrophy in infants with heart failure.[120] The mechanism of their effect on myocardial hypertrophy in hypertensive infants is not known.

β-Adrenoreceptor blocking agents produce a reversible and competitive inhibition of β-adrenergic stimulation. Most of the diseases for which beta-blocking agents are prescribed in adults also occur in the pediatric age group, but not commonly in neonates. Further indications for these drugs in infancy and childhood are tetralogy of Fallot and other conditions associated with dynamic infundibular obstruction.

All β-adrenoreceptors are analogues of the beta stimulator isoproterenol. Beta-blocking agents may be classified according to potency of beta blockade, selectivity, intrinsic sympathomimetic activity, membrane-stabilizing activity, associated class 3 antiarrhythmic properties, associated vasodilatory properties, and lipid solubility. The hemodynamic effects common to all beta-blocking agents are slowing of heart rate; decreases in myocardial contractility, cardiac output, and systemic arterial pressure; and for most beta blockers, an increase in systemic vascular resistance. Beta-blocking agents have side effects specific to each agent as well as side effects common to the whole group. The most famous and hazardous side effect is the oculomucocutaneous syndrome produced by practolol. Side effects common to the whole group result directly from beta blockade and include bradycardia, conduction disturbances, myocardial depression, hypotension, fatigue and bronchoconstriction, central nervous system effects, and aggravation of symptoms of peripheral vascular disease.

Propranolol

Propranolol, the most widely used beta blocker, is a nonselective β-adrenoreceptor blocking agent without intrinsic sympathomimetic activity but with membrane-stabilizing activity. The main indications for propranolol in infants and children are hypertension, tetralogy of Fallot, hypertrophic obstructive cardiomyopathy, arrhythmias, and thyrotoxicosis. In the newborn, propranolol is commonly used for treatment of systemic hypertension, arrhythmias, and also symptomatic hypertrophic obstructive cardiomyopathy seen in infants of diabetic mothers. Propranolol decreases heart rate, myocardial contractility, and systemic arterial pressure.

Effects in Hypertension

Propranolol lowers both systolic and diastolic blood pressure at rest and during exercise. The antihypertensive effect is dose dependent.[123] Although the drug may be used alone, especially in patients with high-renin hypertension,[54] monotherapy is not recommended.

Patients with high-renin hypertension require lower doses of propranolol to control the elevated blood pressure than patients with low-renin hypertension. This therapeutic feature is important to consider in infants and children with coarctation of the aorta and high-renin hypertension. The combination of propranolol and diuretic agents is more effective than the use of either drug alone in the control of hypertension. The mechanism of the antihypertensive effect is the decrease in cardiac output.

Hypertrophic Obstructive Cardiomyopathy

In children, propranolol is the preferred drug for treatment of hemodynamic abnormalities and rhythm disturbances associated with hypertrophic obstructive cardiomyopathy. Propranolol produces significant hemodynamic and symptomatic improvement in patients of all ages with hypertrophic obstructive cardiomyopathy. The suppression of

myocardial contractility, leading to a reduction in the systolic pressure gradient over the left ventricular outflow tract, is considered to be the main hemodynamic effect of propranolol. Propranolol may improve left ventricular compliance and filling in these patients.[116] Patients with mild symptoms and a small or latent gradient have been reported to derive greater benefit from propranolol than those with severe symptoms, which consist mainly of dyspnea and a high pressure gradient.[129]

Gillette and associates studied the effects of propranolol in six infants and children with hypertrophic obstructive cardiomyopathy.[40] Symptoms and abnormal signs were abolished by propranolol in all six patients. None of them required surgical intervention, and none died. Echocardiography showed regression of septal hypertrophy. Shand and coworkers studied an 8-week-old infant with this disease, characterized by a pressure gradient of 120 mmHg across the left ventricular outflow tract and right ventricular gradient with marked hypertrophy of both ventricles and the interventricular septum.[103] With propranolol the patient showed clinical improvement. During a repeat cardiac catheterization at the age of 22 months, performed 24 hours after discontinuance of propranolol, no left ventricular outflow pressure gradient was noted. In newborn infants of diabetic mothers, propranolol has been used to reduce symptomatic left ventricular outflow obstruction.

Tetralogy of Fallot

Administration of propranolol may produce symptomatic relief, may eliminate the need for a shunt, and may allow complete surgical correction to be delayed in older patients with tetralogy of Fallot.

Garson and colleagues reported that the responders to propranolol were older and received higher doses of propranolol than the nonresponders.[38] They studied 35 infants who received propranolol as palliative treatment for hypoxemic spells associated with tetralogy of Fallot. Propranolol effectively abolished spells for at least 3 months in 80 per cent of the patients.

The following mechanisms may account for the beneficial effect of propranolol in tetralogy of Fallot: (1) the negative inotropic effect of propranolol causes a decrease in the extent of the dynamic right ventricular obstruction, mainly at the infundibular level, and (2) propranolol slows the heart rate, and this effect contributes to the decrease in right-to-left shunting.

Symptomatic newborn infants with tetralogy of Fallot usually have fixed valvular rather than dynamic subvalvular pulmonary outflow obstruction. Thus, agents such as propranolol usually have little to offer infants with tetralogy of Fallot requiring intervention in the newborn period.

Electrophysiologic Effects

Yabek and colleagues evaluated the effect of propranolol at doses of 0.1 mg/kg administered intravenously in 10 children.[129] The drug increased the spontaneous sinus cycle length in all patients. The maximum corrected sinus node recovery time increased in nine patients. An inconsistent effect on sinoatrial conduction time was observed. A depressant effect on the atrioventricular node prolongs the P-R and A-H intervals. Propranolol has no significant effect on the anterograde or retrograde effective refractory periods of accessory atrioventricular pathways in adults but was occasionally reported to prolong conduction and refractoriness in children.[3]

Effects in Arrhythmias

Propranolol is effective in termination and prevention of supraventricular tachycardia in older children, but it is not often required in neonates. Intravenous propranolol may be required in neonates with refractory supraventricular tachycardia, but standby ventricular pacing should be available in case severe bradycardia occurs. Oral propranolol is useful in combination with oral digoxin in the chronic suppression of recurrent supraventricular tachycardia unresponsive to oral digoxin alone.

Tingelstad and associates were the first to report that propranolol administered concomitantly with digoxin was particularly helpful in the treatment of persistent supraventricular tachycardia in childhood.[118] Gillette and colleagues[40] studied 30 infants and children with supraventricular tachycardia. Propranolol was effective in treatment of this arrhythmia in six of eight patients with Wolff-Parkinson-White syndrome, in seven of nine patients with concealed anomalous pathway, in six of eight patients with automatic ectopic focus, and in three of five patients with undetermined mechanism.

Propranolol, which crosses the placenta, may be used for treatment of fetal tachycardia during pregnancy.[117] Also, alone or in combination with digixon, it is moderately effective in infants and children with atrial flutter. The limited effect of propranolol should be interpreted keeping in mind the well-known resistance of atrial flutter in these age groups to all forms of treatment.

Propranolol can abolish syncope associated with malignant ventricular arrhythmias in children, but sudden death may nevertheless occur.[126] Propranolol abolishes cardiovascular and other symptoms and reduces the plasma level of the active thyroid hormome T_3. Several investigators have reported that propranolol is useful for treatment of thyrotoxicosis in neonates, infants, and children.[88]

Clinical Pharmacology

Propranolol may be given orally or intravenously. Maximal plasma concentration is reached within 2 hours of administration of a single oral dose. Propranolol undergoes extensive first-pass hepatic metabolism, resulting in systemic bioavailability of 30 to 40 per cent. A significant level of beta blockade is achieved in almost all patients at plasma levels of up to 30 ng/ml.[82,83] In children with tetralogy of Fallot, a correlation between the effect and the dose was found. Propranolol is bound by about 90 per cent to plasma proteins. It is eliminated by hepatic metabolism and renal excretion of the metabolites. The side effects of propranolol are usually predictable because most are related to β-adrenoreceptor blockade.

Dosage and Administration

Doses of 1 to 3 mg/kg/day have been used in infants and children. Children with tetralogy of Fallot who responded to propranolol received a mean dose of 2.6 mg/kg/day.

Atenolol

Atenolol is one of the three most widely used β-adrenoreceptor blockers in adults. It is a β_1-selective adrenoreceptor blocking drug devoid of local anesthetic or intrinsic sympathomimetic activities. In children, the experience is limited to a few patients with hypertension. Neonatal experience is minimal, but atenolol does cross the placenta and reach high plasma levels in the neonate. Liedholm reported that during long-term treatment the plasma levels of atenolol in mothers and neonates were similar.[70] The pharmacodynamic effect is sustained for 24 hours.

Timolol

Timolol is a nonselective β-adrenoreceptor blocking agent devoid of intrinsic sympathomimetic or membrane-stabilizing activity. No pediatric experience with timolol in cardiovascular diseases has been reported, but young patients with glaucoma may be treated with this drug.

ANTIARRHYTHMIC AGENTS

Antiarrhythmic agents are drugs that terminate and/or prevent arrhythmias. They are classified into four groups:

Class I: Agents with membrane-stabilizing (local anesthetic) properties.
Class II: β-adrenoreceptor blocking agents.
Class III: Agents that mainly affect repolarization, such as amiodarone.
Class IV: Calcium antagonists.

Class I antiarrhthymic agents have membrane-stabilizing activity. They thereby affect both cardiac excitability and conductivity and also depress automaticity. Class Ia agents prolong both ventricular and atrial effective refractory periods, and class Ib agents do not alter the atrial effective refractory period.

Quinidine

Quinidine is the most widely used class I antiarrhythmic agent. It is effective in the termination and prevention of almost all ventricular and supraventricular arrhythmias in all age groups. In children, quinidine is used for termination and prevention of supraventricular tachycardia, atrial flutter and fibrillation, and premature ventricular beats and for prevention of malignant ventricular arrhythmias. In neonates, quinidine in combination with digoxin, is sometimes useful in suppression of atrial flutter unresponsive to concomitant digoxin and propranolol. Quinidine is also sometimes useful in neonates with refractory symptomatic ventricular tachycardia unresponsive to propranolol and phenytoin.

In the adult heart, quinidine decreases the maximal rate of rise and the amplitude of phase 0 action potential and decreases the rate of phase 4 action potential, that is, it decreases automaticity.[63] The duration of action potential is not changed, but the refractory periods of Purkinje and myocardial fibers are prolonged. Quinidine increases the spontaneous sinus rate because of its vagolytic effect. It usually delays conduction in the atrioventricular node and usually prolongs the anterograde and retrograde refractory periods of the accessory atrioventricular pathways.[48] It increases the duration of the QRS interval although to a lesser degree than do the class Ic agents. Similar effects are also observed in newborn hearts.

Like other class I antiarrhythmic agents, quinidine has a negative inotropic effect, which can be particularly important in neonates. Quinidine is given almost exclusively orally. In a study of children and young adults aged 4 to 22 years, the peak plasma concentration was achieved within 0.5 to 2.0 hours.[115] The bioavailability is only about 70 per cent.

Quinidine is eliminated mainly by hepatic metabolism. The elimination half-life of it in adults is 4.5 to 6.0 hours. In children, a shorter elimination half-life has been reported.[114] When quinidine is given to patients who are already receiving digoxin, the plasma concentration of digoxin is increased by 20 to 300 per cent.[26] A new steady state is achieved in about a week.

The mechanism of this interaction may involve the displacement of digoxin from tissue binding sites, a decrease in renal and possibly also in nonrenal clearance of digoxin, and an increase in absorption of digoxin from the gastrointestinal tract. Recently, Koren studied 11 children who were treated with a combination of quinidine and digoxin.[64] The addition of quinidine to maintenance digoxin therapy caused an increase of about 100 per cent in the mean digoxin serum concentration. The interaction was observed in 8 of the 11 children. Koren suggested that this higher density of receptor sites in the newborn makes displacement of digoxin by quinidine more difficult.[64]

Side effects of quinidine are syncope, myocardial depression, hypotension, asystole, conduction disturbances, headache, nausea, blurring of vision, ringing in the ears, vertigo, tinnitus, confusion, delirium, diplopia and disturbances of color perception. Intravenous quinidine is not used because of hypotension. In children, oral doses of 15 to 60 mg/kg/day are used. Neonates should be given 4 to 12 mg/kg every 6 hours, orally.

Procainamide

Procainamide is a class I antiarrhythmic drug resembling quinidine. Procainamide is used for treatment of ventricular and supraventricular arrhythmias. As early as 1960, successful control of ventricular tachycardia in children with large doses of procainamide was reported.[81] In infants and children, ventricular or supraventricular arrhythmias resistant to lidocaine and quinidine may respond to procainamide. In neonates, procainamide is useful in the pharmacoconversion of supraventricular tachycardia un-

responsive to intravenous digoxin. Procainamide usually has had no significant effect on the sinus rate. It has been reported not to change or to increase atrial effective refractory periods and has little effect on anterograde conduction and refractoriness in the atrioventricular node. Procainamide can prolong the anterograde effective refractory period of accessory atrioventricular pathways and may even produce a complete anterograde block. It may increase the duration of the QRS interval.

Procainamide may be administered intravenously, intramuscularly, or orally. After oral administration, procainamide is rapidly and completely absorbed from the gastrointestinal tract and undergoes only minimal or no first-pass hepatic metabolism.[57] About 60 per cent of a dose of the drug is excreted unchanged in the urine, and the remainder undergoes hepatic metabolism.

Animal experiments have shown that the pharmacokinetic profile of procainamide in the immature animal may be different from that in adults.[109] Higher or more frequent doses are required in immature animals and probably also in human infants. In neonates, namely, accumulation of procainamide because of delayed elimination resulting from immaturity of the liver and slow hepatic metabolism of the drug may occur.[111] Procainamide frequently produces side effects, the most serious of which are cardiovascular effects and a syndrome resembling systemic lupus erythematosus. In neonates, 1 mg/kg procainamide can be given intravenously over 1 hour; the dose for oral therapy is 3 to 9 mg/kg every 4 hours.

Lidocaine

Lidocaine is a class Ib antiarrhythmic agent. Unavailable orally, lidocaine is used intravenously for rapid suppression of ventricular arrhythmias. In children, lidocaine is used primarily to suppress ventricular arrhythmias after cardiac operations or myocardial injury. In neonates, lidocaine is used to convert or to suppress ventricular tachycardias.

Lidocaine reduces the maximal rate of rise of phase 0 depolarization and reduces the rate of rise of phase 4 depolarization and the duration of the action potential. It does not alter conduction in normal atrioventricular node and Purkinje fibers and increases the threshold for ventricular fibrillation. Lidocaine is at least as effective as phenytoin for ventricular arrhythmias associated with digitalis toxicity.

Lidocaine is administered intravenously, and its onset of action is rapid.[55] Lidocaine is eliminated by hepatic metabolism and urinary excretion of metabolites. Side effects are related to the central nervous system. Cardiovascular effects include depression of myocardial contractility, hypotension, and conduction disturbances.

Phenytoin

Phenytoin is a class Ib antiarrhythmic agent. Its electrophysiologic and antiarrhythmic properties resemble those of lidocaine, but it is also effective orally. In infants and children, phenytoin is used for treatment of arrhythmias associated with digitalis toxicity as well as for treatment of ventricular arrhythmias occurring after surgical procedures for heart disease. Phenytoin appears to be effective in suppressing ventricular arrhythmias in the late postoperative period in patients undergoing corrective operations for congenital heart diseases.[124] In neonates, oral phenytoin is useful in suppression of ventricular tachycardias.

Phenytoin is given either intravenously or orally. In studying children and young adults, Garson and coworkers reported that the mean effective phenytoin concentration was 15.7 µg/ml.[36] It varied from 8.5 to 20.0 µg/ml. Phenytoin is eliminated almost exclusively by hepatic metabolism. Cerebellar and vestibular effects, lethargy, blurring of vision, and nystagmus are the most common side effects of phenytoin. Other side effects are peripheral neuropathy, gingival hyperplasia, and skin rash. A suggested oral regimen for children and young adults is 3 to 3.5 mg/kg twice daily.[124] In neonates similar doses are used.

PHARMACOLOGIC MANIPULATION OF THE DUCTUS ARTERIOSUS

Drugs that shut or reopen the ductus arteriosus are increasingly important in neonatal cardiology because the presence or absence of ductal patency can have large impact on newborn physiology, particularly in critically ill infants who may have significant pulmonary compromise or ductal-dependent congenital heart disease. Indomethacin is used to constrict the ductus;[39,77,80] prostaglandin E_1 is used to reopen it.

Prostaglandin E_1

Prostaglandin E (PGE_1 and PGE_2) has been used since 1975 to maintain the patency of the ductus arteriosus in infants.[28] This concept is supported by findings of in vitro and in vivo studies. In 1972, Elliott and Starling found that prostaglandins dilated the ductus arteriosus in animals.[27] It was later shown that exogenous PGE_1 and PGE_2 relaxed isolated strips of ductal tissue in the presence of low oxygen tension in vitro.[19] Inhibitors of prostaglandin synthesis administered to pregnant animals have constricted the ductus arteriosus in the fetuses.[18,20] PGE_2 has dilated indomethacin-constricted ductus arteriosus in animal experiments.[105] In fetuses, the levels of PGE_2 in the plasma are high. After birth, PGE_2 levels decrease because (1) production is reduced by loss of the placenta, (2) elimination is increased by activation of the pulmonary circulation, and (3) oxygen tension is increased.

These factors contribute to normal closure of the ductus arteriosus early after birth. Abnormalities in pulmonary or hemodynamic status or in oxygenation may sustain postnatal patency of the ductus arteriosus.

Infants with cyanotic anomalies such as pulmonary atresia or severe tetralogy of Fallot are dependent on patency of the dutus for pulmonary blood flow. Infants with aortic arch anomalies are dependent on patency of the ductus arteriosus for systemic blood flow. Infants with transposition of the great vessels and intact ventricular septum are dependent on patency of the ductus arteriosus for adequate mixing and systemic oxygenation. In a large multicenter study of cyanotic and acyanotic patients, Freed and coworkers reported 23 infants with tricuspid atresia who received intravenous infusions of PGE_1.[33] Results were favorable in most of these infants, with an increase in arterial oxygen tension, usually evident within 30 minutes of initiation of the infusion. Beneficial effects were also seen in the majority of 231 infants with pulmonary atresia and in 47 with severe pulmonary stenosis.

Twenty-one infants with complete transposition of the great arteries were included in Freed and coworkers' study.[33] A significant increase in PaO_2 from 22.9 to 31.8 mmHg was observed in infants with transposition of the great arteries. As in other congenital heart diseases, the responsiveness of the patent ductus arteriosus to PGE_1 in infants with transposition is sustained throughout prolonged treatment. Early administration of PGE_1 appears to be especially suitable in transposition when emergency cardiac catheterization and balloon septostomy are not possible.

PGE_1 is also beneficial in infants with ductal-dependent circulation secondary to interruption of the aortic arch or severe coarctation of the aorta. In 1979, Heymann and colleagues first described dilation of the ductus arteriosus in infants with aortic arch abnormalities.[52] In their 1981 report, Freed and associates reported PGE_1 infusion in 107 infants with acyanotic congenital heart diseases and ductal-dependent anomalies.[33] Clinical improvement occurred in about 80 per cent of the infants with aortic arch anomalies. In the infants with interruption of the aortic arch, blood flow to the descending aorta increased, and the pressure differences across the ductus arteriosus decreased. In infants with coarctation of the aorta, blood pressure in the descending aorta increased, and blood pressure in the ascending aorta decreased. In infants in whom the ductus arteriosus was closed before the infusion, PGE_1 had no beneficial effect.[33]

PGE_2 also maintains patency of the ductus arteriosus, and unlike PGE_1, it is effective orally.[106,113] Beitzke and Suppan evaluated the efficacy of intravenous administration of PGE_2 in 15 infants with complete transposition of the great arteries and severe hypoxemia.[7] Fourteen of the infants reponded favorably. Infusion of PGE_2 resulted in significant increases of PaO_2 from 22 ± 3 to 37 ± 5 mmHg within 1 hour of initiation of treatment. PaO_2 remained constantly above 30 mmHg throughout the infusion. Only 1 of the 15 infants failed to respond to PGE_2 treatment.

Several factors may determine the responsiveness of the ductus arteriosus to PGE. Infants under 96 hours of age have responded more favorably than older infants.[33] Heymann and coworkers found a direct relationship between the pretreatment luminal cross-sectional area of the ductus arteriosus and the response to PGE_1.[51] If treatment is initiated soon after functional closure of the ductus arteriosus, a "closed" ductus may reopen. Administration of PGE does not impair the ability of the ductus arteriosus to close spontaneously when PGE is discontinued. The time to onset of effect is longer in infants with acyanotic than cyanotic congenital heart diseases.

In management of critically ill infants suspected of having ductal-dependent congenital heart diseases, treatment is often delayed until diagnosis is confirmed by cardiac catheterization. It is common practice to initiate PGE infusion once such a diagnosis is confirmed. The several hours required for establishing the diagnosis may be critical, however. Heymann suggested that treatment should be initiated in critically ill infants suspected to have a ductal-dependent congenital cardiac anomaly even before confirmation of diagnosis.[53]

One must monitor heart rate, systemic arterial blood pressure, rate of respiration, signs of central nervous system involvement, body temperature, and electrocardiogram carefully during infusion of PGE.

Side effects occasionally occur. Lewis and associates[72] reported on the incidence and types of side effects in 492 infants with congenital cardiac anomalies. These workers reported that 43 per cent of the infants developed at least one adverse effect, but in only about one half of these patients were the effects attributed to treatment with PGE. Cortical hyperostosis is a recently recognized side effect.[119]

Indomethacin

Usage of indomethacin to close the ductus arteriosus is considered in Chapter 54.

References

1. Appelbaum A, Blackstone EH, Kouchoukos NT, Kirklin JW (1977): Afterload reduction and cardiac output in infants early after intracardiac surgery. Am J Cardiol 39:445–451.
2. Arnold SB, Byrd RC, Meister W, Melmon K, Cheitlin MD, Bristow JD, Parmley WW, Chatterjee K (1980): Long-term digitalis therapy improves left ventricular function in heart failure. N Engl J Med 303:1443–1448.
3. Barrett PA, Jordan JL, Mandel WJ, Yamaguchi I, Laks MM (1979): The electrophysiologic effects of intravenous propranolol in the Wolff-Parkinson-White syndrome. Am Heart J 98:213–224.
4. Beekman RH, Rocchini AP, Rosenthal A (1982): Hemodynamic effects of hydralazine in infants with a large ventricular septal defect. Circulation 65:523–528.
5. Beekman RH, Rocchini AP, Dick M II, Crowley DC, Rosenthal A (1984): Vasodilator therapy in children: Acute and chronic effects in children with left ventricular dysfunction or mitral regurgitation. Pediatrics 73:43–51.
6. Bein G, Wolf D (1971): The treatment of supraventricular paroxysmal tachycardia in infants and children with verapamil. Cardiol Pneumol 9:151.
7. Beitzke A, Suppan CH (1983): Use of prostaglandin E₂ in management of transposition of great arteries before balloon atrial septostomy. Br Heart J 49:341–344.
8. Beller GA, Smith TW, Abelmann WH, Haber I, Hooks WB Jr (1971): Digitalis intoxication: A prospective clinical study with serum level correlations. N Engl J Med 284:989–997.
9. Berman W Jr, Ravenscroft PJ, Scheiner LB, Heymann MA, Melmon KL, Rudolph AM (1977): Differential effects of digoxin at comparable concentration in tissue of fetal and adult sheep. Circ Res 41:635–642.
10. Berman W Jr, Musselman J (1979): Myocardial performance in the newborn. Am J Physiol 237:H66–H70.
11. Berman W Jr, Musselman J (1979): The relationship of age to the metabolism and protein binding of digoxin in sheep. J Pharmacol Exp Ther 208:263–266.
12. Berman W Jr, Musselman J, Shortencarrier R (1980): The physiologic effects of digoxin under steady-state drug conditions in newborn and adult sheep. Circulation 62:1165–1171.
13. Bhat R, Fisher E, Raju TNK, Vidyasagar D (1982): Patent ductus arteriosus: Recent advances in diagnosis and management. Pediatr Clin North Am 29:1117–1136.
14. Bifano H, Post EM, Springer J, Williams ML, Streeten DHP (1982): Treatment of neonatal hypertension with captopril. J Pediatr 100:143–146.
15. Case DB, Atlas SA, Laragh JH, Sealey JE, Sullivan PA, McKinstry DN (1978): Clinical experience with blockade of the renin-angiogtensin-aldosterone system by an oral converting-enzyme inhibitor (SQ 14225, Captopril) in hypertensive patients. Prog Cardiovasc Dis 21:195–206.
16. Case DB, Atlas SA, Laragh JH, Sullivan PA, Sealey JE (1980): Use of the first-dose response on plasma renin activity to predict long-term effects of Captopril: Identification of triphasic pattern of blood pressure response. J Cardiovasc Pharmacol 2:339–346.
17. Chan V, Tse TF, Wong V (1978): Transfer of digoxin across the placenta and into breast milk. Br J Obstet Gynaecol 85:605–609.
18. Clyman RI (1980): Ontogeny of the ductus arteriosus response to prostaglandins and inhibitors of their synthesis. Semin Perinatol 4:115–124.
19. Coceani F, Olley PM (1973): The response of the ductus arteriosus to prostaglandins. Can J Physiol Pharmacol 51:220–225.
20. Coceani F, Olley PM (1980): Role of prostaglandins, prostacyclin, and thromboxanes in the control of prenatal patency and postnatal closure of the ductus arteriosus. Semin Perinatol 4:109–113.
21. Dick M, Campbell RM, Rocchini AP, Snider AR, Crowley DC, Spicer RL, Rosenthal A, Portenow D, Patt P, Jenkins JM (1984): A new look at digoxin in supraventricular tachycardia in infants. Circulation 70:206.
22. DiSessa TG, Leitner M, Ti CC, Gluck L, Coen R, Friedman WF (1981): The cardiovascular effects of dopamine in the severely asphyxiated neonate. J Pediatr 99:772–776.
23. Driscoll DJ, Gillette PC, McNamara DG (1978): The use of dopamine in children. J Pediatr 92:309–314.
24. Driscoll DJ, Gillette PC, Duff DF, Nihill MR, Gutgensell HP, Vargo TA, Mullins CE, McNamara DG (1979): Hemodynamic effects of dobutamine in children. Am J Cardiol 43:581–585.
25. Driscoll DJ, Gillette PC, Lewis RM, Hartley CJ, Schwartz A (1979): Comparative hemodynamic effects of isoproterenol, dopamine, and dobutamine in the newborn dog. Pediatr Res 13:1006–1009.
26. Doering W, Kongi E (1978): Anstieg der Digoxinkonzentration in Serum unter Chinidinmedikation. Med Klin 73:1085.
27. Elliott RB, Starling MD (1972): The effects of prostaglandin F₂α in the closure of the ductus arteriosus. Prostaglandins 2:399–403.
28. Elliott RB, Starling MB, Neutze JM (1975): Medical manipulation of the ductus arteriosus. Lancet 1:140.
29. Epstein ML, Keil EA, Victorica E (1985): Cardiac decompensation following verapamil therapy in infants with supraventricular tachycardia. Pediatrics 75:737–740.
30. Fagard R, Amery A, Reybrouck T, Lijnen P, Billiet L (1979): Response of the systemic and pulmonary circulation to alpha-receptor and beta-receptor blockade (Labetalol) at rest and during exercise in hypertensive patients. Circulation 60:1214–1219.
31. Firth J, Pickering D (1980): Timing of indomethacin therapy in persistent ductus. Lancet 2:144.
32. Fouad FM, Ceimo JMK, Tarazi RC, Bravo EL (1980): Contrasts and similarities of acute hemodynamic responses to specific antagonism of angiotensin II ([Sar, Thr A] II) and to inhibition of converting enzyme (Captopril). Circulation 61:163–169.
33. Freed MD, Heymann MA, Lewis AB, Roehl SL, Kensey RC (1981): Prostaglandin E₁ in infants with ductus arteriosus-dependent congenital heart disease. Circulation 64:899–905.
34. Friedman A, Chesney RW, Ball D, Goodfriend T (1980): Effective use of Captopril (angiotensin I–converting enzyme inhibitor) in severe childhood hypertension. J Pediatr 97:664–667.

35. Frishman WH, Klein N, Strom J, Cohen MN, Shamoon H, Willens H, Klein P, Roth S, Iorio L, Lejemtel T, Pollack S, Shonnenblick EH (1982): Comparative effects of abrupt withdrawal of propranolol and verapamil in angina pectoris. Am J Cardiol 50:1191–1195.

36. Garson A, Kugler JD, Gillette PC, Simonelli A, McNamara DG (1980): Control of late postoperative ventricular arrhythmias with phenytoin in young patients. Am J Cardiol 46:290–294.

37. Garson A, Gillette PC, McNamara DG (1981): Supraventricular tachycardia in children: Clinical features, response to treatment, and long-term follow-up in 217 patients. J Pediatr 98:875–882.

38. Garson A, Gillette PC, McNamara DG (1981): Propranolol: The preferred palliation for tetralogy of Fallot. Am J Cardiol 47:1098–1104.

39. Gheorghiade M, Beller GA (1983): Effects of discontinuing maintenance digoxin therapy in patients with ischemic heart disease and congestive heart failure in sinus rhythm. Am J Cardiol 51:1243–1250.

40. Gillette P, Garson A Jr, Eterovic E, Neches W, Mullins C, McNamara DG (1978): Oral propranolol treatment in infants and children. J Pediatr 92:141–144.

41. Gittenberger de Groot AC, van Ertbruggen I, Moulaert AJMG, Harinck E (1980): The ductus arteriosus in the preterm infant: Histologic and clinical observations. J Pediatr 96:88–93.

42. Halliday H, Hirata T, Brady JP (1979): Indomethacin therapy for large patent ductus arteriosus in the very low birth weight infant: Results and complications. Pediatrics 64:154–159.

43. Hernandez A, Burton RD, Pagtakhan RD, Goldring D (1969): Pharmacodynamics of ^{3}H-digoxin in infants. Pediatrics 44:418–428.

44. Harpers HW, Whitford E, Middlebrook K, Federman J, Anderson S, Pitt A (1982): Effects of verapamil on the electrophysiologic properties of the accessory pathway in patients with the Wolff-Parkinson-White syndrome. Am J Cardiol 50:1323–1330.

45. Harris J, Merritt TA, Alexson CG, Longfield L, Manning JA (1982): Parenteral indomethacin for closure of the patent ductus arteriosus. Am J Dis Child 136:1005–1008.

46. Hastreiter AR, Van der Horst RL (1983): Postmortem digoxin tissue concentration and organ content in infancy and childhood. Am J Cardiol 52:330–335.

47. Hastreiter AR, Van der Horst RL (1983): Accidental digoxin overdose in an infant: Postmortem tissue concentration. J Forensic Sci 28:482–488.

48. Hellens HJJ, Durrer D (1974): Effect of procainamide, quinidine and ajmaline in the Wolff-Parkinson-White syndrome. Circulation 50:114–120.

49. Hesslein P, et al (1985): Age-dependent verapamil kinetics effect pediatric oral dose requirements: An abstract submitted to the First International Symposium on Cardiovascular Pharmacology, Geneva, Switzerland.

50. Heymann MA, Rudolph AM, Silverman NH (1976): Closure of the ductus arteriosus in premature infants by inhibition of prostaglandin synthesis. N Engl J Med 295:530–533.

51. Heymann MA, Rudolph AM (1977): Ductus arteriosus dilatation by prostaglandin E_1 in infants with pulmonary atresia. Pediatrics 59:325–329.

52. Heymann MA, Berman W Jr, Rudolph AM, Whitman V (1979): Dilation of the ductus arteriosus by prostaglandin E_1 in aortic arch abnormalities. Circulation 59:169–173.

53. Heymann MA (1981): Pharmacologic use of prostaglandin E_1 in infants with congenital heart disease. Am J Cardiol 101:837–851.

54. Hollifield JW, Sherman K, Zwagg RV, Shand DG (1976): Proposed mechanisms of propranolol's antihypertensive effect in essential hypertension. N Engl J Med 295:68–73.

55. Hollunger G (1960): On the metabolism of lidocaine. II. The biotransformation of lidocaine. Acta Pharmacol Toxicol 17:365–373.

56. Ilbawi MN, Idriss FS, DeLeon SY, Berry TE, Paul MH (1984): Hemodynamic effects of intravenous nitroglycerin in postoperative pediatric cardiac patients (abstr). Circulation (Suppl II) 70:II–25.

57. Karlsson E, Molin L (1975): Polymorphic acetylation of procainamide in healthy subjects. Acta Med Scand 197:299–302.

58. Karpawich PP, Gumbiner CH, Gillette PC, Shih J-Y, Zinner A, Lewis R (1982): Comparative electrophysiologic effects of digoxin in the nonsedated chronically instrumented puppy. Am Heart J 103:1001–1007.

59. Kelliher GH, Roberts J (1976): Effect of age on the cardiotoxic action of digitalis. J Pharmacol Exp Ther 197:10–18.

60. Kim D, Barry WH, Smith TW (1983): Ouabain binding and changes in ^{42}K uptake, sodium content and contractile state in cultured heart cells (abstract). Circulation 68:321.

61. King CR, Mattioli L, Goertzk K, Snodgrass W (1984): Successful treatment of fetal supraventricular tachycardia with maternal digoxin therapy. Chest 85:573–575.

62. Klaassen CD (1972): Immaturity of the newborn rat's hepatic excretory function for ouabain. J Pharmacol Exp Ther 183:520–526.

63. Klein RL, Holland WC, Tinsley B (1960): Quinidine and unidirectional cation fluxes in atria. Circ Res 8:246–252.

64. Koren G (1986): Interaction between digoxin and commonly co-administerd drugs in children. Personal communication.

65. Koren G, Hesslein P, MacLeod SM (1984): Digoxin toxicity associated with amiodarone therapy in children. J Pediatr 104:467–470.

66. Krasula RW, Hastreiter AR, Levitsky S, Yanagi R, Soyka LF (1974): Serum, atrial, and urinary digoxin levels during cardiopulmonary bypass in children. Circulation 49:1047–1052.

67. Lang D, Von Bernuth G (1977): Serum concentration and serum half-life of digoxin in premature and mature newborns. Pediatrics 59:902–906.

68. Lang P, Williams RG, Norwood WI, Castaneda AR (1980): The hemodynamic effects of dopamine in infants after corrective cardiac surgery. J Pediatr 96:630–634.

69. Leibau G, Reigger AJG, Schanzenbächer P, Steilner H, Oehrlein S (1982): Captopril in congestive heart failure. Br J Clin Pharmacol 14:193S–199S.

70. Liedholm H (1983): Transplacental passage and breast milk accumulation of atenolol in humans. Drugs (Suppl 2):217–218.

71. Leier CV, Heban PT, Huss P, Bush CA, Lewis RP (1978): Comparative systemic and regional haemodynamic effects of dopamine and dobutamine in patients with cardiomyopathic heart failure. Circulation 58:466–475.

72. Lewis AB, Freed MD, Heymann MA, Roehl SL, Kensey RC (1981): Side effects of therapy with prostaglandin E_1 in infants with critical congenital heart disease. Circulation 64:893–898.

73. Ligman G, Ohrlander S, Ohlin P (1980): Intrauterine digoxin treatment of fetal paroxysmal tachycardia. Br J Obstet Gynaecol 87:340–342.

74. Loeb H, Bredakis J, Gunnar RM (1977): Superiority of dobutamine over dopamine for augmentation of cardiac output in patients with chronic low output cardiac failure. Circulation 55:375–381.

75. Massie BM, Kramer B, Haughom F (1981): Acute and long-term effects of vasodilator therapy on resting and exercise hemodynamics and exercise tolerance. Circulation 64:1218–1226.

76. McCarthy IS, Zies LG, Gelband H (1978): Age-dependent closure of patent ductus arteriosus by indomethacin. Pediatrics 62:706–721.

77. McDonald RH Jr, Goldberg LI, McNay JL, Tuttle EP Jr (1963): Augmentation of sodium excretion and blood flow by dopamine in man (abstr). Clin Res 11:248.

78. McGoon MD, Seward JB, Vlietstra RE, Choo MH, Reeder GS, Moyer TP (1982): Hemodynamic response to intravenous hydralazine in pulmonary hypertension patients (abstr). Circulation 66:380.

79. McNamara DG, Brewer EJ Jr, Ferry GD (1964): Accidental poisoning of children with digitalis. N Engl J Med 271:1106–1108.

80. Merritt TA, Harris JP, Roghmann K, Wood B, Campanella V, Alexson C, Manning J, Shapiro DL (1981): Early closure of the patent ductus arteriosus in very low birthweight infants: A controlled trial. J Pediatr 99:281–286.

81. Mortimer EA Jr, Rakita L (1960): Ventricular tachycardia in childhood controlled with large doses of procainamide. N Engl J Med 262:615–618.

82. Mullane JF, Kaufman J, Dvornik D, Coelho J (1982): Propranolol dosage, plasma concentration, and beta-blockade. Clin Pharmacol Ther 32:692–700.

83. Nadas AS (1982): Mannheimer lecture. Pediatr Cardiol 3:71–76.
84. Nakazawa M, Takao A, Shimizu T, Chon Y (1983): Afterload reduction treatment for large ventricular septal defects. Dependence of haemodynamic effects of hydralazine on pretreatment systemic blood flow. Br Heart J 49:461–465.
85. Oberfield SE, Case DB, Levine LS, Rapaport R, Rauh W, New MI (1979): Use of the oral angiotensin I–converting enzyme inhibitor (Captopril) in childhood malignant hypertension. J Pediatr 95:641–644.
86. Beekman RH, Rocchini AP, Rosenthal A (1982): Hemodynamic effects of hydralazine in infants with a large ventricular septal defect. Circulation 65:523–528.
87. Park SC, Steinfeld L, Dimich I (1973): Systolic time intervals in infants with congestive heart failure. Circulation 47:1281–1288.
88. Pemberton PJ, McConnell B, Shanks RG (1974): Neonatal thyrotoxicosis treated with propranolol. Arch Dis Child 49:813–815.
89. Perkin RM, Levin DL, Aquino A, Reedy J (1982): Dobutamine: A hemodynamic evaluation in children with shock. J Pediatr 100:977–983.
90. Pinsky WW, Jacobsen JR, Gillette PC, Adams J, Monroe L, McNamara DG (1979): Dosage of digoxin in premature infants. J Pediatr 94:639–642.
91. Plumer LB, Kaplan GW, Mendoza SA (1976): Hypertension in infants—a complication of umbilical arterial catheterization. J Pediatr 89:802–805.
92. Porter CJ, Gillette PC, Garson A Jr, Hesslein PS, Karpawich PP, McNamara DG (1981): Effects of verapamil on supraventricular tachycardia in children. Am J Cardiol 48:487–491.
93. Porter CJ, Garson A Jr, Gillette PC (1983): Verapamil: An effective calcium channel blocking agent for pediatric patients. Pediatrics 71:748–755.
94. Roge CL, et al (1980): Cardiovascular actions of isuprel, dopamine, and dobutamine in mature newborn lambs. In World Congress of Pediatric Cardiology, London, June 2–6.
95. Rosenblum R, Tai AR, Lawson D (1970): Cardiac and renal hemodynamic effects of dopamine in man (abstr). Clin Res 18:326.
96. Rowland TW, Mathew R, Chameides L, Keane JF (1978): Idiopathic atrial flutter in infancy: A review of eight cases. Pediatrics 61:52–56.
97. Sapire DW, O'Riordan AC, Black IFS (1981): Safety and efficacy of short- and long-term verapamil therapy in children with tachycardia. Am J Cardiol 48:1091–1097.
98. Schamroth L, Krikler DM, Garrett C (1972): Immediate effects of intravenous verapamil in cardiac arrhythmias. Br Med J 1:660–662.
99. Schneeweiss A, Shem-Tov A, Neufeld HN (1983): Persistent left ventricular disease in clinically "cured" primary endocardial fibroelastosis. Br Heart J 50:252–256.
100. Schimmel MS, Inwood RJ, Eidelman AI, Eylath U (1980): Toxic digitalis levels associated with indomethacin therapy in a neonate. Clin Pediatr 19:768–769.
101. Shahar E, Barziley Z, Frand M (1981): Verapamil in the treatment of paroxysmal supraventricular tachycardia in infants and children. J Pediatr 98:323–326.
102. Shakibi JG, Kashani IA, Mehranpur M, Yazdanyar A (1979): Electrophysiologic effects of verapamil in children. Jpn Heart J 20:789–801.
103. Shand DG, Sell CG, Oates JA (1971): Hypertrophic obstructive cardiomyopathy in an infant—propranolol therapy for three years. N Engl J Med 285:843–844.
104. Shettigar UR, Hultgren HN, Specter M, Martin R, Davies DH (1976): Primary pulmonary hypertension: Favorable effect of isoproterenol. N Engl J Med 295:1414–1415.
105. Sideris EB (1983): Effects of indomethacin and prostaglandins E_2, I_2, and D_2 on the fetal circulation. Adv Prostaglandin Thromboxane Leukotriene Res 12:477–495.
106. Silove ED, Coe JY, Shiu MF, Brunt JD, Page AJF, Singh SP, Mitchell MD (1981): Oral prostaglandin E_2 in ductus-dependent pulmonary circulation. Circulation 63:682–688.
107. Sinaiko AR, Mirkin BL (1977): Management of severe childhood hypertension with minoxidil: A controlled clinical study. J Pediatr 91:138–142.
108. Sinaiko AR, Mirkin BL, Hendrick DA, Green TP, O'Dea RH (1980): Antihypertensive effect and elimination kinetics of Captopril in hypertensive children with renal disease. J Pediatr 103:799–805.
109. Singh S, et al (1983): The pharmacokinetics of procainamide in the immature canine (abstract). Pediatr Cardiol 4:315A.
110. Soler-Soler J, Permanyer-Miralda G, Sangristá-Savleda J, Noguera L, Larrousse E, Tor nos NP (1983): Electroconversion after verapamil administration. Chest 83:225–227.
111. Sonnhag C, Karlsson E (1979): Comparative antiarrhythmic efficacy of intravenous N-acetylprocainamide and procainamide. Eur J Clin Pharmacol 15:311–317.
112. Spicer RL, Rocchini AP, Crowly DC, Vasiliades J, Rosenthal A (1983): Hemodynamic effects of verapamil in children and adolescents with hypertrophic cardiomyopathy. Circulation 67:413–420.
113. Sone K, Tashoir M, Fujinaga T, Tomomasa T, Tokuyama K, Kuroume T (1980): Long-term low-dose prostaglandin E_1 administration. J Pediatr 97:866–867.
114. Szefler SJ, Picroni DR, Gingell RL, Shen DD (1982): Rapid elimination of quinidine in pediatric patients. Pediatrics 70:370–375.
115. Tabtznik B (1976): Ambulatory monitoring in the late postmyocardial infarction period. Postgrad Med J (Suppl 7)52:56.
116. Teuscher A, Bossi E, Imhof P, Erb E, Stocker FP, Weber JW (1978): Effect of propranolol in fetal tachycardia in diabetic pregnancy. Am J Cardiol 42:304–307.
117. Tingelstad JB, McCue CM, Mauck HP Jr (1968): Propranolol in the management of children with paroxysmal supraventricular tachycardia. Circulation (Suppl VI)38:194.
118. Tuttle PR, Mills J (1975): Dobutamine: Development of a new catecholamine to selectively increase cardiac contractility. Circ Res 36:185–196.
119. Ueda K, Saito A, Nakano H, Aoshima M, Yokota M, Muraoka R, Iwaya T (1980): Cortical hyperostosis following long-term administration of prostaglandin E_1 in infants with cyanotic congenital heart disease. J Pediatr 97:834–836.
120. Unverferth DV, Mehegan JP, Magorien RD, Unverferth BJ, Leier CV (1983): Regression of myocardial cellular hypertrophy with vasodilator therapy in chronic congestive heart failure associated with idiopathic dilated cardiomyopathy. Am J Cardiol 51:1392–1398.
121. Vargo TA, Lewis R, Burdine J, Schwartz A (1974): Comparison between puppies and adult dogs following infusion of digoxin (abstract). Pediatr Res 8:355A.
122. Von Hooff MEJ, Does RJMM, Rahn KH, vaBaak MA (1983): Time course of blood pressure changes after intravenous administration of propranolol or furosemide in hypertensive patients. J Cardiovasc Pharmacol 5:773–777.
123. Webb Kavey RE, Blackman MS, Sondheimer HM (1982): Phenytoin therapy for ventricular arrhythmias occurring late after surgery for congenital heart disase. Am Heart J 104:794–798.
124. Weiner DA, Klein MD (1982): Verapamil therapy for stable exertional angina pectoris. Am J Cardiol 50:1153–1157.
125. Wennevoid A, Sande E (1978): 6–14 years beta-blockade in three children with paroxysmal ventricular fibrillation. In Sande E et al (eds): Management of Ventricular Tachycardia: Role of Mexiletine: Proceedings of a Symposium, Copenhagen, May 25–27, Amsterdam, Excerpta Medica, p 429.
126. White RJ, Chamberlain DA, Howard M, Smith TW (1971): Plasma concentrations of digoxin after oral administration in the fasting and postprandial state. Br Med J 1:380–381.
127. White RD, Lietman PS (1978): Commentary: A reappraisal of digitalis for infants with left-to-right shunts and "heart failure." J Pediatr 92:867–870.
128. Wigle ED, Adelman AG, Felderhof CH (1974): Medical and surgical treatment of the cardiomyopathies. Circ Res (Suppl II)34, 35: 196–207.
129. Yabek SM, Berman W, Dillon T (1982): The physiologic effects of propranolol on sinus node function in children. Am Heart J 104:612–616.

54 MEDICAL TREATMENT OF PATENT DUCTUS ARTERIOSUS IN PREMATURE INFANTS

Ronald I. Clyman

HISTORICAL PERSPECTIVE

In 1939, Burnard[18] noted that murmurs were more commonly observed in infants with respiratory distress and suggested that the ductus arteriosus might be patent in these infants. The presence of a ductal left-to-right shunt, shortly after birth, in normal full-term infants was first inferred from dye dilution studies by Prec and Cassels,[76] and also by cardiac catheterization studies by Adams and Lind[1] and Rowe and James.[80] Twenty years after his initial observations, Burnard[17] described a murmur indicative of a patent ductus arteriosus (PDA) in 10 per cent of premature infants 48 hours after birth; a similar murmur could not be heard in full-term infants more than 10 hours after delivery.

The first-reported catheterization proof of a PDA in premature infants with respiratory distress syndrome was provided by Rudolph and coworkers[81] in 1961. Their findings suggested that near-term infants with minimal or no respiratory distress may have an anatomically open although functionally closed ductus and that premature infants with severe respiratory distress may have a wide-open ductus. Over the ensuing 25 years, in concert with improvements in survival of preterm infants with respiratory distress, the incidence of patent ductus arteriosus has increased.[30,39,53,58,73,74,86,87,95,103]

DIAGNOSIS

Although it has been known for many years that a PDA occurs commonly in premature infants, the exact incidence of the disorder varies from institution to institution and from year to year. These discrepancies probably occur because of differences in diagnostic criteria for PDA and in methods of managing preterm infants. In general, the diagnosis of PDA is based on the presence of a typical harsh murmur that initially is only systolic but may become continuous.[49] However, in 10 to 20 per cent of infants with a large ductus arteriosus, there may be absence of the typical murmur.[30,67] Ellison and colleagues[30] attempted to

evaluate several commonly used criteria for diagnosing a large left-to-right shunt through the PDA by noting the occurrence of each sign before and 36 to 48 hours after surgery in 91 infants who underwent PDA ligation. No single criterion could be taken alone as an indicator of PDA (Fig. 54–1). Although certain signs, such as a continuous murmur or a hyperactive left ventricular impulse, were quite specific for PDA, they were not that sensitive (more than 40 per cent of PDAs were missed). On the other hand, echocardiographic and ventilatory support criteria may be very sensitive but lack specificity for diagnosing a PDA. For example, a left atrial-to-aortic-root ratio (LA/Ao) by M-mode echocardiography of greater than 1.2:1 was present in 86 per cent of infants with a PDA but also in 38 per cent of infants without a PDA; a ratio greater than 1.3:1 was present in 80 per cent with a PDA and in 27 per cent without a PDA; and a ratio greater than 1.5:1 was present in 66 per cent with a PDA and 11 per cent without a PDA.

If an infant with PDA is receiving positive-pressure ventilation for coexistent lung disease, the "typical" radiographic findings of cardiomegaly, pulmonary edema, and increased pulmonary vascularity may be absent.[19,50] In fact, cardiomegaly may be absent in infants with PDA even without positive-pressure ventilation. Those infants with the largest ductal shunts may not have a very wide pulse pressure if systemic flow is low and systemic vascular resistance is elevated. The main adjuncts to diagnosis are echocardiography and Doppler studies. Specificity and sensitivity of M-mode echocardiographic determinations of LA/Ao ratios have been improved with the addition of ventricular dimensions[51,88] and systolic time intervals.[45,46,54] A more definitive test is contrast echocardiography in which saline is injected into an umbilical artery catheter, the tip of which is above the diaphragm; the visualization of microbubbles in the pulmonary artery verifies that there is an aortopulmonary connection.[2,3,96,104] However, it is not clear whether the sudden increase in aortic pressure during the saline injection might not either transiently alter the ductus diameter or have a detrimental effect on cerebral blood flow.

Transcutaneous, continuous wave Doppler measurements have been used to evaluate the degree of left-to-right PDA shunt;[83] however, the accuracy of this technique has been questioned.[47,56] Two-dimensional echocardiographic visualization of the PDA and pulsed Doppler techniques have

I wish to thank Richard Truelove and Paul Sagan for their skillful preparation of this manuscript.

been reported to be very sensitive and specific;[37,82,90] these reports need to be confirmed in other laboratories.

INCIDENCE

Despite discrepancies among the reported incidences of PDA, there is good evidence that the presence of PDA is inversely related to the maturity of the infant.[86] In full-term, healthy newborns, functional closure of the ductus occurs rapidly after birth. Assessment of these infants using pulsed Doppler echocardiography indicates that final functional closure of the ductus has occurred in almost half by 24 hours after birth, in 90 per cent by 48 hours, and in all by 96 hours.[42] In contrast, the ductus of many preterm infants will remain open for many days or weeks. In one study[30] of 1689 infants with birthweights less than 1750 g, a large "hemodynamically significant" PDA was noted in 42 per cent of infants with birthweights less than 1000 g, in 21 per cent of infants weighing between 1000 and 1500 g, and in 7 per cent of those weighing between 1500 and 1750 g.

The incidence of PDA is much higher in infants with respiratory distress syndrome.[58,60,74,86,94,95] Conversely, factors associated with a decreased incidence of respiratory distress syndrome (intrauterine growth retardation, prolonged rupture of the membranes, maternal steroid administration) have been associated with a decreased incidence of PDA.[21,86,92,94,98] Although it has been suggested that these "factors" decrease the PDA shunt owing to their effects on the pulmonary status of the infant, studies suggest that these "factors" act directly on the ductus arteriosus itself.[25,35,93] In fact, therapies that *only* improve the infant's pulmonary condition (e.g., artificial surfactant replacement) can lead to an *increased* incidence of PDA.[24,35]

An increased incidence of symptomatic PDA has been noted in preterm infants who experience perinatal asphyxia. Discriminant analysis suggests that this effect may be independent of both gestational age and respiratory distress syndrome.[27a] In addition, infants born at high altitudes have an increased incidence of PDA.[6] The rate of fluid administration during the initial several days after birth also influences the incidence of symptomatic PDA.[7]

TREATMENT

Definitive treatment of a PDA is closure of the ductus arteriosus. Unless there is a primary defect of the ductus wall, constriction and permanent anatomic closure eventually should occur spontaneously. In order to forestall the use of therapeutic interventions to close the PDA (indomethacin or surgical ligation), other conservative measures (e.g., fluid restriction, diuretics, and digitalis) have been advocated. Although excessive fluid administration has been associated with an increased incidence of PDA,[7] it is unlikely that fluid restriction will cause the ductus to close.[42] In addition, the combination of fluid restriction and diuretics frequently leads to electrolyte abnormalities, dehydration, and, most important, caloric deprivation. Furthermore, furosemide, the most commonly used diuretic,

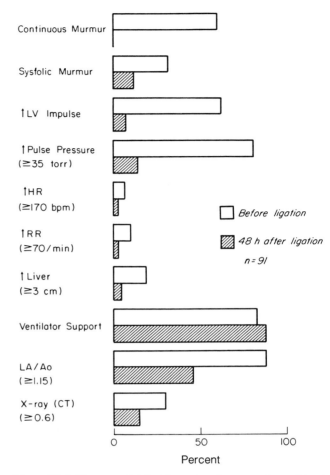

Figure 54–1. Signs associated with a patent ductus arteriosus. (Based on data presented in reference 30.)

in one study has been associated with an increased incidence of PDA.[43] Digitalis, especially in smaller infants weighing less than 1250 g, appears to have little or no beneficial effect and frequently is toxic. One would not expect digitalis to be very useful, because myocardial contractility is increased rather than reduced in infants with PDA.[46] In fact, a controlled study by McGrath failed to show any advantage to digoxin.[68] Finally, there may be an interaction between digoxin and indomethacin that increases the patient's susceptibility to the toxic effects of digoxin.[10,59,100]

The addition of positive end-expiratory pressure has been found to be useful in managing infants with a PDA.[27] When end-expiratory pressure is added, there is a decrease in the amount of left-to-right shunt through the ductus arteriosus; as a result, an increase in effective systemic blood flow occurs.[27] A low hematocrit has been shown to aggravate left-to-right shunting by lowering the resistance to blood flow through the pulmonary vascular bed,[61] leading some to advocate maintaining a hematocrit in the mid 40s. Higher hematocrits diminish excessive shunting through the PDA and help ensure systemic oxygen delivery when

Table 54–1. EFFECTS OF PDA
ON THE PREMATURE INFANT

	Control (n = 15)	Ligation (n = 10)
Birthweight	1006 g	1088 g
Gestation	28.3 weeks	29.0 weeks
Onset of symptoms	2.7 days	2.4 days
Age of randomization	8.4 days	8.6 days
Survivors	12	9
Intubation	30 days	14 days
Necrotizing enterocolitis	3	0
Retrolental fibroplasia (Grades III and IV)	4(2)	1(0)
Time to > 890 cal/kg/day via enteral route	24 days	13 days
Central intravenous line	7	2
Average daily hospital bill	$543	$440

Adapted from data from Cotton RB, et al (1978): Randomized trail of early closure of symptomatic patent ductus arteriosus in small preterm infants. J Pediatr 93:647–651.

perfusion is limited. Similarly, demands on left ventricular output should be minimized in infants with PDA by maintaining adequate oxygenation and by keeping the patient in a neutral thermal environment.

However, such therapies usually only delay, rather than prevent, the ultimate need for PDA closure. Clear justification for therapeutic closure of symptomatic PDA came from Cotton and colleagues,[28] who performed a controlled, randomized study to examine the long-term consequences of large symptomatic PDA in preterm infants. Infants weighing less than 1500 g with congestive heart failure and pulmonary edema (which was controlled with furosemide and digoxin) were randomized either to a "continued medical management" group or to a group that underwent surgical ligation (Table 54–1). Infants who underwent surgical closure were not ventilator dependent as long as infants assigned to the continued medical management group. In addition, the surgical closure group became free of the need of a central venous catheter sooner and was able to tolerate enteral feedings at an earlier age. Necrotizing enterocolitis and retrolental fibroplasia with cicatricial changes occurred less frequently in the surgical closure group, and hospital bills were smaller.[28] Ligation of a symptomatic PDA in premature infants now can be done with low mortality and morbidity.[29,36,72,99]

Based on experimental animal studies, the use of cyclooxygenase inhibitors in an attempt to close the ductus arteriosus was introduced in 1976.[33,48] Since then, a few controlled, and many uncontrolled, studies have been reported using indomethacin as a substitute for conservative medical management.[12] Gersony and associates have reported on the effects of intravenous indomethacin in the largest double-blind, controlled study to date.[38] Infants who received indomethacin were given 0.2 mg/kg for the initial dose. Infants under 48 hours of age at the time of trial entry received 0.1 mg/kg for the second and third doses of the drug. Infants who were 2 to 7 days of age at the time of the first dose received 0.2 mg/kg for the second and third doses, and those infants 8 days or older received 0.25 mg/kg for the second and third doses. Doses were given at 12-hour intervals. For the purposes of the study, infants were considered to have a hemodynamically

significant PDA only if the left-to-right shunt was large enough to compromise cardiorespiratory status. Closure of the ductus arteriosus was achieved without the need for surgical ligation in 79 per cent of the 135 infants given indomethacin versus 35 per cent of the 270 infants who received medical therapy alone (placebo). Closure rates within the indomethacin and placebo groups were *not* significantly related to birthweight, gestational age, gender, or race. Plasma concentrations of indomethacin were not statistically different between infants in whom the ductus closed or remained patent. In addition, Gersony and associates[38] compared the relative risks and benefits of treatment either with indomethacin or with surgical ligation for infants with a hemodynamically significant ductal shunt (Table 54–2). There were no significant differences between the two therapies in the overall mortality or incidence of bronchopulmonary dysplasia, intracranial hemorrhage, necrotizing enterocolitis, sepsis, elevated serum creatinine concentration, duration of mechanical ventilation, or age at discharge. However, the surgical ligation group had a significantly higher incidence of pneumothoraces, initial incidence of grade III and IV retrolental fibroplasia, and thoracotomies than did the indomethacin-treated group.

The best time to treat a premature infant with a PDA is controversial. In all of the studies reported previously, indomethacin or surgery was withheld until a major left-to-right shunt through a PDA was well established. In two controlled studies, early interruption of significant symptomatic ductal shunting decreased the need for assisted ventilation and additional oxygen in the management of respiratory distress syndrome,[55] and also decreased the incidence of bronchopulmonary dysplasia.[70]

A question that has been addressed is whether treatment should be reserved for those infants who have symptomatic ductus or whether small preterm infants should be treated prophylactically. Several trials of "prophylactic" indomethacin treatment of all infants within the first 12 hours after birth showed both a decreased incidence of PDA and prevention of subsequent reopening.[65,77,84,89] However, in these studies, no difference was observed in the subsequent incidence of chronic lung disease or other perinatal

Table 54–2. HOSPITAL COURSE IN INFANTS WITH PDA

	Indomethacin (Per Cent) (n = 75)	Surgery (Per Cent) (n = 79)
Death	23	15
Bronchopulmonary dysplasia	31	39
Intracranial hemorrhage	11	9
Necrotizing enterocolitis	7	6
Sepsis	20	23
Creatinine > 1.8 mg/dl	7	4
Mechanical ventilation (days)	10.0	10.5
Pneumothorax*	15	39
Cicatricial retrolental fibroplasia*	4	15
Surgical ligation*	33	99

*Significant difference at $p < 0.05$ level.
Adapted from data from Gersony WM, et al (1983): Effects of indomethacin in premature infants with patent ductus arteriosus: Results of a national collaborative study. J Pediatr 102:895–906.

morbidity. Treating all small preterm infants at birth involves giving indomethacin to the 50 to 60 per cent who would not develop a significant symptomatic PDA during their hospitalization,[65] which may account for the failure to observe a significant improvement in respiratory status after indomethacin treatment at birth.

It has been observed that 70 to 80 per cent of infants weighing less than 1000 g at birth who develop a systolic murmur will develop a hemodynamically significant left-to-right ductal shunt over the next 5 to 7 days.[65,66,84] Limiting "prophylactic" treatment to this specific group has been associated not only with a decreased incidence of PDA but also with improvement in respiratory status.[66]

In a double-blind, controlled study, Mahony and co-workers[66] treated infants with a PDA as soon as the PDA became apparent but before there were signs of cardio-respiratory compromise. The diagnosis of subclinical PDA was made when a murmur (even transient) was first heard. Despite the lack of clinical evidence (active precordium, bounding pulses, or increased pulmonary vascular markings) or echocardiographic evidence of a major shunt at the time of treatment, "prophylactic" (indomethacin) treatment of infants with birthweights below 1000 g who developed a murmur was associated with fewer subsequent PDA ligations, shorter duration of oxygen therapy and intubation, and fewer days to regain birthweight.[66] These observations suggest that not only do obviously symptomatic PDA shunts increase morbidity but also smaller "subclinical" PDA shunts may present a significant problem for the very low birthweight infant.

Indomethacin Failures

Not all infants who are treated with indomethacin will permanently close their ductus. Treatment failures may be classified into two groups. There may be little or no constrictive effect following administration of the drug, or there may be a recurrence of shunting afer a major constrictive effect.

Brash and colleagues[16] have suggested that plasma indomethacin concentrations need to be above a critical level of 250 ng/ml at 24 hours following drug administration in order to achieve ductus constriction. However, in several other studies, no differences in serum levels were seen at 24 hours in responders and nonresponders.[5,38] The only consistent finding associated with the failure of indomethacin to produce ductus constriction is the time after birth when indomethacin treatment is initiated.[26,52,75] When indomethacin treatment is begun several weeks after birth, often after prolonged conservative medical treatment, ductal closure rate is significantly reduced.

About 30 per cent of ductus that close after indomethacin treatment reopen.[23,38,69] In some infants the reopened ductus either is smaller or produces less disturbance and in time will close spontaneously; in others, all the signs and symptoms of PDA recur. The incidence of ductal reopening after indomethacin treatment is inversely related to birthweight.[23,69] Infants whose ductus reopens after indomethacin treatment frequently remain responsive to indomethacin, which suggests that there is a persistence of ductus responsiveness to prostaglandins in the most immature infants, a persistence that is lost in infants nearer term.[23] As a result, increased production of prostaglandins, as occurs in necrotizing enterocolitis,[22] may cause the ductus to reopen in very premature infants. In addition, premature infants have ductus that are histologically immature with very little development of intimal cushions or fibrosis to prevent reopening.[40] There is good evidence to suggest that early "prophylactic" use of indomethacin may decrease the incidence of later ductus reopening.[23,65,66,77,84,89] Several reports have shown a decreased rate of reopening associated with indomethacin maintenance therapy for 5 to 7 days.[32,85] These studies have shown a decreased incidence of ductal reopening if indomethacin therapy is maintained; however, there was no difference in the final reopening rate once the indomethacin was discontinued.[32,85]

Pharmacokinetics of Indomethacin

Indomethacin is poorly soluble in water or saline but can be dissolved in 0.2M phosphate buffer at pH 7.2.[5] Therefore, those who crush the indomethacin and suspend it in water or saline run the risk of uneven drug dispersion, and thus of uneven dosage when oral or rectal administration is used. Inaccurate dosing may have contributed to the variable results reported in pharmacokinetic studies and may explain some of the reported differences in clinical response to indomethacin.

Indomethacin absorption from the gut is reported to be almost 100 per cent in adults; in preterm infants, indomethacin absorption from the gut has been found to be as low as 10 to 20 per cent in some studies[13,14] but higher in others.[15,97] The peak plasma concentration of indomethacin in premature infants occurs 1 to 4 hours after oral or rectal administration, which is more than twice the time taken in adults.[13–15,97] The time course of plasma indomethacin concentrations is complex after both oral and intravenous administrations. Often, there is an initial rapid fall of concentration followed by a prolonged slow phase; there may even be a late rise in concentration that has led some investigators to postulate an enterohepatic circulation.[91] The slow phase has been reported in some studies to be longer in smaller infants: a half-life of 19 hours for infants below 1500 g birthweight or 32 weeks' gestation compared with 13 hours for those over 1500 g or over 32 weeks' gestation,[13,14] and 20.7 hours for infants under 1000 g birthweight compared with 15.4 hours for those over 1000 g.[101] Furthermore, the half-life appears to be longer in the first week after birth than later, being 21.4 hours compared with 12.2 hours in one study[101] and 28 hours compared with 18 hours in another.[91] However, in other studies, wide patient-to-patient variability and much longer half-lives (30 to 90 hours) have been reported,[16,97] throwing the relationship of indomethacin pharmacokinetics to gestational or postnatal age into question. Decreased plasma clearance of indomethacin probably reflects reduced hepatic metabolism since only minimal amounts of indomethacin are excreted unchanged in urine.

Two hours after intravenous injections of indomethacin, plasma concentrations are similar in all patients; however, 6 and 24 hours later there are 5- and 20-fold variations from highest to lowest indomethacin concentrations.[16] Protein binding (99 per cent) and volume of distribution (0.36 liter/kg) in premature infants have been found to be similar to adult values.[13,14] Studies in adults have shown that plasma concentrations of indomethacin should be above 300 ng/ml to inhibit almost completely prostaglandin E_2 synthesis in platelets, and that total body synthesis of prostaglandin E_2 (measured by the urinary excretion of one of its metabolites) was reduced by 60 per cent when trough plasma concentrations of indomethacin were between 50 and 300 ng/ml.[78] In infants, similar reductions in prostaglandin synthesis have been measured after indomethacin therapy.[63] As mentioned previously, there does not appear to be a good correlation between indomethacin concentration and ductus response.

Complications of Indomethacin

A majority of the infants treated with indomethacin in early studies developed transient diminution in renal function with variable effects on sodium, chloride, and water homeostasis.[11,20,33,44] However, studies have shown conflicting and inconclusive results on the effects of indomethacin on renal function.[31] The effects reported have been a transient decrease in both glomerular filtration rate and urine output, fractional excretion of sodium and chloride, and serum sodium concentration. Under different experimental conditions, indomethacin has been found to alter renal hemodynamics[57,62] and to potentiate the vasopressin-regulated water permeability of the collecting duct.[9]

Giving furosemide with indomethacin may prevent some of the renal side effects.[102] It is important to note that, in most clinical studies, indomethacin has been given after a period of fluid restriction and diuretic therapy; in addition, the presence of a PDA itself will significantly reduce glomerular filtration rate, urine output, and sodium reabsorption.[41]

It has been observed that infants treated within the first hours after delivery do not show a decrease in urine output after indomethacin administration.[65,66] This lack of decrease in urine output may be due to the elevated vasopressin concentrations that are present in the infants even prior to indomethacin treatment.[41] If given to well-hydrated, full-term, newborn lambs, indomethacin has almost no effect on renal blood flow, urine output, or glomerular filtration rate;[8] however, in prematurely delivered lambs with respiratory distress, indomethacin does appear to decrease glomerular filtration rate and sodium reabsorption.[41] Therefore, the renal manifestations of indomethacin may be masked or potentiated by the hemodynamic and hormonal changes that occur during the transitional period.

Initially there was concern that indomethacin would displace bilirubin from albumin and increase the risks of kernicterus in a hyperbilirubinemic infant. This concern has abated because indomethacin, at the plasma concentrations achieved therapeutically, does not displace bilirubin.[79]

Indomethacin, in adequate doses, inhibits platelets from producing cyclooxygenase products and prolongs the bleeding time.[34] This effect lasts 7 to 9 days, until the affected platelets are replaced by new ones not exposed to indomethacin. As a result, there has been concern that indomethacin might either increase the incidence of intracerebral hemorrhage or cause extension of an existing hemorrhage. Controlled clinical trials have failed to show an increase in intracerebral hemorrhage,[38,65,66] and in one study there was a significant decrease in the incidence.[32] Maher and coworkers[64] found that indomethacin did not cause extension of intracranial hemorrhages that existed prior to the treatment.

The National Collaborative Study did observe an increased incidence of occult blood loss from the gastrointestinal tract.[38] No increased incidence of necrotizing enterocolitis, retrolental fibroplasia, or sepsis has been observed.[38,66]

A unique intestinal lesion following indomethacin therapy has been described[4]; however, this lesion has not been observed in any of the controlled trials.

A detailed longitudinal follow-up study of patients receiving indomethacin or undergoing surgical ligation recorded no differences between groups in somatic growth, psychomotor and mental development, neurologic function, hearing, renal function, or vision.[70a,71]

Contraindications to Indomethacin

Most contraindications are relative, and few are beyond dispute.

Poor Renal Function

Many centers do not use indomethacin if the serum creatinine value is above 1.2 to 1.7 mg/dl or if urine output is below 1 ml/kg/hr. The reasoning behind this caveat is that indomethacin may decrease urine output further and cause significant water and electrolyte problems. A critical value of serum creatinine is not available; not only have different upper limits been selected arbitrarily in different studies, but different laboratories may give different values for the same sample. Furthermore, the interpretation of any given serum creatinine concentration will differ according to gestational and postnatal age. Whether giving indomethacin to a patient with moderate renal failure damages the kidney is uncertain; nevertheless, it is prudent to withhold indomethacin in infants who have significant renal failure, however it is defined. In some infants, indomethacin is followed by a markedly decreased urine output that must be allowed for when replacing fluid and electrolyte losses. Simultaneous administration of furosemide may prevent these renal changes.[102]

Bleeding Disorders and Low Platelets

Frank renal or gastrointestinal bleeding are contraindications to the use of indomethacin. Intracranial hemorrhage, however, is not a contraindication.[64] It is customary to withhold indomethacin if the platelet count is under 50,000/mm³, even in the absence of overt bleeding. There seems to be no continuing reason for this ban. Indomethacin in adequate doses abolishes platelet function for 7 to 9 days, no matter how many platelets there are.[34]

Necrotizing Enterocolitis

If infants have signs of early necrotizing enterocolitis, indomethacin is usually contraindicated. Part of the rationale for this caveat is that the necrotizing enterocolitis may be due to bowel ischemia secondary to the ductus arteriosus and that indomethacin may further decrease blood flow to the bowel. A more important reason is that if closing the ductus arteriosus prevents the progression of necrotizing enterocolitis, as many neonatologists believe, then surgical ligation is a more certain and rapid way of achieving ductus closure. Indomethacin may not close the ductus or may take 36 hours to do so, and such a delay may not preserve viability of the bowel.

Sepsis

All anti-inflammatory agents should be withheld if there is sepsis, unless no alternative is available. Thus indomethacin should not be used if sepsis is proven or strongly suspected.

Recommendations for Treatment

Because we believe that the ductus responds better to indomethacin if treated early, and that nonspecific medical treatment is ineffective, prolongs hospital stay, or causes complications (especially water, electrolyte, and nutritional imbalance), we prefer to treat patients early and without prior nonspecific therapy. At Mt. Zion Hospital and Medical Center, infants with birthweights less than 1000 g are treated with indomethacin when signs of a symptomatic or asymptomatic PDA are present. An asymptomatic PDA is defined as the presence of a murmur, even if heard on only one occasion.[66] Infants with birthweights greater than 1000 g are treated with indomethacin only when there are signs of a symptomatic PDA.[66] If the PDA closes and subsequently reopens, and no contraindications to the use of indomethacin exist, we will re-treat the infant with indomethacin. Surgery is reserved for those infants who do not respond to indomethacin or have contraindications to its use or who are believed to need immediate PDA closure because of clinical deterioration.

There are many variations in dosage regimens reported in the literature. We currently recommend an initial dose of lyophilized indomethacin of 0.2 mg/kg by intravenous administration over 20 minutes. Second and third doses are given 12 and 36 hours after the first dose. Infants who weigh less than 1250 mg at birth are given 0.1 mg/kg per dose for the second and third doses (unless they are older than 7 days). Infants weighing more than 1250 g, or older than 7 days, are given 0.2 mg/kg per dose for the second and third doses. In most instances, a single dose has not resulted in persistent constriction of the ductus arteriosus.

With this regimen of treating infants with birthweights lower than 1000 g who have a hemodynamically insignificant PDA, we find that there has not been an increase in the number of infants who are treated compared with the period when we treated infants only if they had a hemodynamically significant PDA; and we have reduced the number of surgical ligations in infants with a PDA from 27 per cent to less than 5 per cent.

References

1. Adams FH, Lind J (1957): Physiologic studies on the cardiovascular status of normal newborn infants (with special reference to the ductus arteriosus). Pediatrics 19:431–437.
2. Allen HD, Goldberg SJ, Valdes-Cruz LM, Sahn DT (1982): Use of echocardiography in newborns with patent ductus arteriosus: A review. Pediatr Cardiol 3:65–70.
3. Allen HD, Sahn DJ, Goldberg SJ (1978): New serial contrast technique for assessment of left to right shunting patent ductus arteriosus in the neonate. Am J Cardiol 41:288–294.
4. Alpan G, Eyal F, Vinograd I, Udassin R, Amir G, Mogle P, Glick B (1985): Localized intestinal perforations after enteral administration of indomethacin in premature infants. J Pediatr 106:277–281.
5. Alpert BS, Lewins MJ, Rowland DW, Grant MJA, Olley PM, Soldin SJ, Swyer PR, Coceani F, Rowe RD (1979): Plasma indomethacin levels in preterm newborn infants with symptomatic patent ductus arteriosus: Clinical and echocardiographic assessments of response. J Pediatr 95:578–582.
6. Alzamora V, Rotta A, Battilana G, Abugattas R, Rubio C,

Bournocle J, Zapata C, Santa-Maria E, Binder T, Subiria R, Paredes D, Pando B, Graham GG (1953): On the possible influence of great altitudes on the determination of certain cardiovascular anomalies. Pediatrics 12:259–262.

7. Bell EF, Warburton D, Stonestreet BS, Oh W (1980): Effect of fluid administration on the development of symptomatic patent ductus arteriosus and congestive heart failure in premature infants. N Engl J Med 302:598–604.

8. Benson D, Lister G, Heymann M, Rudolph A (1977): Effects of indomethacin on renal function in newborn lambs. Circulation (Suppl III)56:192.

9. Berl T, Raz A, Wald H, et al (1977): Prostaglandin synthesis inhibition and the action of vasopressin: Studies in man and rat. Am J Physiol 232:F529–F537.

10. Berman W Jr, Dubynsky O, Whitman V, Friedman Z, Maisels MJ (1978): Digoxin therapy in low-birth-weight infants with patent ductus arteriosus. J Pediatr 93:652–655.

11. Betkcrur MV, Yeh TF, Miller K, et al (1981): Indomethacin and its effects on renal function and urinary kallikrein excretion in premature infants with patent ductus arteriosus. Pediatrics 68:99–102.

12. Bhat R, Fisher E, Raju TNK, Vidyasagar D (1982): Patent ductus arteriosus: Recent advances in diagnosis and management. Pediatr Clin North Am 29:1117–1136.

13. Bhat R, Vidyasagar D, Fisher E, et al (1980): Pharmacokinetics of oral and intravenous indomethacin in preterm infants. Dev Pharmacol Ther 1:101–110.

14. Bhat R, Vidyasagar D, Vadapalli M, et al (1979): Disposition of indomethacin in preterm infants. J Pediatrics 95:313–316.

15. Bianchetti G, Monin P, Marchal F, et al (1980): Pharmacokinetics of indomethacin in the premature infant. Dev Pharmacol Ther 1:111–124.

16. Brash AR, Hickey DE, Graham TP, Stahlman MT, Oates JA, Cotton RB (1981): Pharmacokinetics of indomethacin in the neonate. N Engl J Med 305:67–72.

17. Burnard ED (1959): Discussion on the significance of continuous murmurs in the first few days of life. Proc R Soc Med 52:77–78.

18. Burnard ED (1939): The cardiac murmur in relation to symptoms in the newborn. Br Med J 1:134.

19. Burney B, Smith WL, Franken EA Jr, Smith JA, Klatte EC (1978): Chest film diagnosis of patent ductus arteriosus in infants with hyaline membrane disease. AJR 130:1149–1151.

20. Cifuentes RF, Olley PM, Balfe JW, et al (1979): Indomethacin and renal function in premature infants with persistent patent ductus arteriosus. J Pediatr 95:583–587.

21. Clyman RI, Ballard PL, Sniderman S, Ballard RA, Roth R, Heymann MA, Granberg JP (1981): Prenatal administration of betamethasone for prevention of patent ductus arteriosus. J Pediatr 98:123–126.

22. Clyman RI, Brett C, Mauray F (1980): Circulating prostaglandin E$_2$ concentrations and incidence of patent ductus arteriosus in preterm infants with respiratory distress syndrome. Pediatrics 66:725–729.

23. Clyman RI, Campbell D, Heymann MA, Mauray F (1985): Persistent responsiveness of the neonatal ductus arteriosus in immature lambs: A possible cause for reopening of patent ductus arteriosus after indomethacin-induced closure. Circulation 71:141–145.

24. Clyman RI, Jobe A, Heymann MA, Ikegami M, Roman C, Payne B, Mauray F (1982): Increased shunt through the patent ductus arteriosus after surfactant replacement therapy. J Pediatr 100:101–107.

25. Clyman RI, Mauray F, Roman C, Heymann MA, Ballard PL, Rudolph AM, Payne B (1981): Effects of antenatal glucocorticoid administration on ductus arteriosus of preterm lambs. Am J Physiol 241:H415–H420.

26. Cooke RWI, Pickering D (1979): Poor response to oral indomethacin therapy for persistent ductus arteriosus in very low birth-weight infants. Br Heart J 41:301–303.

27. Cotton RB, Lindstrom DP, Kanarek KS, et al (1980): Effect of positive end expiratory pressure on right ventricular output in lambs with hyaline membrane disease. Acta Paediatr Scand 69:603–606.

27a. Cotton RB, Lindstrom DP, Stahlman MT (1981): Early prediction of symptomatic patent ductus arteriosus from perinatal risk factors: A discriminant analysis model. Acta Paediatr Scand 70:723–727.

28. Cotton RB, Stahlman MT, Berder HW, Graham TP, Catterton WZ, Kover I (1978): Randomized trial of early closure of symptomatic patent ductus arteriosus in small preterm infants. J Pediatr 93:647–651.

29. Edmunds LH Jr, Gregory GA, Heymann MA, Kitterman JA, Rudolph AM, Tooley WH (1973): Surgical closure of the ductus arteriosus in premature infants. Circulation 48:856–863.

30. Elison RC, Peckham GJ, Lang P, Talner NS, Lerer TJ, Lin L, Dooley KJ, Nadas AS (1983): Evaluation of the preterm infant for patent ductus arteriosus. Pediatrics 71:364–372.

31. Feigen LP, Klainer E, Chapnik BM, et al (1976): The effects of indomethacin on renal function in pentobarbital-anesthetized dogs. J Pharmacol Exp Ther 198:457–463.

32. Ferguson MG, Rhodes PG, Joransen JA (1985): Prolonged treatment of patent ductus arteriosus with indomethacin. Pediatr Res 19:341A.

33. Friedman WF, Hirschklau MJ, Printz MP, Pitlick TP, Kirkpatrick SE (1976): Pharmacologic closure of patent ductus arteriosus in the premature infant. N Engl J Med 295:526–529.

34. Friedman Z, Whitman V, Maisels MJ, Berman W Jr, Marks KH, Vessel ES (1978): Indomethacin disposition and indomethacin induced platelet dysfunction in premature infants. J Clin Pharmacol 18:272–279.

35. Fujiwara T, Maeta H, Morita T, Watamabe V, Chida S, Abe T (1980): Artificial surfactant therapy in hyaline membrane disease. Lancet 1:55–59.

36. Gay JH, Daily WJR, Meyer BHP, Trump DS, Cloud DT, Molthan ME (1973): Ligation of the patent ductus arteriosus in premature infants: Report of 45 cases. J Pediatr Surg 8:677–683.

37. Gentile R, Stevenson G, Dooley T, Franklin D, Kawabori I, Pearlman A (1981): Pulsed Doppler echocardiographic determination of time of ductal closure in normal newborn infants. J Pediatr 98:443–448.

38. Gersony WM, Peckham GJ, Ellison RC, Miettinen OS, Nadas AS (1983): Effects of indomethacin in premature infants with patent ductus arteriosus: Results of a national collaborative study. J Pediatr 102:895–906.

39. Girling DJ, Hallidie-Smith KA (1971): Persistent ductus arteriosus in ill and premature babies. Arch Dis Child 46:177–181.

40. Gittenberger-DeGroot AC, Van Ertbruggen I, Moulaert AJMG, Harinck E (1980): The ductus arteriosus in the preterm infant: Histologic and clinical observations. J Pediatr 96:88–93.

41. Gleason C, Clyman RI, Heymann MA, Mauray F, Leake R, Roman C (1988): Indomethacin and patent ductus arteriosus: Effects on renal function in preterm lambs. Am J Physiol 254: F38–F44.

42. Green TP, Thompson TR, Johnson D, Lock JE (1980): Fluid administration and the development of patent ductus arteriosus. N Engl J Med 303:337–338.

43. Green TP, Thompson TR, Johnson DE, Lock JE (1983): Furosemide promotes patent ductus arteriosus in premature infants with the respiratory distress syndrome. N Engl J Med 308:743–748.

44. Halliday HL, Hirata T, Brady JP (1979): Indomethacin therapy for large patent ductus arteriosus in the very low birthweight infant: Results and complications. Pediatics 64:154–159.

45. Halliday HL, Hirata T, Brady JP (1979): Echocardiographic findings of large patent ductus arteriosus in the very low birthweight infant before and after treatment with indomethacin. Arch Dis Child 54:744–749.

46. Heitz F, Fouron J-C, van Doesburg NH, Bard H, Teasdale F, Chessex P, Davignon A (1984): Value of systolic time intervals in the diagnosis of large patent ductus arteriosus in fluid-restricted and mechanically ventilated preterm infants. Pediatrics 74:1069–1074.

47. Henry GW, Keagy BA, Lucas CL, Hsiao HS, Wilcox BR (1983): The validity of ultrasound quantification of ductal flow (abstract). Pediatr Res 17:113A.

48. Heymann MA, Rudolph AM, Silverman NH (1976): Closure of the ductus arteriosus in premature infants by inhibition of prostaglandin synthesis. N Engl J Med 295:530–533.

49. Heymann MA (1977): Patent ductus arteriosus. In Moss AJ, Adams FH, Emmanouilides GC (eds): Heart Disease in Infants, Children and Adolescents. Baltimore, Williams & Wilkins, p 168.

50. Higgins CB, Rausch J, Friedman WF, Hirschklau MJ, Kirkpatrick SE, Goergen TG, Reinke RT (1977): Patent ductus arteriosus in preterm infants with idiopathic respiratory distress syndrome. Pediatr Radiol 124:189–195.

51. Hirschklau MJ, DiSessa TG, Higgins CB, Friedman WF (1978): Echocardiographic diagnosis: Pitfalls in the premature infant with a large patent ductus arteriosus. J Pediatr 92:474–477.

52. Ivey HH, Kattwinkel J, Park TS, Krovetz LJ (1979): Failure of indomethacin to close persistent ductus arteriosus in infants weighing under 1000 grams. Br Heart J 41:304–307.

53. Jegier W, Karn G, Stern L (1968): Operative treatment of patent ductus arteriosus complicating respiratory distress syndrome of the premature. Can Med Assoc J 98:105.

54. Johnson GL, Breart GL, Gewitz MH, Brenner JI, Lang P, Dooley KJ, Ellison RC (1983): Echocardiographic characteristics of premature infants with patent ductus arteriosus. Pediatrics 72:864–871.

55. Kaapa P, Lanning P, Koivisto M (1983): Early closure of patent ductus arteriosus with indomethacin in preterm infants with idiopathic respiratory distress syndrome. Acta Paediatr Scand 72:179–184.

56. Karsdon J, Clyman RI (1983): A comparison of continuous wave Doppler ultrasonography with microsphere measured left-to-right shunt through the patent ductus arteriosus. Crit Care Med 11:556–558.

57. Kirschenbaum MA, White N, Stein HJ, et al (1974): Redistribution of renal cortical blood flow during inhibition of prostaglandin synthesis. Am J Physiol 227:801–805.

58. Kitterman JA, Edmunds LH, Gregory GA, et al (1972): Patent ductus arteriosus in premature infants: Incidence, relation to pulmonary disease and management. N Engl J Med 287:473–477.

59. Koren G, Zarfin Y, Perlman M, MacLeod SM (1984): Effects of indomethacin on digoxin pharmacokinetics in preterm infants. Pediatr Pharmacol 4:25–30.

60. Levitsky S, Fisher E, Vidyasagar D, Hastreiter AR, Bennet EJ, Raja TNK, Roper K (1976): Interruption of patent ductus arteriosus in premature infants with respiratory distress. Ann Thorac Surg 22:131–137.

61. Lister G, Hellenbrand WE, Kleinman CS, et al (1982): Physiologic effects of increasing hemoglobin concentration in left-to-right shunting in infants with ventricular septal defects. N Engl J Med 306:502–506.

62. Lonigro AJ, Itskovitz HP, Crowshow K, et al (1973): Dependency of renal blood flow on prostaglandin synthesis in the dog. Circ Res 32:712–717.

63. Lucas A, Mitchell MD (1978): Plasma-prostaglandins in pre-term neonates before and after treatment for patent ductus arteriosus. Lancet 2:130–132.

64. Maher P, Lane B, Ballard R, Piecuch R, Clyman RI (1985): Does indomethacin cause extension of intracranial hemorrhages: A preliminary study. Pediatrics 75:497–500.

65. Mahony L, Caldwell RL, Girod DA, Hurwitz RA, Jansen RD, Lemons JA, Schreiner RL (1985): Indomethacin therapy on the first day of life in infants with very low birth weights. J Pediatr 106:801–805.

66. Mahony L, Carnero V, Brett C, Heymann MA, Clyman RI (1982): Prophylactic indomethacin therapy for patent ductus arteriosus in very low-birthweight infants. N Engl J Med 306:506–510.

67. McGrath RL, McGuinness GA, Way GL, Wolfe RR, Nova JJ, Simmons MA (1978): The silent ductus arteriosus. J Pediatr 93:110–113.

68. McGrath RL (1978): In general discussion. Session III: Persistent patency of ductus arteriosus in premature infants. Report of the 75th Ross Conference on Pediatric Research. Columbus, Ohio, p 92.

69. Mellander M, Leheup B, Lindstrom DB, Palme C, Graham TP Jr, Stahlman MT, Cotton RB (1984): Recurrence of symptomatic patent ductus arteriosus in extremely premature infants, treated with indomethacin. J Pediatr 105:138–143.

70. Merritt TA, Harris JP, Roghmann K, Wood B, Campanella V, Alexson C, Manning J, Shapiro DL (1981): Early closure of the patent ductus arteriosus in very low birth weight infants: A controlled trial. J Pediatr 99:281–286.

70a. Merritt TA, White CL, Coen RW, et al (1982): Preschool assess-

ment of infants with a patent ductus arteriosus. Am J Dis Child 136:507–512.

71. Merritt TA, White CL, Jacob J, et al (1979): Patent ductus arteriosus treated with ligation or indomethacin: A follow-up study. J Pediatr 95:588–594.

72. Mikhail M, Lei W, Toews W, Synhorst DP, Hawes CW, Hernandez J, Lockhart C, Whitfield J, Pappas G (1982): Surgical and medical experience with 734 premature infants with patent ductus arteriosus. J Thorac Cardiovasc Surg 83:349–357.

73. Moss AJ, Emmanouilides GC, Rettori O, Higashino SM, Adams FH (1966): Postnatal circulatory and metabolic adjustments in normal and distressed premature infants. Biol Neonate 8:177–197.

74. Neal WA, Bessinger FB, Hunt CE, Lucas RV (1975): Patent ductus arteriosus complicating respiratory distress syndrome. J Pediatr 86:127–131.

75. Neal WA, Kyle JM, Mullett MD (1977): Failure of indomethacin therapy to induce closure of patent ductus arteriosus in premature infants with respiratory distress syndrome. J Pediatr 91:621–623.

76. Prec KJ, Cassels DE (1955): Dye dilution curves and cardiac output in newborn infants. Circulation 11:789–798.

77. Puckett CG, Cox MA, Haskins KS, Fisher DJ (1985): Prophylactic indomethacin for the prevention of patent ductus arteriosus. Pediatr Res 19:358A.

78. Rane A, Oelz O, Frohlich JC (1978): Relation between plasma concentration of indomethacin and its effect on prostaglandin synthesis and platelet aggregation in man. Clin Pharmacol Ther 23:658–668.

79. Rasmussen LF, Ahlfors CE, Wennberg RP (1978): Displacement of bilirubin from albumin by indomethacin. J Clin Pharmacol 18:477–481.

80. Rowe RD, James LS (1957): The normal pulmonary arterial pressure during the first year of life. J Pediatr 51:1–3.

81. Rudolph AM, Drorbaugh JE, Auld PAM, Rudolph AJ, Nadas AS, Smith CA, Hubbell JP (1961): Studies on the circulation in the neonatal period. Pediatrics 27:551–566.

82. Sahn DJ, Allen HD (1978): Real time cross sectional echocardiographic imaging and measurement of the patent ductus arteriosus in infants and children. Circulation 58:343–354.

83. Serwer GA, Armstrong BE, Anderson PAW (1982): Continuous wave Doppler ultrasonographic quantitation of patent ductus arteriosus flow. J Pediatr 100:297–299.

84. Setzer ES, Torres Arraut E, Gomez del Rio M, Young ML, Pacheco I, Ferrer PL, Schert RF, Bancalari E (1984): Cardiopulmonary effects of prophylactic indomethacin in the very low birth weight infant (abstract). Pediatr Res 18:346A.

85. Seyberth HW, Rascher W, Hackenthal R, Wille L (1983): Effect of prolonged indomethacin therapy on renal function and selected vasoactive hormones in very-low-birth-weight infants with symptomatic patent ductus arteriosus. J Pediatr 103:979–984.

86. Siassi B, Blanco C, Cabal LA, Goran AG (1976): Incidence and clinical features of patent ductus arteriosus in low-birth-weight infants: A prospective analysis of 150 consecutively born infants. Pediatrics 57:347–351.

87. Siassi B, Emmanouilides GC, Cleveland RJ, Hirose F (1969): Patent ductus arteriosus complicating prolonged assisted ventilation in respiratory distress syndrome. J Pediatr 74:11–19.

88. Silverman NH, Lewis AB, Heymann MA, Rudolph AM (1974): Echocardiographic assessment of ductus arteriosus shunts in premature infants. Circulation 50:821–825.

89. Sola A, Rogido M, Lezama C, Urman JE (1986): Effects of "prophylactic" I.V. indomethacin (P Indo) in VLBW infants with HMD (abstract). Pediatr Res 20:361A.

90. Stevenson JG, Kawabori I, Guntheroth WG (1980): Pulsed Doppler echocardiographic diagnosis of patent ductus arteriosus: Sensitivity, specificity, limitations, and technical features. Cathet Cardiovasc Diagn 6:255–263.

91. Thalji AA, Carr I, Yeh TF, Raval D, Luken JA, Pildes RS (1980): Pharmacokinetics of intravenously administered indomethacin in premature infants. J Pediatr 97:995–1000.

92. Thibeault DW, Emmanouilides GC (1977): Prolonged rupture of fetal membranes and decreased frequency of respiratory distress syndrome and patent ductus arteriosus in preterm infants. Am J Obstet Gynecol 123:43–46.

93. Thibeault DW, Emmanouilides GC, Dodge ME (1978): Pulmonary and circulatory function in preterm lambs treated with hydrocortisone in utero. Biol Neonate 34:238–247.

94. Thibeault DW, Emmanouilides GC, Dodge ME, Lachman RS (1977): Early functional closure of the ductus arteriosus complicating the respiratory distress syndrome in preterm infants. Am J Dis Child 131:741–745.

95. Thibeault DW, Emmanouilides GC, Nelson RJ, Lachman RS, Rosengart RM, Oh W (1975): Patent ductus arteriosus complicating the respiratory distress syndrome in preterm infants. J Pediatr 86:120–126.

96. Valdes-Cruz LM, Dudell GC (1981): Specificity and accuracy of echocardiographic and clinical criteria for diagnosis of patent ductus arteriosus in fluid-restricted infants. J Pediatr 98:298–305.

97. Vert P, Bianchetti G, Marchal F, Monin P, Morselli PL (1980): Effectiveness and pharmacokinetics of indomethacin in premature infants with patent ductus arteriosus. Eur J Clin Pharmacol 18: 83–88.

98. Waffarn F, Siassi B, Cabal L, Schmidt PL (1983): Effect of antenatal glucocorticoids on clinical closure of the ductus arteriosus. Am J Dis Child 137:336–338.

99. Wagner HR, Ellison RC, Zierler S, Lang P, Purohit DM, Behrendt D, Waldhausen JA (1984): Surgical closure of patent ductus arteriosus in 268 preterm infants. J Thorac Cardiovasc Surg 87: 870–875.

100. Wilkerson RD, Glenn TM (1977): Influence of nonsteroidal anti-inflammatory drugs on oubain toxicity. Am Heart J 94:454–459.

101. Yaffe SJ, Friedman WF, Rogers D, Lang P, Rangi M, Saccar C (1980): The disposition of indomethacin in premature babies. J Pediatr 97:1001–1006.

102. Yeh TF, Wilks A, Betkerur M, Lilien L, Pildes RS (1982): Furosemide prevents the renal side effects of indomethacin therapy in premature infants with patent ductus arteriosus. J Pediatr 101:433–437.

103. Zachman RD, Steinmetz GP, Botham RJ, Graven SN, Ledbetter MK (1974): Incidence and treatment of the patent ductus arteriosus in the ill premature neonate. Am Heart J 87:697–703.

104. Zednikova M, Baylen BG, Yoshida Y, Emmanouilides GC (1982): Precordial contrast echocardiographic detection of patent ductus arteriosus in small preterm infants. Pediatr Cardiol 2:271–275.

55 TREATMENT OF PPHNS

Joseph B. Philips, III

Once the diagnosis of persistent pulmonary hypertension of the newborn syndrome (PPHNS) is established, the physician must promptly begin treatment. Most infants with full-blown PPHNS are critically ill, and many will die or be severely damaged if effective interventions are not applied. For unclear reasons, infants with PPHNS do not tolerate the low PaO_2 values often encountered and well-tolerated in infants with cyanotic congenital heart disease. Instead, increasing respiratory distress and metabolic acidosis occur. Low pH levels increase pulmonary vasoconstriction[93] and exacerbate right-to-left shunting, resulting in even lower PaO_2 values. The combination of alveolar hypoxia and severe acidosis lead to a vicious, downhill cycle that must be interrupted, or death may occur.

This chapter examines various treatments for PPHNS and casts a critical eye upon the available literature. Methodologic details for each therapy are presented only when necessary. The reader is referred to previous reviews for further details. Our emphasis here is on the scientific validity of claims of efficacy for various proposed remedies for PPHNS. Presently, there is no general consensus on the best management method(s). Approaches to treatment are currently guided by dogma and personal experience, as the literature contains no studies that unequivocally document the effectiveness or superiority of any particular management method. This situation exists for at least two reasons. First, PPHNS is rare enough that an individual institution would have difficulty amassing a large enough population to perform a controlled clinical trial in a reasonable time period. The rarity of PPHNS is confirmed by data from the National Institute of Child Health and Human Development (NICHD)-sponsored Neonatal Network.* In 1985, the eight member institutions treated an average of 20 cases of PPHNS yearly with a range of 10 to 47 cases

per institution. A controlled trial comparing two competing forms of therapy can detect a statistically significant difference ($\alpha = 0.05$, $\beta = 0.80$) between a 60 per cent response rate for one treatment and an 80 per cent response rate for the other with about 95 subjects per group. Clearly, such a trial cannot be conducted in a single institution in a reasonable time period.

A second and equally important reason for a lack of controlled clinical trials is the "bandwagon" syndrome, wherein a new treatment is developed and enthusiastically promoted. Others jump on the bandwagon, and soon a plethora of similar reports appear. Usually, these are phase I type studies in which the new treatment is applied to all subjects. Results are usually reported as short-term changes in a response variable (e.g., a rise in PaO_2) or are reported in comparison with a historical control group (e.g., survival). Both approaches are acceptable as initial studies, but they can neither scientifically confirm that the new treatment is solely or even partly responsible for the observed effect, nor can they adequately assess the risks and complications of the new treatment. Such studies should be followed by more rigorous phase II and phase III controlled clinical trials in which the new treatment is compared with no treatment or with the previously accepted therapy in terms of efficacy, safety, and long-term outcome. Studies of this type are lacking in the area of PPHNS. Acceptance of preliminary studies as proof of efficacy leads to a dilemma that has been oft debated. FJ Ingelfinger, past editor of The New England Journal of Medicine wrote the following:

> Preconceived opinions concerning the efficacy of a certain treatment, whatever their validity, place immense constraints on attempts at objective evaluation of that treatment.... Popular enthusiasm brooks no randomization, and only decades will tell whether some current treatments established by acclaim rather than hard evidence are really beneficial or whether they, like bloodletting and purging, are but manifestations of the power of faith.[53]

Spodick wrote in the same vein:

> The problem with not beginning with a randomized controlled trial (RCT) is that the apparent success of such "pilot trials" discourages RCTs by raising pseudoethical compulsions not to conduct them, once convinced that the trial treatment works.[105]

We find ourselves precisely in this position when deciding on which of several possible remedies to use in treating critically ill infants with PPHNS.

GENERAL SUPPORTIVE CARE

Infants with PPHNS are notoriously unstable. Anecdotal reports abound that these infants "flip flop" or respond

*The NICHD Neonatal Network consists of the following institutions and investigators:

University of Alabama at Birmingham, Birmingham, AL; Principal Investigator (PI), Joseph B. Philips, III; Co-PI, George Cassady

Rainbow Babies and Childrens Hospital, Cleveland, OH; PI, Avroy A. Fanaroff; Co-PI, Maureen Hack

Southwestern Medical School, Dallas, TX; PI, Jon E.Tyson; Co-PI, Ricardo Vauy

Wayne State University, Detroit, MI; PI, Ronald L. Poland; Co-PI, Seetha Shankaran

University of Tennessee Newborn Center, Memphis, TN; PI, Sheldon B. Korones; Co-PI, Richard Cooke

University of Miami, Miami, FL; PI, Charles R. Bauer; Co-PI, Emmalee Bandstra

University of Vermont, Burlington, VT, and Dartmouth University, Hanover, NH; PI, Jerold F. Lucey; Co-PI, Jeffrey D. Horbar.

negatively to noxious stimuli such as venipuncture, sudden loud noises, and cold drafts. Thus, a hands-off policy is often recommended for infants with PPHNS, meaning that procedures (suctioning, endotracheal tube changes, bathing, and repositioning) should be performed only when clinically indicated rather than according to a preset protocol, that infants with PPHNS should be cared for in the quietest part of the nursery (if such an area exists), and that extreme care and gentleness be employed in performing essential maneuvers. It is common to see a sign posted on these infants' care stations stating "PPHNS—Hands Off!"

There are no controlled studies to support these policies; however, they do seem prudent to this author and are employed in our nursery. Infants with PPHNS should certainly be provided with intravenous fluids and nutrition. Whether intravenous fat should be given is unclear, since these preparations may cause pulmonary dysfunction.[62,85]

Some authors recommend that infants with PPHNS be sedated to blunt their responses to noxious stimuli. Again, there are no studies documenting the appropriateness of this approach, nor is there general agreement as to which agent should be used. Chloral hydrate, morphine, diazepam, and others have been advocated (it must be understood that sedative and not anesthetic doses, which have also been advanced as treatments, are discussed here). It seems reasonable to use sedation in individual cases in which unusual instability is encountered.

TOLAZOLINE HYDROCHLORIDE

Tolazoline is a fascinating drug with diverse pharmacologic actions including α-adrenergic antagonism and agonism, cholinergic antagonism and agonism, and histaminergic agonism.[2,44,95,120,124] Figure 55–1 shows the structures of tolazoline, histamine, epinephrine, and atropine. Each of the other compounds clearly shares structural characteristics with tolazoline. Effects of tolazoline may be primary—due to the drug itself, or secondary—due to release of another vasoactive substance by the tolazoline.[52] Tolazoline causes release of histamine, a pulmonary vasodilator in newborn lambs and probably also in human infants. The pulmonary vasodilator effect of tolazoline in hypoxic newborn lambs is eliminated

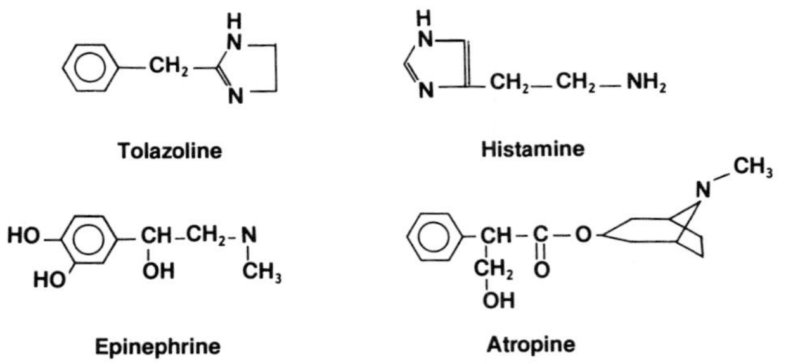

when H_1 and H_2 receptors are blocked.[44] Before its use in PPHNS, tolazoline had been used in the cardiac catheterization laboratory for many years to test for reversibility of pulmonary hypertension in patients with congenital or acquired lesions. Thus, it was logical that tolazoline would be tried early in the discovery phase of the new entity—PPHNS.

One of two patients in the best known early report of PPHNS received tolazoline.[41] An improvement in oxygenation was noted but so was the most significant complication of tolazoline therapy—systemic arterial hypotension. Six years later, Korones et al reported "successful" use of tolazoline in five infants with PPHNS.[59] All five had clinically significant increases in PaO_2, and three had decreases in systemic arterial pressure of 5 to 20 mmHg.

A flood of reports subsequently appeared wherein tolazoline was given to infants with a variety of types of PPHNS. Table 55–1 summarizes the findings of 49 such publications. All share common design characteristics and flaws (the bandwagon syndrome is evident here). Every report, from single patient case reports (n = 6) to those involving several dozen subjects, has a nonrandomized, self-controlled design in which response variables such as oxygenation and systemic arterial pressure are assessed before and after injection of tolazoline. Tolazoline was administered, usually as an intravenous bolus of 1 to 2 mg/kg over 1 minute, and was often followed by a continuous infusion of 0.5 to as much as 10 mg/kg/hr. Studies of this type are important and should constitute phase I in the development of a new therapy. They should be followed by prospective, randomized controlled trials to assess

Table 55–1. SUMMARY OF TOLAZOLINE REPORTS
(563 PATIENTS IN 49 PAPERS)

	Number	Per Cent
Types of reports		
Peer-reviewed	39	79.6
Nonpeer reviewed	4	8.2
Abstract	6	12.2
Randomized, controlled trials	0	0.0
Types of patients		
Hyaline membrane disease	137	24.3
Diaphragmatic hernia	68	12.1
Persistent fetal circulation	64	11.4
Meconium aspiration syndrome	57	10.1
Sepsis	19	3.4
Other or unknown	218	38.7
Initial response to tolazoline[46]*	326/537	60.7 (33 to 92)†
Survival[34]	237/408	58.1 (40 to 100)
Complications		
Systemic arterial hypotension[30]	140/419	33.4 (0 to 71)
Evidence of GI bleeding[13]	66/285	23.2 (0 to 54)
Increased GI secretions[4]	50/120	41.7 (35 to 48)
Decreased urine output[8]	24/169	14.2 (0 to 42)

*Number of reports mentioning the variable.

†Range of prevalence (percentage) in reports of more than 10 patients.

References: 1, 3, 6, 8, 10, 11, 13, 16, 19, 20, 23, 25, 28, 29, 33, 34, 38, 39, 41, 45, 50, 55, 59, 63, 64, 65, 72, 73, 73a, 74, 76, 78, 79, 80, 84, 86, 91, 100, 102, 103, 107, 108, 110, 116, 117, 119, 121, 122, 123.

Figure 55–1. Chemical structures of tolazoline, histamine, epinephrine, and atropine. Note structural similarities of tolazoline to portions of other agents.

accurately the safety and effectiveness of the new treatment. In one study patients were randomized to receive either a single tolazoline bolus or a bolus followed by continuous tolazoline infusion.[73a] *No infant has ever received a tolazoline placebo!* Thus, there is no valid evidence to discount the hypothesis that improvement after tolazoline in these patients actually resulted from volume expansion, temporal factors, or other unspecified cointerventions.

Nevertheless, some information can be gained from the literature on tolazoline—not all of it is good. Overall, 63 per cent of infants given tolazoline were judged to have benefited; response rates ranged from 33 per cent to 92 per cent. Nearly 58 per cent of tolazoline-treated infants ultimately survived, with survival rates varying between 40 per cent and 100 per cent. The reports are diverse in reporting formats, including six abstracts, several letters and brief communications, and a number of peer-reviewed papers. In addition, outcome variables differed widely among reports. Because of these variations, it is difficult to analyze the effects of tolazoline in PPHNS of different etiologies. In general, however, lower response and survival rates are seen in the infants with diaphragmatic hernias, while those with hyaline membrane disease and idiopathic PPHNS (± meconium aspiration) display higher response rates and variable survival. In six reports, survival exceeded the response rate to tolazoline, suggesting that factors other than tolazoline contributed to survival. Thus, it is unclear whether tolazoline is a life saving treatment for PPHNS.

The complication rate for tolazoline approaches 50 per cent overall. About 30 per cent of tolazoline-treated infants in 22 studies were judged to have had significant drops in systemic arterial pressure, while about one fourth developed gastrointestinal bleeding that was severe in some cases. In four reports, tolazoline caused significant increases in gastrointestinal secretions, which in one case contributed to a marked hypochloremic alkalosis.[1] Urine output may be affected by tolazoline because of lowered renal blood flow or through other mechanisms. Many infants with PPHNS may also have acute tubular necrosis or another form of renal dysfunction, making it difficult to differentiate effects of tolazoline from those of other causes. Nevertheless, 14 per cent of infants in eight reports showed decreased urine output in temporal association with tolazoline. Dosing was inadequately described in many reports, while infusion rates varied so much in others that specific conclusions about complication rates in comparison to dosages are not possible. A general feeling emerges, however, that higher doses led to the most significant complications. In the study of McMillan and Sauve, a higher complication rate was seen in the group given a bolus of tolazoline followed by a continuous infusion.[73a]

Until recently, there were no data on tolazoline pharmacokinetics in neonates. Dosage regimens were developed empirically and consequently vary considerably among reports. The most commonly used bolus doses are 1 to 2 mg/kg intravenously over 1 to 5 minutes. Continuous infusion rates range from 0.5 to as high as 25 mg/kg/hr.

Ward developed a microassay method and studied tolazoline pharmacokinetics in 13 infants.[116] He found that

plasma half-life ranged from 1.5–41.2 hours with a median value of 4.4 hours. Since tolazoline is excreted unchanged in the urine via a saturable transport system for organic bases, it is logical to hypothesize that urine output might be related to tolazoline excretion. In fact, Ward found a significant (r = 0.61, p < 0.05) correlation between urine output and tolazoline plasma half-life.

For infants with urine output of 0.9 ml/kg/hr or greater, Ward recommends an infusion rate of 0.16 mg/kg/hr of tolazoline for each 1 mg/kg given in the bolus dose to maintain a steady plasma concentration. This dosage rate is five- to tenfold lower than the most commonly used doses in the literature! Worse yet, infants with urine output less than 0.9 ml/kg/hr should receive only 0.08 mg/kg/hr for each 1 mg/kg of bolus. If most infants with PPHNS have similar pharmacokinetic variables, we can predict that tolazoline accumulated during continuous infusion in most infants reported in the literature. Ward tested his dosage recommendations in two infants and found that tolazoline did not accumulate in their plasma.

More data on tolazoline pharmacokinetics are needed before more precise dosage recommendations can be made. It appears that many of the previous published reports on tolazoline may have described use of inappropriately high maintenance infusion rates. It remains possible that tolazoline, when used in proper dosages, may be a life-saving and comparatively safe treatment in PPHNS.

Largely because of the high complication rate of tolazoline use, enthusiasm for its use has waned. Another apparently effective therapy—mechanical hyperventilation—began replacing tolazoline as the treatment of choice for initial management of PPHNS in most centers. Within the NICHD Neonatal Network, hyperventilation is almost always used before tolazoline. Many neonatologists now reserve tolazline as a "last ditch" drug, giving it only when all other treatments have failed.

HYPERVENTILATION

In 1978, Peckham and Fox published a report documenting impressive reductions in pulmonary artery pressure in infants with PPHNS when the infants were mechanically hyperventilated.[84] Table 55–2 summarizes available reports on the use of hyperventilation in various forms of PPHNS.

In contrast to tolazoline, mechanical hyperventilation therapy has been reported less often, patients are more poorly characterized, and complications are not well documented. The initial response rate is an impressive 91 per cent, although survival is only 67 per cent overall. As with the tolazoline reports, all hyperventilation studies are noncontrolled and nonrandomized. All patients served as their own controls, and the effects of cointerventions and temporal factors were not examined. There are no studies comparing the effectiveness of tolazoline and that of hyperventilation as frontline treatments for PPHNS. Despite a lack of rigorous proof of efficacy, hyperventilation replaced tolazoline as the initial treatment of choice for PPHNS in most intensive care nurseries in the early to

Table 55–2. SUMMARY OF USE OF HYPERVENTILATION IN PPHNS (159 PATIENTS IN 11 REPORTS)

	Number	Per Cent
Types of reports		
Peer-reviewed	9	81.8
Nonpeer reviewed	2	18.2
Randomized, controlled trials	0	0.0
Types of patients		
Meconium aspiration syndrome	19	11.9
Diaphragmatic hernia	13	8.2
Persistent fetal circulation	12	7.5
Hyaline membrane disease	8	5.0
Sepsis	3	1.9
Other or unknown	104	65.4
Initial response to hyperventilation[8]*	118/130	90.8 (87 to 100)[†]
Survival[8]	102/152	67.1 (56 to 85)
Complications		
Pneumothorax[2]	24/59	40.7

*Number of reports mentioning the variable

[†]Range of prevalence (percentage) in reports of more than 10 patients

References: 11, 25, 28, 30, 33, 35, 38, 48, 84, 117, 122

mid 1980s. When queried about this, most neonatologists state that "hyperventilation is safer and more effective than tolazoline." The literature provides hints that hyperventilation is preferable to tolazoline, but firm evidence is lacking.

There is good experimental evidence that pulmonary vascular resistance (PVR) is pH dependent. Rudolph and Yuan showed many years ago that PVR increases as pHa decreases below 7.40, regardless of PaO_2, and that the threshold for exponential increases in PVR occurs at progressively higher PaO_2 values as pHa decreases.[93] Several recent animal studies have shown that alkalosis induced by mechanical hyperventilation attenuates or partially reverses hypoxic pulmonary hypertension.[70,97] This effect appears owing to changes in blood pH, not from changes

in $PaCO_2$. Thus, the primary goal of mechanical hyperventilation is the production of alkalosis.

The paper by Peckham and Fox[84] and another by Drummond et al[25] provide the clinical basis for use of mechanical hyperventilation in PPHNS. Both suggest that a $PaCO_2$ decrease to less than 25 mmHg and a pHa increase above 7.55 to 7.60 will improve distal aortic oxygenation in infants with PPHNS, presumably by relaxing abnormally constricted pulmonary resistance vessels. Figure 55–2 shows the effect of pH on PaO_2 in a single infant with PPHNS.

Because of variations in treatment protocols (some patients received tolazoline only after hyperventilation had failed), selection biases, and outcome criteria, attempted comparisons of cumulative tolazoline and hyperventilation therapy response and survival rates from the current literature are probably invalid. Nevertheless, the initial response rate (an improvement in distal aortic oxygenation) to hyperventilation is much higher than that for tolazoline (91 per cent versus 61 per cent, respectively, χ^2 = 42.4, p < 0.001). Hyperventilation therapy is also associated with a smaller but significant increase in survival (67 per cent versus 59 per cent, χ^2 = 6.38, p = 0.012).

Significant complications can occur with hyperventilation treatment. In one report, 45 per cent of infants developed at least one pneumothorax.[48] Such events often precipitate pulmonary vasospasm and result in severe hypoxemia, which can cause severe morbidity or death if not rapidly reversed. In addition, the high ventilator rates and pressures often needed to achieve the desired effect, combined with the prolonged use of 100 per cent oxygen, may lead to bronchopulmonary dysplasia. Thirty-one per cent of mechanically ventilated PPHNS infants in one follow-up study had chronic lung disease.[99] In this light, it is important to recognize that a "transition phase" may occur in hyperventilated infants wherein continued oxygen and ventilator requirements result not from the PPHNS from which the infant suffered initially, but from the over-

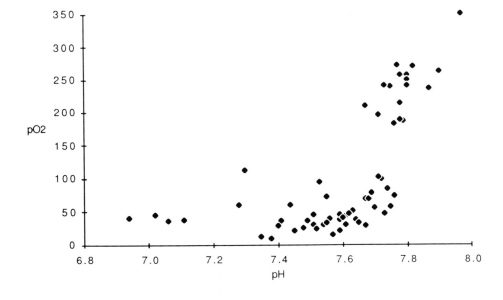

Figure 55–2. Relationship between pH and PaO_2 in a single infant hyperventilated for PPHNS. Data represent all values obtained in the 72 hours following birth. The infant did not receive tolazoline.

lapping, insidious development of chronic lung disease during therapy.[36] It is not known how long hyperventilation therapy should be continued if a favorable initial response is seen. Most neonatologists favor keeping the infant's $PaCO_2$ below Fox's "critical value"[36] for 24 to 48 hours before making significant ventilator changes. Once this waiting period has passed, the physician should periodically reduce ventilator rates and pressures in small decrements, allowing $PaCO_2$ to rise and pHa to fall slightly. If these changes are tolerated, more aggressive ventilator "weaning" should be employed in an effort to minimize barotrauma and oxygen toxicity.

Fox has reported tracheal secretion impactions during hyperventilation therapy.[37] These impactions were apparently due to faulty humidification circuitry (WW Fox, personal communication), but such a possiblilty should certainly be considered in the differential diagnosis of sudden deteriorations in hyperventilated infants.

Profound alkalosis sharply reduces cerebral blood flow and also lowers cerebral oxygen consumption in newborn puppies.[92] Hyperventilation may reduce cardiac output by impeding thoracic blood return. Many fear that cerebral ischemia and hypoxia may occur during hyperventilation. Whether cerebral compromise actually develops in hyperventilated neonates with PPHNS is unknown. Bruce reviewed this subject and found no substantive evidence for hyperventilation-induced cerebral ischemia in PPHNS.[12] However, follow-up studies of hyperventilated infants have shown a high rate of hearing loss (up to 27 per cent) which may have resulted from cerebral ischemia.[82,99] Klesh et al have reported that 9 of 19 infants hyperventilated for PPHNS had cerebral infarctions.[58a] Many of these infants had perinatal asphyxia, and 16 had received tolazoline. Since many infants with PPHNS have had perinatal asphyxia, severe acidosis and hypoxemia, these residua may also be unrelated to the treatments given. Noninvasive metabolic studies of hyperventilated animals and humans using novel methods such as magnetic resonance imaging are needed to help resolve this issue.

PARALYSIS

When hyperventilation is employed, neuromuscular blockade is almost invariably used. Most neonatologists think this treatment facilitates the attainment of systemic alkalosis while minimizing barotrauma resulting from asynchronous breathing efforts by the patient. Henry and associates published preliminary data supporting this hypothesis, but truly convincing data are lacking.[51]

Pancuronium is the most commonly used paralyzing agent. This drug does not release histamine and has little effect on systemic vascular resistance.[112] Many infants treated for several days with pancuronium develop significant peripheral edema, an effect which may be due to impairment of "muscle pumping" on lymphatics or perhaps due to a hormonelike effect, since pancuronium is a steroid based compound.

Curare compounds release histamine, leading to effects other than the primary neuromuscular blockade.[112] Some prefer curare because of this histamine-releasing effect, as histamine is thought to be a pulmonary vasodilator in human infants. Others recommend use of high dose morphine to achieve apnea and sedation simultaneously in the belief that such treatment minimizes both asynchronous breathing and the effects of noxious stimuli. Morphine is also a histamine releaser.[54]

At present, choice of neuromuscular blocking or relaxing agents is at the discretion of the individual physician; data supporting use of any one agent in preference to another are lacking. If neuromuscular blockade is used, the agents should be withdrawn as soon as possible, as there is a report of profound disuse atrophy in two infants treated continuously for 5 weeks with pancuronium.[113] Improvement from severe flaccid paralysis in these patients was very slow.

EICOSANOIDS

There is much evidence that eicosanoids are involved in at least some forms of PPHNS. Group B streptococcus–induced pulmonary hypertension in animals is mediated via products of the cyclooxygenase system and is almost certainly caused by elevations in thromboxane A_2 (TXA_2).[90,94] Stenmark and associates documented increased leukotriene (powerful vasoconstrictors) content in lung lavage fluid of infants with PPHNS but not in infants ventilated for other indications.[106] Hammerman et al found very high levels of TXB_2, the inactive metabolite of TXA_2, in the blood of infants with PPHNS but not in the blood of other infants.[49] Two case reports show very high thromboxane levels in infants with congenital diaphragmatic hernia.[34,109] Thus, it is logical to hypothesize that exogenous vasodilatory eicosanoids or inhibitors of vasoconstrictor synthesis might be helpful in PPHNS.

Prostacyclin (PGI_2) is a potent vasodilator that may have some specificity for the pulmonary circulation.[14,67] In 1979, Lock and colleagues reported the successful use of PGI_2 in an infant with PPHNS.[66] This promising case report was followed by a multicentered trial of PGI_2 in PPHNS. Five of 10 infants responded with improved oxygenation, but nine eventually died, leading to the abrupt discontinuation of the trial (WA Long, personal communication). One of these infants died of a myocardial infarction, which resulted when PGI_2 was abruptly discontinued and then restarted.[24] Kappa et al gave PGI_2 to five infants with PPHNS and reported improvment in all, although only two survived.[56] Two infants had large drops in systemic blood pressure. Thus, PGI_2 use has been reported in 16 PPHNS infants, with 10 (62 per cent) responding but only four (25 per cent) surviving. Based on this small sample, it is impossible to say whether PGI_2 is life-saving in PPHNS, although it does not appear to be a panacea.

Prostaglandin E_1 is a nonspecific pulmonary vasodilator frequently used in maintaining ductus arteriosus patency in infants with congenital heart disease. Five infants did not respond favorably to PGE_1 infusion in the first report documenting its use in PPHNS.[81] Oxygenation did appear to improve in one infant in a case report of PGE_1 use in

PPHNS.[117] Nevertheless, some neonatologists apparently do use PGE$_1$ in PPHNS (WA Long, personal communication). An advantage of PGE$_1$ is its extremely short half-life, which allows for rapid reversal of untoward effects simply by reducing or stopping the infusion. Presently, however, definitive evidence for efficacy of PGE$_1$ in PPHNS is lacking.

Prostaglandin D$_2$ has the unique property of being a specific pulmonary vasodilator in fetal and hypoxic neonatal lambs.[15,87] In fact, bolus doses of PGD$_2$ cause dose-related decreases in pulmonary artery pressure and increases in systemic arterial pressure.[88] Only six PPHNS infants have been reported to have received PGD$_2$ therapy; all had failed maximal conventional treatment before being given PGD$_2$.[104] Only two showed a transient improvement in oxygenation, and two survived. It remains possible that PGD$_2$ could be helpful earlier in the course of PPHNS.

Our current knowledge of the role and use of eicosanoids in PPHNS is rudimentary. Improved understanding of the different forms of PPHNS may eventually lead to more specific remedies. For example, if group B streptococcus–induced PPHNS is mediated via TXA$_2$, then use of a specific inhibitor of thromboxane synthesis could abolish the pulmonary hypertension. Studies in animals have shown that specific inhibition of TX synthesis results in prompt return of pulmonary artery pressure to near normal levels in animals with GBS-induced pulmonary hypertension, despite continued infusion of GBS.[21,111] Systemic arterial pressure was unaffected by thromboxane synthesis inhibition. Other gram-positive organisms, as well as gram-negative bacterial endotoxin, also cause pulmonary hypertension in animals, probably through a similar mechanism.[32,118] Thromboxanes do not appear to mediate the high fetal pulmonary vascular resistance or neonatal hypoxia-induced pulmonary hypertension in animals.[17] Other studies suggest that leukotrienes may help mediate hypoxia-induced pulmonary hypertension, raising the possibility of using leukotriene synthesis inhibitors or receptor blockers in PPHNS.[46,98] More biochemical information is needed on infants with PPHNS in order for rational drug therapies to be developed. One thing is certain, we have not seen the last of use or blockade of eicosanoids in PPHNS.

OTHER DRUGS

Pressors

Dopamine is probably the pressor of choice among neonatologists for use in PPHNS, with dobutamine also widely used. Many infants with PPHNS have myocardial dysfunction from asphyxia and/or hypoxia and present with cardiogenic shock or echocardiographic evidence of reduced myocardial performance. The reader is referred to other sections of this book for discussions on use of these agents for cardiogenic shock and other disorders.

Dopamine is frequently used in PPHNS to counter the hypotensive effects of tolazoline. Drummond and Williams studied the interactions between dopamine and tolazoline in chronically instrumented, conscious lambs and found these interactions to be complex.[26] Newborn animals and humans appear to require higher doses of dopamine than do adults.[42] Little information is available on the hemodynamic effects of dopamine in tolazoline-treated infants with PPHNS. Fiddler reported in 1980 that low dose dopamine infusion was helpful in treating myocardial dysfunction associated with PPHNS.[31] Drummond stated that "dopamine was a very useful pressor" in PPHNS but that doses of 20 to 125 µg/kg/min were needed to elevate systemic pressures; she also showed an example of an infant with PPHNS who was inadvertently given 2000 µg/kg of dopamine as a bolus.[25] Systemic artery pressure increased promptly to a value exceeding pulmonary artery pressure, which was not affected by the dopamine bolus. Meadow et al suggested that treatment aimed at selectively raising systemic pressure, rather than lowering pulmonary pressure, could be an effective treatment for PPHNS.[75] Further work is needed in this area before recommendations can be made.

Once tolazoline dosage and pharmacokinetics are better understood, perhaps the prevalence of tolazoline-induced hypotension will decrease and there will be less need for multiple drug regimens. Additional data are needed in the area of cardiotonic therapy in PPHNS before treatment recommendations can be made with any assurance of safety and efficacy.

Other Vasodilators

Chlorpromazine, a major tranquilizer, is a potent α-adrenergic receptor blocker. Larsson et al reported the use of chlorpromazine in 18 infants with severe hypoxia; 14 (78 per cent) raised their PaO$_2$, and 9 (50 per cent) survived.[61] Mean systemic pressure fell about 30 per cent following the drug, and urine output declined. These and other results suggest that chlorpromazine is no more effective or less hazardous than tolazoline.

Calcium channel blockers are effective vascular smooth muscle relaxers, and their use in PPHNS has been suggested. The effects of one calcium channel blocker, nifedipine, were studied in normoxic and hypoxic newborn lambs.[89] During normoxia, nifedipine reduced systemic pressure in a dose-related fashion, while pulmonary pressure was unaffected; in hypoxia, nifedipine reduced both pressures such that the ratio of pulmonary to systemic pressures did not change. Thus, nifedipine at least appears to be a nonspecific vasodilator and is not a good candidate for use in PPHNS. Verapamil, also a calcium channel blocker, appears to have a similar lack of specificity.[22]

One report states that sodium nitroprusside may be helpful in PPHNS.[7] Infants with PPHNS had a variable response to treatment and only 7 of 15 (47 per cent) survived. As with most other proposed remedies for PPHNS, there simply is not enough experience at present with nitroprusside to make positive or negative recommendations.

Mammel et al reported that amrinone, a nonglycoside, noncatechole cardiotonic agent was a pulmonary vasodilator with a lower threshold for pulmonary than for systemic vasodilation in conscious juvenile lambs.[71] Unfortunately, amrinone was not helpful in human infants with PPHNS (JE Lock, personal communication).

Others have suggested that chronic anesthesia maintained with fentanyl may reduce pulmonary artery pressure in infants with PPHNS.[115] This treatment appears to have become particularly popular among pediatric surgeons in treating or preventing the PPHNS associated with congenital diaphragmatic hernia. As with the other proposed PPHNS remedies, no controlled trials have been conducted, and rigorous proof of efficacy and reliable estimates of safety are unavailable.

Sodium Bicarbonate

Use of this agent in PPHNS is based primarily on anecdotal evidence of efficacy. A single abstract suggests beneficial effects of $NaHCO_3$,[9] while other authors simply suggest that it be used. Both rapid bolus and continuous infusions have been employed.

Rapid injection of 1 to 2 mg/kg of diluted (one part of 1 mEq/ml $NaHCO_3$ to three parts sterile H_2O) is often used in a effort to "open up" the pulmonary circulation. Anecdotally, such infusions are often followed by transient rises in PaO_2. Whether these rises are sustained or allow beneficial ventilator adjustments is unclear. It is uncertain whether the effects are due to the $NaHCO_3$—some or all of the effects may be from the rapid volume expansion also produced by this treatment. Increasing evidence suggests that rapid $NaHCO_3$ infusions may worsen neurologic damage in experimental asphyxia.[47,69] One should therefore be cautious in using this treatment.

Slow, continuous $NaHCO_3$ infusions at the rate of 0.5–1.0 mEq/kg/hr are commonly used in PPHNS, especially when a significant metabolic acidosis is present. Given the effects of pHa on pulmonary vascular resistance, this seems a rational therapy. However, even this therapy can have negative effects, especially fluid and sodium overload in infants with renal dysfunction. There are no studies using aggressive $NaHCO_3$ infusion as a primary treatment for PPHNS.

THE COLUMBIA (WUNG AND ASSOCIATES) APPROACH

In late 1985, Wung and associates of the College of Physicians and Surgeons at Columbia University published their experience in managing PPHNS without hyperventilation.[123] Data were presented for 15 severely ill infants; seven with meconium aspiration, four with hyaline membrane disease, and two with idiopathic PPHNS. Ventilator management was directed at maintaining $PaO_2 \geq 50$ mmHg while minimizing barotrauma. Hypocarbia was avoided, and paralysis was not used. A series of guidelines was given for dealing with various respiratory problems. Tolazoline was given to all but one patient—a point not adequately emphasized by the authors. Sodium bicarbonate was given to infants with base deficits exceeding 10 mEq/liter. Three infants had Neonatal Pulmonary Insufficiency Index scores predicting 90 to 100 per cent

mortality. All 15 patients survived, and only one required oxygen beyond 30 days. This startling report caused many neonatologists to reexamine the aggressive approach to PPHNS by implying that iatrogenic illness is a significant contributor to morbidity and mortality in PPHNS.

Dworetz et al recently reported preliminary data using the Columbia method that showed survival of five of six infants considered to have a ≥ 90 per cent mortality risk.[27] This survival rate compares favorably with that shown for extracorporeal membrane oxygenator therapy using similar entry criteria for patient selection.

The conservative approach advocated by Wung and his associates is becoming more widely used and is the newest trend in management of PPHNS. Although there are no controlled trials using this treatment algorithm, early reports suggest that results compare favorably with hyperventilation and even with extracorporeal membrane oxygenator therapy. In the absence of a clearly superior treatment alternative, the one least likely to produce harm should be employed first. The Columbia approach seems to fit this principle best.

EXTRACORPOREAL MEMBRANE OXYGENATOR THERAPY

Extracorporeal membrane oxygenator (ECMO) therapy offers the ultimate high-tech approach to infants who appear destined to die of reversible respiratory failure. In essence, this procedure involves establishment of cardiopulmonary artery bypass for several days on the assumption that providing the lung with a few days of "rest" will allow return of sufficient pulmonary function so that life will continue to be possible after removal of ECMO therapy. In most cases, use of ECMO therapy requires permanent ligation of the right common carotid artery. Continuous heparinization is required, and large numbers of platelet and blood transfusions are usually needed. Costs of an ECMO therapy "run" averaged $25,000 to $35,000 in the mid 1980s. In spite of these formidable obstacles, over 1000 neonates received this aggressive, costly treatment by the end of 1987 for a variety of conditions, which commonly included PPHNS. As of mid 1987, at least 25 centers in the United States were offering ECMO therapy, with perhaps 6 to 10 new centers opening per year for the next few years. Is this treatment effective? What are its risks and benefits? These and many other questions must be answered before this (or any other) therapy can be generally recommended.

Somewhat better survey data are available about ECMO therapy than for tolazoline and hyperventilation, perhaps because the treatment is so invasive and costly that investigators have been more conscious of the necessity to document the need for and efficacy of ECMO therapy. Table 55–3 summarizes the results of 342 patients in 14 published reports on ECMO therapy. Most papers appeared in peer-reviewed journals, and patients are well characterized as to primary diagnosis. Survival is an impressive 72.5 per cent in a group thought by investigators to have a greater than 80 per cent risk of death. A number

Table 55–3. SUMMARY OF USE OF ECMO IN PPHNS
(342 PATIENTS IN 13 REPORTS)*

	Number	Per Cent
Types of reports		
Peer-reviewed	10	69.2
Nonpeer reviewed	1	15.4
Abstracts	3	23.1
Randomized, controlled trials	1	7.1
Types of patients		
Meconium aspiration syndrome	138	40.4
Diaphragmatic hernia	59	17.3
Hyaline membrane disease	46	13.5
Idiopathic PPHNS	27	7.9
Sepsis	17	5.0
Congenital heart disease	9	2.6
Other or unknown	46	13.5
Survival[10][†]	248/342	72.5 (41 to 89)[‡]
Outcome and complications		
"Normal"[4]	88/183	48.1 (44 to 60)
Intracranial hemorrhage[5]	47/219	21.5 (9 to 36)
Seizures[5]	34/164	20.7 (9 to 42)
Bronchopulmonary dysplasia[4]	22/163	13.5 (6 to 27)
Mechanical problems[3]	12/89	13.5 (3 to 20)
Neurologic deficit[5]	20/157	12.7 (3 to 36)
Bleeding[5]	14/27	11.0 (4 to 13)

*Ten reports used for total patient count, three smaller series used for out-
come and complications when more detail was supplied
[†]Number of reports mentioning the variable
[‡]Range of prevalence (percentage) in reports of more than 10 patients

References: 4, 5, 40, 57, 58, 60, 68, 77, 83, 96, 109, 114, 119

of serious sequelae are seen in survivors, but one should recall that infants must be critically ill in order to qualify for ECMO therapy.

The Neonatal ECMO Data Registry is a voluntary central data base that includes data on 696 infants treated with ECMO therapy as of December 31, 1986 (personal communication, Neonatal ECMO Data Registry). Overall, 566 (81.3 per cent) of ECMO-treated infants have survived, while 84.4 per cent of infants with primary PPHNS lived.

As usual, ECMO therapy was introduced by a series of phase I treatment trials showing that the technique could be employed and that substantial numbers of infants survived with ECMO who were predicted to die based on historical control groups. Unlike the other treatments, one group of investigators undertook a randomized, controlled trial of ECMO versus maximal conventional therapy in neonatal respiratory failure.[4] This study is the only randomized controlled trial of a treatment for PPHNS. Unfortunately, the authors used a novel, controversial patient allocation scheme that resulted in only one control infant, who died, and 11 ECMO treated infants, who all lived. The control infant was among the sickest infants studied. Because of the unusual study design, this study failed to satisfy many critics that ECMO therapy is a truly efficacious remedy.

Amplifying the uncertainty about ECMO therapy are recent reports of high survival rates in two centers using the Columbia approach in infants predicted to have high mortality on historically standardized scoring systems used

as entry criteria for many ECMO programs.[27,101] Thus, as with the other forms of treatment in PPHNS, it is not yet clear whether ECMO therapy is a life-saving remedy. Most neonatologists believe that ECMO therapy will ultimately be shown effective in some forms of severe, but reversible, neonatal pulmonary disease such as PPHNS. It is imperative that properly designed controlled clinical trials of ECMO therapy be conducted before widespread use of this technique occurs. One such trial is currently under way in New England, and a multicentered trial is being contemplated in California. Perhaps the answers will be available in a few years.

SUMMARY AND CONCLUDING REMARKS

The therapeutic history of PPHNS has seen waves of enthusiasm for one management scheme after another. First came tolazoline and then hyperventilation followed by ECMO therapy for conventional treatment failures. The latest treatment concept is the conservative approach of Wung and associates at Columbia University. *Not one convincing randomized, controlled treatment trial in PPHNS has been published!* Despite this fact, many neonatologists and others caring for sick newborns are convinced that they know how to manage PPHNS. The foregoing discussion should cause us to realize that, in the late 1980s, we really have very little idea of the best way to manage PPHNS.

Tolazoline may be helpful in some infants with PPHNS. Most published reports used doses that were probably excessive and that may have accounted for a large portion of the observed rate of adverse reaction. Tolazoline is still widely used, however, despite the fact that we understand its proper use poorly; 483 of the 696 infants in the ECMO Central Registry received tolazoline.

Mechanical hyperventilation is associated with impressive initial response rates in PPHNS and may be a life-saving therapy. This treatment also fits with intensivists' desires to do something aggressive for a critical disorder. However, we have no proof that hyperventilation is a safe, efficacious treatment for PPHNS.

Recent trends away from hyperventilation toward a more conservative use of respirators and a return to the use of tolazoline confirm that we are dissatisfied with the results of hyperventilation. Preliminary reports showing high survival rates in severely ill infants *without* hyperventilation or ECMO therapy argue strongly for a formal comparison of hyperventilation and the more conservative approach (including tolazoline in proper doses) as initial treatments for PPHNS. This task has been identified as a major goal by the NICHD Neonatal Network. First, however, a preliminary trial will be conducted to gather more data on tolazoline pharmacokinetics in human infants with PPHNS. Following this preliminary study, it is hoped that the Neonatal Network will conduct a prospective, randomized controlled trial of hyperventilation versus conservative ventilation with use of appropriate doses of tolazoline. If the issue of ECMO therapy has not been settled at this point, then such a trial would also provide an opportunity to compare ECMO therapy with maximal conventional care.

Thus, the current state of knowledge about management of PPHNS is rudimentary and clouded with uncertainty. There is light in the tunnel, however, as several groups including the NICHD Neonatal Network are at work to help resolve current issues in management of PPHNS. Once solid data begin to appear, a firm foundation will have been set for further scientific studies comparing the established best therapy with what is hypothesized to be a better remedy. Our empirically derived remedies must emerge from the darkness of uncertainty into the spotlight of scientific scrutiny, where they must withstand objective testing before being accepted. Only when we have done this will we know what to do for our patients with PPHNS and why.

References

1. Adams JM, Hyde WH, Procianoy RS, Rudolph AJ (1980): Hypochloremic metabolic acidosis following tolazoline-induced gastric hypersecretion. Pediatrics 65:298–300.
2. Ahlquist RP, Huggins RA, Woodbury RA (1947): The pharmacology of benzyl-imidazoline (Priscol). J Pharmacol Exper Ther 89:271–288.
3. Akesode FA, Sandor GGS, MacNab AJ, Patterson MWH, Ebelt VJ, Tipple M, Pendray MR, Ling E (1981): Respiratory and cardiac effects of tolazoline in persistent fetal circulation (abstr). Clin Res 29:138A.
4. Bartlett RH, Dietrich MD, Roloff MD, Cornell RG, Andrews AF, Dillon PW, Zwischenberger JB (1985): Extracorporeal circulation in neonatal respiratory failure: A prospective randomized study. J Pediatr 76:479–487.
5. Bartlett RH, Gazzaniga AB, Toomasian J, Corwin AG, Roloff D, Rucker R (1986): Extracorporeal membrane oxygenation (ECMO) in neonatal respiratory failure. Ann Surg 204:236–245.
6. Benitz WE, Bloss RS, Turment T, Beardmore HE, Aranda JV (1980): Tolazoline therapy for persistent pulmonary hypertension after congenital diaphragmatic hernia repair. J Pediatr 97:984–988.
7. Benitz WE, Malachowski N, Cohen RS, Stevenson DK, Ariagno RL, Sunshine P (1985): Use of sodium nitroprusside in neonates: Efficacy and safety. J Pediatr 106:102.
8. Bloss RS, Turmen T, Beardmore HE, Aranda JV (1980): Tolazoline therapy for persistent pulmonary hypertension after congenital diaphragmatic hernia repair. J Pediatr 97:984–988.
9. Bolan DL, Ruckerman RN (1979): Acid-base balance in persistent fetal circulation (abstr). Pediatr Res 13:490.
10. Boyle RJ, Oh W (1978): Transcutaneous PO_2 monitoring in infants with persistent fetal circulation who are receiving tolazoline therapy. Pediatrics 63:605–606.
11. Brett C, Dekle M, Leonard CH, Clark C, Sniderman S, Roth R, Ballard R, Clyman R (1981): Developmental follow-up of hyperventilated neonates: Preliminary observations. Pediatrics 68:588–591.
12. Bruce DA (1984): Effects of hyperventilation on cerebral blood flow and metabolism. Clin Perinatol 11:673–680.
13. Bucher HU, Arbenz U, Bucher A (1979): $TcPO_2$ in pediatric cardiology: Application during balloon septostomy, tolazoline administration, and in children with right-to-left shunt. Birth Defects 15:355–362.
14. Cassin S, Winikor I, Tod M, Philips J, Frisinger J, Jordan J, Gibbs C (1981): Effects of prostacyclin on the fetal pulmonary circulation. Pediatr Pharmacol 1:197–207.
15. Cassin S, Tod M, Philips J, Frisinger J, Jordan J, Gibbs C (1981): Effects of prostaglandin D_2 on perinatal circulation. Am J Physiol 240:H755–H760.
16. Chow-Tung E, Fischer JH, Bhat R, Vidyasagar D (1985): Clinical pharmacology of tolazoline in persistent fetal circulation (abstr). Pediatr Res 19:169A.
17. Clozel M, Clyman R, Soifer S, Heymann M (1985): Thromboxane is not responsible for the high pulmonary vascular resistance in fetal lambs. Pediatr Res 19:1254–1257.
18. Cohen RS, Stevenson DK, Malachowski N, Ariango RL, Johnson JD, Sunshine P (1980): Late morbidity among survivors of respiratory failure treated with tolazoline. J Pediatr 97:644–647.
19. Collins DL, Pomerance JJ, Travis KW, Turner SW, Pappelbaum SJ (1977): A new approach to congenital posterolateral diaphragmatic hernia. J. Pediatr Surg 12:149–156.
20. Cotton EK (1964): The use of Priscoline in the treatment of the hypoperfusion syndrome (letter). Pediatrics 36:149.
21. Crouse D, Lyrene R, Tarpey M, Oliver J, Cassady G, Philips J (1987): Furegulate, a thromboxane synthase inhibitor, reverses group B streptococcus induced pulmonary hypertension (abstr). Pediatr Res 21:447A.
22. Dickstein PJ, Trindade O, Goldberg RN, Bancalari E (1984): The effect of calcium antagonists on hypoxic pulmonary hypertension in the piglet. Pediatr Res 18:1262–1265.
23. Dillard RG (1982): Fatal gastrointestinal hemorrhage in a neonate treated with tolazoline. Clin Pediatr 21:761–762.
24. Drummond WH, Williams BJ, Blanchard WB, Bucholz CJ, Bucholz CL (1982): Myocardial infarction after prostacyclin (PGI_2) treatment of neonatal pulmonary hypertension (PH) (abstr). Pediatr Res 16:99A.
25. Drummond WH, Gregory GA, Heymann MA, Phibbs RA (1981): The independent effects of hyperventilation, tolazoline, and dopamine on infants with persistent pulmonary hypertension. J Pediatr 98:603–611.
26. Drummond WH, Williams BJ (1983): Effect of continuous tolazoline infusion on cadiopulmonary response to dopamine in unanesthetized newborn lambs. J Pediatr 103:278–284.
27. Dworetz AR, Mova FR, Sabo B, Gross I (1987): Survival in infants with persistent pulmonary hypertension (PPHTN) without extracorporeal membrane oxygenation (ECMO) (abstr). Pediatr Res 21:360A.
28. Easa D, Herrman K, Holt D (1981): Management of persistent fetal circulation in a neonate. Hawaii Med J 40:355–356.
29. Ein SH, Barker G, Olley P, Shandling B, Simpson JS, Stephens CA, Filler RM (1980): The pharmacologic treatment of newborn diaphragmatic hernia—a 2-year evaluation. J Pediatr Surg 15:384–394.
30. Ferrara TB, Johnson DE, Chang PN, Thompson TR (1984): Efficacy and neurologic outcome of profound hypocapnic alkalosis for treatment of persistent pulmonary hypertension in infancy. J Pediatr 105:457–461.
31. Fiddler GI, Chatrath R, Williams GJ, Walker DR, Scott O (1980): Dopamine infusion for the treatment of myocardial dysfunction associated with a persistent transitional circulation. Arch Dis Child 55:194–198.
32. Fletcher JR, Ramwell PW, Harris RH (1981): Thromboxane, prostacyclin and hemodynamic events in primate endotoxin shock. Adv Shock Res 5:143–148.
33. Fong LV, Pemberton PJ (1985): Congenital diaphragmatic hernia and the management of persistent foetal circulation. Anesth Inten Care 13:375–379.
34. Ford WDA, James MJ, Walsh JA (1984): Congenital diaphragmatic hernia: Association between pulmonary vascular resistance and plasma thromboxane concentrations. Arch Dis Child 59:143–146.
35. Fox WW (1982): Mechanical ventilation in the management of persistent pulmonary hypertension of the neonate (PPHN). In Peckham GJ, Heymann MA (eds): Cardiovascular Sequelae of Asphyxia in the Newborn. Columbus, Ross Laboratories.
36. Fox WW, Duara S (1983): Persistent pulmonary hypertension in the neonate: Diagnosis and management. J Pediatr 103:505–514.
37. Fox WW, Spitzer AR, Smith D, Musci M, Beatty JR, Myerberg DZ (1984): Tracheal secretion inpaction during hyperventilation for persistent pulmonary hypertension of the neonate (abstr). Pediatr Res 18:323A.
38. Gaulin P, Rubin SZ (1983): Persistent fetal circulation in neonates postoperatively: The value of manual ventilation. Can J Surg 26:250–251.

39. German JC, Bartlett RH, Gazzaniga AB, Huxtable RF, Amalie R, Sperling DR (1977): Pulmonary artery pressure monitoring in persistent fetal circulation (PFC). J Pediatr Surg 12:913–919.

40. German JC, Worcester C, Gazzaniga AB, Huxtable RF, Amalie RN, Brahmbhatt N, Bartlett RH (1980): Technical aspects in the management of the meconium aspiration syndrome with extracorporeal circulation. J Pediatr Surg 15:378–383.

41. Gersony WM, Duc GV, Sinclair JC (1969): "PFC" syndrome (persistence of fetal circulation) (abstr). Circulation (Suppl III) 40:87.

42. Godoy G, Lyrene R, Cassady G, Dew A, Philips J (1985): Hemodynamic effects of dopamine (abstr). Pediatr Res 19:171A.

43. Goetzman BW, Milstein JM (1980): Pulmonary vascular histamine receptors in newborn and young lambs. J Appl Physiol Respirat Environ Exer Physiol 49:380–385.

44. Goetzman BW, Milstein JM (1979): Pulmonary vasodilator action of tolazoline. Pediatr Res 13:942–944.

45. Goetzman BW, Sunshine P, Johnson JD, Wennberg RP, Hackel A, Merton DF, Bartoletti AL, Silverman NH (1976): Neonatal hypoxia and pulmonary vasospasm: Response to tolazoline. J Pediatr 89:617–621.

46. Goldberg RN, Suguihara C, Ahmed T, Deseda de Cudemus B, Barrios P, Setzer ES, Bancalari E (1985): Influence of an antagonist of slow–reacting substance of anaphylaxis on the cardiovascular manifestations of hypoxia in piglets. Pediatr Res 19:1201–1205.

47. Graf H, Leach W, Arieff AI (1985): Evidence for a detrimental effect of bicarbonate therapy in hypoxic lactic acidosis. Science 227:754–756.

48. Hageman JR, Adams MA, Gardner TH (1984): Persistent pulmonary hypertension of the newborn. Am J Dis Child 138:592–595.

49. Hammerman C, Lass N, Strates E, Komar K, Bui KC (1987): Prostanoids in neonates with persistent pulmonary hypertension. J Pediatr 110:470–472.

50. Hegyi T, Hiatt IM (1980): Tolazoline and dopamine therapy in neonatal hypoxia and pulmonary vasospasm. Acta Paediatr Scand 69:101–103.

51. Henry GW, Stevens DC, Schreiner RL, Grosfeld JL, Ballantine TVN (1979): Respiratory paralysis to improve oxygenation and mortality in large newborn infants with respiratory distress. J Pediatr Surg 14:761–766.

52. Hughes MJ, O'Brien LJ (1977): Liberation of endogenous compounds by tolazoline. Agents Actions 7:225–230.

53. Ingelfinger FJ (1972): The randomized clinical trial (editorial). N Engl J Med 287:100–101.

54. Jaffe JH, Martin WR (1985): Opioid analgesics and antagonists. In Gilman AG, Goodman LS, Rall TW, Murad F (eds): Goodman and Gilman's The Pharmacologic Basis of Therapeutics. Norwalk, Macmillan, pp 491–531.

55. Johnson GL, Cunningham MD, Desai NS, Cottrill CM, Noonan JA (1980): Echocardiography in hypoxemic neonatal pulmonary diseases. J Pediatr 96:716–720.

56. Kappa P, Koivisto M, Ylikorkala O, Kouvalainen K (1985): Prostacyclin in the treatment of neonatal pulmonary hypertension. J Pediatr 107:951–953.

57. Keszler M, Moront KN, Subramanian S, Smith Y, Molina B, Mehta NR, Dhanireddy R (1987): Pulmonary management during extracorporeal membrane oxygenation (abstr). Pediatr Res 21:456A.

58. Kirkpatrick BV, Krummel TM, Mueller DG, Ormazabal MA, Greenfield LJ, Salzberg AM (1983): Use of extracorporeal membrane oxygenation for respiratory failure in term infants. Pediatrics 72:872–876.

58a. Klesh KLO, Murphy TF, Scher MS, Buchanan DE, Maxwell EP, Guthrie RD (1987): Cerebral infarction in persistent pulmonary hypertension of the newborn. Am J Dis Child 141:852–857.

59. Korones SB, Fabien GA (1975): Successful treatment of "persistent fetal circulation" with tolazoline (abstr). Pediatr Res 9:367A.

60. Krummel TM, Greenfeld LJ, Kirkpatrick BV, Mueller DG, Kerkering KW, Salzberg AM (1982): Extracorporeal membrane oxygenation in neonatal pulmonary failure. Pediatr Annal 11:905–908.

61. Larsson LE, Ekstrom-Jodal B, Hjalmarson O (1982): The effect of chlorpromazine in severe hypoxia in newborn infants. Acta Paediatr Scand 71:399–402.

62. Levene MI, Wigglesworth JS, Desai R (1980): Pulmonary fat accumulation after intralipid infusion in the preterm infant. Lancet 2:815–818.

63. Levin DL, Heymann MA, Kitterman JA, Gregory GA (1976): Persistent pulmonary hypertension of the newborn infant. J Pediatr 88:626–630.

64. Levin DL (1978): Morphologic analysis of the pulmonary vascular bed in congenital left-sided diaphragmatic hernia. J Pediatr 92:805–809.

65. Levy RJ, Rosenthal A, Freed MD, Smith CD, Eraklis A, Nadas AS (1977): Persistent pulmonary hypertension in a newborn with congenital diaphragmatic hernia: Successful management with tolazoline. Pediatrics 60:740–742.

66. Lock JE, Olley PM, Swyer PR, Rowe RD (1979): Use of prostacyclin in persistent fetal circulation (letter). Lancet 1:1343.

67. Lock JE, Olley PM, Coceani F (1980): Direct pulmonary vascular responses to prostaglandins in the conscious newborn lamb. Am J Physiol 238:H631–H638.

68. Loe WA, Graves ED, Ochsner JL, Falterman KW, Arensman RM (1985): Extracorporeal membrane oxygenation for newborn respiratory failure. J Pediatr Surg 20:684–688.

69. Lou HC, Lassen NA, Friis-Hansen B (1978): Decreased cerebral blood flow after administration of sodium bicarbonate in the distressed newborn infant. Acta Neurol Scand 57:239–347.

70. Lyrene RK, Welch KA, Godoy G, Philips JB (1985): Alkalosis attenuates hypoxic pulmonary vasoconstriction in neonatal lambs. Pediatr Res 19:1268–1271.

71. Mammel MC, Einzig S, Kulik TJ, Thompson TR, Lock JE (1983): Pulmonary vascular effects of amrinone in conscious lambs. Pediatr Res 17:720–724.

72. Markstad T, Finne PH (1980): Effect of tolazoline in pulmonary hemorrhage in the newborn. Case report. Acta Paediatr Scand 69:425–426.

73. McIntosh N, Walter RO (1979): Effect of tolazoline in severe hyaline membrane disease. Arch Dis Child 54:105–110.

73a. McMillan DD, Sauve RS (1986): Bolus and continuous infusion of tolazoline in neonates with hypoxemia. Dev Pharmacol Ther 9:192–200.

74. Meadow W, Benn A, Giardini N, Hageman J, Berger S (1986): Clinical correlates do not predict PaO$_2$ response after tolazoline administration in hypoxic newborns. Crit Care Med 14:548–551.

75. Meadow WL, Rudinsky BF, Strates E (1986): Selective elevation of systemic blood pressure by epinephrine during sepsis-induced pulmonary hypertension in piglets. Pediatr Res 20:872–875.

76. Merten DF, Goetzman BW, Wennberg RP (1977): Persistent fetal circulation: An evolving clinical and radiographic concept of pulmonary hypertension of the newborn. Pediatr Radiol 6:74–80.

77. Miller MK, Short BL, Glass P, Lotze A, Anderson KD (1987): Outcome of 100 infants treated with extracorporeal membrane oxygenation (ECMO) (abstr). Pediatr Res 21:369A.

78. Monin P, Vert P (1978): Persistence de la circulation foetale hypertension arterielle pulmonaire neonatale. Effect favorable de la tolazoline. Nouv Presse Med 7:2853–2861.

79. Moodie DS, Kleinberg F, Telander RL, Kaye MP, Feldt RH (1978): Tolazoline as adjuvant therapy for ill neonates with pulmonary hypoperfusion. Chest 74:604–605.

80. Moodie DS, Telander RL, Kleinberg F, Feldt RH (1978): Use of tolazoline in newborn infants with diaphragmatic hernia and severe cardiopulmonary disease. A preliminary report. J Thoracic Cardiovasc Surg 75:725–729.

81. Murphy JD, Freed MD, Lang P, Epstein M, Frantz I (1980): Prostaglandin E$_1$ infusion in persistent pulmonary hypertension (abstr). Pediatr Res 14:606A.

82. Naulty CM, Weiss IP, Herer GR (1984): Sensorineural hearing loss in survivors of persistent fetal circulation (PFC) (abstr). Clin Res 32:918A.

83. O'Rourke PP, Crone RK, Lillehei CW, Vacanti JP (1987): Extracorporeal membrane oxygenation (ECMO) in infants with congenital diaphragmatic hernia (CDH): Why are the outcomes different (abstr)? Pediatr Res 21:462A.

84. Peckham GJ, Fox WW (1978): Physiologic factors affecting pulmonary artery pressure in infants with persistent pulmonary hypertension. J Pediatr 93:1005–1010.

85. Pereira GR, Fox WW, Stanley CA, Baker L, Schwartz JG (1980):

Decreased oxygenation and hyperlipemia during intravenous fat infusions in premature infants. Pediatrics 66:26–30.

86. Perkin RM, Levin DL, Clark R (1980): Serum salicylate levels and right-to-left ductus shunts in newborn infants with persistent pulmonary hypertension. J Pediatr 96:721–726.

87. Philips JB, Lyrene RK, McDevitt M, Perlis W, Satterwhite C, Cassady G (1983): Prostaglandin D_2 inhibits hypoxic pulmonary vasoconstriction in neonatal lambs. J Appl Physiol Respirat Environ Exercise Physiol 54:1585–1589.

88. Philips JB, Lyrene RK, McDevitt M, Leslie G, Cassady G (1983): Bolus prostaglandin D_2 decreases pulmonary and raises systemic arterial pressures in hypoxic newborn lambs (abstr). Pediatr Res 17:153A.

89. Philips JB, Lyrene RK, Leslie GI, McDevitt M, Cassady G (1985): Hemodynamic effects of nifedipine in normoxic and hypoxic newborn lambs. Pediatr Pharmacol 5:23–30.

90. Philips J, Lyrene R, Godoy G, Graybar G, Barefield E, Sams J, Gray B (1985): Effects of inhibitors and antibody on the pulmonary hypertensive effects of group B streptococci in conscious piglets (abstr). Pediatr Res 19:302A.

91. Purohit DM, Pai S, Levkoff AH (1978): Effect of tolazoline on persistent hypoxemia in neonatal respiratory distress. Crit Care Med 6:14–18.

92. Reuter JH, Disney TA (1986): Regional cerebral blood flow and cerebral metabolic rate of oxygen during hyperventilation in the newborn dog. Pediatr Res 20:1102–1106.

93. Rudolph AM, Yuan S (1966): Response of the pulmonary vasculature to hypoxia and H^+ ion concentration changes. J Clin Invest 45:399–411.

94. Runkle B, Goldberg RN, Streitfeld MM, Clark MR, Buron E, Setzer ES, Bancalari E (1984): Cardiovascular changes in group B streptococcal sepsis in the piglet: Response to indomethacin and relationship to prostacyclin and thromboxane A_2. Pediatr Res 18:874–878.

95. Saunders J, Miller DD, Patil PN (1975): Alpha adrenergic and histaminergic effects of tolazoline-like imidazolines. J Pharmacol Exp Ther 195:362–371.

96. Schlesinger AE, Cornish JD, Null DM (1986): Dense pulmonary opacification in neonates treated with extracorporeal membrane oxygenation. Pediatr Radiol 16:448–451.

97. Schreiber MD, Heymann MA, Soifer SJ (1986): Increased arterial pH, not decreased $PaCO_2$ attenuates hypoxia-induced pulmonary vasoconstriction in newborn lambs. Pediatr Res 20:113–117.

98. Schreiber MD, Heymann MA, Soifer SJ (1987): The differential effects of leukotriene C_4 and D_4 on the pulmonary and systemic circulations in newborn lambs. Pediatr Res 21:176–182.

99. Sell EJ, Gaines JA, Gluckman C, Williams E (1985): Persistent fetal circulation. Neurodevelopmental outcome. Am J Dis Child 139:25–28.

100. Shankaran S, Farooki Z, Desai NS (1982): β-Hemolytic streptococcal infection appearing as persistent fetal circulation. Am J Dis Child 136:725–729.

101. Shelton CK, Gonzales F (1987): Patient selection for extracorporeal membrane oxygenation (ECMO). Importance of individual institutional reviews (abstr). Pediatr Res 21:376A.

102. Shochat SJ, Naeye RL, Ford WDA, Whitman V, Maisels MJ (1979): Congenital diaphragmatic hernia. Ann Surg 190:332–341.

103. Slack MR, Desai NS, Cunningham MD (1979): Tolazoline. Limited efficiency in pulmonary vasoreactive hypoxemia (abstr). Pediatr Res 15:681A.

104. Soifer SJ, Clyman RI, Heymann MA (1985): Prostaglandin D_2 does not lower pulmonary arterial pressure or improve oxygenation in infants with persistent pulmonary hypertension syndrome (PPHN) (abstr). Pediatr Res 19:365A.

105. Spodick SJ (1983): Controlled clinical trials (letter). JAMA 249:1434.

106. Stenmark KR, James SL, Voelkel NF, Toews WH, Reeves JT, Murphy RC (1983): Leukotriene C_4 and D_4 in neonates with hypoxemia and pulmonary hypertension. N Engl J Med 309:77–80.

107. Stevens DC, Schreiner RL, Bull MJ, Bryson CO, Lemons JA, Gresham EL, Grosfeld JL, Weber TR (1980): An analysis of tolazoline therapy in the critically ill neonate. J Pediatr Surg 15:964–970.

108. Stevenson DK, Kasting DS, Darnall RA, Ariagno RL, Johnson JD, Malachowski N, Beets CL, Sunshine P (1979): Refractory hypoxemia associated with neonatal pulmonary disease: The use and limitations of tolazoline. J Pediatr 95:595–599.

109. Stolar CJH, Dillon PW, Stalcup SA (1985): Extracorporeal membrane oxygenation and congenital diaphragmatic hernia: Modification of the pulmonary vasoactive profile. J Pediatr 20:681–683.

110. Sumner E, Frank JD (1981): Tolazoline in the treatment of congenital diaphragmatic hernias. Arch Dis Child 56:350–353.

111. Tarpey MM, Graybar GB, Lyrene RK, Godoy G, Oliver J, Gray BM, Philips JB III (1987): Thromboxane synthesis inhibition reverses group B streptococcus-induced pulmonary hypertension. Crit Care Med 15:644–647.

112. Taylor P (1985): Neuromuscular blocking agents. In Gilman AG, Goodman LS, Rall TW, Murad F (eds): Goodman and Gillman's The Pharmacological Basis of Therapeutics. Norwalk, Macmillan, pp 222–235.

113. Torres CF, Maniscalco WM, Agostinelli T (1985): Muscle weakness and atrophy following prolonged paralysis with pancuronium bromide in neonates (abstr). Ann Neurol 18:403A.

114. Trento A, Griffith BP, Hardesty RL (1986): Extracorporeal membrane oxygenation experience at the University of Pittsburgh. Ann Thorac Surg 42:56–59.

115. Vacanti JP, Crone RK (1983): Chronic anesthesia reduces pulmonary artery pressure in newborns with persistent fetal circulation (abstr). Pediatr Res 17:339A.

116. Ward RM, Daniel CH, Kendig JW, Wood MA (1986): Oliguria and tolazoline pharmacokinetics in the newborn. Pediatrics 77:307–315.

117. Watchko JF (1985): Persistent pulmonary hypertension in a very low birthweight preterm infant. Clin Pediatr 24:592–595.

118. Welch KA, Godoy G, Dew A, Gray BM, Lyrene RK, Philips JB (1984): Pulmonary hypertension following bolus infusions of pneumococci, other gram bacteria, and zymosan (abstr). Circulation (Suppl II) 70:425.

119. Wiener ES (1982): Congenital posterolateral diaphragmatic hernia: New dimensions in management. Surgery 92:670–681.

120. Weiner N (1985): Drugs that inhibit adrenergic nerves and block adrenergic receptors. In Gilman AG, Goodman LS, Rall TW, Murad F (eds): Goodman and Gilman's The Pharmacological Basis of Therapeutics. Norwalk, Macmillan, pp 181–214.

121. Wilkinson AR, Aynsley-Green A, Mitchell MD (1979): Persistent pulmonary hypertension and abnormal prostaglandin E levels in preterm infants after maternal treatment with naproxen. Arch Dis Child 54:942–945.

122. Wilson RG, George RJ, McCormick WJ, Raine PAM (1985): Duodenal perforation associated with tolazoline. Arch Dis Child 60:878–879.

123. Wung JT, James LS, Kilchevsky E, James E (1985): Management of infants with severe respiratory failure and persistence of the fetal circulation, without hyperventilation. Pediatrics 76:488–494.

124. Yellin TO, Sperow JW, Buck SH (1975): Antagonism of tolazoline by histamine H_2-receptor blockers. Nature 253:561–563.

56 NEONATAL CATHETER PALLIATIONS

Zuhdi Lababidi

Although use of the term *cardiac catheterization* is well established, the procedure is no longer the simple introduction of the catheter into the heart. Cardiac catheterization has long been a technique for measurement of cardiac pressures, blood flow, and electrical activities and for imaging the different cardiac chambers, arteries, and veins. It can be used to delineate cardiovascular anatomy, quantitate shunts, determine myocardial function, calculate the severity of valvular stenosis and regurgitation, and determine pulmonary vascular resistance. It is now relatively simple and safe, even in sick neonates, to introduce diagnostic catheters percutaneously and to float and maneuver catheters through complex anatomic malformations. Improved knowledge of neonatal circulatory hemodynamics and the anatomy of complex and stenotic congenital cardiac defects is essential not only for accurate diagnosis but also for further advances in the treatment of congenital cardiac defects.

During the past 2 decades there have been outstanding technical advances in catheter and equipment design. The catheter has been reshaped from a simple diagnostic tube for monitoring intracardiac hemodynamics and visualizing cardiac anatomy to a sophisticated and elaborate therapeutic instrument that can be used for the treatment of congenital cardiac defects.

Since a significant percentage of infants with heart disease die during the first month of life,[1] and since surgical mortality is still high during the neonatal period,[55] new approaches to treat symptomatic neonates with congenital heart disease appear to be warranted. Interventional cardiac catheterization can be performed in neonates as soon as accurate diagnosis is established in the catheterization laboratory. Whether interventional cardiac catheterization will prove to be a safer and more effective therapeutic approach than surgery in critically ill neonates with congenital heart disease remains to be established, but initial results are quite promising. Patient safety during interventional procedures in the catheterization laboratory depends on proper monitoring and support of the patient's vital signs, which should begin as soon as the patient arrives at the laboratory. Monitoring rectal temperature continually (with a rectal probe) and using heating pads and radiant heat to prevent hypothermia are essential. Blood pressure should be measured frequently using Doppler studies until establishment of an arterial line permits continuous monitoring. Respiratory and ECG monitoring should take place throughout the catheterization. An intravenous line should be placed before the infant is transported to the laboratory to provide access for emergency medications and fluids.

INTERVENTIONAL CARDIAC CATHETERIZATION

As improvements in noninvasive cardiovascular diagnosis continue, cardiac catheterization is moving from a diagnostic to a therapeutic modality. Since balloon atrial septostomy was reported in 1966,[63] several procedures have been developed to expand cardiac catheterization from a purely investigational and diagnostic procedure to an amazingly effective therapeutic instrument. Such palliative and therapeutic catheterization procedures have been reported in infants and children to achieve the following anatomic or hemodynamic corrections:

1. Creating intracardiac shunts with the use of balloon atrial septostomy[63] in neonates and blade atrial septostomy[59] in infants and children
2. Occluding preexisting harmful shunts with the use of either detachable plugs, balloons, or umbrellas.[18,61,64] Such transcatheter occlusions appear to be effective in children with patent ductus arteriosus, arteriovenous fistulas, surgical aortic-pulmonary shunts, and atrial septal defects. Although promising, occlusion techniques have not yet been scaled down for use in neonates.
3. Retrieving foreign bodies from the right atrium using urologic forceps[37] and baskets.[80] Swan-Ganz balloon catheters have also been used to retrieve nasotracheal tubes inadvertently introduced into the esophagus.[41]
4. Dilating a thrombosed inferior vena cava with the use of a Fogarty balloon catheter[73]
5. Inserting transvenous and transatrial temporary and permanent pacemakers[32]
6. Draining pericardial effusions[43,50] and evacuating pneumopericardia
7. Dilating stenotic arteries and veins (balloon angioplasty)[40,42,65]
8. Dilating stenotic valves (balloon valvuloplasty)[45,46]
9. Ablating refractory cardiac arrhythmias[4]
10. Improving cardiac output and cardiogenic shock with intra-aortic balloon pumps.[76]

Laser catheter therapy has not yet been used in the treatment of congenital cardiac defects[20] but appears to have a promising future.

INTERVENTIONAL BALLOON PROCEDURES

The two most widely used therapeutic balloon procedures in the neonate are balloon atrial septostomy and transluminal balloon angioplasty/valvuloplasty. Balloon atrial septostomy, first reported in 1966,[63] is now a well-established procedure. In several cyanotic congenital cardiac defects, it is a lifesaving procedure, and its use should not be delayed. Balloon angioplasty, originally described by Gruentzig[22] in 1978 for the dilation of coronary artery stenosis in adults, has now come of age for pediatric patients. The genius and dedication of Rashkind[61] and Gruentzig[22] in developing interventional cardiology has prompted us[40,42] and others[17,47] to scale down the balloon dilation procedures for symptomatic neonates with stenotic congenital cardiac defects, thus avoiding thoracotomies in more and more neonates. Many of the complications of interventional balloon procedures are common to diagnostic cardiac catheterization; these include arrhythmias, perforation, thrombosis, hypothermia, acidosis, and knotting of the catheters. Complications unique to interventional balloon procedures include balloon rupture, balloon embolization, temporary obstruction of blood flow, excessive radiation due to the prolongation of the procedure, vascular rupture, and valvular regurgitation.

Balloon Atrial Septostomy

Balloon atrial septostomy was introduced by Rashkind and Miller[63] in 1966, primarily for use in neonates with complete transposition of the great arteries. However, balloon atrial septostomy also provides a prompt means of nonoperative palliation for several other types of cardiac defects[57] and is well tolerated by the critically ill neonate.[61]

TECHNIQUE

A balloon-tipped catheter is advanced from the femoral vein via the inferior vena cava to the right atrium. From there the tip of the catheter is passed across the foramen ovale. The balloon is inflated in the left atrium and then withdrawn from the left to the right atrium with a rapid jerking motion, resulting in a tearing of the valve of the foramen ovale. Pulling of the balloon through the valve of the foramen ovale is repeated until the balloon meets no resistance on traversing the atrial septum.

The introduction of the atrial septostomy catheter can be done under direct visualization via the femoral vein through a cutdown in the right groin, or through a percutaneous insertion using a No. 6 or 7 French (F) sheath.[30] The atrial septostomy catheter can also be introduced via the umbilical vein in the first 4 days of life.[58] Balloon atrial septostomy is usually performed in the catheterization laboratory using fluoroscopy and cineangiography but can be performed in the neonatal intensive care unit with two-dimensional echocardiographic guidance.[3,6] The advantage of the latter technique is that echocardiographic guidance allows passage of a smaller single-lumen catheter safely and accurately into the left atrium without moving the patient, which can be particularly useful in intubated sick neonates who are too unstable to tolerate transportation and hypothermia. In the catheterization laboratory, positioning of the balloon in the left atrium for withdrawal

across the atrial septum can be confirmed fluoroscopically by leftward and posterior positioning of the catheter tip. If a double-lumen catheter is used, documenting arterial saturations in a chamber with atrial pressures can also confirm left atrial position. Confirmation of left atrial catheter position is very important to avoid tearing of the mitral or tricuspid valve apparatus during the jerking of the balloon. If the catheter is in the left atrium but its tip has been inadvertently introduced into a pulmonary vein, damage to the pulmonary vein from balloon distention can be avoided by slow inflation of the balloon, which results in gentle extrusion of the entire catheter tip back into the left atrial cavity.

CLINICAL ROLE

Balloon atrial septostomy improves the circulation and the clinical condition of the neonate by one of the following mechanisms:

1. By increasing bidirectional shunting (mixing) at the atrial level, balloon atrial septostomy improves arterial oxygen saturations when the pulmonary and systemic circuits are operating in parallel rather than in series (i.e., complete transposition of the great arteries). Transposition of the great arteries occurs once every 2130 to 4500 live births.[48] In a study of 655 unpalliated patients with transposition of the great arteries, Liebman and coworkers[48] found that 28.7 per cent were dead by 1 week of age, 51.6 per cent by 1 month of age, and 89.3 per cent by 1 year of age. Palliation with balloon atrial septostomy has allowed the majority of patients with transposition of the great vessels to survive to age 6 months, which is perhaps optimal for venous switching.[63]

2. By increasing left-to-right shunting at the atrial level, balloon atrial septostomy decreases pulmonary venous congestion in patients with severe obstructive left-sided lesions (i.e., hypoplastic left heart syndrome).

3. By increasing right-to-left shunting at the atrial level, balloon atrial septostomy decreases systemic venous congestion in severe right-sided obstruction, (i.e., tricuspid atresia and pulmonary valve atresia with intact septum).

4. By increasing right-to-left shunting at the atrial level, balloon atrial septostomy decreases pulmonary venous congestion in total anomalous pulmonary venous drainage.

Rashkind[61] reported balloon atrial septostomies in 301 patients over a 15-year period. Of these, 192 patients had transposition of the great arteries, 31 patients had total anomalous pulmonary venous drainage, 27 patients had tricuspid atresia, 23 patients had pulmonary atresia with intact ventricular septum, and 29 patients had miscellaneous defects.

LIMITATIONS AND COMPLICATIONS

Balloon atrial septostomy has been shown to be a safe and effective means of immediate palliation in over 70 per cent of infants with transposition of the great arteries,[61] but early favorable results after balloon atrial septostomy

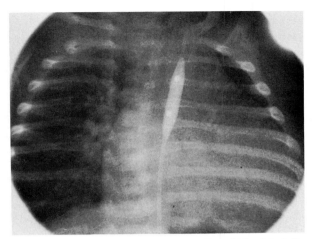

Figure 56–1. Balloon coarctation angioplasty. The middle of the balloon is positioned at the level of the coarctation ridge.

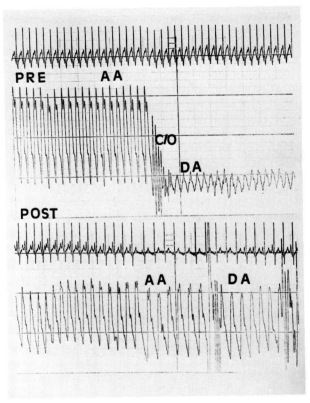

Figure 56–2. Aortic pressure recording of the gradient across the coarctation of the aorta. Upper tracing, preballoon angioplasty; lower tracing, postballoon angioplasty. AA = ascending aorta; C/O = coarctation; DA = descending aorta.

may not necessarily indicate successful long-term palliation. Close observation and continued medical management are essential, since considerable cumulative morbidity and mortality while awaiting definitive surgery have been reported after balloon atrial septostomy for transposition of the great vessels.[26,75]

There is little doubt that the use of larger balloons has contributed appreciably to improved survival,[60] because smaller balloons usually do not create an adequate atrial communication. Balloons under 2 ml in volume may lead to stretching rather than tearing of the atrial septum. On the other hand, very large balloons can result in tears of the atrial wall or interatrial groove.[69] The recommended balloon volume is 3–4 ml.

The complications of balloon atrial septostomy include perforation of the right atrial appendage or pulmonary veins,[62] failure to achieve adequate septostomy,[26] femoral vein tearing,[62] femoral vein thrombosis,[34] inferior vena caval thrombosis,[25] balloon deflation failure,[29] and balloon embolization.[77]

Balloon Angioplasty

Balloon angioplasty is one of the fastest growing and most exciting developments in interventional cardiology. Although balloon dilatation was described by Dotter and Judkins[12] in 1964, its clinical application for coronary stenosis was popularized by Gruentzig[22] in 1978. Similar techniques were also reported in dilating renal,[72] iliac, and femoral artery stenosis.[71]

Recent applications of balloon angioplasty techniques to neonates have included dilatations of neonatal coarctation of the aorta,[17,40] patent ductus arteriosus in a newborn infant with an interrupted aortic arch,[9] obstructed common trunk in total anomalous pulmonary venous drainage,[65] and narrowed venous channels in postoperative patients.[49] Balloon dilatation of pulmonary artery branch stenosis[66] has been reported only in older infants and children, but the possibility exists for similar use in neonates.

Balloon Coarctation Angioplasty

Surgical repair of coarctation of the aorta has undergone several modifications. Crafoord[10] and Gross[21] were the first to report the classic resection with end-to-end anastomosis in 1945. To avoid restenosis, synthetic-patch angioplasty was introduced by Vosschulte[78] in 1957 and subclavian-patch angioplasty was popularized by Waldhausen and Nahrwold[81] in 1966. Although there have been dramatic improvements in the past 40 years, morbidity and mortality rates from surgical repair are still high in the neonates with coarctation of the aorta and congestive heart failure. For infants under 8 weeks of age, an operative mortality ranging from 24 per cent to 67 per cent has been observed.[19,23,68] Recurrent obstruction (restenosis) is common (20 per cent to 35 per cent) after early coarctation repair, especially after end-to-end anastomosis.[24,27] Aneurysm formation at the site of surgical coarctation repair and aortic dissection also occurs.[82] Postoperative hypertension is common in all age groups (but younger patients are less likely to have persistent hypertension at long-term follow-up).[7,56] On the other hand, the outcomes of symptomatic neonates with coarctation treated medically rather than surgically are even worse; mortality ranges from 50 per cent to 86 per cent.[28,36]

In 1979, Sos and coworkers[70] demonstrated the balloon dilatation of the restenosed coarcted segment in postmortem specimens of newborn infants who had undergone coarctation repair. In 1983, my colleagues and I reported neonatal transluminal balloon coarctation angioplasty in a neonate with native coarctation of the aorta.[40]

TECHNIQUE

Immediately after the diagnosis of coarctation is proven angiographically, balloon coarctation angioplasty can be performed via the femoral artery either through a cutdown or a percutaneous approach. Although in older children with coarctation, balloon size is determined by the age of the patient and the diameter of the descending aorta, a No. 5 F catheter and a 4 to 6 mm balloon diameter are quite adequate in all neonates. Balloon coarctation angioplasty permits the neonate with coarctation to grow to an age when either surgical repair can be performed at much lower risk or repeat balloon angioplasty can be attempted using a larger balloon.

A femoral arterial approach is used, and a No. 5 F end-hole catheter is placed in the ascending aorta. A flexible tip 0.028-inch guide wire is inserted, and the catheter is removed, leaving the wire in the ascending aorta. The balloon catheter is then introduced over the guide wire, and the middle of the deflated balloon is placed fluoroscopically at the level of the coarctation ridge. The balloon is then inflated with a diluted mixture of contrast medium (Fig. 56–1). At the start of the inflation, the balloon assumes the shape of an hourglass. The indentation in the middle of the balloon disappears when the coarctation is fully dilated. A pressure of 80 to 100 psi is often needed to fully dilate the coarctation. Full inflations for more than 5 seconds are unnecessary, as are repeated inflations. The balloon is then deflated, pulled back to the femoral artery, and then carefully removed from the groin. Postangioplasty monitoring of these patients is the same as postcardiac catheterization monitoring.

CLINICAL ROLE

Balloon coarctation angioplasty has been used successfully in the treatment of coarctation of the aorta at all ages, ranging from neonates[40] to adults,[44] in native as well as postoperative restenotic coarctations.[42] Immediately after the procedure, the diameter of the coarcted area enlarges and the gradient across the coarctation decreases (Fig. 56–2). Congestive heart failure, tachypnea, cyanosis, and left ventricular ejection fraction improve within 24 hours (Fig. 56–3).

My colleagues and I have now performed balloon coarctation angioplasty successfully on 59 infants and children with no mortality or major complication. The immediate results and our 3-year follow-up data have been gratifying (Fig. 56–4). The predilatation mean gradient was decreased from 45 ± 19 mmHg to 9 ± 6 mmHg. Cardiac catheterization 3 months to 3 years after the dilatation showed the gradient to remain low (15 ± 10 mmHg), indicating persistence of the dilatation. Eleven neonates, aged 4 to 26 days, had balloon angioplasty for native coarctation. The mean gradients were decreased from 45 ± 28 to 11 ± 17

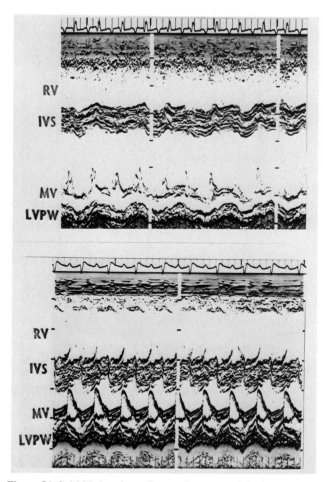

Figure 56–3. M-Mode echocardiogram demonstrated the improvement in left ventricular function after balloon coarctation angioplasty in a neonate with congestive heart failure. Upper panel, preballoon angioplasty; lower panel, postballoon angioplasty. IVS = interventricular septum; LVPW = left ventricular posterior wall; MV = mitral valve; RV = right ventricle.

mmHg. Dilatation is accomplished by tearing of the coarctation ridge and by stretching of the media and the intima in the area adjacent to the coarctation.

The goals of transluminal balloon dilatation and surgical coarctectomy are identical: the relief of obstruction, the alleviation of symptoms, and the elimination of future myocardial dysfunction. Both surgery and balloon dilatation can be used as palliative or definitive procedures, depending on the indication. Although it is not fair to compare the results of 40 years of surgical experience with 4 years of balloon dilatation procedures, the lack of long-range follow-up should not detract from the possible value and merit of balloon dilatation. One advantage of balloon dilatation is that treatment can be started as soon as the diagnosis of coarctation is made in the catheterization laboratory. Unlike surgery, there is no waiting period between diagnosis and therapy with balloon angioplasty; therefore, the chance of further deterioration in critically ill neonates is decreased. Other obvious advantages of balloon dilatation angioplasty in critically ill neonates

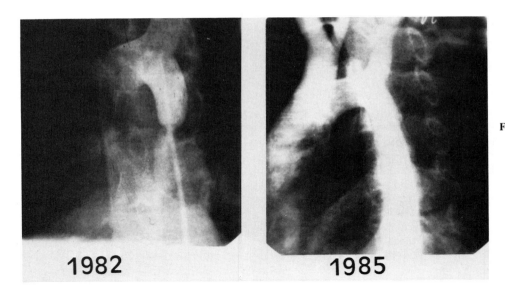

Figure 56–4. Aortography just before balloon coarctation angioplasty (1982) and 3 years later (1985) showing adequate dilation with no evidence of aneurysm formation.

with coarctation include avoidance of general anesthesia and thoracotomy.

LIMITATIONS AND COMPLICATIONS

Although balloon coarctation angioplasty is relatively simple and safe, perforation[17] and aneurysm formation[52] have been reported. The following is a list of precautions that my colleagues and I have found helpful in avoiding complications:

1. Balloons larger than 6 mm in diameter should be avoided in neonates.

2. The object is to dilate the coarctation ridge area and not the narrow isthmus proximal to the ridge.

3. Prolonged balloon inflations should be avoided, since the pressure on the aortic wall may result in necrosis and weakening of the aortic media with resultant aneurysm formation.

4. Manipulation of the catheters and wires in the area that has been freshly dilated should be minimized since intimal tears are common.

5. The intima of the recently dilated area should be protected from the sharp tip of the catheter by leaving the flexible-tip guide wire beyond the catheter tip during subsequent insertions and withdrawals.

6. Contrast injections for cineangiography immediately after the procedure should be performed in the ascending aorta, away from the freshly dilated area (to avoid perforation).

7. Balloon rupture should be avoided in coarctation angioplasty since it may tear and dissect the aortic wall, although balloon rupture in balloon valvuloplasty has been shown to be harmless.[45,46]

Balloon Pulmonary Vein Angioplasty

The experience with balloon pulmonary vein angioplasty has been limited. Although Driscoll and coworkers[13] demonstrated the procedure to be unsuccessful in dilating

individual pulmonary veins, Rey and coworkers[65] have reported successful dilation of a stenotic common pulmonary vein in a 3-month-old infant with total anomalous pulmonary venous drainage.

Balloon Ductus Arteriosus Angioplasty

Balloon dilatation of the ductus arteriosus was reported by Corwin and coworkers[9] in 1981 in a 2-day-old neonate with interrupted aortic arch and in eight piglets (12 to 15 days old) by Lund and coworkers[51] in 1983.

Balloon Valvuloplasty

As an extension of balloon angioplasty, balloon valvuloplasty has been successfully used in dilating stenotic valves, especially the pulmonary and aortic valves.

Balloon Pulmonary Valvuloplasty

In 1982, Kan and coworkers[31] reported the first use of balloon valvuloplasty to treat pulmonary valvular stenosis. Since that report, my coworkers and I[45] and others[38] have reported similar successful pulmonary valve dilatations after balloon valvuloplasty.

TECHNIQUE

Right- and left-sided cardiac catheterizations and cardiac output measurements are usually carried out through the right groin. A pressure recording of the gradient across the pulmonary valve is performed, followed by a right ventricular cineangiogram in the right anterior oblique view. The right-sided cardiac catheter is then replaced by a balloon catheter, introduced percutaneously over a flexible tip guide wire, previously placed in either the right or the left pulmonary artery. The balloon catheter is passed over the guide wire until the middle of the deflated bal-

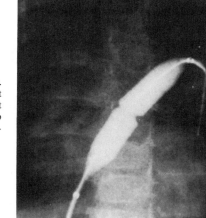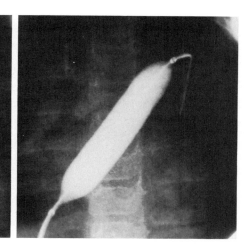

Figure 56–5. Balloon pulmonary valvuloplasty. *A*, hourglass shape of the balloon at the start of inflation. *B*, Full balloon inflation. The left pulmonary artery is protected from the sharp tip of the catheter with a flexible tip guidewire.

loon is positioned fluoroscopically across the pulmonary valve.

The maximum inflatable diameter of the balloon should be equal to or 2 mm larger than the diameter of the pulmonary valve annulus as measured on the cineangiogram monitor. To avoid air embolization in the event of balloon rupture, the balloon is inflated and deflated several times outside the patient with a 50/50 mixture of saline solution and contrast medium until all air bubbles are removed. The balloon is inflated to a pressure of 100 psi for approximately 10 seconds. At the start of the inflation, the balloon assumes an hourglass shape due to the stenotic valve. The indentation in the middle of the balloon disappears as soon as the valve is dilated to the maximum diameter of the balloon (Fig. 56–5). During the inflation, the pulmonary valve obstruction results in a sharp drop in the aortic pressure (Fig. 56–6). The aortic pressure returns to normal as soon as the balloon is deflated. The balloon catheter is then replaced by the previous right-sided cardiac catheter. Cardiac output and gradient across the pulmonary valve

are measured again approximately 15 minutes after the dilatation, when the heart rate and aortic pressures have returned to prevalvuloplasty levels.

CLINICAL ROLE

Pulmonary valve stenosis with intact ventricular septum is a relatively common congenital cardiac lesion with an incidence of 7.5 to 11.6 per cent.[35] Patients with mild to moderate stenosis are asymptomatic. Critical pulmonary valve stenosis presents with symptoms of heart failure, cyanosis from a right-to-left shunt through a patent foramen ovale or atrial septal defect, and severe hypoxia.[2] Untreated critical pulmonary valve stenosis with intact ventricular septum is potentially lethal in infants.[16] The surgical approach includes transpulmonary valvectomy either with hypothermic or normothermic inflow occlusion or cardiopulmonary bypass. The mortality rate of infants subjected to all of these surgical procedures is high. In patients 10 days of age or younger having cardiopulmonary bypass,

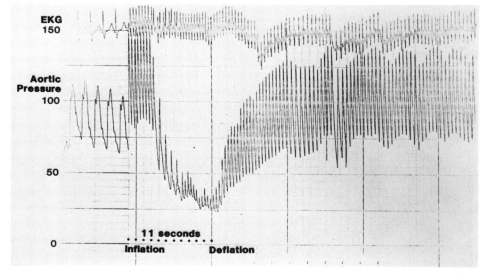

Figure 56–6. Aortic pressure tracing during balloon pulmonary valvuloplasty. Aortic pressure rises at the start of inflation, then drops until the balloon is deflated.

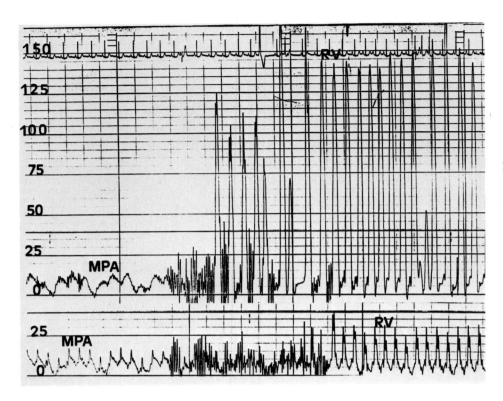

Figure 56–7. Pressure tracings of the gradient across the pulmonary valve. Upper tracing, before balloon pulmonary valvuloplasty; lower tracing, after balloon pulmonary valvuloplasty. MPA = main pulmonary artery; RV = right ventricle.

an operative mortality of 33 per cent has been reported; and among those having an outflow patch, an operative mortality of 60 per cent has been reported.[2] To reduce the operative mortality and improve survival significantly, perioperative prostaglandin E_1 therapy is currently used at a dosage of 0.1 μg/kg/min.[8]

Balloon pulmonary valvuloplasty has been used to dilate pulmonary valves in infants with isolated pulmonary valvular stenosis and infants with complex cyanotic cardiac defects associated with severe pulmonary valvular stenosis (e.g., tetralogy of Fallot). The decrease in pressure gradient across the pulmonary valve is often dramatic

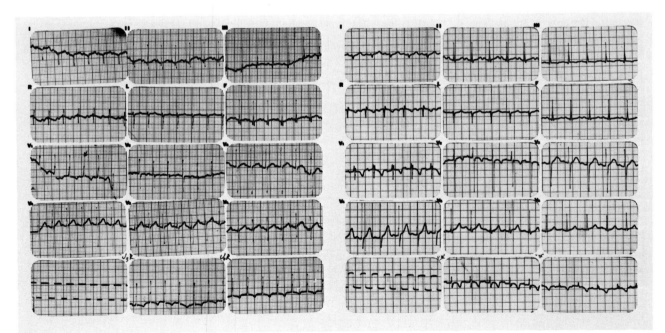

Figure 56–8. Electrocardiograms in an infant with valvular pulmonary stenosis. Left panel, severe right ventricular hypertrophy before balloon pulmonary valvuloplasty; right panel, normal ECG 1 year after the procedure.

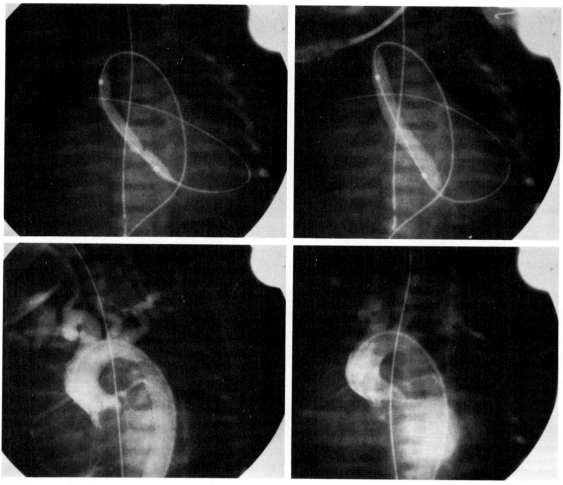

Figure 56–9. Balloon aortic valvuloplasty in a neonate with critical aortic stenosis and mitral regurgitation. Upper left panel, balloon at the start of inflation; upper right panel, balloon at full inflation, with the guidewire advanced out of the tip of the catheter and through the mitral valve into the left atrium; lower left panel, aortogram showing the stenotic domed aortic valve prevalvuloplasty; lower right panel, the widely open aortic valve with aortic regurgitation postvalvuloplasty.

(Fig. 56–7). In the past 4 years, my colleagues and I have performed balloon pulmonary valvuloplasty on 75 infants and children with pulmonary valvular stenosis. The mean gradient was decreased from 76 ± 34 to 22 ± 15 mmHg. Follow-up cardiac catheterization 6 months to 3 years later showed persistence of dilatation. The mean gradient on follow-up was 23 ± 19 mmHg. In three neonates with critical pulmonary valvular stenosis, the mean gradient across the pulmonary valve was decreased from 67 ± 33 mmHg to 21 ± 15 mmHg. Noninvasive follow-up with two-dimensional echocardiography, Doppler studies, and electrocardiography (Fig. 56–8) has shown dramatic and sustained clinical improvements.

LIMITATIONS AND COMPLICATIONS

Other than transient bradycardia, hypotension, and premature ventricular beats during the inflation, balloon pulmonary valvuloplasty has been free of major complications. It is often difficult to maneuver the stiff and straight bal-

loon catheter into the right ventricle and pulmonary artery. Placing a 200-cm exchange wire into the left pulmonary artery through an end-hole Gensini catheter, and then passing the balloon catheter over the wire, can help guide the stiff balloon catheter through the tricuspid and pulmonary valves. In neonates, serial dilatations with Nos. 5, 6 and 7 F end-hole catheters may be needed before a balloon catheter can be passed through a tight pulmonary valve. To maintain pulmonary blood flow, such neonates require prostaglandin E_1 infusions to keep the ductus open during catheter obstruction of the pulmonary valve.

Balloon Aortic Valvuloplasty

Successful balloon aortic valvuloplasty was first introduced by my colleagues and me[46] in 1983. Waller and associates[79] reported an unsuccessful balloon aortic valvuloplasty in a neonate. The patient died a few hours after operative repair. At necropsy, an aortic tear was shown to be due to the use of an oversized balloon. Rupprath and

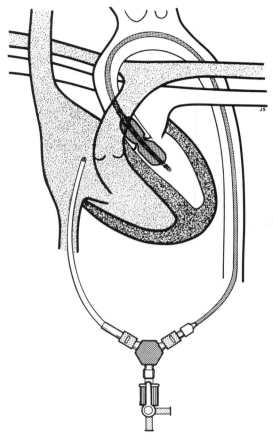

Figure 56–10. The left ventricular–right atrial shunt when the inflated balloon occludes the aortic valve orifice. The arterial and venous catheters are connected outside the groin.

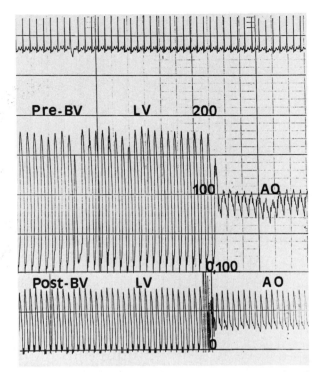

Figure 56–11. Pressure tracing of the gradient across the aortic valve. Upper tracing, preballoon aortic valvuloplasty gradient; lower tracing, postballoon valvuloplasty with no gradient. AO = aorta; LV = left ventricle.

Neuhaus[67] have reported successful balloon aortic valvuloplasty in three infants aged 4 to 6 weeks.

TECHNIQUE

The technique for balloon aortic valvuloplasty is similar to that for balloon pulmonary valvuloplasty. In neonates with critical aortic stenosis, a No. 5 F Cook balloon catheter with balloon dimensions of 5 to 6 mm by 30 mm can be used to dilate the aortic valve. Larger balloons and catheters should not be used in neonates because of the small femoral artery. The balloon catheter is introduced into the left ventricle over a 0.028-inch J flexible-tip guide wire. In infants with mitral regurgitation, which often accompanies critical aortic stenosis, the guide wire can be maintained inside the balloon catheter throughout the dilatation procedure; the presence of mitral regurgitation permits spontaneous decompression of the left ventricle during balloon inflation. The aortic valve dilatation is carried out similarly to the pulmonary valve dilatation considered earlier (Fig. 56–9). In patients without mitral regurgitation, the guide wire should be removed and the balloon catheter should be connected to the venous catheter during the dilatation to permit left ventricular decom-

pression (Fig. 56–10). The balloon diameter should be equal to or 1 to 2 mm less than the aortic valve annulus. The balloon inflation should not last more than 5 seconds to avoid cerebral ischemia.

CLINICAL ROLE

The incidence of valvular aortic stenosis among children with congenital heart disease is 5 per cent.[35] The natural hemodynamic history of aortic stenosis is one of progressive obstruction, due usually to increased flow (as a result of somatic growth) across a fixed obstruction. In a few patients with aortic stenosis, actual narrowing of the valve orifice contributes to progressive obstruction.[15] Critical valvular aortic stenosis usually presents in early infancy as congestive heart failure. In neonates with critical valvular aortic stenosis, medical treatment is only briefly effective.[54] Newborns with symptomatic aortic stenosis require urgent or emergency valvulotomy, which carries a high risk. In infants 1 month of age or younger, the mortality has ranged from 29 per cent to 86 per cent.[11,14,33,39] Aortic valvulotomy has been performed by an open method with and without cardiopulmonary bypass,[32] by a closed method with a transventricular blunt dilator through an incision in the left ventricular apex,[74] and more recently, by a transventricular balloon catheter after thoracotomy.[5] Transluminal balloon aortic valvuloplasty has been increasingly considered as an alternative to surgical aortic valvulotomy in severe congenital valvular aortic stenosis.[46] In the past 3 years my colleagues and I have successfully performed balloon aortic valvuloplasty in 48 children, two of whom were neonates (6 and 7 days of age). The mean gradient across the aortic valve in the 48 patients was decreased from 102 ± 44 mmHg to 26 ± 15 mmHg; and on 3-month to 3-year follow-up, the gradient was still low (33 ± 21 mmHg). Successful aortic valve dilatation is immediately evident by dramatic reduction in the pressure gradient across the valve (Fig. 56–11).

LIMITATIONS AND COMPLICATIONS

Although the small femoral artery in the neonate limits the use of larger balloons, we have found that 5- to 6-mm balloons create an adequate neonatal aortic valve opening. Larger balloons can be used during repeat valvuloplasty when the patient is older and larger. Although balloon aortic valvuloplasty is performed percutaneously in older patients, open femoral arteriotomy is preferable in the neonate, so that the femoral artery can be carefully repaired after the procedure.

To avoid excessive increase in left ventricular pressure during balloon inflation, decompressing the left ventricle may be necessary in critical aortic stenosis,[46] particularly in neonates with severe cardiac dysfunction. Unlike balloon pulmonary valvuloplasty, during which the large and stiff balloon catheter probably makes the tricuspid valve insufficient (thus decompressing the right ventricle during balloon occlusion of the pulmonary valve), the catheter does not pass through the mitral valve during aortic valvuloplasty. Unless mitral regurgitation is present, the arterial and venous catheters are connected outside the body (thus creating a left ventricular–right atrial communication) during balloon inflation in aortic valvuloplasty, but the value of this approach remains unproven.

Aortic regurgitation, a common finding after surgical aortic commissurotomy, is also often seen after the balloon aortic valvuloplasty. Aortic regurgitation can be minimized or avoided by using a balloon smaller than the aortic valve annulus.

Advantages of Transluminal Balloon Dilatations

Transluminal balloon angioplasty and valvuloplasty offer an attractive alternative to open-heart surgery for a rapidly growing list of congenital cardiac defects. Transluminal balloon dilatations are probably safer and definitely less expensive than surgery, and the long-term results are extremely promising. No general anesthesia is required; no blood products are needed to prime a heart-lung machine. Since neither sternotomy nor thoracotomy is required, no intrathoracic adhesions develop, which makes any future intrathoracic repair less complicated. In addition, morbidity and length of hospitalization after successful transluminal dilatation are much less than after cardiac surgery.

The emergence of therapeutic cardiac catheterization in the 1980s has placed a greater than ever demand on the pediatric cardiologist, who has an ongoing responsibility for the well-being of neonates and infants with congenital cardiac defects. The demands are greater because the therapeutic weapon at hand is powerful and, to some extent, dangerous in inexperienced hands. Angioplasty is not the same as angiography. The stress, manipulation, and risks are greater. Therefore, balloon dilatation in the neonate must be wisely and selectively used for the well-being of the patient.

References

1. Adams FH (1957): The early definitive diagnosis of patients with congenital heart disease. J Pediatr 52:202–206.
2. Awariefe SO, Clarke DR, Pappas G (1964): Surgical approach to critical pulmonary valve stenosis in infants less than six months of age. J Thorac Cardiovasc Surg 85:375–385.
3. Baker EJ, Allan LD, Tynan MJ, Jones ODH, Joseph MC, Deverall PB (1984): Balloon atrial septostomy in the neonatal intensive care unit. Br Heart J 51:377–378.
4. Belhassen B, Miller HI, Laniado S (1985): Catheter ablation of incessant ventricular tachycardia refractory to external cardioversions. Am J Cardiol 55:1637–1639.
5. Brow JW, Robinson RJ, Waller BF (1985): Transventricular balloon catheter aortic valvulotomy in neonates. Ann Thorac Surg 39:376–378.
6. Bullaboy CA, Jennings RB, Johnson DH, Fulcher CW (1984): Bedside balloon atrial septostomy using echocardiographic monitoring. Am J Cardiol 53:971.
7. Clarkson PM, Nicholson MR, Barrett-Boyes BG, Neutze JM, Whitlock RM (1983): Results after repair of coarctation of the aorta beyond infancy: A 10 to 18 year follow-up with particular reference to late systemic hypertension. Am J Cardiol 51:1481–1488.
8. Cole JG, Freedom RM, Olley PM, Coceani F, Williams WG, Trusler GA, (1984): Surgical management of critical pulmonary stenosis in the neonate. Ann Thorac Surg 38:458–465.
9. Corwin RD, Singh AK, Karlson KE (1981): Balloon dilatation of ductus arteriosus in a newborn with interrupted aortic arch and ventricular septal defect. Am Heart J 102:446–447.
10. Crafoord C, Nylin G (1945): Congenital coarctation of the aorta and its surgical treatment. J Thorac Surg 14:347–361.
11. Dobell ARC, Bloss RS, Gibbons JE, Collins GE (1981): Congenital valvular aortic stenosis. J Thorac Cardiovasc Surg 81:916–921.
12. Dotter CT, Judkins MP (1964): Transluminal treatment of arteriosclerotic obstruction. Description of a new technique and a preliminary report of its application. Circulation 30:654–670.
13. Driscoll DJ, Husslein PS, Mullins CE (1982): Congenital stenosis of individual pulmonary veins: Clinical spectrum and unsuccessful treatment by transvenous balloon dilatation. Am J Cardiol 49:1767–1772.
14. Edmunds LV, Wagner HR, Heyman MA (1980): Aortic valvulotomy in neonates. Circulation 61:421–427.
15. El-Said G, Galioto FM, Mullins CE, McNamara DG (1972): Natural hemodynamic history of congenital aortic stenosis in childhood. Am J Cardiol 30:6–12.
16. Engle MA, Ito T, Goldberg HP (1964): The fate of the patient with pulmonic stenosis. Circulation 30:554–561.
17. Finley JP, Beaudien RG, Nanton MA, Roy DL (1983): Balloon catheter dilatation of coarctation of the aorta in young infants. Br Heart J 50:411–415.
18. Florentine M, Wolfe RR, White RI (1984): Balloon embolization to occlude a Blalock-Taussig shunt. J Am Coll Cardiol 3:200–202.
19. Gersony WM (1983): Coarctation of the aorta. In Adams FH, Emmanouilides GC (eds): Moss' Heart Disease in Infants, Children and Adolescents. Baltimore, Williams & Wilkins, pp 188–199.
20. Gessman LJ, Reno CW, Chang KS, MacMillan RM, Maranho V (1984): Feasibility of laser catheter valvulotomy for aortic and mitral stenosis. Am J Cardiol 54:1375–1377.

21. Gross RE (1945): Surgical correction for coarctation of the aorta. Surgery 18:347–352.

22. Gruentzig A (1978): Transluminal dilatation of coronary artery stenosis. Lancet 1:263.

23. Hamilton DI, Di Eusanio G, Sandrasagra FA, Donnelly RJ (1978): Early and late results of aortoplasty with a left subclavian flap for coarctation of the aorta in infancy. J Thorac Cardiovasc Surg 75:699–704.

24. Hartman AF, Goldring D, Hernandez A, Behrer MR, Schad N, Ferguson T, Burford T (1970): Recurrent coarctation of the aorta after successful repair in infancy. Am J Cardiol 25:405–410.

25. Hawker RE, Celermajer JM, Cartmill TB, Bowdler JD (1971): Thrombosis of the inferior vena cava following balloon septostomy in transposition of the great arteries. Am Heart J 82:593–595.

26. Hawker RE, Krovetz LJ, Rowe RD (1974): An analysis of prognostic factors in the outcome of balloon atrial septostomy for transposition of the great arteries. Johns Hopkins Med J 134:95–106.

27. Hesslein PS, Gutgessel HP, McNamara DG (1983): Prognosis of symptomatic coarctation of the aorta in infancy. Am J Cardiol 51:299–303.

28. Hesslein PS, McNamara DG (1981): Surgical intervention in infants with isolated coarctation of the aorta. J Thorac Cardiovasc Surg 82:640–641.

29. Hohn AR, Webb HM (1972): Balloon deflation failure. A hazard of medical atrial septostomy. Am Heart J 83:389–391.

30. Hurwitz RA, Girod DA (1976): Percutaneous balloon atrial septostomy in infants with transposition of the great arteries. Am Heart J 91:618–622.

31. Kan JS, White RI, Mitchell SE (1982): Percutaneous balloon valvuloplasty: A new method for treating congenital pulmonary valve stenosis. N Engl J Med 370:540–542.

32. Kanpawich PP, Parker S, Anato JJ, Khan MAA (1985): Emergency transvenous pacing in infants. Am Heart J 109:385–386.

33. Keane JF, Bernhard WF, Nadas AS (1975): Aortic stenosis in infancy. Circulation 52:1138–1143.

34. Keane JF, Lang P, Newburger J, Fyler DC (1980): Iliac vein–inferior caval thrombosis after cardiac catheterization in infancy. Pediatr Cardiol 1:257–260.

35. Keith JD, Rowe RD, Vlad P (1978): Heart Disease in Infancy and Childhood. 3rd ed. New York, Macmillan, pp 3–13.

36. Kilman JW, Williams TE Jr, Breza TS, Craenen J, Hosier DM (1972): Reversal of infant mortality by early surgical correction of coarctation of the aorta. Arch Surg 105:865–868.

37. King JF, Manley JC, Zeft HJ, Auer JE (1976): Nonsurgical removal of foreign body from right heart. J Thorac Cardiovasc Surg 71:785–786.

38. Kveselis DP, Rocchini AP (1984): Long term results of balloon valvuloplasty of the pulmonary valve (abstract). Pediatr Res 18:423A.

39. Lakier JB, Lewis AB, Heyman MA, Stonzer P, Hoffman JIE, Rudolph AM (1974): Isolated aortic stenosis in the neonate. Circulation 50:801–806.

40. Lababidi Z (1983): Neonatal transluminal balloon coarctation angioplasty. Am Heart J 106:752–753.

41. Lababidi Z, Bland H, James E (1978): Retrieval of an endotracheal tube from the esophagus. Am Heart J 93:1025.

42. Lababidi Z, Daskalopoulos D, Stoeckle H (1984): Transluminal balloon coarctation angioplasty: Experience with 27 patients. Am J Cardiol 54:1288–1291.

43. Lababidi Z, Hakami N, Almond C (1977): Chronic granulomatous disease associated with acute pericarditis with tamponade. Miss Med 5:170–171.

44. Lababidi Z, Madigan N, Wu JR, Murphy TJ (1984): Balloon coarctation angioplasty in an adult. Am J Cardiol 53:350–351.

45. Lababidi Z, Wu JR (1983): Percutaneous balloon pulmonary valvuloplasty. Am J Cardiol 52:560–562.

46. Lababidi Z, Wu JR, Walls JT (1984): Percutaneous balloon aortic valvuloplasty. Am J Cardiol 53:194–197.

47. Lezo JS, Fernandez R, Sancho M, Concha M, Arizon J, Franco M, Alemany F, Barcones F, Lopez-Rubio F, Valles F (1984): Percutaneous transluminal angioplasty for aortic isthmic coarctation in infancy. Am J Cardiol 54:1147–1149.

48. Liebman J, Cullum L, Belloc NB (1969): Natural history of transposition of the great arteries: Anatomy and birth and death characteristics. Circulation 40:237–262.

49. Lock JE, Bass JL, Castañeda-Zuniga W, Fuhrman BP, Rashkind WJ, Lucas RV (1984): Dilation angioplasty of congenital or operative narrowings of venous channels. Circulation 70:457–464.

50. Lock JE, Bass JL, Kulik TJ, Fuhrman BP (1984): Chronic percutaneous pericardial drainage with modified pigtail catheter in children. Am J Cardiol 53:1179–1182.

51. Lund G, Rysavy J, Cragg A, Salomanowitz E, Vlodaver Z, Zuniga WC, Amplatz K (1984): Long-term patency of the ductus arteriosus after balloon dilatation: An experimental study. Circulation 69:772–774.

52. Marvin WJ, Mahoney LT (1985): Balloon angioplasty of unoperated coarctation of the aorta in young children (abstr). J Am Coll Cardiol 5:405A.

53. Mitchell SC, Korones SB, Berendes HW (1971): Congenital heart disease in 56,109 births. Circulation 43:323–332.

54. Mody MR, Nadas AS, Bernhard WF (1967): Aortic stenosis in infants. N Engl J Med 276:832–838.

55. Nadas AS, Fyler DC, Castañeda AR (1973): The critically ill infant with congenital heart disease. Mod Concepts Cardiovasc Dis 42:53–58.

56. Nanton MA, Olley PM (1976): Residual hypertension after coarctectomy in children. Am J Cardiol 37:769–772.

57. Neches WH, Mullins CE, McNamara DG (1973): Balloon atrial septostomy in congenital heart disease in infancy. Am J Dis Child 125:371–375.

58. Newfeld EA, Purcell C, Paul MH, Cole RV, Muster AJ (1974): Transumbilical balloon atrial septostomy in 16 infants with transposition of the great arteries. Pediatrics 54:495–498.

59. Park SC, Neches WH, Zuberbuhler JR, Lenox CC, Mathews RA, Fricker FJ, Zoltan RA (1978): Clinical use of blade atrial septostomy. Circulation 58:600–606.

60. Powell TG, Dewey M, West CR, Arnold R (1984): Fate of infants with transposition of the great arteries in relation to balloon atrial septostomy. Br Heart J 51:371–376.

61. Rashkind WJ (1983): Transcatheter treatment of congenital heart disease. Circulation 67:711–716.

62. Rashkind W (1971): Palliative procedures for transposition of the great arteries. Br Heart J 33:69–72.

63. Rashkind WJ, Miller WW (1966): Creation of an atrial septal defect without thoracotomy: Palliative approach to complete transposition of the great arteries. JAMA 196:991–992.

64. Reidy JF, Jones ODH, Tynan MJ, Baker EJ, Joseph MC (1985): Embolization procedures in congenital heart disease. Br Heart J 54:184–192.

65. Rey C, Marache P, Francart C, Dupuis C (1985): Percutaneous balloon angioplasty in an infant with obstructed total anomalous pulmonary vein return. J Am Coll Cardiol 6:894–896.

66. Ring JC, Bass JL, Marvin W, Fuhrman BP, Kulik TJ, Foker JE, Lock JE (1985): Management of congenital stenosis of a branch pulmonary artery with balloon dilation angioplasty. J Thorac Cardiovasc Surg 90:35–44.

67. Rupprath G, Neuhaus K (1985): Percutaneous balloon valvuloplasty for aortic valve stenosis in infancy. Am J Cardiol 55:1655–1656.

68. Shinebourne EA, Tam ASY, Elseed AM, Panelli M, Lennox SC, Cleland WP, Lincoln C, Joseph MC, Anderson RH (1976): Coarctation of the aorta in infancy and childhood. Br Heart J 38:375–380.

69. Sondheimer H, Havey RW, Blackman MS (1982): Fatal overdistension of an atrioseptostomy catheter. Pediatr Cardiol 2:255–257.

70. Sos T, Sniderman KW, Rettek-Sos B (1979): Percutaneous transluminal dilation of coarctation of thoracic aorta postmortem. Lancet 2:970–971.

71. Spence RK, Friedman DB, Gratenby R (1981): Long term results of transluminal angioplasty of the iliac and femoral arteries. Arch Surg 116:1377–1386.

72. Tegtmeyer CJ, Dyer R, Teates CD (1980): Percutaneous transluminal dilatation of the renal arteries. Radiology 135:589–599.

73. Thompson IM, Schneider H, Lababidi Z (1974): Thrombectomy for neonatal renal vein thrombosis. Trans Am Assoc Genitourinary Surg 66:177–180.

74. Trinkle JK, Grover FL, Arom KU (1978): Closed aortic valvulotomy in infants. J Thorac Cardiovasc Surg 76:198–201.

75. Tynan M (1971): Survival of infants with transposition of the great arteries after balloon atrial septostomy. Lancet 1:621–623.

76. Veasy LG, Blalock RC, Orth JL, Boucek MM (1983): Intra-aortic balloon pumping in infants and children. Circulation 68:1095–1100.

77. Vogel JHK (1970): Balloon embolization during atrial septostomy. Circulation 42:155–156.

78. Vosschulte K (1957): Surgical correction of coarctation of the aorta by an Isthmusplastik. Thoraxchirugie 4:433–436.

79. Waller BF, Girod DA, Dillon JC (1984): Transverse aortic wall tears in infants after balloon angioplasty for aortic valve stenosis. J Am Coll Cardiol 4:1235–1241.

80. Wahi PL, Talwar KK, Sapru RP (1980): Nonsurgical extraction of a broken catheter sheath lodged in the right atrium, using a Dorma ureteral stone dislodger. Br Heart J 44:349–351.

81. Waldhausen JA, Nahrwold DL (1966): Repair of coarctation of the aorta with a subclavian flap. J Thorac Cardiovasc Surg 51:532–533.

82. White CW, Zoller RP (1973): Left aortic dissection following repair of coarctation of the aorta. Chest 63:573–577.

57 CONGENITAL HEART SURGERY: PRESENT AND FUTURE

Francisco J. Puga

The rapid development of techniques for the surgical treatment of congenital heart defects has been astounding even to the casual lay observer. The epoch–making contributions of Gross, Blalock and Taussig, and Gibbon[1,2,3] all dating back no more than 45 years, provided the basis for innumerable contributions that have radically modified the dismal prognosis of children born with developmental cardiovascular defects.

Speculation on the future of this surgical specialty is fraught with risk. Indeed, it would have been impossible to predict 15 years ago that the use of a percutaneous, balloon-tipped catheter would make surgery for pulmonary valve stenosis obsolete. Even more startling was the rebuke suffered by the noted surgeon, Sir Stephen Paget, who, near the turn of the century, stated: "In the heart, surgery meets the limits imposed by nature. No new method or discovery will overcome the natural difficulties imposed by a cardiac wound." Only a year later, Rehn[4] reported the first successful suture of a cardiac wound with survival of the patient.

Rather than simple elucubration on the future of congenital heart surgery and instead of awed recollections on what has been achieved thus far, it would seem better to dedicate this chapter to an appraisal of what has been left undone and of the persistent problems that affect the welfare of patients with congenital heart disease, whether operated or not. It is clear that some of our future activities must concentrate on the resolution of these problems.

A list of present, unresolved problems affecting patients with congenital heart disease could be similar to the one shown in Table 57–1. Some of these problems are common to all cardiac surgical patients (behavior of implanted prosthesis, fate of palliative procedures), while others are peculiar to the pediatric population (effects of extracorporeal circulation in infants and small children, effects of growth on anastomosis).

Unfortunately, the problems are not only biologic but also economic and even ethical. Thus, there exists a discrepancy in the magnitude of resources allocated for research and development in the area of pediatric cardiac surgery compared with that expended for the adult patient with cardiac disease. New advances in products such as valves or pacemakers are usually geared for the adult population and simply scaled down for use in pediatric surgery. In comparison, less money is dedicated by the medical industrial complex for the development of products and devices necessary for the repair of congenital heart defects. Such is the case of extracardiac pulmonary conduits, a mainstem in the treatment of many complex anomalies.

Cost effectiveness is often used as the rationale behind this apparent neglect, yet for society at large, the repair of truncus arteriosus in an infant with an otherwise essentially normal life expectancy must be as cost effective as the replacement of a calcified aortic valve in a 70-year-old individual whose average life expectancy is only 6 years. As medical technology becomes more costly, development of such products has migrated from university surgical laboratories to research and development laboratories sponsored by commercial companies, where research efforts are heavily influenced by marketability of products and potential for profit. Such gauges of the merit of innovations in medical technology seem inappropriate in view of the needs of individual patients.

Access to expensive, sophisticated medical care is becoming more difficult for patients in the pediatric age group. Bureaucratic apportioning of funds may fail to discriminate the peculiar needs of this group of patients. Thus, children can be referred for complicated cardiac surgical repair to centers that do not have sufficient experience in the management of complex congenital heart anomalies. Results of such endeavors may be less satisfactory than those demanded by the state of the art of care.

As the cost of surgical care of these patients increases, the access to this type of care is becoming limited to those families able to supplement the limited payments of public or third party contributors. Such dilemmas are particularly painful in developing nations, where the cost of surgical technology can be prohibitive, so that large numbers of patients are simply left untreated.

The growth and development of cardiac surgery, firmly based on physiologic principles explored during the nineteenth century and early years of the twentieth century, was sadly interrupted by the artificial demands imposed by two world wars. Economic resources were stressed and preferentially diverted to the war effort, with the resulting drain of human and material wealth from Western societies. Indeed, cardiac surgery required more than a bold surgeon invading yet uncharted areas of human pathology. Investment in sophisticated technology and economic resources were also indispensable, and these were suddenly available in the postwar years. Such investment was necessary to aid the transition of cardiac surgery from the anecdotal achievement to the realities of daily clinical practice. Interestingly, the financing for such ventures was favored by a sociopolitical attitude that defined health and access to medical care as a right and not only a privilege

Table 57–1. FACTORS LIMITING SUCCESS OF SURGERY FOR CONGENITAL HEART DISEASE

I. Behavior of implanted prosthetics
  A. Patches (contraction and scarring)
  B. Valves (degeneration and/or thromboembolism)
  C. Conduits (calcification and obstruction)
  D. Pacemakers (lead failure, displacement)

II. Effect of growth on reconstructed structures
  A. Vascular anastomosis (coarctation)
  B. Repaired valves (atrioventricular septal defect)

III. Surgically induced pathology
  A. Pulmonary artery scarring from shunts (Waterston)
  B. Ventricular failure from palliative procedures
  C. Untoward effects of pulmonary artery banding
  D. Mediastinal scarring
  E. Pulmonary insufficiency (tetralogy of Fallot)

IV. Future of patients with "definitive palliation"
  A. Inflow procedures for transposition of great arteries
  B. Fontan procedure and modifications

V. Deleterious effects of extracorporeal circulation in infants

VI. Consequences of circulatory arrest

VII. Inadequate present techniques
  A. Hypoplastic left-heart syndrome
  B. Hypoplastic mitral annulus

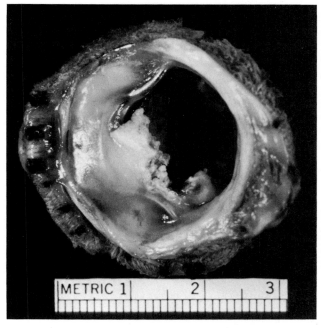

Figure 57–1. Explanted disk valve. Thrombosis resulting from inadequate anticoagulation.

of the public. In addition, the economic and political power of the patient as a consumer of medical care strongly favored the enactment of legislation, allowing appropriation of funds to help defray the growing cost of medical care. Furthermore, this availability of funds has promoted the unrestricted proliferation of medical products not necessarily justified by medical needs. Examples of such proliferation can be found in the multiplicity of available pacemakers, cardiac valves, and oxygenators. Unfortunately, significant differences among such products are hard to demonstrate clinically. Such duplication represents one more example of waste of resources, which are best directed to the resolution of pressing clinical problems. Intellectually, such resources would be best applied to the search of truly new solutions and not to the perpetuation of old problems.

For better or worse, economic factors have had a strong influence in the explosive growth of cardiac surgical procedures and must be fully understood in the present era of cost containment imposed by restrictions in public funding or in payment by third party insurers. Predictably, reductions in health care funding are affecting preferentially the most vulnerable group of patients. The weakness of the pediatric population as a consumer group is manifested in the increasing difficulty of finding adequate funding for their surgical care.

Accomplishments of cardiac surgery in the treatment of congenital heart disease have been impressive, and yet objective evaluation of such results must lead to sobering appraisal of what has been left undone. The impact of evolving medical technology on traditional medical thought has resulted in the loss of the mystique associated with biologic phenomena. Indeed, manipulation of biologic phe-

nomena has become commonplace in all areas of medicine. The initial applications of technology to biologic systems were by necessity simplistic and ignored the magnificent complexity inherent in these systems. It was relatively simple to manipulate the basic functions of the cardiovascular system with replacement or modifications of its altered mechanical functions: the pump function of the heart, the crude replacement of the arterial wall, and the implantations of simple valvular mechanisms. But as experience has repeatedly demonstrated, significant properties of these structures were ignored until the price was paid by the operated patients in the form of thrombosed, degenerated cardiac valves (Figs. 57–1 and 57–2), clogged arterial conduits (Fig. 57–3), and, lately, incapacitated patients perfused by mechanical "hearts," all of these surrounded by the public exposure normally reserved for the politician or the actor.

In the competitive race to achieve dramatic clinical goals, we have left behind the prudent assessment of all aspects of the interventions that may affect the long-term wellness of our patients. We continue to explore new avenues—cardiac transplantation in children, intrauterine interventions—without a thorough understanding of the long-term effects of such manipulations. Attempts are made to diagnose and even to treat fetal malformations, and yet simultaneously, sacrifice of normal embryos and fetuses continues based on ephemeral and sometimes capricious social dictates.

In the future, those involved in the care of patients with congenital heart disease must strive for solutions to these problems. The modern provision of care for complex cardiac surgical patients is becoming a multidisciplinary activity with varied contributions from several medical specialists

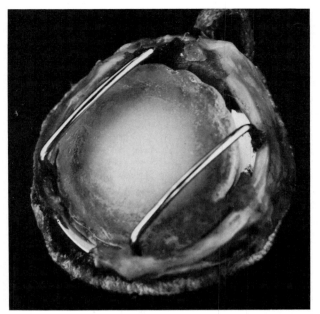

Figure 57–2. Explanted disk valve. Deformed plastic disk occluded, resulting in valve failure.

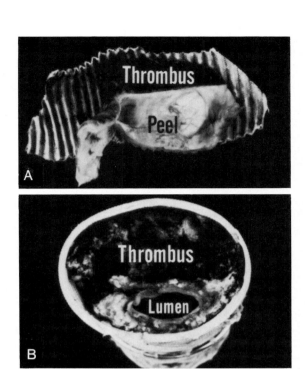

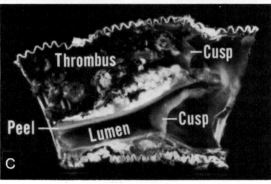

Figure 57–3. Explanted extracardiac pulmonary conduit. Inadequate behavior of implanted Dacron conduits.

(surgeons, anesthesiologists, diagnosticians, critical care specialists). Furthermore, in the provision of such care, other disciplines come into play (social workers, hospital administrators, specialized nurses, physician assistants). All of these individuals, dedicated to the welfare of the patient and integrated in their particular roles, must become involved in solving the economic, medical, and scientific problems presented by these patients.

International efforts are sorely needed in congenital heart disease. Assistance to developing economies is required not only in terms of money but also in transfer of technology, education, and training of medical teams. Particularly important is vigilant surveillance of the quality of medical products exported to countries with inadequate agencies for the regulation of such products.

Traditionally, the medical community at large has been content in responding only to the individual patient who presents for care but has conveniently avoided addressing the social, economic, and ethical impacts of its activities. Such lack of attention has created a vacuum now filled by interfering agencies, whose rulings are many times in disagreement with the best care of the patient. Thus, the individual physician has lost his traditional mantle of humanism and dedication as a public servant.

The remarkable triumphs achieved in the treatment of congenital heart disease are obvious to all. The remaining problems require deeper insight and, perhaps, the humility of the scientist in search for further improvements. DRG's, multihospital corporations, and cost effectiveness are all new concepts in the arena of medical care. The incorporation of such concepts with the traditional medical mission is urgent and indispensable. Furthermore, the confidence of the patient in the physician and the health care system must be fully restored not only because of the fear of litigation and because of the respect and admiration due their roles in society, but also because such trust is integral to healing.

The future will undoubtedly bring new technical feats in the treatment of patients with congenital heart disease. For the total success of these new activities, maturation in our approach to the patient in response to new economic realities must occur. A balance must be struck between the needs of the aging population, the needs of the investor in the medical industrial complex, and the needs of children with congenital heart disease. Social responsibility must be exercised by all of us who, armed with the powerful modern tools of medical technology, strive to apply them to the care of patients. Only through such a process will the confused adolescence of this new surgical specialty, cardiac surgery, be able to enter adulthood and realize its full potential.

References

1. Blalock A, Taussig HB (1945): The surgical treatment of malformations of the heart in which there is pulmonary stenosis or pulmonary atresia. JAMA 128:189–202.
2. Gibbon JH Jr (1953): Application of a mechanical heart and lung apparatus to cardiac surgery. Recent advances in cardiovascular physiology and surgery. Minneapolis, University of Minnesota, pp 107–113.
3. Gross RE, Hubbard JP (1939): Surgical ligation of a patent ductus arteriosus. Report of first successful case. JAMA 112:729–731.
4. Rehn L (1897): Überpenetirende Herzwuden und Herznacht. Arch Klin Chir 55:315.

58 ANESTHESIA FOR NEONATAL CARDIAC SURGERY

Neal H. Cohen

Care of the newborn with congenital heart disease presents special challenges to the anesthesiologist. Surgical intervention is usually done on an emergency, life-saving basis; the anesthesiologist involved in the care of these infants must be attuned to their special needs in addition to understanding the consequences of the cardiac surgical procedure and cardiopulmonary bypass (CPB). Approaches to the anesthetic management of the neonate undergoing palliative and definitive repair of congenital cardiac anomalies are outlined in this chapter, and some of the special needs of the premature and term infant are reviewed.

HISTORICAL PERSPECTIVE

As the understanding of the pharmacology and physiologic sequelae of anesthesia has increased, the anesthesiologist has been able to tailor the intraoperative management of the infant with complex cardiac anomalies to improve operative outcome. These improvements in anesthetic management have progressed in parallel with the development of surgical techniques to repair the congenitally abnormal heart.

History of Anesthesia

The origins of anesthesia date to the 1500s when Valerius Cordus prepared diethyl ether. It was initially used by Paracelsus, a Swiss physician and alchemist, to sweeten the feed of fowl.[78] Subsequently, nitrous oxide was obtained by Priestley from nitric oxide in 1774.[101,115]

These agents were first used clinically in the mid 1800s. Humphrey Davy,[36] a chemist and physiologist, breathed nitrous oxide to relieve a headache and pain from an erupting third molar. Davy described the effects of nitrous oxide as "thrilling and an uneasiness swallowed up in pleasure." Surgical anesthesia using ether was probably first administered by Crawford W. Long, a general practitioner in Georgia, in the late 1830's. Subsequently, the first successful public demonstration illustrating the benefits of inhalation anesthesia was performed at the Massachusetts General Hospital, on October 16, 1846, when William T.G. Morton anesthetized a patient for removal of a congenital venous malformation.[78]

The use of intravenous anesthetic agents has its origin as far back as 1665 when Harvey's studies of the circulation enabled Percival Christopher Wren and Daniel Johann Major to suggest injection of medicinal agents into the bloodstream. The development of hollow hypodermic needles and glass syringes around the 1850s facilitated administration of drugs into the circulation. They also allowed injection of medications into the vicinity of nerves, providing the foundation for regional anesthesia.

Although these approaches to surgical anesthesia were significant, most of the important advances in anesthetic management for the critically ill neonate have been made over the past 30 years. The development of new inhalation anesthetics and potent intravenous agents, such as the synthetic narcotics, have provided the anesthesiologist with more control over myocardial function and hemodynamics. Advances in hemodynamic monitoring techniques allow the anesthesiologist to optimize care to the critically ill infant. New nondepolarizing muscle relaxants with more rapid onset, shorter duration, and minimal cardiovascular effects are now available. These advances, combined with improvements in neonatal respiratory care, including continuous positive airway pressure and improved ventilatory support, make it feasible for the newborn with congenital heart disease to undergo major surgical procedures with minimal stress.

History of Cardiac Surgery

Although the Egyptian *Book of the Dead*[15] warned that the heart, as the seat of intellect and emotion, should not be touched, and Bilroth suggested that "a surgeon who would attempt such an operation should lose the respect of his colleagues,"[12] repair of the injured heart dates back to the late 1800s.[104] Surgical repair of congenital heart disease has more recent origins. Successful ligation of a patent ductus arteriosus was accomplished in 1938 by Gross and Hubbard.[59] Beginning in the early 1940s and 1950s, palliative shunt procedures were used to increase pulmonary blood flow in children with cyanotic congenital heart disease.[43]

Development of surgical techniques to allow open cardiac procedures, including repair of valvular lesions and intracardiac communications became possible as techniques for extracorporeal perfusion and myocardial preservation were developed. Total CPB was first successfully used by Gibbon in 1953 to facilitate repair of an atrial septal defect.[55] Although the clinical uses of CPB have expanded greatly since that time, Gibbon's success represented a major advance in the evolution of corrective procedures for congenital heart disease. Subsequently, surgical repair of the most complex lesions, including transposition of the great arteries, truncus arteriosus, and atrioventricular septal defect has been possible. Further advances in the care of the neonate with congenital heart disease will be possible as we acquire a better understanding of the physiologic alterations imposed by CPB, profound hypothermia, total circulatory arrest, and the interaction between these interventions and anesthesia.

GENERAL CONSIDERATIONS

Special Problems of the Newborn and Premature Infant

During the last 3 months of gestational life, most organ systems undergo significant structural and functional maturation. When an infant is born prematurely, before 36 weeks' gestational age or with a weight of under 2500 g, multiple functional abnormalities may exist. Some of the problems of concern to the anesthesiologist include difficulty with temperature regulation,[14] impaired nutritional status, respiratory distress syndrome, necrotizing enterocolitis, coagulation abnormalities, and central nervous system disorders.

The anesthesiologist must be attuned to the special needs of the premature infant. Exposure hypothermia during surgery and transport to and from the operating room increases metabolic rate and oxygen consumption.[63] The premature infant has a large surface area relative to body weight, so heat loss can be significant. During transport of the patient from the neonatal intensive care unit to the operating room, the infant's body, including the head, must be covered. Radiant warmers are commonly used to maintain body temperature. In addition, inspired gases should be warmed and fully humidified at 34°C to 37°C.

The premature infant can easily become dehydrated.[64] Adequate intravascular volume must be maintained to prevent hypotension during anesthetic induction. Intravenous fluid should be administered to ensure adequate intravascular volume, since oral intake should be avoided within 4 to 6 hours of surgery.

Because of diminished nutrient stores, the newborn, particularly the premature infant, is at risk for hypoglycemia. In addition to the well-recognized neurologic sequelae of hypoglycemia, temperature regulation is more difficult for the hypoglycemic infant. Glucose-containing fluids should be administered and blood sugar followed closely prior to and during surgery.

Premature infants, particularly those born at 24 to 30 weeks' gestational age, commonly develop respiratory distress. Although the infant with respiratory distress syndrome is unlikely to undergo a corrective cardiac surgical procedure, ligation of a patent ductus arteriosus or palliative procedure may be required. Under these circumstances, ventilatory management must be optimized prior to transferring the patient to the operating room and during the surgical procedure. Because of changes in chest wall and lung compliance that accompany intraoperative position changes and surgical compression of the lung, meticulous attention must be paid to ventilatory support and gas exchange.

Another respiratory problem that may develop in the preterm infant is bronchopulmonary dysplasia, which may occur as a result of recurrent respiratory infections or as a sequela of positive-pressure ventilation.[97] Ventilatory support must be carefully managed to optimize ventilation-perfusion relationships. Cautious intraoperative use of positive end-expiratory pressure is often required.

The preterm infant commonly has episodes of periodic breathing or apnea.[32,51] The etiology of these altered respiratory patterns is unclear, although both patterns are associated with various metabolic abnormalities, altered thermoregulation, and poor control of respiration.[113] Apneic episodes commonly occur postoperatively in preterm infants. The premature infant who has a surgical procedure within the first 6 months after birth must be closely monitored postoperatively for periodic breathing or apneic episodes. Some of these infants will require postoperative mechanical ventilation.

The development of retrolental fibroplasia (retinopathy of prematurity) is of concern to the anesthesiologist who cares for any preterm infant who receives supplemental oxygen.[60,102] Hyperoxia causes constriction of the retinal arterioles and capillary endothelial degeneration; retinal ischemia can develop. The resultant neovascularization and retinal detachment can cause blindness. Retrolental fibroplasia usually occurs in infants under 30 weeks' gestational age, although it can occur in more mature infants.[60,91] Retrolental fibroplasia is often associated with PaO_2 greater than 100 mmHg for prolonged periods of time, although the exact level of PaO_2 at which retrolental fibroplasia develops is variable.

When caring for the sick neonate with congenital heart disease, the anesthesiologist must weigh the risk of retrolental fibroplasia against the risk imposed by potential hypoxemia during surgery. Retrolental fibroplasia can usually be avoided by maintaining PaO_2 between 50 and 70 mmHg during anesthesia for the infant under 35 weeks' gestational age or under 1500 g.[19] Vitamin E, when administered until retinal vascularization is complete, is protective.[70]

Associated Congenital Anomalies

As many as 25 per cent of newborns with cardiac disease may have associated congenital anomalies (see Chapter 50), many of which have significance to the anesthesiologist. Airway abnormalities can make intubation difficult. The presence of a tracheoesophageal fistula or abnormal tracheal anatomy will affect airway management and anesthetic selection. Abnormal lung development or respiratory distress syndrome can account for significant intraoperative gas exchange abnormalities, superimposed on problems related to the cardiac defect. Such pulmonary pathology can alter airway pressures during positive-pressure ventilation and influence approaches to management of hypoxemic and hypercarbic episodes.

The normal newborn infant has a low glomerular filtration rate.[124] Congenital renal anomalies may further impair renal function. Diminished renal function can significantly affect drug clearance and therefore influence intra-operative drug selection and dosing.

A number of gastrointestinal abnormalities are associated with congenital cardiac defects. Esophageal atresia and tracheoesophageal fistula (including VATER association) predispose to recurrent aspiration and altered pulmonary function. Abdominal wall defects, including omphalocele and diaphragmatic hernia, affect lung development. Biliary atresia may impair hepatic metabolism or biliary clearance of some anesthetic agents.

Many premature infants develop necrotizing enterocolitis, which appears to occur as a result of decreased cardiac output or a patent ductus arteriosus, both of which affect bowel perfusion. Necrotizing enterocolitis has also been associated with early feeding of a hyperosmolar formula to the premature infant. The most significant anesthetic implication of necrotizing enterocolitis is hypovolemia; infants with necrotizing enterocolitis usually require large fluid volumes during anesthesia and surgery. In addition, if air is present in the bowel wall, nitrous oxide must be avoided, because any air-containing spaces increase in size during nitrous oxide anesthesia.[44]

Polycythemia may be present in neonates who require cardiac surgery. High hematocrits are associated with coagulation abnormalities, including clotting factor deficiencies, fibrinolysis and platelet dysfunction. Preoperative red cell pheresis may be required to correct the coagulation deficits.

Central nervous system (CNS) damage is a serious complication of prematurity. Hypoglycemia and hyperglycemia are often associated with CNS abnormalities. Intracranial hemorrhage, which is occasionally associated with rapid administration of sodium bicarbonate, also occurs. Sodium bicarbonate increases intravascular volume and CO_2 production. If bicarbonate is to be administered, it should be infused at a rate no faster than 1 mEq/kg/min. For the child who has sustained an intracranial hemorrhage, $PaCO_2$ and pH should be carefully controlled to normalize intracranial pressure and cerebral perfusion. Hypocarbia and alkalosis decrease cerebral perfusion, which can reduce intracranial pressure, but at the price of reducing brain oxygen delivery; hypercarbia and acidosis increase cerebral perfusion and volume and exacerbate increased intracranial pressure.

Preoperative Assessment

Prior to defining an anesthetic plan for the neonate in need of cardiac surgery, the anesthesiologist must thoroughly evaluate the infant's clinical status. The assessment includes a review of the pathophysiology of the cardiac anomaly, as well as the usual preoperative evaluation for the newborn undergoing anesthesia and surgery.

History

The anesthesiologist must review the history and presenting characteristics of the cardiac anomaly. The history most often identifies the presenting feature. The neonate with decreased pulmonary blood flow may have profound cyanosis from birth or intermittent cyanotic episodes associated with crying or agitation. For the neonate who presents with increased pulmonary blood flow and signs of congestive heart failure, the history may include poor

feeding and respiratory insufficiency. A review of the medications, including diuretics or inotropic agents, helps the anesthesiologist estimate the magnitude of the underlying physiologic abnormality. For the infant receiving medications preoperatively, assessment of intravascular volume status and serum potassium concentration are essential prior to induction of anesthesia.

The results of laboratory and diagnostic studies should also be reviewed. Ideally, the patient should be metabolically stable with normal electrolyte values prior to induction of anesthesia. When emergency procedures such as shunts or pulmonary artery bands are required, stabilization of the patient prior to surgery may not be possible.

Cardiac catheterization and echocardiography will identify the cardiac anomaly. The catheterization data also provide information about systemic oxygen saturation, myocardial performance, and magnitude of any intracardiac shunt.

Physical Examination

A careful physical examination can provide evidence of the patient's general condition, as well as identify specific abnormalities that may be of concern during anesthetic and postoperative management of the neonate. Routine evaluation of the head and neck can guide intraoperative airway management. Assessment of cardiovascular function is facilitated by examination of the heart to determine location and magnitude of murmurs, peripheral pulses and perfusion, and capillary filling. Intravascular volume status can be indirectly assessed by palpation of the fontanelle and liver edge relative to the right costal margin. When the venous system is full, both the fontanelle and liver will pulsate. If the fontanelle is sunken or liver size is small, intravascular volume depletion should be suspected. Peripheral perfusion may also be a manifestation of decreased intravascular volume, if myocardial performance is adequate. In the presence of poor myocardial performance or a significant left-to-right shunt, systemic perfusion may be poor, as manifested by pallor, decreased peripheral pulses, and cool extremities.

General assessment of the patient's status should also include evaluation of the infant's pulmonary function. The neonate with increased lung water due to congestive heart failure will be tachypneic and have grunting respirations, nasal flaring, and intercostal retractions. Bronchospasm due to peribronchiolar edema is common. The neonate with florid congestive heart failure will often be inactive.

Neonates with lesions resulting in decreased pulmonary blood flow may present with intermittent or continuous cyanosis. For the neonate with intermittent cyanosis, alterations in systemic or pulmonary vascular resistance as a result of anesthetic management may result in changes in the magnitude of the right-to-left shunt. Anesthetic induction and intraoperative management must be tailored to avoid interventions that worsen the shunt.

Premedication

In general, neonates do not require sedative premedication; they do not anticipate surgery, and so are not apprehensive. In addition, analgesia is rarely required preoperatively.

Premedication does have potential advantages for some infants. Oxygen consumption is reduced. If crying and agitation are avoided, the risk of hypoxemia and cyanosis in the infant with a right-to-left intracardiac shunt is minimized.

When performing painful procedures on the infant prior to induction of general anesthesia, analgesics may be required. Morphine sulfate (0.1 to 0.15 mg/kg) or meperidine (1 to 3 mg/kg) will provide satisfactory analgesia. Because these drugs cause significant respiratory depression in the sick neonate, close monitoring of the respiratory status is required whenever the infant is not intubated and mechanically ventilated. In general, if the anesthesiologist elects to administer a premedicant, the infant must be constantly observed prior to and during transport to the operating room.

Some neonates receive sedatives, narcotics, or muscle relaxants preoperatively in the newborn intensive care unit. The anesthesiologist should review the doses and responses to these drugs. This information can help guide selection of agents to be used intraoperatively.

Anticholinergic agents are occasionally given preoperatively to decrease secretions and produce vagal blockade; such agents are useful in a number of clinical situations. Instrumentation of the airway can result in bradycardia and hypotension unless an anticholinergic agent is given.[110] Administration of succinylcholine can also cause bradycardia if it is not preceded by administration of an anticholinergic agent. Halothane can cause a fall in heart rate and cardiac output, which is reversed with atropine.[3]

The anticholinergic agents that are commonly used include atropine or scopolamine (0.01 to 0.02 mg/kg, minimum dose 0.1 mg) or glycopyrrolate (0.005 mg/kg). Atropine has fewer antisialogogue effects but produces more vagal blockade than scopolamine.[2] Scopolamine has some sedating effect, because it more effectively crosses the blood-brain barrier. Glycopyrrolate may have an advantage over the other agents in the neonate at risk for aspiration, because it decreases gastric volume and increases the pH of gastric contents.

Despite these potential advantages, the routine use of anticholinergic premedication is debatable.[132] The dry mouth and vasodilated skin caused by these drugs may make the infant irritable. In addition, the laryngeal reflexes may not be as brisk in the immediate newborn as in slightly older infants. Many anesthesiologists prefer to administer anticholinergic agents intravenously in the operating room under controlled conditions only when clinically necessary rather than as a routine practice.

INTRAOPERATIVE ANESTHETIC MANAGEMENT

Anesthesia Equipment

Prior to transporting the infant from the nursery to the operating room, careful preparation of the room and anes-

thesia equipment is essential. Once the patient is transported, full attention should be paid to optimizing the patient's care and not searching for supplies or repairing faulty equipment.

The anesthesia machine should be carefully checked. A mechanical ventilator with low compliance tubing appropriate to provide positive pressure ventilation for the infant must be available. Mechanical ventilatory support is usually provided using pressure-limited, time-cycled ventilation. Volume-cycled ventilation is less effective for pediatric patients because of the relatively large compression volume of the anesthesia circuit and the changing lung and chest wall compliance associated with position changes and surgical manipulation.

A variety of breathing circuits is available for use during anesthesia for the infant. T-piece systems include the Bain circuit and the Jackson-Rees modification of the Ayres T-piece (Mapleson D systems). These systems are advantageous because they are simple, are lightweight, and have no valves. They are continuous-flow devices. A high fresh gas flow (approximately two times minute ventilation) is required to prevent rebreathing. Because of the high gas flow, an added humidifier is often necessary.

The anesthesia circle system can also be used for the neonate. Because it has unidirectional valves, rebreathing is avoided. If low gas flows are used, humidification is usually satisfactory without the need for an auxiliary humidifier.

Appropriate laryngoscope blades and endotracheal tubes of multiple sizes must be available. For all pediatric patients, including neonates, some leak around the endotracheal tube is desirable to prevent laryngeal trauma. For the neonate undergoing a thoracic surgical procedure, however, the leak around the endotracheal tube must be minimized. The lungs are compressed during surgery to obtain adequate exposure. They are also not ventilated during CPB. Post-bypass lung compliance is therefore often markedly reduced. If a large leak exists around the endotracheal tube, reexpansion of the lungs may be difficult.

An uncuffed endotracheal tube is preferred for neonates. For the infant undergoing a thoracotomy during which lung compliance may be poor, a relatively large endotracheal tube with minimal leak can be used intraoperatively and replaced with a smaller tube with an appropriate leak at the end of the procedure to facilitate postoperative ventilatory support. If a smaller tube is used intraoperatively, the pharynx can be packed with gauze to obliterate the air leak when higher airway pressures are required after CPB. To provide adequate gas exchange while minimizing laryngeal trauma, a small cuffed endotracheal tube can be used as an alternative. A leak should occur when the peak inspiratory pressure is approximately 20 cm H_2O with the cuff deflated. If higher airway pressures are required to optimize ventilation, the cuff of the endotracheal tube can be inflated. As lung compliance improves, the cuff is deflated to prevent laryngeal edema.

Intravenous access must be ensured prior to or immediately after induction of anesthesia. Many neonates with complex cardiac anomalies will have venous access established prior to transfer to the operating room. Intravenous access should be of appropriate size to allow adequate volume administration and blood replacement during and after the surgical procedure. No matter when the catheter is placed, care must be taken to prevent air from entering the tubing. The risk of systemic air embolization is high when any intracardiac shunt is present.

Monitoring

During induction of anesthesia, the patient is usually monitored electrocardiographically, with a precordial stethoscope and with a noninvasive blood pressure monitor. If the patient has an existing arterial catheter prior to anesthetic induction, the blood pressure should be transduced to follow beat-by-beat variation in blood pressure during induction.

After induction of anesthesia and intubation of the trachea, an arterial catheter is placed to continuously monitor blood pressure and provide access for blood sampling. A 20- or 22-gauge Teflon catheter is placed in the radial, ulnar, dorsalis pedis, or posterior tibial artery. It is usually placed percutaneously but may require placement by cutdown in the very small infant. For the infant with a patent ductus arteriosus the arterial catheter must be placed proximal to the ductus (right radial artery), if the PaO_2 is to reflect the oxygen tension of the blood perfusing the brain and retinal vessels.

A five-lead ECG system is usually used to facilitate monitoring of rhythm and ST-segment changes suggestive of cardiac ischemia (due to coronary artery disruption or air embolization).

Central venous access is rarely obtained prior to surgical repair. Central venous pressure monitoring is not usually required during or after induction of anesthesia. Since right atrial pressure does not necessarily correlate with clinical evidence of congestive heart failure,[95] right atrial pressure measurements do not provide information beyond that available from clinical assessment. A central venous catheter may be necessary before the surgical repair is complete, however, for drug and fluid administration to the sick neonate with inadequate peripheral venous access.

After completion of the surgical procedure, many surgeons insert right atrial and left atrial or pulmonary artery catheters to provide continuous monitoring of right- and left-sided myocardial performance postoperatively. The information obtained is used to optimize fluid administration and maximize inotropic and vasopressor support.

Temperature must be closely monitored during the surgical procedure. Nasopharyngeal temperature reflects brain temperature and provides direct information about adequacy of cooling and rewarming during CPB. Nasopharyngeal temperature is preferred over esophageal temperature, because esophageal temperature may more directly reflect the temperature of blood in the arterial cannula used for CPB, rather than cerebral temperature. Rectal temperature is also monitored during CPB as a reflection of core body temperature and is useful in assessing adequacy of rewarming prior to termination of CPB.

The most appropriate monitor of oxygenation during induction of anesthesia and prior to CPB is a pulse oxim-

eter, which provides direct evidence of adequacy of oxygen delivery before and after CPB, as well as an indirect index of perfusion (based on the adequacy of the pulsations). Unfortunately, when peripheral perfusion is poor, the pulse oximeter may not provide clinically useful information.

A transcutaneous oxygen electrode is also a useful monitor of oxygenation for some infants. When skin perfusion is adequate, the transcutaneous oxygen tension ($PtcO_2$) correlates well with the PaO_2. As perfusion deteriorates, the $PtcO_2$ no longer reflects arterial oxygenation, although it can provide an indirect trend of myocardial function and oxygen delivery during periods of impaired perfusion.[4]

Monitoring of end tidal carbon dioxide tension ($P_{ET}CO_2$) documents adequacy of ventilatory support and facilitates careful titration of positive pressure ventilation. A comparison of $PaCO_2$ and $P_{ET}CO_2$ provides indirect evidence of adequacy of pulmonary blood flow. If pulmonary blood flow is reduced, the difference between $PaCO_2$ and $P_{ET}CO_2$ increases. For infants with cyanotic congenital heart disease, a widening of the gradient between $PaCO_2$ and $P_{ET}CO_2$ represents further compromise in pulmonary blood flow. Such reductions in pulmonary flow may occur secondary to a fall in systemic vascular resistance (due to anesthesia) or a rise in pulmonary vascular resistance (as may occur with high airway pressures). A mass spectrometer is also a useful monitor of alveolar oxygen, carbon dioxide, and anesthetic level, when using inhaled anesthetic agents.

Anesthetic Management

Induction of Anesthesia

Anesthetic induction is a critical time for the newborn about to undergo cardiac surgery. Most of the procedures are performed urgently in critically ill neonates.[114] As a result, attempts should be made to optimize gas exchange and hemodynamic status, if possible, prior to transport to the operating room. Surgery should not be unduly delayed, however, since medical management alone is often inadequate in correcting the abnormal physiology.

Maintenance of the airway is essential during induction of anesthesia; awake intubation or administration of continuous positive airway pressure by mask are useful in this regard. Unless the anesthesiologist is confident that the patient's airway patency can be maintained, no drugs that compromise airway competence should be administered.

An awake oral intubation is the procedure most often used to secure the airway in the newborn. Using this technique avoids the need for respiratory depressants and potential airway obstruction. Unfortunately, manipulation of the airway without adequate anesthesia can result in bradycardia, owing to stimulation of the recurrent laryngeal nerve and the potential for laryngospasm with manipulation of the vocal cords. If the endotracheal tube passes easily, this technique is well tolerated. If multiple attempts at laryngoscopy are required, hemodynamic and gas exchange abnormalities can result, particularly if laryngospasm occurs.

During laryngoscopy and anesthetic induction, oxygenation must be ensured, which can be particularly difficult in neonates who are already hypoxemic due to cyanotic heart disease. Newborns have high oxygen consumptions relative to functional residual capacity (FRC) (so oxygen reserve is minimal),[85] and FRC is further reduced by anesthesia.[39] Hypoxemia is, therefore, a recognized complication of anesthetic induction even in neonates with normal hearts and lungs. Pulse oximeters can be used to continuously monitor oxygen saturation during induction of anesthesia and during airway manipulation.

Hemodynamic instability can also occur during anesthetic induction. Of particular concern is a drop in heart rate. In neonates, high heart rates are required to maintain adequate cardiac output, because stroke volume is relatively fixed. Laryngoscopy, hypoxemia, or an anesthetic overdose can result in severe hypotension for the newborn if bradycardia develops; in such cases chronotropic agents such as atropine or isoproterenol may be necessary. If the heart rate falls precipitously, the low cardiac output will prevent circulation of any drugs; external cardiac massage may be necessary.

Prior to induction of anesthesia, adequate intravascular volume must be ensured. The hypovolemic infant will become hypotensive during induction of anesthesia, particularly if inhalation anesthetic agents are used. A fall in blood pressure is poorly tolerated, because in the anesthetized neonate the heart rate does not increase in response to hypotension due to blunted baroreceptor responses.[58] Superimposed positive-pressure ventilation can decrease venous return and compound the physiologic manifestations of intravascular volume depletion.

Drug selection for anesthesia induction is determined by the pharmacologic properties of the available agents and the anesthesiologist's experience in using particular induction techniques. Anesthetic induction can be accomplished using inhalation agents or drugs administered intramuscularly, intravenously,[82] or rectally.

Anesthetic induction with an inhalation agent such as halothane or isoflurane is usually well tolerated by the newborn, but the heart rate and blood pressure can fall significantly.[53,54] Pretreatment with atropine can prevent the bradycardia. If the child cries and struggles during induction, increases in pleural pressure and pulmonary vascular resistance may result in increased right-to-left intracardiac shunting. In addition, hypoxemia may result from breath holding. If low concentrations of inhalation anesthetics are administered in combination with muscle relaxants to facilitate intubation, inhalation induction is usually well tolerated. Inhalation induction with isoflurane can be associated with significant airway irritability and laryngospasm,[123] limiting its use during anesthetic induction.[54]

For the child with decreased pulmonary blood flow due to right-to-left intracardiac shunting, the induction of anesthesia using an inhalation agent may be prolonged.[123] This prolongation is of minimal clinical significance, since the child will generally lose consciousness and tolerate intubation without clinically significant delay.

Intravenous induction of anesthesia can be accomplished with a number of sedative-hypnotic agents. If venous access has been obtained prior to transfer to the operating room, this route is commonly used in combination with muscle relaxants to initiate anesthesia and allow rapid control of the airway. Inhalation or additional intravenous anesthesia can then be used for anesthetic maintenance. If intravenous access is not available prior to arrival in the operating room, a 25-gauge needle can often be quickly introduced into a peripheral vein and facilitate intravenous induction.

The most commonly used parenteral induction agents include sodium thiopental (4 to 6 mg/kg), ketamine, and narcotics, such as morphine (0.05 mg/kg) or fentanyl (20 to 50 mg/kg). Midazolam (0.025 to 0.1 mg/kg IV) and methohexital (30 mg/kg per rectum) have also been used, although rarely for the neonate.

Ketamine is a useful anesthetic induction agent because hemodynamic stability is usually ensured.[67,94] Ketamine can be given intramuscularly (5 to 10 mg/kg) or intravenously (1 to 2 mg/kg). The intramuscular route is useful for induction of anesthesia in the infant with no intravenous access.

Because of infrequent hemodynamic effects, ketamine is preferred by some anesthesiologists for induction of anesthesia, particularly for the infant with decreased pulmonary blood flow.[103] Ketamine does, however, have potential deleterious cardiovascular effects. It has potent sympathomimetic actions due primarily to direct central nervous system stimulation.[134] In the absence of autonomic control, ketamine has direct myocardial depressant properties.[130,134] If ketamine is administered to the sick neonate with depleted catecholamine stores, severe hypotension can occur.

Some studies indicate that ketamine increases pulmonary vascular resistance,[118,129] which could potentiate right-to-left shunting in cyanotic newborns. However, ketamine-induced increases in pulmonary vascular resistance, which are secondary to the effect of ketamine on ventilation and oxygenation,[67] appear to be modest.[94] If oxygenation and ventilation are ensured, ketamine is a safe induction agent.

To facilitate laryngoscopy, intubation, and positive-pressure ventilation, muscle relaxants are also often required. The usual relaxant for use during laryngoscopy is succinylcholine (1 to 2 mg/kg intravenously, 2 to 4 mg intramuscularly). Because succinylcholine has been associated with severe bradycardia, it is often administered with atropine (0.01 mg/kg). Nondepolarizing muscle relaxants such as pancuronium (0.05 to 0.1 mg/kg) and vecuronium (0.05 to 0.1 mg/kg) have also been used to provide relaxation during induction of anesthesia and intubation. Both drugs have prolonged effects in the neonate, as compared with older children or adults,[10,49] although for cardiac procedures long duration of effects is rarely significant. Pancuronium can also produce hemodynamic changes, including tachycardia and hypertension.[7,9] These effects may be minimal in the sick neonate.[24,29] Vecuronium is without hemodynamic effects.[57]

Anesthetic Agents

Following induction of anesthesia and intubation, the goal of anesthetic maintenance is to provide safe surgical conditions with minimal interference in gas exchange or hemodynamics.

INHALATION AGENTS

Nitrous Oxide. Nitrous oxide is commonly used as an adjunct to inhalation or narcotic anesthesia. Nitrous oxide has a moderate depressant effect on systemic hemodynamics. Arterial blood pressure and cardiac index fall. Pulmonary vascular resistance does not change in infants with both normal and elevated pulmonary pressures.[69] For most stable infants, therefore, nitrous oxide is well tolerated during induction and maintenance of anesthesia, even in the presence of an intracardiac shunt and high pulmonary vascular resistance. In the severely compromised neonate, however, even minimal hemodynamic effects are not tolerated and nitrous oxide should be avoided.[34]

The use of nitrous oxide has other limitations. When nitrous oxide is used, the inspired oxygen concentration must be reduced. For the hypoxemic child, high inspired oxygen concentrations may be required to overcome the effects of ventilation-perfusion mismatch on PaO_2. In addition, nitrous oxide promotes expansion of air-containing spaces. The volume of gas in the air spaces increases as nitrous oxide enters faster than nitrogen (which has a lower solubility) is removed.[44] As a result, small air bubbles in blood or the pleural space will increase in size in a nitrous oxide–containing environment.

Volatile Anesthetics. Inhaled anesthetic agents are commonly used for anesthetic maintenance prior to and during CPB. Although all of the inhalation agents can be safely used, the concentration delivered must be carefully titrated for the sick neonate.

Some studies have suggested that the inhalation agents should not be used for anesthetic maintenance for children with cyanotic heart disease. In these patients with decreased pulmonary blood flow, inhalation anesthesia uptake is slow and, as importantly, elimination is prolonged.[18] Despite these concerns, inhalation anesthesia has been safely used for these infants.[82]

Halothane and isoflurane are the commonly used inhaled anesthetic agents. Both agents depress myocardial function, reducing cardiac index and blood pressure.[3,13,52–54,58,84,107,109] As the infant is anesthetized, oxygen consumption falls. This decrease in oxygen requirement results in an appropriate (matched) reduction in oxygen delivery.[13]

The inhalation anesthetic agents also obliterate the baroreceptor response in the newborn.[13,58,107,109] The heart rate does not increase as blood pressure falls. In the infant with poor ventricular compliance, severe hypotension can result if the inhalation agent is not carefully titrated.

PARENTERAL AGENTS

Ketamine. As described previously, ketamine is commonly used during anesthesia for cardiac surgery in the newborn period. Although ketamine has been advocated because of its infrequent cardiovascular side effects,[134] it has not been demonstrated to be superior to inhaled agents. Ketamine is useful for anesthetic induction and to provide sedation during cardiac catheterization. Ketamine is not a useful maintenance anesthetic agent.

Narcotics. Narcotics are commonly used for anesthetic maintenance for the sick infant undergoing cardiac surgery. Morphine has frequently been used to provide anesthesia during repair of congenital cardiac defects because of its good analgesia and sedation. However, morphine causes histamine release, and marked hypotension can occur; as a result, synthetic narcotics, which have minimal hemodynamic effects, are often preferred.

The synthetic narcotics fentanyl and sufentanil have been studied in a variety of clinical settings, including ligation of patent ductus arteriosus[108] and repair of complex cardiac defects.[35,66] In combination with oxygen and pancuronium, both fentanyl and sufentanil are safe and effective analgesics and have minimal hemodynamic effects. Sufentanil may be somewhat more effective in blocking systemic hemodynamic responses to surgical stimuli than fentanyl. Nonetheless, both drugs provide adequate anesthesia and surgical conditions.

One disadvantage of both fentanyl and sufentanil during rapid intravenous administration is the stiffening of the chest, which can interfere with adequate ventilation; muscle relaxants will reverse this effect.

Studies in adults give conflicting information about the effect of the narcotics on pulmonary vascular resistance.[37,117] Some improvement in oxygenation is noted when narcotics are used to anesthetize cyanotic neonates with right-to-left shunts.[66]

All narcotics are significant respiratory depressants, and neonates may be especially sensitive to narcotic-induced respiratory depression.[81] When high narcotic doses are used intraoperatively, postoperative mechanical ventilation is usually required. The variable, but prolonged elimination half-lives of morphine and fentanyl[79,81,120] make these agents particularly likely to cause postoperative respiratory depression.

MUSCLE RELAXANTS

Muscle relaxants are used to facilitate intubation and as adjuncts to anesthesia for the infant undergoing cardiac surgery. They also facilitate mechanical ventilation, prevent diaphragmatic motion, and provide satisfactory surgical conditions when low concentrations of inhalation anesthetics are used.

Premature and full-term infants have decreased neuromuscular function compared with older children and adults.[56,80] They manifest considerable variation in response to nondepolarizing relaxants, probably because of differences in neuromuscular development at birth. Responses to the muscle relaxants are therefore unpredictable.

Pancuronium and vecuronium are commonly used to provide muscle relaxation. Pancuronium bromide (0.05 to 0.01 mg/kg) produces neuromuscular blockade for 30 to 35 minutes.[7,9] Although in older children and adults it can raise the heart rate and blood pressure, its hemodynamic effects in the sick neonate are usually minimal.[24,29] Vecuronium, another nondepolarizing muscle relaxant, is now frequently used because it has minimal cardiovascular effects.[57] Its duration of action is about 20 minutes.

Other nondepolarizing agents such as *d*-tubocurarine, atracurium, and metocurine have also been used as adjuncts to general anesthesia. Although *d*-tubocurarine (0.3 mg/kg) has the same duration of action in neonates and adults, it can produce prolonged neuromuscular blockade with repeated doses.[89] Hypotension due to histamine release can also occur after administration of *d*-tubocurarine. Atracurium has similar hemodynamic effects, but it is shorter acting. Metocurine has minimal heart rate and blood pressure effects in the adult, although the hemodynamic effects in the infant are not defined.

Anesthetic Management for Cardiopulmonary Bypass

The anesthesiologist is responsible for maintaining an adequate level of anesthesia during CPB, while ensuring hemodynamic stability.

Initiation of CPB

ANTICOAGULATION

Before initiating CPB, anticoagulation is accomplished using heparin. Prior to administration of heparin, a control activated clotting time or partial thromboplastin time is obtained. The usual control level of activated clotting time ranges between 90 and 150 seconds. Heparin is administered prior to placement of the arterial and venous cannulae. The usual initial dose of heparin is 300 units/kg, administered through a well-running venous cannula. Beef lung heparin appears to have better anticoagulant properties than pork mucosal heparin.[48] Adequate anticoagulation is confirmed when the activated clotting time is about three times normal or greater than 400 seconds.[46]

Inadequate anticoagulation may result from heparin administration through a poorly running venous catheter or relative heparin resistance (for which a larger dose of heparin must be administered).[21,45] The per kilogram heparin dosage required for neonates may be greater than that required for adults.[33] The etiology for this increased dosage requirement is unclear, but lower antithrombin III levels in the newborn may be responsible.[90] Other studies confirm that reduced circulating antithrombin III levels prevent anticoagulation with heparin.[6,116] Administration of fresh frozen plasma with a high antithrombin III activity may reverse this process and ensure adequate anticoagulation after the administration of heparin. Since higher doses of heparin might be required for the neonate, appropriate monitoring of activated clotting time or partial thromboplastin time prior to and after administration of heparin is essential to confirm adequate anticoagulation throughout cardiopulmonary bypass.

In addition to inadequate anticoagulation after administration of heparin, heparin-associated thrombocytopenia[22] and bleeding can occur. Since many patients are thrombocytopenic after CPB, it is clinically difficult to determine the incidence of heparin-associated thrombocytopenia in patients who have undergone cardiac surgery.

HEMODYNAMIC CHANGES

A variety of problems can occur during manipulation of the heart to prepare for CPB. During placement of the venous cannula(e), supraventricular arrhythmias can occur but pharmacologic conversion is rarely necessary at this point in the surgical procedure (unless blood pressure falls). In addition, blood pressure may fall after placement of the arterial cannula. The hypotension has two causes. First, resistance to aortic outflow is increased and blood pressure measured distally is reduced after cannula placement. Second, a substantial volume of blood can be lost during cannula placement. Volume can be easily administered through the arterial cannula to treat hypotension prior to initiation of CPB.

Management During Cardiopulmonary Bypass

With the initiation of CPB, the arterial blood pressure falls. The fall in blood pressure is probably due primarily to acute vasodilation secondary to changes in blood viscosity and decreases in blood temperature. The mean arterial pressure gradually rises over several minutes and is usually maintained between 30 and 50 mmHg. Although some neonates will remain hypotensive during CPB with mean arterial pressures as low as 20 to 30 mmHg, vasopressors are rarely required if flow is maintained at normal levels.

Some surgeons use cardioplegic solution for myocardial protection during repair of congenital cardiac abnormalities.[16] If crystalloid cardioplegia is used, it may contain a high concentration of potassium chloride (20 mEq/liter); infusion into the root of the aorta results in ventricular relaxation.[83] High potassium concentrations in the cardioplegic solution may account for hyperkalemia at the termination of bypass and interfere with myocardial function as the heart is required to resume function. If a significant volume of crystalloid cardioplegia is used, it may also contribute to a low hematocrit after CPB. At the end of CPB, red blood cell volume may be low despite adequate intravascular volume, and diuresis and blood replacement may be necessary in the post-bypass period. Hemodilution can be avoided without apparent difference in outcome by the use of blood cardioplegia or intermittent cross-clamping with topical cooling of the heart.[16,26]

During CPB, anesthesia is maintained using inhalation anesthetic agents or fixed agents such as narcotics and sedatives. The selection of anesthetic technique during CPB depends on the patient's hemodynamic status during bypass, as well as on planned post-bypass management.

When inhaled agents are used during CPB, a flow-compensated vaporizer is inserted into the inspiratory side of the oxygenator. Uptake of anesthesia is dependent on oxygen flow through the oxygenator and pump flow. The inhalation anesthetic agents will usually cause some peripheral vasodilation and lower the blood pressure.

Narcotics are also frequently used during CPB. Minimal hemodynamic changes result. Adequate levels of anesthesia can be achieved with morphine sulfate, fentanyl, or sufentanil. The use of narcotics during CPB may necessitate postoperative ventilation for respiratory depression.

Since most newborns undergoing correction of congenital cardiac anomalies are mechanically ventilated during the early postoperative period anyway, narcotic-induced respiratory depression is of minimal clinical significance. Additional sedatives, including diazepam or midazolam, can be used during cardiopulmonary bypass.

Since respiratory efforts could result in air entrainment into the circulation when the heart is open, respiratory movements should be prevented. Adequate levels of anesthesia are usually effective in abolishing breathing movements, but muscle relaxants are often also given to prevent any diaphragmatic or other respiratory motions.

Discontinuation of CPB

After completion of the surgical repair, management is directed toward facilitating return to normal circulatory physiology. Prior to discontinuation of CPB, the patient is rewarmed to 37°C. Ventilation of the lungs is reinitiated. Bilateral lung expansion can be confirmed by direct visualization. Once the lungs are reexpanded, ventilation is controlled using positive pressure and 100 per cent oxygen or an oxygen/air mixture.

After rewarming, the neonate usually regains a sinus rhythm. Occasionally, supraventricular tachycardia or ventricular ectopy must be corrected prior to weaning from CPB; electrical cardioversion is commonly used.

Once ventilation has been ensured and the patient has a satisfactory heart rate and rhythm, weaning from CPB begins. During weaning from CPB, volume is administered to the patient from the bypass circuit until cardiac ejection begins. During this time, intravascular volume can be assessed by inspecting cardiac chamber filling, by monitoring intravascular pressures, and indirectly by palpation of the fontanelle.

If the patient remains hypotensive despite adequate volume replacement, inotropic support may be necessary. If hypotension persists after discontinuation of bypass, calcium chloride (10 to 20 mg/kg) is the drug of choice. Thereafter, other inotropic agents, particularly dopamine, are titrated to maintain adequate blood pressure.[100] If the heart rate is low after discontinuation of bypass, atrial distention must be considered. When intravascular volume is appropriate but the heart rate is low, atropine (0.01 to 0.04 mg/kg) should be administered. Isoproterenol can also be used for its inotropic and chronotropic effects. Isoproterenol infusion can be titrated to obtain satisfactory heart rate and blood pressure.

During weaning from CPB, the inhalation anesthetic is usually discontinued. When the patient has been successfully weaned, additional inhaled or intravenous agents can be given as needed. Nitrous oxide should be avoided after CPB, because of concern about potential enlargement of loculated air bubbles in the heart or great vessels.[44]

After satisfactory discontinuation of CPB and assurance of adequate intravascular volume, anticoagulation is reversed using protamine. The protamine dose is 3 to 4.5 mg/kg (1 to 1.5 mg/100 units of heparin).[72] Some studies suggest that smaller doses of protamine may be sufficient

to reverse the anticoagulant effects of heparin.[41,131] In calculating the total heparin dose, the amount of heparin added to the CPB prime must be included, particularly for the neonate. Two thousand five hundred units of heparin are often added to the CPB prime solution for each unit of blood used. This dose is often greater than the dose given to the neonate prior to initiating CPB.

Protamine has significant side effects. Protamine-induced hypotension, although rare in the newborn, occurs with variable magnitude secondary to peripheral vasodilation.[72,77,92] Volume administration will usually reverse protamine-induced hypotension. When hypotension persists, calcium chloride (20 to 50 mg/kg) or other vasopressors may be necessary. If the hypotension is refractory, reinstitution of CPB after administration of additional heparin may be necessary. Hypoxemia,[76] fulminant noncardiogenic pulmonary edema,[98] and anaphylaxis[93] have also been reported. An additional consequence of protamine administration is severe pulmonary vasoconstriction.[86,93] For the neonate with a persistent intracardiac communication, increases in pulmonary vascular resistance can cause increased right-to-left shunting and marked hypoxemia.[86]

Management During Total Circulatory Arrest

For some surgical procedures, deep hypothermic circulatory arrest is used to facilitate surgical management. Hypothermia decreases metabolic rate and protects vital organs from ischemia during total circulatory arrest (TCA). TCA is generally restricted to those infants weighing under 10 kg having complex surgical procedures, particularly those involving the atria, including repair of transposition of the great arteries or atrioventricular septal defect. When TCA is anticipated, some surgeons prefer initial surface cooling with ice.[5] If this technique is used, surface cooling is initiated after induction of anesthesia and intubation of the trachea. During surface cooling, additional heat loss can be achieved using inhaled anesthetics, which act as superficial vasodilators and permit more rapid cooling. Surface cooling is usually continued until the rectal temperature is approximately 28°C. Thereafter cooling is achieved using CPB. TCA is initiated when the rectal temperature is 12 to 15°C.

During cooling, metabolic demands are decreased. As a result, carbon dioxide production is less. Mechanical ventilatory support must be reduced to normalize $PaCO_2$ and prevent severe respiratory alkalosis, which might precipitate arrhythmias and alter cerebral blood flow.

As core temperature falls, rhythm changes occur. Initially the heart rate slows; subsequently the PR interval increases. Ventricular ectopy rarely occurs, unless the temperature falls below 28°C. When ventricular fibrillation occurs, defibrillation is rarely effective. CPB should be initiated immediately.

The duration of hypothermic TCA that is safe is poorly defined. Studies of neurologic and psychologic sequelae of TCA suggest that no definite safe period can be ensured,[125,133] although TCA has been maintained for as long as 60 minutes with minimal neurologic impairment in some infants.[61]

The role of anesthesia during TCA is also poorly understood. Anesthetics can significantly alter metabolic demands and reduce CNS electrical activity. The appropriate anesthetic agents to use and the depth of anesthesia to maintain are as yet undefined.

POSTANESTHETIC MANAGEMENT

Mechanical Ventilatory Support

Postoperative mechanical ventilatory support is required for most neonates undergoing palliative and corrective cardiac surgical procedures.[88,111] Early postoperative ventilatory support ensures adequate gas exchange, while allowing time for normalization of intravascular volume, administration of vasopressors as needed, and assurance that bleeding has ceased. Once hemodynamic stability is ensured and bleeding controlled, weaning from ventilatory support can be initiated.[62,88,111]

Mechanical ventilation may be required for longer periods of time for younger infants[88] with preoperative pulmonary edema,[135] pulmonary hypertension,[62] and prolonged CPB times for more complex surgical repairs.[62] The use of total circulatory arrest alone is not a predictor of prolonged mechanical ventilatory requirement,[88] although many of these infants become edematous and develop decreased lung-thorax compliance postoperatively.

Anesthetic management may dictate the need for postoperative mechanical ventilation. High-dose narcotic anesthesia will depress ventilatory drive and prevent the infant from sustaining adequate spontaneous ventilatory effort.[79,81] The premature infant may have a periodic breathing pattern after narcotic anesthesia for which positive-pressure ventilation may be required.[32,51] Residual muscle relaxation can also interfere with successful weaning.

Weaning from Mechanical Ventilation

Mechanical ventilatory support is discontinued when the patient is hemodynamically stable and can maintain normal spontaneous ventilation. Fixed sedatives and narcotics are discontinued prior to weaning from ventilatory support. When narcotics are used for sedation, reversal of the narcotic-induced respiratory depression can be achieved with naloxone, if necessary. When muscle relaxants are administered postoperatively, the neuromuscular blockade should be carefully antagonized with an anticholinesterase drug.[30] Care must be taken in the administration of the antagonist to avoid hemodynamic effects, particularly bradycardia and hypotension.

Specific methods of weaning vary from institution to institution. Most patients are weaned from positive-pressure ventilation using intermittent mandatory ventilation. The infant is weaned by reducing the mechanical ventilatory rate until full spontaneous respirations are achieved and gas exchange is satisfactory. If, at that time, the child is awake, is alert, and can maintain an adequate airway, the endotracheal tube is removed. For some infants, breathing spontaneously through a small endotracheal tube results in high airway resistance. Under these circumstances, extubation will be attempted without a prolonged weaning trial.

Hemodynamic Support

Intravascular volume is the mainstay of hemodynamic support after cardiac surgery. Volume is administered cautiously, as necessary. Monitoring includes clinical signs (fontanelle, liver size, peripheral perfusion), as well as central hemodynamic measurements of central venous pressure, pulmonary artery pressure, and left atrial pressure, when available. Urine output may poorly reflect intravascular volume in the neonate.[96] Inotropic and vasopressor agents are used to improve cardiac output only after intravascular volume is adequate.

The selection of inotropic and vasopressor agents depends on the clinical condition of the patient. Dopamine is commonly used to improve cardiac output and blood pressure in the critically ill newborn.[100] A dose of 1 to 8 µg/kg/min administered in a titrated fashion will often result in improved left ventricular performance. Tachycardia and increased pulmonary vascular resistance can occur with administration of higher doses of dopamine. Careful titration can often avoid severe tachycardia. Isoproterenol has also been used for the newborn with congenital heart disease, particularly when the heart rate is low. Its chronotropic effects often improve heart rate and blood pressure without concomitant increases in pulmonary vascular resistance.

A fixed-ratio infusion of norepinephrine and phentolamine has also been used for inotropic support after repair of congenital cardiac anomalies.[1] Titration of a combination of norepinephrine and phentolamine result in improved cardiac output and mean arterial pressure with only mild increases in systemic and pulmonary vascular resistance.

The effects of other inotropic agents, such as dobutamine, have not been studied in the neonate undergoing repair of congenital cardiac anomalies.[136] Dobutamine either alone or in combination with dopamine has been effective in improving myocardial performance and mean arterial pressure in adults with myocardial dysfunction.[105] Dobutamine may be of benefit for the neonate when inotropy and afterload reduction are required to facilitate myocardial performance postoperatively.

Combinations of inotropic agents and vasodilators have been used in children after cardiac surgery. Dopamine and nitroprusside administered simultaneously improved cardiac index significantly, while systemic and pulmonary vascular resistances fell.[121] Unfortunately, tachycardia may limit the usefulness of this combined therapy for some infants. Epinephrine and nitroprusside have also been used to improve postoperative myocardial performance in children;[11] the effectiveness of this combination in neonates is not known.

MANAGEMENT OF SPECIFIC CARDIAC LESIONS

Patent Ductus Arteriosus

As pulmonary vascular resistance falls after birth, pulmonary blood flow increases. For the premature infant whose ductus arteriosus remains patent, pulmonary edema may result. The increased pulmonary blood flow interferes with gas exchange and often necessitates mechanical ventilatory support. In addition, systemic blood flow may be compromised, because pulmonary vascular resistance falls below systemic vascular resistance, shifting blood to the pulmonary circulation. As a result, peripheral perfusion may be poor, manifested as renal and hepatic insufficiency and bowel ischemia.

Initially the premature infant with a patent ductus arteriosus is managed medically with fluid restriction and diuresis,[27] mechanical ventilatory support to facilitate gas exchange, and pharmacologic attempts at closure of the ductus using indomethacin.[65] Although for most premature infants ductal constriction occurs with indomethacin treatment, reopening frequently occurs. Surgical ligation of the ductus is commonly required.

When surgical ligation of the patent ductus arteriosus is required, the anesthesiologist is presented significant challenges. The premature infant may weigh as little as 500 g, have clinical manifestations of congestive heart failure, and be intravascularly volume depleted. Prior to induction of anesthesia, adequate intravascular volume must be ensured. Some of these infants will require fluid resuscitation with as much as 10 to 20 ml/kg of crystalloid solution in spite of the increased lung water, particularly when inhaled anesthetics are used. Although inhaled anesthetics have been used to provide anesthesia for these premature infants,[47] the preferred method of anesthesia is intravenous narcotics (usually 20 to 50 μg/kg of fentanyl) and muscle relaxation with pancuronium or succinylcholine.[25,108]

Mechanical ventilatory support is required for patent ductus ligation. The surgical approach is usually through a left posterolateral thoracotomy (see Chapter 61). Ventilation of the left lung may therefore be altered. Supplemental oxygen is used in combination with air. To optimize oxygen delivery during surgery, a pulse oximeter or transcutaneous oxygen electrode is essential. These monitors allow careful titration of oxygen to ensure a safe PaO_2, while minimizing the risk of retrolental fibroplasia.

Because of the unstable clinical condition of many of these infants, careful control of ventilation and close monitoring is essential during transport to the operating room. Some anesthesiologists and surgeons now prefer using a specially designed transport/operating table to transfer the patient from the neonatal intensive care unit to the operating room. This device allows the patient to be positioned prior to transfer and to undergo the surgical procedure on the same bed without the need to transfer the infant to and from an operating room table. Other centers ligate the ductus in the nursery without moving the infant at all (see Chapter 61).

Since most of these infants have persistent pulmonary edema due to increased interstitial lung water and significant atelectasis as a result of the surgical approach, positive-pressure ventilatory support is usually continued for at least 24 hours postoperatively. Weaning from ventilatory support is begun after the pulmonary edema resolves.

Coarctation of the Aorta

Coarctation of the aorta in the newborn is usually due to generalized aortic isthmus narrowing. Coarctation is usually manifest as severe left-sided outflow obstruction and congestive heart failure presenting within the first few days of life. Systemic perfusion is poor, and most of these infants have a severe metabolic acidosis.

Coarctation of this type is often associated with other intracardiac anomalies (see Chapter 37). Commonly, these infants will have intracardiac communications at the ventricular level and significant left-to-right shunting. The combination of aortic narrowing and ventricular septal defect results in increased pulmonary blood flow and potentiation of the systemic hypoperfusion. Surgical correction is generally directed at relieving the aortic narrowing. If associated anomalies require correction, these are often deferred until the infant is stabilized after coarctation repair (see Chapter 62).

For the newborn with severe coarctation, anesthesia is usually maintained with an inhaled anesthetic. The inspired oxygen concentration is high to prevent hypoxemia during thoracotomy and lung compression. Blood pressure control is essential during and after repair of the coarctation. Inhalation anesthetic agents, ganglionic blocking drugs,[8] and drugs with alpha- and beta-blocking properties[74] have been used to control hypertension.

Although most older children undergoing repair of coarctation can be weaned from mechanical ventilatory support postoperatively, the sick neonate who presents with severe coarctation often has associated intracardiac anomalies and requires postoperative ventilatory support.

Palliative Procedures

Although in general many surgeons now prefer attempting total corrections of congenital cardiac lesions at an early age,[127] some infants require palliative procedures, usually pulmonary artery bands or shunts (see Chapter 60).

Pulmonary Artery Banding

A pulmonary artery band procedure is performed when pulmonary blood flow is high and refractory congestive heart failure develops, or the risk of early pulmonary vascular disease is substantial. Under these circumstances, banding the pulmonary artery can reduce or eliminate congestive heart failure as well as protect the pulmonary circulation from progressive pulmonary hypertension and resultant pulmonary vascular disease. The common lesions for which a pulmonary artery band is placed include truncus arteriosus, large ventricular septal defects with increased pulmonary blood flow, and atrioventricular septal defects.

The patients undergoing a band procedure have pulmonary edema with decreased lung compliance due to increased lung water. They often require high airway pressures to ensure adequate chest expansion. At the time of endotracheal intubation, the endotracheal tube must be of adequate size to prevent significant leak that would interfere with ventilation with high airway pressures. Increased airway resistance, manifested as wheezing, may also accompany the peribronchiolar edema resulting from the increased lung water. Bronchodilators are occasionally of benefit, although the primary management is directed at decreasing pulmonary blood flow.[71,119]

Either inhalation anesthesia or narcotic-relaxant techniques can be used during the banding procedure. Of most concern is appropriate monitoring of oxygenation using a pulse oximeter to guarantee that oxygen saturation remains adequate after band placement. If the pulmonary artery band decreases pulmonary artery blood flow too much, oxygen saturation will fall significantly. Use of a pulse oximeter can therefore help guide the surgeon during band placement.

Postoperatively, many of these patients remain intubated and ventilated because of increased lung water. Weaning from ventilatory support can begin after lung compliance improves with resolution of the pulmonary edema.

Shunt Procedures

When pulmonary blood flow is inadequate, palliative shunt procedures are performed to improve pulmonary blood flow and promote growth of the hypoplastic pulmonary circulation. Palliative shunts are placed as an interim procedure until later total correction for lesions such as severe pulmonary stenosis, pulmonary atresia, severe tetralogy of Fallot, and tricuspid atresia.

A variety of shunt procedures have been described (see Chapter 60). These include Blalock-Taussig shunt from the subclavian artery to the pulmonary artery, Waterston shunt from the ascending aorta to the right pulmonary artery, and Potts shunt from the descending aorta to the left pulmonary artery. The Glenn shunt from the superior vena cava to the pulmonary artery is rarely placed in the neonatal period. Although each of these procedures results in improved pulmonary blood flow, a central shunt from the aorta to the main pulmonary artery is preferred by some surgeons.[127] The central shunt procedure using a Gore-Tex graft results in symmetrical growth of the pulmonary arteries bilaterally. In addition, this central shunt can be most easily removed at the time of total correction.

Because of decreased pulmonary blood flow and resultant cyanosis, high concentrations of supplemental oxygen are usually used during shunt placement. Either inhaled agents or intravenous narcotics can be used for anesthesia.

Similar anesthetic considerations apply to both palliative procedures and total corrective procedures for reduced pulmonary blood flow. Although uptake of inhalation anesthetics in the child with decreased pulmonary blood flow

is reduced,[123] this reduction is of little clinical significance. Infants with decreased pulmonary blood flow may not reach deep levels of anesthesia quickly, but anesthetic induction using inhalation agents is rarely difficult. Of more concern is the inability to eliminate the anesthetic agent via the the lungs should too great an anesthetic depth be achieved. Hypotension from inhaled anesthetics may be prolonged when pulmonary blood flow is low, and countermeasures may be required.

Pulmonary vascular resistance can change rapidly as a result of anesthetic management. Ventilatory maneuvers, including high airway pressures, excessive hyperventilation with increased mean airway pressure, and positive end-expiratory pressure may increase pulmonary vascular resistance. In addition, inadequate anesthesia with significant catecholamine release may increase pulmonary vascular resistance out of proportion to systemic vascular resistance. Hypoxia and hypercarbia are also profound pulmonary vasoconstrictors and may worsen the right-to-left shunt. The anesthesiologist must maintain adequate ventilation and oxygenation by using the lowest peak airway pressures necessary to maintain adequate chest expansion. Minute ventilation is controlled by adjusting the respiratory rate.

During the surgical manipulation of the central circulation and with cross-clamping of the pulmonary artery, pulmonary blood flow will be severely compromised. This further reduction in pulmonary blood flow may worsen the preexisting hypoxemia and result in bradycardia and cardiac arrest. Good communication between the surgeon and anesthesiologist is essential during manipulation of the pulmonary artery to ensure good surgical exposure with the shortest possible disruption of flow through the pulmonary circulation.

Lesions Associated with Increased Pulmonary Blood Flow

Ventricular Septal Defect

Infants with a large ventricular septal defect may have significant symptoms from birth, particularly if other lesions are present as well (see Chapter 35). Such infants can present with early and severe congestive heart failure and pulmonary edema. The increased lung water due to increased pulmonary blood flow results in decreased lung compliance. As a result, such infants feed poorly and are severely growth retarded. In spite of aggressive medical management with digoxin and furosemide, congestive heart failure can prove quite refractory. Whenever technically feasible, surgical closure of the ventricular septal defect is currently undertaken at the time of presentation in many centers in an attempt to surgically cure congestive heart failure and prevent subsequent or further compromise of growth and development.

Infants with ventricular septal defect and refractory congestive heart failure will usually require intubation and mechanical ventilatory support preoperatively. Both inhalation and intravenous anesthetic techniques are acceptable during repair of a ventricular septal defect. To facilitate intraoperative gas exchange, the mechanical ventilatory technique should include use of a long inspiratory time.[99]

Postoperative mechanical ventilation is required for these infants. To facilitate postoperative ventilation some intravenous sedation should be administered prior to transport from the operating room to the neonatal intensive care unit. Subsequent management will require additional sedation and muscle relaxation to facilitate ventilatory support.

Atrioventricular Septal Defect

The atrioventricular septal defect has physiologic manifestations similar to a large ventricular septal defect, but congestive heart failure is often more severe because of accompanying atrioventricular valve dysfunction (see Chapter 35). Right and left ventricular outflow are dependent on vascular resistance relationships. Although medical management is initially attempted for this lesion, early surgical intervention is often required (see Chapter 65). In the newborn period a palliative banding procedure is often preferred,[127] although some surgeons are attempting total correction at an early age.

Because of the involvement of the tricuspid and mitral valves, surgical repair of atrioventricular septal defect is more difficult than closure of ventricular septal defect. Atrioventricular valve insufficiency, which is common preoperatively, is often exacerbated postoperatively.

Anesthetic management is similar to that for ventricular septal defect. Common problems during and immediately after repair include poor lung compliance (from increased lung water) and arrhythmias. Pharmacologic control of rhythm disturbances may be necessary.

Atrioventricular septal defects are commonly associated with Down syndrome (see Chapter 48). The Down Syndrome child may have significant upper airway abnormalities, including small mandible and relatively large tongue size. Airway obstruction can occur during the induction of anesthesia. For the newborn undergoing surgical repair of the atrioventricular septal defect, awake intubation is preferred. In addition, close observation of the airway is essential at the time of extubation because postextubation airway obstruction and respiratory compromise are common. Most neonates undergoing surgical correction of the atrioventricular septal defect require postoperative ventilatory support with positive end-expiratory pressure because of increased lung water and poor lung compliance.

Truncus Arteriosus

Truncus arteriosus results from incomplete septation of the aorta and pulmonary artery (see Chapter 46). The anomalies represent a spectrum of defects, although the clinical presentation is similar for most infants with truncus arteriosus.[104] The infant with truncus arteriosus has signs of severe congestive failure due to high flow in the pulmonary circulation at systemic pressures. The magnitude of pulmonary flow is dependent on the relationship between pulmonary and systemic vascular resistances. As pulmonary vascular resistance falls in the neonate, pulmonary blood flow increases. Signs of congestive heart failure usually occur earlier and are more severe in the infant with truncus arteriosus than the infant with a ventricular septal defect or patent ductus arteriosus. The runoff of blood into the pulmonary circulation accounts for a fall in diastolic pressure and reduced coronary blood flow. The truncal valve that usually overrides a ventricular septal defect may be incompetent, causing progressive diastolic ventricular overload.[38]

To prevent pulmonary vascular changes secondary to high pulmonary blood flow at high pressures, surgical correction is performed at an early age.[42,75,106,127] If pulmonary vascular changes develop prior to surgical repair, the child becomes cyanotic due to inadequate pulmonary blood flow. This physiology precludes successful surgical repair.

The infant with a truncus arteriosus is generally growth retarded and feeds poorly. Peripheral perfusion is poor, skin is pallid, and pulses are weak, collapsing due to preferential blood flow into the pulmonary circulation. Metabolic acidosis is common. Depending on the magnitude of pulmonary blood flow, the infants are tachypneic and have congestive heart failure with reduced lung compliance.

Anesthetic management for these extremely ill infants is a challenge. Induction of anesthesia is usually accomplished without difficulty, although intravenous and arterial access are often difficult. Low concentrations of inhaled anesthetics in combination with oxygen and muscle relaxants are usually well tolerated.

Total surgical correction of truncus arteriosus usually includes placement of a conduit from the right ventricle to the pulmonary artery and closure of the ventricular septal defect. In the infant the conduit is small and may cause restriction to outflow. When the chest is closed the conduit can become partially occluded and further obstruct pulmonary blood flow. Other postoperative problems include bleeding, persistent pulmonary hypertension with right ventricular failure, and respiratory failure. Most neonates require prolonged ventilatory support after repair of truncus arteriosus due to small size, poor nutritional status, and persistent pulmonary edema.[111]

Anomalous Pulmonary Venous Drainage

Anomalous pulmonary venous drainage can be partial or complete (see Chapter 34). The signs, symptoms, and timing of surgical repair depend on the amount of pulmonary blood flow directed to the right side of the heart. Most often total anomalous pulmonary venous drainage presents as congestive heart failure early, whereas symptoms due to partial anomalous pulmonary venous drainage do not develop until adulthood.

The clinical presentation depends on the presence of a right-to-left shunt, either an atrial septal defect or patent ductus arteriosus. Occasionally, a ventricular septal defect is associated with anomalous pulmonary venous drainage as a manifestation of asplenia syndrome.

The symptomatic neonate with total anomalous venous drainage usually has inadequate right-to-left shunting due to restriction of flow through a septal defect or closure of the ductus. The infant may be cyanotic and acidotic and have poor systemic perfusion. Early surgical repair (see Chapter 67) is essential for this group of patients.[128] If systemic flow is ductal dependent, prostaglandin E_1 infusion can be used to maintain flow until surgical repair can be accomplished.

Anesthetic management usually includes low concentrations of inhaled anesthetics in combination with an air/oxygen mixture. Because high oxygen tension may encourage closure of the ductus prior to surgical repair, hyperoxia should be avoided, while maintaining normal oxygen saturation.

Positive-pressure ventilation with positive end-expiratory pressure is necessary intraoperatively and postoperatively to optimize gas exchange in the infant with pulmonary edema. Pulmonary venous obstruction can persist postoperatively due to kinking or thrombosis at the site of repair. If the pulmonary edema does not resolve with medical management and ventilatory support, repeat catheterization may be necessary. Supraventricular arrhythmias can also occur postoperatively, owing to cardiac manipulation during the surgical repair.

Lesions With Decreased Pulmonary Blood Flow

Pulmonary Stenosis

Congenital pulmonary stenosis is either valvular or infundibular (see Chapter 45). Infundibular pulmonary stenosis is often associated with a ventricular septal defect (tetralogy of Fallot). The infant with valvular pulmonary stenosis usually has few symptoms, unless the pulmonary outflow tract is critically stenotic. When critical pulmonary stenosis is present, adequate pulmonary blood flow is dependent on the presence of a patent ductus arteriosus. Symptoms appear in these infants as ductal flow decreases. Cyanotic episodes associated with feeding or crying dictate the need for surgical intervention. Prostaglandin E_1 is commonly administered preoperatively to maintain flow through the ductus arteriosus, increasing pulmonary blood flow until surgical intervention (see Chapter 63) can be accomplished.[40]

For the infant with tetralogy of Fallot, the pulmonary outflow obstruction may be more dynamic (see Chapter 46). Cyanosis will develop if the outflow tract narrows due to increased right ventricular contractility or alterations in pulmonary or systemic vascular resistances. As pulmonary vascular resistance increases with crying or struggling, or if systemic vascular resistance falls, right-to-left shunting and cyanosis worsen.

During surgery for tetralogy of Fallot (see Chapter 64), anesthetic management depends on an understanding of the etiology of the pulmonary outflow obstruction and the effects of pharmacologic manipulations on pulmonary blood flow. For the infant with severe infundibular stenosis, beta-blocking agents may be used preoperatively to decrease right ventricular contractility and reduce the pulmonary outflow obstruction. Vasopressors may also be administered to increase systemic vascular resistance and

improve flow through the pulmonary circulation. If cyanosis is severe preoperatively, supplemental oxygen and sedation may be necessary to improve systemic oxygen saturation.

During induction of anesthesia, management should be directed at maintaining pulmonary blood flow. Anesthesia is often induced using ketamine and succinylcholine intramuscularly.[67] Although uptake of inhaled anesthetic agents may be delayed in the infant with decreased pulmonary blood flow,[123] inhalation agents can also be safely used for anesthetic induction if carefully administered.[53,54] The reduction in myocardial contractility from the inhaled anesthetic agents probably causes a decrease in infundibular outflow obstruction, thereby improving pulmonary blood flow and anesthetic uptake in the child with infundibular stenosis. In addition, the decrease in oxygen consumption secondary to adequate anesthesia results in an increase in mixed venous oxygen content and improved systemic oxygenation.

Postoperatively the patients usually do relatively well. Mechanical ventilatory support may be necessary if pulmonary blood flow increases markedly and causes gas exchange abnormalities, or if hemodynamic instability develops due to persistent right ventricular failure. Otherwise these infants will tolerate spontaneous ventilation within 24 hours of surgical repair.[88,111]

Tricuspid Atresia

Tricuspid atresia is usually manifest by marked reduction in pulmonary blood flow and arterial hypoxemia (see Chapter 43). The neonate with tricuspid atresia often requires surgical intervention to increase pulmonary blood flow. Although the Fontan procedure, surgically connecting the right atrium to the pulmonary artery, has been performed in small infants, staged procedures are probably advisable.[23,31] A classic shunt procedure is most commonly performed in the neonatal period to increase pulmonary blood flow followed by a Fontan procedure at a later time. For the infant with tricuspid atresia and increased pulmonary blood flow, early pulmonary artery banding may be necessary.

Anesthetic management depends on the clinical manifestations of the lesion. The plan will vary depending on the amount of pulmonary blood flow. Management must attempt to minimize pulmonary vascular resistance and optimize left-to-right shunting. For the infant who undergoes a Fontan procedure, pulmonary blood flow is dependent on a high systemic venous pressure. After the Fontan procedure, early extubation should be considered to decrease the effects of positive-pressure ventilation on systemic venous return.[112]

Aortic Stenosis

The infant with critical congenital aortic stenosis requires early surgical intervention (see Chapter 36). Medical treatment is rarely successful. When the aortic outflow obstruction is severe, aortic valvulotomy using CPB is attempted (see Chapter 62).

The infant with critical aortic stenosis presents with very poor peripheral perfusion and congestive failure. Anesthetic management depends on maintenance of systemic blood pressure during induction. Patients with congenital aortic valvular or supravalvular stenosis may not tolerate inhalation agents as well as narcotic-relaxant anesthetics.

Transposition of the Great Arteries

Transposition of the great arteries results in complete separation of the pulmonary and systemic circulations (see Chapter 46). Neonates with transposition of the great arteries present with profound arterial hypoxemia due to inadequate interatrial mixing. These children usually undergo balloon atrial septostomy (Rashkind procedure) in the cardiac catheterization laboratory to improve atrial mixing. If oxygenation improves, surgical repair can be delayed. If the atrial septostomy is unsuccessful in producing adequate mixing, emergency surgical intervention is necessary. Although atrial septectomy (Blalock-Hanlon procedure) has been used in the past (see Chapter 60), many surgeons now prefer a corrective procedure.[87] Either an intra-atrial baffling operation to redirect flow (Mustard or Senning procedure) or an arterial switch procedure with coronary artery reimplantation (Jatene procedure) may be performed (see Chapter 66).

Anesthetic induction can be accomplished most easily with ketamine intramuscularly or intravenously and a muscle relaxant. Drugs given intravenously will be rapidly distributed to the systemic circulation (heart, brain) without passing through the lungs. In contrast, onset of anesthesia with inhaled agents is markedly delayed due to ineffective communication between the pulmonary and systemic circulations. Subsequent anesthesia is provided with narcotics or an inhaled anesthetic, such as halothane or isoflurane. A high FiO_2 is recommended, so nitrous oxide is usually avoided.

For the infant with transposition of the great arteries and ventricular septal defect, the presentation is more complicated. These infants are cyanotic with pulmonary edema. As a result, lung compliance is poor. Airway pressures during positive-pressure ventilation tend to be high. The high airway pressures may further compromise pulmonary blood flow and compound the impaired gas exchange. Under these circumstances, close monitoring of gas exchange is essential to ensure adequate oxygenation with minimal impairment of pulmonary or systemic perfusion.

For the newborn undergoing total correction, the procedure is performed using profound hypothermia and total circulatory arrest. Postoperative complications after total circulatory arrest include bleeding and intravascular volume depletion due to significant third space losses. Arrhythmias, including atrioventricular blocks and junctional tachyarrhythmias, are also common. Occasionally, myocardial dysfunction can result in impaired perfusion with postoperative renal failure. Seizures have also been described.

Complications of the intra-atrial baffle include supraventricular rhythm disturbances,[17,50] superior vena cava obstruction,[28] and phrenic nerve palsy.[122] After the intra-atrial operations, the right ventricle continues to function as the systemic ventricle. Right ventricular failure and tricuspid valve incompetence are long-term complications.[126]

Although the Jatene arterial switch procedure has a higher initial surgical mortality, long-term outcome may be better than after intra-atrial operations, because the left ventricle functions as the systemic ventricle.[20,73] A recognized complication of the Jatene procedure is pulmonary stenosis, which may require subsequent surgical repair.

CONCLUSION

The newborn with congenital heart disease presenting for surgery represents a major challenge to the anesthesiologist. Until recently, the neonate was managed medically until the child grew sufficiently to tolerate surgical repair. Those infants who could not be stabilized required early surgical intervention. In recent times, physiologic repair at the time of presentation has become the favored approach for many surgical lesions, even if presentation is in the newborn period.

Appropriate anesthetic management is an important determinant of surgical outcome at any age. The anesthesiologist must have a clear understanding of the anatomic abnormality and pathophysiology, as well as the pharmacology of the available anesthetic agents. Careful planning of anesthetic management preoperatively, intraoperatively, and postoperatively can optimize surgical conditions and outcome[67] and avoid potential complications.

References

1. Armstead V, Lynn AM (1987): Hemodynamic effects of norepinephrine and phentolamine in children after repair of congenital heart defects (abstr). Western Anesthesia Residents' Conference.
2. Bachmann L, Freeman A (1961): Cardiac rate and rhythm in infants during induction of anesthesia with cyclopropane. J Pediatr 59:922–927.
3. Barash PG, Glanz S, Katz JK, Taunt RT, Talner NS (1978): Ventricular function in children during halothane anesthesia: An echocardiographic evaluation. Anesthesiology 49:79–85.
4. Barker SJ, Tremper KK (1985): Transcutaneous oxygen tension: A physiologic variable for monitoring oxygenation. J Clin Monit 1:129–134.
5. Barrat-Boyes BG, Simpson MJ, Neutze JM (1971) Intracardiac surgery in neonates and infants using deep hypothermia and limited cardiopulmonary flow. Circulation 25 (suppl 1):43–44.
6. Barrowcliffe TW, Johnson EA, Thomas D(1978): AT-III and heparin. Br Med Bull 34:143–150.
7. Bennett EJ, Bowyer DE, Giesecke AH, Stephen CR (1973): Pancuronium bromide: A double-blind study in children. Anesth Analg 52:12–18.
8. Bennett EJ, Dalal FY (1974): Hypotensive anaesthesia for co-arctation: A method of prevention of post-operative hypertension. Anaesthesia 29:269–271.
9. Bennett EJ, Daughety MJ, Bowyer DE, Stephen CR (1971): Pancuronium bromide: Experiences in 100 pediatric patients. Anesth Analg 50:798–807.
10. Bennett EJ, Ramamurthy S, Dalal FY, Salem MR (1975): Pancuronium and the neonate. Br J Anaesth 47:75–78.
11. Benzing G III, Helmsworth JA, Schreiber JT, Kaplan S (1979): Nitroprusside and epinephrine for treatment of low output in children after open-heart surgery. Ann Thorac Surg 27:523–528.

12. Bilroth T, cited by Jeger E (1913): Die Chirurgie der Blutgefasse und des Herzens. Berlin, A Hirschwald.
13. Brett CM, Teitel DF, Heymann MA, Rudolph AM (1987): The cardiovascular effects of isoflurane in lambs. Anesthesiology 67:60–65.
14. Bruck K (1961): Temperature regulation in the newborn infant. Biol Neonatol 3:65–119.
15. Budge EW (1910): The Book of the Dead. London, Kegan, Paul, Trench, Trübner and Co, Ltd.
16. Bull C, Cooper J, Stark J (1984): Cardioplegic protection of the child's heart. J Thorac Cardiovasc Surg 88:287–293.
17. Byrum CJ, Bove EL, Sondheimer HM, Kavey R-EW, Blackman MS (1986): Hemodynamic and electrophysiologic results of the Senning procedure for transposition of the great arteries. Am J Cardiol 58:138–142.
18. Caldwell TB III, Almond A (1973): Anesthetic management of infants having surgery on the heart or great vessels: Report on 33 cases under one year of age. South Med J 66:1003–1010.
19. Campbell PB, Bull MJ, Ellis FD, Bryson CQ, Lemons JA, Schreiner RL (1983): Incidence of retinopathy of prematurity in a tertiary newborn intensive care unit. Arch Ophthalmol 101:1686–1688.
20. Castañeda AR, Norwood WI, Jonas RA, Colon SD, Sanders SP, Lang P (1984): Transposition of the great arteries and intact ventricular septum: Anatomic repair in the neonate. Ann Thorac Surg 38:438–443.
21. Chung F, David TE, Watt J (1981): Excessive requirement for heparin during cardiac surgery. Can Anaesth Soc J 28:280–282.
22. Cines DB, Kaywin P, Bina M, Tomaski A, Schreiber AD (1980): Heparin-associated thrombocytopenia. N Engl J Med 303:788–795.
23. Cleveland DC, Kirklin JK, Naftel DC, Kirklin JW, Blackstone EH, Pacifica AD, Bargeron LM (1984): Surgical treatment of tricuspid atresia. Ann Thorac Surg 38:447–457.
24. Cohen NH (1980): Hemodynamic effects of pancuronium in critically ill children (abstr). Anesthesiology 53:S139.
25. Collins C, Koren G, Crean P, Klein J, Roy WL, MacLeod SM (1985): Fentanyl pharmacokinetics and hemodynamic effects in preterm infants during ligation of patent ductus arteriosus. Anesth Analg 64:1078–1080.
26. Corno AF, Bethencourt DM, Laks H, Haas GS, Bhuta S, Dartyan HG, Flynn WM, Drinkwater DC, Laidig C, Chang P (1987): Myocardial protection in the neonatal heart: A comparison of topical hypothermia and crystalloid and blood cardioplegic solutions. J Thorac Cardiovasc Surg 93:163–172.
27. Cotton RB, Stahlman MT, Kovar I, Catterton WZ (1978): Medical management of small preterm infants with symptomatic patent ductus arteriosus. J Pediatr 92:467–473.
28. Coulson JD, Pitlick PT, Miller DC, French JW, Marshall WH, Fryer AD, Shumway NE (1984): Severe superior vena cava syndrome and hydrocephalus after the Mustard procedure: Findings and a new surgical approach. Circulation 70 (suppl I):47–53.
29. Crone RK, Favorito J (1980): The effects of pancuronium bromide on infants with hyaline membrane disease. J Pediatr 97:991–993.
30. Cronnelly R, Morris RB (1982): Antagonism of neuromuscular blockade. Br J Anaesth 54:183–194.
31. Crupi G, Alfieri O, Locatelli G, Villani M, Parenzan L (1979): Results of systemic-to-pulmonary artery anastomosis for tricuspid atresia with reduced pulmonary blood flow. Thorax 34:290–293.
32. Daily WJR, Klaus M, Meyer HB (1969): Apnea in premature infants: Monitoring incidence, heart rate changes and an effect of environmental temperature. Pediatrics 43:510–518.
33. Dauchot PJ, Berzina-Moetlus L, Rabinovitch A, Ankeney JL (1983): Activated coagulation and activated partial thromboplastin times in assessment and reversal of heparin-induced anticoagulation for cardiopulmonary bypass. Anesth Analg 62:710–719.
34. Davidson JR, Chinyanga HM (1982): Cardiovascular collapse associated with nitrous oxide anaesthetic: A case report. Can Anaesth Soc J 29:484–488.
35. Davis PJ, Cook DR, Stiller RL, Davin-Robinson KA (1987): Pharmacodynamics and pharmacokinetics of high-dose sufentanil in infants and children undergoing cardiac surgery. Anesth Analg 66:203–208.
36. Davy H (1800): Researchs, Chemical and Philosophical; Chiefly Concerning Nitrous Oxide, or Dephlogisticated Nitrous Air, and its Respiration. London, J Johnson.
37. deLange S, Stanley TH, Boscoe MJ (1980): Comparison of sufentanil-O_2 and fentanyl-O_2 anesthesia for coronary artery surgery (abstr). Anesthesiology 53:S64.
38. DiDonato RM, Fyfe DA, Puga FJ, Danielson GK, Ritter DH, Edwards WD, McGoon DC (1985): Fifteen-year experience with surgical repair of truncus arteriosus. J Thorac Cardiovasc Surg 89:414–422.
39. Dobbinson TL, Nisbet HIA, Pelton DA, Levison H, Volgyesi G (1973): Functional residual capacity (FRC) and compliance in anaesthetized paralyzed children. II. Clinical results. Can Anaesth Soc J 20:322–333.
40. Donahoo JS, Roland JM, Kan J, Gardner TJ, Kidd BSL (1981): Prostaglandin E_1 as an adjunct to emergency cardiac operations in neonates. J Thorac Cardiovasc Surg 81:227–231.
41. Dutton DA, Hothersall AP, McLaren AD, Taylor KM, Turner MA (1983): Protamine titration after cardiopulmonary bypass. Anaesthesia 38:264–268.
42. Ebert PA, Turley K, Stanger P, Hoffman JIE, Heymann MA, Rudolph AM (1984): Surgical treatment of truncus arteriosus in the first 6 months of life. Ann Surg 200:451–456.
43. Edmonds LH (1979): A Historical Review of Shunts for Cyanotic Congenital Heart Disease: First Clinical Conference on Congenital Heart Disease. Tucrer BL, Lindesmith GG, eds. New York, Grune & Stratton.
44. Eger EI II, Saidman LJ (1965): Hazards of nitrous oxide anesthesia in bowel obstruction and pneumothorax. Anesthesiology 26:61–66.
45. Esposito RA, Culliford AT, Colvin SB, Thomas SJ, Lackner H, Spencer FC (1983): Heparin resistance during cardiopulmonary bypass: The role of heparin pretreatment. J Thorac Cardiovasc Surg 85:346–353.
46. Esposito RA, Culliford AT, Colvin SB, Thomas SJ, Lackner H, Spencer FC (1983): The role of the activated clotting time in heparin administration and neutralization for cardiopulmonary bypass. J Thorac Cardiovasc Surg 85:174–185.
47. Finucane BT, Symbas PN, Braswell R (1981): Ligation of patent ductus arteriosus in premature neonates: Anesthetic management. South Med J 74:21–23.
48. Fiser WP, Read RC, Wright FE, Vecchio TJ (1983): A randomized study of beef lung and pork mucosal heparin in cardiac surgery. Ann Thorac Surg 35:615–620.
49. Fisher DM, Miller RD (1983): Neuromuscular effects of vecuronium (ORG NC45) in infants and children during N_2O, halothane anesthesia. Anesthesiology 58:519–523.
50. Flinn CJ, Wolff GS, Dick M II, Campbell RM, Borkat G, Casta A, Hordof A, Hougen TJ, Kavey R-E, Kugler J, Liebman J, Greenhouse J, Hees P (1984): Cardiac rhythm after the Mustard operation for complete transposition of the great arteries. N Engl J Med 310:1635–1638.
51. Flores-Guevara R, Plouin P, Curzi-Dascalova L, Radvanyi M-F, Guidasci S, Pajot N, Monod N (1982): Sleep apneas in normal neonates and infants during the first 3 months of life. Neuropediatrics 13 (suppl):21–28.
52. Friesen RH, Henry DB (1986): Cardiovascular changes in preterm neonates receiving isoflurane, halothane, fentanyl, and ketamine. Anesthesiology 64:238–242.
53. Friesen RH, Lichtor JL (1982): Cardiovascular depression during halothane anesthesia in infants: A study of three induction techniques. Anesth Analg 61:42–45.
54. Friesen RH, Lichtor JL (1983): Cardiovascular effects of inhalation induction with isoflurane in infants. Anesth Analg 62:411–414.
55. Gibbon JH (1954): Application of a mechanical heart and lung approaches to cardiac surgery. Minn Med 37:171–180.
56. Goudsouzian NG (1980): Maturation of the neuromuscular junction in the infant. Br J Anaesth 52:205–214
57. Goudsouzian NG, Martyn JJA, Liv LMP, Gionfriddo M (1983): Safety and efficacy of vecuronium in adolescents and children. Anesth Analg 62:1083–1088.
58. Gregory GA (1982): The baroresponses of preterm infants during halothane anaesthesia. Can Anaesth Soc J 29:105–107.
59. Gross RE, Hubbard JP (1939): Surgical ligation of a patent ductus

arteriosus: Report of first successful case. JAMA 112:729–731.

60. Gunn TR, Easdown J, Outerbridge EW, Aranda JV (1980): Risk factors in retrolental fibroplasia. Pediatrics 65:1096–1100.

61. Haka-Ikse K, Blackwood MJA, Steward DJ (1978): Psychomotor development of infants and children after profound hypothermia during surgery for congenital heart disease. Dev Med Child Neurol 20:62–70.

62. Heard GG, Lamberti JJ Jr, Park SM, Waldman D, Waldman J (1985): Early extubation after surgical repair of congenital heart disease. Crit Care Med 13:830–832.

63. Hey EN (1969): The relation between environmental temperature and oxygen consumption in the newborn baby. J Physiol 200:589–603.

64. Hey EN, Kofy G (1969): Evaporative water loss in the newborn baby. J Physiol 200:605–619.

65. Heymann MA, Rudolph AM, Silverman NH (1976): Closure of the ductus arteriosus in premature infants by inhibition of prostaglandin synthesis. N Engl J Med 295:530–533.

66. Hickey PR, Hansen DD (1984): Fentanyl- and sufentanil-oxygen-pancuronium anesthesia for cardiac surgery in infants. Anesth Analg 63:117–124.

67. Hickey PR, Hansen DD, Cramolini GM, Vincent RN, Lang P (1985): Pulmonary and systemic hemodynamic responses to ketamine in infants with normal and elevated pulmonary vascular resistance. Anesthesiology 62:287–293.

68. Hickey PR, Hansen DD, Norwood WI, Castaneda AR (1984): Anesthetic complications in surgery for congenital heart disease. Anesth Analg 63:657–664.

69. Hickey PR, Hansen DD, Stratford M, Thompson JE, Jonas RE, Mayer JE (1986): Pulmonary and systemic hemodynamic effects of nitrous oxide in infants with normal and elevated pulmonary vascular resistance. Anesthesiology 65:374–378.

70. Hittner HM, Godio LB, Rudolph AJ, Adams JM, Garcia-Prats JA, Friedman Z, Kautz JA, Monaco WA (1981): Retrolental fibroplasia: Efficacy of vitamin E in a double-blind clinical study of preterm infants. N Engl J Med 305:1365–1371.

71. Hordof AJ, Mellins RB, Gersony WM, Steeg CN (1977): Reversibility of chronic obstructive lung disease in infants following repair of ventricular septal defect. J Pediatr 90:187–191.

72. Horrow JC (1985): Protamine: A review of its toxicity. Anesth Analg 64:348–361.

73. Jatene AD, Fontes VF, Souza LCB, Paulista PP, Neto CA, Sousa JEMR, Zerbini EJ (1982): Anatomic correction of transposition of the great arteries. J Thorac Cardiovasc Surg 83:20–26.

74. Jones SEF (1979): Coarctation in children. Controlled hypotension using labetalol and halothane. Anaesthesia 34:1052–1055.

75. Juaneda E, Haworth SG (1984): Pulmonary vascular disease in children with truncus arteriosus. Am J Cardiol 54:1314–1320.

76. Kim YD, Michalik TE (1985): Protamine induced arterial hypoxaemia: The relationship to hypoxic pulmonary vasoconstriction. Can Anaesth Soc J 32:5–11.

77. Kirklin JK, Chenoweth DE, Naftel DC, Blackstone EH, Kirklin JW, Bitran DD, Curd JG, Reves JG, Samuelson PN (1986): Effects of protamine administration after cardiopulmonary bypass on complement, blood elements, and the hemodynamic state. Ann Thorac Surg 41:193–199.

78. Kitz RJ, Vandam LD (1985): A history and the scope of anesthetic practice. In Miller RD (ed): Anesthesia. New York, Churchill Livingstone, pp 3–25.

79. Koehntop DE, Rodman JH, Brundage DM, Hegland MG, Buckley JJ (1986): Pharmacokinetics of fentanyl in neonates. Anesth Analg 65:227–232.

80. Koenigsberger MR, Patten B, Lovelare RE (1973): Studies of neuromuscular function in the newborn: I. A comparison of myoneural function in the full term and premature infant. Neuropediatrics 4:350–361.

81. Koren G, Butt W, Chinyanga H, Soldin S, Tan Y-K, Pape K (1985): Post-operative morphine infusion in newborn infants: Assessment of disposition characteristics and safety. J Pediatr 107:963–967.

82. Laishley RS, Burrows FA, Lerman J, Roy WL (1986): Effect of anesthetic induction regimens on oxygen saturation in cyanotic congenital heart disease. Anesthesiology 65:673–677.

83. Lazar HL, Roberts AJ (1985): Recent advances in cardiopul-
monary bypass and the clinical application of myocardial protection. Surg Clin North Am 65:455–476.

84. Lerman J, Robinson S, Willis MM, Gregory GA (1983): Anesthetic requirements for halothane in young children 0–1 months and 1–6 months of age. Anesthesiology 59:421–424.

85. Lister G, Walter TK, Versmold HJ, Dallman PR, Rudolph AM (1979): Oxygen delivery in lambs: Cardiovascular and hematologic development. Am J Physiol 237:H668–H675.

86. Lowenstein E, Johnston WE, Lappas DG, D'Ambra MN, Schneider RC, Daggett WM, Akins CW, Philbin DM (1983): Catastrophic pulmonary vasoconstriction associated with protamine reversal of heparin. Anesthesiology 59:470–473.

87. Mahoney L, Turley K, Ebert P, Heymann MA (1982): Long-term results after atrial repair of transposition of the great arteries in early infancy. Circulation 66:253–258.

88. Manners JM, Monro JL, Edwards JC (1980): Corrective cardiac surgery in infants: A review of 136 patients including the contribution of postoperative ventilation. Anaesthesia 35:1149–1156.

89. Matteo RS, Lieberman IG, Salanitre E, McDaniel DD, Diaz J (1984): Distribution, elimination, and action of d-tubocurarine in neonates, infants, children, and adults. Anesth Analg 63:799–804.

90. McDonald MM, Hathaway WE, Reeve EB, Leonard BD (1982): Biochemical and functional study of antithrombin III in newborn infants. Thromb Haemostas 47:56–58.

91. Merritt JC, Kraybill EN (1986): Retrolental fibroplasia: A five-year experience in a tertiary perinatal center. Ann Ophthalmol 18:65–67.

92. Michaels IAL, Barash PG (1983): Hemodynamic changes during protamine administration. Anesth Analg 62:831–835.

93. Moorthy SS, Pond W, Rowland RG (1980): Severe circulatory shock following protamine (an anaphylactic reaction). Anesth Analg 59:77–78.

94. Morray JP, Lynn AM, Stamm SJ, Herndon PS, Kawabori I, Stevenson JG (1984): Hemodynamic effects of ketamine in children with congenital heart disease. Anesth Analg 63:895–899.

95. Moss AJ, Duffie ER (1962): Congestive heart failure in infancy: Significance of the venous pressure. J Pediatr 60:346–351.

96. Nash MA, Edelmann CM Jr (1974): The developing kidney: Immature function or inappropriate standard. Nephron 11:71–90.

97. Northway WH Jr, Rosan R, Porter D (1967): Pulmonary disease following respirator therapy of hyaline-membrane disease: Bronchopulmonary dysplasia. N Engl J Med 276:357–368.

98. Olinger GN, Becker RM, Bonchek LI (1985): Noncardiogenic pulmonary edema and peripheral vascular collapse following cardiopulmonary bypass: Rare protamine reaction? Ann Thorac Surg 29:20–25.

99. Olsson A-K, Lindahl SGE (1987): Spontaneous versus controlled ventilation in anaesthetized children with congenital cardiac malformations. Acta Anaesthesiol Scand 31:87–92.

100. Padbury JF, Agata Y, Baylon BG, Ludlow JK, Polk DH, Goldblatt E, Pescetti J (1987): Dopamine pharmacokinetics in critically ill newborn infants. J Pediatr 110:293–298.

101. Priestly J (1775): Experiments and Observations on Different Kinds of Air. 2nd ed. London, J Johnson.

102. Purohit DM, Ellison RC, Zierler S, Miettinen OS, Nadas AS (1985): Risk factors for retrolental fibroplasia: Experience with 3,025 premature infants. Pediatrics 76:339–344.

103. Radnay PA, Hollinger I, Santi A, Nagashima H (1976): Ketamine for pediatric cardiac anesthesia. Anaesthetist 25:259–265.

104. Rashkind WJ (1982): Historical aspects of surgery for congenital heart disease. J Thorac Cardiovasc Surg 84:619–625.

105. Richard C, Ricome JL, Rimailho A, Bottineau G, Auzepy P (1983): Combined hemodynamic effects of dopamine and dobutamine in cardiogenic shock. Circulation 67:620–626.

106. Richardson JV, Doty DB, Rossi NP, Ehrenhaft JL (1979): The spectrum of anomalies of aortopulmonary septation. J Thorac Cardiovasc Surg 78:21–27.

107. Robinson S, Gregory GA (1980): Circulatory effects of anesthesia in developing sheep: I. Halothane (abstr.). Anesthesiology 53:S330.

108. Robinson S, Gregory GA (1981): Fentanyl-air-oxygen anesthesia for ligation of patent ductus arteriosus in preterm infants. Anesth Analg 60:331–334.

109. Robinson S, Gregory GA, Fisher DM, Hoffman JIE, Rudolph AM (1980): Circulatory effects of anesthesia in developing sheep: II. Enflurane (abstr). Anesthesiology 53:S331.

110. Sagarminaga J, Wynands JE (1963): Atropine and the electrical activity of the heart during induction of anesthesia in children. Can Anaesth Soc J 10:328–342.

111. Schuller JL, Bovill JG, Nijveld A, Patrick MR, Marcelletti C (1984): Early extubation of the trachea after open heart surgery for congenital heart disease. Br J Anaesth 567:1101–1108.

112. Schuller JL, Sebel PS, Bovill JG, Marcelleti C (1980): Early extubation after Fontan operation: A clinical report. Br J Anaesth 52:999–1004.

113. Schulte FJ, Albani M, Schnizer H, Bentele K (1982): Neuronal control of neonatal respiration: Sleep apnea and the sudden death syndrome. Neuropediatrics 13(suppl):3–14.

114. Schweiss JF, Pennington DG (1981): Anesthetic management of neonates undergoing palliative operations for congenital heart defects. Cleve Clin Quart 48:153–165.

115. Smith WDA (1982): Under the influence: A History of Nitrous Oxide and Oxygen Anaesthesia. London, Macmillan.

116. Soloway HB, Christiansen TW (1980): Heparin anticoagulation during cardiac surgery in an AT-III deficient patient. Am J Clin Pathol 73:723–725.

117. Sonntag H, Larsen R, Hilfiker O, Kettler D, Brockschneider B (1982): Myocardial blood flow and oxygen consumption during high-dose fentanyl anesthesia in patients with coronary artery disease. Anesthesiology 56:417–422.

118. Spotoff H, Korshin JD, Sorenson MB, Skovsted P (1979): The cardiovascular effects of ketamine used for induction of anesthesia in patients with valvular heart disease. Can Anaesth Soc J 26:463–467.

119. Stanger P, Lucas RV, Edwards JE (1969): Anatomic factors causing respiratory distress in acyanotic congenital cardiac disease. Pediatrics 43:760–769.

120. Stanley TH, Lathrop GD (1976): Urinary morphine excretion during and after morphine anaesthesia for open-heart surgery in children. Can Anaesth Soc J 23:640–647.

121. Stephenson LW, Edmunds LH Jr, Raphaely R, Morrison DF, Hoffman WS, Rubis LJ (1978): Effects of nitroprusside and dopamine on pulmonary arterial vasculature in children after cardiac surgery. Circulation 60(suppl 1): I104–I110.

122. Stewart S, Alexson C, Manning J (1986): Bilateral phrenic nerve paralysis after the Mustard procedure: Experience with four cases and recommendations for management. J Thorac Cardiovasc Surg 92:138–141.

123. Stoelting RK, Longnecker DE (1972): The effect of right-to-left shunt on the rate of increase of arterial anesthetic concentration. Anesthesiology 36:352–356.

124. Stonestreet BS, Oh W (1978): Plasma creatinine levels in low-birth weight infants during the first three months of life. Pediatrics 61:788–789.

125. Treasure T, Naftel DC, Conger KA, Garcia JH, Kirklin JW, Blackstone EH (1983): The effect of hypothermic circulatory arrest time on cerebral function morphology and biochemistry. J Thorac Cardiovasc Surg 86:761–776.

126. Trusler GA, Williams WG, Izukawa T, Olley PM (1980): Current results with the Mustard operation in isolated transposition of the great arteries. J Thorac Cardiovasc Surg 80:381–389.

127. Turley K, Tucker WY, Ebert PA (1980): The changing role of palliative procedures in the treatment of infants with congenital heart disease. J Thorac Cardiovasc Surg 79:194–201.

128. Turley K, Tucker WY, Ullyot DJ, Ebert PA (1980): Total anomalous pulmonary venous connection in infancy: Influence of age and type of lesion. Am J Cardiol 45:92–97.

129. Tweed WA, Minuck M, Mymin D (1972): Circulatory responses to ketamine anesthesia. Anesthesiology 37:613–619.

130. Tweed WA, Mymin D (1974): Myocardial force-velocity relations during ketamine anesthesia at constant heart rate. Anesthesiology 41:49–52.

131. Umlas J, Taff RH, Gauvin G, Swierk P (1983): Anticoagulant monitoring and neutralization during open heart surgery: A rapid method for measuring heparin and calculating safe reduced protamine doses. Anesth Analg 62:1095–1099.

132. Vivori E, Bush GH (1977): Modern aspects of the management of newborns undergoing operation. Br J Anaesth 49:51–57.

133. West FC, Coghill S, Caplan HC, Lincoln C, Kirklin JW (1983): Duration of circulatory arrest does influence the psychological development of children after cardiac operation in early life. J Thorac Cardiovasc Surg 86:823–831.

134. White PF, Way WL, Trevor AJ (1982): Ketamine: Its pharmacology and therapeutic uses. Anesthesiology 56:119–136.

135. Yates AP, Lindahl SGE, Hatch DJ (1987): Pulmonary ventilation and gas exchange before and after correction of congenital cardiac malformations. Br J Anaesth 59:170–178.

136. Zaritsky A, Charnow B (1984): Use of catecholamines in pediatrics. J Pediatr 105:341–350.

59 NEONATAL CARDIOPULMONARY BYPASS

James K. Kirklin

Cardiopulmonary bypass (CPB) is the basic support technique for nearly all open intracardiac operations in the neonate as well as older patients. Special modifications of this methodology have unique applications to the neonate. To optimize visualization in a very small operative field, the techniques of low-flow perfusion and total circulatory arrest (TCA) have evolved to provide a nearly bloodless field for the performance of an efficient and accurate repair. In addition, proper neonatal myocardial protection during the global ischemic period required for intracardiac repair is necessary for early and late survival to equal or exceed results obtained in infants and older children.

HISTORICAL PERSPECTIVE

After Gibbon's first successful open heart operation (closure of an atrial septal defect) with a pump oxygenator in 1953,[18] the wide application of open-heart surgery to the correction of congenital heart defects became possible. In 1954 Warden, Cohen, Read, and Lillehei began a historic series of open-heart operations for congenital heart disease using controlled cross-circulation.[40] The following year, J.W. Kirklin and colleagues performed the first series of open-heart operations using a mechanical pump oxygenator.[27]

The safe application of total circulatory arrest (TCA) as an adjunct to CPB in the surgical treatment of congenital heart disease had much of its origins in the experimental studies in dogs by Bigelow and colleagues in 1950.[4] Early clinical success with this methodology was reported by Weiss[42] and J.W. Kirklin.[26]

The evolution of neonatal open-heart surgery was a gradual process occurring over the ensuing 10 to 15 years in many institutions. Encouraging results for neonatal and infant cardiac surgery were reported by many groups in the 1960s and early 1970s[3,10,21,26] that generally employed the methods of deep hypothermia, limited CPB, and TCA.

CARDIOPULMONARY BYPASS

The general principles of CPB as applied to neonates are similar to those for larger patients. Perfusion flow rate, perfusion and patient temperature, the arterial input pressure wave, systemic venous pressure, pulmonary venous pressure, the hematocrit, and composition of the oxygenator prime must all be decided by the surgeon and perfusionist and are called *externally controlled variables*. In order to improve exposure for intracardiac repairs, hypothermic

perfusion is used in nearly all neonatal cardiac operations to provide effective organ and microvascular perfusion at lower flow rates. At normothermia, perfusion flow rates of 2.2 to 2.5 liter/min/m^2 are desirable to maximize whole body oxygen consumption (an indirect assessment of the effectiveness of perfusion to the microcirculation) (Fig. 59–1).[24]

In order to benefit from the flexibility of CPB as a tool for maximizing surgical exposure as well as preserving organ function, low flow perfusion during hypothermia is widely practiced. Flow rates of 1.2 to 1.6 liter/min/m^2 are well tolerated at a nasopharyngeal temperature of 20°C (Fig. 59–1), and low flow perfusion at 0.5 liter/min/m^2 for 30 to 45 minutes at 20°C has been shown clinically to be safe. In monkey experiments, oxygen consumption of the brain is well maintained as flow is reduced from 1.5 to 0.5 liter/min/m^2 on bypass at 20°C (Table 59–1).[14] The resistance to blood flow during reduction of flow is unchanged in the brain but progressively increases in the remainder of the body (Table 59–2),[14] thus acting to preserve cerebral perfusion.

The damaging effects of perfusion with CPB in the neonate may be greater than those in older patients,[25] although there are no established data on this point. Abnormal events associated with CPB include exposure of blood to the *shear stresses* generated by the blood pumps, suction devices, and cavitation around the end of the arterial cannula; the *incorporation of abnormal substances* such as air bubbles, fibrin debris, platelet thrombi, and defoaming agents; and *exposure to nonphysiologic surfaces* (Fig. 59–2).[24] CPB is known to activate complement[6] as well as the coagulation,[2] fibrinolytic,[2] and kallikrein[34] cascades. The exposure of blood to the non-physiologic surfaces of the pump-oxygenator system results in a complex activation of these cascades, known collectively as the humoral amplification system. The result is a whole body inflammatory response, which produces variable degrees of increased capillary permeability, extravascular extravasation of plasma, increased interstitial fluid, fever, vasoconstriction, leukocytosis, and a generalized bleeding diathesis.[24]

Complement activation during CPB may provide some index of the intensity of activation of the humoral amplification system. The alternative pathway of complement is activated at the initiation of CPB (presumably related to exposure of blood to the nonendothelial surfaces of the oxygenator system) with elaboration of the anaphylatoxins C3a and C5a.[6] Specific C5a-binding sites exist on granulocytes,[7] and the C5a-leukocyte complex undergoes sequestration in the lung[6] as well as in other organs during

CPB. This phenomenon promotes endothelial injury, increased capillary permeability, and extravasation of fluid into the interstitial spaces.[32] Such events may partially explain the pulmonary dysfunction that is occasionally seen after CPB in neonates and infants undergoing intracardiac operations.

A prospective clinical study has shown that morbidity after CPB, including postoperative cardiac, pulmonary, renal, and coagulation dysfunction, is related to higher C3a levels 3 hours after CPB, longer duration of CPB, and younger age at operation.[25]

Despite these deleterious physiologic responses to CPB, which may be more pronounced in the neonate, intracardiac repair of many cardiac malformations can now be safely performed in the first few weeks after birth.

In order to prevent severe hemodilution and its possibly contributory effect in promoting accumulation of extravascular fluid, my colleagues and I generally add sufficient packed red cells to the pump prime to keep the mixed patient-machine hematocrit about 30 during CPB. No established data are currently available to recommend pulsatile over nonpulsatile perfusion in the neonate or to recommend a membrane versus bubble oxygenator.

TOTAL CIRCULATORY ARREST

The safety of total circulatory arrest (TCA) as a support technique depends on the relationship between hypothermia and oxygen consumption ($\dot{V}O_2$). According to the Arrhenius equation, the logarithm of the rate of a chemical reaction is inversely proportional to the reciprocal of the absolute temperature. At physiologic temperatures, a more linear relationship exists (Van't Hoff's law) that states that the logarithm of the rate of a chemical reaction is directly related to the temperature.[20] Even at temperatures approaching 0°C, however, there is ongoing oxygen consumption, which is partially related to maintenance of cellular integrity.[36]

The precise safe (without structural or functional brain damage) period of TCA during deep hypothermia to 18 to 20°C has long been debated. Animal studies indicate that 30 minutes of TCA with the brain at 19 to 20°C is nearly always associated with no structural or functional damage.[11-13,29,44] Structural and functional changes become

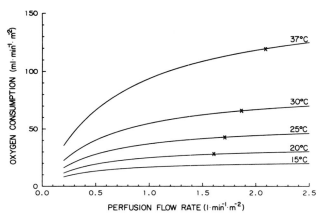

Figure 59–1. Nomogram of an equation expressing the relation of oxygen consumption to perfusion flow rate and temperature. The small x's represent the perfusion flow rates used by us at these temperatures. (Reproduced by permission from Kirklin JK et al [1985]: Cardiopulmonary bypass. In Arciniegas E [ed]: Pediatric Cardiac Surgery. Chicago, Year Book Medical Publishers, pp 67–77.)

increasingly common when arrest time exceeds 45 to 60 minutes.[11,29,39] The metabolic and biochemical factors that determine the safe period of TCA are only partially understood. The reduction in metabolic rate during hypothermia is a critical factor, but other important factors include the "no-reflow" lesion seen after prolonged circulatory arrest[1] and alterations in extracellular pH in brain tissue.[33]

Human studies have provided variable findings. At 18 to 20°C, periods of TCA exceeding 40 minutes are generally accompanied by longer post-TCA intervals before EEG recovery occurs.[41] Seizures may be a manifestation of damage from TCA, but a precise relationship is difficult to establish,[5,8] and seizures are also occasionally seen in neonates and infants after CPB without TCA. Major neurologic events (choreoathetosis, coma, or severe brain damage) occurred only when TCA exceeded 45 minutes at 18 to 20°C among a series of neonates, infants, and children undergoing intracardiac operations at the University of Alabama at Birmingham (Fig. 59–3).[23] There is no clear evidence to suggest that neonates are either more or less susceptible to such damage than are older infants and children.

Table 59–1. OXYGEN CONSUMPTION DURING PROFOUNDLY HYPOTHERMIC, NONPULSATILE, HEMODILUTED CARDIOPULMONARY BYPASS IN THE MONKEY

Organ	Oxygen consumption (ml·min⁻¹·100 g⁻¹)			p Value
	1.5[†]	1.0[†]	0.5[†]	
Whole body	0.119 ± 0.0077 (17.3 ± 1.16)*	0.086 ± 0.0045 (12.5 ± 0.65)*	0.057 ± 0.0029 (8.3 ± 0.44)*	< 0.0001
Brain	0.51 ± 0.095	0.47 ± 0.076	0.45 ± 0.113	0.5
Whole body minus brain	0.114 ± 0.0074	0.081 ± 0.0085	0.0518 ± 0.00176	< 0.0001

*The numbers in parentheses are the whole body oxygen consumption expressed in ml/min/m².
[†]Perfusion flow rate (l·min⁻¹·m⁻²)
(Reproduced with permission from Fox LS, et al [1984]: Relationship of brain blood flow and oxygen consumption to perfusion flow rate during profoundly hypothermic cardiopulmonary bypass: An experimental study. J Thorac Cardiovasc Surg 87:658–664.)

Table 59–2. BLOOD FLOW RESISTANCE IN BRAIN,
AND BODY MINUS THE BRAIN, AT VARIOUS PERFUSION FLOW RATES

Organ	Resistance (units·100 g)							p Value
	*1.75**	*1.5**	*1.25**	*1.0**	*0.75**	*0.5**	*0.25**	
Brain	1.2 ± 0.51	0.80 ± 0.080	0.8 ± 0.22	0.78 ± 0.126	1.05 ± 0.165	0.80 ± 0.117	1.02 ± 0.173	0.4
Whole body minus brain	2.8 ± 0.157	3.3 ± 0.22	3.3 ± 1.21	3.9 ± 0.24	4.6 ± 0.077	5.1 ± 0.49	9.5 ± 0.70	< 0.0001

*Perfusion flow rate ($1 \cdot min^{-1} \cdot m^{-2}$)
(Reproduced with permission from Fox LS, et al [1984]: Relationship of brain blood flow and oxygen consumption to perfusion flow rate during profoundly hypothermic cardiopulmonary bypass: An experimental study. J Thorac Cardiovasc Surg 87:658–664.)

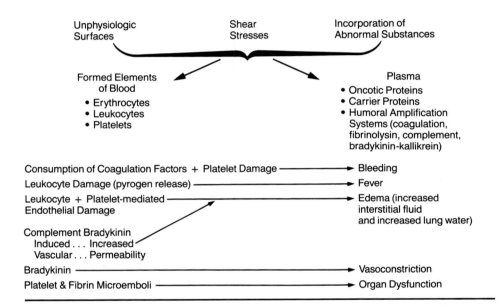

Figure 59–2. Schematic representation of a current concept of the damaging effects of cardiopulmonary bypass in terms of the exposure of blood to abnormal events. (Reproduced with permission from Kirklin JK et al [1985]: Cardiopulmonary bypass. In Arciniegas E [ed]: Pediatric Cardiac Surgery. Chicago, Year Book Medical Publishers, pp 67–77.)

Figure 59–3. The relation between the probability of a major neurologic event occurring postoperatively and the total circulatory arrest (TCA) time in 219 patients (eight events) undergoing open intracardiac operations at the University of Alabama at Birmingham. Among the 211 without such events, TCA time was 42 ± 14.0 (SD) minutes versus 59 ± 10.2 for the eight with such events (P = 0.0008). The equation for the nomogram is: Logistic equation is Z = − 7.3 ± 1.56 + 0.08 ± 0.026 ·TCA. P (intercept) < 0.0001; P (TCA) = 0.002. (Reproduced by permission from Kirklin JK al [1985]: Deep hypothermia and total circulatory arrest. In Arciniegas E [ed]: Pediatric Cardiac Surgery. Chicago, Year Book Medical Publishers, pp 79–85.)

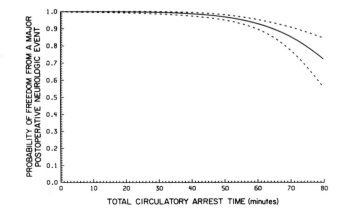

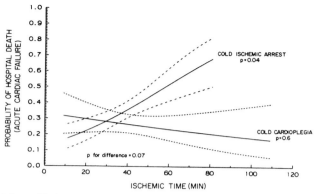

Figure 59–4. Nomogram of equation from a univariate logistic analysis of the probability of death from acute cardiac failure with and without cold cardioplegia according to ischemic time in patients less than 3 months of age undergoing intracardiac surgery. The solid lines indicate the point estimate, the dashed lines the 70 per cent confidence limits. (Reproduced with permission from Kirklin JK et al [1981]: Intracardiac surgery in infants under age 3 months: Incremental risk factors for hospital mortality. Am J Cardiol 48:500–506.)

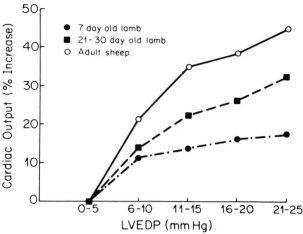

Figure 59–5. Changes induced by the continuous infusion of saline (5 ml/kg/min) in conscious, unsedated newborn lambs and adult sheep. The left ventricular end-diastolic pressure (LVEDP) response to the volume infusion is on the abscissa. With heart rate constant, limited cardiac reserve in the youngest newborn lambs is evidenced by their inability to augment cardiac output at much lower filling pressures compared with the older newborn lambs or the adult. (Reproduced with permission from Friedman WF [1986]: Physiological properties of the developing heart. In Marcelletti C et al [eds]: Pediatric Cardiology. Vol 6. Edinburgh, Churchill Livingstone, pp 3–12.)

The effect of TCA on intellectual and psychomotor development has been studied, with conflicting results reported. Several studies suggest that intellectual and psychomotor development is usually not impaired when TCA is less than about 60 minutes at 18 to 20°C.[19,31,38] However, a more recent study indicates that late intellectual impairment may occur with TCA time exceeding about 50 minutes.[43]

MYOCARDIAL PROTECTION

The most common mode of death following intracardiac surgery in the neonate is acute cardiac failure.[22] Furthermore, indirect evidence suggests that the duration and magnitude of the damaging effects of CPB may be reduced in the presence of robust cardiac performance early postoperatively.[25] Thus, an understanding of the etiology of postrepair low cardiac output and its possible prevention by optimal intraoperative myocardial protection is a central feature in successful neonatal cardiac surgery.

The probability of death among infants (and likely neonates) after intracardiac surgery rises rapidly when the early postoperative cardiac index (at normothermia) falls below about 1.5 liter/min/m².[35] In order to reduce the probability of death from low cardiac output, the general principles of hypothermia and cardioplegia (arrest of the heart in the diastolic phase of the cardiac cycle to maximize substrate preservation) have generally been applied to myocardial protection of the neonatal heart. In patients less than 3 months of age, the duration of cardiac ischemic time is a risk factor for death from acute cardiac failure when cold ischemic arrest is employed. The use of cold cardioplegia appears to neutralize the deleterious effect of the *duration* of global ischemia out to about 100 minutes (Fig. 59–4).[22] However, in comparison to older patients, less is known about the tolerance of the neonatal

heart to ischemia and the effectiveness of potassium cardioplegia in preserving the rather limited reserves of the neonatal heart.

Animal studies indicate that both diastolic and systolic cardiac reserves are limited in the newborn in comparison to the infant or adult (Fig. 59–5).[15] Additionally, even in the absence of stress, the neonatal heart functions nearer its peak performance to satisfy the body's metabolic demands (Fig. 59–6); overall oxygen consumption per surface area in neonates is greater than during adult life.[15]

There is also a reduced contractile response to direct myocardial stimulation with inotropic drugs.[15] The cardiac sympathetic nerves and the adrenergic system in general are underdeveloped in the newborn heart.[16,17]

Both clinically and experimentally,[30] the additional stress of acute hypoxia and acidosis is particularly deleterious to neonatal left ventricular function. Cardioplegia is even less effective in this setting.[30] Patients with cyanotic congenital heart disease have the additional problem of an extensive bronchial collateral circulation[28] as well as increased coronary-bronchial collaterals.[45] This collateral circulation acts rapidly to wash out cardioplegic solution and to produce early rewarming unless deep hypothermia is employed. The presence of chronic hypoxemia may also render the heart more susceptible to ischemic damage.[37]

The limited cardiac reserves of the neonate underscore the importance of optimizing methods of myocardial protection during neonatal open cardiac surgery. In contrast to adult cardiac surgery, there is a paucity of evidence to demonstrate superiority of cold cardioplegia over other methods of myocardial protection in neonatal cardiac surgery. Despite indirect clinical evidence that cold cardioplegia extends

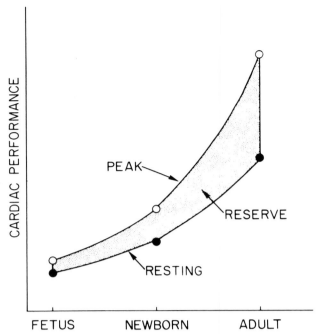

Figure 59–6. Schematic representation of the principle of reduced cardiac reserve in the fetal and newborn heart when compared with the adult. In the younger hearts, resting cardiac performance is close to the peak, or ceiling, of ventricular function because of limitations on preload, systolic, and heart rate reserves. (Reproduced with permission from Friedman WF [1986]: Physiological properties of the developing heart. In Marcelletti C et al [eds]: Pediatric Cardiology. Vol 6. Edinburgh, Churchill Livingstone, pp 3–12.)

the safe ischemic period in neonatal cardiac surgery,[22] experimental studies have failed to show superiority of cold cardioplegia over deep hypothermia, limited total circulatory arrest, and topical hypothermia for myocardial protection.[30] Recent studies by Davtyan and colleagues from the University of California at Los Angeles suggest that an intracellular-based solution for cardioplegia and storage may provide superior extended preservation of the neonatal heart.[9]

References

1. Ames A III, Wright RL, Kowada M, et al (1968): Cerebral ischemia. II. The no-reflow phenomenon. Am J Pathol 52:437–447.
2. Bachmann F, McKenna R, Cole ER, et al (1975): The hemostatic mechanism after open-heart surgery. I. Studies on plasma coagulation factors and fibrinolysis in 512 patients after extracorporeal circulation. J Thorac Cardiovasc Surg 70:76–85.
3. Barratt-Boyes BG, Simpson MM, Neutze JM (1970): Intracardiac surgery in neonates and infants using deep hypothermia (abstract). Circulation (Suppl III) 41,42:73.
4. Bigelow WG, Callaghan JC, Hopps JA (1950): General hypothermia for experimental intracardiac surgery. Ann Surg 132:531–539.
5. Brunberg JA, Reilly EL, Doty DB (1974): Central nervous system consequences in infants of cardiac surgery using deep hypothermia and circulatory arrest. Circulation (Suppl II) 49,50:60–66.
6. Chenoweth DE, Cooper SW, Hugli TE, et al (1981): Complement activation during cardiopulmonary bypass: Evidence for generation of C3a and C5a anaphylatoxins. N Engl J Med 304:497–503.
7. Chenoweth DE, Hugli TE (1978): Demonstration of specific C5a receptor on intact human polymorphonuclear leukocytes. Proc Natl Acad Sci USA 75:3943.–3947
8. Clarkson PM, MacArthur BA, Barratt-Boyes BG, et al (1980): Developmental progress after cardiac surgery in infancy using profound hypothermia and circulatory arrest. Circulation 62:855–861.
9. Davtyan HG, Corno AF, Laks H, Bhuta S, Flynn WM, Laidig C, Drinkwater DC (1988): Long-term neonatal heart preservation. J Thorac Cardiovasc Surg 94:44–53.
10. Dillard DH, Mohri H, Hessel EA II, et al (1967): Correction of total anomalous pulmonary venous drainage in infancy utilizing deep hypothermia with total circulatory arrest. Circulation (Suppl I)35,36:105–110.
11. Fisk GC, Wright JS, Hicks RG, et al (1976): The influence of duration of circulatory arrest at 20°C on cerebral changes. Anaesth Intensive Care 4:126–134.
12. Fisk GC, Wright JS, Turner BB, et al (1974): Cerebral effects of circulatory arrest at 20°C in the infant pig. Anaesth Intensive Care 2:33–42.
13. Folkerth TL, Angell WW, Fosburg RG, et al (1975): Effect of deep hypothermia, limited cardiopulmonary bypass, and total arrest on growing puppies. In Roy P-E, Ronna G (eds): The Metabolism of Contraction. Baltimore, University Park Press, pp 411–421.
14. Fox LS, Blackstone EH, Kirklin JW, Bishop SP, Bergdahl LAL, Bradley EL (1984): Relationship of brain blood flow and oxygen consumption to perfusion flow rate during profoundly hypothermic cardiopulmonary bypass: An experimental study. J Thorac Cardiovasc Surg 87:658–664.
15. Friedman WF (1986): Physiological properties of the developing heart. In Marcelletti C, Anderson RH, Becker AE, Corno A, diCarlo D, Mazzera E (eds): Pediatric Cardiology. Vol 6. New York, Churchill Livingstone, pp 3–12.
16. Friedman WF, Pool PE, Jacobowitz D, Seagren S, Braunwald E (1968): Sympathetic innervation of the developing rabbit heart: Biochemical and histochemical comparisons of foetal, neonatal, and adult myocardium. Circ Res 23:25–32.
17. Geis WP, Tatooles CJ, Priola DV, Friedman WF (1975): Factors influencing neurohumoral control of the heart in the newborn dog. Am J Physiol 228:1685–1689.
18. Gibbon JH (1953): Application of a mechanical heart and lung apparatus to cardiac surgery. In Recent Advances in Cardiovascular Surgery. Minneapolis, University of Minnesota, pp 107–113.
19. Haka-Ikse K, Blackwood MJA, Steward DJ (1978): Psychomotor development of infants and children after profound hypothermia during surgery for congenital heart disease. Dev Med Child Neurol 20:62–70.
20. Harris EA, Seelye ER, Squire AW (1971): Oxygen consumption during cardiopulmonary bypass with moderate hypothermia in man. Br J Anaesth 43:1113–1120.
21. Horiuchi T, Koyamada K, Matano I, et al (1963): Radical operation for ventricular septal defect in infancy. J Thorac Cardiovasc Surg 46:180–190.
22. Kirklin JK, Blackstone EH, Kirklin JW, McKay R, Pacifico AD, Bargeron LM Jr (1981): Intracardiac surgery in infants under age 3 months: Incremental risk factors for hospital mortality. Am J Cardiol 48:500–506.
23. Kirklin JK, Kirklin JW, Pacifico AD (1985): Deep hypothermia and total circulatory arrest. In Arciniegas E (ed): Pediatric Cardiac Surgery. Chicago, Year Book Medical Publishers, pp 79–85.
24. Kirklin JK, Kirklin JW, Pacifico AD (1985): Cardiopulmonary bypass. In Arciniegas E (ed): Pediatric Cardiac Surgery. Chicago, Year Book Medical Publishers, pp 67–77.
25. Kirklin JK, Westaby S, Blackstone EH, Kirklin JW, Chenoweth DE, Pacifico AD (1983): Complement and the damaging effects of cardiopulmonary bypass. J Thorac Cardiovasc Surg 86:845–857.
26. Kirklin JW, Dawson B, Devloo RA, et al (1961): Open intracardiac operations: Use of circulatory arrest during hypothermia induced by blood cooling. Ann Surg 154:769–776.
27. Kirklin JW, DuShane JW, Patrick RT, et al (1955): Intracardiac surgery with the aid of a mechanical pump-oxygenator system (Gibbon type): Report of eight cases. Proc Staff Meet Mayo Clinic 30:201–206.
28. Kirklin JW, Karp RB (1970): The Tetralogy of Fallot From a Surgical Viewpoint. Philadelphia, WB Saunders.

29. Kramer RS, Sanders AP, Lesage AM, et al (1968): The effect of profound hypothermia on preservation of cerebral ATP content during circulatory arrest. J Thorac Cardiovasc Surg 56:699–709.

30. Laks H, Milliken J, Haas G (1986): Myocardial protection in the neonatal heart. In Marcelletti C, Anderson RH, Becker AE, Corno A, diCarlo D, Mazzera E (eds): Pediatric Cardiology. Vol 6. New York, Churchill Livingstone, pp 13–27.

31. Messmer BJ, Schallberger U, Gattiker R, et al (1976): Psychomotor and intellectual development after deep hypothermia and circulatory arrest in early infancy. J Thorac Cardiovasc Surg 72:495–502.

32. Muller-Eberhard HJ (1975): Complement. Am Rev Biochem 44:697–724.

33. Norwood WI, Norwood CR, Castaneda AR (1979): Cerebral anoxia: Effect of deep hypothermia and pH. Surgery 86:203–209.

34. Pang LM, Stalcup SA, Lipset JS, et al (1979): Increased circulating bradykinin during hypothermia and cardiopulmonary bypass in children. Circulation 60:1503–1507.

35. Parr GVS, Blackstone EH, Kirklin JW (1975): Cardiac performance and mortality early after intracardiac surgery in infants and young children. Circulation 51:867–874.

36. Rosomoff HL, Holaday DA (1954): Cerebral blood flow and cerebral oxygen consumption during hypothermia. Am J Physiol 179:85–88.

37. Silverman NA, Kohler J, Levitsky S, Pavel DG, Fang RB, Feinberg H (1984): Chronic hypoxemia depresses global ventricular function and predisposes to the depletion of high-energy phosphates during cardioplegic arrest: Implications for surgical

38. Stevenson JG, Stone EF, Dillard DH, et al (1974): Intellectual development of children subjected to prolonged circulatory arrest during hypothermic open heart surgery in infancy. Circulation (Suppl II)49,50:54–59.

39. Treasure T, Naftel DC, Conger KA, et al (1983): The effect of hypothermic circulatory arrest time on cerebral function, morphology, and biochemistry. J Thorac Cardiovasc Surg 86:761–770.

40. Warden HE, Cohen M, Read RC, Lillehei CW (1954): Controlled cross circulation for open intracardiac surgery. J Thorac Surg 28:331–343.

41. Weiss M, Weiss J, Cotton J, et al (1975): A study of the electroencephalogram during surgery with deep hypothermia and circulatory arrest in infants. J Thorac Cardiovasc Surg 70:316–329.

42. Weiss M, Piwnica A, Lenfant C, et al (1960): Deep hypothermia with total circulatory arrest. Trans Am Soc Artif Intern Organs 6:227–239.

43. Wells FC, Coghills S, Caplan HL, et al (1983): Duration of circulatory arrest does influence the psychological development of children after cardiac operation in early life. J Thorac Cardiovasc Surg 86:823–831.

44. Wolin LR, Massopust LC Jr, White RJ (1960): Behavioral effects of autocerebral perfusion, hypothermia with total circulatory arrest. Trans Am Soc Artif Intern Organs 6:227.

45. Zureikat HY (1980): Collateral vessels between the coronary and bronchial arteries in patients with cyanotic congenital heart disease. Am J Cardiol 45:599–603.

repair of cyanotic congenital heart defects. Ann Thorac Surg 37:304–308.

60 NEONATAL SURGICAL PALLIATIONS

Donald B. Doty

Patients with serious congenital cardiac anomalies may present for medical attention during the first month of life with symptoms suggesting heart failure, such as feeding difficulty and rapid respirations, or with signs of a heart defect, such as cardiomegaly, hepatomegaly, tachypnea, or cardiac murmur. The age of the patient will give a clue to the diagnosis. Obstructive lesions of the right or left side of the heart present in the first week of life, whereas septal defects with left-to-right shunt present at 2 or 3 weeks after natural decline of pulmonary vascular resistance. Clinical evaluation of these patients includes the usual history, physical examination, ECG, and chest radiograph. Definitive diagnosis often is obtainable by two-dimensional echocardiography, and in some cases operative intervention is recommended entirely on the basis of noninvasive evaluation. In some of the more complex anomalies, cardiac catheterization with angiography is indicated for complete evaluation of the morphology of the defect and therapeutic planning, which may include operative intervention.

When operative intervention is indicated, the morphology of some congenital cardiac malformations or the condition of the patient may make complete repair of the defect either impossible or impractical at that point in time. Palliative operations are designed to alter the hemodynamic physiology so that symptoms are relieved and growth and development can occur. These palliative procedures have become established and accepted forms of therapy in the treatment of infants with congenital heart disease, especially in the first month of life. The role of palliative procedures[84] has changed as corrective operations in the first year of life have become more frequent. Palliative procedures are now used almost exclusively in the treatment of complex lesions in the first month of life, or for other lesions less amenable to early correction.

Blalock and Taussig[8] reported the first successful operation for palliation of congenital cardiac defects. Since that time, several ingenious and useful operations have been described and used.[69]

OPERATIONS TO INCREASE PULMONARY BLOOD FLOW

The classic operation described by Blalock and Taussig in 1945[8] has become the standard by which all shunt operations are compared. During the early years in which the operation was employed, the subclavian artery-to-pulmonary artery anastomosis was used for a number of anatomic variations in which pulmonary blood flow was decreased by the presence of congenital pulmonic stenosis.[6] The most common condition treated was tetralogy of Fallot. The early experience provided data that the operation should be performed on the side opposite to that on which the aorta descends (on the side opposite that of the aortic arch) and that the preferred anastomosis was between the end of the subclavian artery and the side of the pulmonary artery. Taussig reported a unique seven-part long-term follow-up study of the consecutive series of patients operated on between 1944 and 1951. The thrust of these articles was that palliative operations do indeed provide for increased survival and useful exercise tolerance; some patients remained in good condition 15 years after operation.[73-79] Some patients developed bacterial endocarditis during follow-up; brain abscess occurred in about 5 per cent of the patients.

The advantage the Blalock-Taussig shunt has over shunts is that the blood flow to the pulmonary artery may be increased without producing excessive flow; there is little risk of obstructive pulmonary vascular disease. The Blalock-Taussig shunt is also the easiest of all shunts to take down at the time of definitive repair of the cardiac defect. In the early years, the best results were obtained in patients over 2 years of age, apparently because of difficulty in obtaining a satisfactory anastomosis between the small subclavian artery and the pulmonary artery in younger patients. Current practice with monofilament suture material and optical magnification now permits reliable construction of Blalock-Taussig shunts in the neonatal period. The details of the operation are shown in Figures 60–1 and 60–2. The side branches of the subclavian artery are ligated and divided, and it is freed from beneath the vagus nerve. Thorough mobilization of the subclavian artery and the common carotid artery allows sufficient length to approximate the right pulmonary artery. Fine monofilament suture material is used to construct an end-to-side anastomosis of the subclavian artery to the right pulmonary artery.

Other procedures were devised to connect the aorta directly to the pulmonary artery. These operations are seldom performed in current practice but are not simply of historical interest, however, because there are many patients currently living who have been successfully palliated by these methods. These patients survive because of these operations but also have the consequences of the procedures. Subsequent treatment must be provided with an understanding of the hemodynamic properties of their

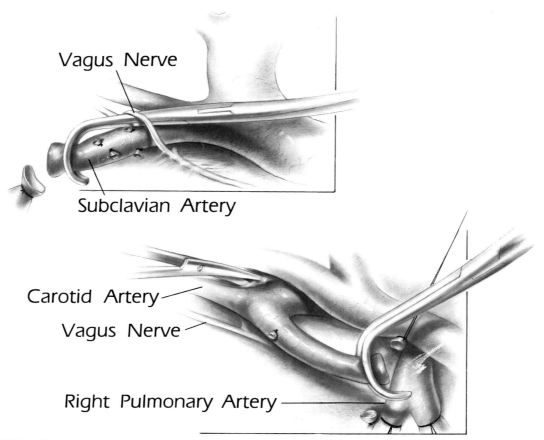

Figure 60–1. Blalock-Taussig shunt. The branches of the subclavian artery are ligated, and the artery is freed from beneath the vagus nerve. Mobilization of the subclavian and carotid arteries allows the end of the subclavian artery to reach the pulmonary artery. (Reproduced with permission from Doty DB [1986]: Cardiac Surgery: A Loose Leaf Workbook and Update Service. Chicago, Year Book Medical Publishers, p. VII Palliat 2.)

palliated condition and the anatomic arrangements altered by the shunt.

Potts and associates[62] described anastomosis of the descending thoracic aorta to the left pulmonary artery in 1946. The early experience demonstrated this anastomosis could be successfully performed in infants under 1 year of age.[61] Later, it became evident that one of the principal disadvantages of this shunt was the difficulty of closing it. The most established methods of closing the Potts shunt at the time of corrective operation involved the use of total circulatory arrest under deep hypothermia so that the shunt could be approached through the opened pulmonary artery.[39] Another disadvantage of the Potts shunt was the difficulty in controlling the size of the anastomosis and thus the amount of pulmonary blood flow. As a result, pulmonary hypertension was frequent after the Potts procedure.

Waterston[86] described anastomosis of the ascending aorta to the right pulmonary artery in 1962. Cooley and Hallman[13] and Edwards and associates[22] later used similar shunt procedures. The Waterston shunt had particular usefulness in neonates. Compared with the Potts operation, the Waterston shunt was easy to take down at later operation via a transaortic approach; however, control of pulmonary blood flow was inconsistent and pulmonary hypertension commonly occurred. Kinking of the right pulmonary artery at the point of anastomosis is a frequently recognized complication of ascending aorta-to-right pulmonary shunt procedures.[82] Rotation of the anastomosis appears to result in stenosis or occlusion of the right pulmonary artery. The tendency for right pulmonary artery obstruction is probably reduced by performing the anastomosis posterior to the superior vena cava. Another mechanism of pulmonary artery obstruction could be the "drum head" effect produced by making the anastomosis of the side of the aorta to a tiny right pulmonary artery with flattening of the circumference of the pulmonary artery over the anastomotic opening. Several approaches to correction of the stenotic right pulmonary artery at the time of definitive repair operations have been described.[21,77,87] In spite of drawbacks, the Waterston operation was successfully used in large series of patients requiring palliative shunt procedures.[4,57,71,85]

All of the standard shunt procedures share a tendency for preferential blood flow to one lung even though the intent is to achieve bilateral flow. To provide blood flow to both lungs (in hopes that symmetrical and bidirectional flow may promote growth and enlargement of small pulmonary arteries), Gazzaniga and associates[26] used a microporous expanded polytetrafluoroethylene (PTFE) prosthesis to create a shunt between the ascending aorta and the main

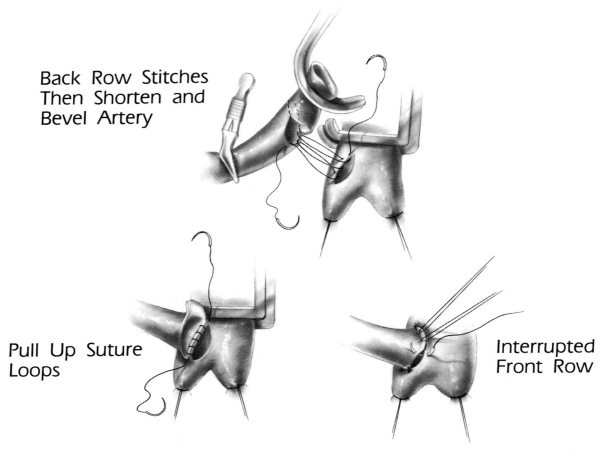

Back Row Stitches Then Shorten and Bevel Artery

Pull Up Suture Loops

Interrupted Front Row

Figure 60–2. Blalock-Taussig shunt. The end of the subclavian artery is anastomosed to the side of the pulmonary artery. (Reproduced with permission from Doty DB [1986]: Cardiac Surgery: A Loose Leaf Workbook and Update Service. Chicago, Year Book Medical Publishers, p. VII Palliat 4.)

pulmonary artery. A 4-mm prosthesis was used exclusively in two large series,[27,45] and a 4- or 5-mm prosthesis was successfully employed in another series.[18] Early results were encouraging, but these shunts proved to be of value for only short periods when 4-mm prostheses were used because of thrombosis or inadequate volume of pulmonary blood flow as the patient grew. When 5-mm prostheses were used, the chance of creating too much pulmonary blood flow increased. Current practice, however, seems to indicate that 5-mm prostheses are useful and results predictable for most patients.

The modified Blalock-Taussig operation was proposed by de Leval and associates[14] to overcome some of the problems encountered with the so-called central shunts. This operation interposes the larger prosthesis (5-mm PTFE) between the subclavian artery and the pulmonary artery. The modified Blalock-Taussig operation was devised because of the notion that the Blalock-Taussig shunt offers the best palliation because the diameter of the subclavian artery is especially suitable for proper control of pulmonary blood flow. A prosthesis of greater diameter than that of the subclavian artery is sutured end to side to the undivided subclavian artery; such shunts should theoretically allow for increased pulmonary blood flow with growth of the patient. In practice, a 5-mm PTFE prosthesis has proven optimal in neonates. The anastomosis is generally performed on the same side as the aortic arch, in other words, from the subclavian artery that originates from the aorta rather than from the side of the innominate artery (as in the classic Blalock-Taussig operation). The operation, however, may be performed on either side of the aortic arch. An end-to-side anastomosis of the prosthesis to the subclavian artery is performed using continuous stitches of fine monofilament suture material. An end-to-side anastomosis of the prosthesis to the pulmonary artery is then performed. Overall patency has been good but duration of palliation has not been long. There was inadequate palliation in two thirds of patients by 2 years when a 4-mm prosthesis was used in the series of de Leval and coworkers. The modified Blalock-Taussig shunt must be viewed as temporary and used for patients in whom early corrective operation is anticipated. Take down of the modified Blalock-Taussig shunt is somewhat more difficult than for the classic Blalock-Taussig anastomosis because a fibrous reaction occurs in response to the prosthetic material. However, take down of the modified Blalock-Taussig shunt is certainly less complicated than that for direct anastomosis of the aorta to the pulmonary artery. Closure of the prosthetic shunt is probably best accomplished by metal clip ligature to flatten the tubular prosthesis rather than by suture ligature.

The choice between the classic Blalock-Taussig operation and the modified operation with interposed PTFE graft remains controversial. The modified operation is certainly easier to perform and is probably more reproducible in the hands of the average thoracic surgeon and probably produces less distortion of the pulmonary artery during growth of the patient. The modified Blalock-Taussig shunt, however, is a little less predictable than the classic Blalock-Taussig anastomosis in terms of shunt size because it is more dependent on the diameter of the prosthesis than on the size of the subclavian artery to which it is attached. Furthermore, thrombosis of the graft remains an undesirable and unpredictable fact of its use. The classic Blalock-Taussig operation still retains an important place in the treatment of patients requiring palliative intervention. Some investigators have suggested that the Blalock-Taussig operation is the procedure of choice for systemic-pulmonary anastomoses in infancy because of the predictability and duration of palliation.[2,31,43,53] Even the problems of performing subclavian artery to pulmonary artery anastomosis on the same side as the aortic arch (ipsilateral) have largely been overcome by the subclavian arterioplasty described by Laks and Castañeda.[42] The vascular consequences, however, of subclavian artery transection required to perform the classic Blalock-Taussig operation must always be considered. Arm and hand ischemia following subclavian artery transection are rare, occurring in about 1 per cent of patients having classic Blalock-Taussig operations.[1] Permanent reduction of the blood pressure in the operated arm appears to be uniform and limb growth is significantly less, but there is no evidence of altered manual preference[46] Taken in balance, it appears that the most popular operation in current practice is the modified procedure with interposed prosthetic graft.

Most patients with decreased pulmonary blood flow could be treated by complete correction of the defect. Condition of the patient, age, or technical factors such as small pulmonary arteries may make early operation inadvisable. These patients can be benefited by creating a shunt between the aorta or one of its branches and the pulmonary artery to increase pulmonary blood flow. The conditions most often treated by this approach include tetralogy of Fallot, pulmonary atresia with intact septum or ventricular septal defect, transposition of the great vessels with pulmonary stenosis, and tricuspid atresia. Severe hypoxemia with cyanosis, dyspnea, and growth failure are the main indications for operative intervention. Patients with cyanosis often have polycythemia so that an increasing hematocrit is another frequent indication for operation. Hypoxic spells with loss of consciousness and dyspnea may occur in patients with tetralogy of Fallot. These spells are an indication for emergency operation.

Systemic artery-to-pulmonary artery shunts increase not only pulmonary blood flow but also the total blood flow that the systemic ventricle must pump. A common complication of these shunt procedures is congestive cardiac failure. Generally, the failure is temporary and responds well to medical management. Occasionally, an operation to reduce the size of the shunt is required.

A shunt between a systemic vein and the pulmonary artery increases only effective pulmonary blood flow without adding to the load on the systemic ventricle. Experimental superior vena cava-to-right pulmonary artery anastomosis was reported by Carlon and associates in 1951,[11] and the operation was successfully applied clinically by Glenn in 1958.[29] The anastomosis of the end of the right pulmonary artery to the side of the superior vena cava with ligation of the superior vena cava below the anastomosis is the most commonly employed form of the operation. This anastomosis has had its greatest use in patients with tricuspid atresia.[16,83] Long-term evaluation of patients with cavopulmonary artery shunts have shown good initial palliation but a tendency for late deterioration due to decreased flow through the shunt as pulmonary resistance increased and collateral blood flow pathways to the inferior vena cava developed.[44,49] Best results have been obtained in patients older than 1 year of age. Pulmonary arteriovenous malformations have been reported to develop after the Glenn shunt,[50] but Pennington and associates[60] have shown that these pulmonary abnormalities are not necessarily the consequence of systemic vein–pulmonary artery shunts. Take down and reconstruction of the cavopulmonary anastomosis for later corrective operation is difficult but possible.[56,66] This shunt should probably be reserved for selected cases with tricuspid atresia as a part of staged complete diversion of pulmonary blood flow with subsequent Fontan procedure.[25] At present there seem to be few, if any, indications for this shunt procedure in the neonatal period.

A more direct palliative procedure to increase pulmonary blood flow caused by right ventricular outflow tract obstruction was devised by Brock in 1948,[9] who used closed pulmonary valvotomy and infundibular dilation or resection to enlarge the right ventricular outflow tract. The results in 100 cases of tetralogy of Fallot in which this approach was used were encouraging.[10] The Brock procedure has enjoyed considerable enthusiasm in centers in Europe, but only a few centers in the United States have used it as the initial palliation of tetralogy of Fallot.[24] Kirklin and associates[39] have reviewed the reported experience in 903 patients with tetralogy of Fallot who underwent a palliative Brock procedure and concluded that the mortality risk of the closed Brock procedure for initial palliation of the tetralogy of Fallot is about 16 per cent. The mortality risk of later repair does not appear to be adversely affected by a closed Brock procedure, and presumably good palliation can often be achieved. The mortality risk of the initial procedure itself seemed to be inordinately high compared with that of shunting operations. The operation appears to have greatest application in patients with pulmonary atresia with intact ventricular septum (hypoplastic right-heart syndrome). In these patients, closed pulmonary valvotomy combined with shunting procedures seems to be the operation most favored, and results are reasonably good.[17,51] Diminutive right ventricles have actually been shown to grow and dilate if a reasonable passageway is formed from right ventricle to pulmonary artery.[17,59]

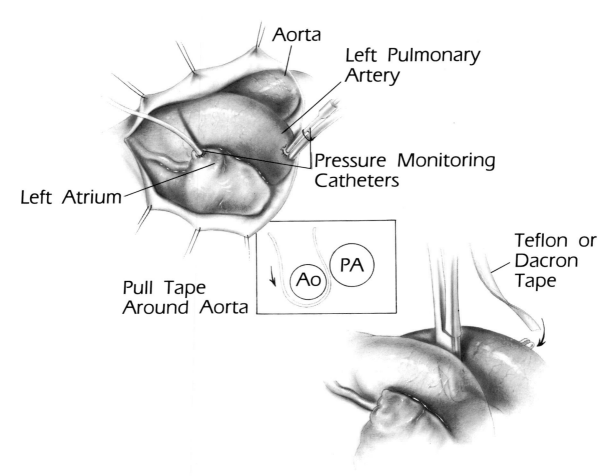

Figure 60–3. Banding of the pulmonary artery. Teflon or Dacron tape is passed around the aorta after placement of appropriate monitoring catheters in the pulmonary artery, left atrium, and peripheral systemic artery. (Reproduced with permission from Doty DB [1986]: Cardiac Surgery: A Loose Leaf Workbook and Update Service. Chicago, Year Book Medical Publishers, p. VII Palliat 12.)

The concept that blood flow will bring about growth of hypoplastic blood vessels or cardiac chambers is the basis for central shunt operations such as aorta-to-main pulmonary shunts, right ventricular outflow patches, and occasionally pulmonary arterial conduits.[84] Experience with right ventricular outflow patches is limited but in some cases very encouraging; significant enlargement of even diminutive pulmonary arteries has been observed.[28] Some ingenious techniques for placement of the right ventricular outflow patch without cardiopulmonary bypass have been reported.[12,15,63]

OPERATIONS TO REDUCE PULMONARY BLOOD FLOW

Constriction or banding of the pulmonary artery to create pulmonary stenosis was introduced in 1952 by Muller and Dammann[52] as a palliative procedure designed to limit pulmonary blood flow in congenital cardiac malformations with unrestricted pulmonary blood flow. Subsequently, studies were published showing the effectiveness of this mode of therapy for infants and young patients with refractory congestive heart failure due to large ventricular septal defect[35,36,70] and complex congenital cardiac defects,[55] such as atrioventricular septal defects,[23,68,80] truncus arteriosus,[3] and tricuspid atresia.[81] Good results in terms of patient mortality were generally experienced for isolated ventricular septal defect, whereas considerably higher mortality was the rule for complex defects. There were some problems induced by mechanical constriction of the pulmonary artery that became evident at second-stage operations.[30,38] In spite of problems with the procedure, pulmonary artery banding continues as a valuable therapeutic intervention for complex defects even during the era of total correction of congenital cardiac anomalies during infancy.[19,48,72]

The operation is performed through a left anterolateral thoracotomy. Dissection between the aorta and pulmonary artery opens a plane for passage of a right-angle clamp between the great vessels. The clamp is first passed around the aorta, and the banding tape is pulled through between the aorta and pulmonary artery (Fig. 60–3). The clamp is then passed through the transverse sinus, and the end of the tape

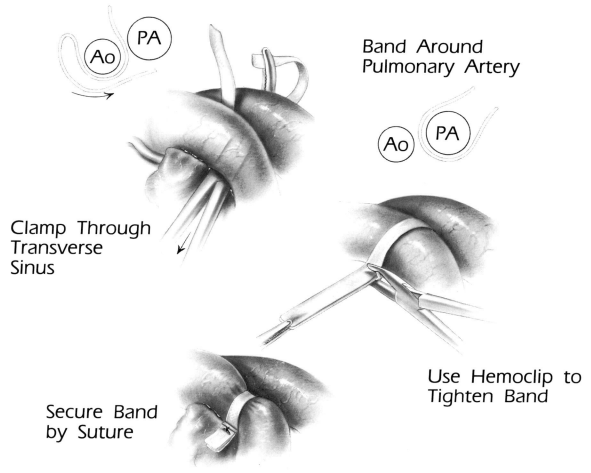

Ao PA

Band Around Pulmonary Artery

Ao PA

Clamp Through Transverse Sinus

Use Hemoclip to Tighten Band

Secure Band by Suture

Figure 60–4. Banding of the pulmonary artery. A clamp is passed through the transverse sinus, and the banding tape is pulled through so that it surrounds the pulmonary artery. The band is tightened around the pulmonary artery to reduce the blood flow into it. A hemoclip is used to secure the band temporarily while the hemodynamics are adjusted to bring the pulmonary artery pressure distal to the band to about one half that of systemic artery pressure. Final securing of the band is by suture. (Reproduced with permission from Doty DB [1986]: Cardiac Surgery: A Loose Leaf Workbook and Update Service. Chicago, Year Book Medical Publishers, p. VII Palliat 13.)

is pulled through around the pulmonary artery, thus avoiding direct dissection of the more delicate pulmonary artery (Fig. 60–4). Teflon tape is the most popular banding material, but umbilical tape, silk suture, and other synthetic materials have been used. The band is tightened around the pulmonary artery to achieve a balance of pulmonary and aortic flow. The band is temporarily secured with a hemoclip and finally secured by suture after verifying satisfactory hemodynamics. Pressure in the pulmonary artery distal to the band should drop to about one half of aortic pressure, which should rise slightly. Left atrial pressure should drop slightly as the pulmonary blood flow is decreased. A rise in right atrial pressure implies too much afterload resistance on the right ventricle, and the band should be loosened.[20]

Evaluation of the long-term results of pulmonary banding must include the sum of the medical and operative interventions that ultimately achieve correction of the cardiac defect. To the initial mortality of 5 to 26 per cent for pulmonary banding itself must be added the mortality for medical therapy between the time of banding and the time of second-stage operation, as well as the mortality for operative correction of the congenital cardiac defect. The operative risk of pulmonary artery banding is a function of the age of the patient (with the highest risk for pulmonary banding being in patients under 3 months of age) and of the complexity of the cardiac defect. Mahle and associates[47] studied 63 patients who had pulmonary artery banding during the period of modern postoperative intensive care (1968 to 1975) and followed half of the survivors through the corrective period. The problem of cumulative mortality is evident from their data. The operative mortality for pulmonary artery banding for ventricular septal defect was only 7 per cent, but additional medical mortality and the deaths at second-stage operations brought the total mortality to 33 per cent. The situation in more complex anomalies is even more difficult, with 40 to 71 per cent cumulative mortality.

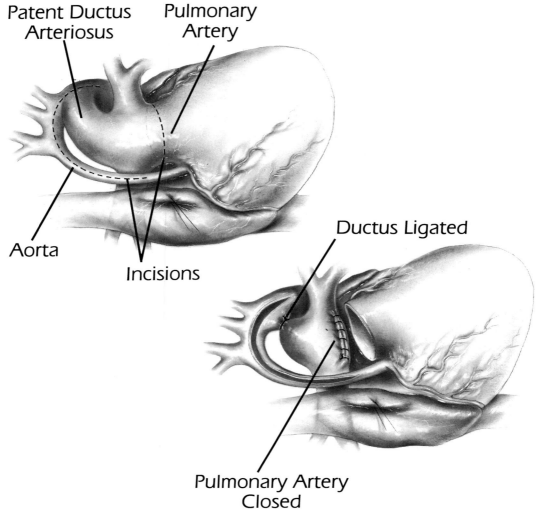

Figure 60–5. Norwood operation. The pulmonary artery is divided and the aorta opened from ascending portion through the arch and past any point of coarctation in the upper descending portion. The ductus arteriosus is ligated and the distal end of the pulmonary artery closed. (Reproduced with permission from Doty DB [1986]: Cardiac Surgery: A Loose Leaf Workbook and Update Service. Chicago, Year Book Medical Publishers, p. VI Hypo-LV1.)

At present, assuming experience and expertise for closure of ventricular septal defect during infancy, there is probably no longer a need to band the pulmonary artery in patients with large ventricular septal defects unless there is some major technical problem, such as multiple septal defects, complex coarctation of the aorta, or other complex associated anomaly. For complete atrioventricular septal defect, truncus arteriosus, and complex malpositions of the great arteries with ventricular septal defect, including double-outlet right ventricle, the choice of total repair or banding of the pulmonary artery depends on local experience and preference. For those miscellaneous high-risk lesions, including single ventricle (univentricular heart) and tricuspid-mitral atresia, in which complete repair of the defect is not at present feasible during infancy, pulmonary banding to control excessive pulmonary blood flow and achieve balance in the circulation is the preferred method of treatment.

OPERATIONS TO INCREASE SYSTEMIC-PULMONARY MIXING

Survival of patients with transposition of the great arteries depends on an effective mixing of the blood from the systemic and pulmonary circulations at some point across the atrial or ventricular septum. The foramen ovale remains somewhat patent for variable periods after birth and may temporarily sustain the patient. If a ventricular septal defect is present, there may be no need for palliative intervention. If there is no effective communication point in either septum, the atrial septum must be opened by operation. The first successful atrial septectomy was reported by Blalock and Hanlon in 1948.[7] The procedure was closed in that cardiopulmonary bypass was not required. The operation soon became standardized, and by 1964, Hallman and Cooley[32] had operated on 100 patients using this procedure.

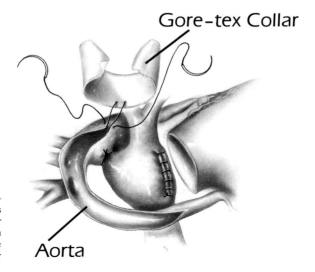

Gore-tex Collar

Aorta

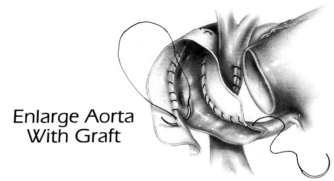

Enlarge Aorta
With Graft

Figure 60–6. Norwood operation. The aorta and pulmonary artery are joined by anastomosis. This is facilitated by interposition of a prosthetic collar (PTFE–Gore Tex). (Reproduced with permission from Doty DB [1986]: Cardiac Surgery: A Loose Leaf Workbook and Update Service. Chicago, Year Book Medical Publishers, p. VI Hypo-LV2.)

The operation is performed via a right thoracotomy. The pericardium is opened just anterior to the right pulmonary veins. The right pulmonary artery and veins are temporarily occluded while a vascular clamp is applied to exclude a portion of each atrium and the intra-atrial septum. Parallel incisions are made in each atrium near the intra-atrial septum, and the portion of the septum between the incisions is excised. The right atrial incision is then closed to the left atrial incision. The operation is very effective in achieving a large intra-atrial communication. Its main deficiencies include requirement for thoracotomy in an infant who may be critically ill and placement of the vascular clamp on a tiny heart that may impede venous return and cause hemodynamic collapse. Nevertheless the Blalock-Hanlon operation has been favored in some centers up to very recently.[5,33]

In order to avoid thoracotomy, Rashkind devised a technique of catheter balloon atrial septostomy.[65] His initial report was followed by a series of 45 patients with transposition of the great arteries treated by balloon atrioseptostomy; 90 per cent had effective immediate palliation that was maintained long term in 80 per cent.[64] These excellent results have made this catheter procedure the standard for early palliation of transposition of the great arteries. There are some anatomic limitations, however, to the opening in the atrial septum that can be achieved by

balloon septostomy.[41] The actual size of the fossa ovalis and the thickness of the limbus of the fossa determine the results since only the membrane of the fossa is ruptured by balloon septostomy. Park and associates[58] reported the use of a blade catheter to actually cut through the atrial septum when a larger opening is desired or when the atrial septum is thick or intact.

In spite of these truly effective catheter techniques to open the atrial septum, a few infants with transposition of the great arteries cannot be effectively palliated with catheter therapy. The Blalock-Hanlon procedure has been used for failure of catheter balloon atrioseptostomy, but the results are unpredictable. In some centers, operations to effect intra-atrial transposition of venous return have been favored to achieve correction of the defect when operative intervention is required. Here again, the results have been unpredictable in newborns. There has been great interest in some centers to eliminate all palliative forms of treatment and proceed directly to total anatomic correction of transposition of the great arteries in the neonatal period. Jatene and associates[37] described an operation in which the aorta and pulmonary artery were divided and their positions switched. The coronary arteries were removed from the aortic sinuses and transferred to the remaining base of the proximal pulmonary artery. Subsequent successful application of this procedure in patients

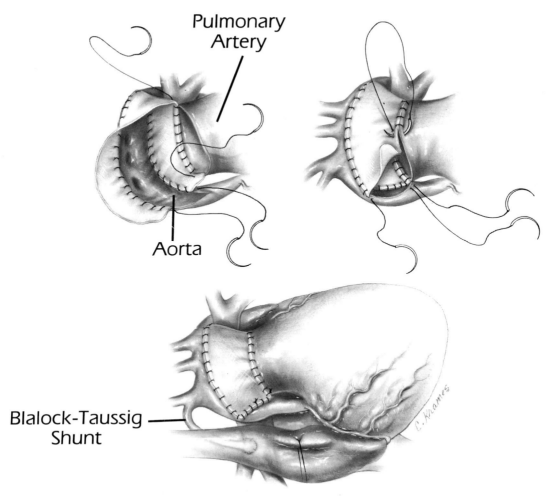

Figure 60–7. Norwood operation. The aorta-to-pulmonary anastomosis is completed, providing unobstructed systemic blood flow from the right ventricle. Pulmonary blood flow is controlled by establishing a subclavian artery–to–pulmonary artery anastomosis (Blalock-Taussig shunt). (Reproduced with permission from Doty DB [1986]: Cardiac Surgery: A Loose Leaf Workbook and Update Service. Chicago, Year Book Medical Publishers, p. VI Hypo-LV 3.)

during the first month of life is based on the premise that the left ventricle in transposition of the great arteries is of normal thickness at birth and until about 30 days of life.[34] Thereafter, the left ventricle becomes thin like a pulmonary ventricle as pulmonary vascular resistance naturally declines. Thus, in some centers, palliative operations for transposition of the great arteries in the newborn period have been replaced by definitive repair of the defect (see Chapter 66).

OPERATIONS TO BALANCE SYSTEMIC AND PULMONARY BLOOD FLOW

Aortic atresia and other forms of hypoplastic left-heart syndrome are the most common cause of death due to congenital cardiac anomalies in the first week of life. Palliation and correction of these defects have largely eluded the best efforts of pediatric cardiologists and surgeons.

Occasional successful cases have been reported in which a combination of known palliative operations have been used to balance the systemic and pulmonary circulations. The operation that is currently in vogue and that has received the most attention was described by Norwood and associates.[54] This operation represents an evolution of operations that had led to successful palliation of a number of patients. Even this operation appears to be evolving by continuing slight modifications. It consists of totally rearranging the configuration of the aorta and pulmonary arteries. The pulmonary artery is divided above the sinus rim (Fig. 60–5). The ductus arteriosus is ligated, and the distal end of the pulmonary artery is closed. The aorta is opened by a long incision extending from the ascending portion, around the arch, and past any area of coarctation in the upper descending portion. The proximal pulmonary artery is anastomosed to the aorta. This anastomosis is facilitated by interposition of a collar of polytetrafluoro-ethylene (GoreTex-PTFE) graft (Figs. 60–6 and 60–7), which provides for unobstructed systemic blood flow from the single ventricle (right ventricle). A controlled amount of pulmonary blood flow is provided by a subclavian artery to pulmonary artery anastomosis. Pulmonary venous return is directed to the right ventricle by excision of the atrial septum. If palliation is successful with this operation, it is expected that ultimate repair will be achieved by the Fontan operation. About half of patients with hypoplastic left-heart syndrome have been successfully palliated by this approach in a few centers with extensive experience. Unfortunately, other centers have not been able to duplicate these results. It may be that transplantation of the human heart may be a better form of palliation for this otherwise fatal condition.

CONCLUSION

Palliative operations remain important in the effective treatment of patients with complex congenital cardiac malformations. More frequent use of corrective operations in the first year of life has somewhat diminished the use of the classic palliative operations. Palliative operations are now reserved for the treatment of complex conditions that do not lend themselves well to total correction at an early age. Palliative operations, therfore, are most used during the neonatal period when the most complex conditions often present and require operative intervention. The choice of palliative operation is influenced not only by the nature of the lesion but also by factors that affect the ultimate operative repair, especially those factors related to inducing symmetrical growth and development of the cardiac chambers and the great vessels.

References

1. Arciniegas E, Blackstone EH, Pacifico AD, Kirklin JW (1979): Classic shunting operations as part of two-stage repair for tetralogy of Fallot. Ann Thorac Surg 27:514–518.
2. Arciniegas E, Farooki ZQ, Hakimi M, Perry BL, Green EW (1982): Classic shunting operations for congenital cyanotic heart defects. J Thorac Cardiovasc Surg 84:88–96.
3. Armer RM, DeOliveira PE, Lurie PR (1961): True truncus arteriosus: Review of seventeen cases and report of surgery in seven patients (abstr). Circulation 24:878.
4. Azzolina G, Russo PA, Mafei G, Marchese A (1982): Waterston anastomosis in two-stage correction of severe tetralogy of Fallot: Ten years of experience. Ann Thorac Surg 34:413–421.
5. Behrendt DM, Kirsh MM, Orringer MB, Perry V, Sigmann J, Stern A, Sloan H (1975): The Blalock-Hanlon procedure: A new look at an old operation. Ann Thorac Surg 20:424–432.
6. Blalock A (1948): Surgical procedures employed and anatomic variations encountered in treatment of congenital pulmonic stenosis. Surg Gynecol Obstet 87:385–409.
7. Blalock A, Hanlon CR (1950): Surgical treatment of complete transposition of the aorta and pulmonary artery. Surg Gynecol Obstet 90:1–15.
8. Blalock A, Taussig HB (1945): The surgical treatment of malformations of the heart in which there is pulmonary stenosis or pulmonary atresia. JAMA 128:189–202.
9. Brock RC (1948): Pulmonary valvulotomy for relief of congenital pulmonary stenosis. Br Med J 1:1121–1126.
10. Campbell M, Deucher DC, Brock RC (1954): Results of pulmonary valvotomy and infundibular resection in 100 cases of Fallot's tetralogy. Br Med J 2:111–122.
11. Carlon CA, Mondini PG, DeMarchi R (1951): Surgical treatment of some cardiovascular diseases (a new vascular anastomosis). J Int Coll Surg 16:1–10.
12. Clarke DR, Amato JJ (1982): Discussion of Puga FJ, Uretzky G: Establishment of right ventricle-hypoplastic pulmonary artery continuity without the use of extracorporeal circulation. J Thorac Cardiovasc Surg 83:79–80.
13. Cooley DA, Hallman GL (1966): Intrapericardial aortic-right pulmonary arterial anastomosis. Surg Gynecol Obstet 122:1084–1086.
14. de Leval MR, McKay R, Jones M, Stark J, Macartney F (1981): Modified Blalock-Taussig shunt: Use of subclavian artery orifice as flow regulator in prosthetic systemic-pulmonary artery shunts. J Thorac Cardiovasc Surg 81:112–119.
15. Diaz FA, Salvador JC, Zurdo GC (1982): Letter: Partial reconstruction of right ventricular outflow tract without cardiopulmonary bypass. J Thorac Cardiovasc Surg 83:149–150.
16. di Carlo D, Williams WG, Freedom RM, Trusler GA, Rowe RD (1982): The role of cava-pulmonary (Glenn) anastomosis in the palliative treatment of congenital heart disease. J Thorac Cardiovasc Surg 83:437–442.
17. Dobell ARC, Grignon A (1977): Early and late results in pulmonary atresia. Ann Thorac Surg 24:264–274.
18. Donahoo JS, Gardner TJ, Zahka K, Kidd BSL (1980): Systemic-pulmonary shunts in neonates and infants using microporous expanded polytetrafluoroethylene: Immediate and late results. Ann Thorac Surg 30:146–150.
19. Dooley KJ, Parisi-Buckley L, Fyler DC, Nadas AS (1975): Results of pulmonary arterial banding in infancy: Survey of 5 years' experience in the New England Regional Infant Cardiac Program. Am J Cardiol 36:484–488.
20. Doty DB (1983): Pulmonary artery banding. In Glenn WWL (ed): Thoracic and Cardiovascular Surgery. 4th ed. Norwalk, Appleton-Century-Crofts, pp 681–687.
21. Ebert PA, Gay WA Jr, Oldham HN (1972): Management of aorta-right pulmonary artery anastomosis during total correction of tetralogy of Fallot. Surgery 71:231–234.
22. Edwards WS, Mohtashemi M, Holdefer WF (1966): Ascending aorta to right pulmonary artery shunt for infants with tetralogy of Fallot. Surgery 59:316–318.
23. Epstein ML, Moller JH, Amplatz K, Nicoloff DM (1979): Pulmonary artery banding in infants with complete atrioventricular canal. J Thorac Cardiovasc Surg 78:28–31.
24. Flege JB, Ehrenhaft JL (1967): Transventricular pulmonary valvotomy and infundibular resection for tetralogy of Fallot. Dis Chest 52:727–731.
25. Fontan F, Baudet E (1971): Surgical repair of tricuspid atresia. Thorax 26:240–248.
26. Gazzaniga AB, Elliott MP, Sperling DR, Dietrick WR, Eisenman JI, McRae M, Bartlett RH (1976): Microporous expanded polytetrafluoroethylene arterial prosthesis for construction of aortopulmonary shunts: Experimental and clinical results. Ann Thorac Surg 21:322–327.
27. Gazzaniga AB, Lamberti JJ, Siewers RD, Sperling DR, Dietrick WR, Arcilla RA, Replogle RL (1976): Arterial prosthesis of microporous expanded polytetrafluoroethylene for construction of aorta-pulmonary shunts. J Thorac Cardiovasc Surg 72:357–363.
28. Gill CC, Moodie DS, McGoon DC (1977): Staged surgical management of pulmonary atresia with diminutive pulmonary arteries. J Thorac Cardiovasc Surg 73:436–442.
29. Glenn WWL (1958): Circulatory bypass of the right side of the heart. IV. Shunt between superior vena cava and distal right pulmonary artery: Report of a clinical application. N Engl J Med 259:117–120.
30. Griepp R, French JW, Shumway NE, Baum D (1974): Is pulmonary artery banding for ventricular septal defects obsolete? Circulation (Suppl 2)49,50:14–19.
31. Guyton RA, Owens JE, Waumet JD, Dooley KJ, Hatcher CR Jr, Williams WH (1983): The Blalock-Taussig shunt: Low risk, effective palliation, and pulmonary artery growth. J Thorac Cardiovasc Surg 85:917–922.
32. Hallman GL, Cooley DA (1964): Complete transposition of great vessels: Results of surgical teatment. Arch Surg 89:891–898.
33. Herrmann V, Laks H, Kaiser GC, Barner HB, Willman VL (1975): The Blalock-Hanlon procedure: Simple transposition of the great arteries. Arch Surg 110:1387–1390.
34. Huhta JC, Edwards WD, Feldt RH, Puga FJ (1982): Left ventricular

wall thickness in complete transposition of the great arteries. J Thorac Cardiovasc Surg 84:97–101.

35. Hunt CE, Formanek G, Levine MA, Castañeda A, Moller JH (1971): Banding of the pulmonary artery. Results in 111 children. Circulation 43:395–406.

36. Idriss FS, Riker WL, Paul MH (1968): Banding of the pulmonary artery: A palliative surgical procedure. J Pediatr Surg 3:465–474.

37. Jatene AD, Fontes VF, Paulista PP, Souza LCB, Neger F, Galantier M, Sousa JEMR (1976): Anatomical correction of transposition of great vessels. J Thorac Cardiovasc Surg 72:364–370.

38. Kirklin JW (1971): Pulmonary arterial banding in babies with large ventricular septal defects (editorial). Circulation 43:321–322.

39. Kirklin JW, Devloo RA (1961): Hypothermic perfusion and circulatory arrest for surgical correction of tetralogy of Fallot with previously constructed Potts anastomosis. Dis Chest 39:87–91.

40. Kirklin JW, Nojek CA, Vanini V (1979): "The Brock operation" as initial palliation for the tetralogy of Fallot (editorial). Thorac Cardiovasc Surg 27:2–4.

41. Korns ME, Garabedian HA, Lauer RM (1972): Anatomic limitations of balloon atrial septostomy. Hum Pathol 3:345–349.

42. Laks H, Castañeda AR (1975): Subclavian arterioplasty for the ipsilateral Blalock-Taussig shunt. Ann Thorac Surg 19:319–321.

43. Laks H, Marco JD, Willman VL (1975): The Blalock-Taussig shunt in the first six months of life. J Thorac Cardiovasc Surg 70:687–691.

44. Laks H, Mudd JG, Standeven JW, Fagan L, Willman VL (1977): Long-term effect of the superior vena cava-pulmonary artery anastomosis on pulmonary blood flow. J Thorac Cardiovasc Surg 74:253–260.

45. Lamberti JJ, Campbell C, Replogle RL, Anagnostopoulos C, Lin CY, Chiemmongkoltip P, Arcilla R (1979): The prosthetic (Teflon) central aortopulmonary shunt for cyanotic infants less than three weeks old: Results and long-term follow-up. Ann Thorac Surg 28:568–577.

46. Lodge FA, Lamberti JJ, Goodman AH, Kirkpatrick SE, George L, Mathewson JW, Waldman JD (1983): Vascular consequences of subclavian artery transection for the treatment of congenital heart disease. J Thorac Cardiovasc Surg 86:18–23.

47. Mahle S, Nicoloff DM, Knight L, Moller JH (1970): Pulmonary artery banding: Long-term results in 63 patients. Ann Thorac Surg 27:216–224.

48. Marco JD, Laks H, Barner HB, Willman VL (1977): Intracardiac repair after previous pulmonary artery banding. Vasc Surg 11:8–13.

49. Mathur M, Glenn WWL (1973): Long-term evaluation of cavapulmonary artery anastomosis. Surgery 74:899–916.

50. McFaul RC, Tajik AJ, Mair DD, Danielson GK, Seward JB (1977): Development of pulmonary arteriovenous shunt after superior vena cava-right pulmonary artery (Glenn) anastomosis: Report of four cases. Circulation 55:212–216.

51. Moulton AL, Bowman FO, Edie RN, Hayes CJ, Ellis K, Gersony WM, Malm JR (1979): Pulmonary atresia with intact ventricular septum: Sixteen-year experience. J Thorac Cardiovasc Surg 78:527–536.

52. Muller WH Jr, Dammann JF Jr (1952): The treatment of certain congenital malformations of the heart by creation of pulmonic stenosis to reduce pulmonary hypertension and excessive pulmonary blood flow: A preliminary report. Surg Gynecol Obstet 95:213–219.

53. Neches WH, Naifeh JG, Park SC, Lenox CC, Zuberbuhler JR, Siewers RD, Pontius RG, Bahnson HT (1975): Systemic-pulmonary artery anastomoses in infancy. J Thorac Cardiovasc Surg 70:921–927.

54. Norwood WI, Lang P, Hansen DD (1983): Physiologic repair of aortic atresia–hypoplastic left-heart syndrome. N Engl J Med 308:23–26.

55. Oldham HN Jr, Kakos GS, Jarmakani MM, Sabiston DC Jr (1972): Pulmonary artery banding in infants with complex congenital heart defects. Ann Thorac Surg 13:342–350.

56. Pacifico AD, Kirklin JW (1975): Take-down of cava-pulmonary artery anastomosis (Glenn) during repair of congenital cardiac malformations: Report of 5 cases. J Thorac Cardiovasc Surg 72:272–277.

57. Parenzan L, Alfieri O, Vanini V, Bianchi T, Villani M, Tiraboschi R, Crupi G, Locatelli G (1981): Waterston anastomosis for initial palliation of tetralogy of Fallot. J Thorac Cardiovasc Surg 82:176–181.

58. Park SC, Neches WH, Mullins CE, Girod DA, Olley PM, Falkowski G, Garibjan VA, Mathews RA, Fricker FJ, Beerman LB, Lenox CC, Zuberbuhler JR (1982): Blade atrial septostomy: Collaborative study. Circulation 66:258–266.

59. Patel RG, Freedom RM, Moes CAF, Bloom KR, Olley PM, Williams WG, Trusler GA, Rowe RD (1980): Right ventricular volume determinations in 18 patients with pulmonary atresia and intact ventricular septum: Analysis of factors influencing right ventricular growth. Circulation 61:428–440.

60. Pennington DG, Nouri S, Ho J, Secker-Walker R, Patel B, Sivakoff M, Willman VL (1981): Glenn shunt: Long-term results and current role in congenital heart operations. Ann Thorac Surg 31:532–539.

61. Potts WJ (1948): Aortic-pulmonary anastomosis for pulmonary stenosis. J Thorac Surg 17:223–231.

62. Potts WJ, Smith S, Gibson S (1946): Anastomosis of aorta to pulmonary artery: Certain types in congenital heart disease. JAMA 132:627–631.

63. Puga FJ, Uretzky G (1982): Establishment of right ventricle-hypoplastic pulmonary artery continuity without the use of extracorporeal circulation. J Thorac Cardiovasc Surg 83:74–80.

64. Rashkind WJ (1971): Palliative procedures for transposition of the great arteries. Br Heart J (Suppl)33:69–72.

65. Rashkind WJ, Miller WW (1966): Creation of an atrial septal defect without thoracotomy: A palliative approach to complete transposition of the great arteries. JAMA 196:991–992.

66. Rohmer J, Quaegebeur JM, Brom AG (1977): Takedown and reconstruction of cavopulmonary anastomosis. Ann Thorac Surg 23:129–134.

67. Sade RM, Sloss L, Treves S, et al (1977): Repair of tetralogy of Fallot after aortopulmonary anastomosis. Ann Thorac Surg 23:32–38.

68. Somerville J, Agnew T, Stark J, et al (1967): Banding of the pulmonary artery for common atrioventricular canal. Br Heart J 29:816–828.

69. Sperling DR, Connolly JE (1970): Palliative procedures in congenital heart disease in infants. Am Fam Physician/GP 1:92–97.

70. Stark J, Aberdeen E, Waterston DJ, Bonham-Carter RE, Tynan M (1969): Pulmonary artery constriction (banding): A report of 146 cases. Surgery 65:808–818.

71. Stewart S, Harris P, Manning J (1978): Current results with construction and interruption of the Waterston anastomosis. Ann Thorac Surg 25:431–436.

72. Stewart S, Harris P, Manning J (1980): Pulmonary artery banding: An analysis of current risks, results, and indications. J Thorac Cardiovasc Surg 80:431–436.

73. Taussig HB, Crocetti A, Eshaghpour E, Keinonen R, Yap KN, Bachman D, Momberger N, Kirk H (1971): Long-time observations on the Blalock-Taussig operation. I. Results of first operation. Johns Hopkins Med J 129:243–257.

74. Taussig HB, Crocetti A, Eshaghpour E, Keinonen R, Yap KN, Bachman D, Momberger N, Kirk H (1971): Long-time observations on the Blalock-Taussig operation. II. Second operations, frequency and results. Johns Hopkins Med J 129:258–273.

75. Taussig HB, Crocetti A, Eshaghpour E, Keinonen R, Yap KN, Bachman D, Momberger N, Kirk H (1971): Long-time observations on the Blalock-Taussig operation. III. Common complications. Johns Hopkins Med J 129:274–289.

76. Taussig HB, Kallman CH, et al (1975): Long-time observations on the Blalock-Taussig operation. VIII. 20 to 28 year follow-up on patients with tetralogy of Fallot. Johns Hopkins Med J 137:13–19.

77. Taussig HB, Keinonen R, Momberger N, Kirk H (1973): Long-time observations on the Blalock-Taussig operation. IV. Tricuspid atresia. Johns Hopkins Med J 132:135–145.

78. Taussig HB, Keinonen R, Momberger N, Kirk H (1974): Long-time observations on the Blalock-Taussig operation. VII. Transposition of the great vessels and pulmonary stenosis. Johns Hopkins Med J 135:161–170.

79. Taussig HB, Momberger N, Kirk H (1973): Long-time observations on the Blalock-Taussig operation. VI. Truncus arteriosus type IV. Johns Hopkins Med J 133:123–147.

80. Thomson NB Jr, Niguidula FN, Hohn A (1966): Correction of complete atrioventricular canal defect in patients with previous pulmonary artery banding. Am J Cardiol 18:769–776.

81. Tingelstad JB, Lower RR, Howell TR, Eldredge WJ (1971): Pulmonary artery banding in tricuspid atresia without transposed great arteries. Am J Dis Child 121:434–437.

82. Trusler GA, MacGregor D, Mustard WT (1971): Cavopulmonary anastomosis for cyanotic congenital heart disease. J Thorac Cardiovasc Surg 62:803–809.

83. Trusler GA, Miyamura H, Culham JAG, Fowler RS, Freedom RM, Williams WG (1981): Pulmonary artery stenosis following aortopulmonary anastomoses. J Thorac Cardiovasc Surg 82:398–406.

84. Turley K, Tucker WY, Ebert PA (1980): The changing role of palliative procedures in the treatment of infants with congenital heart disease. J Thorac Cardiovasc Surg 79:194–201.

85. Vetter VL, Rashkind WF, Waldhausen JA (1978): Ascending aorta-right pulmonary artery anastomosis: Long-term results in 137 patients with cyanotic congenital heart disease. J Thorac Cardiovasc Surg 76:115–125.

86. Waterston WJ (1962): Treatment of Fallot's tetralogy in infants under the age of 1 year. Rozhl Chir 41:181–183.

87. Yamamoto N, Reul GJ Jr, Kidd JN, Cooley DA, Hallman GL (1976): A new approach to repair of pulmonary branch stenosis following ascending aorta-right pulmonary artery anastomosis. Ann Thorac Surg 21:237–242.

61 NEONATAL PATENT DUCTUS SURGERY

James K. Kirklin

Patent ductus arteriosus (PDA) results from the failure of normal closure of the ductus arteriosus after birth. The complete failure of ductal closure is termed *persistent PDA*, whereas delayed closure of the ductus is termed *prolonged patency of PDA*.

Among term newborns, the incidence of isolated persistent PDA is approximately 1 in 2000 live births,[29] accounting for 5 to 10 per cent of congenital heart disease. Persistent PDA may have a genetic component in some cases but is particularly common when the mother is afflicted with rubella during the first trimester of pregnancy.

In the premature neonate with PDA, the overall incidence of prolonged patency beyond the third day of life is approximately 35 per cent and is related to decreasing gestational age (Table 61–1)[24,35] and lower birthweight (Table 61–2).[35]

HISTORICAL PERSPECTIVE

The earliest anatomic description of the ductus arteriosus is attributed to Galen (born in AD 131).[24] Harvey demonstrated the physiologic importance of the ductus in the fetal circulation, and Munro demonstrated in a cadaver the possibility of dissecting and ligating a PDA.[31] In 1937, Graybial and coworkers attempted surgical closure of a PDA in a patient with severe "endocarditis," but the patient died 4 days after operation.[18] The first successful closure of a PDA was performed in 1938 by Gross in a 7-year-old girl at the Boston Children's Hospital.[20] The first reported case of successful ligation of a PDA in a premature neonate appears to be that of DeCancq in 1963, in which Mahoney ligated the ductus of a 1417-g premature infant with congestive heart failure and pneumonitis.[11]

MORPHOLOGY AND PHYSIOLOGY OF DUCTAL CLOSURE

The ductus arteriosus develops from the distal portion of the sixth aortic arch and enters the descending thoracic aorta 5 to 10 mm distal to the left subclavian artery. The ductus is normally 5 to 10 mm in diameter.[21] When the aortic arch is left sided, the ductus is on the left side, connecting the proximal left pulmonary artery to the descending aorta (Fig. 61–1).[3] When the arch is right sided, the ductus is still usually left sided, connecting the proximal left pulmonary artery to the proximal left subclavian artery or left innominate artery.[25] Rarely, there is a bilateral ductus.

The histology of the ductus differs from that of the adjoining aorta and pulmonary artery, in which the media has circumferential layers of elastic fibers. In contrast, the media of the ductus contains dense layers of smooth muscle with a spiral orientation. The intima of the ductus is thicker than that of the aorta or pulmonary artery and contains increased amounts of mucoid substance.[17,19] The medial components join with intimal swellings termed *cushions* that contain mucoid substance and longitudinally oriented smooth muscle cells.[36]

Normally, ductal closure occurs in two stages.[4] In full-term infants, the initial stage is complete within 10 to 15 hours after birth[30,33] and consists of contraction of the smooth muscle components of the media (and resultant shortening of the ductus and thickening of the walls) with approximation of the intimal cushions and their protrusion into the lumen.[17] This process occurs most prominently at the pulmonary end of the ductus.

The second stage is normally completed by 2 to 3 weeks of age. The intima undergoes fibrous proliferation with occasional hemorrhage into the ductal wall and necrosis of the inner layer of media.[4] The result is complete obliteration of the lumen and formation of the fibrous ligamentum arteriosum.[17] The ductus is completely closed by 8 weeks in about 90 per cent of infants without other cardiac anomalies.[5]

The precise mechanism responsible for ductal closure in early postnatal life is not fully understood but probably involves an interplay between PO_2,[6,7,14,15] certain circulating vasoconstrictive substances, and prostaglandins. The sensitivity of ductal constriction to increasing levels of PO_2 is partly a function of gestational age, with newborns of greater gestational age being more sensitive to the effect of PO_2 on ductal closure (Fig 61–2).[21,22,27] Prostaglandin E_2 (PGE_2) and prostacyclin (PGI_2) are formed within the ductal wall and probably have a direct local effect in maintaining ductal patency by dilating ductal smooth muscle.[6–8] Additional prostaglandins are produced in the placenta.[6–8] At birth, the placenta is removed, and, in addition, circulating prostaglandins have less effect on ductal patency as gestational age advances.[6,7] The release of vasoactive substances (such as acetylcholine, bradykinin, and endogenous catecholamines) soon after birth may also contribute to ductal closure.[22,27,33]

OPERATIVE TECHNIQUE

Surgical closure of a PDA in the premature neonate should be accomplished with an operating room mortality that approaches 0 per cent. The procedures can be safely

Table 61-1. APPROXIMATE INCIDENCE OF NEWBORNS WITH PROLONGED PDA ACCORDING TO GESTATIONAL AGE

Gestational Age (wks)	Prolonged PDA (Per Cent)
28–30	75
31–32	50
33–34	35
35–36	25

Data from Kirklin JW, Barratt-Boyes BG (1985): Cardiac Surgery. New York, John Wiley & Sons, pp 679–697; and Siassi B, et al (1976): Incidence and clinical features of patent ductus arteriosus in low-birthweight infants: A prospective analysis of 150 consecutively born infants. Pediatrics 57:347–351.

Table 61-2. APPROXIMATE INCIDENCE OF NEWBORN INFANTS WITH PROLONGED PDA ACCORDING TO BIRTHWEIGHT

Birthweight (g)	Prolonged PDA (Per Cent)
<1000	85
1000–1500	50
1500–2000	25

Data from Siassi B, et al (1976): Incidence and clinical features of patent ductus arteriosus in low-birthweight infants: A prospective analysis of 150 consecutively born infants. Pediatrics 57:347–351.

performed in either the neonatal intensive care unit or the operating room. Safe transport and efficient, safe surgical care require close coordination between members of the neonatal unit, the anesthesia team, and the surgical team. Specific protocols for anesthetic and surgical management are effective and likely reduce the probability of human error.

The premature infant is intubated in the neonatal unit, and proper position of the endotracheal tube is verified by chest radiograph. An intravenous line is placed. The infant is transported to the operating room in a prewarmed transport isolette with the body temperature controlled at 37°C. Fresh frozen plasma and packed red cells are brought to the operating room with the infant.

The operating room is prewarmed to 85 to 90°F, and the infant is transferred from the isolette to a special small operating table with overhead radiant heaters (Baker Operating Bed, Ohio Neonatal Care Center) and a servocontrol set at 37°C skin temperature.

The patient is generally anesthetized with fentanyl and paralyzed with pancuronium. Routine intraoperative surveillance includes ECG monitoring, transcutaneous PO_2 monitoring, and continuous measurement of nasopharyngeal and skin temperature. Nasopharyngeal temperature is maintained near 37°C throughout the procedure.

The operation is performed through a limited left lateral thoracotomy incision about 3 cm in length. The chest is entered through the fourth intercostal space. A small chest spreader is positioned, and the lung is gently retracted with a single 2.5-cm malleable retractor. Great care must be exercised by the assistant to avoid excessive pressure on the lungs or downward pressure on the aorta during retraction, both of which can cause prompt hemodynamic deterioration.

The ductus arteriosus is located, taking care to identify the distal aortic arch and left subclavian artery above it. The mediastinal pleura is incised at the superior and inferior aspect of the ductus, adjacent to the aorta. A fine right-angled clamp is used to dissect the tissue plane along the superior and inferior aspect of the ductus for placement of an occluding clip (Liga Clip LC-200, [medium size], Ethicon). The dissection must be deep enough to allow the clip applicator to include the full depth of the ductus to ensure complete ductal occlusion. Note that circumferential dissection is not necessary with this method, thus reducing the likelihood of perforation of the posterior ductal wall.

The ductus is now partially occluded with forceps while the surgical clip is positioned on the ductus adjacent to the aorta (to avoid injury to the recurrent laryngeal nerve). The ductus is then accurately and completely occluded with the clip (Fig. 61-3).[40] A surgical clip that is much longer than the diameter of the ductus should be avoided because of the possible impingement on the underlying left bronchus.

The area of dissection is then carefully examined for hemostasis and a No. 10 chest tube (Argyle trocar 10 F catheter HRI 8888-561019) is placed in the left pleural cavity and attached to a Heimlich valve (Bard-Parker Heimlich chest drain valve 3460) for drainage. The chest tube is generally removed in 24 to 48 hours. The ribs are approximated with two pericostal sutures, and the muscles

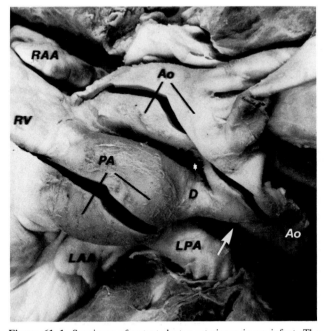

Figure 61-1. Specimen of patent ductus arteriosus in an infant. The superior border of the ductus (asterisk) enters the descending aorta at an acute angle, and the inferior ductal border (arrow) enters the aorta at an obtuse angle. Ao = aorta; D = ductus; LAA = left atrial appendage; LPA = left pulmonary artery; PA = pulmonary artery; RAA = right atrial appendage; RV = right ventricle. (From Calder AL et al [1984]: Pathology of the ductus arteriosus treated with prostaglandins: Comparisons with untreated cases. Pediatr Cardiol 5:85. Copyright © 1984 by John Wiley & Sons, Inc. Reprinted by permission of John Wiley & Sons, Inc.)

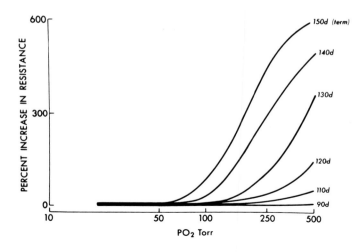

Figure 61–2. The relationship between blood oxygen tension and the increase in resistance across the isolated perfused ductus arteriosus in fetal lambs of differing gestational ages. With increasing gestational age, there is a greater constrictor response in the ductus for a given pO_2. (Reproduced with permission from Heymann MA: Patent ductus arteriosus. In Adams FH and Emmanouilides GC [eds]: Heart Disease in Infants, Children and Adolescents. 3rd ed. © 1983, Williams & Wilkins Co, Baltimore, p 168.)

are approximated with a single layer of continuous absorbable suture. The skin is closed with continuous proline or nylon. Operative time is generally 15 to 20 minutes using this technique.

The infant is then returned to the isolette (which has been maintained at an appropriate temperature during the surgical procedure) for transport back to the neonatal intensive care unit. Once stabilized in the neonatal unit, the pancuronium paralysis is reversed with atropine and neostigmine, and ventilator support is tapered as rapidly as possible.

RESULTS OF SURGERY

Early Results

Surgical closure of PDA in premature infants can be safely performed with proper surgical technique and anesthetic management. The reported mortality resulting from perioperative events is less than 2 per cent.[1,10,12,13,26,28,42] In a collective review of 21 published reports, Edmunds noted six deaths among 361 premature infants undergoing surgical PDA closure to be directly related to the operative procedure (6/361 = 1.6 per cent; confidence limits = 1 to 3 per cent). Correlates of death in 4 infants dying early after operation included intraoperative hemorrhage (n =

2), pneumothorax (n = 1), and mistaken ligation of left pulmonary artery (n = 1). Two late deaths were associated with chylothorax in 1 infant and left phrenic nerve paralysis in 1 infant.[12]

The overall hospital survival of premature infants undergoing surgical closure of PDA is 70 to 85 per cent,[26,28,34,39,41] and the survival at the University of Alabama at Birmingham has been representative (Tables 61–3 and 61–4). Much of the early mortality relates to complications of idiopathic respiratory distress syndrome (IRDS) or necrotizing enterocolitis.

Direct comparisons of surgical closure, closure with indomethacin (an inhibitor of prostaglandin synthesis) administration, or traditional medical treatment of prolonged ductal patency in the premature infant are difficult because of the paucity of large-scale randomized studies, differing indications for intervention, and the numerous additional variables that affect both early and late survival.

Available studies suggest that surgical closure has the following advantages over medical therapy in the treatment of premature infants with IRDS and ventilator dependence or congestive heart failure (CHF) associated with PDA early after birth:

1. A lower incidence of necrotizing enterocolitis is noted if surgical closure of PDA is performed early in the course of IRDS or CHF.[28,37] At the University of Alabama at Birmingham, a randomized trial of premature infants

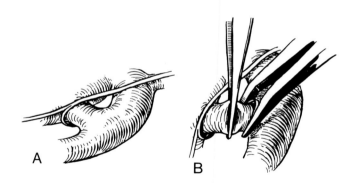

Figure 61–3. Application of the surgical clip for closure of patent ductus arteriosus (PDA) in the premature neonate. *A,* Anatomic configuration. *B,* Technique of clip application after dissection of the superior and inferior border of the PDA (see text for details). (Reproduced with permission from Traugott RC et al [1980]: A simplified method of ligation of patent ductus arteriosus in premature infants. Ann Thorac Surg 29:263.)

Table 61–3. HOSPITAL MORTALITY
AFTER SURGICAL CLOSURE OF PATENT
DUCTUS ARTERIOSUS IN PREMATURE INFANTS
(AT THE UNIVERSITY OF ALABAMA AT
BIRMINGHAM, 1974 TO 1978 AND 1982 TO 1985)

Year of Operation	n	Mortality* No.	Per Cent	70 Per Cent CL†
1974	4	0	0	
1975	2	1	50	7–93
1976	3	1	33	4–76
1977	8	2	25	9–50
1978	26	6	23	14–35
1982	21	5	24	14–37
1983	40	7	18	11–26
1984	36	4	11	6–19
1985	50	11	22	16–30
Total	190	37	19	16–23

*P-(X^3) = 0.75
†CL = confidence limits

Table 61–4. DAY OF DEATH AFTER SURGICAL CLOSURE
OF PATENT DUCTUS ARTERIOSUS IN PREMATURE
INFANTS (AT THE UNIVERSITY OF ALABAMA AT
BIRMINGHAM, 1974 TO 1978 AND 1982 TO 1985)

Postoperative Day	No. of Deaths
0–day of surgery	1*
1	5
2	5
3	1
4–10	6
11–20	4
>20	15
Total	37

*Operation 1975

with PDA who required supplemental oxygen after birth (medical therapy versus surgical PDA closure within 24 hours of birth) revealed a significant reduction in the incidence of necrotizing enterocolitis in the surgical group.[37] Animal studies suggest that systemic hypoperfusion occurs when PDA is associated with prematurity,[1] likely related to a large left-to-right shunt and left ventricular failure. The resultant decrease in gastrointestinal perfusion may predispose to the development of necrotizing enterocolitis.

2. More rapid gastrointestinal function and weight gain.[9]

3. More rapid weaning from ventilator support (Fig. 61–4).[9,28]

4. Decrease in left ventricular volume overload as evidenced by a decrease in left atrial-to-aortic ratio by two-dimensional echocardiography.[2]

5. Shorter hospitalization.[9]

In addition, studies at the University of Alabama at Birmingham have shown no relationship between surgical PDA closure and the incidence and severity of intraventricular central nervous system hemorrhage.[38]

Some risk factors have been identified (although not rigorously) for premature infants who undergo surgical

PDA closure (presumably the same risk factors would also apply to other modes of therapy for PDA):

1. Smaller birth weight (particularly less than 1000 g). Mavroudis and colleagues noted a 4 per cent mortality in the first month of postnatal life after PDA closure when the birthweight was greater than 1000 g compared with 17 per cent when it was less than 1000 g ($p < 0.02$).[26]

2. Associated IRDS (as opposed to isolated CHF).[2] In the presence of IRDS, reported hospital survival is only 60 to 80 per cent,[26,32] but in its absence, 85 to 90 per cent of infants survive the hospital period.[2,12]

3. Preoperative pneumothorax[26] (perhaps an indicator of more severe IRDS).

Analysis of the University of Alabama at Birmingham data (Table 61–5) indicates that the interval between birth and operation (in contrast to birthweight) is not a risk factor for surgical PDA closure. This observation suggests that PDA surgical closure can be safely performed anytime after birth.

Late Results

The late results after surgical closure of PDA in premature infants are dependent primarily on the severity of

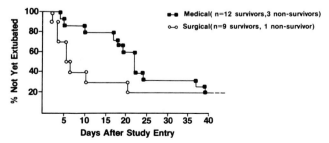

Figure 61–4. Duration of ventilator dependence in a randomized trial of medical versus surgical treatment of symptomatic patent ductus arteriosus in premature infants. (Reproduced with permission from Cotton RB et al [1978]: Randomized trial of early closure of symptomatic patent ductus arteriosus in small preterm infants. J Pediatr 93:647–651.)

Table 61–5. HOSPITAL MORTALITY
AFTER SURGICAL CLOSURE OF PATENT
DUCTUS ARTERIOSUS IN PREMATURE INFANTS
(AT THE UNIVERSITY OF ALABAMA AT
BIRMINGHAM, 1974 TO 1978 AND 1982 TO 1985)

Age at Operation (Days)	n	Mortality* No.	Per Cent
0	1	0	0
1	9	3	33
2	6	2	33
3	5	2	40
4	9	0	0
5	9	3	33
6	4	1	25
7–13	25	3	12
14–20	21	7	33
21–45	15	1	7
Total	104	22	21

*P-(X^2) = 0.28

associated lesions. There are no known late effects of the operation itself or the anesthetic agents with follow-up to 10 years, except for the rare instance of recurrent laryngeal nerve injury or phrenic nerve trauma at surgery.[12] Although early surgical therapy has provided improved late survival compared with medical therapy for PDA in ventilator-dependent premature infants,[9] one study noted only 50 per cent of hospital survivors to be normal 1 to 5 years later.[2] About one third of survivors had radiographic evidence of bronchopulmonary dysplasia, with variable symptoms. Approximately one sixth of survivors had more severe complications, including retrolental fibroplasia, blindness, cerebral palsy, mental retardation, and hydrocephaly.[2]

Comparison with Indomethacin Therapy

Indomethacin is reported to effect closure of PDA within 24 hours in 70 to 80 per cent of premature infants.[12,43] Its effectiveness is increased if administered in the first 10 days of postnatal life.[16,23,43] Disadvantages of indomethacin therapy include mild (and usually transient) renal dysfunction, hyponatremia, and occasional subsequent ductal reopening.[12] Relative contraindications to the use of indomethacin in neonates include hyperbilirubinemia, renal dysfunction, sepsis, and coagulopathies.[12] Mavroudis and colleagues[26] compared indomethacin with surgical therapy in 168 premature infants (nonrandomized) with PDA, IRDS, and ventilator dependence. The surgical group had a lower hospital mortality (17 per cent versus 39 per cent, $p = 0.001$), and a lower incidence of necrotizing enterocolitis (10 per cent versus 26 per cent; $p = 0.008$). This retrospective, nonconcurrent comparison, however, does not provide secure conclusions about the superiority of either therapy.

INDICATIONS FOR OPERATION

Although the precise indications for operation vary among institutions, surgery is generally indicated for premature infants with CHF or IRDS who remain ventilator dependent after the first several days of postnatal life despite "appropriate" medical therapy[12,24,26,32] and have a PDA documented by echocardiography with Doppler studies or by radionucleotide scanning for Qp:Qs. Operation in the first few days after birth is particularly effective in improving survival and reducing morbidity for such infants when the birthweight is less than 1000 g.[39] Because of the suggested relationship between high levels of inspired oxygen within the early hours after birth and the severity of IRDS[43] as well as the favorable effect of PDA closure on the incidence of necrotizing enterocolitis,[28,37] some institutions also recommend urgent operation for premature infants weighing less than 1000 g with a demonstrated PDA who are ventilator dependent during the first 24 to 48 hours after birth.

A policy of more liberal use of surgical closure of PDA can be justified only if the morbidity and mortality related to the operation are extremely low. The precise role of an indomethacin trial before surgery currently depends on the trade-off between the likelihood of prompt ductal closure with each method and the associated morbidity and mortality.

References

1. Baylen BG, Ogata H, Ikegami M, Jacobs HC, Jobe AH, Emmanouilides GC (1983): Left ventricular performance and regional blood flows before and after ductus arteriosus occlusion in premature lambs treated with surfactant. Circulation 67:837–843.
2. Brandt B, Marvin WJ, Ehrenhaft JL, Heintz S, Doty DB (1981): Ligation of patent ductus arteriosus in premature infants. Ann Thorac Surg 32:166–172.
3. Calder AL, Kirker JA, Netuze JM, Starling MB (1984): Pathology of the ductus arteriosus treated with prostaglandins: Comparisons with untreated cases. Pediatr Cardiol 5:85–92.
4. Cassals DE (1973): The Ductus Arteriosus. Springfield, Charles C Thomas, p 75.
5. Christie A (1930): Normal closing time of the foramen ovale and the ductus arteriosus. Am J Dis Child 40:323–326.
6. Clyman RI (1980): Ontogeny of the ductus arteriosus response to prostaglandins and inhibitors of their synthesis. Semin Perinatol 4:115–124.
7. Clyman RI, Heymann MA (1981): Pharmacology of the ductus arteriosus. Pediatr Clin North Am 28:77–93.
8. Coceani F, Olley PM (1980): Role of prostaglandins, prostacyclin, and thromboxanes in the control of prenatal patency and postnatal closure of the ductus arteriosus. Semin Perinatol 4:109–113.
9. Cotton RB, Stahlman MT, Bender HW, Graham TP, Catterton WZ, Kovar I (1978): Randomized trial of early closure of symptomatic patent ductus arteriosus in small preterm infants. J Pediatr 93:647–651.
10. Crafoord G (1947): Discussion of paper by RE Gross: Complete division for the patent ductus arteriosus. J Thorac Surg 16:314–322.
11. DeCancq HE Jr (1963): Repair of patent ductus arteriosus in a 1417-g infant. Am J Dis Child 106:402–410.
12. Edmunds LH Jr (1978): Operation or indomethacin for the premature ductus. Ann Thorac Surg 26:586–589
13. Emmanouilides GC (1977): Persistent patency of the ductus arteriosus in premature infants. In Seventy-fifth Ross Conference on Pediatric Research, Palm Beach, Florida, December 4–7.
14. Fay FS (1972): Guinea pig ductus arteriosus. I. Cellular and metabolic basis for oxygen sensitivity. Am J Physiol 221:470–479.
15. Fay FS, Jobsis FF (1972): Guinea pig ductus arteriosus. III. Light absorption changes during response to O_2. Am J Physiol 223:588–595.
16. Friedman WF, Kurlinski J, Jacob J, DiSessa TG, Gluck L, Merritt TA, Feldman BH (1980): The inhibition of prostaglandin and prostacyclin synthesis in the clinical management of patent ductus arteriosus. Semin Perinatol 4:125–133.
17. Gittenberger-De Groot AC, Van Ertbruggen I, Moulaert AJMG, Harinck E (1980): The ductus arteriosus in the preterm infant: Histologic and clinical observations. J Pediatr 96:88–93.
18. Graybial A, Strieder JW, Boyer NH (1938): An attempt to obliterate the patent ductus arteriosus in a patient with subacute bacterial endarteritis. Am Heart J 15:621–624.
19. Gregory GA, Kitterman JA, Phibbs RH, Tooley WH, Hamilton WK (1971): Treatment of the idiopathic respiratory distress syndrome with continuous positive airway pressure. N Engl J Med 284:1333–1340.
20. Gross RE, Hubbard JP (1939): Surgical ligation of a patent ductus arteriosus: Report of first successful case. JAMA 112:729–731.
21. Heymann MA (1983): Patent ductus arteriosus. In Adams FH, Emmanouilides GC (eds): Moss' Heart Disease in Infants, Children and Adolescents. 3rd ed. Baltimore, Williams & Wilkins, p. 168.
22. Heymann MA, Rudolph AM (1975): Control of the ductus arteriosus. Physiol Rev 55:62–78.
23. Hoffman JIE (1978): The abnormal pulmonary circulation. In Scarpelli EM, Auld PAM, Goldman HS (eds): Pediatric Pulmonary Physiology and Disease. Philadelphia, Lea & Febiger, pp. 235–253.

24. Kirklin JW, Barratt-Boyes BG (1985): Cardiac Surgery: Morphology, Diagnostic Criteria, Natural History, Techniques, Results, and Indications. New York, John Wiley & Sons, pp 679–697.
25. Knight L, Edwards JE (1974): Right aortic arch: Types and associated cardiac anomalies. Circulation 50:1047–1051.
26. Mavroudis C, Cook LN, Fleischaker JW, Nagaraj HS, Shott RJ, Howe WR, Gray LA Jr (1983): Management of patent ductus arteriosus in the premature infant: Indomethacin versus ligation. Ann Thorac Surg 36:561–566.
27. McMurphy DM, Heymann MA, Rudolph AM, Melmon KL (1972): Developmental change in constriction of the ductus arteriosus: Response to oxygen and vasoactive substances in the isolated ductus arteriosus of the fetal lamb. Pediatr Res 6:231–238.
28. Mikhail M, Lee W, Toews W, Synhorst DP, Hawes CR, Hernandez J, Lockhart C, Whitfield J, Pappas G (1982): Surgical and medical experience with 734 premature infants with patent ductus arteriosus. J Thorac Cardiovasc Surg 83:349–357.
29. Mitchell SC, Korones SB, Berendes HW (1971): Congenital heart disease in 56,109 births. Incidence and natural history. Circulation 43:323–332.
30. Moss AJ, Emmanouilides GC, Duffie ER Jr (1963): Closure of the ductus arteriosus in the newborn infant. Pediatrics 32:25–30.
31. Munro JC (1907): Surgery of the vascular system: Ligation of patent ductus arteriosus. Ann Surg 46:335.
32. Nelson RJ, Thibeault DW, Emmanouilides GC, Lippmann M (1976): Improving the results of ligation of patent ductus arteriosus in small preterm infants. J Thorac Cardiovasc Surg 71:169–178.
33. Oberhansli-Weiss I, Heymann MA, Rudolph AM, Melmon KL (1972): The pattern and mechanisms of response to oxygen by the ductus arteriosus and umbilical artery. Pediatr Res 6:693–700.
34. Salomon NW, Anderson RM, Copeland JG, Allen HD, Goldberg SJ, Sahn DJ (1979): A rational approach to ligation of patent ductus arteriosus in the neonate. Chest 75:671–674.
35. Siassi B, Blanco C, Cabal LA, Coran AG (1976): Incidence and clinical features of patent ductus arteriosus in low-birthweight infants: A prospective analysis of 150 consecutively born infants. Pediatrics 57:347–351.
36. Silver MM, Freedom RM, Silver MD, Olley PM (1981): The morphology of the human newborn ductus arteriosus: A reappraisal of its structure and function with special reference to prostaglandin E_1 therapy. Hum Pathol 12:1123–1136.
37. Strange M, Cassady G, Phillips J, Kirklin JK, Pacifico AD (1986): Unpublished data.
38. Strange M, Myers G, Kirklin JK, Pacifico AD, Cassady G (1983): Lack of effect of patent ductus arteriosus ligation on intraventricular hemorrhage in preterm infants. Clin Res 31:913A.
39. Thibeault DW, Emmanouilides GC, Nelson RJ, Lachman RS, Rosengart RM, Oh W (1975): Patent ductus arteriosus complicating the respiratory distress syndrome in preterm infants. J Pediatr 86:120–126.
40. Traugott RC, Will RJ, Schuchmann GF, Treasure RL (1980): A simplified method of ligation of patent ductus arteriosus in premature infants. Ann Thorac Surg 29:263.
41. Wilkerson SA, Fleischaker J, Mavroudis C, Cook L (1985): Developmental sequelae in premature infants undergoing ligation of patent ductus arteriosus. Ann Thorac Surg 39:541–546.
42. Williams WH, Gelband H, Bancalari E, Bauer C, Garcia O, Tamer D, Kaiser GA (1976): The ductus debate: Ligation in prematurity? Ann Thorac Surg 22:151–156.
43. Yeh TF, Luken JA, Thalji A, Raval D, Carr I, Pildes RS (1981): Intravenous indomethacin therapy in premature infants with persistent ductus arteriosus: A double-blind controlled study. J Pediatr 98:137–145.

62 NEONATAL LEFT VENTRICULAR OUTFLOW TRACT SURGERY

S. Kenn Beeman
John W. Hammon, Jr.

Although somewhat broad and general, left ventricular outflow obstruction remains a conceptually useful term for both diagnostic and therapeutic purposes. The precise anatomic variations and their respective pathophysiologic features that comprise this subdivision of congenital heart disease are as varied as the patients who present with these anomalies. Strictly speaking, however, the associated anatomic defects within this class can be assigned to three basic subgroups of abnormalities: (1) lesions of the left ventricular outflow tract proper (proximal to the aortic valve), (2) a continuum of lesions resulting from dysgenesis or agenesis of the aortic valve itself, and (3) the spectrum of defects occurring in the aortic arch and proximal descending aorta (distal to the aortic valve).

Overall, the lesions that present with epidemiologically important frequency and clinical significance in the neonatal period are confined to the latter two subsets. Coarctation of the aorta and arch interruption represent the two extremes of the continuum of defects occurring distal to the aortic valve. Within the range of anomalies between discrete valvular aortic stenosis and frank aortic atresia exists hypoplastic left heart syndrome.

To remain true to the spirit and orientation of this text, the discussion of the surgical management of left ventricular outflow obstruction in the neonate will focus on the guidepost topics of these four lesions: valvular aortic stenosis, coarctation of the aorta, interrupted aortic arch, and aortic atresia (hypoplastic left-heart syndrome).

HISTORICAL PERSPECTIVE

Within the scope of cardiovascular surgery, operative intervention to relieve left ventricular outflow tract obstruction in the neonate is a relatively recent event. Crafoord and Nylin and Gross in 1944 and 1945, respectively, are acknowledged to have performed the first clinical coarctation repair by excision of the coarctation and primary end-to-end anastomosis.[11,16] It remained, however, for Mustard and colleagues in 1953 to perform the first successful neonatal repair of coarctation—thus, the first successful repair of any form of neonatal left ventricular outflow obstruction—in a 3-week-old infant.[33]

Before the use of synthetic material in coarctation repair in 1960, aortic homografts were used exclusively in replacing the defect of coarctectomy in those cases not repairable by primary end-to-end anastomosis. In 1966,

Waldhausen and Nahrwold[51] introduced the subclavian flap aortoplasty; with some important modifications, their clinical repair emulated the experimental method reported by Blalock and Park in 1944.

Pertinent to the treatment of congenital valvular aortic stenosis, Tuffier successfully digitally dilated a stenotic aortic valve in 1913.[49] In 1952, Bailey et al reported a series of patients systematically treated with closed transventricular valvulotomy/dilation.[1] Swan and Kortz[45] and Lewis et al[27] independently in 1956 reported the first open valvulotomy under moderate hypothermia and inflow stasis. While the literature credits Spencer and colleagues in 1958[44] with the first accurate valvulotomies using cardiopulmonary bypass, essentially the same procedure had been performed at the Mayo Clinic as early as 1956.[14]

In 1955, Merrill, Webster, and Samson first successfully treated an aortic arch interruption (type A in a 3-year-old girl) by a ductal–left subclavian arterial anastomosis.[28] Thirteen years elapsed before a neonatal survivor of operative repair, carried out by Sirak et al, of interrupted arch was reported in 1968.[43] In 1970, operation by Barratt-Boyes et al on an 8-day-old neonate with a type A interruption, a ventricular septal defect, and total anomalous pulmonary venous drainage represented the first successful simultaneous repair of aortic arch interruption and all intracardiac defects.[2]

Cayler and colleagues in 1969 successfully palliated a neonate with a less severe form of hypoplastic left-heart syndrome by creating a shunt from the ascending aorta to the right pulmonary artery and by using bilateral pulmonary artery banding.[9] In 1976 Freedom et al reported the palliation of a neonate with aortic atresia, a ventricular septal defect, and a normal-sized left ventricle.[15] Successful correction of aortic atresia (with interrupted arch and ventricular septal defect) was first reported by Norwood and Stellin in 1981; they utilized placement of a valved conduit from the apex to the descending aorta, a graft conduit between the ascending and descending aorta, and pulmonary artery banding.[35] And in 1983 Norwood, Lang, and Hansen reported an infant who had undergone successful two-stage correction of aortic atresia and hypoplastic left-heart syndrome.[37]

The techniques of cardiopulmonary bypass, circulatory arrest, and profound hypothermia have played an indispensible role in the progression of actual operative therapy for neonatal left ventricular outflow obstruction. No historical review, however, would be complete without citing the advent of prostaglandin E_1 as adjunctive therapy for left ventricular outflow obstruction. In 1976, the remarkable immediate preoperative improvement in the setting of aortic arch interruption, as a consequence of ductal dilation by prostaglandin E_1, was reported.[39] The use of prostaglandin E_1 was subsequently extended to the other forms of left ventricular outflow obstruction.

INDICATIONS FOR OPERATION

Patients with left ventricular outflow tract obstruction who present with symptoms in infancy are usually critically ill. Symptoms begin with ductus closure and ordinarily reflect congestive heart failure, low cardiac output, or both. Infants manifest extreme shortness of breath, a dusky skin color, and decreased urinary output. Physical signs include cardiomegaly, a systolic murmur heard in the aortic area or over the back, coarse rales or wheezes, and decreased or absent peripheral pulses. Cardiac catheterization and/or two-dimensional echocardiography should be performed on an emergent basis. More patients are now managed with echocardiography alone.

Valvular Aortic Stenosis

Operation is indicated emergently once the diagnosis of critical valvular aortic stenosis is made. Such a neonate manifests signs of congestive heart failure, radiographic evidence of pulmonary edema and/or cardiomegaly, and/or electrocardiographic evidence of left ventricular hypertrophy or strain. A valve area of less than 0.5 cm²/M² is indicative of severe stenosis. While a large peak systolic ejection gradient (50 to 75 mmHg) supports the diagnosis of critical obstruction, a lower value is often observed in severe stenosis, particularly with hypoplasia of the left ventricle or with left ventricular failure (elevated left ventricular end-diastolic pressure and/or depressed ejection fraction). In the case of the moribund neonate with extremely poor systemic perfusion and significant metabolic acidosis, operation can be delayed up to 12 hours to allow for medical stabilization (with prostaglandin E_1, bicarbonate, digoxin, and diuretic therapy) of the patient's condition.

Coarctation of the Aorta

With symptomatic isolated coarctation, it is ideal to delay operation on the neonate until he is at least 6 months old. If the neonate with severe coarctation (diminished femoral pulses and reduction in the luminal diameter by greater than 50 per cent at the site of the constriction) presents with congestive heart failure, intensive medical therapy is initiated. If the failure resolves completely, permitting reduction and ultimately discontinuation of decongestive therapy, operation can be postponed until the optimal age is attained. If, on the other hand, congestive heart failure does not respond to a 24 to 48 hour trial of medical therapy, immediate coarctation repair is indicated. In the neonate with severe coarctation whose lower body perfu-

sion is ductal dependent, prostaglandin E_1 infusion and emergent operation are indicated.

When coarctation complicates the presence of a ventricular septal defect, urgent operation is indicated. If the ventricular septal defect is solitary and small, only a coarctation repair need be performed. When the ventricular septal defect is large or is multiple, several approaches may be considered. We elect to repair the coarctation and to band the pulmonary artery—delaying (or possibly obviating) ultimate ventricular septal defect repair. Banding the pulmonary artery reduces congestive heart failure and makes the convalescence from the coarctation repair markedly easier. In our experience, the neonate who has had coarctation repair and continues to have congestive heart failure because of a large ventricular septal defect is a poor operative candidate because of poor nutrition and the possibility of infection from long-term tracheal intubation and intravenous catheterization. If the ventricular septal defect does not spontaneously close, operation for debanding and ventricular septal defect closure is undertaken at 3 months of age. In this short period of time, pulmonary artery scarring does not occur, and pulmonary artery reconstruction is unnecessary.[17] If the ventricular septal defect closes, the band is removed through the same incision 3 to 6 months later.

Other surgeons only repair the coarctation at the original operation. If the patient is not extubated and is not making good progress at 48 hours postoperatively, then repair of the ventricular septal defect is performed without delay.

When coarctation is associated with more complicated intracardiac anomalies other than ventricular septal defect, urgent repair of the coarctation alone is almost always proper. However if the underlying malady is the Taussig-Bing malformation, then pulmonary artery banding should also be performed initially.[38] If after 72 hours the patient is not making progressive recovery (off intravenous inotropic or vasoactive drugs and extubated), then the associated lesions should be surgically addressed.

Interrupted Aortic Arch

Operation for interrupted aortic arch is indicated on an urgent basis. Operation should follow patient presentation by only the length of time necessary to permit medical stabilization with prostaglandins.

If the associated intracardiac lesions are correctable in a single stage, such as ventricular septal defect, aorticopulmonary (A-P) window, or truncus arteriosus, then primary complete repair of the complex should be pursued. Otherwise, repair of the interruption via a left thoracotomy and palliation of the associated lesion(s) with pulmonary artery banding are the preferred courses.

Left Heart Atresia

Only in those neonates with severe metabolic acidosis and hypoperfusion, (refractory to PGE_1 and bicarbonate infusion), with bleeding diatheses, or with coexistent severe extracardiac anomalies is operation for left heart atresia currently contraindicated. Despite historically poor surgical results, such an aggressive approach to these neonates stems from several considerations: (1) hypoplastic left-heart syndrome is a common congenital cardiac defect (the fourth most common in some series), (2) without surgery the condition is uniformly fatal, (3) as many as 25 per cent of cardiac deaths in the first week of life are due to this syndrome, and (4) these patients have a very low incidence of associated extracardiac defects.[12,34] Operation should rarely, however, be performed emergently. Instead, it should be delayed, as long as several days, until vigorous medical management has allowed amelioration of renal and hepatic function.[42]

PREOPERATIVE CARE

The nature of the lesions comprising left ventricular outflow obstruction in the neonate presupposes that the infant presents in a critically ill condition. Except in a small subset of patients with isolated coarctation of the aorta, in whom perfusion of the lower body is *not* ductal dependent, neonates with left ventricular outflow obstruction come to operation either emergently or urgently. Depending on the individual infant's condition, care of the patient—from the time of suspicion of the presence of the lesion, through confirmation of the diagnosis, and until the time of operation—may include endotracheal intubation with mechanical ventilation and oxygen supplementation, balloon atrioseptostomy (hypoplastic left-heart syndrome with mitral atresia), intensive invasive monitoring, and digoxin, diuretic, bicarbonate, and/or prostaglandin E_1 therapy. The delivery of this care must be streamlined and goal directed. This intensive preoperative management must optimize the patient's medical condition to mitigate the very great attendant risks of perioperative morbidity and mortality in these patients. Without causing undue or excessive delay in definitive operative intervention, this care should yield amelioration of congestive heart failure and alveolar-arterial gas exchange and improvement in peripheral perfusion as manifest by increases in systemic blood pressure, pulses, urinary output, and arterial pH.

To this end, prostaglandin E_1 deserves particular comment. The use of constant intra-arterial or intravenous infusion of prostaglandin E_1, at beginning doses of 0.025 to 0.1 µg/kg/min, throughout the preoperative period into the operating room is advantageous in any neonate with left ventricular outflow obstruction in whom systemic perfusion is limited by a restrictive ductus arteriosus. The dose can be increased to 0.5 µg/kg/min. Prostaglandin E_1 is likely to be more effective in those neonates in whom the ductus has not already closed anatomically. Thus, prostaglandin E_1 efficacy is somewhat age dependent, although less so in patients with acyanotic lesions than in those with cyanotic heart disease.

The beneficial results of prostaglandin E_1 infusion—namely partial cardiac decongestion, improved oxygenation, and optimized peripheral perfusion—are primarily due to its ductal and pulmonary vascular relaxant properties. As a consequence of increased right-to-left ductal flow, renal perfusion improves, with a resultant enhancement of the kidney's ability to respond appropriately to volume overload and metabolic acidosis. Moreover, in localized juxtaductal coarctation, prostaglandin E_1 will lower the pressure gradient between the ascending and descending aorta. This effect may be a reflection of relaxation of ductal tissue in the lumen of the aorta at the site of coarctation or dilation of the aortic end of the ductus.[25]

The side effects of prostaglandin E_1 infusion are negligible. Certainly, no death has ever been attributed to its use. Any number of mild cardiovascular, neurologic, respiratory, metabolic, gastrointestinal, and hematologic findings have been *associated* with critically ill neonates receiving prostaglandin E_1 infusion. No frank causal relation between prostaglandin E_1 and these intercurrent medical events, however, has been established. Respiratory depression, apnea, hypotension, and bradycardia are the the most consequential correlates. To be sure, these events are more likely to occur in neonates weighing less than 2 kg, but otherwise they do not seem to be age related. The cardiovascular events seem to be more prominent when the duration of prostaglandin E_1 infusion exceeds 48 hours.[26]

Some infants who would have died preoperatively now, because of prostaglandin E_1 therapy, survive to operation. Still many others, whose condition would have been grave at operation without preoperative prostaglandin E_1, now have significant improvement in their clinical condition at the time of operation. Indeed, short-term preoperative prostaglandin E_1 infusion is associated with a significant reduction in early surgical mortality in these critically ill neonates.[25] In view of this very low risk–to–benefit ratio, treatment with prostaglandin E_1 is recommended for any neonate with left ventricular outflow obstruction in which systemic perfusion is limited by a restrictive ductus.[23]

SURGICAL MANAGEMENT

Valvular Aortic Stenosis

The preferred operative therapy for valvular aortic stenosis in the neonate is valvulotomy, which is palliative. There is, however, a divergence of opinion among surgeons over whether an open or a closed approach should be used. Open valvulotomy can be performed with either profound hypothermia and circulatory arrest or modest hypothermia and cardiopulmonary bypass. Through an ascending aortotomy, a sharp commissurotomy is performed, adopting the limited objective of maximal relief of stenosis with minimal creation of regurgitation. In general, very deliberate, staged commissural incisions are made to prevent incompetence. Incision in any rudimentary raphe is virtually always eschewed, lest almost certain aortic insufficiency should result. It is rarely possible by valvulotomy to fashion a tricuspid valve. Occasionally, myxomatous nodules or fibrous thickening on the ventricular surface of the cusps can be shaved and debrided.

Alternatively, closed valvulotomy can be performed through median sternotomy or left thoracotomy with insertion of a valvulotome, Hegar dilator, or Gruntzig catheter through a controlled apical left ventricular stab wound. Valvotomy is then performed blindly and titrated to a palpable "pop."

Proponents of open valvulotomy emphasize the advantages of direct visualization of the valve during performance of the commissurotomy, which should attenuate the incidence of iatrogenic incompetence. Furthermore, advocates of open valvulotomy with hypothermia and cardiopulmonary bypass assert that the myocardial protection afforded by the latter techniques are crucial in this setting in which myocardial ischemia and extreme ventricular irritability are so common and can be so unforgiving. (The closed technique requires a period of total left ventricular outflow obstruction, which is not always well tolerated.)

On the other hand, closed valvulotomy can be performed through a left thoracotomy, preserving a virginal median sternotomy route for future operative approach. This technique avoids the deleterious effects of cardiopulmonary bypass on the sick neonate, which can be profound. (Our preference is for the open technique whenever possible.)

Coarctation of the Aorta

To relieve obstruction and to avoid restenosis are the goals of operative intervention in neonatal coarctation. Principles of management include (1) preservation and avoidance of intercostal vessels, which are often friable; (2) awareness of the precarious nature of the vascular supply to the anterior spinal column; and (3) adequate repair, which it is hoped will avoid residual coarctation or recoarctation.

Performed through a left thoracotomy, subclavian flap aortoplasty and patch angioplasty are the most popular methods of repair. Atraumatic vascular clamps are placed in such a manner so as to minimize the amount of aorta and arch vessels included, yet to allow for complete exposure of the coarctation.

Subclavian flap aortoplasty is accomplished by division of the left subclavian artery just proximal to the origin of the vertebral artery, which is ligated separately. The proximal subclavian stump is then incised longitudinally along its inferoposterior margin. This incision is extended onto the aorta, completely across the coarctation. Any intimal shelf in the aortic lumen at the coarctation site is carefully excised. The newly created flap is turned down and trimmed as necessary to be interposed between the borders of the longitudinal defect produced in the aorta. Sutures are carefully placed using running 6- or 7-0 polydioxone suture material. After the distal clamp is removed and a hemostatic suture line is confirmed (Fig. 62–1), the proximal clamp is slowly removed (Fig. 62–2). Slight arterial hypertension is maintained, and sodium bicarbonate is administered for about 5 minutes to protect against the development of ventricular fibrillation (so-called declamping syndrome).[46] A residual systolic gradient across the repair exceeding 10 mmHg mandates refashioning of the repair. A small chest tube is placed laterally and inferiorly in such a way to avoid injury to vulnerable intercostal arteries.

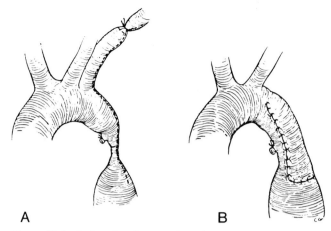

Figure 62–1. *A*, Juxtaductal coarctation of the aorta. The ductus arteriosus has been ligated and transected; the left subclavian artery has been ligated proximal to the origin of the vertebral artery. The proposed location and extent of incision in the proximal subclavian artery and aorta are depicted. *B*, Subclavian flap coarctation repair. The proximal subclavian artery has been transected. After excision of any intimal shelf at the coarctation site, the incised subclavian stump has been fashioned into a turned-down flap and has been interposed within the longitudinal defect created by the aortic incision.

Patch angioplasty is performed in a similar manner with pericardium or polytel (polytetrafluoroethylene), which is the preferred substitute. A large patch is used so that the new lumen is at least 1.5 to 2 cm in diameter to avoid recoarctation. Careful resection of the internal shelf is always recommended (Fig. 62–3).

Proponents of both subclavian flap aortoplasty and patch angioplasty believe their respective *methods* of repair, in their hands, are associated with less recoarctation. Moreover, opponents of subclavian flap aortoplasty emphasize the sacrifice of the antegrade inflow to the left subclavian artery if it is not anastomosed to the left common carotid artery. This latter procedure is extremely technically difficult through a left thoracotomy and would greatly extend the operation time. It, therefore, is not routinely done; instead, the vertebral artery is ligated at its origin to prevent subclavian steal. Without reattachment of the left subclavian artery, the development of a shortened, slightly weakened left arm is possible over the course of the patient's life. Even when this phenomenon has developed, it has not been functionally significant.

The disadvantage to patch angioplasty is the development of aneurysms at the operative site, sometimes many years after operation.[3] In addition, this technique, when performed with synthetic materials, places the patient at risk for the remainder of his or her life for development of subacute bacterial endocarditis at the operative site.

Resection and end-to-end anastomosis should be reserved for the very favorable anatomic situation in which the arch and ascending aorta are large. It is very important to mobilize the aorta so that the anastomosis is performed under minimal tension (Fig. 62–4). The recurrence rate will be higher with this technique because of failure of

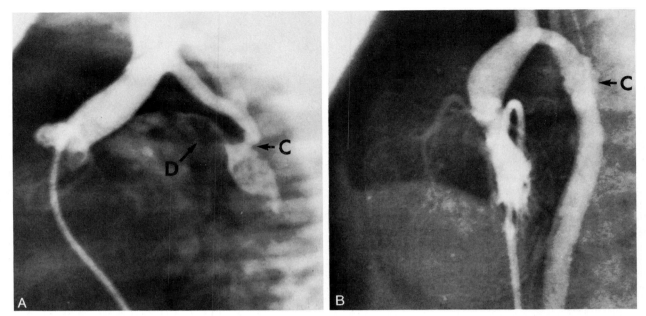

Figure 62–2. *A*, This preoperative arteriogram demonstrates juxtaductal coarctation of the aorta. C = coarctate segment; D = ductus arteriosus. *B*, The postoperative arteriogram illustrates the dramatic dilation to an optimal luminal diameter at the site of the former coarctation, obtained by subclavian aortoplasty. C = site of coarctation repair.

growth of the anastomosis despite the suture technique or type of suture employed.

Special Circumstances

Coarctation *proximal* to the left subclavian artery can be repaired by a reverse subclavian flap aortoplasty or resection. For a management strategy pertinent to coarctation complicated by other cardiac lesions, please refer to the earlier section on surgery for coarctation of the aorta.

Interrupted Aortic Arch

Aortic arch interruptions can be repaired by direct anastomosis, by use of an endogenous vessel for conduit, or by interposed tube grafts. These methods can be performed with profound hypothermia and circulatory arrest through either a median sternotomy or a left thoracotomy (Fig. 62–5). Occasionally, when graft interposition is elected, a combined left lateral and anterior approach is utilized, so that the distal anastomosis is fashioned through the left thoracotomy and the proximal anastomosis is completed via the anterior approach—again with profound hypothermia and circulatory arrest.

In general, the mediastinal approach is reserved for repair of interrupted arch in those neonates who have associated intracardiac lesions, such as ventricular septal defect and aorticopulmonary window, that can be corrected concomitantly. This approach has the distinct advantage of complete resolution of all hemodynamic abnormalities in one procedure. The left lateral approach to repair of the interruption is employed when only palliation (typically, pulmonary artery banding) of associated intracardiac defects is possible.

Left Heart Atresia

The principles that guide conventional operative therapy for lesions comprising the hypoplastic left-heart syndrome include (1) maintenance of adequate systemic perfusion, (2) normalization of pulmonary blood flow, and (3) relief of pulmonary venous obstruction. Classical aortic atresia–hypoplastic left-heart syndrome has required staged repair. In the initial operation, utilizing profound hypothermia and circulatory arrest, the precarious ductus is ligated. To provide an unobstructed path from the right ventricle to the aorta, synthetic or homograft conduits have been applied between the right ventricle or proximal pulmonary artery and the aorta. Though often more difficult, an oblique anastomosis of the transected proximal pulmonary artery to the vestigial ascending aorta is currently preferable.[24] To control pulmonary flow, only pulmonary bands need to be placed, unless the pulmonary artery has been divided for creation of continuity between the right ventricle and the aorta. In that instance, a classic Blalock-Taussig shunt or Gore-Tex shunt between the innominate artery and the right pulmonary artery must be constructed. Finally, an atrial septectomy is performed, regardless of whether balloon septostomy has already been performed. Additional discussion and illustrations of these palliative procedures are found in Chapter 60.

At 6 to 24 months of age, survivors of palliation undergo a Fontan-type repair. If a shunt was fashioned at palliation, it is removed. A direct anastomosis between the right atrium and the right pulmonary artery is created. If pulmonary bands are present, they are removed. Finally an atrial baffle is constructed to direct caval flow through the right atrial–pulmonary arterial anastomosis and to direct pulmonary venous return across the tricuspid valve.

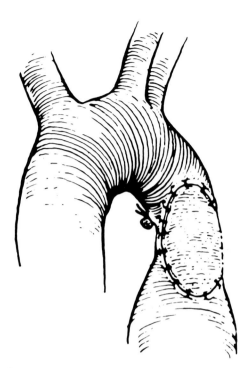

Figure 62–3. Patch angioplasty coarctation repair. The ductus arteriosus has been ligated and transected. The angioplasty has been completed, utilizing a relatively large patch to yield a new luminal diameter of 1.5 cm or more.

In the special circumstance of aortic atresia with a large ventricular septal defect and a normal-sized left ventricle, repair is still staged and is similar in many respects to the approach outlined above. In this instance, operative therapy in stage I is also oriented toward decompressing an often hypertensive left ventricle. The ductus is closed, and a conduit or direct side-to-side anastomosis is constructed between the undivided proximal pulmonary artery and the aorta. Pulmonary artery banding is performed. (No Blalock-Taussig or innominate-to-pulmonary arterial shunt is made.) For survivors, the stage II procedure consists of ventricular septal defect closure, release of the pulmonary arterial bands (with any necessary pulmonary arterioplasty), and removal of the pulmonary arterial-aorta anastomosis/conduit. Finally, systemic circulation is restored with the placement of a valved conduit between the left ventricular apex and the descending aorta.

As experience with pediatric cardiac transplantation is amassed, the current operative management of left heart atresia, as outined above, may well be supplanted in the coming years by orthotopic (or heterotopic) transplantation.

POSTOPERATIVE CARE

Of course, the preoperative patient profile and events occurring in the operating room are crucial determinants of the ultimate success of palliative or curative operations for

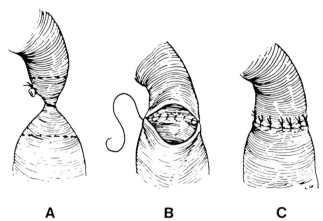

Figure 62–4. *A,* Coarctation repair using end-to-end anastomosis. The ductus arteriosus has been ligated and transected. The proposed sites of aortic transection and the extent of coarctectomy are depicted. The adequate but conservative margins of resection reflect the need to negotiate competing interests: to maximize the luminal diameter at the site of eventual anastomosis without producing excessive anastomotic tension. *B,* The coarctectomy has been accomplished. The "back" wall of the anastomosis has been performed with a continuous suture technique. *C,* The end-to-end anastomosis has been completed. Note the interrupted suture technique utilized in the "front" wall.

neonatal left ventricular outflow obstruction. This observation, however, in no way lessens the importance of appropriately aggressive postoperative care (see Chapter 68).

In the immediate postoperative period, the neonate, whose condition before operation was most often critical, must not only deal with possible residual cardiac disease but also new, often extensive alterations in cardiopulmonary anatomy and physiology. Superimposed on this gargantuan task is the requirement to recover from the insults inherent to the techniques that allowed such aggressive invasion and manipulation in the first place—cardiac

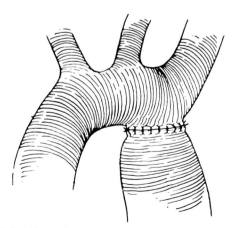

Figure 62–5. A Type A interruption of the aortic arch has been repaired with primary end-to-end anastomosis of the descending aorta to the transverse arch. Again, note that at least the front wall of the anastomosis has been performed with an interrupted suture technique to facilitate circumferential growth at the anastomotic site.

anesthesia, cardiopulmonary bypass, profound hypothermia, and/or circulatory arrest.

Postoperative care may be relatively simple and straightforward, as in the uncomplicated repair of isolated coarctation of the aorta. The patient, for example, may be admitted to the recovery area with neither an endotracheal tube or a chest tube. In other cases, however, such as with left heart atresia or interrupted arch, postoperative care may be extremely complex.

In general, all neonates in the immediate postoperative period will require at a minimum the following:

1. Warming and attention to temperature stability.
2. Supplemental oxygen and/or humidified air.
3. Assisted pulmonary toilet.
4. Frequent assessment of vital signs and constant electrocardiographic monitoring.
5. Consideration and attention to nutritional needs (enteral or parenteral) within the first 6 to 12 hours.
6. Frequent assessment of gross neurologic function (particularly in the perioperative settings in which right-to-left shunts and prolonged periods of low-to-no flow may pertain).
7. Chest radiographs for evaluation of lung fields; heart size; mediastinal width; and the positions of the endotracheal tube, central lines, and mediastinal or thoracostomy tubes.
8. Serial hematocrits until chest tube output is less than 50 ml/day, blood loss from phlebotomy for other laboratory determinations is minimal, and the actual hematocrit assumes a stable value.
9. Frequent observation of input and urinary and chest tube output.
10. Continuation of parenteral antibiotic prophylaxis (begun immediately before operation and adjusted for age, weight, and hepatic and renal function).

As the condition of the infant and the magnitude of the operative insult dictate, additional intervention for monitoring physiologic function and responses to therapeutic interventions may be required as follows:

1. Central venous access for drug delivery and right heart functional indices.
2. Pulmonary arterial catheters for preload and left-heart diastolic function assessments—although data derived from these catheters may have less meaning in the face of native or created shunts.
3. Arterial blood gases.
4. Coagulation studies (prothrombin time, partial thromboplastin time, platelet count, bleeding time, fibrinogen concentration, fibrin degradation products).
5. Serum creatinine and potassium determinations. (Because hyperkalemia, exacerbated by possible persistent acidosis, low cardiac output, and marginal renal function, is so much more life-threatening in the neonate than hypokalemia, potassium replacement in the early postoperative period is avoided. Only when serum potassium level is below 2.5 mEq/liter [below 3.0 mEq/liter if the patient is on digoxin] or when arrhythmias can be attributed to hypokalemia is potassium replaced at 0.2 mEq/kg/hr.)
6. Serum calcium assay (particularly important in patients with interrupted arch because of the frequent association with DiGeorge syndrome).

7. Medications (diuretics, digoxin, antihypertensive agents, intravenous vasoactive drugs, and intravenous inotropic agents).
8. Blood products for blood loss and coagulopathy.
9. Sonography to assess the integrity of the phrenic nerves.

Prerequisites for extubation include an intact cough, an ability to clear the airway, adequate oxygenation on an FiO_2 of 0.4, cardiovascular stability, and adequate cardiac output. Mediastinal and thoracostomy tubes are removed in the absence of an air leak when the drainage is less than 50 ml/24 hr.

Special Features of Postoperative Care Peculiar to Particular Lesions

Coarctation of the Aorta

Systemic arterial hypertension is usually present after coarctation repair, although it ordinarily is not significant enough to require antihypertensive medication. Some centers, however, follow a protocol of vigorous treatment of even mild hypertension to prevent any possibility of the development of necrotizing arteritis. Should postoperative abdominal distention and hypoactive bowel sounds occur beyond the second postoperative day, treatment should include bowel decompression via a naso/orogastric tube connected to low intermittent wall suction, an intravenous histamine-2 receptor antagonist, intravenous hydration, and antihypertensive therapy with reserpine, hydralazine, or sodium nitroprusside. It is extremely rare for neonates to develop this entity, and as a rule they never require laparotomy.

Milky thoracostomy tube drainage is probably chyle. The chest tube should remain in place until such drainage abates. If the chest tube is in place on the sixth postoperative day because of chylothorax, total parenteral nutrition is indicated to reduce thoracic duct flow. A chest radiograph is obtained about day 7, since chylothorax can develop late. If there is evidence of an unexplained pleural effusion, it should be aspirated. Repeat aspiration may be required. Reoperation is indicated for any reaccumulation following a third aspiration.

Interrupted Aortic Arch

DiGeorge syndrome is associated with interrupted arch as frequently as 68 per cent of the time.[50] Absence of thymic tissue can be noted at operation. Repeat serum calcium determinations in the postoperative period should be standard, and hypocalcemia should be treated (100 mg $CaCl_2$/kg/24 hr). Parathyroid hormone levels and immunologic evaluation can be carried out at a later time.

RESULTS

Valvular Aortic Stenosis

Early Results

In the decade between 1974 and 1984, operative mortality in the neonate at open valvulotomy declined from almost 100 per cent to as low as 9 per cent. Messina and colleagues, who reported the 9 per cent neonatal mortality, attribute this result to prompt recognition and diagnosis followed by emergent operation, use of moderate hypothermia and cardiopulmonary bypass, brief cross-clamp time, and conservative valvulotomy to avoid development of significant aortic insufficiency.[29] Trinkle's results indicate 100 per cent survival after closed valvulotomy in three neonates.[47] Mortality from closed valvulotomy in the Toronto experience has been reported to be 39 per cent.[21]

In contrast to surgery for other forms of congenital heart disease, operative mortality after neonatal aortic valvulotomy almost always occurs early, within 48 hours of operation. The historically high neonatal operative mortality has been related to the critical preoperative condition, very young age, the degree of valvular morphologic dysplasia, and coexistence of other intracardiac lesions (left-heart hypoplasia [LVEDV less than 30 ml/M^2], endocardial fibroelastosis, mitral valvular disease, and left ventricular hypertrophy).

Late Results

Of 17 early survivors of open valvulotomy reported in two series since 1980, only one patient died within the mean follow-up period of 2.5 years.[13,29] All three of Trinkle's early survivors of closed valvulotomy were still alive at least 3 years postoperatively.[48]

About 35 per cent of these patients will undergo repeat aortic valve operation within 15 to 20 years of the original valve operation. Young age at valvulotomy, however, does not seem to add increased risk for reoperation, certainly within the early or intermediate term. Moreover, for those patients who had valvulotomy as a neonate and who require reoperation, frequently a repeat valvulotomy is satisfactory.

Aortic incompetence is a rare complication of open valvulotomy performed properly (conservatively). Aortic regurgitation, instead, is more common after closed valvulotomy, particularly if a cutting valvulotome is employed. The incidence of bacterial endocarditis is not lessened by valvulotomy; in fact, the operation may enhance the incidence.

Coarctation of the Aorta

Early Results

The early mortality in neonates who are older than 4 days at the time of coarctation repair and who do not have significant associated intracardiac lesions now approaches zero. Most operative mortality is associated with acute cardiac failure. Occasionally, death occurs in the operating room, temporally related to removal of the proximal cross-clamp (acute declamping syndrome). Prolonged preoperative ventilatory support seems to be an additional correlate to operative mortality. Poor preoperative condition also adds increased risk for early death. Bergdahl and colleagues believe failure to adopt subclavian flap aortoplasty as the method of repair is associated with increased hospital mortality.[4]

The incidence of postoperative paraplegia in the setting of neonatal coarctation also approaches zero. This observation is surprising, since very young age is a predisposing factor for poor collateral formation and thus very tenuous anterior spinal vascular supply. Further risk for paraplegia development arises when (1) the coarctation is proximal to the left subclavian artery, (2) the ductus supplies the descending thoracic aorta, (3) there is stenosis at the origin of the left subclavian artery, (4) the right subclavian artery originates distal to the coarctation, and (5) the coarctation is less than severe. The incidence of necrotizing arteritis in neonates also is negligible.

Late Results

Intermediate mortality after neonatal coarctation repair over a mean follow-up of 2 to 3 years has been reported as 0 to 14 per cent.[8,30,31] The mode of late death is usually related to recoarctation or associated cardiac lesions awaiting definitive treatment.

When the resting peak systolic pressure gradient across the repair exceeds 10 mmHg, persistent or recurrent coarctation exists. Recurrence after end-to-end anastomosis can be due to lack of growth of the suture line (particularly if a continuous suture was employed) and to damage to the aorta from cross-clamping. Recurrence may also result from residual ductal tissue or the presence of abnormal mesodermal tissue that proliferates as well as from abnormal concentrations of certain mucopolysaccharides (chondroitin sulfate) in the aortic wall (with subsequent deterioration in wall compliance), which can lead to restenosis.[5,7,20,32,40] Of course, technical factors at the time of repair (insufficient resection and anastomotic tension) contribute to "residual" coarctation.

The incidence of recurrent or persistent coarctation in neonates after end-to-end anastomosis is as high as 50 per cent in some centers.[21] (The reoperation rate is, naturally, much lower.) The rate of recoarctation after subclavian flap aortoplasty in the experience of surgeons at the University of Maryland and at Hershey Medical Center approaches zero.[8,31] In fact, in the report by Campbell and associates, neonates in whom interrupted suture or absorbable suture was used have no gradient at all.[8] Contrary to these latter findings, however, Metzdorff and colleagues have experienced a greater incidence of reoperation for recurrence in infants under 2 months of age when subclavian flap aortoplasty was used instead of end-to-end anastomosis.[30]

The incidence of recoarctation after patch aortoplasty repair has been less in some series and equivalent in others when compared with end-to-end anastomoses.[10,19,41] The comparison between subclavian flap and patch aortoplasty has not been reported.

Having coarctation repair in the neonatal period (compared with later childhood, adolescence, or adulthood) is somewhat protective against the late development of upper body arterial hypertension in the absence of a significant resting gradient. This protection, obviously, is not conferred on those neonates who have hypertension at the time of discharge; indeed, they are more likely to remain hypertensive or redevelop elevated blood pressure at a later date.

Late aneurysm formation is a problem in patients with patch angioplasty repair as neonates. Based on their experience in somewhat older patients, Bergdahl and Ljungqvist discourage use of patch aortoplasty because of its association with late aneurysm development.[3]

When coarctation repair is performed in *infants* without other complex cardiac lesions, as many as 7 per cent of these patients will require subsequent operation within childhood for subvalvular or valvular aortic stenosis. Moreover, repair of neonatal coarctation will not alter the predilection for bacterial endocarditis in patients with bicuspid aortic valves.

Interrupted Arch

Early Results

In the single-stage repair of interrupted aortic arch and correctable coexisting lesions (ventricular septal defect, aorticopulmonary window), recent reports of the early results have been promising. Hammon and colleagues[18] obtained eight of eight neonatal survivors; Norwood had 10 of 13 survivors.[36] Alternatively, when only arch repair and palliation of the lesions are accomplished initially, the operative mortality can range from 30 per cent to 80 per cent or more.

Late Results

Intermediate survival among hospital survivors of single-stage repair of interrupted arch is 75 to 85 per cent for a follow-up period of 1 to 9 years. Among those patients who survive initial interruption repair and palliation of other lesions and later undergo definitive repair, intermediate survival is about 60 per cent. Consideration of these combined early and late findings has led to the following formulation: Whenever possible, interruption and coexisting cardiac lesions should be repaired concomitantly.

Data on the development of anastomosis or conduit stenoses are limited and inconclusive. An early impression is that pressure gradients are going to be natural occurrences as the child grows, regardless of the method of repair (interposed synthetic tube graft, direct anastomosis, or turned-down endogenous vascular tissue conduit). Although mixed results have been realized with use of endogenous vessel or direct end-to-end anastomosis repair, Kron believes these anastomoses *can* grow in older survivors.[22]

Intermediate survivors of interruption repair are at moderate risk for the development of subvalvular aortic stenosis. In one of the largest series reported by Norwood and colleagues, of nine intermediate survivors undergoing follow-up catheterization 1 to 3 years after repair, six had subvalvular aortic stenosis. The gradients in two patients were mild (that is, less than 20 mmHg); in four patients they were severe (greater than 50 mmHg), necessitating reoperation.[36]

Left Heart Atresia

At least in the short-intermediate–term, left heart atresia is no longer necessarily a uniformly lethal disease. Lang and Norwood report a 63 per cent hospital mortality associated with stage I repair (palliation). Of four patients who underwent the final (stage II) repair, two survivors were alive 1 year later.[24] Operative mortality, even in experienced hands, remains high and justifies a continued search for the proper surgical therapy for this lesion. The encouraging early results with cardiac allotransplantation offers another therapeutic avenue for the treatment of this severe anomaly.

CONCLUSION

Suffering from cardiopulmonary congestion, the neonate presenting with left ventricular outflow obstruction is virtually always critically ill. Congestive heart failure worsens, and systemic hypoperfusion results, with closure of the ductus arteriosus.

Any reasonable expectation of a successful outcome is predicated on early collaboration among the neonatologist, pediatric cardiologist, and surgeon. The likelihood of a good result is directly and inextricably related to the infant's condition at the time of operation. Preoperative care, including definitive diagnostic tests, must be delivered in an efficient, streamlined, and decisive manner in order to optimize the newborn's medical condition. Owing its pivotal therapeutic role to its peculiar ductal and pulmonary vascular relaxant properties, infusion of prostaglandin E_1 has been an indispensable adjunctive therapy. Indeed, prostaglandin E_1 has been crucial in the advancement of surgical management and thus in the improvement of survival.

Although the precise procedure of choice, in some instances, is controversial, definitive therapy of the various forms of neonatal left ventricular outflow obstruction remains surgical. Depending on the nature of the lesion and the existence of other complicating cardiac anomalies, primary operation or staged surgical intervention may be curative or just palliative. Moreover, just as left ventricular outflow obstruction as a class represents a spectrum of diseases, likewise the results of surgical management for the various defects distribute themselves fairly evenly along the continuum between high hospital mortality and excellent late survival. Fortunately, operation on these infants, in general, has yielded acceptably modest morbidity. These patients are not placed at undue disadvantage, as a rule, from surgical intervention just because they are neonates!

In short, and in relative terms, surgical management of neonatal left ventricular outflow obstruction is yet in its formative stage. While substantial progress has been made, much remains to be accomplished (particularly in the sphere of left heart atresia). To be sure, there is good reason to be encouraged.

References

1. Bailey CP, Redondo Ramirez HP, Larzelere HB (1952): Surgical treatment of aortic stenosis. JAMA 150:1647–1652.
2. Barratt-Boyes BG, Nicholls TT, Brandt PWT, Neutze JM (1972): Aortic arch interruption associated wth patent ductus arteriosus, ventricular septal defect, and total anomalous pulmonary venous connection. J Thorac Cardiovasc Surg 63:367–373.
3. Bergdahl L, Ljungqvist A (1980): Long-term results after repair of coarctation of the aorta by patch grafting. J Thorac Cardiovasc Surg 80:177–181.

4. Bergdahl LAL, Blackstone EH, Kirklin JW, Pacifico AD, Bargeron LM (1982): Determinants of early success in repair of aortic coarctation in infants. J Thorac Cardiovasc Surg 83:736–742.

5. Berry CL, Tawes RL Jr (1970): Mucopolysaccharides of the aortic wall in coarctation and recoarctation. Cardiovasc Res 4:224–227.

6. Blalock A, Park EA (1944): The surgical treatment of experimental coarctation (atresia) of the aorta. Ann Surg 119:445–456.

7. Brom AG (1965): Narrowing of the aortic isthmus and enlargement of the mind. J Thorac Cardiovasc Surg 50:166–180.

8. Campbell DB, Waldhausen JA, Pierce WS, Fripp R, Whitman V (1984): Should elective repair of coarctation of the aorta be done in infancy? J Thorac Cardiovasc Surg 88:929–938.

9. Cayler GG, Smeloff EA, Miller GE (1970): Surgical palliation of hypoplastic left side of the heart. N Engl J Med 282:780–783.

10. Connor TM, Baker WP (1981): A comparison of coarctation resection and patch angioplasty using postexercise blood pressure measurements. Circulation 64:567–572.

11. Crafoord C, Nylin G (1945): Congenital coarctation of the aorta and its surgical treatment. J Thorac Surg 14:347–361.

12. Doty DB (1980): Aortic atresia. J Thorac Cardiovasc Surg 79:462–463.

13. Edmunds LH, Wagner HR, Heymann MA (1980): Aortic valvulotomy in neonates. Circulation 61:421–427.

14. Ellis FH, Kirklin JW (1962): Congenital valvular aortic stenosis: Anatomic findings and surgical technique. J Thorac Cardiovasc Surg 43:199–202.

15. Freedom RM, Williams WG, Dische MR, Rowe RD (1976): Anatomical variants in aortic atresia: Potential candidates for ventriculoaortic reconstitution. Br Heart J 38:821–826.

16. Gross RE (1945): Surgical correction for coarctation of the aorta. Surgery 18:673–678.

17. Hammon JW Jr, Graham TP Jr, Boucek RJ, Bender HW Jr (1985): Operative repair of coarctation of the aorta in infancy: Results with and without ventricular septal defect. Am J Cardiol 55:1555–1559.

18. Hammon JW Jr, Merrill WH, Prager RL, Graham TP, Bender HW Jr (1986): Repair of interrupted aortic arch and associated malformations in infancy: Indications for complete or partial repair. Ann Thorac Surg 42:17–21.

19. Hesslein PS, McNamara DG, Morriss MJH, Hallman GL, Cooley DA (1981): Comparison of resection versus patch aortoplasty for repair of coarctation in infants and children. Circulation 64:164–168.

20. Khoury GH, Hawes CR (1968): Recurrent coarctation of the aorta in infancy and childhood. J Pediatr 72:801–806.

21. Kirklin JW, Barratt–Boyes BG (1986): Cardiac Surgery. New York, John Wiley and Sons, pp 988, 1061.

22. Kron IL, Rheuban KS, Carpenter MS, Nolan SP (1983): Interrupted aortic arch. J Thorac Cardiovasc Surg 86:37–40.

23. Lang P, Freed MD, Rosenthal A, Castaneda AR, Nadas AS (1977): The use of prostaglandin E$_1$ in an infant with interruption of the aortic arch. J Pediatr 91:805–807.

24. Lang P, Norwood WI (1983): Hemodynamic assessment after palliative surgery for hypoplastic left heart syndrome. Circulation 68:104–108.

25. Leoni F, Huhta JC, Douglas J, MacKay R, de Leval MR, Macartney FJ, Stark J (1984): Effect of prostaglandin on early surgical mortality in obstructive lesions of the systemic circulation. Br Heart J 52:654–659.

26. Lewis AB, Freed MD, Heymann MA, Roehl SL, Kensey RC (1981): Side effects of therapy with prostaglandin E$_1$ in infants with critical congenital heart disease. Circulation 64:893–898.

27. Lewis FJ, Shumway NE, Niazi SA, Benjamin RB (1956): Aortic valvulotomy under direct vision during hypothermia. J Thorac Surg 32:481–492.

28. Merrill DL, Webster CA, Samson PC (1957): Congenital absence of the aortic isthmus. J Thorac Surg 33:311–320.

29. Messina LM, Turley K, Stanger P, Hoffman JIE, Ebert PA (1984): Successful aortic valvotomy for severe congenital valvular aortic stenosis in the newborn infant. J Thorac Cardiovasc Surg 88:92–96.

30. Metzdorff MT, Cobanoglu A, Grunkemeier GL, Sunderland CO, Starr A (1985): Influence of age at operation on late results with subclavian flap aortoplasty. J Thorac Cardiovasc Surg 89:235–241.

31. Moulton AL, Brenner JI, Roberts G, Tavares S, Ali S, Nordenberg A, Burns JE, Ringel R, Berman MA, McLaughlin JS (1984): Subclavian flap repair of coarctation of the aorta in neonates. J Thorac Cardiovasc Surg 87:220–235.

32. Mulder DG, Linde LM (1959): Recurrent coarctation of the aorta in infancy. Am Surg 25:908–911.

33. Mustard WT, Rowe RD, Keith JD, Sirek A (1955): Coarctation of the aorta with special reference to the first year of life. Ann Surg 141:429–436.

34. Norwood WI, Kirklin JK, Sanders SP (1980): Hypoplastic left heart syndrome: Experience with palliative surgery. Am J Cardiol 45:87–91.

35. Norwood WI, Stellin GJ (1981): Aortic atresia with interrupted aortic arch. J Thorac Cardiovasc Surg 81:239–244.

36. Norwood WI, Lang P, Castaneda AR, Hougen TJ (1983): Reparative operations for interrupted aortic arch with ventricular septal defect. J Thorac Cardiovasc Surg 86:832–837.

37. Norwood WI, Lang P, Hansen DD (1983): Physiologic repair of aortic atresia–hypoplastic left heart syndrome. N Engl J Med 308:23–26.

38. Parr GVS, Waldhausen JA, Bharati S, Lev M, Fripp R, Whitman V (1983): Coarctation in Taussig-Bing malformation of the heart. J Thorac Cardiovasc Surg 86:280–287.

39. Radford DJ, Bloom KR, Coceani F, Fariello R, Olley PM (1976): Prostaglandin E$_1$ for interrupted aortic arch in the neonate (letter). Lancet 2:95.

40. Rodbard S (1958): Physical factors in the progression of stenotic vascular lesions. Circulation 17:410–417.

41. Sade RM, Taylor AB, Chariker EP (1979): Aortoplasty compared with resection for coarctation of the aorta in young children. Ann Thorac Surg 28:346–353.

42. Sade RM, Crawford FA, Fyfe DA (1986): Letters to the Editor. J Thorac Cardiovasc Surg 91:937–939.

43. Sirak HD, Ressallat M, Hosier DM, deLorimier AA (1968): A new operation for repairing aortic arch atresia in infancy. Circulation 37, 38 (Suppl II):45–50.

44. Spencer FC, Neill CA, Bahnson HT (1958): The treatment of congenital aortic stenosis with valvotomy during cardiopulmonary bypass. Surgery 44:109–124.

45. Swan H, Kortz AB (1956): Direct vision trans-aortic approach to the aortic valve during hypothermia: Experimental observations and report of successful clinical case. Ann Surg 144:205–214.

46. Tawes RL, Aberdeen E, Waterston DJ, Carter REB (1969): Coarctation of the aorta in infants and children. Circulation 39, 40 (Suppl I):173–184.

47. Trinkle JK, Norton JB, Richardson JD, Grove FL, Noonan JA (1975): Closed aortic valvotomy and simultaneous correction of associated anomalies in infants. J Thorac Cardiovasc Surg 69:758–762.

48. Trinkle JK, Grover FL, Arom KV (1978): Closed aortic valvotomy in infants: Late results. J Thorac Cardiovasc Surg 76:198–201.

49. Tuffier T (1913): Etat actuel de la chirurgie intrathoracique. Tr Internat Cong Med Sect VIII Surg, pt 2, p 249.

50. Van Mierop LHS, Kutsche LM (1986): Cardiovascular anomalies in DiGeorge syndrome and importance of neural crest as a possible pathogenetic factor. Am J Cardiol 58:133–137.

51. Waldhausen JA, Nahrwold DL (1966): Repair coarctation of the aorta with a subclavian flap. J Thorac Cardiovasc Surg 51:532–533.

63 NEONATAL SURGERY FOR CRITICAL PULMONARY STENOSIS

John G. Coles
George A. Trusler

Critical pulmonary stenosis with an intact ventricular septum presenting in the neonatal period is a deceptively lethal disorder. The clinical course of patients with critical pulmonary stenosis resembles that of pulmonary atresia with intact ventricular septum much more than it does the more benign course associated with isolated pulmonary stenosis in older infants and children. These infants are critically ill and ductus dependent and require urgent evaluation and surgical treatment in the first few days of life.

HISTORICAL PERSPECTIVE

Blalock was the first surgeon to report the results of surgical treatment in a series of patients having congenital valvular pulmonary stenosis.[2] The surgical technique used in that series was a closed transventricular approach described earlier by Brock[3] in patients with tetralogy of Fallot; Brock, in turn, credited Doyen with the original application of this approach. In 1913, Doyen attempted pulmonary valvotomy using a tenotomy knife introduced into the infundibulum of the right ventricle; the patient, a 20-year-old girl who probably had tetralogy of Fallot, died several hours later.[5] Mustard and Trusler, in 1960[9] and later in 1968,[8] described the results of surgical treatment of critical pulmonary stenosis in the neonatal period using transarterial pulmonary valvotomy with inflow occlusion.

CLINICAL FEATURES

Morphologically, infants with critical pulmonary stenosis typically have a minute pulmonary valve orifice associated with a variable degree of maldevelopment of the right ventricle, consisting of concentric hypertrophy with cavitary hypoplasia. The pulmonary annulus may be small and tends to be commensurate in size with the right ventricular infundibulum. In contrast to pulmonary atresia with an intact ventricular septum, the right ventricle in critical pulmonary stenosis is nearly always tripartite and coronary sinusoids are rare. Cardiac catheterization almost invariably demonstrates suprasystemic right ventricular pressures associated with functional tricuspid incompetence. A patent foramen ovale or a secundum atrial septal defect and a patent ductus arteriosus are usual. Experience suggests that the diagnosis of critical pulmonary stenosis

and its differentiation from pulmonary atresia with intact ventricular septum can be reliably confirmed on the basis of two dimensional echocardiography with continuous-wave Doppler interrogation.

SURGICAL MANAGEMENT

A previous study from the Hospital for Sick Children, Toronto, based on 36 neonatal infants with critical pulmonary stenosis, demonstrated the limitations of pulmonary valvotomy as an isolated therapeutic measure. Review of that experience indicated that provision of an extracardiac source of pulmonary blood flow, accomplished by a systemic-pulmonary shunt or prostaglandin E_1 (PGE_1) infusion continued postoperatively, was the most important determinant of early survival. This conclusion has been substantiated by a more recent analysis of the complete experience, including 51 infants (all under 14 days of age) with this disorder (January 1967–January 1986).

Management protocols have varied but can be summarized on the basis of inclusion of either a surgical shunt or perioperative PGE_1 infusion as an adjunct to pulmonary valvotomy (Table 63–1). Logistic regression analysis confirms that the use of either of these adjuncts to pulmonary valvotomy yields a significantly higher early survival rate.

SURGICAL TECHNIQUE

Several surgical approaches have evolved to accomplish pulmonary valvotomy, including transarterial pulmonary valvotomy with or without inflow occlusion, closed transventricular pulmonary valvotomy, and open pulmonary valvotomy supported by cardiopulmonary bypass. Our experience involving each of these methods indicates that the specific technique used to perform pulmonary valvotomy has not influenced the early results (Table 63–2).

We concur with others[4,6,7,10] in recommending a transventricular pulmonary valvotomy that can generally be performed with less blood loss than open techniques and readily allows the simultaneous creation of a modified Blalock-Taussig shunt through a single operative approach. An extended left fourth anterolateral intercostal thoracotomy provides good exposure of the right ventricle and allows insertion of an interposition Gore-Tex shunt between the undivided left subclavian artery and the left pulmonary artery immediately distal to the ductal insertion. Alternatively, the right ventricular outflow tract can be approached through a right thoracotomy, which allows creation of a right-sided modified Blalock shunt. With either the right- or left-sided approach, more direct access to the axis of the right ventricular outflow tract is afforded with the surgeon positioned on the right side of the operating table. To perform pulmonary valvotomy, a stab incision is made within a pledget-reinforced pursestring suture controlled by tourniquets placed in the anterior wall of the right ventricle just proximal to the infundibulum. The pulmonary valve is opened using a Pott or Himmelstein valvulotome, or valvotomy may simply be accomplished using graduated Hegar dilators, starting with a 2- or 3-mm diameter dilator and progressing to the estimated diameter of the pulmonary annulus. It is important that PGE_1 infusions be routinely administered preoperatively and intraoperatively and continued postoperatively until patency of the surgical shunt is ensured, and for longer periods in patients in whom a concomitant shunt is not performed. We have generally preferred to proceed with a concomitant shunt, especially in the presence of moderate or severe right ventricle hypoplasia, in order to avoid the need for prolonged periods of PGE_1 therapy.

RESULTS

The operative risk remains rather high even in the more favorable groups managed by perioperative PGE_1 infusion or a surgical shunt in addition to pulmonary valvotomy (see Table 62–1). Preoperative and postoperative two dimensional echocardiograms demonstrate the rather consistent finding of systolic closure of the right ventricular infundibulum producing obstruction at a subvalvular level. This subvalvular obstruction appears to be associated with some degree of residual stenosis at the valve level, results in important residual gradients across the right ventricular outflow tract and in right ventricular hypertension, and has been documented to persist as a conspicuous finding for several weeks in some cases. Right ventricular infundibular obstruction may result from the sudden afterload reduction effect of pulmonary valvotomy, and whether anatomical or dynamic, it probably contributes to the se-

Table 63–1. HOSPITAL DEATHS AFTER SURGICAL TREATMENT OF CRITICAL PULMONARY STENOSIS (1967 TO 1986)

	Treatment Group	No. of Patients	No. of Deaths	Per Cent	70 Per Cent CL
I	Valvotomy only	22	12	55	44–66
II	Valvotomy + shunt	8	2	25	9–41
III	Valvotomy + PGE_1*	13	3	23	11–35
IV	Miscellaneous†	5	3	60	27–93
	Total	48	20	42	33–50

Groups II + III vs I: p (logistic) = 0.026
*Includes patients receiving PGE_1 therapy before, during, and after surgery.
†Includes four delayed shunts (two deaths) and one shunt only (died).
CL = Confidence limits.

vere and sometimes fatal right ventricular failure occurring in the postoperative period.

The late results among hospital survivors of pulmonary valvotomy in the neonatal period have been good. Repeat cineangiography in 16 patients performed at 38 ± 8 months postoperatively demonstrated consistent growth of the right ventricle as well as the pulmonary annulus and pulmonary arteries. Tricuspid incompetence was absent at the time of recatheterization in 81 per cent of patients, whereas this finding had been almost invariably present in the neonatal period. Late reoperation to repair residual right ventricular outflow tract obstruction was required in more than 25 per cent of patients at 5 years and in more than 50 per cent of patients at 10 years postoperatively and was significantly more common among patients with a hypoplastic infundibulum on the initial angiographic study (Fig. 63–1). In patients requiring reoperation, the obstruction was at the valve level but was usually associated with subvalvular infundibular obstruction necessitating a transannular patch repair. The results of late reoperation have been favorable (Table 63–3).

PERCUTANEOUS BALLOON PULMONARY VALVE ANGIOPLASTY

Our experience with balloon pulmonary valve angioplasty is limited to three patients and has yielded mixed

Table 63–2. HOSPITAL DEATHS AFTER SURGICAL TREATMENT OF CRITICAL PULMONARY STENOSIS (1967 TO 1986)

Technique of Pulmonary Valvotomy	No. of Patients*	No. of Deaths	Per Cent	70 Per Cent CL
Transarterial, inflow occlusion	18	7	39	27–51
Transarterial, no inflow occlusion	8	2	25	9–41
Transventricular	10	4	40	24–56
Cardiopulmonary bypass†	10	5	50	34–66

*Excludes two patients having combined transventricular and transarterial pulmonary valvotomy (neither survived).
†Includes three patients undergoing profoundly hypothermic circulatory arrest.
CL = confidence limits.

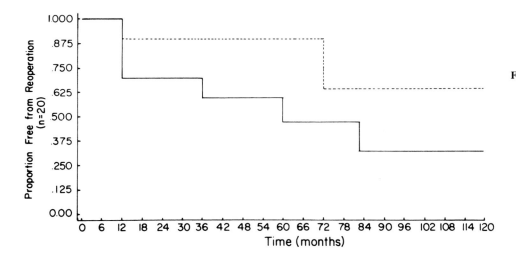

Figure 63–1. Actuarial freedom from reoperation according to the morphological status of the right ventricular infundibulum among 20 hospital survivors with critical pulmonary stenosis. Ten patients had a normal infundibulum (- - - -), and 10 had a hypoplastic infundibulum (——). Regression coefficient (Cox) for this variable = 0.9161; $p = 0.07$ (Wilcoxon).

results. The technique was successful in one patient with a well-developed right ventricle, was unsuccessful in another because the catheter guide wire could not be negotiated across the pulmonary valve, and resulted in right ventricular infundibular rupture in the third patient that eventuated in successful repair at operation. Although the preliminary results of balloon valvuloplasty in the treatment of congenital valvular pulmonary stenosis in infants and children have been favorable, further experience is required to determine the efficacy of this method in neonates with critical pulmonary stenosis.[1] This topic is further considered in Chapter 56.

CONCLUSIONS

Further improvements in the management of critical pulmonary stenosis are required. The frequent finding of residual right ventricular outflow tract obstruction in the early (as well as late) postoperative period suggests a role for performing open pulmonary valvotomy using bypass in conjunction with an infundibular pericardial patch as a more rational initial procedure. Although we have not yet employed this approach, it presumably would allow a more complete valvotomy and relief of subvalvular obstruction, while preserving some degree of pulmonary valve competence. A primary transannular patch is probably inadvisable since it results in the coexistence of severe pulmonary and tricuspid incompetence in the neonatal period[6] and is unnecessary since consistent growth of the pulmonary annulus has been demonstrated on late reevaluation. Whether the potential benefits resulting from simultaneous correction of infundibular obstruction in addition to pulmonary valvotomy justify the risks attendant to the use of bypass and a procedure of slightly greater magnitude remains to be determined.

Table 63–3. SECONDARY AND TERTIARY PROCEDURES

Type of Reoperation	No. of Patients	Hospital Deaths	Per Cent CL
ASD closure	1	0	
Pulmonary valvotomy + ASD closure	2	0	
Transannular patch	1	0	
Transannular patch + ASD closure	3*	0	
Transannular patch + ASD closure + Potts closure	1	1†	
Total	8	1	12 (70% CL: 2–36%)

*One patient subsequently underwent successful insertion of a pulmonary valve.
†Operative death.
ASD = atrial septal defect; CL = confidence limits
Reproduced with permission fom Coles JG et al (1984): Ann Thorac Surg 38:458–465.

References

1. Awariefe SO, Clarke DR, Pappas G (1983): Surgical approach to critical pulmonary valve stenosis in infants less than six months of age. J Thorac Cardiovasc Surg 85:375–387.
2. Blalock A, Keiffer RF (1950): Valvotomy for the relief of congenital valvular pulmonary stenosis with intact ventricular septum: Report of 19 operations by the Brock method. Ann Surg 132:496–516.
3. Brock RC (1948): Pulmonary valvotomy for the relief of congenital pulmonary stenosis: Report of 3 cases. Br Med J 1:1121–1126.
4. Daskalopoulos DA, Pieroni DR, Gingell RL, Rowland JM, Subramanian S (1982): Closed transventricular pulmonary valvotomy in infants. J Thorac Cardiovasc Surg 84:187–191.
5. Dumont J (1913): Chirurgie des malformations congenitales ou acquisés du coeur pres. Presse Med 21:860.
6. Kveselis DA, Rocchini AP, Snider R, Rosenthal A, Crowley C, Dick M II (1985): Results of balloon valvuloplasty in the treatment of congenital valvar pulmonary stenosis in children. Am J Cardiol 56:527–532.
7. Milo S, Yellin A, Smolinsky A, Blieden LC, Neufeld HN, Goor DA (1980): Closed pulmonary valvulotomy in infants under six months of age: Report of fourteen consecutive cases without mortality. Thorax 35:814–818.
8. Mustard WT, Jain SC, Trusler GA (1968): Pulmonary stenosis in the first year of life. Br Heart J 30:255–257.
9. Mustard WT, Rowe RD, Firor WB Jr (1960): Pulmonic stenosis in the first year of life: Results of surgery. Surgery 47:678–684.
10. Srinivasan V, Konyer A, Broda JJ, Subramanian S (1982): Critical pulmonary stenosis in infants less than three months of age: A reappraisal of closed transventricular pulmonary valvulotomy in infants. J Thorac Cardiovasc Surg 85:375–387.

64 NEONATAL REPAIR OF TETRALOGY OF FALLOT

Aldo R. Castañeda

Richard A. Jonas

HISTORICAL PERSPECTIVE

The surgical treatment of tetralogy of Fallot was initiated by Blalock and Taussig in 1945 with the establishment of a subclavian artery-to-pulmonary artery anastomosis.[3] Two years later, Potts and associates introduced the descending aorta-to-left pulmonary artery shunt, a technique primarily designed for infants.[15] Waterston's ascending aorta-to-right pulmonary artery anastomosis,[21] and other modifications,[8,11] provided an important alternative to the Blalock-Taussig and Potts operations. Sellors[19] and Brock[5] introduced a different palliative approach by focusing on the right ventricular outflow tract obstruction directly, performing a pulmonary valvotomy and closed infundibulectomy and leaving the ventricular septal defect open.

In a brilliant and daring effort, Lillehei and coworkers, in 1955, performed the first intracardiac repair of tetralogy of Fallot using controlled cross-circulation.[12] The operation included closure of the ventricular septal defect and relief of the right ventricular outflow tract obstruction under direct vision. Lillehei and coworkers also recognized early the need to enlarge the right ventricular outflow tract with a patch.[13] The interposition of a right ventricular to pulmonary artery (nonvalved) prosthetic conduit for patients with tetralogy of Fallot and pulmonary atresia was first reported by Klinner and Zenker in 1964.[10] One year later, Rastelli and colleagues fashioned a pericardial conduit for the same purpose.[17] In 1966, Ross and Somerville first reported the use of a valved homograft to bridge the gap between the right ventricle and the pulmonary arteries.[18]

Although during the early experience with cross-circulation at the University of Minnesota, several infants underwent successful repair of tetralogy of Fallot, because of the higher mortality and morbidity with primary repair of tetralogy of Fallot in infants and young children, a two-stage approach, that is, a systemic artery-to-pulmonary artery shunt followed later by takedown of the shunt and repair of tetralogy of Fallot became more widely favored. In 1971, Barratt-Boyes and colleagues at Green Lane Hospital in New Zealand reintroduced the idea of primary repair of tetralogy of Fallot in infants,[2] a policy that we also adopted.[6,14]

Fallot's original concept (1888) of four coexisting defects (i.e., pulmonary outflow tract stenosis, ventricular septal defect, dextroposition of the aorta, and right ventricular hypertrophy) has been challenged by Van Praagh and colleagues, who favor the notion that tetralogy of Fallot is a monology, resulting principally from the underdevelopment or hypoplasia of the right ventricular infundibulum or conus.[20] The infundibular septum, which normally follows a posterior inferior and rightward course, is deviated superiorly and anteriorly in tetralogy of Fallot, thus contributing importantly to the obstruction of the right ventricular outflow tract. By remaining anterior and superior, the infundibular septum also fails to occupy the space above the ventricular septum between the left anterosuperior and right posteroinferior limbs of the septal band, resulting in the typical large malaligned ventricular septal defect, which is posterior and inferior to the infundibular septum. This primary infundibular hypoplasia is particularly evident in the neonate and young infant with tetralogy of Fallot, in whom the malpositioned infundibular septum, the septal band, and the right ventricular free wall have not yet undergone secondary hypertrophic changes.

INDICATIONS FOR PRIMARY SURGICAL REPAIR

Approximately 70 per cent of patients with tetralogy of Fallot require an operation during the first year of life because of either hypoxic spells or persistent severe hypoxemia (resting oxygen saturation less than 70 per cent). In our experience with repair of tetralogy of Fallot in 175 infants, the mean age at operation was 5.8 months; 14 per cent of these patients required an operation within the first month of life. Anatomically, this group of symptomatic neonates with tetralogy of Fallot generally has either diffuse right ventricular outflow tract hypoplasia (9 patients [36 per cent]) or congenital pulmonary atresia (16 patients [64 per cent]) (Fig. 64–1).

Diffuse infundibular hypoplasia in the neonate is almost invariably associated with a hypoplastic valve annulus and pulmonary arteries. However, in our experience, these hypoplastic pulmonary arteries prove in most instances to be quite distensible and therefore dilate significantly once right ventricular to pulmonary artery continuity has been established. Nevertheless, it is important preoperatively to identify localized areas of stenosis within the pulmonary vascular tree. The most common site of segmental obstruction is close to the origin of the left pulmonary artery, seemingly related to the entrance site of the ductus arteriosus.

In congenital pulmonary atresia, the infundibular septum is commonly fused with the anterior free wall and the pulmonary valve is reduced to a fibrous diaphragm. Beyond the atretic segment, the main pulmonary artery is often in continuity and pulmonary flow is supplied in approximately 50 per cent of the patients by a patent ductus arteriosus. If there is anatomic (long segment) discontinuity between the right ventricle and the right and left pulmonary arteries, or in the even more rare instance of absence of either central and hilar portions of one or both pulmonary arteries, primary repair is not advised in the neonate at this time. These patients commonly have large direct or indirect aortopulmonary collaterals.

Preoperative studies should include biplane cineangiography. For adequate planning of surgical repair, the area of bifurcation of the pulmonary trunk, the left and right pulmonary arteries, and the intraparenchymal distribution of the pulmonary artery branches must be visualized. It is critical to identify areas of localized stenosis within the pulmonary arteries. The cranially tilted frontal view, commonly referred to as "sitting up position," provides an ideal view of these areas.[1] We also insist on a left ventriculogram to rule out additional ventricular septal defects and also to visualize the origin and course of coronary arteries, particularly anomalous origin of the anterior descending coronary artery from the right coronary artery, which is present in approximately 5 per cent of patients with tetralogy of Fallot.[9]

Presently, primary repair of tetralogy of Fallot, irrespective of age or weight, is preferred to a two-stage approach in neonates and infants with hypoxic spells and/or persistent hypoxemia. Systemic artery-to-pulmonary artery shunts are reserved for those rare infants with tetralogy of Fallot and an anomalous origin of the anterior descending coronary artery from the right coronary artery, or for patients with tetralogy of Fallot and long segment discontinuity between the right ventricle and the pulmonary arteries.

Although propranolol has been used to decrease right ventricular outflow tract obstruction with the expectation of postponing surgery, particularly in the younger infant, our experience with propranolol is limited. However, 15 per cent of the infants who had repair of the defect were referred to us from other centers because of failure of propranolol (up to 2.5 mg/kg/day) to provide adequate palliation. Parenthetically, the risk of repair did not increase in infants who were being treated with propranolol.

The one-stage repair avoids the cumulative risk of two operations, eliminates the common complications of shunts performed in the neonate and during early infancy, and significantly decreases the psychological and economic burden on the family. In our experience, the superiority of the one-stage approach has been substantiated by the early and late postoperative outcome.[4,7] Because of these encouraging results with repair of Fallot's tetralogy in infancy, we have also steadily decreased the age of elective repair, primarily to avoid the secondary hypertrophic changes of the infundibular septum and the right ventricular free wall and also the development of heavy trabeculations binding the parietal and septal bands to the right ventricular free wall. We now carry out elective repair in asymptomatic infants within the second year of life. With the availability of homografts, repair is postponed to 3 or 4 years of age in patients requiring a valved conduit.

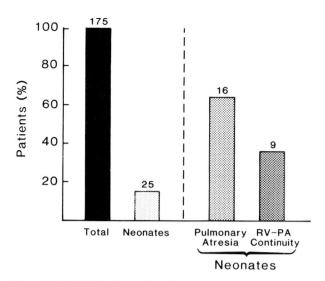

Figure 64–1. Of 175 patients who underwent tetralogy of Fallot (TOF) repair in infancy, 25 were neonates. Of this group of symptomatic neonates with TOF, 16 patients (64 per cent) had pulmonary valve atresia.

SURGICAL TECHNIQUE

Anesthesia

Because of the presence of a right-to-left shunt in patients with tetralogy of Fallot, a sudden or significant decrease in systemic peripheral resistance must be avoided; anesthesia is therefore induced with ketamine (1 to 2 mg/kg) intravenously. Succinylcholine or curare (0.5 mg/kg) is given to facilitate intubation, and the patient is subsequently maintained on nitrous oxide, oxygen, and curare.

A 22-gauge plastic cannula is placed in the radial artery by cutdown. A 20-gauge catheter is placed in a central vein, either transcutaneously or by cutdown to a peripheral vein. Temperature probes are placed in the nasopharynx, esophagus, and rectum, and the bladder is catheterized using a No. 8 or 10 F catheter. Pulse oximetry prior to anesthesia induction is now a useful monitoring adjunct.

Operation

Through a median sternotomy, cardiopulmonary bypass is instituted using an ascending aortic cannula (10 F) and a venous (16 F) cannula placed through the right atrial appendage. The oxygenator prime combines Ringer's lactate solution with heparinized bank blood (3000 units/500 ml) in the proportion required to produce a final hematocrit of 20 per cent during bypass. During core cooling the main pulmonary artery and the right pulmonary artery are dissected free from the ascending aorta. The ductus arteriosus, if patent, is ligated, and a rectangular segment of pericardium is excised for subsequent use in the reconstruction of the right ventricular outflow tract. At 20°C rectal temperature, the aorta is cross-clamped and cardioplegic solution is infused. The circulation is stopped, and the right atrial cannula is removed.

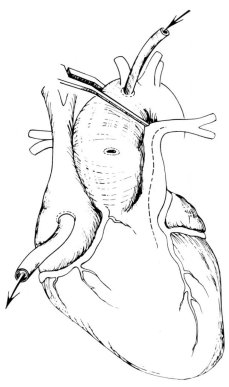

Figure 64–2. Tetralogy of Fallot repair. Vertical incision through right ventricular outflow tract, pulmonary valve annulus, main pulmonary artery, and stenosed origin of left pulmonary artery. Ascending aortic cannula (10 F) and right atrial venous return cannula (16 F) in place. Aorta is cross-clamped.

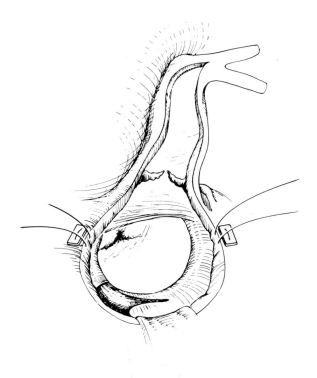

Figure 64–3. Tetralogy of Fallot repair. View of ventricular septal defect, bordered superiorly by the hypoplastic infundibular septum, on the left by the anterosuperior limb of the septal band, and inferiorly by the right posteroinferior limb of the septal band and the fibrous confluency of tricuspid valve tissue and aortic annulus. Note dysplastic pulmonary valve leaflets.

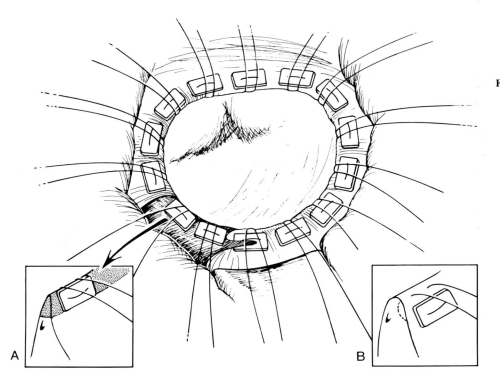

Figure 64–4. Tetralogy of Fallot repair. All interrupted and pledgeted sutures in place within the rim of the ventricular septal defect (VSD). *A,* Inferoposterior border of the VSD capped by dense fibrous rim formed by the confluence of aortic valve annulus and tricuspid valve tissue. The more superficially located conduction bundle is protected by placing stitches within the tough fibrous tissue. *B,* Inferoposterior border of the VSD formed by well-developed muscle of the posteroinferior limb of the septal hand. In this case the bundle of His is imbedded within muscle and is more closely related to the left ventricular aspect of the ventricular crest.

A vertical incision is made in the free wall of the infundibulum. If the pulmonary valve annulus is hypoplastic or the dysplastic leaflets are obstructive, the incision is extended through the annulus to the bifurcation of the main pulmonary artery (Fig. 64–2). The pulmonary leaflets, if thickened, are excised. Not uncommonly, there is a localized stenosis within the proximal left pulmonary artery, in which case the incision must extend beyond the obstruction into the distal left pulmonary artery. Proximally the incision is limited to the level of the infundibular septum. Deep hypothermia and cardioplegia render the heart quite flaccid, facilitating intracardiac exposure and hence allowing for a shorter ventriculotomy. Since in the neonate there is virtually no hypertrophy of the infundibular septum, nor are there yet heavily muscular trabeculations, resection of muscle from the outflow tract is avoided. Excision of infundibular septum and free ventricular wall muscle may well weaken function of the right ventricle postoperatively. We, in fact, make only a small tangential incision where the infundibular septum fuses with the anterior right ventricular free wall (infundibuloventricular fold) to facilitate exposure of both the posteroinferior and posterosuperior margin of the ventricular septal defect (Fig. 64–3). The malalignment-type ventricular septal defect is closed with a Dacron patch using interrupted horizontal mattress sutures (6-0 Teflon-coated Dacron), reinforced by Teflon pledgets (Fig. 64–4). We place the first suture into the midportion of the infundibular septum and progress clockwise. Each subsequent suture helps in exposing the margin of the defect. Once the level of the papillary muscle of the conus is reached, the septal and anterior leaflets of the tricuspid valve are retracted inferiorly. Depending on the type of anatomy, sutures are either placed within the muscular posteroinferior limb of the septal band (Fig. 64–4B) approximately 3 mm from the rim of the defect using shallow bites in the septum or, if the posteroinferior rim of the defect is fibrous, the stitches are anchored within this tough tissue (Fig. 64–4A). The use of Teflon pledgets permits a more shallow placement of sutures, which decreases the risk of encircling and damaging the bundle of His while at the same time avoiding suture line disruption. Once all sutures are in place, a Dacron patch is tailored to the contours of the ventricular septal defect, the sutures are then placed through the Dacron patch and tied (Fig. 64–5). Next, the ventricular septum is searched for additional defects. The muscular portion anterior to the septal band is particularly suspect. If a muscular ventricular septal defect is present, we prefer to use a patch instead of primary closure to avoid tearing of this often very friable tissue.

In our experience, 85 per cent of infants under 3 months of age and 100 per cent of the neonates required a transannular right ventricular outflow tract patch because of hypoplasia of the pulmonary valve annulus. This high incidence of transannular outflow patches reflects the severity and the nature of the outflow tract obstruction in patients requiring surgery at such an early age. As mentioned previously, the right ventricular outflow patch is quite often carried across the junction of the main and left

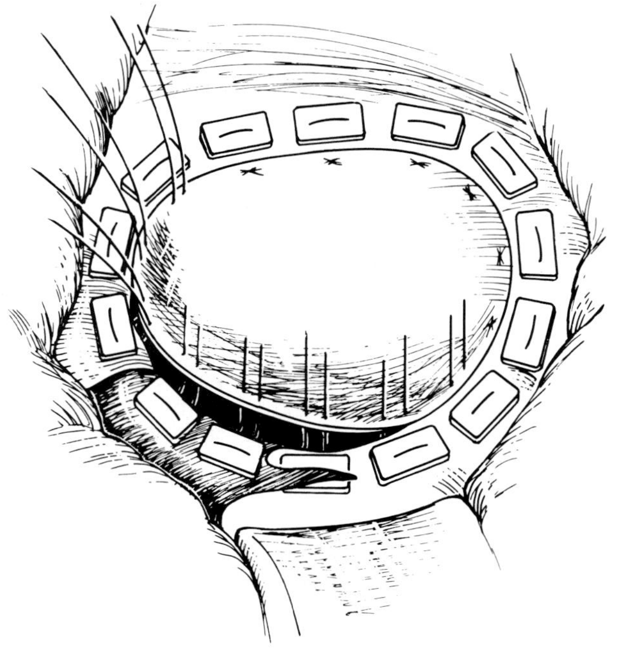

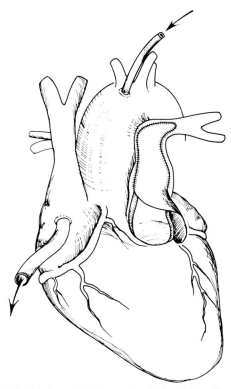

Figure 64–6. Tetralogy of Fallot repair. Pericardial outflow patch is sutured across the right ventricular outflow tract, the hypoplastic pulmonary valve annulus, the main pulmonary artery, and the stenosed orifice of the left pulmonary artery.

Figure 64–5. Tetralogy of Fallot repair. Sutures placed through appropriately tailored Dacron patch and tied.

pulmonary arteries. The rectangular segment of pericardium is secured with a continuous 5-0 prolene suture to the edges of the pulmonary artery and right ventriculotomy incision (Fig. 64–6).

Before the pericardial patch is entirely secured, a pursestring suture is placed in the epicardium of the right ventricular free wall close to the distal end of the ventriculotomy incision and a 20-gauge catheter is guided into the distal pulmonary artery for postoperative monitoring (Fig. 64–7). Once the pericardial outflow patch is completely sutured in place, the right atrium is opened through a small incision to close any coexisting atrial septal defect or large patent foramen ovale (PFO). Small PFOs are left open in order to allow right-to-left decompression during the early postoperative course and also to facilitate transseptal left-sided heart catheterization studies 1 year after surgery.

Repair of Tetralogy of Fallot With Pulmonary Valve Atresia

The vertical ventriculotomy is carried through the area of the atretic infundibular septum and atretic pulmonary valve (diaphragm), extending the incision into the widening main pulmonary artery to its point of bifurcation. Severe narrowing at the atretic area is the rule. To obtain uniform widening of the right ventricular outflow tract, particularly at its narrowest point, a specially tailored patch is sutured (Fig. 64–8) to neighboring areolar tissue surrounding this area rather than along the free edge of

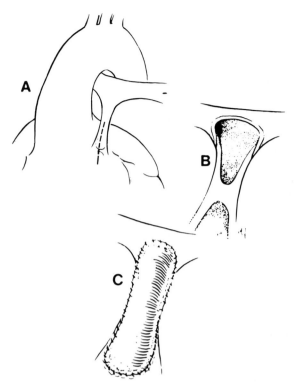

Figure 64–8. Tetralogy of Fallot with pulmonary valve atresia. *A,* Incision through atretic valve area. *B,* Ventricular-pulmonary artery discontinuity caused by atretic segment. Note normal distal PA lumen. *C,* Dacron patch in place. In the area of the atretic segment, the patch is sutured to neighboring areolar tissue.

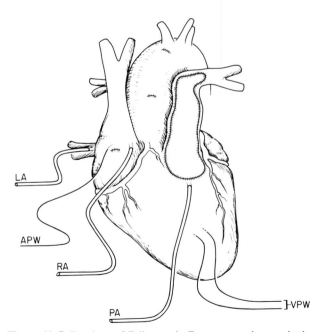

Figure 64–7. Tetralogy of Fallot repair. For postoperative monitoring, 20-gauge catheters are left within the left atrium (LA), right atrium (RA), and pulmonary artery (PA). Atrial (APW) and ventricular (VPW) temporary pacemaker wires are also sutured to the epicardium.

the incision. Uniform widening of the entire length of the right ventricular outflow tract is essential.

POSTOPERATIVE MANAGEMENT

The endotracheal tube is connected to a volume-cycled respirator for at least 24 hours. The neonate is then weaned from the mechanical ventilator using progressively lower intermittent mandatory ventilation rates. The child is extubated when a rate of 4 is tolerated. Intracardiac catheters (left atrial, right atrial, pulmonary artery) facilitate postoperative monitoring, volume replacement, and quantitation of intracardiac shunts (if present), as well as measurement of right ventricular-pulmonary artery pressure gradients during the immediate postoperative period.

Patients do not routinely receive positive inotropic support. Dopamine is used only when low cardiac output is documented.

RESULTS

Three of the 25 neonates died after operation (Table 64–1). However, similar to our experience with other types of corrective operations in neonates and infants,

Table 64–1. REPAIR OF TETRALOGY OF FALLOT IN NEONATES USING DEEP HYPOTHERMIC CIRCULATORY ARREST (JANUARY 1973 TO JANUARY 1986)

Age (days)	No. of Patients	Mortality	
		Hospital	*Late*
0 < 8	9	1 (11.0%)	0
8 < 15	11	1 (9.0%)	0
15 < 31	5	0	1 (20.0%)
Total	**25**	**2 (8.0%)**	**1 (4.0%)**

deaths after repair of tetralogy of Fallot were determined principally by associated conditions or metabolic state rather than by the age or weight of the infants per se. The two neonates who died early had a complex form of absent pulmonary valve syndrome. In both instances the aneurysmal dilatation of the pulmonary arteries extended into the hilar branches with consequent obliteration of pulmonary alveoli.[16] The third patient died suddenly after a viral illness 16 months after the operation. No autopsy was performed.

Hemodynamic studies done 24 hours and 1 year after surgery (16 patients) revealed one residual ventricular shunt (Qp:Qs > 1.5). Four neonates had residual right ventricular outflow tract gradients of greater than 40 mmHg. All four initially had tetralogy of Fallot and pulmonary atresia.

Abolition of intracardiac right-to-left shunting and relief of right ventricular outflow tract obstruction, the principal aims of surgical repair of tetralogy of Fallot, were accomplished in the majority of these neonates. The hemodynamic results after early repair of tetralogy of Fallot were in general very satisfactory, including assessment of left ventricular function. Although the use of transannular patches did not increase the risk of the procedure, an important remaining issue is whether the high incidence of transannular right ventricular outflow patches, used so early in life, will contribute to hemodynamic dysfunction at a later date. This question remains controversial and demands serious long-term evaluation.

References

1. Bargeron LM Jr, Elliott LP, Soto B, Bream PR, Curry GC (1977): Axial cineangiography in congenital heart disease: I. Concept, technical and anatomic considerations. Circulation 56:1075–1083.
2. Barratt-Boyes BG, Simpson M, Neutze JM (1971): Intracardiac surgery in neonates and infants using deep hypothermia with surface cooling and limited cardiopulmonary bypass. Circulation 43,44(suppl 1):25–30.
3. Blalock A, Taussig HB (1945): The surgical treatment of malformations of the heart in which there is pulmonary stenosis or pulmonary atresia. JAMA 128:189–202.
4. Borow KM, Green LH, Castañeda AR, Keane JF (1980): Left ventricular function after repair of tetralogy of Fallot and its relationship to age at surgery. Circulation 61:1150–1158.
5. Brock RC (1948): Pulmonary valvulotomy for relief of congenital pulmonary stenosis: Report of 3 cases. Br Med J 1:1121–1126.
6. Castañeda AR, Freed MD, Williams RG, Norwood WI (1977): Repair of tetralogy of Fallot in infancy: Early and late results. J Thorac Cardiovasc Surg 74:372–381.
7. Castañeda AR, Norwood WI (1983): Fallot's tetralogy. In Stark J, de Leval N (eds): Surgery for Congenital Heart Defects. London, Grune & Stratton, pp 321–329.
8. de Leval MR, McKay R, Jones M, Stark J, Macartney FJ (1981): Modified Blalock-Taussig shunt: Use of subclavian artery orifice as flow regulator in prosthetic systemic-pulmonary artery shunts. J Thorac Cardiovasc Surg 81:112–119.
9. Fellows KE, Freed MD, Keane JR, Van Praagh R, Bernhard WF, Castañeda AC (1975): Results of routine preoperative coronary angiography in tetralogy of Fallot. Circulation 51:561–566.
10. Klinner W, Zenker R (1965): Experience with correction of Fallot's tetralogy in 178 cases. Surgery 57:353–357.
11. Laks H, Castañeda AR (1975): Subclavian arterioplasty for the ipsilateral Blalock-Taussig shunt. Ann Thorac Surg 19:319–321.
12. Lillehei CW, Cohen M, Warden HE, Read RC, Aust JB, DeWall RA, Varco RL (1955): Direct vision intracardiac surgical correction of the tetralogy of Fallot, pentalogy of Fallot, and pulmonary atresia defects: Report of first ten cases. Ann Surg 142:418–442.
13. Lillehei CW, Levy MJ, Adams P, Anderson RC (1964): Corrective surgery for tetralogy of Fallot: Long-term follow-up by postoperative recatheterization in 69 cases and certain surgical considerations. J Thorac Cardiovasc Surg 48:556–576.
14. Murphy JD, Freed MD, Keane JF, Norwood WI, Castañeda AR, Nadas AS (1980): Hemodynamic results after intracardiac repair of tetralogy of Fallot by deep hypothermia and cardiopulmonary bypass. Circulation 62(I):168.
15. Potts WJ, Smith S, Gibson S (1946): Anastomosis of the aorta to a pulmonary artery. JAMA 132:627–634.
16. Rabinovitch M, Grady S, David I, Van Praagh R, Sauer U, Buhlmeyer K, Castañeda AR, Reid LM (with technical assistance of Silva DK) (1982): Compression of intrapulmonary bronchi by abnormally branching pulmonary arteries associated with absent pulmonary valves. Am J Cardiol 50:804–813.
17. Rastelli GC, Ongley PA, Davis GD, Kirklin JW (1965): Surgical repair for pulmonary valve atresia with coronary-pulmonary artery fistula: Report of case. Mayo Clin Proc 40:521–527.
18. Ross DN, Somerville J (1966): Correction of pulmonary atresia with a homograft aortic valve. Lancet 2:1446–1447.
19. Sellors TH (1948): Surgery of pulmonary stenosis: A case in which the pulmonary valve was successfully divided. Lancet 1:988–989.
20. Van Praagh R, Van Praagh S, Nebesar RA, Muster AJ, Sinha SN, Paul MH (1970): Tetralogy of Fallot: Underdevelopment of the pulmonary infundibulum and its sequelae. Am J Cardiol 26:25–33.
21. Waterston DJ (1962): Treatment of Fallot's tetralogy in children under one year of age. Rozhl Chir 41:181–183.

65 REPAIR OF ATRIOVENTRICULAR SEPTAL DEFECTS

Mark E. Sand
Albert D. Pacifico

Atrioventricular (AV) septal defects (atrioventricular canal defects) are characterized by deficiency or absence of septal tissue and usually result in an ostium primum type atrial septal defect immediately above the AV valves and a scooped-out deficiency of the inlet ventricular septum below the AV valves. When the valve leaflets fail to attach to the crest of the ventricular septum, an interventricular communication (VSD) results. The common AV valve may be thought of as a six-leaflet structure (Fig. 65–1).[27] There is great variability in the completeness of each commissure and the leaflet sizes and positions relative to the ventricular septum. Also, the normal "wedged position" of the aorta between the AV valves is absent,[21] and a foreshortened left ventricular inlet and elongated and sometimes (in approximately 1 per cent of patients) a significantly narrowed left ventricular outflow tract are present.[22]

AV septal defect encompasses an anatomic spectrum. The simplest type is the partial form, in which there is an ostium primum atrial septal defect, usually no ventricular septal defect, and a connection between the left superior leaflet and the left inferior leaflet, resulting in two separate left AV valve orifices. The complete form lacks this connection between the left-sided bridging leaflets, resulting in a common valve orifice. The atrial septal defect is accompanied by a ventricular septal defect of variable size and position. Each of the components of AV septal defects has a spectrum as well: size of interatrial communication, size and position of interventricular communication, degree of left superior and left inferior leaflet connection, and degree of bridging of the left superior and left inferior leaflets, respectively.[27] Less common valve abnormalities such as accessory orifices, single papillary muscle (parachute), and leaflet perforations may further complicate surgical repair.[7]

NATURAL HISTORY

Pulmonary vascular resistance usually remains high for the first 2 to 3 months after birth, which limits the magnitude of left-to-right shunting through the interatrial or interventricular defects and makes symptomatic presentation in the neonatal period uncommon. In the absence of major associated cardiac anomalies, only 1 of 140 patients with partial AV canal and 7 of 97 with complete AV septal defect required operation under 3 months of age between 1967 and 1982 at the University of Alabama at Birmingham.[27] Severe heart failure in a newborn infant with AV septal defects is most likely due to severe AV valve incompetence or the presence of associated major cardiac anomalies such as patent ductus arteriosus, coarctation, double-outlet right ventricle without pulmonary stenosis, multiple ventricular septal defects, or other lesions.

The natural history and symptomatic presentation are dependent on the morphologic and functional details of the individual's malformation. Patients without interventricular communications or important AV valve incompetence (approximately 25 per cent of the spectrum of patients) have a natural history similar to those with an isolated type of atrial septal defect (ASD). These patients usually develop symptoms in their second, third, or fourth decade, and only a relatively small number will develop important pulmonary vascular disease. Individuals with a complete form of AV septal defect have the most unfavorable natural history. In the absence of available prospective data, an approximation of the natural history has been derived from two autopsy series.[2] These data predict a 50 per cent chance of survival beyond 6 months and a 30 per cent chance of survival beyond 1 year; 80 per cent of patients without operation will die by 2 years of age. Patients with complete AV septal defects surviving the first year of life have a progressive risk of developing severe pulmonary vascular disease. Newfeld and colleagues have shown that histologically advanced pulmonary vascular disease may occur even in the first year of life.[26] After age 1 year, nearly 90 per cent of cases had histologic evidence of pulmonary vascular disease.

HISTORICAL PERSPECTIVE

The partial form of AV septal defect was successfully repaired in 1954 using the atrial well technique initially described by Gross and then elaborated by others.[9,28] In 1955, Kirklin and associates began repairing these defects using cardiopulmonary bypass methods.[10,24] Lillehei and colleagues in 1954 first successfully repaired the complete form of AV septal defect using cross-circulation by directly suturing the rim of the atrial septum to the crest of the ventricular septum.[12] The early experience with repair of the complete form was associated with a high incidence of surgically induced complete heart block until 1958 when Lev described the location of the bundle of

Figure 65–1. Diagrammatic representation of the atrioventricular (AV) valves. *A,* Normal, with anterior (ALMV) and posterior (PLMV) mitral valve leaflets and septal (SLTV), anterior (ALTV), and posterior (PLTV) tricuspid valve leaflets. *B,* The leaflets in AV septal defects with two AV valve orifices and no interventricular communications. The left superior (LSL), left inferior (LIL), and left lateral (LLL) leaflets form the left AV valve; the right superior (RSL), right inferior (RIL), and right lateral (RLL) leaflets form the right AV valve. *C,* The leaflets in AV septal defects with common AV valve orifice are similar to those in *B.* However, the LSL and LIL are not connected. The LIL usually bridges to some degree (grade 1 or 2 on the basis of 1 through 5) across the crest of the ventricular septum. The LSL may bridge little or not at all (grade 0 or 1, Rastelli type A), moderately (grade 2 or 3, Rastelli type B), or severely (grade 4 or 5, Rastelli type C). (Reproduced with permission of Studer M et al [1982]: Determinants of early and late results of repair of atrioventricular septal [canal] defects. J Thorac Cardiovasc Surg 84:523–542.)

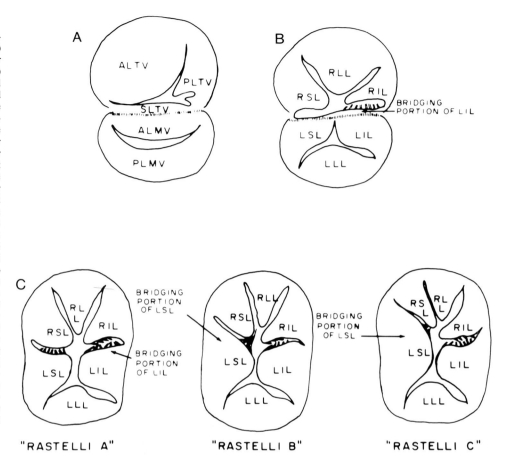

INDICATIONS FOR OPERATION

Some centers still advocate selective use of palliative pulmonary artery banding for small patients.[17,29] We and others have adopted a policy of primary complete repair for AV septal defect in part because of high mortality and unpredictable results associated with pulmonary artery banding.[1,3,4,13,15] Symptomatic patients usually undergo primary repair at the time of initial presentation. Presentation in the neonatal period should prompt a search for other lesions or disease processes before repair is recommended at this age. For patients with ventricular septal defect (complete AV canal) we recommend elective repair between 3 and 6 months of age because of the propensity to develop pulmonary vascular disease. We believe that patients without VSD (partial AV canal) should be electively repaired during the first few years of life.

His. This discovery permitted the development of reparative methods designed to avoid injury to the specialized conduction tissue. In the late 1950s and early 1960s, the modern type of repair evolved, which consisted of patch closure of the interventricular and interatrial defects with suspension of the AV valve leaflets to the patch.[6,14,23]

SURGICAL MANAGEMENT

The goals of repair include (1) closure of the ASD, (2) closure of the interventricular communication if present, (3) avoidance of injury to the AV node or bundle of His, and (4) maintenance or creation of two competent and nonstenotic AV valves.[11,18]

Partial Form

A median sternotomy is made, and a portion of pericardium is cleaned, excised, and placed on a trimmed towel soaked with saline. It remains adherent to the towel, improving its handling quality, and later, after both the towel and the pericardium are simultaneously trimmed to the final shape, suturing is begun by peeling the working edge of the pericardium away from the towel. The heart is externally inspected to assess chamber size, anomalies of systemic or pulmonary venous connection, and patency of the ductus arteriosus. A fine polyvinyl catheter is placed into the left atrium through a purse-string suture on the right superior pulmonary vein, and left atrial pressure is continuously monitored.

Cardiopulmonary bypass is established with ascending aortic perfusion, and direct bicaval cannulation is accomplished using thin-walled angled cannulae.[19] When a left superior vena cava is present, generally it is not cannulated directly, and the return is drained by an intracardiac sump sucker. Perfusate temperature is initially profoundly reduced, and after the aorta is cross-clamped, it is adjusted to 28°C. Cold cardioplegic solution is injected into the ascending aorta. The right atrium is opened longitudinally from the midportion of the right atrial appendage and extended inferiorly medial to the inferior caval cannula. Four stay sutures are placed to secure the edges of the atriotomy to the subcutaneous tissue or the pericardial edges. A sump tip sucker is placed through the foramen ovale, or if it is not present, a stab wound in this location is deliberately made. The anatomy is best inspected with the aorta cross-clamped and residual blood aspirated from the cardiac chambers.

Cold saline is injected into the left ventricle, floating the left AV valve to its closed position to assess valve architecture, the extent of septal commissure, and the location and presence of incompetence and jet lesions. The septal commissure, if competent, is left untouched. If there is incompetence of this commissure, it is usually best treated by repair. A 6-O polypropylene suture is first placed to approximate the left superior and inferior leaflets nearest their septal attachment, which serves as a commissuroplasty and brings the leaflets closer together. Saline is reinjected into the ventricle, and if persistent incompetence is present, two or three additional interrupted sutures are placed to approximate the "kissing edges" of the leaflet (Fig. 65–2A). Care is exercised to avoid excessive

closure of the commissure, which can further distort the leaflets and possibly create a stenotic orifice. The pathology of the left AV valve in this malformation may include incompetence of the anterolateral or posterolateral commissures in addition to an incompetent septal commissure. There may be elongation of the chordae tendineae, with leaflet prolapse or annular dilation with resultant central incompetence. Saline is again injected into the left ventricle, and these additional but less frequently found abnormalities are sought. Should prolapse of the leaflet because of elongated chordae be present and be responsible for persistent incompetence, shortening of the involved chordae is accomplished by the technique shown in Fig. 65–2B and C. Central incompetence from annular dilation is repaired by local annuloplasty at the anterolateral and posterolateral commissures as described in Fig. 65–2D. Localized incompetence at the anterolateral or posterolateral commissure is repaired by a single commissuroplasty at the appropriate site. Final valve architecture and competency are reviewed by injecting saline into the left ventricle.

The patch of pericardium is trimmed to size, oriented with its smooth surface leftward, and is sutured to close the interatrial defect with continuous double-armed 4-O polypropylene. The suture line is placed on the base of the left superior and inferior leaflets and begins at the inferior aspect of the left superior leaflet adjacent to the septal commissure. It continues anteriorly to the junction of the atrial septum with the AV valve annulus. A rubber-shod clamp is placed on this suture, and the other end is used to attach the patch to the base of the left inferior leaflet (Fig. 65–3). The conduction tissue lies on the atrial wall just above the crux cordis and is in the area between the coronary sinus and the junction of the left and right in-

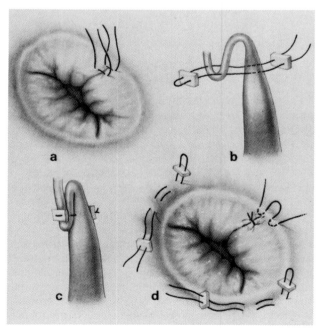

Figure 65–2. Mitral valve repair in ostium primum atrioventricular septal defect. *A,* The incompetent septal commissure is repaired by interrupted sutures placed in the coapting edges of the superior and inferior leaflets. *B* and *C,* Elongated chordae tendineae are shortened by the method shown. *D,* Method of constructing anterolateral and posterolateral commissuroplasty. (Reproduced with permission of Pacifico AD [1983]: Atrioventricular septal defects. In Stark J, de Leval M [eds]: Surgery for Congenital Heart Defects. Orlando, Grune & Stratton, p 288.)

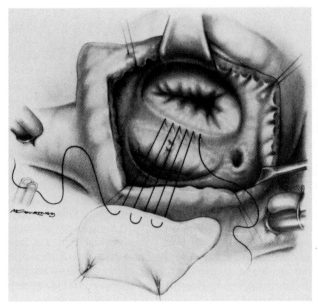

Figure 65–3. Ostium primum atrioventricular septal defect. Initial suturing of pericardial patch to close ostium primum defect. (Reproduced with permission of Pacifico AD [1983]: Atrioventricular septal defects. In Stark J, de Leval M [eds]: Surgery for Congenital Heart Defects. Orlando, Grune & Stratton, p 289.)

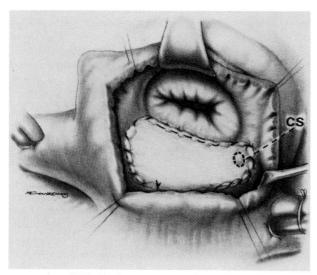

Figure 65–4. Ostium primum atrioventricular septal defect. Completed closure of ostium primum defect. CS = coronary sinus. (Reproduced with permission of Pacifico AD [1983]: Atrioventricular septal defects. In Stark J, de Leval M [eds]: Surgery for Congenital Heart Defects. Orlando, Grune & Stratton, p 289.)

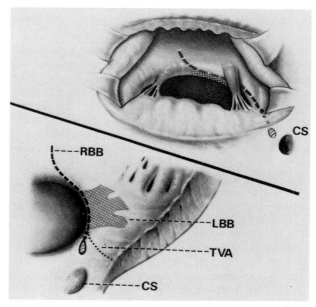

Figure 65–5. Complete atrioventricular septal defect. The location of the specialized conduction tissue in the complete form. CS = coronary sinus; RBB = right bundle branch; LBB = left bundle branch; TVA = tricuspid valve annulus. (Reproduced with permission of Pacifico AD [1983]: Atrioventricular septal defects. In Stark J, de Leval M [eds]: Surgery for Congenital Heart Defects. Orlando, Grune & Stratton, p 291.)

ferior leaflets, extending on the crest of the septum and dividing into bundle branches before the septal commissure. Nearing the posterior junction of the left inferior leaflet and the AV valve annulus, the suture line continues anteriorly on the base of the right inferior leaflet for about 1 cm then anteriorly around the coronary sinus, leaving it and the conduction tissue leftward. Closure is completed by suturing the patch to the remaining free edge of the ostium primum defect (Fig. 65–4). The foramen ovale is directly closed with a separate polypropylene suture, evacuating air from the left atrium by inflating the lungs prior to completion. Rewarming is commenced, and the aortic cross-clamp is released, with the usual debubbling technique employed. The right atriotomy is then closed. Bypass is discontinued when nasopharyngeal temperature reaches 37°C. It is important, especially in infants, to maintain left atrial pressure at levels less than 10 to 14 mmHg throughout the procedure to prevent injury to the pulmonary capillaries and to the left ventricle.

Complete Form

Repair of complete AV septal defects consists of closure of the interventricular communication with a Dacron patch, attachment of the common AV valve to the crest of this patch, and closure of the atrial septal defect with a patch of pericardium. The repair is planned so as to disturb the valve apparatus as little as possible, which gives the best chance for a competent valve after repair. The two-patch technique is employed to aid in achieving this goal, and the bridging portions of the left superior and inferior leaflets and their chordae are only rarely incised. Prosthetic valve replacement can be avoided in the overwhelming majority of cases.

Specialized techniques of intraoperative electrophysiologic mapping are not employed, since the location of the conduction tissues has been well defined, and our operative techniques have not resulted in surgical heart block. The location of the specialized conduction tissue in the complete form of atrioventricular septal defect is similar to the partial form and is shown in Figure 65–5. The AV node lies in the atrial wall just above the crux cordis. The penetrating bundle then passes through the tricuspid valve annulus (TVA) and divides into the left bundle branch (LBB) and right bundle branch (RBB).

Bypass and support techniques are similar to those employed for the repair of the partial form. Cold cardioplegic myocardial protection is likewise employed and facilitates optimal operating conditions in the soft-arrested heart. The right atrium is opened as is done in the partial form. Cold saline is injected into the ventricles to approximate the AV valve in its closed position. The anatomy of the valve leaflets, presence of accessory orifice, size and location of the interatrial and interventricular defects, location of the coronary sinus, and possible presence of pulmonary or systemic venous anomalies are specifically discerned. The position of the common AV valve relative to the plane of the ventricular septum is determined to ensure that repair will leave adequate orifices to each ventricle. When this adequacy is in doubt, it is helpful to relate the diameters of these orifices to the normal mitral and tricuspid dimensions described by Rowlatt et al and measured in the operating room with Hegar dilators (Table 65–1).[25] The morphology of the left superior leaflet is studied to determine its position relative to the crest of the ventricular septum, to the origin and insertion of its

Table 65–1. MEAN
NORMAL DIAMETER OF
ATRIOVENTRICULAR VALVES

BSA (m)	Mitral* (mm)	Tricuspid* (mm)
0.25	11.2	13.4
0.30	12.6	14.9
0.35	13.6	16.2
0.40	14.4	17.3
0.45	15.2	18.2
0.50	15.8	19.2
0.60	16.9	20.7
0.70	17.9	21.9
0.80	18.8	23.0
0.90	19.7	24.0
1.0	20.2	24.9
1.2	21.4	26.2
1.4	22.3	27.7
1.6	23.1	28.9
1.8	23.8	29.1
2.0	24.2	30.0

*The approximate standard deviations (±) are mitral
< 0.3 m² = 1.9 mm, > 0.3 m² = 1.6 mm; tricuspid < 1.0
m² = 1.7 mm, > 1.0 m² = 1.5 mm.
(Modified from Rowlatt UF et al (1963): The quantitative anatomy of the normal child's heart. Pediatr Clin North Am 10:499–588.)

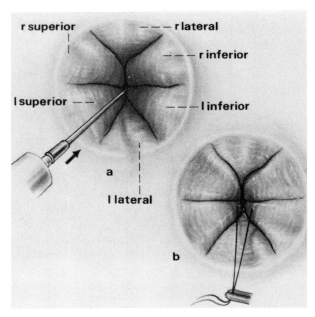

Figure 65–6. Repair of complete atrioventricular septal defect. *A*, Initial inspection of the common AV valve by injection of saline into the ventricle. *B*, The placement of the initial suture approximating the coapting edges of the left superior and inferior leaflets above the crest of the septum. r = right, l = left. (Reproduced with permission of Pacifico AD [1983]: Atrioventricular septal defects. In Stark J, de Leval M [eds]: Surgery for Congenital Heart Defects. Orlando, Grune & Stratton, p 292.)

chordal connections, to the amount of its tissue, and to the size of the underlying interventricular communication. We believe it is best to consider the anatomy of the AV valve as a continuous pathologic spectrum rather than within the limited classification as proposed by Rastelli (see Fig. 65–1).[23]

Cold saline is injected into the ventricles, and the valve architecture is studied in the closed position. The surgeon must identify the precise site of coaptation of the left superior and inferior leaflets above the crest of the septum. A 6-O polypropylene suture is placed through each leaflet at this coaptation site to mark the position of separation of the common AV valve into the mitral and tricuspid components. This site will later become the apex of the septal commissure of the newly created left AV valve (Fig. 65–6). The suture is left untied and is secured by a rubber-shod clamp. When there is no rightward bridging of the left superior leaflet (type A), this suture is usually, but not always, placed at the medial corner of this leaflet. When the left superior leaflet bridges leftward (type C), this suture is usually placed at a site directly above the crest of the ventricular septum. Hegar dilators are then placed through the left and right orifices to measure the size of the mitral and tricuspid portions, comparing them with the normal valve of a similar-sized patient (see Table 65–1). At times, it may be necessary to accept an orifice size smaller than normal, but it must never be smaller than two standard deviations from the mean normal value. Often, adjustment of the position of the initial coapting suture will result in normal-sized orifices, and this is preferred. Mild traction is placed on this suture, and saline is again reinjected to ascertain that the natural leaflet coaptation has not been disturbed and that valve incompetency has not been created or worsened. This important initial step sets the stage for a proper repair.

Stay sutures (5-O silk) are placed in the right superior and inferior leaflets to permit gentle traction to expose the defect in the ventricular septum. When there is marked rightward bridging of the left superior leaflet, one stay suture is placed on its rightward edge, instead of on the right superior leaflet. When the ventricular septal deficiency extends beneath the left inferior leaflet, the leaflet is not incised, but if troublesome secondary chordae attaching it to the right side of the ventricular septal crest are present, they are divided to permit complete exposure of the right side of the crest of the septum. This chordal division is sometimes necessary to improve exposure and to aid the surgeon in avoiding injury to the conduction tissue. When the left inferior leaflet is attached to the crest of the underlying septum by a membrane or by many closely placed chordae permitting only tiny communications, they are left undisturbed, recognizing that they will remain to the left of the Dacron ventricular patch. Similarly, when chordae are present, attaching either the left superior leaflet to the right side of the crest of the septum, or the left superior leaflet to an anomalously placed right ventricular papillary muscle (Rastelli, type B), and interfere with placement of the ventricular patch, they are divided.[20]

The next step in the procedure is to close the defect of the ventricular septum with the Dacron velour patch (Fig. 65–7). Initially, the distance between the AV valve annulus over the septum, superiorly and inferiorly, is measured. This measurement is used to mark the width of the Dacron patch (Fig. 65–7*B*). The height of the patch is

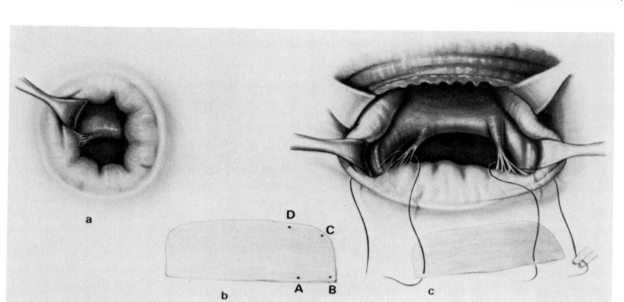

Figure 65–7. Repair of complete atrioventricular septal defect. Closure of the interventricular defect in the complete form (see text for details). (Reproduced with permission of Pacifico AD [1983]: Atrioventricular septal defects. In Stark J, de Leval M [eds]: Surgery for Congenital Heart Defects. Orlando, Grune & Stratton, p 293.)

judged by floating the leaflets to their closed position by injecting cold saline into the ventricles and by making a second measurement, which is marked on the Dacron patch. The shape of the defect in the ventricular septum is studied and translated to the Dacron patch by marking it with a sterile pen. It is important to note that the defect of the septum may extend more anteriorly than the position of the annulus, as is the rule when tetralogy of Fallot or double-outlet right ventricle is an associated condition. The above measurements are very important and useful. If the patch width is too narrow, then the superior and inferior aspects of the AV valve annulus will later be brought closer together. If there was marked central incompetence of the AV valve, using a narrow patch width to bring the superior and inferior aspects of the AV valve annulus closer might be useful (and sometimes is purposely done), as in effect it represents a type of annuloplasty. Otherwise, too narrow a patch will inappropriately narrow the new circumference of the mitral and tricuspid valves and later result in leaflet prolapse. When the size and shape of the desired Dacron patch has been obtained, it is further extended 1 cm in its posterior aspect (Fig. 65–7B). This posterior extension allows additional width to the patch, which can later be folded at this point (Fig. 65–7B, points A to D) in a 90-degree angle and attached to the base of the right inferior leaflet or the bridging portion of the left inferior leaflet, so as completely to avoid suturing in the area of the conduction tissue. Double-armed 4-O polypropylene sutures are passed through the Dacron patch at the appropriate sites and then through the respective points of the AV valve annulus superiorly and inferiorly (Fig. 65–7C). The Dacron patch will be continuously sutured with a 4-O double-armed prolene suture beginning at the posterior annulus (Fig. 65–8A). The patch is initially held away

from the heart and the suture that has been placed through the patch posteriorly is used to suture the patch to the base of the leaflet overlying the right side of the posterior septal crest (Fig. 65–8A, point A–B). This technique is similar to the one used for repair of an isolated perimembranous ventricular septal defect. The objective of this maneuver is to bring the suture line completely away from the area of the conduction tissue. When the corner of the patch is reached (Fig. 65–8A, point B), it is lowered in place. Placement of points A, B, C, and D of the patch on the heart are illustrated in Figure 65–8A. Figure 65–8B shows this part of the patch completed. Suturing then continues anteriorly, keeping initially on the mural right ventricular wall and then on to the right side of the ventricular septum until the superior aspect of the annulus is reached. Here the suture is brought through the annulus into the atrium, tied to the previously placed and tied double-armed suture and secured with a rubber-shod clamp.

The height of the patch is evaluated and appropriately contoured and trimmed if necessary (Fig. 65–8C). If properly done, the patch should not interfere in any way with the contour of the closed AV valve. The patch must not be too short, as excessive displacement of the valve into the ventricle can result in subaortic obstruction. The next step in the procedure is to attach the valve leaflets to the crest of the Dacron patch. This attachment is accomplished using interrupted 6-O prolene sutures placed at intervals of approximately 2 to 3 mm (Fig. 65–9). One of these sutures will replace the earlier-placed coapting suture. The entire group is left long and secured by a rubber-shod clamp.

The pericardial patch is next fashioned after measuring the distance necessary for it to close the atrial septal defect and also to leave the coronary sinus leftward (Fig.

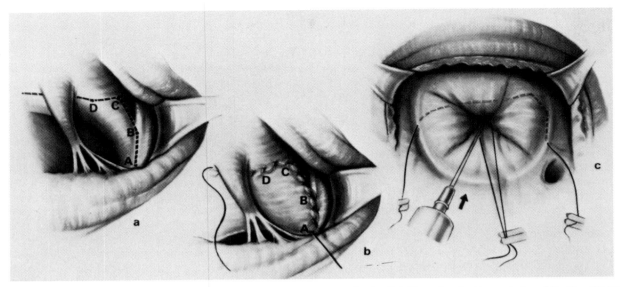

Figure 65–8. Closure of the interventricular defect in the complete form. (See text for details.) (Reproduced with permission of Pacifico AD [1983]: Atrioventricular septal defects. In Stark J, de Leval M [eds]: Surgery for Congenital Heart Defects. Orlando, Grune & Stratton, p 294.)

65–10A). Suturing begins superiorly at the annulus and continues as a simple over-and-over suture, which incorporates both the AV valve leaflet (L) and the underlying crest of the Dacron ventricular patch (D) as well as the pericardial patch (P), as shown in Figure 65–10B. Placement of traction on the previously placed interrupted sutures in sequence aids in inclusion of the Dacron patch into this suture line. When the inferior aspect of the AV valve annulus is reached, the suture line continues an-

teriorly, incorporating the base of the right-sided leaflet and its underlying Dacron patch before continuing around and rightward of the coronary sinus and around the inferior and posterior edges of the atrial septal defect. Prior to completion (Fig. 65–10C) the interrupted sutures are cut, and saline is injected into the left ventricle through the mitral valve to assess again its degree of competency. If additional valvuloplasty is indicated, it is now performed as shown in Figure 65–2.

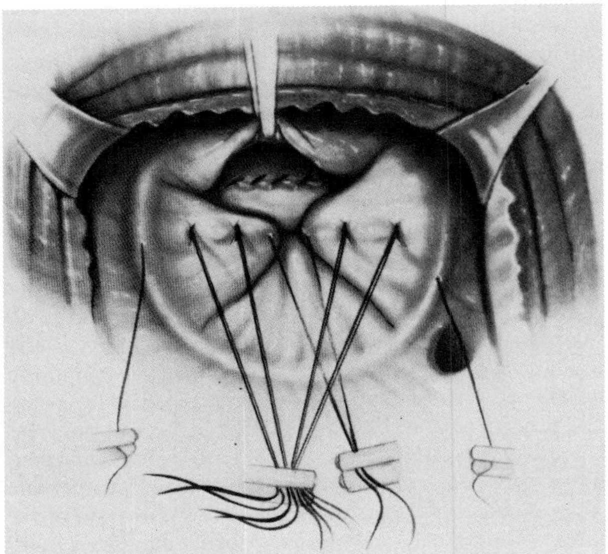

The type of patch material and whether a single patch or separate patches are used to close the defects in the atrial and ventricular septae remain controversial. We prefer separate patches because they allow the surgeon to avoid any significant alteration of the AV valve and also completely to avoid suturing near the conduction tissue. A pericardial patch is preferred for closure of the atrial defect to avoid the small risk of severe postoperative hemolysis, which can result from a jet of residual mitral incompetence striking the patch.

RESULTS

Studer et al have analyzed the 310 patients undergoing repair of all forms of AV septal defects at the University of Alabama at Birmingham between 1967 and 1982.[27] With our current methods, repair of isolated partial AV septal defect carries a very low hospital mortality, estimated to be 0.6 per cent (70 per cent confidence limits [CL] of 0.2 per cent to 1.4 per cent). The risk is higher, 4 per cent (CL of 2 percent to 7 percent) when severe left AV valve incompetence is present preoperatively in patients with partial AV septal defect.[27] For patients with complete AV septal defect, the estimated risk for hospital death currently is 2 per cent (CL of 0.3 per cent to 8 per cent).[8] Multivariate analysis of this experience shows that

Figure 65–9. Repair of complete atrioventricular septal defect. Attachment of the left superior and inferior leaflets to the crest of the Dacron patch (see text). (Reproduced with permission of Pacifico AD [1983]: Atrioventricular septal defects. In Stark J, de Leval M [eds]: Surgery for Congenital Heart Defects. Orlando, Grune & Stratton, p 295.)

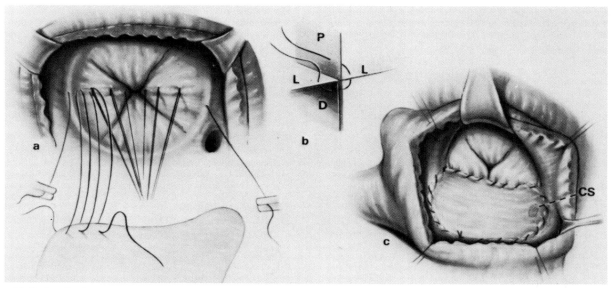

Figure 65–10. Repair of complete atrioventricular septal defect. Closure of the ostium primum defect in the complete form (see text). (Reproduced with permission of Pacifico AD [1983]: Atrioventricular septal defects. In Stark J, de Leval M [eds]: Surgery for Congenital Heart Defects. Orlando, Grune & Stratton, p 295.)

the results in all categories have improved with time. For example, the risk of young age (small size) on hospital death was neutralized by improved techniques and increased experience after the year 1976. The results of repair continue to improve, but severe ventricular dominance (hypoplasia of the right or left ventricle), increasing severity of AV valve incompetence, increased functional disability (as based on the New York Heart Functional Class descriptions), the presence of a ventricular septal defect, accessory valve orifice, or associated major cardiac anomalies remain risk factors.[8,27]

Late results after repair of AV septal defect can be expected to be good unless there is failure of AV valve repair with residual or recurrent severe AV valve incompetence or significant pulmonary vascular disease. Eighty-eight per cent of long-term survivors were in New York Heart Functional Class I or II.[11] Actuarial survival at 12.5 years was 84 per cent for hospital surviors (CL of 76 per cent to 90 per cent). Incremental risk factors for late death include severe preoperative AV valve incompetence, poor preoperative functional status, the presence of an accessory AV valve orifice, and the presence of Down syndrome.[27]

AV valve failure occurred in approximately 10 per cent of partial AV septal defect repairs and 10 per cent of complete AV septal defect repairs.[11] Failure is more likely to occur when severe preoperative AV valve incompetence is present. Use of the current reinforced repair technique has reduced the incidence of valve repair failure. When the postoperative course of a patient is suboptimal, residual left AV valve incompetence should be considered as an explanation. Early Doppler echocardiography or left ventriculography are indicated to quantitate the magnitude of incompetence. Prompt reoperation should be considered when severe left AV valve incompetence is present, since AV valve insufficiency contributes importantly to death

during the first postoperative year.[11] When left AV valve replacement is necessary, a low profile device is preferred, and consideration should be given to the need for extending the "aortic mitral annulus" with a crescent-shaped Dacron patch to minimize the left ventricular outflow tract obstruction.[16] Sutures should be placed in the leaflet remnants rather than in the annulus inferiorly and anteriorly to avoid injury to the AV node and bundle of His.

References

1. Bender HW Jr, Hammon JW Jr, Hubbard SG, Muirhead J, Graham TP (1982): Repair of atrioventricular canal malformation in the first year of life. J Thorac Cardiovasc Surg 84:515–522.
2. Berger TJ, Blackstone EH, Kirklin JW, Bargeron LM Jr, Hazelrig JB, Turner ME Jr (1978): Survival and probability of cure without and with operation in complete atrioventricular canal. Ann Thorac Surg 27:104–111.
3. Berger TJ, Kirklin JW, Blackstone EH, Pacifico AD, Kouchoukos NT (1978): Primary repair of complete atrioventricular canal in patients less than 2 years old. Am J Cardiol 41:906–913.
4. Chin AJ, Keane JF, Norwood WI, Castaneda AR (1982): Repair of complete common atrioventricular canal in infancy. J Thorac Cardiovasc Surg 84:437–445.
5. Epstein ML, Moller JH, Amplatz K, Nicoloff DM (1979): Pulmonary artery banding in infants with complete atrioventricular canal. J Thorac Cardiovasc Surg 78:28–31.
6. Gerbode F (1962): Surgical repair of endocardial cushion defect. Ann Chir Thorac Cardio-Vasculaire 1:753–755.
7. Ilbawi MN, Idriss FS, DeLeon SY, Riggs TW, Muster AJ, Berry TE, Paul MH (1983): Unusual mitral valve abnormalities complicating surgical repair of endocardial cushion defects. J Thorac Cardiovasc Surg 85:697–704.
8. Kirklin JW, Blackstone EH, Bargeron LM Jr, Pacifico AD, Kirklin JK (1986): The repair of AV canal defects in infancy. Inter J Cardiol 13:333–360.
9. Kirklin JW, Daugherty GW, Burchell HB, Wood EH (1955): Repair of the partial form of persistent common atrioventricular canal: So-called ostium primum type of atrial septal defect with interventricular communication. Ann Surg 142:858–862.

10. Kirklin JW, DuShane JW, Patrick RT, Donald DE, Hetzel PS, Harshbarger HG, Wood EH (1955): Intracardiac surgery with the aid of a mechanical pump-oxygenator system (Gibbon type): Report of eight cases. Proc Staff Meet Mayo Clin 30:201–206.

11. Kirklin JW, Pacifico AD, Kirklin JK (1985): The surgical treatment of atrioventricular canal defects. In Arciniegas E (ed): Pediatric Cardiac Surgery. Chicago, Yearbook Medical Publishers, pp 155–170.

12. Lillehei CW, Cohen M, Warden HE, Varco RL (1955): The direct vision intracardiac correction of congenital anomalies by controlled cross circulation: Results in thirty-two patients with ventricular septal defects, tetralogy of Fallot, and atrioventricularis communis defects. Surgery 38:11–29.

13. Mair DD, McGoon DC (1977): Surgical correction of atrioventricular canal during the first year of life. Am J Cardiol 40:66–69.

14. Maloney JV Jr, Marable SA, Mulder DG (1962): The surgical treatment of common atrioventricular canal. J Thorac Cardiovasc Surg 43:84–96.

15. Mavroudis C, Weinstein G, Turley K, Ebert PA (1982): Surgical management of complete atrioventricular canal. J Thorac Cardiovasc Surg 83:670–679.

16. McGrath LB, Kirklin JW, Soto B, Bargeron LM Jr (1985): Secondary left atrioventricular valve replacement in atrioventricular septal (AV canal) defect: A method to avoid left ventricular outflow tract obstruction. J Thorac Cardiovasc Surg 89:632–635.

17. Newfeld EA, Sher M, Paul MH, Nikaidoh R (1977): Pulmonary vascular disease in complete atrioventricular canal defect. Am J Cardiol 39:721–726.

18. Pacifico AD (1983): Atrioventricular septal defects. In Stark J, de Leval M (eds): Surgery for Congenital Heart Defects. London, Grune & Stratton, pp 285–300.

19. Pacifico AD (1984): Low flow bypass: the University of Alabama technique. In Moulton AL (ed): Congenital Heart Surgery: Current Techniques and Controversies. Pasadena, Appleton Davies, Inc, pp 187–192.

20. Pacifico AD, Kirklin JW (1973): Surgical repair of complete atrioventricular canal with anterior common leaflet attached to an anomalous right ventricular papillary muscle. J Thorac Cardiovasc Surg 65:727–730.

21. Piccoli GP, Gerlis LM, Wilkinson JL, Lozsadi K, Macartney FJ, Anderson RH (1979): Morphology and classification of atrioventricular defects. Br Heart J 42:621–632.

22. Piccoli GP, Ho SY, Wilkinson JL, Macartney FJ, Gerlis LM, Anderson RH (1982): Left-sided obstructive lesions in atrioventricular septal defects: An anatomic study. J Thorac Cardiovasc Surg 83:453–460.

23. Rastelli GC, Ongley PA, Kirklin JW, McGoon DC (1968): Surgical repair of complete form of persistent common atrioventricular canal. J Thorac Cardiovasc Surg 55:299–308.

24. Rastelli GC, Weidman WH, Kirklin JW (1965): Surgical repair of the partial form of persistent common atrioventricular canal, with special reference to the problem of mitral valve incompetence. Circulation 31,32(Suppl I):31–35.

25. Rowlatt UF, Rimoldi HJA, Lev M (1963): The quantitative anatomy of the normal child's heart. Pediatr Clin North Am 10:499–588.

26. Silverman N, Levitsky S, Fisher E, DuBrow I, Hastreiter A, Scagliotti D (1983): Efficacy of pulmonary artery banding in infants with complete atrioventricular canal. Circulation 68(Supp 2): 148–153.

27. Studer M, Blackstone EH, Kirklin JW, Pacifico AD, Soto B, Chung GKT, Kirklin JK, Bargeron LM Jr (1982): Determinants of early and late results of repair of atrioventricular septal (canal) defects. J Thorac Cardiovasc Surg 84:523–542.

28. Watkins E Jr, Gross RE (1955): Experiences with surgical repair of atrial septal defects. J Thorac Cardiovasc Surg 30:469–491.

29. Williams WH, Guyton RA, Michalik RE, Plauth WH Jr, Zorn-Chelton S, Jones EL, Rhee KH, Hatcher CR Jr (1983): Individualized surgical management of complete atrioventricular canal. J Thorac Cardiovasc Surg 86:838–844.

66 NEONATAL REPAIR OF TRANSPOSITION OF THE GREAT ARTERIES

Aldo R. Castañeda

John E. Mayer, Jr.

Transposition of the great arteries (TGA) denotes a congenital cardiac condition in which atrioventricular connection is concordant and ventriculoarterial connection is discordant. The ventricular septum can be intact or is considered essentially intact when there is only a small hemodynamically inconsequential ventricular septal defect. Approximately 75 per cent of children born with TGA have an intact or essentially intact ventricular septum. The remainder have either associated hemodynamically significant ventricular septal defects or associated pulmonary or subpulmonary stenosis. TGA is the second most common congenital cardiac defect causing critical heart disease in infancy and the most common cardiac lesion in infants requiring medical or surgical management during the first 3 months of life.[12]

HISTORICAL PERSPECTIVE

Surgical treatment for TGA was initiated in 1950 by Blalock and Hanlon, who devised an ingenious closed method of excising part of the interatrial septum to facilitate mixing of pulmonary and systemic venous blood at the atrial level.[5] To ensure obligatory rerouting of pulmonary venous blood into the aorta, Edwards and associates[9] modified the Blalock-Hanlon concept in 1964 by reattaching the atrial septum in such a way that all right pulmonary venous blood was diverted exclusively into the right atrium. Two years later, Rashkind and Miller[27] significantly improved initial palliation of neonates with TGA by introducing balloon atrial septostomy. In 1975, Park and associates[25] extended the usefulness of this procedure by developing blade septostomy, a technique applicable to children beyond the neonatal period.

Lillehei and Varco, in 1953, introduced the concept of partial physiologic correction of TGA by transposing the right pulmonary veins into the right atrium and the inferior vena cava directly into the left atrium.[21] Baffes modified this operation by interposing a segment of aortic homograft between the inferior vena cava and the left atrium.[3]

In 1954, Albert advocated the intriguing principle of complete physiologic repair of TGA by rerouting and separating pulmonary and systemic venous blood at the atrial level.[1] He proposed the use of the atrial septum to channel both the superior and the inferior vena cava return into the left ventricle and the pulmonary venous return into the right ventricle. Using this principle, Senning, in

1959, accomplished the first physiologic correction of TGA using autogenous tissue, including right atrial wall and atrial septum.[29] However, despite several modifications of the Senning operation, operative mortality remained high until 1964 when Mustard described the use of an intra-atrial pericardial baffle to redirect systemic and pulmonary venous blood after excision of the atrial septum.[22] This important modification was found to be more easily reproducible by surgeons in general and was soon adopted worldwide. However, because of late complications following the Mustard repair,[10,14,15] the Senning technique has enjoyed a successful renaissance in many centers.[24,26]

Since the intracardiac structures are essentially normal in TGA with intact ventricular septum, it is not surprising that as soon as cardiopulmonary bypass became available clinically, surgeons attempted to repair this lethal malformation by switching the aorta and the pulmonary artery. In 1954, Mustard, in addition to switching the great arteries, also transferred the left coronary artery, leaving, however, the right coronary artery attached to the pulmonary circuit.[23] These attempts, as well as other reported[17,19] and perhaps many more unreported trials, did not succeed. Fortunately, Jatene and colleagues in São Paolo, Brazil, persisted in these efforts, and eventually in 1975 they achieved the first successful arterial switch operation in an infant with TGA and ventricular septal defect.[18] Although Aubert's attempts at retaining the left ventricle as the systemic ventricle in TGA without anatomically transferring the coronary arteries were successful,[2] the Jatene technique has retained its original appeal and is being used with increasing frequency.

In the initial report, Jatene limited the arterial switch concept to patients with TGA and a ventricular septal defect. He realized that in patients with TGA and an intact ventricular septum the left ventricle would soon adapt to the low resistance of the pulmonary circuit and thus be unable to function when faced with systemic resistance. However, since approximately 75 per cent of patients with TGA have an intact ventricular septum it would clearly be desirable to apply the arterial switch principle to this group of patients as well. In order to "prepare" the left ventricle for a subsequent arterial switch procedure, Yacoub and associates[31] first proposed banding the pulmonary artery in patients with TGA and an intact ventricular septum and performing the arterial switch procedure as a second-stage several months later. To accomplish the same goal, that is, to offer an arterial switch operation to patients with TGA and an intact ventricular septum, we based our approach on the fact that intrauterine pulmonary and systemic resistances are nearly equal and that if the arterial switch operation were performed during the neonatal period, the left ventricle should still be prepared to carry a systemic work load.[8]

WHY ARTERIAL RATHER THAN ATRIAL SWITCH?

Much anatomic and physiologic data support the idea that the left ventricle is better suited than the right ventricle to function as a systemic pump. For example, the normal right ventricular cavity is crescent-shaped and has a large internal surface area-to-volume ratio; its bellows-like contraction pattern seems ideally suited for pumping large volumes of blood against the low resistance pulmonary circuit. In contrast, the more ellipsoid-shaped and concentrically contracting normal left ventricle favors pressure work.[28] The right ventricle in TGA is similar to the normal right ventricle, and therefore from a strictly anatomic point of view it seems less well adapted to function as a systemic pump. Also, the late physiologic results of the anatomic right ventricle functioning as a systemic ventricle after atrial inversion procedures for TGA are of some concern. Right ventricular end-diastolic and end-systolic volumes, right ventricular ejection fractions, and the response to afterload stress have all been found to be distinctly abnormal after atrial inversion procedures.[7,16] Also, tricuspid valvular regurgitation occurs as a late complication in as many as 5 per cent of the cases.[30] Finally, arrhythmias and sudden death are being reported late after atrial inversion procedures.[11]

INDICATIONS FOR THE ARTERIAL SWITCH OPERATION IN TGA WITH INTACT VENTRICULAR SEPTUM

Untreated, approximately 80 per cent of infants with TGA and an intact ventricular septum die within the first 2 months of life. Therefore, intervention is necessary very early in life. Until recently, this intervention generally consisted of a balloon atrial septostomy during the first few days of life, followed by an elective atrial inversion operation within the first year of life. The timing of operation must be altered when the arterial switch operation is contemplated because of anatomic and physiologic adaptive changes that occur in the left ventricle soon after birth.

Of critical importance is the condition of the left ventricle in neonates with TGA and an intact ventricular septum, since the left ventricle must be capable of pumping against the resistance of the systemic circuit after the operation. In patients with TGA and an intact ventricular septum, the left ventricular free-wall thickness is normal at birth and begins to decrease rapidly, paralleling the normal postnatal decrease in pulmonary vascular resistance.

Baño-Rodrigo and associates measured at autopsy left and right ventricular free-wall thickness of patients with or without TGA.[4] In TGA patients, the postnatal increase in right ventricular free-wall thickness parallels the postnatal increase in left ventricular free-wall thickness of patients with normally related great arteries. In contrast, by 4 months of age the left ventricle in TGA infants becomes statistically significantly thinner than in normal hearts. It should be recalled that ventricular wall stress is directly proportional to intraventricular pressure and diameter and inversely proportional to wall thickness. Consequently, a dilated and thin-walled ventricle will be subject to high wall stress when faced with the increased afterload presented by the systemic circuit following an arterial switch procedure. For a patient with TGA and an intact ventricular septum undergoing an arterial switch operation, the timing of the procedure therefore becomes critical.

The limits of age and left ventricular wall thickness or left ventricular pressure beyond which the left ventricle can be predicted to fail after arterial switch in infants with TGA have not been clinically defined with certainty. Nevertheless, we have developed some tentative criteria. During the first 10 days of life virtually all patients have adequate left ventricular function after an arterial switch operation regardless of the preoperative left ventricular pressure. After this age we have arbitrarily chosen a left ventricular to right ventricular pressure ratio of 0.6 as the lower limit of acceptable left ventricular pressure. Two-dimensional echocardiography can provide a noninvasive index of relative left and right ventricular pressures by outlining the ventricular septal position. When the ventricular septum bows towards the left, the ventricular pressure is almost certainly low, and after 10 days of age these patients are considered unfavorable candidates for the arterial switch operation unless the left ventricular to right ventricular pressure ratio measured at catheterization or in the operating room exceeds 0.6.

Beyond this physiologic assessment of left ventricular function, anatomic contraindications also exist. For example, organic left ventricular outflow tract obstructions caused by subvalvular or valvular abnormalities preclude the arterial switch operation in most instances. Hemodynamically significant mitral atrioventricular valve abnormalities may coexist in some patients with TGA and an intact ventricular septum, and these abnormalities also contraindicate an arterial switch operation.

The pattern of coronary artery origin and distribution is somewhat variable in TGA and an intact ventricular septum.[13] Few of these anatomic variants constitute contraindications to the operation. Most commonly, the right coronary artery arises from the right facing sinus, and the left coronary artery, including the circumflex branch, arises from the left facing sinus. In the second most common variant the circumflex coronary artery arises from the right coronary artery. In this case the surgeon must be careful to avoid kinking of the circumflex coronary artery. Coronary artery transfer can prove difficult whenever the right coronary artery arises from the left facing cusp (single left-sided origin) and passes anterior to the aorta or likewise when the anterior descending coronary artery originates from the right facing cusp. Coronary transfer can also prove somewhat more problematic when the aortopulmonary artery relationship is side by side rather than anteroposterior.

PREOPERATIVE ASSESSMENT

Detailed preoperative diagnosis of this defect is essential in order to achieve a successful outcome. Two-dimensional echocardiography can accurately define the diagnosis of TGA and can provide additional data about the presence of associated defects such as mitral valve or left ventricular outflow tract abnormalities, the position of the ventricular septum, and coronary arterial patterns. Nevertheless, at this stage of our experience, we still perform cardiac catheterizations in all patients, mostly to obtain direct measurements of right and left ventricular pressures and to help exclude other defects. An aortic root injection is helpful in outlining the coronary arteries, but the final decision on their suitability for an arterial switch operation is made in the operating room. The indication for a balloon atrial septostomy at catheterization depends largely on the patient's metabolic condition and the projected timing of the operation. When acidosis is present or if operating time is not immediately available, a balloon atrial septostomy is performed and prostaglandin E_1 may be started to maintain ductal patency and improve oxygenation.

INTRAOPERATIVE MANAGEMENT

The anesthetic technique for an arterial switch operation is similar to that used for other neonatal cardiac operations. A synthetic narcotic with muscle paralysis is generally used. After anesthesia is induced and the neonate is intubated, an arterial catheter is placed into the radial artery unless an umbilical artery catheter has been placed preoperatively. Two large intravenous lines (at least 22-gauge), a urinary catheter, and rectal, esophageal, and tympanic temperature probes are also inserted. During bypass, left and right atrial pressure monitoring lines and temporary pacing wires are placed to facilitate postoperative management.

OPERATIVE TECHNIQUE

The heart is exposed through a median sternotomy. A strip of pericardium is harvested for use as patches to fill the explanted coronary artery sites. The aorta and the pulmonary artery are cleared from each other, the ductus arteriosus is dissected, and the branches of the right and left pulmonary arteries are completely mobilized well out into the hilum to the first pulmonary artery branches to reduce tension on the eventual pulmonary artery anastomosis (Fig. 66–1). The arterial cannula is inserted as far distally in the ascending aorta as possible, to gain adequate length for the aortic anastomosis as well as aortic

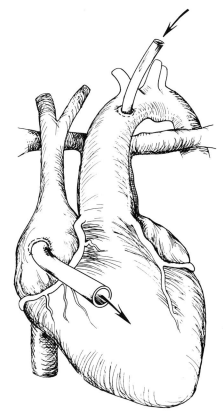

Figure 66–1. Cannulation sites for cardiopulmonary bypass. Arterial cannula inserted far distally in the ascending aorta; single venous cannula placed through the right atrial appendage.

cross-clamps. A single venous cannula is inserted through the right atrial appendage. Core cooling to rectal temperatures of 20°C is then carried out. During cooling the pulmonary artery dissection is completed and the ductus arteriosus is divided.

At 20°C rectal temperature, the aorta is clamped as far distally as possible, cardioplegic solution is injected into the proximal aorta, and the circulation is stopped. Then the aorta is transected approximately 10 mm distal to the coronary arteries. The left coronary artery is excised first (Fig. 66–2). The incision is begun at the free edge of the proximal aorta and is then carried toward the base of the coronary sinus, well below the coronary ostium. As large a button of aortic sinus wall is excised as possible without damage to the valve leaflets. After excision of the coronary arteries from the proximal aorta, the proximal portions of the left and right coronary artery are mobilized to allow a tension-free transfer to the posteriorly positioned pulmonary artery (neoaorta). Small conal branches encountered during this dissection should be divided between suture ligatures. Then the main pulmonary artery is transected proximal to its bifurcation (Fig. 66–3). The distal pulmonary artery segment is transferred anterior to the distal aorta (Lecompte maneuver)[20] and is held in place by a second aortic cross-clamp placed proximal to the initial aortic clamp. A V-shaped excision of the pulmonary

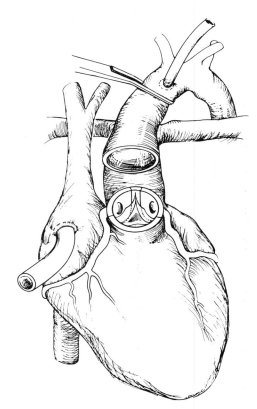

Figure 66–2. Division of ascending aorta approximately 1 cm distal to valve commissures. Patent ductus arteriosus divided.

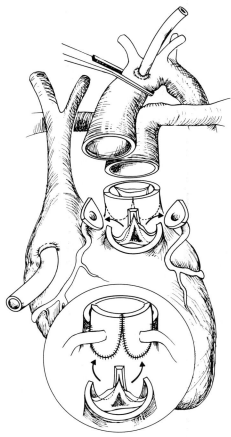

Figure 66–3. Excision of left and right coronary arteries with generous patch of aortic wall. Division of main pulmonary artery. Excision of segments of pulmonary artery wall (see inset), transfer of coronary arteries, and anastomosis of both left and right coronary arteries into neoaorta.

artery wall is then made into the left anterior (facing) sinus of the neoaorta (i.e., the sinus facing the left posterior cusp of the aorta). The incision must not extend deeply into the sinus, since this increases the distance across which the mobilized coronary artery must reach; this downward displacement of either the transferred left or right coronary artery can cause a kink and interfere significantly with coronary perfusion. The left coronary artery with its surrounding aortic wall is then sewn into this incision within the neoaorta with continuous absorbable monofilament suture. A similar technique is used to transfer the right coronary artery into the right anterior sinus of the neoaorta. When the circumflex coronary artery arises from the right coronary artery (the second most common variant), the site of implantation is kept slightly higher to avoid kinking of the circumflex coronary artery. The proximal neoaorta is then sewn end to end to the distal aorta with continuous monofilament absorbable suture (Fig. 66–4). When the distal aorta is considerably smaller than the proximal neoaortic segment, the anterior wall of the distal aorta is incised. We also like to use excess aortic wall tissue from the transferred coronary flap to tailor the neoaortic anastomosis, compensating for size discrepancies of the two vascular segments. After completion of the aortic anastomosis, a strip of Gelfoam is treated with fibrin glue and wrapped around all anastomoses. Cardiotomy suction is then discontinued to prevent aspiration of fibrin into the oxygenator. Then, the atrial septal communi-

cation (if present) is closed through a right atrial incision. At this stage, and depending on the length of circulatory arrest time, the venous cannula can be reinserted, the circulation restarted, and the aorta unclamped. Air should be vented through a separate stab incision in the distal aorta. All regions of the myocardium should be inspected early after the removal of the aortic clamp to ensure coronary patency and myocardial perfusion.

The next step is the reconstruction of the neopulmonary artery. The coronary donor sites in the neopulmonary artery are filled with autologous pericardium (Fig. 66–5). The handling of these patches is improved by 10-minute fixation in 0.6 per cent glutaraldehyde. Subsequently, the distal pulmonary artery is sewn to the proximal segment (neopulmonary artery) with continuous monofilament suture.

Rewarming to 36°C rectal temperature is carried out on bypass. During the rewarming phase, the left atrial pressure monitoring line is inserted through a pursestring suture in the right superior pulmonary vein and a right atrial pressure monitoring line is inserted through the right atrial appendage. Temporary ventricular pacing wires are placed on the right ventricular surface.

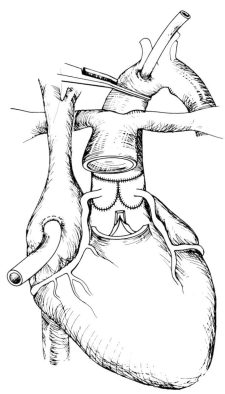

Figure 66–4. Distal pulmonary artery is brought anterior to the ascending aorta (LeCompte maneuver). Anastomosis of proximal neoaorta to distal aorta.

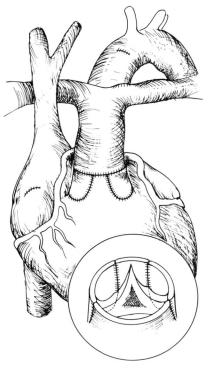

Figure 66–5. Coronary donor site from neopulmonary artery filled with pericardial patches (see inset). End-to-end anastomosis between the proximal neopulmonary artery segment and the distal pulmonary artery. The branch pulmonary arteries were extensively mobilized at the beginning of the procedure.

POSTOPERATIVE CARE

Heart rate and left atrial pressure are monitored and the blood pressure supported to levels of 60 mmHg systolic if necessary with calcium and vasopressors. Myocardial perfusion and performance have occasionally been critically dependent on the aortic root pressure, which may well overcome minor deformities of the coronary arteries after the transfer. The use of fresh whole blood is important to minimize postoperative bleeding.

After transfer of the neonate to the cardiac intensive care unit, these patients are managed in a fashion similar to other neonates undergoing cardiac surgery. Mechanical ventilation is used at least during the first 24 hours after surgery, or until the infant is hemodynamically stable. During this period all neonates are heavily sedated with intravenous narcotics and muscle relaxants. Arterial blood gas, electrolyte, calcium, and glucose levels and the hematocrit are monitored frequently.

Cardiac output is judged by measuring hourly urine output and by evaluating the strength of the distal pulses, leg temperature, and the rapidity of capillary refill. Hemodynamic support, when necessary, is provided by positive inotropic agents such as dopamine (5 to 10 µg/kg/min) and afterload reduction with nitroprusside (0.5 to 1.0 µg/kg/min). The phosphodiesterase inhibitor amrinone has also been used on occasion with beneficial effects.

Early postoperative two-dimensional echocardiography and cardiac catheterization are used liberally to exclude surgically remediable anatomic problems such as coronary artery compromise or previously unsuspected atrial or ventricular septal defects.

RESULTS AND COMPLICATIONS

In general, the results of the arterial switch operation for TGA with intact ventricular septum have been favorable (Table 66–1). The majority of the early deaths have been attributed to technical factors such as hemorrhage

Table 66–1. RESULTS OF ARTERIAL SWITCH OPERATION IN NEONATES WITH TRANSPOSITION OF THE GREAT ARTERIES AND INTACT VENTRICULAR SEPTUM (JANUARY 1983 TO AUGUST 1986)

Age (days)	No. of Patients	Mortality	
		Hospital	*Late*
0 < 8	37	2 (5.4%)	0
8 < 15	9	2 (22.2%)	0
15 < 31	10	3 (30.0%)	0
Total	56	7 (12.5%)	0

and obstructed branches of the coronary arteries causing left ventricular failure. In two other neonates, left ventricular failure with patent coronary arteries caused the death of the patients. In one, the preoperative echocardiogram showed deviation of the ventricular septum into the left ventricle, although the left ventricular pressure 1 week earlier was equal to systemic. Two other deaths were due to pulmonary hemorrhage that occurred despite low left atrial pressures. The incidence of perioperative myocardial infarction has been difficult to determine, since neither the ECG, pyrophosphate scans, nor serum enzyme levels have been sufficiently sensitive or specific to prove reliable. The most favorable results have been achieved in neonates under 10 days of age.

Recatheterization 12 months after operation has been carried out in 28 patients. Both coronary arteries were patent in 27 of the 28 patients. One asymptomatic patient had an occluded left anterior descending artery; in this patient the right coronary and circumflex arteries arose from the right cusp. For all patients, left ventricular function was normal, including left ventricular end-systolic and end-diastolic pressures and volumes and left ventricular ejection fractions. Hemodynamically significant main pulmonary artery stenosis was present in 5 patients, four of whom required reoperation, and the fifth patient underwent a balloon dilation. Our impression is that with more extensive mobilization of the pulmonary arteries, the incidence of main pulmonary artery stenosis can be avoided or at least importantly reduced. No significant supravalvular aortic stenosis has been identified in any of the patients we studied, and there has been no aortic (semilunar) valve regurgitation. All patients are in sinus rhythm.

On the basis of our experience thus far and the reports of others,[6] the arterial switch operation in the first few weeks of life can be recommended for children born with TGA and an intact ventricular septum. With additional experience, the indices by which to judge the ability of the left ventricle to support the systemic circulation should become better defined. We continue to perform early operations in neonates, preferably during the first 2 weeks of life, before the left ventricle loses its capacity to function as a systemic pump.

References

1. Albert HM (1954): Surgical correction of transposition of the great vessels. Surg Forum 5:74–77.
2. Aubert J, Pannetier A, Couvelly JP, Unal D, Rouault F, Delarue A (1978): Transposition of the great arteries: New technique for anatomical correction. Br Heart J 40:204–208.
3. Baffes TG (1956): A new method for surgical correction of transposition of the aorta and the pulmonary artery. Surg Gynecol Obstet 102:227–233.
4. Baño-Rodrigo A, Quero-Jiménez M, Moreno-Granado F, Gamallo-Amat C (1980): Wall thickness of ventricular chambers in transposition of the great arteries: Surgical implications. J Thorac Cardiovasc Surg 79:592–597.
5. Blalock A, Hanlon CR (1950): The surgical treatment of complete transposition of aorta and the pulmonary artery. Surg Gynecol Obstet 90:1–15.
6. Borow KM, Arensman FW, Webb C, Radley-Smith R, Yacoub MH (1984): Assessment of left ventricular contractile state after anatomic correction of transposition of the great arteries. Circulation 69:106–112.
7. Borow KM, Keane JF, Castañeda AR, Freed MD (1981): Systemic ventricular function in patients with tetralogy of Fallot, ventricular septal defect and transposition of the great arteries repaired during infancy. Circulation 64:878–885.
8. Castañeda AR, Norwood WI, Jonas RA, Colon SD, Sanders SP, Lang P (1984): Transposition of the great arteries and intact ventricular septum: Anatomical repair in the neonate. Ann Thorac Surg 38:438–443.
9. Edwards WS, Bargeron LM, Lyons C (1964): Reposition of right pulmonary vein in transposition of the great vessels. JAMA 188:522–523.
10. Egloff LP, Freed MD, Dick M II, Norwood WI, Castañeda AR (1978): Early and late results with the Mustard operation in infancy. Ann Thorac Surg 26:474–484.
11. Flinn CJ, Wolff GS, MacDonald D II, Campbell RM, Borkat G, Casta A, Hordof A, Hougen TJ, Kavey R-G, Kugler J, Liebman J, Greenhouse J, Hees P (1984): Cardiac rhythm after the Mustard operation for complete transposition of the great arteries. N Engl J Med 310:1635–1638.
12. Fyler DC (1980): Report of the New England Regional Infant Cardiac Program. Pediatrics 65(suppl):377–461.
13. Gittenberger-de Groot AC, Sauer U, Oppenheimer-Dekker A, et al (1983): Coronary arterial anatomy in transposition of the great arteries: A morphologic study. Pediatr Cardiol 4(suppl 1):15–24.
14. Graham TP Jr, Atwood GF, Boucek RJ, Boerth RC, Bender HW Jr (1975): Abnormalities of right ventricular function following Mustard's operation for transposition of the great arteries. Circulation 52:678–684.
15. Graham TP Jr, Burger J, Bender HW, Hammon JW, Boucek RJ, Appleton S (1985): Improved right ventricular function after intraatrial repair of transposition of the great arteries. Circulation 72(suppl II):45–51.
16. Hagler DJ, Ritter DG, Mair DD, Tajik AJ, Seward JB, Fulton RE, Ritman EL (1979): Right and left ventricular function after the Mustard procedure in transposition of the great arteries. Am J Cardiol 44:276–283.
17. Idriss FS, Goldstein IR, Grana L, French D, Potts WJ (1961): A new technique for complete correction of transposition of the great vessels: An experimental study with a preliminary clinical report. Circulation 24:5–11.
18. Jatene AD, Fontes VF, Paulista PP, et al (1975): Successful anatomic correction of transposition of the great arteries: A preliminary report. Arq Bras Cardiol 28:461–464.
19. Kay EB, Cross FS (1955): Surgical treatment of transposition of the great vessels. Surgery 38:712–716.
20. Lecompte Y, Zannini L, Hazan E, Jarreau MM, Bex JP, Tu TV, Neveux JY (1981): Anatomic correction of transposition of the great arteries: New technique without use of a prosthetic conduit. J Thorac Cardiovasc Surg 82:629–663.
21. Lillehei CW, Varco RL (1953): Certain physiologic, pathologic and surgical features of complete transposition of the great vessels. Surgery 34:376–400.
22. Mustard WT (1964): Successful two-stage correction of transposition of the great vessels. Surgery 55:469–472.
23. Mustard WT, Chute AL, Keith JD, et al (1954): A surgical approach to transposition of the great vessels with extracorporeal circuit. Surgery 36:39–51.
24. Otero-Coto E, Norwood WI, Lang P, Castañeda AR (1979): Modified Senning operation for treatment of transposition of the great arteries. J Thorac Cardiovasc Surg 78:721–729.
25. Park SC, Zuberbuhler JR, Neches WH, Lenox CC, Zoltun RA (1975): A new atrial septostomy technique. Cathet Cardiovasc Diagn 1:195–201.
26. Quaegebeur JM, Rohmer J, Brom AG, Tinkelenberg J (1977): Revival of the Senning operation in the treatment of transposition of the great arteries: Preliminary report on recent experience. Thorax 32:517–524.
27. Rashkind WJ, Miller WW (1966): Creation of an atrial septal defect without thoracotomy: A palliative approach to complete transposition of the great arteries. JAMA 196:991–992.

28. Rushmer RF (1976): Cardiovascular Dynamics. 4th ed. Philadelphia, WB Saunders, p 91.
29. Senning A (1959): Surgical correction of transposition of the great vessels. Surgery 45:966–980.
30. Trusler GA, Williams WG, Izukawa T, Olley PM (1980): Current results with Mustard operation in isolated transposition of the great arteries. J Thorac Cardiovasc Surg 80:381–388.
31. Yacoub MH, Radley-Smith R, Maclaurin R (1977): Two-stage operation for anatomical correction of transposition of the great arteries with intact interventricular septum. Lancet 1:1275–1278.

67

NEONATAL REPAIR OF TOTAL ANOMALOUS PULMONARY VENOUS CONNECTION

Martin J. Elliott

Jaroslav Stark

Surgery for total anomalous pulmonary venous connection (TAPVC) in the neonate is usually urgent, may be technically demanding, and often requires aggressive pre- and postoperative intensive care. Yet despite these difficulties, the long-term results of surgery make TAPVC one of the most rewarding conditions on which to operate. The development of operations for TAPVC must represent one of the greatest surgical success stories of the past 30 years. However, there remains a significant mortality associated with surgery, and some would argue that the risks are greater in the neonate than in the older child. In this chapter we shall review our current surgical management of TAPVC in the neonate and discuss the results of such procedures.

HISTORICAL PERSPECTIVE

Total anomalous pulmonary venous connection was probably first described by Wilson almost 200 years ago[61] from the autopsy material of a 7-day-old neonate with pulmonary venous drainage direct to a right superior vena cava. Techniques to correct TAPVC were not, however, developed until 150 years later. Muller[40] in 1951 reported partial correction of an unobstructed, probably infradiaphragmatic, TAPVC in a 4-year-old child. In the operation described, Muller anastomosed the left pulmonary vein to the left atrial appendage, approaching the vessels via a left thoracotomy. The first "open" repair of TAPVC (using moderate hypothermia induced by surface cooling and inflow occlusion), was reported in a 5-year-old child by Lewis and colleagues in 1956.[37] In that same year Burroughs and Kirklin,[9] then at the Mayo Clinic, reported the successful correction of TAPVC using cardiopulmonary bypass in two children aged 6½ months and 8½ years, respectively. Cooley and Oschner[12] also reported the successful repair of TAPVC using cardiopulmonary bypass. This operation was probably performed earlier than that of Burroughs and Kirklin.

The first report of successful repair of TAPVC in a neonate was probably in Sloan and colleagues' review of their experience, published in 1962,[49] whereas the next report of surgery for TAPVC was from Jegier et al of Montreal, in 1967,[30] who described a 6-day-old girl with infracardiac TAPVC.

During the late 1960s, a number of groups must have been attempting to repair TAPVC in neonates as evidenced by the rush of publications emerging in the early 1970s.[3–5,7,8,20,21,26,31,44] Repair of TAPVC using cardiopulmonary bypass was reported by Friedli et al,[20] who were also from Montreal. Cardiopulmonary bypass was also used in the repairs performed on the patients described in the reports of Behrendt et al[5] from London, and Higashimo et al[26] from Oakland. Behrendt et al reported the results of surgery for TAPVC in 37 children, of whom seven were neonates. Operative mortality was 100 per cent in that subgroup. Higashimo[26] reported the results of surgery in six neonates with infracardiac TAPVC, of whom three died (50 per cent). These series are important, since they described, perhaps more accurately than the previous scattered case reports, the state of affairs existing prior to the introduction of the deep hypothermic circulatory arrest techniques first proposed by the Kyoto University group.[27] The use of this technique for TAPVC was first described by Joffe et al[31] from Cape Town, and 3 months later in a keynote publication from Barratt-Boyes et al[4] describing a much more extensive experience from Green Lane Hospital, Auckland. As we shall describe later, the utilization of deep hypothermic circulatory arrest has, in most centers, radically improved the results of surgery for TAPVC in neonates.

PREOPERATIVE DIAGNOSIS

The clinical diagnosis of TAPVC can be confirmed in the majority of patients by cross-sectional echocardiography and/or color flow Doppler echocardiography. If the diagnosis of TAPVC and/or associated cardiac anomalies is not completely clear from cross-sectional echocardiography, then cardiac catheterization and angiocardiography are indicated. (For diagnostic details see Chapter 34.) Neonates presenting with TAPVC are frequently in a perilous state of low cardiac output, acidosis, and occasionally renal failure. Under these circumstances cardiac catheterization should, wherever possible, be avoided, but as we shall describe, it is important to confirm the diagnosis accurately, and thus catheterization may be necessary.

That TAPVC may be diagnosed with accuracy by echocardiography[45,50] and by color flow Doppler techniques[58] has been confirmed, and surgery has been performed successfully on the basis of echocardiographic diagnosis alone.[53] During the past few years, the proportion of patients with TAPVC operated on during the neonatal period *without* preceding catheterization has increased in our own experience.

So what does the surgeon need to know? In our view these factors may be listed as follows:

1. Confirm the diagnosis of TAPVC.
2. Define the connection of each pulmonary vein.
3. Define the presence of other intracardiac anomalies and, in addition, the presence of a patent ductus arteriosus or coarctation of the aorta.

In the majority of neonates with TAPVC, echocardiography alone will satisfy these criteria. However, if any of these factors cannot clearly be defined or if there is a "mismatch" between the clinical findings and the history and echocardiograhic findings, then cardiac catheterization is advisable.[53] Such an approach to investigation demands a high degree of cooperation between physician and surgeon. In addition, the *exact* threshold for cardiac catheterization will vary from unit to unit.

Since most children with TAPVC presenting as neonates will have obstructed venous drainage, the use of cardiac catheterization to perform balloon atrial septostomy, as suggested by Mullins et al,[41] is rarely necessary, since surgery usually follows semiurgently. However, as Ward et al[59] point out, there are a number of patients in whom neonatal surgery may be deemed inappropriate, and in whom balloon atrial septostomy (BAS) may provide the time required until they can safely undergo surgery. They suggest that BAS may still be appropriate in a very select group of patients with severe hemodynamic compromise because of a restrictive interatrial communication, in patients with mixed TAPVC and a very small pulmonary venous confluence, in patients who are the progeny of Jehovah's Witnesses, or in patients presenting in areas where the risk of neonatal surgery is high. In our experience, restrictive atrial septal defect or patent foramen ovale is very rare. Early in our experience we saw some deterioration of the clinical condition of patients with TAPVC even in the presence of a large atrial septal defect, and therefore it is our current policy to advise early surgery.

PREOPERATIVE PREPARATIONS

Many neonates presenting with TAPVC in the first few days of life are in critical condition and require intensive resuscitation. Since so many patients with TAPVC are in a significant degree of respiratory failure, endotracheal intubation and ventilation are usually required. Insertion of arterial and central venous cannulae usually follows, allowing monitoring of blood pressure and arterial blood gases and safe infusion of vasoactive agents. The patient is always sedated and may require paralysis. Renal impairment is frequent in patients with TAPVC and is managed initially by an intravenous infusion of dopamine given at 4 to 6 μg/kg/min and supplemented, if necessary, by diuretics and mannitol. Occasionally, peritoneal dialysis proves necessary and should not be delayed. Acidosis *must*

be corrected. The above measures frequently contribute to the correction of acid-base balance, but infusion of sodium bicarbonate may also be required. In our recent experience, prostacyclin (PGI$_2$) in a dose of 5 to 20 ng/kg/min intravenously has proven an effective supplementary aid to the reversal of acidosis. As we have stated previously,[51] the majority of patients respond well to such intensive treatment within 6 to 12 hours. In the exceptional patient, in whom such measures fail, surgery should not be further delayed, since acute and fatal deterioration can follow, especially if pulmonary venous obstruction is present.

SURGICAL TECHNIQUES

Anesthesia and Monitoring Devices

The technique of anesthesia for neonates with TAPVC does not differ from the techniques used for neonates with other congenital heart defects. Generally, we use atropine at a dose of 0.02 mg/kg for premedication. All neonates also receive vitamin K prior to the operation. Anesthesia is induced with a cyclopropane/oxygen mixture and maintained with nitrous oxide and oxygen, with intermittent fentanyl given at 3 to 5 μg/kg and pancuronium given at 0.1 to 0.2 mg/kg. Patients are usually intubated with a nasotracheal tube so that the tube does not have to be changed at the end of the procedure.

A 20- to 22-gauge cannula is inserted percutaneously, usually into the radial artery; brachial or femoral arteries are our other choices. Sixteen-gauge cannulae are inserted into the internal jugular vein. We prefer to use two cannulae, so that one can be used exclusively for catecholamines while the other is used for central venous pressure monitoring, injection of drugs, and crystalloid and colloid infusion. A urinary catheter is placed, and temperature probes are inserted into the nasopharynx and esophagus.

Currently, we do not use surface cooling, although others continue to use it. The patient is prepared and draped and the lines from and to the heart lung machine are placed on the table, debubbled, cut, and prepared for cannulation. We prefer to take this step before opening the sternum.

Antibiotic Prophylaxis

Gentamicin (2 mg/kg body weight) and floxacillin (12.5 mg/kg body weight) are given intravenously as soon as an intravenous access becomes available after induction of anesthesia, and they are repeated after discontinuation of cardiopulmonary bypass. Further doses are given at 6-hour (floxacillin) or 8-hour (gentamicin) intervals for up to 24 hours after operation.

Operation

A midline sternotomy is performed, and the pericardium is opened and sutured to the edges of the wound. It is important not to tie the stay sutures too tightly because resultant distortion of the ascending vertical vein (in the

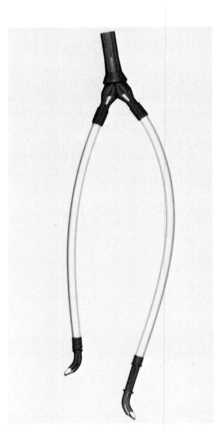

Figure 67–1. Photograph showing the thin-walled metal venous cannula used for venous cannulation.

supradiaphragmtic type) may cause venous obstruction and thus acute pulmonary edema. We inject 3 to 5 ml of 1 per cent lidocaine into the pericardial cavity to reduce irritability of the heart during dissection and cannulation. Neonates with TAPVC are often in critical condition; therefore, we limit dissection to an absolute minimum. Pursestring sutures (4-0 ethibond) are placed on the ascending aorta and on the right atrial appendage. If the patient is stable, the persistent ductus arteriosus (PDA) or ligamentum arteriosus is dissected, and a thick ligature is passed around it. If there is any instability, the PDA is dissected and ligated *after* cardiopulmonary bypass has been established. We search for a PDA in *every* patient with TAPVC irrespective of whether the diagnosis was made by echocardiography or angiocardiography. If the pulmonary artery pressure is at a systemic level, the PDA can be missed even on a good quality aortogram. The dangers of leaving the arterial duct patent during bypass are as follows: (1) The PDA can flood and damage the lungs, and systemic perfusion may become suboptimal. (2) If circulatory arrest is used, air may enter the arterial system through the PDA. (3) In the postoperative period, a residual PDA may be very troublesome, causing or contributing to heart failure.

Heparin (3 mg/kg body weight) is then given, the aorta is cannulated with a Bardik or thin-walled metal cannula (usually a 10 Bardik or 2-mm metal cannula), and one straight venous cannula (4 or 5 Portex) is placed into the right atrium.

Alternatively, it is possible to cannulate the superior and inferior venae cavae directly and to perform the operation using a low flow cardiopulmonary bypass. Thin-walled metal cannulae (Fig. 67–1) facilitate such cannulation in neonates and young infants. However, in neonates we feel that for precise anastomosis, circulatory arrest with a completely bloodless field is preferable. If we wish to shorten the period of circulatory arrest, we cannulate the right atrium through the right atrial appendage, as described above, with one straight venous cannula. When the anastomosis between the confluence of the pulmonary veins and the left atrium is completed, a venous cannula can be advanced to the inferior vena cava, and a sump sucker or another cannula can be placed through the open right atrium into the superior vena cava. Bypass is then restarted, and the patient is rewarmed while the atriotomy is being closed.

Perfusion is started with a perfusate temperature of 25°C then lowered progressively to 14 to 15°C. The patient is cooled to a nasopharyngeal temperature of 18 to 20°C. As soon as the cooling begins, one must be careful to avoid distention of the heart. In addition to ligating the PDA, we make a stab wound in the confluence of the pulmonary veins and place a sump sucker there. During the cooling period, ventilation is stopped, and dissection of the superior vena cava, inferior vena cava, pulmonary veins, pulmonary confluence, and ascending/descending vertical vein is carried out. Another pursestring suture for cardioplegia is placed into the root of the aorta. During the dissection, we are careful not to dislocate the heart too much because the coronary arteries may be kinked and temporily occluded. If any difficulty is encountered, we prefer to leave the dissection behind the heart until after the aorta has been cross-clamped. When dissecting the ascending vertical vein, care must be taken not to damage the left phrenic nerve, which usually runs on its anterolateral aspect. To avoid pulmonary venous distention, the ascending/descending vertical vein is never occluded before cardiopulmonary bypass is discontinued. When the desired temperature (nasopharyngeal temperature of 18 to 20°C) is reached (usually in 10 to 15 minutes), the aorta is cross-clamped, and blood is drained into the oxygenator to achieve a completely bloodless field. The superior vena cava and inferior vena cava are snared as well as the ascending/descending vertical vein.

Controversy exists about the use of cardioplegia in neonates. Some surgeons feel that deep hypothermia provides adequate myocardial protection. It is our belief that stopping the heart immediately after cross-clamping is beneficial. We therefore inject/infuse St. Thomas' Hospital No. 2 cardioplegic solution into the root of the aorta. Because of the additional benefit of systemic hypothermia, we do not use a full dose of 30 ml/kg as in older infants. In general we give 10 to 15 ml/kg.

Supracardiac TAPVC

The pulmonary veins join an ascending vertical vein and drain into the innominate vein (most commonly) or directly into the superior vena cava (rarely). If the connection is to the left vertical vein, we currently favor the su-

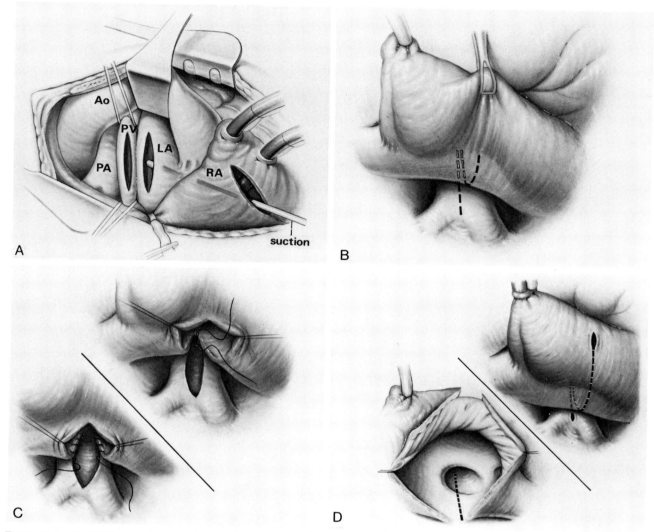

Figure 67–2. *A* to *H*, Diagrams demonstrating techniques of surgery for supracardiac TAPVC. For description see text. (Reproduced with permission from Stark J [1983]: Anomalies of the pulmonary venous return. In Stark J, de Leval MR [eds]: Surgery for Congenital Heart Defects. London, Grune & Stratton, pp 237–239.)

Illustration continued on following page

perior approach as used by Tucker et al.[54] During cooling, the right and left pulmonary veins are identified and dissected. The pulmonary venous confluence usually lies just above and in close proximity to the roof of the left atrium and below the right pulmonary artery. When perfusion is stopped and circulatory arrest is induced, a longitudinal incision is made in the roof of the left atrium with a corresponding incision in the confluence of the pulmonary veins (Fig. 67–2*A*). Through the incision in the left atrium it is sometimes possible to inspect the atrial septal defect/patent foramen ovale and to close it. If, however, we cannot identify the edges of the defect safely from this approach, we do not hesitate to make a small right atriotomy and to close the atrial septal defect/patent foramen ovale through this more familiar route.

Another approach to supracardiac TAPVC is from the right side.[35] The right atrium is grasped with forceps and retracted to the left. An incision is then made into the left atrium from behind the interatrial groove; it is then extended behind the heart toward the base of the left atrial appendage (Fig. 67–2*B*). A long incision is then made on the pulmonary venous confluence. The posterior wall of the left atrium is sutured to the incision in the pulmonary veins using a running stitch of 6-0 or 7-0 prolene or PDS (absorbable monofilament [Ethicon Ltd., Edinburgh, Scotland]) (Fig. 67–2*C*). The atrial septal defect/patent foramen ovale can again be closed from the left atrium, but if we are not sure about the anatomy from this side of the atrial septum, we do not hesitate to make a short incision in the right atrium and to close the defect this way.

The third approach is the transatrial approach suggested by Schumacher,[48] which we have used for many years. The incision gives an excellent approach, and the structures to be joined together lie in close proximity, which avoids the possibility of distorting the anastomosis. The drawback of this technique is that the biatrial incision is

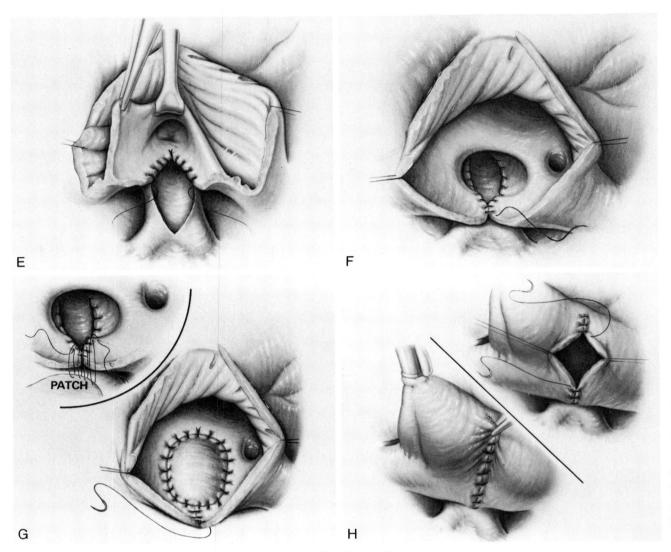

Figure 67–2 *Continued*

extensive, and therefore the construction of the anastomosis, the reconstuction of the atrial septum, and the closure of the atrium take longer. It is also easy to narrow the right pulmonary veins at the point at which the left atrium with the pulmonary anastomosis meets the atrial septum and right atrial incision.

The biatrial incision (Fig. 67–2D) starts on the right atrium and is carried across the atrial septum to the posterior wall of the left atrium. Figure 67–2E shows the beginning of the anastomosis, which is performed with a running over-and-over 6-0 or 7-0 stitch. The anastomosis is completed (Fig. 67–2E) and the right atrial closure is started (Fig. 67–2F). The atrial septal defect can be closed by direct suture or with a patch (Fig. 67–2G). Complete closure of the right atrium is illustrated in Figure 67–2H.

Direct Connection to the Superior Vena Cava

The pulmonary veins are rarely connected directly to the superior vena cava. The ascending channel may be joining the posteromedial aspect of the superior vena cava from the left. We have also seen the ascending channel to be running almost in an intrapulmonary direction on the right side and then join the posterolateral aspect of the superior vena cava. Any technique described above for the repair of supracardiac TAPVC can be applied to this variety. Great care should be taken not to damage the confluence between the ascending vertical vein and the superior vena cava. In most of our cases this confluence was very dilated, and the wall of the vessel was very thin. This varicose vein–like structure can be easily damaged, and bleeding from it may be troublesome. Vargas and Kreutzer[57] have recently described an ingenious technique for correction of anomalous pulmonary venous connection to the superior vena cava (Fig. 67–3). As can be seen from Figure 67–3, this technique involves the utilization of a J-shaped atriotomy to create an autogenous atrial flap to redirect the anomalous pulmonary venous drainage from the superior vena cava through to the left atrium via the atrial septal defect. The superior vena cava is then transected above

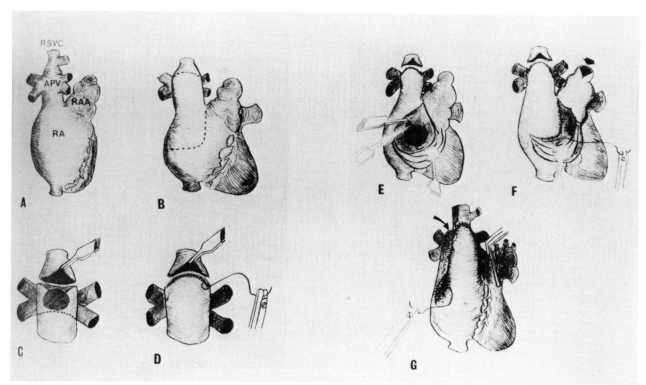

Figure 67–3. Operative technique. *A*, Anomalous right and left pulmonary veins (APV) drain separately into upper right superior vena cava (RSVC). Common pulmonary vein is absent. *B*, Broken lines illustrate both the RSVC incision and the J-shaped atriotomy. *C*, RSVC has been divided just above the site of drainage of the pulmonary veins. *D*, The proximal end of RSVC is closed with a continuous suture. RAA = right atrial appendage; RA = right atrium. *E*, Through the right atriotomy, the laminae of the fossa ovalis is removed, and the atrial defect is enlarged upward and posteriorly. *F*, The posterior flap of the atriotomy is sutured to the atrial septum from the base of the right atrial appendage, following the anterior and inferior edge of the atrial septal defect to the posterior wall of the right atrium. The pulmonary venous return has been directed into the left atrium in this way. The tip of the right atrial appendage has been opened widely (arrow). *G*, The right atrial–RSVC continuity has been reestablished by an anastomosis between the distal end of RSVC and the previously opened right atrial appendage. The right atrium is finally closed by suturing the remaining anterior edge of the atriotomy along the suture line of the posterior flap. Azygos vein must be ligated as described to avoid systemic desaturation. Arrow points to the channel of drainage of the pulmonary venous return. (Reproduced with permission from Vargas F, Kreutzer G [1985]: A surgical technique for correction of total anomalous pulmonary venous drainage. J Thorac Cardiovasc Surg 90:410–413.)

the pulmonary venous connection, where its inferior margin is oversewn and the superior vena cava at its point of transection is then spatulated and reanastomosed to the right atrial appendage. This technique seems more attractive and less prone to potential obstruction than the one described by Kawashima et al.[34]

Before the repair is completed, the perfusionist rewarms the blood to 28°C. The left heart is filled with saline and then perfusion is restarted. An aortic needle vent is placed, and the aortic cross-clamp is removed. When the heart starts beating, the de-airing procedure is carefully repeated. The heart is shaken, the left atrial appendage is inverted, and the lungs are inflated. The aorta is temporarily clamped, and a needle vent is kept on full suction. The patient is now completely rewarmed. During rewarming, atrial and ventricular pacemaker wires are placed, and if a left atrial monitoring catheter is to be used, it is inserted into the left atrial appendage. Alternatively, the anesthetist can place a longer catheter through the superior vena cava, and when the right atrium is opened, this catheter is guided under direct vision to the left atrium. When the patient is completely rewarmed (37°C), perfusion is gradually discon-

tinued. It is advisable to accept as low a central venous pressure (or right atrial pressure) as is compatible with adequate cardiac output. If the patient is transfused to a higher central venous pressure, the blood pressure and the cardiac output may improve, but the child is more likely to develop pulmonary edema. Pulmonary edema prolongs mechanical ventilation and delays extubation. When the patient is hemodynamically stable, the atrial cannula is removed. The aorta may be quite small in TAPVC, and thus even a small cannula may be partially obstructive. The aortic cannula may therefore have to be removed soon after discontinuation of perfusion. If the cardiac output is considered suboptimal at the time of discontinuation of perfusion, we start low dose dopamine (4 to 5 µg/kg/min). Protamine is given, and the chest is closed in the usual manner.

Occasionally, the heart is enlarged at the end of the procedure, and if the left atrial pressure is elevated, one gains the impression that the heart will not fit into the chest of the child. If there is any doubt as to whether the chest can be safely closed without compromising the cardiac output, we leave the sternum open and close only the

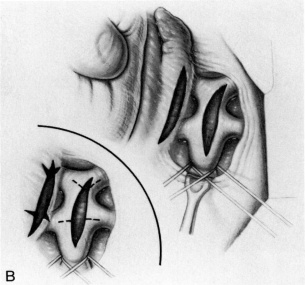

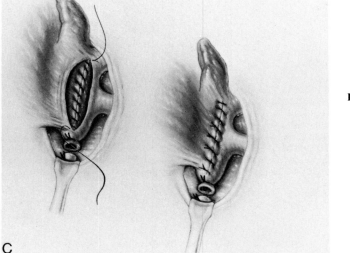

Figure 67–4. *A* to *C*, Diagrams demonstrating techniques of surgery for infracardiac TAPVC. For description see text. (Reproduced with permission from Stark J [1983]: Anomalies of the pulmonary venous return. In Stark J, de Leval MR [eds]: Surgery for Congenital Heart Defects. London, Grune & Stratton, pp 241–242.)

skin. Usually it is possible to close the sternum a few days later without any difficulty. We believe that delayed sternal closure is a useful maneuver; early in our experience we lost some sick neonates when we insisted that the chest had to be closed at the end of the procedure.

Infracardiac TAPVC

The pulmonary veins may connect to the portal vein, inferior vena cava, or hepatic vein. The technique of cannulation and bypass is identical to that described for the supracardiac connection. Most patients with infracardiac TAPVC present in a severe condition in the first week of life. Pulmonary venous drainage is almost always obstructed. We are therefore very particular about decompressing the pulmonary veins. As soon as cardiopulmonary bypass is established, we lift the heart gently, identify the descend-

ing vertical vein, make a stab incision, and place a sump sucker into it. When the aorta is cross-clamped and the circulation is arrested, the heart is lifted upward and to the right. An incision is made from the left upper pulmonary vein into the descending vertical vein (Fig. 67–4*A*). When the incision is made on the left atrium, we make an attempt to visualize how this incision will come into apposition with the pulmonary veins when the heart is replaced into the pericardial cavity. Such visualization is an important step in orienting the incisions so that distortion of the anastomosis can be avoided. If the length of the incisions seems to be short, we can make cuts into the origin of each pulmonary vein with corresponding incisions in the left atrium. These stellate incisions[11] enable us to create a larger anastomosis (Fig. 67–4*B*). On a few occasions the confluence of the pulmonary veins seemed to be located rather low toward the diaphragm. The distance between the confluence and the left atrium was quite long. As we were concerned about the possible tension or kinking of the anastomosis in such cases, we have ligated and divided the vertical descending vein (Fig. 67–4C). This approach has enabled us to construct a tension-free anastomosis.

Ligation of the Ascending/Descending Communicating Vein

In 1962 Mustard[42] suggested that repair be performed in two stages: (1) constructing an anastomosis between the pulmonary veins and the left atrium and (2) ligating the communicating vein. Subsequently, most centers have decided to perform a complete repair in one stage. During the past 2 to 3 years, we have treated several infants in whom the left atrial pressure remained unacceptably high following repair. We can only speculate on the reasons for this persistent left atrial hypertension, as an adequate anastomosis was constructed, and no anomaly of the mitral valve or left ventricle was seen on echocardiography or angiocardiography. As soon as the ligature on the ascending/descending vein was released, the pressure in the left atrium was reduced to normal or at least to acceptable levels. For these reasons, we do not tie the communicating vein at the beginning of perfusion but only snare it. After repair, when bypass is discontinued, we carefully measure the pressures, and if left atrial hypertension is present, the snare is released. The descending vein is left open in most patients on the assumption that the descending vertical vein usually enters the portal vein, which provides more resistance to the flow than the anastomosis between the pulmonary veins and the left atrium. The descending vein always closes spontaneously later. If the ascending vein does not close spontaneously, we may consider closing it with a detachable balloon during recatheterization or, alternatively, ligating it through a left thoracotomy.

TAPVC to the Coronary Sinus

Cannulation and bypass techniques for this condition are the same as those for a supra- or infradiaphragmatic type connection. It is, however, easier to opt for bicaval cannulation and repair on low flow hypothermic bypass in this condition as compared with supra- or infracardiac TAPVC.

When the right atrium is opened, the anatomy is carefully examined. The septum between the coronary sinus and the left atrium is carefully excised (Fig. 67–5A and B). A patch of pericardium is then sutured around the coronary sinus and the atrial septal defect so that the blood from the pulmonary veins and the coronary sinus is diverted into the left atrium. Care is taken to avoid the anterior rim of the coronary sinus so that the tail of the AV node is not injured. Before the patch is completed, the left atrium and left ventricle are filled with saline; perfusion is then restarted, and rewarming is completed in the same way as described previously.

An alternative technique for repair of TAPVC to the coronary sinus was described by Van Praagh and colleagues (Fig. 67–6). The root of the coronary sinus (septum

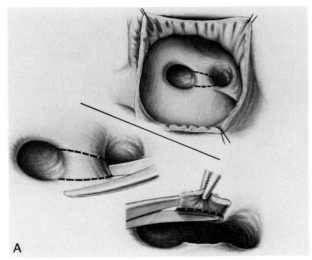

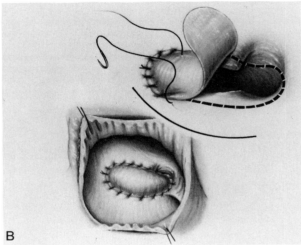

Figure 67–5. *A* and *B*, Diagrams showing surgical techniques for TAPVC to coronary sinus. For description of technique see text. (Reproduced with permission from Stark J [1983]: Anomalies of the pulmonary venous return. In Stark J, de Leval MR [eds]: Surgery for Congenital Heart Defects. London, Grune & Stratton, p 240.)

between the coronary sinus and the left atrium) is excised (Fig. 67–6B and C), creating a large opening between the coronary sinus and the pulmonary veins through the left atrium (Fig. 67–6D). The coronary sinus is then closed with a fine monofilament suture (Fig. 67–6E), and finally the atrial septal defect/patent foramen ovale is also closed (Fig. 67–6F).

TAPVC Directly to the Right Atrium

If the pulmonary veins connect directly into the right atrium, the atrial septal defect is usually enlarged, and the opening of the pulmonary veins is connected to the left atrium via the atrial septal defect with a generous pericardial patch.

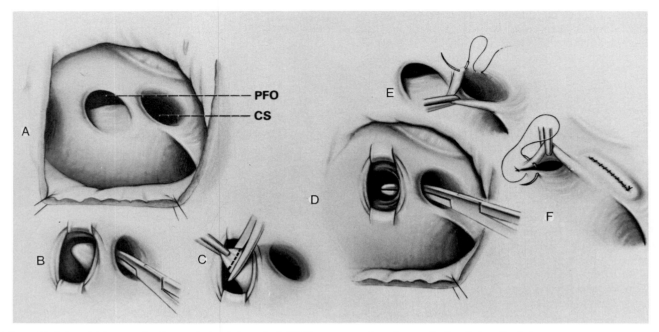

Figure 67–6. *A* to *F*, Diagrams showing surgical techniques for TAPVC to coronary sinus. See text for description of technique.

Connection of the Right Pulmonary Veins into the Right Atrium/Inferior Vena Cava (Scimitar Syndrome)

Infant and adult forms of scimitar syndrome were recognized by Dupuis.[17] If an infant with scimitar syndrome presents with severe heart failure, surgery may be indicated even in the neonatal period. Most infants with scimitar syndrome also have major aortopulmonary collaterals, usually originating from the descending thoracic or abdominal aorta.[1] It is often not necessary to perform the complete repair, including redirection of the right pulmonary veins into the left atrium, at this stage. The heart failure is much improved when the collaterals are occluded, either with coils at the time of cardiac catheterization or by a ligature through a thoracotomy. Complete repair, which involves anastomosis of the right pulmonary veins to the left atrium or tunneling within the inferior vena cava,[52] can then be delayed until the child is older. The repair is technically easier on a bigger heart, and the procedure is less risky.

Anomalous Connection of Left Pulmonary Veins to the Innominate Vein

Often, the left upper pulmonary vein only is connected to the innominate vein. It is our opinion that repair of this lesion is not required whether it is an isolated lesion or whether associated cardiac anomalies are present. A shunt from one isolated lobe is usually not excessive and is well tolerated unless the patient is living at high altitude. If the whole left lung connects to the innominate vein, a shunt of approximately 2:1 can be expected. Repair of this ex-

tremely rare anomaly is achieved by anastomosing the left pulmonary veins to the left atrium.[52]

Mixed Type of TAPVC

Different lobes of the lungs can be connected to the different parts of the venous system. Often, the connection from all parts of the lung is not visualized before the operation. The risk of repair of mixed TAPVC is considered higher[2,32] than that for the other types. The operative techniques depend on the exact anatomy, and all the techniques described in the preceding discussion may have to be used.

POSTOPERATIVE MANAGEMENT

The overall management of patients after surgery for TAPVC does not differ from that of other neonates after open-heart surgery. However, certain features do warrant special mention. Neonates with TAPVC are particularly prone to develop pulmonary edema in the early postoperative period, even in the absence of any anastomotic obstruction.[51] In addition, and in association with preexisting pulmonary venous hypertension, it is known that there is increased arteriolar musculature in the pulmonary vascular bed.[24,25] This new muscle may be reactive, resulting in prolonged pulmonary hypertension and/or acute pulmonary hypertensive crises[29] in which there is a paroxysmal rise in pulmonary artery pressure associated with a fall in systemic blood pressure and thus cardiac output as flow through the lungs acutely falls and right ventricular pressure rises. Thus, the special features of TAPVC requiring specific postoperative treatment are pulmonary edema and pulmonary hypertensive crises.

Fluid Balance

The tendency for these patients to develop severe postoperative pulmonary edema makes accurate fluid balance control mandatory. Fluid retention occurs after any operation is performed using cardiopulmonary bypass. However, operations performed in the neonatal period seem to predispose to fluid retention even more so than is apparent in the older child. Fluid restriction to 20 ml/M^2/hr is routine during the first 24 hours. However, in our experience peritoneal dialysis has often proved necessary to resolve the problem of fluid retention and to reduce associated pulmonary edema, even in the presence of a urine output greater than 1 ml/kg/hr. Recently, we have been encouraged by the effect of ultrafiltration toward the end of bypass in apparently reducing postoperative fluid retention. Ultrafiltration may also be practicable postoperatively if hemodynamics remain stable.

Ventilation

All neonates with TAPVC require intermittent positive pressure ventilation (IPPV) for some amount of time postoperatively, usually for at least 24 to 48 hours. The addition of modest (approximately 5 cm H_2O) positive end-expiratory pressure (PEEP) is frequently helpful, especially if pulmonary edema does indeed develop. Adequate control of ventilation also plays a crucial part in the prevention and management of acute pulmonary hypertensive crises (see the following).

Hemodynamics

The presence of both right and left atrial pressure monitoring lines is very helpful, since, as we have implied, there may be differential "reactivity" of pulmonary and systemic vascular beds, resulting in apparently disparate changes in vascular resistance and thus ventricular afterload. Until recently, we have not used a left atrial line routinely, although a right atrial or systemic venous pressure line has always been inserted in our practice. However, it has recently been established[28] that control of the vascular beds may be best achieved by the selective infusion of vasoactive agents into the right atrium for maximum pulmonary effect and into the left atrium for maximum systemic effects. Thus, it is our current opinion that both right atrial and left atrial pressure lines should be inserted.

As with all patients after open-heart surgery, preload should be optimized,[18] after which attempts should be made to minimize afterload and, if necessary, to increase myocardial contractility. First, we will discuss the pharmacologic manipulation of the systemic vascular bed.

Systemic Vascular Resistance

Reduction of systemic vascular resistance is best achieved by the infusion of vasodilators into the left atrium. Frequently, however, there is a concomitant need to reduce the pulmonary vascular resistance, and vasodilators must be infused into the pulmonary circulation. Although there is significant deactivation of most vasoactive agents in the lung,[28] sufficient vasodilator activity always remains to have a measurable effect upon the systemic vascular bed, and in the context of TAPVC, venous administration of vasodilators is usually sufficient to decrease systemic vascular resistance adequately. If there is no evidence of pulmonary hypertension, then sodium nitroprusside (0.5 to 5.0 µg/kg/min) or nitroglycerin (0.5 to 5.0 µg/kg/min) remains the vasodilator of choice. If longer therapy is required, we switch later to hydralazine (750 µg/kg/24 hours in four divided doses) or captopril (0.3 to 3 mg/day).

Myocardial Contractility

Many of the inotropes normally used in postoperative management may also increase pulmonary vascular resistance. Dopamine is safe to use as long as the dose is maintained at less than 6 µg/kg/min. (Low dose dopamine also has the advantage of preserving renal blood flow.) If we are genuinely concerned about the reactivity of the pulmonary vascular bed, we prefer to use dobutamine in similar doses. Isoproterenol (0.01 to 0.1 mg/kg/min) functions as a pulmonary vasodilator in low doses and thus may be beneficial as an inotrope, if its chronotropic effects are not detrimental. We try to avoid the use of epinephrine (adrenaline).

Pulmonary Vascular Resistance

We have recently reported our experience with the management of acute pulmonary hypertensive crises,[29] and much of this section is drawn from those data. As with most things in medicine, prevention is better than cure. Unfortunately, we still do not know in which patients pulmonary hypertensive crises are likely to occur and why pulmonary hypertensive crises do occur in these patients. However, there are a number of ways in which acute pulmonary hypertensive crises may be held at bay, largely by suppressing the factors that are known to produce pulmonary vasoconstriction. For this reason, we now leave a right ventricular (RV) or pulmonary artery (PA) pressure catheter in the patient at the time of operation in order to monitor the fluctuations in RV or PA pressure. Acidosis *must* be prevented using all the means at ones disposal (bicarbonate, prostacyclin, dialysis). Particularly, the arterial PCO_2 must be kept low (we aim for around 30 mmHg) by hyperventilation, as recommended by Drummond et al in 1981.[16] Similarly, the prevention of hypoxia should be routine, with the use of high FiO_2 values if necessary. Unnecessary endotracheal suction should be avoided, since hypoxia is frequent. If such suction is required, then preoxygenation with 100 per cent oxygen is mandatory. Similar comments on prevention apply to the use of chest physiotherapy. To help clear airway secretions, we believe that physiotherapy should be started soon after the patient is returned to the intensive care unit; any delay in commencement of physiotherapy may be detrimental. Physiotherapy must, of course, be extremely gentle in contrast to other procedures and age groups. These patients may develop pulmonary hypertensive crises in association with even minor physical or environmental disturbances. For this reason, we as well as many other units[36] often maintain a degree of light anesthesia by the continuous infusion of fentanyl (4 to 8 µg/kg/hr) frequently together with a muscle relaxant such as atracurium (8 µg/kg/hr).

Occasionally, and despite the above preventive measures, full-blown acute pulmonary hypertensive crises do develop, and therapeutic measures must be introduced. The first most important, and often the most successful, method of treatment is immediate hand-ventilation with 100 per cent oxygen. If hand ventilation fails to break the hypertensive cycle in a few moments or if the frequency of attacks increases, then pharmacologic agents should be introduced. These agents should be infused directly into the pulmonary artery if a pulmonary arterial manometer line was inserted at surgery; if not, they should be infused into the right atrium. The sensitivity of the pulmonary vasculature to the various agents varies markedly, both in terms of drug and dosage. Thus, to some extent, the management of pulmonary hypertensive crises, and the order in which the drugs are tried, is a matter of trial and error. However, as a guideline, Table 67–1 gives a list of drugs that may be used together with appropriate dose ranges.

As usual, it is easier to start therapy than to stop it, and one of the difficulties that we and other groups have had is determining how to wean the patient from the therapeutic and prophylactic support of pulmonary hypertensive managment. As a general (but not rigid) rule, we attempt to withdraw supportive therapy after 2 to 3 days, starting with the anesthetic agents; FiO$_2$ is reduced prior to withdrawing the other pharmacologic agents. As implied, manipulation of the pulmonary vasculature may take up a disproportionate time in the postoperative management of TAPVC.

Other Aspects of Postoperative Care

Diminished renal function is fairly frequent (see the section Results) after repair of TAPVC and warrants ag-

gressive treatment according to the standard rules. Peritoneal dialysis should not be delayed if determined to be necessary. We have lost one child from intestinal perforation following nasogastric calcium resonium for hyperkalemia, which may well have been better treated by peritoneal dialysis.

The incidence of paralyzed diaphragm (presumably from direct phrenic nerve injury) also seems fairly frequent. It is clearly important to take careful measures to prevent damage to the phrenic nerve, particularly in relation to the pulmonary venous confluence, to a vertical vein, and to any dissection of the thymus gland. Diathermy may be particularly important in this context. Thus, one must initially suspect a paralyzed diaphragm whenever a child proves difficult to wean from a ventilator or later when feeding difficulties or recurrent chest infections occur. Plication of the affected diaphragm may be necessary to prevent further deterioration or a prolonged inhospital stay. Pulmonary infection with or without diaphragmatic paralysis is frequent and must be vigorously treated if unnecessary postoperative deaths are to be prevented.

RESULTS

Without surgery, the outlook for patients with TAPVC is grim, with only approximatly 20 per cent surviving the first year of life.[33] Although scattered reports of survival into adulthood do occur,[47] they are rare. Surgery is thus imperative, but how do the results of surgery in the neonatal period compare with both the natural history and the results of surgery in the older child?

Reports of surgery for TAPVC concerning purely the neonatal period are rare,[8] although as indicated earlier, scattered case reports exist from the early 1960s. Thus, we have abstracted data from more comprehensive series to compile Tables 67–2 and 67–3. Table 67–2 demonstrates the accumulated data available on neonates with TAPVC operated on before the use of deep hypothermic circulatory arrest. The literature records a total of 21 neonates operated on by simple bypass techniques, with 14 (67 per cent) operative deaths and a single late death (although follow-up was short or absent in each of the published series). Two of the seven survivors of operations developed anastomotic stricture, and in one (the late death) this complication proved fatal; the other patient required two additional operations to correct the problem. Thus, overall mortality for TAPVC prior to the acceptance of deep hypothermic circulatory arrest was in excess of 75 per cent, with the best results in a selected (infracardiac) series[26] representing a 50 per cent risk.

Let us now consider the results of surgery *since* the advent of deep hypothermic circulatory arrest (Table 67–3). Since we shall describe the experience of The Hospital for Sick Children, London, a little later in this section, we have excluded all references from our hospital in the following summary of data.

Seventy-two neonatal TAPVC procedures were reported in the literature (other than from the Hospital for Sick Children). There were 17 operative deaths (24 per cent).

Table 67–1. DRUGS USED IN THE MANAGEMENT OF ESTABLISHED PULMONARY HYPERTENSIVE CRISIS*

| Drug | Dose (IV) | |
	Bolus	*Infusion*
Tolazoline	1 mg/kg	1 to 4 mg/kg/hr
Nitroglycerin	–	0.5 to 2.0 µg/kg/min
Prostacyclin	–	5 to 50 ng/kg/min
Phenoxybenzamine	1 to 2 mg/kg	–

*Since writing this chapter, prostacyclin has become our drug of choice for treatment of *established* crises. Phenoxybenzamine is initiated b.i.d. for 4 days as a preventive measure.

Table 67–2. SUMMARY OF PUBLICATIONS REPORTING SURGERY FOR TAPVC IN NEONATES WITHOUT THE USE OF DEEP HYPOTHERMIC CIRCULATORY ARREST

Author	Location	Date	Era	Number of Neonates Reported	Type of TAPVC*				Hospital Mortality	Causes	Late Mortality	Causes	Overall Mortality	Follow-up Period	Comments
					Supra	Infra	Cardiac	Mixed							
Jegier et al	Montreal	1967	1965	1	–	1	–		–	–	–	–	0	2 years	
Friedli et al	Montreal	1970	1970	1	–	1	–		–	–	–	–	0	2 years	This child had two reoperations for anastomotic stenosis.
Behrendt et al	London	1972	1963–70	7/37	Not Described				100%	Low cardiac output	–	–	100%	–	First published series of neonates.
Hagashimo et al	Oakland	1974	1967–71	6	–	6	–		50%	Low cardiac output	–	–	50%	None reported	
Duff et al	Baylor, Houston	1977	1957–75	6/9	–	6	–		67%	Low cardiac output	17%	Anastomotic stricture	84%	None reported	

*Type of TAPVC: Often in larger series, the distribution of TAPVC type is not mentioned separately for the neonatal group.
Total neonates reported equals 21, operative deaths equal 14, late deaths equal 1 (> 75% overall mortality).
Anastomotic stricture occurred in two of the seven operative survivors.

There were four late deaths, including two from anastomotic strictures. Further, two patients were reported to have been successfully reoperated on for anastomotic stricture. These results (overall mortality 29 per cent) demonstrate a considerable improvement over the data compiled before deep hypothermic circulatory arrest was a viable technique.

At The Hospital for Sick Children, London, since 1971 (when the technique of deep hypothermic circulatory arrest was introduced) 49 neonates have undergone surgery for TAPVC. Of these, 22 had infracardiac drainage, 18 supracardiac, and two mixed. The mean ages and weights of these children are shown in Table 67–4. The experience of The Hospital for Sick Children represents the largest series of neonates available for analysis.

The mortality figures for this group of patients are shown in Table 67–5, from which it can be seen that the hospital mortality was 43 per cent and the late mortality 6 per cent, giving an overall mortality of 49 per cent. Since these figures are somewhat worse than the other, although

Table 67–3. SUMMARY OF PUBLICATIONS REPORTING SURGERY FOR TAPVC IN NEONATES WITH THE USE OF DEEP HYPOTHERMIC CIRCULATORY ARREST

Author	Location	Date	Era	Number of Neonates Reported	Type of TAPVC*				Hospital Mortality	Causes	Late Mortality	Causes	Overall Mortality	Follow-up Period	Comments
					Supra	Infra	Cardiac	Mixed							
Joffe et al	Cape Town	1971	1969	1	–	1	–		–	–	–	–	0	–	First reported use of deep hypothermic arrest for repair of TAPVC.
Barratt-Boyes et al	Auckland	1971	1969–70	2	–	1	1		–	–	50% (6)	Tracheal stenosis	50%	1	
Gersony et al	New York	1971	?–1971	1/10	–	–	1		–	–	–	–	0	<39 months	
Barratt-Boyes et al	Auckland	1971	1971	1	–	–	1		0	–	–	–	0	–	Patient also had interrupted aortic arch and ventricular septal defect.
Buckley	Boston	1971	1967–71	3*	1	1	1		33% (1)	Low cardiac output	0	–	33%	–	Two of the patients (including the one who died) had simple cardiopulmonary bypass.
Parr et al	Birmingham	1974	1972–73	5/11	1	4 (4)	–		80%	Low cardiac output	–	–	80%	Not reported	
Kawashima et al	Osaka	1976	1976	1/3	–	1	–		100% (1)	Low cardiac output	–	–	100%	Not reported	
Sparrow et al	Ann Arbor	1976	1975	1	1	–	–		–	–	–	–	0	9 months	To that date the smallest child was 2.5 kg.
Whight et al	Auckland	1977	1967–76	8/23	1 (1)	5 (2)	2 (1)		25%	Low cardiac output	25% (2)	1—tracheal stenosis; 1—anastomotic stricture (cardiac)	50%	<6 years	
Fleming et al	Omaha	1978	1975–77	4	–	4	–		–	–	25% (1)	Anastomotic stricture	25%	<2 years	
Turley et al	San Francisco	1979	1975–79	12/22	Not Described				17% (2)	1—low cardiac output; 1—LVF	–	–	17%	Not reported	
Byrum et al	Ann Arbor	1982	1977–81	8/14*	2	5	1		13% (1)	Low cardiac output	–	–	13%	<13 years	Two patients reoperated on for anastomotic stricture.
Dickinson et al	Liverpool	1982	1970–81	13/44	3	7 (1)	1	2 (1)	15% (2)	Low cardiac output	–	–	15%	<10 years	
Hawkins et al	Iowa City	1983	–1983	6/20	2	4 (1)	–	–	17% (1)	Low cardiac output	–	–	17%	<10 years	
Mazzucco et al	Padova	1983	1971–81	9/20	Not Described				44% (4)	Low cardiac output	–	–	44%	<10 years	

Abbreviations: DOT = died on the operating table; LVF = left ventricular failure.
*Type of TAPVC: Often in larger series, the distribution of TAPVC type is not mentioned separately for the neonatal group. Total neonates reported equals 72, operative deaths equal 17, late deaths equal 4 (29 per cent overall mortality). Anastomotic strictures occurred in four patients, two of whom survived.

Table 67–4. NUMBERS, AGES, AND WEIGHTS OF NEONATES UNDERGOING SURGERY FOR TAPVC AT THE HOSPITAL FOR SICK CHILDREN, GREAT ORMOND STREET, 1971–1986

	Number	Age (days)*	Weight (kg)*
All types	49	8 ± 1	3.0 ± 0.5
Infracardiac	22	9 ± 1	2.8 ± 0.1
Supracardiac	18	5 ± 1	3.1 ± 0.1
Cardiac	7	15 ± 2	3.2 ± 0.2
Mixed	2	5, 8	2.8, 3.7

* Values represent mean ± SEM.

Table 67–6. CAUSES OF HOSPITAL DEATHS AMONG 49 NEONATES UNDERGOING SURGERY FOR TAPVC AT THE HOSPITAL FOR SICK CHILDREN, GREAT ORMOND STREET, 1971–1986

Cause	No. of Deaths
Low cardiac output (early postoperative)	7
Bronchopneumonia (four with septicemia)*	6 (4 with pseudomonas, 1 with *S. aureus*, 1 with cytomegalovirus)
Died on table (low cardiac output)	3
Technical (SVC obstruction)†	2 (1 cardiac, 1 supracardiac)
Pulmonary hypertensive crisis	1 (patient had additional VSD)
Subarachnoid hemorrhage	1
Intestinal perforation (calcium resonium)	1

*Four patients had preceding low cardiac output.
†One SVC damaged during control of bleeding vertical vein; one SVC obstructed by postoperative thrombus.

smaller, published series, we should consider the causes of these deaths.

The causes of the hospital deaths in our series are shown in Table 67–6. Ten patients died of low cardiac output either on the operating table or in the early postoperative period, which is a proportion similar to that reported in other series. The remaining deaths may (perhaps) be defined as potentially preventable: six from bronchopneumonia, two from technical superior vena caval obstruction (see Table 67–6), one from pulmonary hypertensive crises in a child with an additional small ventricular septal defect, one from intestinal perforation after nasogastric calcium resonium, and one from subarachnoid hemorrhage.

The causes of the late deaths are shown in Table 67–7. Note that only one child had anastomotic obstruction, a relatively low incidence compared with other published series (Table 67–8). Cardioplegic techniques were used in our institution after 1978. However, cardioplegia does not seem to have altered mortality significantly. Before 1978, 12 of 22 patients died compared with 12 of 27 since 1978.

Morbidity

Consideration of perioperative morbidity has received scant attention in most published series. However, Table 67–9 shows the morbidity figures in our patients since 1971. Forty per cent of the patients developed some sort of complication, and several developed more than one. Renal failure, cerebral damage, and paralyzed diaphragms were the most serious complications observed. These data suggest that continued research into perfusion during and after surgery is indicated and that surgeons should be

Table 67–5. MORTALITY AMONG NEONATES UNDERGOING SURGERY FOR TAPVC AT THE HOSPITAL FOR SICK CHILDREN, GREAT ORMOND STREET, 1971–1986

Type	n	Hospital Deaths	Late Deaths	Total Deaths
Infracardiac	22	9	0	9 (41%)
Supracardiac	18	8	2	10 (56%)
Cardiac	7	3	1	4 (57%)
Mixed	2	1	0	1 (50%)
Total	49	21 (43%)	3 (6%)	24 (49%)

especially aware of the proximity of the phrenic nerve to the pulmonary venous pathways in TAPVC.

Risk Factors for Hospital Death

As Kirklin points out,[36] multivariate analysis of risk factors has not been undertaken to date in TAPVC, largely because of its relative rarity. However, a number of potential risk factors have been mentioned in previous sections, and examination of published data allows one to infer certain conclusions. It is, however, important to realize that these inferences are based on data from *all* patients operated on for TAPVC and not simply neonates.

Age

Does the very fact of being a neonate modify the patient's chances of survival? In the combined Birmingham and Green Lane experience,[36] young age was only a possible risk factor. Turley et al[55] did not find age to be a risk factor; nor did Dickinson et al.[15] However, our data[51] would lend support to those of Mazzucco et al,[39] which suggest that young age does adversely affect survival.

Poor Preoperative Condition

There seems little doubt that poor preoperative condition is an important factor influencing survival,[36,51] particularly if acidosis is present.[6,13,23,55] Thus, it is worth restating that vigorous attempts at improving preoperative condition are worth pursuing for 6 to 12 hours; however, if no improvement ensues, surgery must not be further delayed for fear of acute deterioration.

Associated Cardiac Anomalies

Associated cardiac anomalies have been said[39] to increase mortality. However, other than patent ductus arteriosus, associated cardiac anomalies are but rarely reported in the neonatal population.[3,14] It is extremely important to

Table 67–7. CAUSES OF LATE DEATHS AMONG 49 NEONATES UNDERGOING SURGERY FOR TAPVC AT THE HOSPITAL FOR SICK CHILDREN, GREAT ORMOND STREET, 1971–1986

Cause	No. of Deaths
At reoperation for obstruction of pulmonary venous pathway by adherent ADS patch (1 month after first operation [supracardiac])	1
Cardiopulmonary collapse, severe multiple anomalies (7 months after first operation [supracardiac])	1
Viral pneumonia (21 months after first operation [cardiac])	1

[ ] = site of anomalous pulmonary venous connection.

ligate the patent ductus arteriosus at the time of repair, since late left ventricular failure and even death may ensue if it is not tied off.[7,19] An additional risk of leaving the ductus patent is the possibility of air embolism if deep hypothermic circulatory arrest is utilized in the operative technique.

Small Left Ventricle

It has been suggested[22,32] that small left ventricular volume may be an important risk factor. The combined Green Lane and Birmingham experience only hints at this possibility.[36] However, a recent study by Oliveira Lima et al[43] addressing the problem both echocardiographically and with postmortem data in a small group of patients supports the view that an increased right ventricle–left ventricle dimension ratio is associated with a poor prognosis. A small left atrium is also probably an important risk factor.

Long-Term Functional Results

Unless pulmonary venous obstruction ensues, long-term functional results are excellent. Of the 25 survivors in our series, all are in New York Heart Association Functional Class I, and none are on any medications. Our long-term results are similar to the long-term results presented by others.[10,15,36,39] The very long-term results are awaited with interest.

Long-Term Hemodynamic Results

Pulmonary arterial pressure may be expected to be normal after repair, provided pulmonary venous obstruction is relieved.[23,36,44] Right ventricular volume, left ventricular end-diastolic volume, and left ventricular systolic function should also return to normal after surgery.[23]

Anastomotic Stricture/Pulmonary Vein Stenosis

The incidence of postoperative anastomotic pulmonary venous obstruction is relatively low (see Table 67–8), but if it occurs, it can be very difficult and dangerous to manage.[7] If suspected (by dyspnea, tachypnea, and pulmonary venous congestion on chest radiograph), investigation and

Table 67–8. REPORTED INCIDENCE OF LATE STENOSIS OF THE PULMONARY VEINS/ANASTOMOSIS

Author	Reference	Number	Survivors	Incidence
Dickinson et al	15	4	36	11%
Byrum et al	10	1	10	10%
Whight et al	60	3	20	15%
Stark	51	2	26	6%
G.O.S. (neonates)	This chapter	1	28	4%

G.O.S. = Great Ormond Street.

therapy must be performed urgently. The number of patients with small and clinically insignificant transanastomotic pressure gradients is not known, since only symptomatic patients are investigated.[36] However, if obstruction is confirmed, it should be relieved by surgery.

Infrequently, the pulmonary venous orifices become stenotic.[19,20,36] The obvious operation would seem to be patch angioplasty, but repair can be quite difficult, and results have not been good. The pathology of the disease seems to consist of extensive and obstructive endothelial fibrosis of the pulmonary ostia. Simple resection of this ostial fibrosis from within, as pioneered by Louhimo in Helsinki[38] for congenital pulmonary venous stenosis, has proved effective both for him and for one case of TAPVC at the University of Alabama.[36] Judging the adequacy of pulmonary veins has proved difficult in the past, but the recent publication of a range of normal values by the Helsinki group[46] should help surgeons in planning or assessing corrective procedures.

FUTURE PROSPECTS

There remains an unacceptably high mortality of between 15 and 50 per cent associated with surgery for TAPVC in the neonate. The most "resistant" cause of death remains

Table 67–9. MORBIDITY* AMONG 49 NEONATES UNDERGOING REPAIR OF TAPVC AT THE HOSPITAL FOR SICK CHILDREN, GREAT ORMOND STREET, 1971–1986

Morbidity	No. of Patients
Early	
Acute renal failure (PD)	8
Paralyzed hemidiaphragm (Left)	4 (2 with plication)
(Right)	1
Septicemia	4
Cerebral damage†	6
Junctional tachycardia	1
Chylothorax	1
Necrotizing enterocolitis	1
Pulmonary hypertensive crisis	1
Late	
Residual neurologic signs	1

* Several patients suffered more than one complication.
† Five patients developed seizures after episodes of low cardiac output early postoperatively. All but one have completely recovered. One patient developed seizures after a cardiac arrest 12 days postoperatively. The patient is also normal now.
PD = peritoneal dialysis.

perioperative low cardiac output, and it is to the etiology of this complication that attention must be turned. Despite detailed analysis by many teams, no reliable prognostic factor has been defined. Perhaps pooling the clinical data will allow meaningful multivariate analysis to be performed.

In the meantime, rigorous perioperative management is likely to reap the best reward. We would encourage units to continue to publish both the immediate and late results of surgery and to strive to reduce this residual mortality in what should be a completely correctable lesion.

References

1. Alivizatos P, Cheatle T, de Leval MR, Stark J (1985): Pulmonary sequestration complicated by anomalies of pulmonary venous return. J Pediatr Surg 20:76–79.
2. Arciprete P, McKay R, Watson GH, Hamilton DI, Wilkinson JL, Arnold RM (1986): Double connections in total anomalous pulmonary venous connection. J Thorac Cardiovasc Surg 92:146–152.
3. Barratt-Boyes BG, Nicholls TT, Brandt PWT, Neutze JM (1972): Aortic arch interruption associated with patent ductus arteriosus, ventricular septal defect, and total anomalous pulmonary venous connection. J Thorac Cardiovasc Surg 63:367–373.
4. Barratt-Boyes BG, Simpson M, Neutze JM (1971): Intracardiac surgery in neonates and infants using deep hypothermia with surface cooling and limited cardiopulmonary bypass. Circulation 43,44(Suppl I):25–30.
5. Behrendt DM, Aberdeen E, Waterston DJ, Bonham-Carter RE (1972): Total anomalous pulmonary venous drainage in infants. I. Clinical and hemodynamic findings, methods, and results of operation in 37 cases. Circulation 46:347–356.
6. Bove EL, de Leval MR, Taylor JF, Macartney FJ, Szarnicki RJ, Stark J (1981): Infradiaphragmatic total anomalous pulmonary venous drainage. Surgical treatment and long term results. Ann Thorac Surg 31:544–550.
7. Breckenridge IM, de Leval MR, Stark J, Waterston DJ (1973): Correction of total anomalous pulmonary venous drainage in infancy. J Thorac Cardiovasc Surg 66:447–453.
8. Buckley MJ, Behrendt DM, Goldblatt A, Laver MB, Austen WG (1972): Correction of total anomalous pulmonary venous drainage in the first month of life. J Thorac Cardiovasc Surg 63:269–274.
9. Burroughs JT, Kirklin JW (1956): Complete surgical correction of total anomalous pulmonary venous connection: Report of three cases. Proc Mayo Clin 31:182–188.
10. Byrum CJ, Dick M, Behrendt DM, Rosenthal A (1982): Repair of total anomalous pulmonary venous connection in patients younger than 6 months old. Late postoperative hemodynamic and electrophysiologic status. Circulation 66(Suppl I):208–214.
11. Clarke DR, Paton BC, Stewart JR (1979): Surgical treatment of total anomalous pulmonary venous drainage. Adv Cardiol 26:129–137.
12. Cooley DA, Ochsner A Jr (1957): Correction of total anomalous pulmonary venous drainage. Surgery 42:1014–1021.
13. Cooper DKC, Stark J (1979): Factors contributing to the mortality associated wtih open-heart surgery in infants. In Rickham PP, Hecker WCh, Prevot J (eds): Causes of Postoperative Death in Children: Analysis and Therapeutic Implications. Baltimore, Urban & Schwarzenberg, pp 115–129.
14. de Leval MR, Stark J, Bonham-Carter RE (1973): Total anomalous pulmonary venous drainage to superior vena cava associated with preductal coarctation of aorta: Successful correction in a 12-day-old infant. Br Heart J 35:1098–1100.
15. Dickinson DF, Parimelazhagan KM, Tweedie MCK, West CR, Piccoli GP, Musumeci F, Hamilton DI (1982): Total anomalous pulmonary venous connection: Repair using deep hypothermia and circulatory arrest in 44 consecutive infants. Br Heart J 48:249–254.
16. Drummond WH, Gregory GA, Heymann MA, Phibbs RA (1981): The independent effects of hyperventilation, tolazoline, and dopamine on infants with persistent pulmonary hypertension. J Pediatr 98:603–611.
17. Dupuis C (1977): The scimitar syndrome in infants and children (Preliminary report of a cooperative study; 81 cases: 64 children and adolescents, and 17 newborns and infants) (abstr). Europ J Cardiol 5:302–303.
18. Elliott MJ (1987): The postoperative care of the paediatric cardiac surgical patient: Lessons for paediatricians. In Hunter S (ed): Perspectives in Paediatric Cardiology (in press).
19. Fleming WH, Clark EB, Dooley KJ, Hofschire PJ, Ruckman RN, Hopeman AR, Sarafian L, Mooring PK (1979): Late complications following surgical repair of total anomalous pulmonary venous return below the diaphragm. Ann Thorac Surg 27:435–439.
20. Friedli B, Davignon A, Stanley P (1971): Infradiaphragmatic anomalous pulmonary venous return. Surgical correction in a newborn infant. J Thorac Cardiovasc Surg 62:301–306.
21. Gersony WM, Bowman FO, Steeg CN, Hayes CJ, Jesse MJ, Malm JR (1971): Management of total anomalous pulmonary venous drainage in early infancy. Circulation 43,44(Suppl I):19–24.
22. Graham TP Jr, Jarmakani JM, Canent RV Jr (1972): Left heart volume characteristics with a right ventricular volume overload: Total anomalous pulmonary venous connection and large atrial septal defect. Circulation 45:389–396.
23. Hammon JW Jr, Bender HW Jr, Graham TP Jr, Boucek RJ Jr, Smith CW, Erath HG Jr (1980): Total anomalous pulmonary venous connection in infancy: Ten years' experience including studies of postoperative ventricular function. J Thorac Cardiovasc Surg 80:544–551.
24. Haworth SG (1982): Total anomalous pulmonary venous return: Prenatal damage to pulmonary vascular bed and extrapulmonary veins. Br Heart J 48:513–524.
25. Haworth SG, Reid L (1977): Structural study of pulmonary circulation and of heart in total anomalous pulmonary venous return in early infancy. Br Heart J 39:80–92.
26. Higashino SM, Shaw GG, May IA, Ecker RR (1974): Total anomalous pulmonary venous drainage below the diaphragm: Clinical presentation, hemodynamic findings, and surgical results. J Thorac Cardiovasc Surg 68:711–718.
27. Hiakasa Y, Shirotani H, Satomura K, Muraoka R, Abe K, Tsushimi K, Yokota Y, Miki S, Kawai J, Mari A, Okamoto Y, Koie H, Ban T, Kanzaki Y, Yokota M, Mori C, Kamiya T, Tamura T, Nishii A, Asawa Y (1967): Open heart surgery in infants with an aid of hypothermic anesthesia. Archiv fur japanische chirurgie 36:495.
28. Hochberg MS, Gielchinsky I, Parsonnet V, Hussain SM, Fisch D (1986): Pulmonary inactivation of vasopressors following cardiac operations. Ann Thorac Surg 41:200–203.
29. Hopkins RA, Bull C, Sumner E, Haworth SG, de Leval MR, Stark J (1987): Pulmonary hypertensive crises following surgery for congenital heart defects in children. Circulation (submitted for publication).
30. Jegier W, Charrette E, Dobell AR (1967): Infradiaphragmatic anomalous pulmonary venous drainage: Normal hemodynamics following operation in infancy. Circulation 35:396–400.
31. Joffe HS, O'Donovan TG, Glaun BP, Chesler E, Schrire V (1971): Subdiaphragmatic total anomalous pulmonary venous drainage: Report of a successful surgical correction. Am Heart J 81:250–254.
32. Katz NM, Kirklin JW, Pacifico AD (1978): Concepts and practices in surgery for total anomalous pulmonary venous connection. Ann Thorac Surg 25:479–487.
33. Kauffman SL, Ores CN, Anderson DH (1962): Two cases of total anomalous pulmonary venous return of the supracardiac type with stenosis simulating infradiaphragmatic drainage. Circulation 25:376–382.
34. Kawashima Y, Nakano S, Matsuda H, Miyamoto T, Manabe H (1973): Successful correction of total anomalous pulmonary venous drainage with a new surgical technique. J Thorac Cardiovasc Surg 66:959–964.
35. Kirklin JW (1973): Surgical treatment of total anomalous pulmonary venous connection in infancy. In Barratt-Boyes BG, Neutze JM, Harris EA (eds): Heart Disease in Infancy, Diagnosis and Surgical Treatment. Edinburgh, Churchill Livingstone, p 89.
36. Kirklin J, Barratt-Boyes B (1986): Total anomalous pulmonary venous connection. In Kirklin JW, Barratt-Boyes BG (eds): Cardiac Surgery: Morphology, Diagnostic Criteria, Natural History, Techniques, Results, and Indications. New York, John Wiley & Sons, pp 499–523.

37. Lewis FJ, Varco RL, Traufic M, Niazi SA (1956): Direct vision repair of triatrial heart and total anomalous pulmonary venous drainage. Surg Gynecol Obstet 102:713–720.

38. Louhimo I (1985): IV. Actualites des Chirurgie Cardiovasculaire de l'hospital Broussais. Presentation at Marseille.

39. Mazzucco A, Rizzoli G, Fracasso A, Stellin G, Valfré C, Pellegrino P, Bortolotti U, Gallucci V (1983): Experience with operation for total anomalous pulmonary venous connection in infancy. J Thorac Cardiovasc Surg 85:686–690.

40. Muller WH Jr (1951): The surgical treatment of transposition of the pulmonary veins. Ann Surg 134:683–693.

41. Mullins CE, El-Said GM, Neches WH, Williams RL, Vargo TA, Nihill MR, McNamara DG (1973): Balloon atrial septostomy for total anomalous pulmonary venous return. Br Heart J 35:752–757.

42. Mustard WT, Keith JD, Trusler GA (1962): Two-stage correction for total anomalous pulmonary venous drainage in childhood. J Thorac Cardiovasc Surg 44:477–485.

43. Oliveira Lima C, Valdes-Cruz LM, Allen HD, Horowitz S, Sahn DJ, Goldberg SJ, Vargas Barron J, Grenadier E (1983): Prognostic value of left ventricular size measured by echocardiography in infants with total anomalous pulmonary venous drainage. Am J Cardiol 51:1155–1159.

44. Parr GVS, Kirklin JW, Pacifico AD, Blackstone EH, Lauridsen P (1974): Cardiac performance in infants after repair of total anomalous pulmonary venous connection. Ann Thorac Surg 17:561–573.

45. Sahn DJ, Allen HD, Lange LW, Goldberg SJ (1979): Cross-sectional echocardiographic diagnosis of the sites of total anomalous pulmonary venous drainage. Circulation 60:1317–1325.

46. Sairanen H, Louhimo I, Tolppanen E-M (1986): Pulmonary vein diameter in normal children. Pediatr Cardiol 6:259–261.

47. Schamroth CL, Sareli P, Klein HO, Davidoff R, Barlow JB (1985): Total anomalous pulmonary connection with pulmonary venous obstruction: Survival into adulthood. Am Heart J 109:1112–1114.

48. Shumacker HB Jr, King H (1961): A modified procedure for complete repair of total anomalous pulmonary venous drainage. Surg Gynecol Obstet 112:763–765.

49. Sloan H, Mackenzie J, Morris JO, Stern A, Sigmann J (1962): Open-heart surgery in infancy. J Thorac Cardiovasc Surg 44:459–476.

50. Smallhorn JF, Sutherland GR, Tommasini G, Hunter S, Anderson RH, Macartney FJ (1981): Assessment of total anomalous pulmonary venous connection by two-dimensional echocardiography. Br Heart J 46:613–623.

51. Stark J (1985): Anomalies of pulmonary venous return. World J Surg 9:532–542.

52. Stark J (1983): Anomalies of the pulmonary venous return. In Stark J, de Leval MR (eds): Surgery for Congenital Heart Defects. London, Grune & Stratton, pp 235–251.

53. Stark J, Smallhorn J, Huhta J, de Leval MR, Macartney FJ, Rees PG, Taylor JFN (1983): Surgery for congenital heart defects diagnosed with cross-sectional echocardiography. Circulation 68(Suppl II):129–138.

54. Tucker BL, Lindesmith GG, Stiles QR, Meyer BW (1976): The superior approach for correction of the supracardiac type of total anomalous pulmonary venous return. Ann Thorac Surg 22:374–377.

55. Turley K, Tucker WY, Ullyot DJ, Ebert PA (1980): Total anomalous pulmonary venous connection in infancy: Influence of age and type of lesion. Am J Cardiol 45:92–97.

56. Van Praagh R, Harken AH, Delisle G, Ando M, Gross RE (1972): Total anomalous pulmonary venous drainage to the coronary sinus: A revised procedure for its correction. J Thorac Cardiovasc Surg 64:132–135.

57. Vargas FJ, Kreutzer G (1985): A surgical technique for correction of total anomalous pulmonary venous drainage. J Thorac Cardiovasc Surg 90:410–413.

58. Vitarelli A, Scapato A, Sanguigni V, Caminiti MC (1986): Evaluation of total anomalous pulmonary venous drainage with cross-sectional colour-flow Doppler echocardiography. Eur Heart J 7:190–195.

59. Ward KE, Mullins CE, Huhta JC, Nihill MR, McNamara DG, Cooley DA (1986): Restrictive interatrial communication in total anomalous pulmonary venous connection. Am J Cardiol 57:1131–1136.

60. Whight CM, Barratt-Boyes BG, Calder AL, Neutze JM, Brandt PWT (1978): Total anomalous pulmonary venous connection. Long-term results following repair in infancy. J Thorac Cardiovasc Surg 75:52–63.

61. Wilson J (1798): A description of a very unusual formation of the human heart. Philos Trans R Soc Lond 88:346.

68 NEONATAL POSTOPERATIVE CARDIAC INTENSIVE CARE

Susan W. Denfield

G. William Henry

I believe all children's good,
Ef they're only understood,—
Even bad ones 'pears to me
'S jes' as good as they kin be!
The Hired Man's Faith in Children,
James Whitcomb Riley

The most common clinically significant complication following neonatal cardiovascular surgery is heart failure. The most common complication leading to death in a newborn following cardiovascular surgery is heart failure. Perhaps the least discussed aspect of pediatric cardiac care, and, fortunately, the least common clinical outcome of the care of such children is the death of the child. Thus, the focus of this chapter on postoperative management of the neonate following heart surgery will be directed at these two highly significant and directly related clinical problems: (1) the recognition and treatment of heart failure, and (2) death of a newborn following cardiac surgery.

The newborn who undergoes cardiovascular surgery is typically cared for in a newborn intensive care unit by intensive care nurses, neonatologists, pediatric cardiologists, pediatric intensivists, pediatric cardiac anesthesiologists, and pediatric cardiac surgeons, with each bringing their areas of expertise to the coordinated care of the infant. The complexity of the clinical care of such infants demands such interdisciplinary cooperation to achieve the most favorable outcome for the infant and family. Nothing substitutes for clinical excellence.

HISTORICAL PERSPECTIVE

Three significant advances in medical management of newborns with suspected congenital heart disease have dramatically changed the preoperative condition of neonates requiring cardiovascular surgery and the spectrum of patients undergoing operative intervention.

First, the pharmacologic manipulation of the ductus arteriosus has led to improved medical management. The appropriate use of prostaglandin inhibitors, such as lyophilized indomethacin, to close the ductus arteriosus in premature infants with severe respiratory distress can obviate the need for surgical intervention (see Chapter 54). More importantly, maintenance of ductal patency using a continuous parenteral infusion of prostaglandin E_1 or E_2 has served to palliate newborns with significant congenital heart disease during transfer to an appropriate diagnostic unit, during evaluation, and while arranging for surgical intervention when necessary (see Chapter 53).

Second, advances in cross-sectional echocardiography have led to excellent anatomic description and functional assessment of the heart and great vessels of infants with suspected congenital heart disease, obviating the need for diagnostic cardiac catheterization (see Chapter 25). Magnetic resonance imaging shows promise of providing significantly better anatomic detail than cross-sectional echocardiography and will be particularly useful in delineation of vascular structures.

Finally, application of therapeutic cardiac catheterization, particularly with balloon catheter techniques, has obviated the need for surgery in selected circumstances, such as critical semilunar valve stenosis (see Chapter 56).

Recent advances in intraoperative management of infants undergoing cardiovascular surgery include improved monitoring methods and improved myocardial preservation.[30] In recent years, neonatal cardiac surgery has gravitated toward corrective rather than palliative procedures. The basic indications have not changed, but for selected lesions the surgical approach has changed (e.g., neonatal arterial switch for transposition of the great arteries rather than neonatal balloon septostomy and venous switch repair during the first year).[45]

INDICATIONS FOR CARDIOVASCULAR SURGERY

Postoperative care and outcome are largely dictated by the native physiology and anatomy preoperatively and by the results of the attempted palliation[11] or correction. What are the physiologic indications for consideration of heart surgery in a neonate with congenital heart disease? In the most basic physiologic terms, two indications exist: heart failure and hypoxemia/hypoxia.

Heart failure as a physiologic consequence of structural heart disease in a neonate is associated with high, immediate mortality necessitating emergent diagnosis and therapy. Hypoxemia is no less an emergency whether cardiac or respiratory in etiology; if a cardiac cause is found, urgent intervention is often required.

Obviously, surgery is undertaken when the risks of medical management of the lesion causing the symptoms are greater than the risks of operative intervention. Thus, accurate diagnosis is critical in the choice and timing of therapy. This statement cannot be overemphasized and applies to the postoperative period as well. For example, if a neonate's postoperative course is complicated by heart failure, evaluation must be as thorough and as emergent as the initial evaluation.[39]

HEART FAILURE FOLLOWING NEONATAL CARDIAC SURGERY

We use a simple physiologic approach to postoperative heart failure in newborns following cardiac surgery that focuses on the determinants of ventricular function (Table 68–1). We define heart failure as the inability or inefficiency of the heart in supplying sufficient blood flow for metabolic needs.

Neonatal Ventricular Function

The basic determinants of ventricular function are the same regardless of the patient's age. However, intrinsic physiologic differences in the neonatal myocardium limit neonatal cardiac reserve; these differences must be considered when evaluating cardiac function and treating dysfunction. Ventricular function is determined by preload or diastolic filling, afterload or systolic loading, contractility, and heart rate and rhythm. These four factors can serve as a framework for the evaluation of postoperative cardiac dysfunction, since significant compromise in any one or a combination of these factors can result in heart failure in the newborn.[12,62]

Preload is, in the simplest terms, the load to which a muscle is subjected before shortening. When preload is optimal, the greatest number of muscle filaments can interact, resulting in an increased contractile force (the Starling relationship). Clinically, preload is the diastolic filling condition of the heart and is usually related to the left ventricular end-diastolic pressure, which usually reflects the left ventricular end-diastolic volume and, thus, is related to the average precontraction myocardial fiber length. Measurements that reflect preload include the left ventricular end-diastolic pressure and/or pulmonary capillary wedge pressure. Factors affecting preload include venous return, total blood volume and its distribution, and atrial contraction.

Afterload is defined in the intact ventricle as the tension, force, or stress acting on the fibers in the ventricular wall after the onset of shortening. It is the tension that must be developed to overcome the forces that oppose ventricular ejection. Increase in afterload may decrease stroke volume and cardiac output. In the intact organism, the forces opposing ventricular ejection include peripheral vascular resistance, arterial compliance, and aortic input impedance.

Contractility and its effect on ventricular performance can also be considered independently from preload and afterload. Defined most simply, contractility is the ability of the cardiac muscle to develop tension. If cardiac con-

Table 68–1. DETERMINANTS OF VENTRICULAR FUNCTION

Preload
Contractility
Afterload
Heart rate and rhythm

tractility is augmented without a change in preload, cardiac performance will be improved. The converse is also true. Factors affecting contractility include the sympathetic nervous system, endogenous and exogenous catecholamines/inotropes, physiologic and pharmacologic depressants, loss of contractile mass, and intrinsic properties of the contractile unit.

Finally, heart rate and rhythm can have a profound effect on cardiac output, particularly in the newborn, by altering ventricular filling. If stroke volume remains constant, reductions in heart rate reduce cardiac output proportionally.

Obviously, when preload, contractility, afterload, and heart rate and rhythm are interacting optimally, cardiac function will be optimal. Adverse changes in one or more of these factors can precipitate heart failure when cardiac functional reserve and adaptive mechanisms are exhausted. The concept of cardiac reserve is important, particularly in neonates in whom it is limited compared with older children and adults. Cardiac reserve may be thought of as the properties of the heart that allow it to compensate for stresses on the cardiovascular system. Compensatory changes incurred by heart failure are not necessarily beneficial to myocardial performance. Neonatal cardiac reserve is limited by several factors.[12,14,19,34,35,53,68,76,83,84,87,92] First, myofilament numbers are decreased, although their function is comparable to myofilaments in the mature myocardium. Second, the neonatal ventricle is less compliant, thus limiting its capacity to compensate for increasing volume loads. Third, oxygen consumption, cardiac output, and resting heart rate are greater in the neonate. As a consequence, neonatal cardiac performance is near maximal even in the absence of stress. When abnormalities of preload, afterload, contractility or significant arrhythmia occur, the neonatal myocardium may be unable to compensate, and heart failure may develop, particularly in the postoperative period.

Disorders of Preload or Diastolic Filling

Preload may cause postoperative heart failure in neonates as a result of suboptimal volume status, inadequate systemic venous return, or residual shunts. Both hypovolemia and hypervolemia can cause inadequate tissue perfusion. Hypovolemia may be secondary to inadequate volume replacement of previous deficits or ongoing losses. Blood loss may result from inadequate mechanical hemostasis at surgical sites (anastomoses, ligations) or impairment of clotting from coagulation factor deficiencies, thrombocytopenia, or other coagulation abnormalities following cardiopulmonary bypass. Incomplete reversal of heparinization should also be considered. When there is a falling hematocrit without an identifiable source of blood loss, hemolysis should always be considered when postoperative blood loss or anemia is observed.

Hypovolemia is also encountered when venous return is obstructed. Venous obstruction can result from a variety of problems, ranging from excessive positive end-expiratory pressure to tension pneumothorax to atrial baffle obstruction. Cardiac tamponade may result from inadequate hemostasis, catheter perforation, or later in the postoperative period as a result of postpericardiotomy syndrome effusions.

Excessive volume with real or relative anemia may also lead to heart failure. The newborn who is in heart failure prior to surgery may be volume overloaded before any iatrogenic volume manipulation. Subsequent fluid administration may exacerbate the problem. Other disorders that may lead to volume overload in the postoperative period include valvular insufficiency following valvotomy, residual congenital shunts or excessive therapeutic shunts, and renal insufficiency.

Disorders of Afterload or Systolic Loading

Postoperatively, elevations in afterload can persist from residual obstruction following repair of coarctation or aortic or pulmonic stenosis. Systemic vascular resistance also reflects afterload and cardiac function; sympathomimetic/vasoconstrictive infusions must be evaluated continuously postoperatively. Hypothermia must be corrected. If systemic resistance is low with a high output state, sepsis should always be considered.

Disorders of Contractility

Drugs and sepsis may also affect myocardial contractility. Gram-negative and group B streptococcal sepsis have been reported to depress myocardial contractility and must be considered in the neonate with fever postoperatively. Acidosis and hypoxia are myocardial depressants. Intraoperative ischemia and reperfusion injury after prolonged cardiopulmonary bypass may depress myocardial contractility. Depending on the type of pump prime used and the volumes of blood products given, hypocalcemia and hypophosphatemia may contribute to reduced myocardial contractility.

Disorders of Heart Rate and Rhythm

The final major factors affecting myocardial performance are heart rate and rhythm disturbances. Postoperative hypoxia and acidosis may initially be heralded by sinus tachycardia. Unless the hypoxia and acidosis are recognized and treated, sinus tachycardia may be followed by significant bradycardia. Hypokalemia, hyperkalemia, and hypocalcemia may also lead to significant rhythm disturbances. Drug toxicities should also be considered. Relatively uncommon causes of postoperative arrhythmias include surgical damage to the conducting pathways, sometimes seen after placement of intra-atrial baffles. Supraventricu-

lar tachycardia, sick sinus syndrome, and atrioventricular conduction blocks may occur and result in hemodynamic compromise.[1]

Clinical Assessment

The newborn with serious congenital heart disease can pose major diagnostic difficulties for the examining physician, since the classic findings associated with structural heart disease and heart failure may not be present. Infants with significant structural lesions may present without a heart murmur, whereas other infants with loud murmurs have no significant structural defects. In the postoperative period, heart failure can be even more difficult to recognize. Mechanical ventilation, paralysis, catecholamine infusions, and a myriad of other factors can obscure the often subtle findings of neonatal heart failure.

Besides the history and physical examination, the initial evaluation of the postoperative newborn doing poorly should include chest radiographs, ECG, arterial blood gas analysis, serum electrolyte studies, glucose and calcium determinations, a complete blood count, and blood cultures (in the stressed infant). Echocardiography can demonstrate postoperative cardiac anatomy and function quite readily; cardiac catheterization is reserved for postoperative infants in whom better anatomic delineation is required or in whom the explanation for clinical deterioration remains obscure.

When a neonate is doing poorly in the postoperative period, supportive measures should be initiated whether or not heart failure is identified. General supportive measures should not be overlooked such as correction of electrolyte, acid-base, glucose, calcium, and temperature imbalance. In the appropriate setting, anticongestive measures and/or further medical manipulation of the ductus arteriosus should be considered. If supportive measures are effective, the infant may be managed medically. However, if operative intervention has not successfully corrected or palliated the infant's cardiac anatomy, even the most excellent postoperative care cannot alter the eventual outcome. Immediate reoperation should always be considered in the postoperative infant doing poorly for unexplained reasons.

Clinical Setting and Preoperative Status

The postoperative management must not be separated from considerations of the preoperative clinical setting. The neonate who was stable preoperatively on prostaglandin E_1 for inadequate pulmonary blood flow in whom an aortopulmonary shunt was placed poses different problems from the critically ill newborn with obstructed total anomalous pulmonary venous drainage who has undergone total circulatory arrest during physiologic repair.

The preoperative hemodynamic status of the newborn obviously affects intraoperative and postoperative morbidity and mortality, particularly as it relates to palliative procedures. Therefore, it is incumbent on those responsible for the postoperative care to have an understanding of the events leading to the operating room. Mundane issues such as specific pharmacologic therapy prior to surgery can have profound consequences in the operating room and intensive care unit (e.g., the preoperative use of a digitalis glycoside with intraoperative or postoperative arrhythmia). Specifically, if the child underwent cardiac catheterization, knowledge of the hemodynamic findings and review of the angiography is essential to anticipate potential postoperative problems.

Intraoperative Repair

Complete communication regarding the events in the operating room are essential to appropriate postoperative care. Anesthetic issues deserving specific comment include method of anesthesia; ventilation issues; metabolic and fluid therapy; coagulation status; presence and therapy of any arrhythmias; method, site, and type of line placement and significant hemodynamic events. Surgical issues warranting specific comment include the intraoperative diagnosis and an explicit description of the repair, the duration of cardiopulmonary bypass, and, most important, the length of ischemic time and type of arrest (e.g., total hypothermic circulatory arrest). Whenever possible the cardiologist is well advised to see the intraoperative anatomy and the surgical approach to the repair, particularly as it relates to atrioventricular valve anatomy. If the surgery has been in the area of the sinoatrial or atrioventricular nodes, specific comments should be made regarding the possibility of injury to the conduction system and the potential access for electrical pacing.

Postoperative Physical Examination

The signs of postoperative heart failure in the neonate may not be as obvious or specific as those seen in the older child or neonate who has not had surgery. Therefore, a high index of suspicion must be maintained in the postoperative infant who is "just not doing well."

When examining the infant, the general appearance of the awake, unparalyzed patient can give important clues regarding the child's overall well-being. Infants who are "doing well" will have periods of time in which they are very alert, interested in their environment, and spontaneously move all extremities. They will also have strong startle (Moro reflex) responses to loud noises, jarring of the bed, or abrupt position changes. The ability to cry vigorously is evidence for relatively good cardiac reserve. Conversely, the postoperative infant who is not very interactive or becoming less interactive with his environment or who cries with less vigor should be observed more closely, as should the infant who is excessively fussy or irritable.

The postoperative infant's tone can also be an indicator of general medical status. If the infant is not unconscious, deeply asleep, or paralyzed, he will generally lie with extremities flexed. If the examiner attempts to straighten an extremity he will meet resistance, which generally increases as the infant's level of alertness increases. An awake but relative "floppy" infant should raise the physician's level of concern.

The appearance of the skin should also be included in the general assessment. Normal postoperative infants may have pale-appearing skin and, when crying, perioral cyanosis, but the lips and mucosa remain pink. Although nonspecific, pallor or cyanosis that is also violet in the mucosa and a gray color or mottling of the skin should prompt further evaluation for other evidence of a decreased cardiac output. Skin temperature should also be noted. Cool extremities may indicate a low output state.

Examination of the extremities may quickly provide further evidence of a decreased cardiac output.[54] Capillary refill should be evaluated. In the normothermic postoperative patient, capillary refill should be less than 2 seconds; progressive delay in refill suggests hypoperfusion. Delayed capillary refill is a nonspecific finding but should alert the physician to evaluate the patient more closely. Extremities may feel cool and appear cyanotic. Edema of the extremities may be seen postoperatively, but it is not usually a sign of congestive heart failure in the neonate. Edema is more likely to be a consequence of the increased fluid that is frequently required intraoperatively. Edema is often seen in paralyzed infants.[75]

Respiratory distress is a common sign of postoperative heart failure in the infant. Visual inspection may reveal nasal flaring, intercostal and subcostal retractions, and tachypnea. If the infant is extubated, grunting with exhalation may also be present. On auscultation, wheezing or rales may be noted. However, rales are often heard after cardiopulmonary bypass. Wheezing is common when airway secretions have accumulated. Therefore, the examiner should not be misled by either normal breath sounds or wheezing and rales.

The most frequent indication of inadequate cardiac output is tachycardia. Rhythm disturbances should be noted. Gallop rhythms are common in all infants with heart failure. Distant heart sounds may signify a significant pericardial effusion causing a low output state. Peripheral pulses may be weak and the blood pressure decreased.

Palpation of the abdomen frequently reveals an enlarged liver with a dull liver margin, reflecting passive venous congestion. The liver may be pulsatile. Splenomegaly is an inconsistent finding.

Evaluation of the jugular venous distention is difficult in newborns due to their short necks. If jugular venous distention is noted, increased systemic venous pressure is present.

In summary, the most common signs of heart failure in the postoperative newborn are nonspecific. The following constellation of signs should make the examiner suspect the diagnosis of heart failure: listlessness, pallor, grunting respirations, tachycardia, hepatomegaly, and weight gain out of proportion to caloric intake. Finally, the absence of rales and/or a gallop rhythm does not rule out the diagnosis of heart failure in the postoperative newborn.

Radiography

Chest radiographs can be helpful in the recognition of postoperative heart failure. A systematic approach to the evaluation of the chest radiograph is essential. Cardiomegaly is almost always present in the postoperative patient with congestive heart failure. The cardiomegaly may be generalized, or specific chamber enlargement may occur. The normal-sized heart is less than or equal to six-tenths the largest transverse diameter of the chest. If cardiac enlargement is predominantly of left ventricular origin, the apex of the heart will be displaced downward on a posteroanterior view, whereas right ventricular enlargement will displace the heart upward on the same view. In a lateral view the retrosternal air space will be obliterated if significant right ventricular enlargement is present, a finding more easily read after knowing the cardiac catheterization results.

Heart failure can also result from pericardial effusion; in such cases a large cardiac silhouette is seen on the chest radiograph. Classically, the silhouette looks like a "bag of water"; pericardial effusion should be considered if the heart sounds are muffled and the patient deteriorates rapidly. Similarly, pneumopericardium with cardiac tamponade (see Chapter 29) should be considered if the infant is on mechanical ventilation.

The pulmonary vasculature should be assessed. Evidence for increased pulmonary blood flow includes visible pulmonary vessels in the lateral third of the lung fields and in the apices. Prominent vessels visible through the diaphragm also suggest increased vascularity. The pulmonary veins become hazy and indistinct when there is pulmonary venous congestion.

Examination of the lung fields may reveal patchy, fluffy densities radiating from the hila. Kerley B lines may be seen at the lung periphery. Evaluation of the pleural space may reveal blunting of the costophrenic angles from pleural effusions.

Cardiomegaly and the classic lung field changes may not be present if the infant is ventilated with high positive end-expiratory pressures. Conversely, increasing heart size and increasing density of the lung fields may merely be the result of decreasing mechanical ventilation without any change in cardiac function.

If the "usual" chest radiograph findings are absent in the infant with a low cardiac output, it is especially important to consider specific etiologic factors. The level of positive end-expiratory pressure, the location of the endotracheal tube in the intubated child, and the location of any central lines require assessment. The presence of a pneumothorax should not be overlooked; a pneumothorax may be more difficult to recognize on a portable radiograph of a supine patient. Differential lucency of a hemidiaphragm or lung field should increase the observer's index of suspicion.

The mediastinum should also be assessed. Changes in the width of the mediastinum should alert the clinician to possible complications. Central lines may perforate vessels or cardiac chambers. Ventilator complications such as pneumomediastinum or pneumopericardium may occur. Anatomic sites or suture lines involving the heart or great vessels may be a source of bleeding.

Finally, diaphragmatic paralysis should always be considered in the child unable to have a sufficient reduction in mechanical support to ventilate without assistance.[67,85]

Echocardiography

Cross-sectional echocardiography can offer a complete anatomic description of the heart and great vessels following cardiac surgery. Cross-sectional (including contrast injections), M-mode, and Doppler (including color flow techniques) studies can offer a detailed assessment of the functional consequences of the surgical intervention.

The most important diagnosis that can be made echocardiographically is cardiac tamponade. Cross-sectional echocardiography can easily demonstrate large pericardial effusions. Echocardiography also can be very useful during insertion of pericardial catheters for drainage of pericardial fluid.

Ventricular function can be assessed qualitatively and somewhat quantitatively.[42,46] Commonly determined echocardiographic measurements include left ventricular shortening fraction, left ventricular ejection fraction, right and left systolic time intervals, mean velocity of circumferential fiber shortening, and pressure drops across stenotic sites. Left ventricular shortening fraction requires the measurement of transverse left ventricular systolic and diastolic dimensions obtained by an M-mode image from a cross-sectional echocardiogram in a parasternal long axis position. Left ventricular shortening fraction (SF_{LV}) is simply the fractional shortening of the left ventricular diastolic (LVDD) and systolic (LVSD) dimensions:

$$SF_{LV} = (LVDD - LVSD)/LVDD$$

Left ventricular shortening fraction is meaningful only in the absence of regional wall motion abnormalities and when left ventricular shape is normal. Left ventricular ejection fraction can be determined using geometric assumptions of the left ventricular shape and volume. The left ventricle is assumed to be a prolate ellipse; systolic and diastolic volume measurements are derived from planimetered M-mode or cross-sectional images. Methods for estimating right ventricular ejection fractions have been published from planimetered cross-sectional images in the short and long axes of the right ventricle. The values are less accurate than those for the left ventricle, because the more complex shape of the right ventricle is more difficult to model. Reports of more complex computer-aided models for estimating ventricular ejection fractions are increasingly common. Systolic time intervals (STI) relate mechanical events to electrical events and are derived commonly from measurements of the interval from onset of the QRS complex to the opening of a semilunar valve (pre-ejection period [PEP]) and the interval of semilunar valve opening (ejection time [ET]) and commonly expressed as a ratio for the respective ventricle:

$$RVSTI = RVPEP/RVET$$
$$and$$
$$LVSTI = LVPEP/LVET$$

Mean velocity of circumferential fiber shortening (VCF) normalizes shortening fraction with respect to ventricular ejection time, a measure of the chronotropic effects on myocardial function and is defined as follows:

$$VCF = SF/ET$$

VCF has been reported to be useful in differentiating depressed myocardial performance from the increased myocardial function found in volume load states from left-to-right shunts. Finally, pulsed, continuous-wave, and color-flow Doppler techniques can identify and estimate the pressure gradient across stenotic sites. The simplified Bernoulli equation is commonly used to estimate the gradient; the pressure gradient (P_{grad}) is equal to four times the square of the maximal velocity (V_{max}) measured on the downstream side of the obstruction:

$$P_{grad} = 4(V_{max})^2$$

The reader is referred to the more complete discussion of echocardiography in Chapter 25.

Monitoring Techniques

Blood Chemistry Studies

Postoperative cardiac dysfunction may either cause or result from biochemical imbalance. Careful monitoring of electrolyte, glucose, calcium, and occasionally phosphorus levels is mandatory in the critical care setting.

Hypoglycemia, hypocalcemia, and hypophosphatemia can cause or contribute to postoperative cardiac dysfunction. These substances are all readily measurable, and deficiencies are relatively simple to correct.

Metabolic acidosis may also either cause or result from postoperative myocardial dysfunction. Serum bicarbonate levels should be measured serially. A low serum bicarbonate level, even as an isolated finding, should always alert the physician to evaluate the postoperative infant more closely. Postoperative newborns occasionally will look surprisingly stable just prior to deterioration. A low serum bicarbonate level may be the initial tip-off to the clinician that the postoperative infant's cardiac status is not as well compensated as it appears. In most cases the infant should be carefully evaluated, and the serum bicarbonate level should be reassessed, as should the arterial blood gas values. If serum acidosis is documented, the underlying cause should be identified and treated.

The serum sodium value should also be measured. Hyponatremia is a frequent finding in heart failure. In such cases the total body sodium level is actually normal or slightly elevated, but the serum value is low secondary to free water retention. The renal perfusion is poor in heart failure, despite hypervolemia; as a result, the kidneys conserve sodium, and urine sodium will be low unless diuretics have been given. As the heart failure is controlled, a rise in serum and urine sodium values will occur.[82]

Central Venous Pressure

Central venous catheters are useful adjuncts in postoperative neonatal care for monitoring central venous pressure

(CVP) and providing intravenous therapy.[26] Access to the central venous system is generally most easily attained via the femoral vein. The umbilical vein may also be accessed in the newborn. External and internal jugular veins may also be used. A No. 3 F catheter is a reasonable size for the newborn weighing less than 4 kg. The catheter tip should be in the thoracic cavity, preferably at the caval–right atrial junction. The catheter tip position should be documented radiographically.

Right atrial pressure reflects the right ventricular preload or end-diastolic volume and the ability of the right ventricle to pump the systemic venous return. In infants with normal hearts and lungs, CVP is closely related to pulmonary wedge pressure and, therefore, to left-sided preload. However, in infants with congenital heart disease, and particularly in postoperative infants, the relationship between CVP and left-sided heart filling pressure does not always apply. Such discrepancies do not mean CVP measurements are not useful, but one must be aware of their limitations. In general, serial CVP measurements are more useful than isolated measurements. If the CVP is low or declining and cardiac output is low, the infant is probably hypovolemic and a volume challenge is warranted. Elevated CVP measurements are subject to more errors in interpretation. If the ventilator is applying high levels of positive end-expiratory pressure, the CVP may be falsely elevated. Positive end-expiratory pressure may impair systemic venous return, reduce cardiac output, and elevate CVP. If the patient is stable and breathing spontaneously, more accurate CVP measurements can be obtained by briefly disconnecting the patient from the ventilator.

Hypervolemia, right-sided myocardial dysfunction (following surgery involving the right side of the heart), right-sided obstructive lesions, pulmonary hypertension, and left ventricular failure with elevated pulmonary venous pressure also cause postoperative CVP elevations. CVP line complications are similar to those encountered with arterial catheters and include thromboembolism, infection, and hemorrhage. In addition, arrhythmias may occur due to an intracardiac catheter. Hemopericardium from catheter perforation is a rare complication.

Arterial Blood Pressure Monitoring and Lines

Numerous noninvasive and invasive techniques are available for measuring blood pressure.[31] In the postoperative intensive care unit setting, continuous measurement of the blood pressure is frequently necessary. Indications for the insertion of an arterial cannula include hypotension and/or myocardial dysfunction requiring continuous infusion of vasoactive drugs, hypertensive crises, and need for frequent arterial blood gas measurements to adjust the ventilator settings. The ability to sample blood without disturbing the child is an important reason for establishing an indwelling arterial line. Oxygenation may decline significantly when a compromised infant is crying and struggling during repeated arterial or venous punctures.

Most commonly in the immediate neonatal period, umbilical arteries are cannulated using a No. 3.5 F or 5.0 F catheter and appropriate aseptic technique. The umbilical catheter is placed at the level of the diaphragm or in the interspace between the L3 and L4 vertebrae, below the origin of the renal and mesenteric arteries. A position in the thoracic aorta may be associated with fewer observed complications, but the complications tend to be more severe and often involve the abdominal viscera and kidneys. Emboli from catheters positioned in the lumbar area may also result in areas of ischemia, but the skin and muscle of the lower extremities are affected instead.[73] The lumbar position is preferred at most institutions.

When the umbilical arteries are no longer available, more peripheral arteries are used. The artery of choice is the right radial artery, since most infants will have sufficient collateral circulation to the hand. The adequacy of the collateral circulation must be verified prior to cannulation of the radial artery. The Allen test may be performed to document the dual arterial supply. The ulnar artery is more difficult to cannulate than the radial artery but may be used if the Allen test is positive and the radial artery is not accessible.[72] However, the arteries in the foot are usually easier to cannulate than the ulnar artery. The dorsalis pedis artery is relatively superficial, is straight, and usually courses between the second and third metatarsals. The dorsalis pedis artery may be cannulated after documentation of adequate collateral blood supply to the foot from the posterior tibial artery using a modified Allen test. The posterior tibial artery is used less frequently due to its proximity to the posterior tibial nerve and more winding course, making it more difficult to cannulate. Although easy to palpate, the brachial and temporal arteries are generally not used in the intensive care unit setting for continuous monitoring. The brachial artery does not have adequate collateral circulation for this use, and the temporal artery site has been associated with devastating cerebral infarcts.[80,93] The femoral artery should be used only as a last resort during severe hypotension or resuscitation efforts when no other pulses are palpable.

After placement of the arterial catheter, the system must be properly calibrated to obtain accurate blood pressure measurements. Errors in measurement may occur if the system is dampened. Causes of dampening include air bubbles, thrombus formation at the catheter tip, or the use of very compliant tubing in the system. Compliant tubing results in artificial lowering of the systolic blood pressure and an increase in the diastolic pressure; mean blood pressure is relatively unaffected. The waveform may also be dampened by vasoconstriction from low flow states. The systolic blood pressure may be artifactually raised and the diastolic pressure lowered by the resonance phenomena, another physical property of the system. Resonance can be recognized by an overshoot of the waveform on the monitor. When the blood pressure measurement is suspect, it is common practice to check the blood pressure with a cuff. A difference between cuff and invasive monitor pressure is frequently found. Part of the difference is real, and part is artifactual. Hydrostatic pressure differences account for part of the difference. If the cuff is not at the same level as the zero point of the transducer, a pressure gradient will occur. In addition, the invasive monitor measures both kinetic and static pressure components. The cuff measures only the static pressure exerted on the

lateral walls of the blood vessels, without the flow or velocity component of the blood. Therefore, the invasive monitor will read the systolic pressure 8 to 16 mmHg higher than the cuff under normal conditions.

Observation of the waveform can be useful during patient evaluation. If the waveform is not dampened, the upstroke of the pressure wave can give information about myocardial contractility. Observation of the pulse pressure provides information about the stroke volume. A pulsus paradoxus may be seen in a patient with a pericardial effusion.

Complications seen with systemic arterial catheters include infection, thrombosis, ischemia, and embolism. Hemorrhage may occur at the time of catheter placement; hematomas may result in vascular compromise. If the tubing disconnects, exsanguination may occur. Thus for each indwelling arterial line placement, benefits to the patient should clearly outweigh the potential hazards.[28,100]

Pulmonary Artery Pressure

Monitoring postoperative pulmonary arterial pressure following neonatal cardiac surgery can be lifesaving. Paroxysmal pulmonary hypertensive crises characterized by sudden increases in pulmonary arterial systolic pressure to systemic or suprasystemic levels frequently complicate neonatal cardiac surgery. Such episodes are medical emergencies. Postoperative monitoring of pulmonary artery pressure by an indwelling catheter permits early recognition and treatment of this life-threatening complication. Attendant risks of an indwelling pulmonary artery catheter are listed in Table 68–2. One problem associated with such indwelling lines that is not commonly discussed in textbooks is the short length of time that these lines remain functional (24 to 72 hours). Several types of lines and access routes are used. Multiple-port No. 4 and 5 F catheters inserted via a peripheral vein at the time of cardiac catheterization, during surgery, or at the bedside[79] following surgery permit measurements of additional pressures (e.g., central venous, balloon occlusion wedge), continuous pulmonary artery oximetry, cardiac output (using thermodilution, green dye techniques, or Doppler ultrasound techniques), as well as institution of electrical pacing. An additional option is insertion of a No. 2.5 F Silastic pulmonary artery catheter at surgery via a transventricular, transthoracic approach.

Although pulmonary hypertensive crises can complicate any neonatal cardiac surgery, they are more common after repair of certain defects. Obstructed total anomalous pulmonary venous drainage is a notorious cause of postoperative episodic pulmonary hypertensive crises (see Chapter 67).

Left Atrial Pressure

Direct measurement of left atrial pressure is obtained by the placement of a catheter during the operative procedure. Left atrial pressure reflects left ventricular end-diastolic, just as CVP reflects right ventricular end-diastolic pressure. Determination of left atrial pressure offers an independent assessment of left ventricular function that is superior to the indirect assessment from a central venous catheter and is more accurate and reproducible than pulmonary artery wedge pressure. Evaluation of atrial a, v, and c pressure waves can offer valuable insight to ventricular compliance and the integrity of the left atrioventricular valve. Like the central venous pressure line, the left atrial line can be used to obtain an atrial electrocardiogram, which is useful in distinguishing supraventricular from ventricular tachycardia. The judicious use of the left atrial catheter for obtaining blood gas values and saturations can offer estimations of right-to-left atrial shunts.

Left atrial catheters typically are placed in the right posterior portion of the left atrium in the vicinity of the atrial septum and the entry sites of the right pulmonary veins. Although left atrial pressure measurements can greatly simplify evaluation of left ventricular function, two highly significant risks must be considered. First, the risk of systemic arterial embolization, particularly to the coronary arteries and brain, demands meticulous care to avoid introduction of air into left atrial catheters. Second, the risk of bleeding, including cardiac tamponade, must be remembered, particularly if the catheter was placed transthoracically. When transthoracic left atrial catheters are removed, blood and echocardiography (the latter to assess cardiac tamponade) should be readily available. Less commonly, atrial arrhythmias can be initiated mechanically by left atrial catheters; rarely, catheter migration into the ventricle occurs, and ventricular ectopy can result.

Cardiac Output Measurements

Blood flow is the volume of blood passing a given point per unit time. Cardiac output generally refers to the volume of blood ejected into the aorta by the left ventricle. Qualification of this assumption to specify pulmonary blood flow and systemic blood flow is frequently necessary in patients with congenital heart disease with intracardiac and extracardiac shunts. Accurate, reproducible measurements of cardiac output in newborn infants are difficult. Indirect measurements such as arteriovenous oxygen differences use assumptions that can introduce considerable error.

Invasive techniques for blood flow measurements include Fick measurements of oxygen consumption, indicator dilution, thermodilution, and velocity determinations by Doppler ultrasound or electromechanical flow devices. The Fick method, green dye, and thermodilution techniques incorporate the same general principle of indicator dilution; oxygen, green dye, and heat are the respective indicators.[7,32,37,95,98]

In 1870, Fick[29] suggested that cardiac output could be calculated if oxygen consumption and the arteriovenous oxygen content difference were known. The limiting feature of the Fick method is obtaining an accurate measurement of oxygen consumption. However, the Fick method is useful for determining relative flows such as the pulmonary to systemic flow ratio. A principal assumption of the Fick method is that a steady-state equilibrium exists between the oxygen being taken up by the body and oxygen being extracted from inhaled air. A practical point and

Table 68–2. POTENTIAL COMPLICATIONS OF PULMONARY ARTERY CATHETERS

Venous thrombosis
Endocarditis
Noninfectious thrombotic
Infectious
Cardiac arrhythmias
Hemorrhage
Pulmonary infarction
Atrial perforation
Pulmonary perforation
Pulmonary embolism
Catheter knotting
Arteriovenous fistula formation

a potential source of error is that the sampled blood must be mixed adequately.

$$\frac{\text{Cardiac output}}{\text{(liters/min/m}^2)} = \frac{O_2 \text{ consumption (ml/min/m}^2)}{\text{Arteriovenous } O_2 \text{ difference (ml/liter)}}$$

This method for determining cardiac output is most accurate in low flow states when the $a\bar{v}O_2$ difference is large. Significant errors can be introduced when small changes in $a\bar{v}O_2$ differences represent large changes in the cardiac output.

Thermodilution techniques have become widely used even in newborns.[32] Simply stated, the change in temperature of a distal thermister after injection of a standard quantity of iced saline is proportional to the blood flow. This relationship is defined mathematically by the following equation (which represents a modification of the Stewart-Hamilton equation[50,94]):

$$\text{Cardiac output} = \frac{V_i(T_B - T_i)S_iC_i60k}{S_B C_B \int_o^\infty \Delta T_B(t)dt}$$

V = volume

i = injectate

B = blood

T = temperature

S = specific gravity

C = specific heat

t = time

k = correction factor for heat transfer from injection site to proximal port

Multiple-port, balloon-tipped thermister catheters with a proximal port for fluid injection and display of central venous pressure are used frequently in pediatric intensive care units. The catheter can be placed intraoperatively or postoperatively with the distal catheter tip in a branch pulmonary artery and the proximal port in a consequent central venous location. Computer-aided calculations of cardiac output can be generated easily and frequently. Several assumptions are used. The most notable assumption is that the temperature at the site of the thermister in the branch pulmonary artery is representative of the temperature at all sites in the cross-sectional plane of the artery.[43] Intracardiac and extracardiac shunts and regurgitant intracardiac flows significantly diminish the accuracy of thermodilution cardiac outputs. Complications from using pulmonary arterial catheters are summarized in Table 68–2.

Indicator dilution techniques are based on a 1929 modification by Kinsman and colleagues[50] of a technique described by Stewart in 1897.[94] The most commonly used dye is indocyanine green. Cardiac output is defined by the following relationship:

$$Cardiac\ output = \frac{Amount\ of\ dye\ injected}{\int_0^\infty c(t)dt}$$

$$Cardiac\ output = \frac{(Injectate)(60)}{C \times t}$$

Cardiac output = systemic flow (liters/min)

Injectate = amount of injected dye (mg)

C = mean dye concentration (mg/liter)

t = duration of primary curve (sec)

60 = seconds/minute (sec/min)

Simply stated, blood flow is proportional to the change in concentration of a distally measured dye. Typically, following dye injection into a central venous site (e.g., pulmonary artery), blood is withdrawn from a distal arterial site at a constant rate while dye is measured spectrophotometrically and a concentration curve is plotted. Computer-aided digital curve averaging has simplified the technique, but the technique is limited by the amount of blood withdrawn and the dye recirculation. Left-to-right and right-to-left shunts can be detected with this method, but the downslope of the dye curve can be obliterated in newborns due to the fast recirculation time. The indocyanine green method is least accurate in low cardiac output states.

Invasive measurement of cardiac output using catheters equipped to measure blood velocity by Doppler or electromagnetic methods has been used widely in research but less frequently clinically. With both Doppler and electromagnetic techniques, knowledge of the cross-sectional area and the velocity profile of the vessel is required for accurate measurements. The cross-sectional area is usually determined by echocardiography, angiography, or direct intraoperative measurement. Generally, the velocity profile has been assumed to be flat in the proximal great arteries, although this assumption is poorly established for the pulmonary artery.[43]

A final invasive method for continuous cardiac output measurement that incorporates Doppler techniques has been developed at the University of North Carolina. A small Silastic probe containing a piezoelectric crystal is attached to the adventitia of the ascending aorta during the operative procedure. Small copper wires connect the crystal via a transthoracic exit to an ultrasound generator. The ultrasound output is amplified, and its analog signal is converted to a digital readout. The digital output is processed by a bedside minicomputer using software that averages the changes in vessel cross-sectional area during the cardiac cycle. Cardiac output is plotted each minute on a continuous computer tracing; hemodynamic calculations such as systemic vascular resistance, stroke volume, stroke index, left ventricular stroke work index, and so on can be retrieved from a simple computer menu. The procedure has proved safe and reliable. Following a satisfactory postoperative course, the device is removed transthoracically, much like pacing wires.[47,48,66]

Noninvasive methods for determining pulmonary and systemic blood flow use ultrasound techniques to determine the velocity of blood flow in the main pulmonary artery and proximal aorta. Cross-sectional areas are calculated using diameters obtained from M-mode or cross-sectional echocardiographic images. Assumptions made in using such techniques have been mentioned previously and include a flat transaxial velocity profile, spherical shape of the vessel, and no changes in cross-sectional area during the cardiac cycle. Despite the assumptions, such techniques have been reported as reliable, although extensive experience and expensive equipment are required.

Cardiac output is usually normalized to body surface area. A useful approximation of surface area can be estimated by the following equation:

$$Surface\ area\ (m^2) = \frac{4\ wt\ (kg) + 7}{wt\ (kg) + 90}$$

Systemic Vascular Resistance Calculations

The determination of systemic vascular resistance (SVR) requires the measurement of central venous and systemic arterial pressures and cardiac output. Obviously, any such calculation is only as accurate as the pressure and flow measurements. SVR is a hydraulic resistance based on Ohm's law and as such is artificially applied to pulsatile flow in compliant blood vessels. However, SVR measurements are widely used and do provide some clinically useful information. Recollection of Poiseuille's equations is useful in emphasizing the importance of vessel radius in the calculation of SVR:

$$Q = \frac{(\Delta P)r^4}{8\ nl}$$

$$R = \frac{P}{Q} = \frac{8\ nl}{r^4}$$

Q = blood flow

P = pressure difference

n = viscosity

l = length

r = radius

R = resistance

Pressure measurements can be obtained quite accurately, but cardiac output determinations are subject to a myriad of potential sources of error.

$$SVR = \frac{\text{Cardiac output (liters/min)}}{\text{Mean arterial pressure (mmHg)} - \text{mean central venous pressure (mmHg)}}$$

SVR as calculated above is expressed in Wood units (liters/min/mmHg). To convert SVR expressed in Wood units into metric units of dynes·sec·cm^{-5}, multiply the Wood unit result by 80. Although this brief description has been directed at the SVR, analogous comments can be made regarding pulmonary vascular resistance when the appropriate flow and pressure measurements are available.

Cardiac Catheterization

Cross-sectional and Doppler ultrasound techniques have reduced the need for postoperative cardiac catheterization but not eliminated it. Despite the obvious risks associated with performing cardiac catheterization in a critically ill infant following cardiac surgery, not determining the cause of a poor postoperative clinical course has even higher risks.

Therapy

Once the physiologic etiology of the postoperative heart failure is identified (whether preload, afterload, contractility, rate, rhythm, or a combination is responsible), therapeutic interventions aimed at correcting the underlying physiologic problem are attempted.[61,65] Often the physician is unable to determine prospectively whether a particular therapeutic intervention will be effective and worth the attendant risks. Provocative therapeutic trials are used with appropriate emphasis on obtaining objective feedback. General comments are offered here for the purpose of review and discussion. However, there is no substitute for experience, and the presence of an experienced physician at the bedside is often the critical difference after difficult neonatal surgery.[2,88]

Preload

The adequacy of ventricular preload is often difficult to assess, even with central venous and left atrial (or pulmonary artery wedge) pressures. High ventricular end-diastolic pressures do not necessarily mean hypervolemia; if ventricular compliance is diminished, filling pressures can be elevated in euvolemic or even hypovolemic patients, and even higher end-diastolic pressures may be required for adequate cardiac output.

Debate over the advantages of crystalloid or colloid continues. We approach this issue quite simply. Often a newborn requires blood transfusion to replace ongoing losses from chest-tube losses, mediastinal tube losses, or losses from blood sampling, even prior to a measured drop in the central hematocrit. When one considers that optimizing peripheral oxygen delivery is the goal, using blood for volume replacement is our preference unless polycythemia is present. We attempt to correct clotting abnormalities with appropriate blood products and use colloid judiciously to replace nonblood losses from chest tubes and mediastinal tubes. We measure serum proteins with regularity and use the results in choosing replacement products.

Following cardiopulmonary bypass, quite often the newborn weighs more than he did preoperatively, has an elevated central venous pressure, and has peripheral edema. If cardiac output is normal either by direct measurement or by indirect signs (e.g., normal blood pressure, adequate renal output, normal peripheral temperature), the question of volume status is relatively moot. However, if cardiac output is inadequate by direct or indirect assessment, augmentation of preload by a volume challenge is still quite appropriate despite signs of volume overload since cardiopulmonary bypass causes third spacing (edema and weight gain) and myocardial dysfunction (high atrial pressure).[96] Close monitoring of such a provocative trial of volume loading is essential. Depending on the position on the volume-pressure atrial compliance curve, a significant quantity of fluid may have little effect on atrial pressure while significantly elevating a low systemic arterial pressure or cardiac output. Conversely, minimal amounts of fluid may exacerbate right-sided and/or left-sided heart failure with dramatic increases in atrial pressures. During such volume challenges, close monitoring of the patient's clinical and hemodynamic status is essential.

Contractility

Contractility can be improved pharmacologically, but when contractility is impaired, attention should first be turned to correction of any acid-base imbalances (respiratory or metabolic acidosis) and any metabolic disorders (e.g., hypocalcemia, hypoglycemia).

Inotropes, although used extensively, enhance ventricular performance less well in the newborn (see also Chapters 2 and 53). A brief description of inotropes commonly used in postoperative heart failure is presented. In addition, the reader is referred to Tables 68–3 and 68–4 for summary information.

Digoxin is a complicated cardiac glycoside compound consisting of an aglycone moiety with three molecules of digitoxose.[58,81] Digoxin is a commonly used inotrope that exerts its effect through a poorly understood pathway involving sarcolemmal Na$^+$, K$^+$–adenosine triphosphatase inhibition and intracellular calcium release. Digoxin can be administered orally, intramuscularly, or intravenously. Prior to use of the short-acting catecholamines, digitalis glycosides were used commonly to improve contractility both acutely and chronically. In recent years short-acting catecholamine infusions have replaced digoxin in the intensive care unit, particularly in critically ill newborns.

Table 68–3. CATECHOLAMINES

Catecholamine	Receptor Activity			
	β_1	β_2	α	δ
Dopamine	+	+	+	+
Epinephrine	+	+	+	
Isoproterenol	+	+		
Dobutamine	+			

Table 68–4. COMMONLY USED CATECHOLAMINES

Catecholamine	Predominate Receptor Site	Dose (µg/kg/min)	How Supplied
Dopamine	δ	1–5	200 mg/5-ml ampule
	β	5–10	
	α	>10	
Dobutamine	β_1	1–20	250-mg vial
Epinephrine	β	0.01–1.0	1 mg/1-ml ampule
	α	>1.0	
Isoproterenol	β	0.01–2.0	1 mg/5-ml ampule

We rarely use digoxin for its inotropic properties in postoperative heart failure but often use it postoperatively for control of arrhythmias.[16,59]

Digoxin use following postoperative neonatal surgery has significant potential for toxicity. In patients receiving digoxin, toxicity should be suspected whenever an arrhythmia occurs, particularly ventricular ectopy and atrial slowing, including atrioventricular block. Medications used to reverse digoxin toxicity include phenytoin, lidocaine, propranolol, and more recently FAB fragments.

Sympathomimetic amines are a group of compounds with similar structures and broad, overlapping hemodynamic actions (see Chapter 53).

Dopamine, the direct precursor of norepinephrine in the *in vivo* catecholamine cascade, is the most commonly used catecholamine for postoperative neonatal heart failure. Dopamine has been extensively reviewed in the pediatric intensive care literature.[17,20,21,23,24,52,57,59,64,77,78,81] Dopamine has α, β, and "dopaminergic" receptor activity. Dopamine exerts a direct β_1-effect by stimulation of the myocardial β_1-receptors and causes release of endogenous norepinephrine from myocardial nerve endings. Low doses of dopamine increase renal perfusion, medium doses are inotropic, and high doses increase systemic vascular resistance as a result of α-effects. Dopamine has both inotropic and chronotropic activity. Despite the concern about the tachyarrhythmiagenic effects, we have rarely had to decrease the dopamine dose because of severe tachycardia or ventricular arrthythmia. Two important points warrant emphasis. First, through its α-vasoconstrictive effects, dopamine can raise pulmonary artery pressure and pulmonary vascular resistance, a potentially serious adverse effect in infants with compromised right ventricular dysfunction. Second, at higher doses, dopamine's combination of increasing myocardial oxygen consumption (because of its inotropic activity) and increasing afterload (because of systemic vasoconstriction) could theoretically compromise cardiac output. However, laboratory experience and modest clinical experience suggest that improvement in cardiac output continues at much higher dopamine doses than commonly used (e.g., 20 to 100 µg/kg/min).

Dopamine is commonly used, and such familiarity can lead to inattention; it is desirable to check the dose actually being administered at the bedside. Flowsheets are usually adequate, but the use of a standard dopamine concentration allows one to double-check the flowsheet or to prescribe an accurate dose readily. We typically mix dopamine at a concentration of 0.8 µg/ml (200 µg/250 ml D$_5$W). Therefore, 0.375 × wt (kg) gives the infusion rate in milliliters per hour to achieve a dose of 5 µg/kg/min.

Dobutamine, a synthetic catecholamine, was designed chemically to be a pure inotrope.[77,78,81,90] Dobutamine's inotropic activity is quite similar to dopamine's in directly stimulating myocardial β_1-receptors; however, dobutamine does not stimulate myocardial norepinephrine release. Furthermore, unlike dopamine, dobutamine has no α-vasoconstrictive effects, nor any selective dopaminergic renal effects. Dobutamine does exert β_2-effects, commonly reducing SVR. As a result, one must be ready to infuse volume in infants receiving dobutamine if arterial hypotension develops. The β_2-vasodilator effects can be advantageous if mild afterload reduction is indicated. In addition, pulmonary artery pressure and pulmonary vascular resistance are modestly reduced at higher doses of dobutamine. Dobutamine does have chronotropic activity. It also increases myocardial oxygen consumption; the combination of reducing diastolic blood pressure and increasing myocardial oxygen consumption has the potential for exacerbating myocardial ischemia.[10,22]

Epinephrine, a naturally occurring catecholamine, exerts α-, β_1-, and β_2-effects, with the β-effects predominating at lower doses and the α-vasoconstrictor effects predominating at higher doses. Epinephrine increases cardiac output through a combination of inotropic and chronotropic effects. It raises pulmonary, systemic, and renal vascular resistances at higher doses and predisposes to significant tachyarrhythmias, including ventricular arrhythmias. Epinephrine can be administered as a bolus endotracheally during cardiopulmonary resuscitation (like atropine).

Isoproterenol is a pure β-agonist. Commonly used previously, isoproterenol has been superseded by other catecholamines such as dopamine and dobutamine in many centers. Isoproterenol has chronotropic effects and is useful in the treatment of bradycardia. It reduces pulmonary artery pressure and pulmonary vascular resistance, which is desirable in newborns with increased right ventricular afterload.[69] However, as a result of its β_2-effects, isoproterenol can blunt hypoxia-induced pulmonary vasoconstriction and exacerbate right-to-left intrapulmonary shunting. Thus, use of isoproterenol in the presence of significant lung disease warrants close observation of arterial blood gases. Similarly, isoproterenol's β_2-induced reduction in SVR is a double-edged sword: although cardiac output may increase as a result of afterload reduction, myocardial ischemia may be exacerbated by reduction in diastolic pressure with concomitant increases in myocardial oxygen consumption. Furthermore, much of isoproterenol's increase in cardiac output can be directed to nonessential vascular beds (e.g., splanchnic) at the expense of more vital organs, which is an undesired perfusion "steal" phenomenon. Therefore, patients treated with isoproterenol may demonstrate improvement in measured cardiac output while peripheral perfusion to vital organs and acid-base balance deteriorate.

Norepinephrine is the most maligned of the catecholamines ("Levophed leaves 'em dead"). This drug has α- and β-agonist activity. With all the attention on norepinephrine's powerful α-vasoconstrictive properties, its β-inotropic effects are often forgotten. In some circumstances, norepinephrine infusions can be quite useful. For example, combining norepinephrine with an α-antagonist such as phentolamine can provide powerful inotropic effects without systemic vasoconstriction. As another example, short-term norepinephrine infusions can maintain coronary perfusion pressure following catastrophic volume loss while volume replacement is initiated.[51,81]

A new class of inotrope, the bipyridine nonglycoside, nonsympathomimetic compounds, specifically amrinone and milrinone, have been introduced recently, although very little literature is available on pediatric usage. The mechanism of action of the bipyridines is not clear. The effects of these drugs include dose-dependent inotropic activity and decreases in both pulmonary vascular resistance and SVR. In adult patients in heart failure receiving digitalis preparations, these agents will increase cardiac output while lowering left ventricular end-diastolic pressure and SVR.[36]

Afterload

Reduction in ventricular afterload should be considered in every newborn with heart failure. Vascular resistance is commonly elevated in heart failure and further diminishes ventricular stroke volume.[60] However, the response to afterload reducing agents in newborns is quite variable and severe hypotension can occur. Hence, continuous hemodynamic monitoring capability is essential for safe afterload reduction in postoperative infants.[4,8,18,86]

Attention to afterload in postoperative newborns includes attention to right ventricular afterload, since pulmonary vascular resistance is normally high in neonates and can rapidly rise to even higher levels (see Chapter 7). One of the best methods for right ventricular afterload reduction in newborns is hyperventilation. Pharmacologic reduction in right ventricular afterload is best approached with the capacity to measure pulmonary vascular resistance or at least pulmonary artery pressure. Selective use of pulmonary vasodilating agents can cause profound improvement of right-sided heart failure. Table 68–5 is a partial list of agents known to act as pulmonary vasodilators. Unfortunately, none is particularly selective for the pulmonary circulation; thus, during use of pulmonary vasodilators, measurement of SVR and close monitoring of blood gases and peripheral oximetry are important to identify increased right-to-left shunting.

Table 68–5. PROPOSED PULMONARY VASODILATORS

Prostaglandin E_1
Prostaglandin I_2
Tolazoline
Isoproterenol
Nifedipine
Nitroglycerin
Nitroprusside

Left ventricular afterload reduction can be lifesaving in cases of residual left atrioventricular valve incompetence (e.g., atrioventricular septal defect) or systemic arterial hypertension (e.g., postoperative repair of aortic coarctation). Continuous infusions of nitroprusside (more vasoactive on systemic arterioles) and nitroglycerin (reported to be more vasoactive on venous capacitance vessels) and intravenous administration of hydralazine are commonly used to reduce systemic resistance. If nitroprusside is used for an extended period and/or at a high dose, specific attention should be directed to cyanide toxicity, which can be difficult to assess in the infant already prone to severe metabolic acidosis. Diazoxide, a direct arteriolar smooth muscle relaxant administered intravenously, is used in hypertensive crises but should be used carefully due to its relatively long half-life and its hyperglycemic effects. Less commonly, trimethaphan camsylate, a ganglionic blocking agent administered as a continuous intravenous infusion, has been used. Oral agents are less commonly used in an intensive care unit setting for obvious reasons; however, the use of the converting enzyme inhibitor captopril is becoming more common.[70,81]

Heart Rate and Rhythm

Manipulation of heart rate is often neglected. As discussed previously, neonatal cardiac output is particularly heart rate dependent because of the higher position on the Frank-Starling curve. Therefore, any physiologic change that interferes with an appropriate heart rate response to stress can be quite deleterious in the newborn. Similarly, sinus rhythm is equally important in maintaining cardiac output in stressed newborns. Therefore, in the postoperative newborn, maintaining sinus rhythm and adequate heart rate are very important.

Bradycardia is tolerated particularly poorly by stressed neonates. Every effort should be made to rule out a treatable metabolic etiology. In postoperative patients without external temporary pacemaker leads, persistent bradycardia should be treated with temporary transvenous ventricular pacing, which usually can be accomplished quickly. In postoperative patients with temporary pacing wires, the pacemaker should be activated. We favor the placement of atrial and ventricular pacing wires in any patient undergoing cardiopulmonary bypass to provide atrioventricular pacing if postoperative bradycardia and/or atrioventricular block should occur. In addition to the pacing capability, temporary cardiac leads can be immensely helpful in identifying arrhythmias.[97,99]

Sinus tachycardia at rates below 200 beats per minute (bpm) is usually well tolerated. However, in postoperative infants with cardiac compromise, heart rates above 200 bpm are frequently associated with decreased cardiac output. Obviously, the rhythm should be identified if possible. If paroxysmal atrial tachycardia is diagnosed, sinus rhythm should be restored.[38,40] Medications that might adversely affect ventricular performance, such as propranolol, should be avoided. We favor immediate cardioversion, although other centers favor transesophageal overdrive pacing. Intravenous verapamil should not be used in neonates, because of the risk of atrioventricular block and severe bradycardia. Once sinus rhythm has been restored, suppressive therapy can be begun. Wide QRS tachycardia is quite ominous, and efforts to localize a nodal or ventricular origin are at times impossible. We cardiovert wide QRS tachycardia immediately if any further cardiac compromise is noted; a 1-mg/kg bolus of lidocaine is given intravenously prior to cardioversion. On rare occasions, lidocaine administration has converted wide QRS tachycardia, suggesting a ventricular origin for the arrhythmia.

Future Trends

Identifying advances that can be expected to improve care of newborns requiring cardiovascular surgery is not difficult. The role of cardiac transplantation in the treatment of newborns with cardiac defects not palliable by present techniques will become better defined. Elucidation of the mechanism of ischemic injury during cardiopulmonary bypass will significantly improve the rather crude current techniques directed toward preservation of myocardial integrity. Significant progress can be expected in the understanding of and therapy for pulmonary hypertension. Further improvements in diagnostic techniques will occur rapidly. New inotropes and antiarrhythmics will continue to become available. Interventional catheterization will increasingly replace surgical intervention. Finally, advances in the understanding of the molecular etiologic mechanisms responsible for structural heart disease will eventually put all of us into a happy retirement. In short, the future is bright.

DEATH OF A NEWBORN WITH CONGENITAL HEART DISEASE

> *Children—take'm as they run—*
> *You kin bet on, ev'ry one!—*
> *Treat'm right and reco'nize*
> *Human souls is all one size.*
>
> **The Raggedy Man on Children,**
> **James Whitcomb Riley**

The advances in the management of newborns with heart disease, particularly the surgical successes, have been reported extensively in the media. Parents, when confronted with the news of suspected or confirmed heart disease in their newborn, have high expectations despite the ever-present fear of the child's death. Unfortunately, neonates still die of heart disease. The setting is most likely to be in an intensive care unit of a tertiary care medical center. If parents of children who have died should be the judge, no event ever equals the intensity of the feelings of pain, helplessness, and sorrow from the death of a child, whether the death was expected or not and regardless of the child's age.

We start with the premise that the physician's commitment to the family and staff does not end with the death of the child. Although this premise is rarely debated, actual physician involvement is often haphazard beyond conveying the information at the time of the child's death. The reasons for this lack of involvement are many and include avoidance behavior from a sense of failure or pain, competing priorities for time and energy, assumptions that someone else is involved, a lack of training in this area, and, finally, a lack of discussion about the need and importance of this endeavor. In a splendidly written and exhaustingly complete 1505-page textbook of pediatric intensive care published in 1987, death has no listing in the index and is not discussed except to state that deaths in pediatric intensive care units contribute to the stress to the personnel.[89] To our knowledge, no textbook of pediatric cardiology has any specific discussion regarding the need and scope of follow-up after a child with heart disease dies. Only rarely has any time been devoted to this topic in the many professional meetings devoted to pediatric cardiology and pediatric cardiac surgery.

We recommend that each medical center that cares for newborns with heart disease examine its current approach to infants who die. Each center needs to determine if adequate emphasis and resources are directed to follow-up. This examination of current follow-up practices need not be a cumbersome, formal policy-type review but rather a review simply to determine if coordinated efforts by the staff are devoted to the family and to the staff following the death of a child. Such reviews are particularly important for training programs where residents and fellows participate significantly in the care of such infants.

The essence of management following the death of a child can be summed up in one word—communication. In a sense, everyone is a survivor. However, our remarks are directed toward communication among those survivors most directly involved: the family, the community, the hospital staff, and the physician (Table 68–6).[25,44,55]

The Family

Once a child dies, the family should be informed in person in a private setting. Euphemisms such as "passed away" or "slipped away" should be avoided. The child died, and this fact needs to be provided to the parents in a noneuphemistic, frank, but compassionate manner. The physician recognized by the family as the most senior physician responsible for decision making should be available to the family as soon as possible to discuss the infant's death in simple, brief terms. This physician needs

Table 68–6. SURVIVORS

Family
  Parents
  Siblings
  Extended family
Community
  Family friends
  Local physicians
  Schoolteachers
  Child care providers
  Clergy
Hospital
  Nurses
  House staff
  Physicians
  Other parents

to be available to other family members and be willing to address each person's concerns.

The parents should be allowed time to be alone, even from other family members, in a quiet setting. A hospital chaplain can be called if desired by the parents. Subsequently, the parents should be encouraged to be alone with their child. Despite the temptation to have to face only one conversation, requests for autopsy permission are best deferred for a few minutes. While the parents are with the child, other family members can be directed to think about notification of a funeral home and preparations for a funeral or memorial service; such plans should be settled later in consultation with the parents. If an autopsy is desired, the parents should be approached without other family members or friends in attendance. (In our experience, we have found that every parent who has denied permission for an autopsy has regretted their decision at the subsequent follow-up visit.) Beyond simple factual explanations and brief expressions of sorrow, simply being present is statement enough for most families. The referral and family physicians should be notified promptly of the child's death.

What is the role of the physician once the family has left the hospital? Although this role may be debated vigorously, a working goal is to help the family accept the child's death. The physician serves as a monitor of the family's grief reaction and attempts to ensure that it proceeds to resolution. It should never be assumed that the local physician will follow up. In a previous study of 35 families following the death of a child from congenital heart disease, only two families received any physician follow-up from the local physician. The grief process proceeds normally in most family members and rarely requires intervention to achieve resolution. Furthermore, no data exist that the physician can (or should attempt to) shorten mourning. Why then should the physician continue a relationship with the family? The most important reason is that the parents expect it and consider it important. Subsequent follow-up should be discussed with the family prior to their leaving the hospital. The purpose, approximate time, and location of the follow-up should be quite clear to the parents and local physicians. A tele-

phone call to the parents several days after the child's death has been described as being most helpful and appreciated by parents and other family members. During this early period, relationships established between the parents and other parents of hospitalized children and with the hospital staff should be facilitated as desired by the parents.[15,27,33,41,44,49,63,91]

We recommend follow-up at the hospital (if geographically practical) within 6 to 8 weeks following the child's death. In the past 8 years no parent has refused the opportunity for follow-up. When we have neglected to arrange for such follow-up, often the parents have requested it.

The agenda of the meeting from the physician's perspective is summarized in Table 68–7. Listening and answering parental questions are the principal ingredients of a successful meeting. Autopsy findings can be discussed simply but in sufficient detail to answer as many questions as possible. Young parents may never have experienced the death of a significant person in their lives prior to the death of their child. To such parents the grief reaction can be frightening. A simple summary of what other parents have described will usually provide much reassurance. Generally, parents have described their early feelings of shock and detachment and "going through the motions" for days to weeks. Feelings of anger and intense guilt are often described. Subsequently, sadness and depression lasting for several months are typically described. Flashbacks of intense feelings occur with decreasing regularity. As one parent reflected: "It hurts every day. I think about him every day. But I accept it. I have learned to live with it. I am comfortable again with myself."

The grief reactions of surviving children should be reviewed with the parents as well.[55,71,74] We always mention guilt, whether expressed or not, and address all other concerns. Recurrence risks for future pregnancies should be introduced and discussed if requested, including issues of prenatal diagnosis. Referral for more sophisticated counseling is made if appropriate. As one brings the meeting to a close, subsequent follow-up should be discussed and arranged; usually a telephone call several months later will suffice to meet most parents' needs. Finally, the local physicians should be informed of the meeting and the arrangement for further follow-up.[5,6,9,15]

Table 68–7. OBJECTIVES OF PHYSICIAN FOLLOW-UP INTERVIEW

1. Provide emotional support to the family
2. Answer questions spontaneously raised
3. Discuss autopsy findings
4. Discuss parental grief reaction
5. Discuss surviving children's grief reaction
6. Identify and assess use of support mechanisms
7. Discuss recurrence risks for future pregnancies
8. Establish future follow-up (telephone, visit)
9. Arrange appropriate physician referral
10. Communicate with local physician

From Henry GW, Taylor CA (1982): Reactions of families to the death of a child with congenital heart disease. South Med J 75:988–994.

The Community

The referring physician should be called immediately and informed of the child's death. The documentation of this phone call should be explicit in the chart for subsequent review purposes. The referring physician can identify other local physicians who also need to be contacted. These physicians are vitally important, because they can immediately identify local sources of support available to the family, including themselves. It seems children often die in the middle of the night, but the time of day should not deter one from initiating the appropriate telephone calls. When the local physician's first news of his patient's death is several distraught (or angry) family members on his office doorstep in the morning, the first opportunity for initiation of local support to the family has been lost.

Subsequent follow-up can be coordinated with the appropriate local physicians, who should be provided the autopsy report and how the autopsy information will be shared with the family. A special comment regarding autopsy reports is warranted. The final autopsy report is often prepared by a pathology resident with no experience in the pathophysiology of congenital heart disease for signature by an attending pathologist. Some statements regarding the clinical events are only understood at a superficial level and can confuse parents and local physicians. Being present at the autopsy and being available to the pathologists for comments as they prepare the autopsy report will help the clinicians to avoid having to explain to local physicians or parents inaccurate or confusing autopsy statements.

Survivors in the community are many, and some need to be identified for receipt of appropriate information. Two often forgotten sources of extensive support are the mother's obstetrician and any school-age siblings' schoolteacher(s). The obstetrician may be the most important physician provider, at least to the mother. In our experience the obstetrician often has been invaluable as a source of support to both parents and in monitoring the parental grief reaction. The schoolteacher of a sibling is often forgotten but is uniquely positioned to monitor the grief reactions in surviving school-age siblings. School counseling services are available in most school districts and can be identified by the teacher when appropriate. In most families, both parents work outside the home. Surviving siblings, if not school age, often have some day-care activities. The parents should be reminded to inform the day-care providers of the family's loss and the surviving siblings' comprehension of and reactions to the tragedy. Day-care providers can provide insights and observations on the siblings' grief reaction.

Friends of parents and friends of siblings often exhibit avoidance behavior. The parents need to be aware how often they will have to initiate what before a death was common social interaction. That it becomes the parents' responsibility to initiate such interaction is often misinterpreted as a lack of caring rather than a desire not to intrude.

The Hospital Staff

The interdisciplinary nature of pediatric cardiac intensive care, particularly in a training center setting, requires sensitivity to a variety of staff needs when a newborn dies.

A resident or fellow may not be able to draw from his or her own personal family experience to sort out feelings evoked at the time of a newborn's death. No previous significant family member or friend may have ever died. Hence, the resident or fellow may be thrust into managing a clinical situation with no experience from which to draw. Few studies have been directed at this problem, but the few that are published have pointed out the extreme feelings of depression, guilt, and inadequacy experienced by the house officer. At the University of North Carolina we hold a survivor's conference attended by the attending staff, house staff, nurses, and social workers; the survivor's conference is coordinated by a child psychiatrist. Family needs are anticipated, and responsibility for specific follow-up is delineated. One important purpose of the conference is to offer all concerned the opportunity to discuss their own feelings. Surprisingly, quite candid comments are the norm.

The collective toll of such intensely draining experiences on all the medical personnel must be recognized. High turnover rates, inadequate staff, and the amount of work necessary to care for a single child in an intensive care unit are poorly appreciated by pediatric and surgical chairmen and especially poorly appreciated by hospital administrators. The senior medical staff needs to devote time to discussing these issues, despite the often inadequate resources to reduce the stresses on nurses, house officers, themselves, and other medical personnel.

The Physician

There is no substitute for competence. If the senior physician does not feel competent and comfortable in working with families and staff after the death of a child, often no one else will take the lead to ensure that this process is initiated. It is unimportant whether the surgeon, cardiologist, neonatologist, or intensivist is in charge of follow-up, but it is important that someone assume that responsibility and that others know who has assumed it. Assignment of follow-up responsibility can easily be established shortly after the child dies, because the parents may readily make known their choice of physicians with whom they wish to talk.

The senior physician often devotes so much energy to the family and staff that his or her own needs are not met. The death of a child for whom one is caring is very traumatic, regardless of one's experience. Death is physically and emotionally draining, and one must admit that to oneself. One must be honest in attempts to recognize resultant behavior not in one's best interest or one's family's best interests. The cumulative effects of repeated stress caused by intense clinical responsibilities must be recognized and addressed personally. The privilege of being allowed to care for intensely ill children in a setting of multidisciplinary expertise can be offset entirely by the chronic physical, mental, and emotional burdens incurred by such work. However, to participate competently and effectively in the follow-up care of a family after the death of a child, while tending to the needs of other survivors, can be a source of renewal as well as a quiet source of professional and personal pride.[3,13,36,56]

Epilogue

I ain't, ner don't p'tend to be,
Much posted on philosofy;
But thare is times, when all alone,
I work out idees of my own.
And of these same thare is a few
I'd like to jest refer to you—
Pervidin' that you don't object
To listen clos't and rickollect.

My doctern is to lay aside
Contentions, and be satisfied:
Jest do your best, and praise er blame
That follers that, counts jest the same.
I've allus noticed grate success
Is mixed with troubles, more er less,
And it's the man who does the best
That gits more kicks than all the rest.

My Philosofy,
James Whitcomb Riley

References

1. Abe T, Komatsu S (1983): Conduction disturbances and operative results after closure of ventricular septal defects by three different surgical approaches. Jpn Circ J 47:328–335.
2. Agarwala BN (1982): Postoperative management of open heart surgery in infants and children. Hosp Pract 17:40C–40R.
3. Aires P (1981): The Hour of Our Death. New York, Alfred A. Knopf.
4. Appelbaum A, Blackstone EH, Kouchoukos NT, Kirklin JW (1977): Afterload reduction and cardiac output in infants early after intracardiac surgery. Am J Cardiol 39:445–451.
5. Aradine CR (1976): Books for children about death. Pediatrics 57:372–378.
6. Arnold JH, Gemma PB (1983): A Child Dies: A Portrait of Family Grief. London, Aspen Systems Corporation.
7. Barry WH, Grossman W (1984): Cardiac catheterization. In Braunwald E (ed): Heart Disease: A Textbook of Cardiovascular Medicine. 2nd ed. Philadelphia, WB Saunders, pp 289–294.
8. Benson LN, Bohn D, Edmonds JF, Fortune RL, Price SA, Williams WG, Rowe RD (1979): Nitroglycerin therapy in children with low cardiac index after heart surgery. Cardiovasc Med 4:207.
9. Blinder BJ (1972): Sibling death in childhood. Child Psychiatry Hum Dev 2:169–175.
10. Bohn DJ, Poirier CS, Edmonds JF, Barker GA (1980): Hemodynamic effects of dobutamine after cardiopulmonary bypass in children. Crit Care Med 8:367–371.
11. Bove EL, Sondheimer HM, Byrum CJ, Kavey REW, Blackman MS (1984): Pulmonary hemodynamics and maintenance of palliation following polytetrafluoroethylene shunts for cyanotic congenital heart disease. Am Heart J 108:366–368.
12. Braunwald E, Sonnenblick EH, Ross J Jr (1984): Contraction of the normal heart. In Braunwald E (ed): Heart Disease: A Textbook of Cardiovascular Medicine. 2nd ed. Philadelphia, WB Saunders, pp 430–438.
13. Buscaglia L (1982): The Fall of Freddie the Leaf. Thorofare, Charles B. Slack.
14. Casella ES, Rogers MC, Zahka KG (1987): Developmental physiology of the cardiovascular system. In Rogers MC (ed): Textbook of Pediatric Intensive Care. Baltimore, Williams & Wilkins, pp 329–365.
15. Clayton P, Desmarais L, Winokur G (1968): A study of normal bereavement. Am J Psychiatry 125:168–178.
16. Collins-Nakai RL, Ng PK, Beaudry MA, Ocejo-Moreno R, Schiff D, VanPetten GR (1982): Total body digoxin clearance and steady-state concentrations in low birth weight infants. Dev Pharmacol Ther 4:61–70.
17. Crone RK (1980): Acute circulatory failure in children. Pediatr Clin North Am 27:525–538.
18. Davies DW, Greiss L, Kadar D, Steward DJ (1975): Sodium nitroprusside in children: Observations on metabolism during normal and abnormal responses. Can Anaesth Soc J 22:553–560.
19. Dawes GS, Mott J (1959): The increase in oxygen consumption of the lamb after birth. J Physiol 146:295–315.
20. DiSessa TG, Leitner M, Ti CC, Gluck L, Coen R, Friedman WF (1981): The cardiovascular effects of dopamine in the severely asphyxiated neonate. J Pediatr 99:772–776.
21. Driscoll DJ, Gillette PC, McNamara DG (1978): The use of dopamine in children. J Pediatr 92:309–314.
22. Driscoll DJ, Gillette PC, Duff DF, Nihill MR, Gutgesell HP, Vargo TA, Mullins CE, McNamara DG (1979): Hemodynamic effects of dobutamine in children. Am J Cardiol 43:581–585.
23. Driscoll DJ, Gillette PC, Lewis RM, Hartley CJ, Schwartz A (1979): Comparative hemodynamic effects of isoproterenol, dopamine, and dobutamine in the newborn dog. Pediatr Res 13:1006–1009.
24. Drummond WH, Gregory GA, Heymann MA, Phibbs RA (1981): The independent effects of hyperventilation, tolazoline, and dopamine on infants with persistent pulmonary hypertension. J Pediatr 98:603–611.
25. Easson WM (1981): The Dying Child: The Management of the Child or Adolescent Who is Dying. Springfield, Charles C Thomas.
26. Edmonds JF, Barker GA, Conn AW (1980): Current concepts in cardiovascular monitoring in children. Crit Care Med 8:548–553.
27. Elliott BA, Hein HA (1978): Neonatal death: Reflections for physicians. Pediatrics 62:96–100.
28. Fait CD, Wetzel RC, Dean JM, Schleien CL, Giola FR (1985): Pulse oximetry in critically ill children. J Clin Monit 1:232–235.
29. Fick A (1897): Uber die Messung des Blutquantums in den Herzventrikeln. Sitz der Physik Med Ges Wurzburg, p 16.
30. Finlayson DC, Kaplan JA (1979): Cardiopulmonary bypass. In Kaplan JA (ed): Cardiac Anesthesia. New York, Grune & Stratton, p 416.
31. Finnie KJ, Watts DG, Armstrong PW (1984): Biases in the measurement of arterial pressure. Crit Care Med 12:965–968.
32. Freed MD, Keane JF (1978): Cardiac output measured by thermodilution in infants and children. J Pediatr 92:39–42.
33. Freud S (1917): Mourning and Melancholia. In The Standard Edition of the Complete Psychological Works of Sigmund Freud, 1957. London, Hogarth Press, pp 243–258.
34. Friedman WF (1973): The intrinsic physiologic properties of the developing heart. In Friedman WF, Lesch M, Sonnenblick EM (eds): Neonatal Heart Disease. New York, Grune & Stratton, p 21.
35. Friedman WF (1972): The intrinsic physiologic properties of the developing heart. Prog Cardiovasc Dis 15:87–111.
36. Friedman WF, George BL (1984): New concepts and drugs in the treatment of congestive heart failure. Pediatr Clin North Am 31:1197–1227.
37. Ganz W, Donoso R, Marcus HS, Forrester JS, Swan HJC (1971): A new technique for measurements of cardiac output by thermodilution in man. Am J Cardiol 27:392–396.
38. Garson A Jr, Gillette PC, McNamara DG (1981): Supraventricular tachycardia in children: Clinical features, response to treatment, and long-term follow-up in 217 patients. J Pediatr 98:875–882.
39. Graham TP Jr, Bender HW Jr (1980): Preoperative diagnosis and management of infants with critical congenital heart disease. Ann Thorac Surg 29:272–288.
40. Greco R, Musto B, Arienzo V, Alorino A, Garofalo S, Marsico F (1982): Treatment of paroxysmal supraventricular tachycardia in infancy with digitalis, adenosine-5'-triphosphate, and verapamil: A comparative study. Circulation 66:504–508.
41. Green M, Solnit AJ (1964): Reactions to the threatened loss of a child: Vulnerable child syndrome. Pediatrics 33:58–66.
42. Henry GW (1984): Noninvasive assessment of cardiac function and pulmonary hypertension in persistent pulmonary hypertension of the newborn. Clin Perinatol 11:627–640.

43. Henry GW, Johnson TA, Ferreiro JI, Hsiao HS, Lucas CL, Keagy BA, Lores ME, Wilcox BR (1984): Velocity profile in the main pulmonary artery in a canine model. Cardiovasc Res 18:620–625.

44. Henry GW, Taylor CA (1982): Reactions of families to the death of a child with congenital heart disease. South Med J 75:988–994.

45. Jatene AD, Fontes VF, Souza LC, Paulista PP, Neto CA, Sousa JE (1982): Anatomic correction of transposition of the great arteries. J Thorac Cardiovasc Surg 83:20–26.

46. Johnson GL, Cunningham MD, Desai NS, Cottrill CM, Noonan JA (1980): Echocardiography in hypoxemic neonatal pulmonary disease. J Pediatr 96:716–720.

47. Keagy BA, Lucas CL, Hsiao HS, Wilcox BR (1983): A removable extraluminal Doppler probe for continuous monitoring of changes in cardiac output. J Ultrasound Med 2:357–362.

48. Keagy BA, Wilcox BR, Lucas CL, Hsiao HS, Henry GW, Baudino M, Bornzin G (1987): Constant postoperative monitoring of cardiac output after correction of congenital heart defects. J Thorac Cardiovasc Surg 93:658–664.

49. Kennell JH, Slyter H, Klaus MH (1970): The mourning response of parents to the death of a newborn infant. N Engl J Med 283:344–349.

50. Kinsman JM, Moore JW, Hamilton WF (1929): Studies on the circulation: I. Injection method. Physical and mathematical considerations. Am J Physiol 89:322–330.

51. Kirsh MM, Bove E, Detmer M, Hill A, Knight P (1980): The use of levarterenol and phentolamine in patients with low cardiac output following open-heart surgery. Ann Thorac Surg 29:26–31.

52. Kliegman R, Fanaroff AA (1978): Caution in the use of dopamine in the neonate. J Pediatr 93:540–541.

53. Klopfenstein H, Rudolph AM (1978): Postnatal changes in the circulation and responses to volume loading in sheep. Circ Res 42:839–845.

54. Knight RW, Opie JC (1981): The big toe in the recovery room: Peripheral warm-up patterns in children after open-heart surgery. Can J Surg 24:239–242.

55. Kubler-Ross E (1983): On Children and Death. New York, Macmillan.

56. Kushner HS (1981): When Bad Things Happen to Good People. New York, Schocken.

57. Lang P, Williams RG, Norwood WI, Castaneda AR (1980): The hemodynamic effects of dopamine in infants after corrective cardiac surgery. J Pediatr 96:630–634.

58. Langer GA (1981): Mechanism of action of the cardiac glycosides on the heart. Biochem Pharmacol 30:3261–3264.

59. Larese RJ, Mirkin BL (1974): Kinetics of digoxin absorption and relation of serum levels to cardiac arrhythmias in children. Clin Pharmacol Ther 15:387–396.

60. Levin DL, Heymann MA, Kitterman JA, Gregory GA, Rhibbs RH, Rudolph AM (1976): Persistent pulmonary hypertension of the newborn infant. J Pediatr 89:626–630.

61. Levin DL, Perkin RM (1984): Postoperative care of the pediatric patient with congenital heart disease. In Shoemaker WC, Thompson WL, Holbrook PR (eds): Textbook of Critical Care. Philadelphia, WB Saunders, pp 395–403.

62. Little RC, Little WC (1982): Cardiac preload, afterload and heart failure. Arch Intern Med 142:819–822.

63. Lindemann E (1944): Symptomatology and the management of acute grief. Am J Psychiatry 101:141–148.

64. Lister G (1984): Management of the pediatric patient after cardiac surgery. Yale J Biol Med 57:7–27.

65. Lister G, Talner NS (1981): Management of respiratory failure of cardiac origin. In Gregory G (ed): Respiratory Failure in the Child. New York, Churchill Livingstone, pp 67–87.

66. Lucas CL, Keagy BA, Hsiao HS, Johnson TA, Henry GW, Wilcox BR (1984): The velocity profile in the canine ascending aorta and its effects on the accuracy of pulsed Doppler determinations of mean blood velocity. Cardiovasc Res 18:282–293.

67. Lynn AM, Jenkins JG, Edmonds JF, Burns JE (1983): Diaphragmatic paralysis after pediatric cardiac surgery: A retrospective analysis of 34 cases. Crit Care Med 11:280–282.

68. McPherson RA, Kramer MF, Covell JW, Friedman WF (1976): A comparison of the active stiffness of fetal and adult cardiac muscle. Pediatr Res 10:660–664.

69. Mentzer RM Jr, Alegre CA, Nolan SP (1976): The effects of dopamine and isoproterenol on the pulmonary circulation. J Thorac Cardiovasc Surg 71:807–814.

70. Miller RR, Fennell WH, Young JB, Palomo AR, Quinones MA (1982): Differential systemic arterial and venous actions and consequent cardiac effects of vasodilator drugs. Prog Cardiovasc Dis 24:353–374.

71. Mills GC (1979): Books to help children understand death. Am J Nursing 79:291–295.

72. Miyasaka K, Edmonds JF, Conn AW (1976): Complications of radial artery lines in the pediatric patient. Can Anaesth Soc J 23:9–14.

73. Mokrohisky ST, Levine RL, Blumhagen JD, Wesenberg RC, Simmons MA (1978): Low positioning of umbilical-artery catheters increases associated complications in newborn infants. N Engl J Med 299:561–564.

74. Ordal CC (1983/1984): Death as seen in books suitable for young children. Omega 14:249–277.

75. Palmisano BW, Fisher DM, Willis M, Gregory GA, Ebert PA (1984): The effect of paralysis on oxygen consumption in normoxic children after cardiac surgery. Anesthesiology 61:518–522.

76. Park MK, Sheridan PH, Morgan WW, Beck N (1980): Comparative inotropic response of newborn and adult rabbit papillary muscles to isoproterenol and calcium. Dev Pharmacol Ther 1:70–82.

77. Perkin RM, Levin DL (1982): Shock in the pediatric patient: I. J Pediatr 101:163–169.

78. Perkin RM, Levin DL (1982): Shock in the pediatric patient: II. Therapy. J Pediatr 101:319–332.

79. Pollack MM, Reed TP, Holbrook PR, Fields A (1982): Bedside pulmonary artery catheterization in pediatrics. J Pediatr 96:274–276.

80. Prian GW, Wright GB, Rumack CM, O'Meara OP (1978): Apparent cerebral embolization after temporal artery catheterization. J Pediatr 93:115–118.

81. Roberts RJ (1984): Cardiovascular drugs. In Roberts RJ (ed): Drug Therapy in Infants. Philadelphia, WB Saunders, pp 138–225.

82. Roberts RJ (1984): Diuretics. In Roberts RJ (ed): Drug Therapy in Infants. Philadelphia, WB Saunders, pp 226–249.

83. Romero T, Covell J, Friedman WF (1972): A comparison of pressure-volume relations of the fetal, newborn and adult heart. Am J Physiol 222:1285–1290.

84. Romero TO, Friedman WF (1979): Limited left ventricular response to volume overload in the neonatal period: A comparative study with the adult animal. Pediatr Res 13:910–915.

85. Rousou JA, Parker T, Engelman RM, Breyer RH (1985): Phrenic nerve paresis associated with the use of iced slush and the cooling jacket for topical hypothermia. J Thorac Cardiovasc Surg 89:921–925.

86. Rubis LJ, Stephenson LW, Johnston MR, Nagaraj S, Edmunds LH Jr (1981): Comparison of effects of prostaglandin E_1 and nitroprusside on pulmonary vascular resistance in children after open-heart surgery. Ann Thorac Surg 32:563–570.

87. Rudolph AM (1980): High pulmonary vascular resistance after birth: I. Pathophysiologic considerations and etiologic classification. Clin Pediatr 19:585–590.

88. Sade RM, Cosgrove DM, Castaneda AR (1977): Infant and Child Care in Heart Surgery. Chicago, Year Book Medical Publishers.

89. Schleien CL, Zahka KG, Rogers MC (1987): Principles of postoperative management in the pediatric intensive care unit. In Rogers MC (ed): Textbook of Pediatric Intensive Care. Baltimore, Williams & Wilkins, pp 411–458.

90. Schranz D, Stopfkuchen H, Jungst BK, Clemens R, Emmrich P (1982): Hemodynamic effects of dobutamine in children with cardiovascular failure. Eur J Pediatr 139:4–7.

91. Schreiner RL, Gresham EL, Green M (1979): Physician's responsibility to parents after the death of an infant. Am J Dis Child 133:723–726.

92. Sheldon CA, Friedman WF, Sybers HD (1976): Scanning electron microscopy of fetal and neonatal cardiac cells. J Mol Cell Cardiol 8:853–862.

93. Simmons MA, Levine RL, Lubchenco LO, Guggenheim MA (1978): Warning: Serious sequelae of temporal artery catheterization (letter). J Pediatr 92:284.

94. Stewart GN (1897): Researches on the circulation time and on the influences which affect it. IV. The output of the heart. J Physiol 22:159.

95. Swedlow DB, Cohen DE (1986): Invasive assessment of the failing circulation. In Swedlow DB, Raphaely RG (eds): Cardiovascular Problems in Pediatric Critical Care. New York, Churchill Livingstone, pp 129–168.

96. Vincent RN, Lang P, Elixson EM, Gamble WJ, Fulton DR, Fellows KE, Norwood WI, Castaneda AR (1984): Measurement of extravascular lung water in infants and children after cardiac surgery. Am J Cardiol 54:161–165.

97. Waldo AL, Henthorn RW, Plumb VJ (1984): Temporary epicardial wire electrodes in the diagnosis and treatment of arrhythmias after open-heart surgery. Am J Surg 148:275–283.

98. Wetzel RC, Rogers MC (1980): Pediatric hemodynamic monitoring. In Shoemaker WC, Thompson L (eds): Critical Care: State of the Art. Fullerton, Society of Critical Care Medicine, pp 1–78.

99. Yabek SM, Akl BF, Berman W Jr, Neal JF, Dillon T (1980): Use of atrial epicardial electrodes to diagnose and treat postoperative arrhythmias in children. Am J Cardiol 46:285–289.

100. Yelderman M, New W Jr (1983): Evaluation of pulse oximetry. Anesthesiology 59:349–352.

INDEX

Note: Page numbers in *italics* refer to illustrations; page numbers followed by t refer to tables.

Propranolol *(Continued)*
  for hypertrophic cardiomyopathy, 503, *503*
  for premature ventricular contractions, 516
  for right ventricular outflow tract obstruction, 775
  for ventricular tachycardia, 517
  to prevent atrial flutter recurrence, 515
Propylthiouracil (PTU), in pregnancy, 151
Prostacyclin, effect of, on ductus arteriosus closure, 754
  on pulmonary circulation, *409*, 409–410
  on pulmonary vascular tone, 90, *90*
  for acidosis, in TAPVC, 797
  for PPHNS, 637–638, 695
  for pulmonary hypertension crisis management, 806t
Prostaglandin D$_2$, as pulmonary vasodilator and vasoconstrictor, 658
  for PPHNS, 696
Prostaglandin E$_1$, for coarctation of aorta, 483–484
  for Ebstein anomaly, 546
  for interruption of aortic arch, 490
  for left ventricular outflow obstruction, preoperative administration of, 762
  for PPHNS, 695–696
  for pulmonary atresia with intact ventricular septum, 556
  for pulmonary valve stenosis, 553
    postoperative administration of, 770, 771
  for total anomalous pulmonary venous drainage, 449
  for transposition of great arteries, 563
  for tricuspid atresia, 536
  for valvular aortic stenosis, 470
  patency of ductus arteriosus with, maintenance of, 678–679
  prior to balloon pulmonary valvuloplasty, 708
Prostaglandin E$_2$, effect of, on ductus arteriosus closure, 754
  patency of ductus arteriosus with, maintenance of, 678–679
Prostaglandins, affecting pulmonary vascular tone, 90, *90*
  ductus patency and, 65
  source of, in regulation of ductus arteriosus, 66
  to stimulate labor, 150
Prosthesis, polytetrafluoroethylene, to increase bilateral pulmonary blood flow, 743–744
Protein, N, 46–47
  thin filament of, 22, 34–35
Protein isoform expression, developmental changes in, 34–35
Pseudoephedrine, in pregnancy, 151
Pseudoglandular period, of postembryonic lung development, 101
Pseudotruncus arteriosus, 565
Pseudo-Turner syndrome, 258
Pseudo–Wilson-Mikity syndrome, 254
Psychiatric drugs, effect of, on fetal cardiovascular system, 150
PTA (percutaneous transluminal angioplasty), for coarctation of aorta, 484
PtcO$_2$ (end tidal carbon dioxide tension), monitoring of, during anesthesia, 722
Pterygium colli, in Noonan syndrome, 604
  in Turner syndrome, 587
P-tricuspidale, 530
PTU (propylthiouracil), in pregnancy, 151
Pulmonary. See also *Lung(s)*.
Pulmonary agenesis, radiographic diagnosis of, 256, *257*
Pulmonary artery, development of, *52*
  hypoplasia of, 552

Pulmonary artery *(Continued)*
  muscular, electron micrographs of, *57, 60*
  muscular and elastic, changes in relative radius of, *61*
Pulmonary artery banding, anesthetic management in, 728–729
  as palliation in tricuspid atresia, 537
  material used in, 747
  mortality rate in, 583
  to reduce pulmonary blood flow, *746–747*, 746–748
Pulmonary artery catheter, complications of, 818, 819t
Pulmonary artery hypertension, in asphyxiated newborns, 502
Pulmonary artery pressure, Doppler echocardiographic measurement of, 325–326
  M-mode echocardiography of, 306–307
  postoperative monitoring of, 818, 819t
  two-dimensional echocardiographic estimation of, 316–317, *317*
Pulmonary artery sling, 256, *257*
Pulmonary baroreceptors, reflexes initiated by, 83
Pulmonary circulation, adult, direct autonomic influences in, 86–87
  chemical mediators and messengers in, 89–91
  decreased, in heart disease, 264–265, *264–265*
  developmental physiology of, 76–91
  effects of bronchopulmonary dysplasia on, 405–406
  effects of prostacyclin on, *409*, 409–410
  fetal, 76
    direct autonomic influences in, 85–86
    vs. adult, 76
  historical perspective of, 76–77
  in tricuspid atresia, 528
  neonatal, 76, 76–91
    direct autonomic influences in, 86–87
  physiologic factors altering vascular tone and, 77–88
Pulmonary diffusion capacity, 105
Pulmonary disease, associated with PPHNS, 637t, 637–638
  during pregnancy, 140
Pulmonary edema, causes of, 253t
  in bronchopulmonary dysplasia, 405
  pathogenesis of, 402–403
  radiographic diagnosis of, 253–255, *254–255*
Pulmonary function, in neonate, 101–108
Pulmonary hypertension. See also *Persistent pulmonary hypertension of newborn syndrome (PPHNS)*.
  alveolar hypoxia-induced, effects of chemodenovation on, 83–84, *84*
  in asphyxiated newborns, 502
  phlebotomy for, 80
  postoperative management of, TAPVC repair and, 805–806, 806t
  tracheal fluid-induced, 84
Pulmonary hypertensive crises, after total anomalous pulmonary venous drainage, 450, *450*
Pulmonary hypoplasia, radiographic diagnosis of, 256, *257*
Pulmonary lymphangiectasia, classification of, 255, *255*
Pulmonary maturity studies, in nonimmune hydrops fetalis, 212
Pulmonary oligemia, in tricuspid atresia, 528
Pulmonary plethora, in tricuspid atresia, 528–529
Pulmonary responses, to left-to-right PDA shunt, 71–72
Pulmonary sequestration, 256–257
  total anomalous pulmonary venous drainage and, 440t